CRITICAL
SURGICAL
ILLNESS

Edited By

James D. Hardy, M.D., F.A.C.S.

Professor of Surgery and Chairman of the Department,
University of Mississippi School of Medicine
Surgeon-in-Chief to the University Hospital

W. B. SAUNDERS COMPANY
Philadelphia • London • Toronto

W. B. Saunders Company: West Washington Square
Philadelphia, Pa. 19105

12 Dyott Street
London, WC1A   1DB

833 Oxford Street
Toronto 18, Ontario

Critical Surgical Illness   ISBN   0-7216-4510-0

Print No.:   9   8   7   6   5   4

*To all those surgeons who strive for perfection
in clinical care.*

CONTRIBUTORS

ROBERT J. ALBO, M.D., F.A.C.S.

Assistant Clinical Professor of Surgery, University of California (S.F.); Instructor in Surgery, University of California (Berkeley); Chief of General Surgical Division, Peralta Hospital, Oakland, California.

FRED ALLISON, JR., M.D.

Edgar Hull Professor and Head of the Department of Internal Medicine, Louisiana State University School of Medicine; Physician-in-Chief, L.S.U. Division, and Senior Attending Physician, Charity Hospital of Louisiana, New Orleans, Louisiana.

WILLIAM A. ALTEMEIER, M.D.

Christian R. Holmes Professor of Surgery and Chairman of the Department, University of Cincinnati College of Medicine; Director of Surgical Services, Cincinnati General Hospital; Surgeon-in-Chief, Children's Hospital and Holmes Hospital, Cincinnati, Ohio

WILEY F. BARKER, M.D., F.A.C.S.

Professor of Surgery, University of California (Los Angeles); Attending Surgeon, University of California Hospital, Los Angeles; Consultant in Surgery, Sepulveda Veterans Hospital, Sepulveda, California.

WILLIAM OSCAR BARNETT, M.D., F.A.C.S.

Professor of Surgery, University of Mississippi School of Medicine; Attending Surgeon, The Hospital of the University of Mississippi Medical Center, Jackson, Mississippi.

EDWARD J. BERKICH, M.D.

Instructor in Surgery, University of Cincinnati College of Medicine; Assistant Attending Surgeon, Cincinnati General Hospital, Cincinnati, Ohio

EMIL BLAIR, M.D.

Professor of Surgery, University of Colorado Medical Center; Chairman, Department of Surgery, General Rose Memorial Hospital; Attending Surgeon, General Rose Memorial Hospital, Denver General Hospital, Colorado General Hospital, and Children's Hospital, Denver, Colorado.

THOMAS H. BURFORD, M.D.

Clinical Professor of Thoracic and Cardiovascular Surgery, Washington University School of Medicine; Barnes and Allied Hospitals, St. Louis, Missouri.

JAMES R. CALLISON, M.D.

Associate Professor of Plastic Surgery, Johns Hopkins University School of Medicine; Plastic Surgeon, Johns Hopkins Hospital; Consultant Plastic Surgeon: U.S. Public Health Hospital, Baltimore City Hospitals, Greater Baltimore Medical Center, Baltimore, Maryland.

LARRY C. CAREY, M.D.

Associate Professor of Surgery, University of Pittsburgh School of Medicine; Presbyterian-University Hospital, Veterans Hospital of Oakland, and Children's Hospital of Pittsburgh, Pittsburgh, Pennsylvania.

CARLOS M. CHAVEZ, M.D., F.A.C.S., F.C.C.P.

Assistant Professor, Department of Surgery, University of Mississippi Medical Center; Attending Surgeon, University Hospital and Staff Surgeon, Veterans Administration Hospital, Jackson, Mississippi.

CHARLES G. CHILD III, M.D.

Professor of Surgery and Chairman of the Department, University of Michigan Medical School; University of Michigan Medical Center; Consultant, Wayne County General Hospital; Ann Arbor Veterans Administration Hospital, Ann Arbor, Michigan.

J. HAROLD CONN, M.D.

Professor of Surgery, University of Mississippi School of Medicine; Chief of Surgery, Veterans Administration Center, Jackson, Mississippi.

GORDON K. DANIELSON, M.D., F.A.C.S.

Assistant Professor of Surgery, Mayo Graduate School of Medicine (University of Minnesota); Consultant, Section of Thoracic, Cardiovascular and General Surgery, Mayo Clinic, Rochester, Minnesota.

ROBERT S. DEANE, M.D., B.CH.

Assistant Professor of Anesthesia, University of Vermont Medical College; Director Intensive Care Unit, Director of Respiratory Therapy, Assistant Attending in Anesthesiology: Medical Center Hospital of Vermont, Burlington, Vermont.

STANLEY J. DUDRICK, M.D.

Associate Professor of Surgery, University of Pennsylvania School of Medicine; Attending Surgical Staff, Hospital of the University of Pennsylvania; Chief of Surgery, University of Pennsylvania Service, Philadelphia Veterans Administration Hospital; Assistant Attending Surgeon, Philadelphia General Hospital, Philadelphia, Pennsylvania.

J. ENGLEBERT DUNPHY, M.D.

Professor and Chairman, Dept. of Surgery, University of California (S.F.); Chief of Surgical Service, University of California Hospitals and Clinics, University of California (S.F.), San Francisco, California.

MILTON T. EDGERTON, M.D., F.A.C.S.

Professor of Plastic Surgery, Chairman of Department of Plastic Surgery, University of Virginia; Plastic Surgeon in Charge, University of Virginia Hospital; Consultant Plastic Surgeon, Salem Veterans Administration Hospital, Salem, Virginia.

F. HENRY ELLIS, JR., M.D., PH.D., F.A.C.S.

Professor of Surgery, Mayo Graduate School of Medicine, University of Minnesota; Consultant, Section of Thoracic, Cardiovascular and General Surgery, Mayo Clinic, Rochester, Minnesota.

EDWIN H. ELLISON, M.D.

Professor of Surgery, Marquette School of Medicine, Milwaukee, Wisconsin.

THOMAS B. FERGUSON, M.D.

Associate Clinical Professor of Thoracic and Cardiovascular Surgery, Washington University School of Medicine; Barnes and Allied Hospitals, St. Louis, Missouri.

JAMES H. FOSTER, M.D., F.A.C.S.

Chief of Surgical Service, Hartford Hospital, Hartford, Connecticut.

STEPHEN E. HEDBERG, M.D., F.A.C.S.

Clinical Assistant in Surgery, Harvard Medical School; Assistant Surgeon, Massachusetts General Hospital, Boston, Massachusetts.

ROBERT H. JONES, M.D.

Scholar in Academic Surgery, Duke University Medical Center, Durham, North Carolina.

CARL M. KJELLSTRAND, M.D.

Assistant Professor of Medicine and Surgery, University of Minnesota School of Medicine; University of Minnesota Hospitals, Minneapolis, Minnesota.

HAROLD LAUFMAN, M.D., PH.D., F.A.C.S.

Professor of Surgery, Albert Einstein College of Medicine, New York; Director, Institute for Surgical Studies, and Attending Surgeon, Montefiore Hospital and Medical Center, New York, New York.

S. MARTIN LINDENAUER, M.D.

Associate Professor of Surgery, University of Michigan Medical School; Chief, Surgery Service, Veterans Administration Hospital, Ann Arbor, Michigan; Staff Surgeon, University of Michigan Medical Center; Attending Surgeon, Wayne County General Hospital, Eloise, Michigan.

WILLIAM P. LONGMIRE, JR., M.D.

Professor and Chairman, Department of Surgery, UCLA School of Medicine; Chief of Surgery, UCLA; Consultant in Surgery, Los Angeles County Harbor General Hospital, Torrance, California; Consultant in Surgery, Wadsworth Hospital, Veterans Administration Center, Los Angeles, California.

J. D. MARTIN, JR., M.D.

Professor and Chairman, Department of Surgery, Emory University School of Medicine; Chief of Surgery, Grady Memorial Hospital; Chief of Surgical Service, Emory University Hospital; Chief of Surgery, Henrietta Egleston Hospital for Children, Emory, Georgia.

JOHN ARTHUR MONCRIEF, M.D.

Professor of Surgery, Medical University of South Carolina; Attending Surgeon at Medical University Hospital, Veterans Hospital, and Charleston County Hospital, Charleston, South Carolina.

FRANCIS D. MOORE, M.D.

Moseley Professor of Surgery, Harvard Medical School; Surgeon-in-Chief, Peter Bent Brigham Hospital, Boston, Massachusetts.

JOHN S. NAJARIAN, M.D.

Professor and Chairman of Surgery, University of Minnesota School of Medicine; University of Minnesota Hospitals, Minneapolis, Minnesota.

THOMAS FRANCIS NEALON, JR., M.D.

Professor of Clinical Surgery, New York University School of Medicine; Director, Department of Surgery, St. Vincent's Hospital and Medical Center of New York, New York.

BASIL A. PRUITT, JR., LIEUTENANT COLONEL, MC

Commander and Director, U.S. Army Institute of Surgical Research, Brooke Army Medical Center, Ft. Sam Houston, Texas; ACS Pre- and Postoperative Care Committee; Army Representative to NIH Surgical Study Section B; Assistant Clinical Professor of Surgery, University of Texas Medical School at San Antonio, Texas.

HENRY THOMAS RANDALL, M.D., F.A.C.S.

Professor of Medical Science (Surgery), Division of Biological and Medical Science, Brown University; Surgeon-in-Chief, Rhode Island Hospital, Providence, Rhode Island.

JONATHAN E. RHOADS, M.D., D.SC. (SURG.), F.A.C.S.

John Rhea Barton Professor of Surgery and Chairman of the Department of Surgery and the Harrison Dept. of Surgical Research, University of Pennsylvania School of Medicine; Chief of Surgery, Hospital of the University of Pennsylvania; Senior Surgeon Visiting Staff, Children's Hospital of Philadelphia; Consultant in Surgery, Veterans Administration Hospital, Philadelphia, Pennsylvania.

DAVID C. SABISTON, JR., M.D.

Professor and Chairman, Department of Surgery, Duke University Medical Center, Durham, North Carolina; Consultant in Surgery, National Institutes of Health, Bethesda, Maryland.

NEIL J. SHERMAN, M.D.

Major, USAF, MC, Surgical Service, Department of the Air Force, Headquarters 852D Medical Group (SAC), Castle Air Force Base, California.

RICHARD L. SIMMONS, M.D.

Associate Professor of Surgery and Microbiology, University of Minnesota School of Medicine; University of Minnesota Hospitals, Minneapolis, Minnesota.

HILARY H. TIMMIS, M.D., F.A.C.S.

Associate Professor of Surgery, University
of Mississippi School of Medicine;
Attending Surgeon, University of
Mississippi, Jackson, Mississippi.

CEMALETTIN TOPUZLU,

Assistant Professor of Surgery, University of
Vermont College of Medicine, Burlington,
Vermont.

JEREMIAH G. TURCOTTE, M.D.

Associate Professor of Surgery, University of
Michigan Medical School; University of
Michigan Medical Center, Ann Arbor
Veterans Administration Hospital, and
Wayne County General Hospital, Ann
Arbor, Michigan.

THOMAS T. VOGEL, M.D., PH.D.

Instructor, Department of Surgery, The
Ohio State University College of Medicine;
Senior Resident, Department of Surgery,
The Ohio State University Hospitals,
Columbus, Ohio.

CLAUDE E. WELCH, M.D., F.A.C.S.

Clinical Professor of Surgery, Harvard
Medical School; Visiting Surgeon,
Massachusetts General Hospital, Boston,
Massachusetts.

ROGER D. WILLIAMS, B.S., M.M.SC.,
M.D.

Clinical Professor of Surgery, University of
Miami; Active Staff, Broward General
Hospital and Holy Cross Hospital,
Fort Lauderdale, Florida.

ROBERT M. ZOLLINGER, M.D., F.A.C.S.,
HON F.R.C.S. (ENG.), HON F.R.C.S.
(EDIN.).

Regents Professor and Chairman,
Department of Surgery, Ohio State
University College of Medicine; Director of
Surgical Services. The Ohio State
University Hospitals, Columbus, Ohio.

PREFACE

This is a book about treatment. It had its inception in the belief that the vast array of important new concepts and techniques available for the management of the critically ill surgical patient should be focused upon and presented in one place. It was clear that the range and depth of the clinical experience required to develop such a volume could be achieved only by a number of authors who are leaders in their respective fields. These contributors have recognized that there is no separation between knowledge of pathophysiology and metabolism, surgical technique, and moral acceptance of total responsibility for the patient's welfare.

The titles for the thirty chapters were also selected with care. The specific therapeutic requirements of the major common problems in general surgery, as well as metabolic principles underlying management, were to be included. The subjects chosen represent the principal causes of major morbidity and mortality on most surgical services. These include "shock," peritonitis with abscesses, abdominal and thoracic trauma, "respiratory insufficiency," fluid imbalance, wound sepsis and evisceration, massive burns with stress ulcer, thrombophlebitis with pulmonary embolism, esophageal perforation with mediastinitis, massive gastrointestinal hemorrhage, suppurative cholangitis and postoperative jaundice with hepatic failure, postgastrectomy problems and recurrent peptic ulceration, necrotizing pancreatitis, strangulation obstruction and high-output small bowel fistula, toxic megacolon, endocrine crises, acute aortic occlusion and infected arterial grafts, sepsis in kidney transplantation, low cardiac output syndromes and ventricular arrhythmia, postoperative coma, intravenous hyperalimentation, and a number of other topics of much interest and significance. All these subjects were selected with a view to providing insight and guidance in still other overlapping and related problems. In selecting for discussion only the most severe surgical illnesses, it was assumed that the management of the early stages of these conditions, or of similar ones, would be apparent through inference.

In every chapter the authors set for themselves the objective of providing the essence of the diagnostic and therapeutic requirements. Thus, it has been possible to present a vast amount of clinical knowledge in a volume of convenient length. Publication of this work, devoted to getting the individual patient well, comes at a time when major philosophical interest in this country is being focused on applied therapy and the overall distribution of medical care.

The editor expresses his sincere appreciation to each contributor. These outstanding surgeons extracted from their heavy schedules the time necessary to develop chapters which in every instance comprise truly significant contributions. The editorial assistance of Miss Jane E. Peters and Mrs. Virginia W. Keith is also warmly acknowledged. Finally, the continuous contributions of Mr. Robert B. Rowan, Carroll C. Cann, and John L. Dusseau of the Saunders Company have been invaluable.

JAMES D. HARDY, M.D.

PUBLISHER'S FOREWORD

Considering that this is a book on the management of desperately ill patients, the ability of the contributors to apply sophisticated, in-depth analysis to their own experience, often in the most difficult situations, became a vital criterion for their selection. On this account, Dr. Hardy has elected to present at the beginning of each chapter a brief biographical sketch of its author.

The observant reader will notice that one sketch is missing, and the publisher would like to take this opportunity to supply it.

James D. Hardy was born in Birmingham, Alabama, and received his undergraduate education at the University of Alabama. He came north in 1938 to medical school and received his medical degree at the University of Pennsylvania in 1942. He served a medical residency at the University of Pennsylvania Hospital from 1943 to 1944, became a resident in general surgery in 1946 after service in the United States Army, and was Chief Resident in General Surgery in 1948–1949 under Dr. I. S. Ravdin and a resident in thoracic surgery in 1949–1951 under Dr. Julian Johnson.

In 1954, after three years as Director of Surgical Research at the University of Tennessee, he accepted his present appointment as Professor and Chairman of the Department of Surgery and Director of Surgical Research at the University of Mississippi Medical Center.

His principal area of investigation has been the pathophysiology of surgical disease, and he has been one of the most significant of modern contributors to the elucidation of surgical physiology. He has also done pioneering work in the new field of transplantation of organs and has also had extensive experience in vascular surgery. He is a past President of the Society of University Surgeons and of the Society for Surgery of the Alimentary Tract.

CONTENTS

CHAPTER 1

POST-TRAUMATIC PULMONARY INSUFFICIENCY

by FRANCIS D. MOORE, M.D.

Francis D. Moore was born in Illinois and received his college and medical education at Harvard. Almost immediately after serving his residency at the Massachusetts General Hospital he was appointed Moseley Professor of Surgery at Harvard and Surgeon-in-Chief to the Peter Bent Brigham Hospital. Thus he was early recognized as a superior clinical surgeon, teacher, and investigator, and subsequent years have proved this recognition ever more prophetic. He went on to become possibly the foremost surgical biologist of his time, and several of his books and many articles have become standard reference works throughout the world. His ability to present basic surgical physiology to postgraduate surgical audiences is unexcelled. Dr. Moore was among the first fully to recognize the large role played by various types of respiratory insufficiency in surgical morbidity and mortality, and the following discussion attests his deep learning and understanding of this field.

TERMINOLOGY

The term "post-traumatic pulmonary insufficiency" refers to a variety of cases of pulmonary failure after trauma, exhibiting a wide range of severity, and each one presenting a slightly different balance among several etiologic factors.

When a single cause is predominant, an appropriate diagnosis should be made. This includes particularly those cases in which pulmonary edema predominates (on the basis of either fluid overload or congestive heart failure), and those patients in whom there has been little disturbance until a bacterial process spreads as lobar pneumonia or bronchopneumonia. Patients who die of post-traumatic pulmonary insufficiency show both the histologic and bacteriologic evidences of widespread pulmonary infection, yet the pathologic changes indicate that other processes antedated the infection. The clinical history also bears out the supposition that pulmonary injury was present and severe prior to infection.

Other specific causes of pulmonary difficulty after injury, including primary asthmatic bronchospasm, aspiration pneumonitis, pneumothorax, pulmonary embolism, fat embolism, and mediastinal emphysema, should likewise be differentiated. This clarification of diagnosis is mentioned at the outset because many of the benefits in clinical management that have accrued from identification of the syndrome of post-traumatic pulmonary insufficiency (as distinct from these other forms of pulmonary failure) will be vitiated if the diagnosis becomes a wastebasket for all pulmonary diseases occurring in a traumatized patient.

Despite this multiplicity of causes, and variation in detailed behavior, the syndrome has specific characteristics. It follows severe trauma, often extrathoracic, with early spontaneous hyperventilation and a mixed alkalosis, which leads to a free interval of apparently good pulmonary and circulatory function. This is then followed by the progressive development of pulmonary insufficiency insensitive to increased oxygen tensions in the airway with severe shunting (i.e., venoarterial admixture). The ultimate outcome is predictable on the basis of the biochemical severity of the shunt and the anatomic extent of pulmonary involvement. The terminal event is a severe mixed acidosis, anoxia, hypercapnia, and then cessation of the heartbeat.

1

INCIDENCE

The characteristic setting for this syndrome is a person of young or middle age with no identifiable pulmonary disease prior to his injury or operation. In some cases a heavy smoking history is notable and seems to make the patient more vulnerable. Within this setting, severe injury or extensive operation is followed by a normal initial pattern of resuscitation appropriate to the injury. The disorder then progresses slowly to a stage in which pulmonary disease is predominant—in the clinical picture, in the therapeutic challenge, and, if lethal, as the cause of death.

There are few data on the statistical incidence of this syndrome. It was originally estimated from the material in our Intensive Care Unit that about one-third of those patients who died exhibited this syndrome (Moore et al., 1969). The other two-thirds were approximately equally divided between patients who died of primary visceral failure other than of the lungs (usually heart or kidneys) and those who died with acute overwhelming infection, usually a bacteremia with gram-negative bacilli. With certain steps in prevention and treatment (as indicated in the later sections of this chapter) the incidence of this syndrome in our own Intensive Care Unit has been decreased markedly. Other hospitals in this country that have isolated critically ill patients into some sort of an intensive care or "shock unit" have likewise reported a high incidence of pulmonary failure, with some improvement upon adoption of better procedures in respiratory care. This is noteworthy in the material of Shoemaker, Weil (1967), and MacLean (1967); several reports on studies of the Vietnam casualties likewise emphasize the importance of this syndrome (Conference on Pulmonary Effects of Nonthoracic Trauma, 1968). From none of these reports are any simple statistical analyses available. In the group most severely ill after extensive injury or operation, a fatality is rare unless there is some component of pulmonary failure. Before the development of effective methods for dialysis, death from pure renal failure was commonplace, with but little pathologic pulmonary change other than pulmonary edema. As renal failure has been effectively treated for longer periods of time, and as cardiopulmonary resuscitation has become more effective in the early

phases of injury, post-traumatic pulmonary insufficiency has emerged as a more important cause of death. The frequent combination with renal failure is particularly noteworthy because of the high mortality of renal failure when it occurs as a complication of extensive injury, massive surgery, or burns. In this group of cases recovery from renal failure is the exception rather than the rule; dialysis serves to prolong life effectively for days or weeks, but the combination with severe tissue injury (or the need for continuing massive transfusions, as in ruptured aortic aneurysm) makes recovery most unusual. In all these cases, pulmonary insufficiency enters as a critically important lethal factor commencing three to five days prior to death.

Thus, though statistical incidence has little over-all significance here, there is good justification for the view that pulmonary insufficiency predominates as a cause of death in most patients who die after injury if their survival has been initially maintained for more than five days by conventional methods of resuscitation or by dialysis.

CLINICAL AND CHEMICAL BEHAVIOR; PATHOPHYSIOLOGY

Four clinical stages

INJURY PHASE. This is the initial period after injury or operation. It is characterized by therapy directed toward initial resuscitation, and in all cases includes intravenous infusion of liberal quantities of blood, salt solution, and colloid. As the patient emerges from this period the circulation is stabilized (as indicated by good perfusion of the central organs and the extremities), there is a return of urine output to normal or high levels, and there is restoration of the normal mental state. Cardiac output is normal or high. There is mixed respiratory and metabolic alkalosis.

In this apparently resuscitated period (leading to the "free interval") danger signals can arise, indicating the possibility of future severe pulmonary difficulty. These are maintained spontaneous hyperventilation (as indicated by carbon dioxide tensions below 30 mm. Hg), spotty areas of pathologic change in the lung (on auscultation or x-ray) or the historical fact that the patient's injury involved sudden compression or decompres-

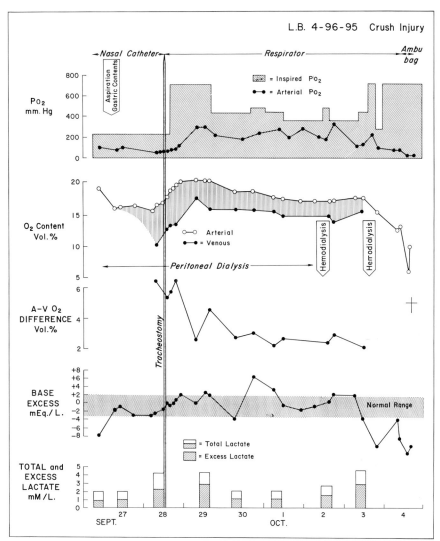

Figure 1-1. Crush injury. The inspired oxygen tension, arterial oxygen tensions, oxygenation data, and acid-base findings are shown here. Initial shunting, as demonstrated by the sluggish response to high oxygen tensions on September 28th and 29th, almost completely disappeared by October 1st, when with inspired oxygen tensions of approximately 380 mm. Hg the arterial oxygen tension approached 300 mm. Hg. Thereafter there was a marked deterioration and finally, in the last 36 hours, despite continuous presentation of high oxygen tensions in the inspired air, the arterial oxygen level progressively fell. Calculation of shunt at this time showed a figure approaching 50 per cent of cardiac output. The acid-base data showed a typical triphasic curve of lactate change, with an early rise, then a fall with improving circulation and oxygenation, followed finally by a terminal rise to a total of 5 mM per liter of which approximately 60 per cent was excess lactate.

sion of the lung itself or inhalation of noxious fumes. This may result from nearby explosions, smoke or fire, from steering wheel injuries to the anterior thorax (even though rib fractures are absent); it may occur in sudden blows to the abdomen even though no viscera are ruptured. This type of injury, even without pulmonary changes in the first 36 hours, is regularly followed by a delayed-onset pulmonary lesion. When the chest wall has lost its integrity, either through multiple rib fractures or rupture of the diaphragm, or by penetrating missile wounds, then the likelihood of pulmonary insufficiency is greatly increased.

FREE INTERVAL. This period usually occupies from one to five days following the initial resuscitation. The patient's recovery now appears superficially to be progressing nicely. There is good blood pressure, cardiac output (which is often grossly increased), urine flow, peripheral perfusion, color, and

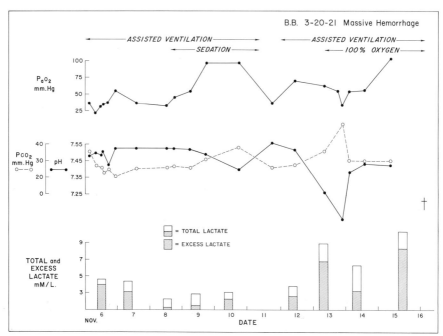

Figure 1-2. Data from a patient with massive hemorrhage followed by pulmonary insufficiency. Arterial oxygen tensions, carbon dioxide tensions, and acid-base data are shown. There is persistent inability to achieve adequate oxygenation, with very low terminal arterial oxygen tensions despite ventilation with 100 per cent oxygen. There was a persistent mild alkalosis with hypocarbia and, on November 13th, a drastic acid-base change produced by the infusion of 88 mEq. of sodium bicarbonate. Although acid-base data were superficially improved thereby, with some improvement in circulation as shown by a drop in the lactate level, diffuse anaerobiosis soon returned, as demonstrated by the high terminal lactate value.

mentation. Indeed, the patient may go on to complete recovery from this phase with no serious pulmonary impairment.

In those for whom further trouble is in store, there is a subtle progression characterized by maintained spontaneous hyperventilation with an inappropriately low carbon dioxide tension long after pain, apprehension, or direct pulmonary injury could be its cause. There is a beginning difficulty of oxygenation, initially very mild, with oxygen tensions above 80 mm. Hg on room air. Test inhalation of 100 per cent oxygen for 20 to 30 minutes, using some type of mask to assure good airway closure (or using a cuffed tracheostomy or endotracheal tube if such has already been necessary because of the original injury) will demonstrate an alveolar-arterial oxygen difference that is greater than normal (see the following section). Thus, though the patient is not yet cyanotic nor is he severely anoxic, he may already show early manifestations of the characteristic respiratory lesion: hypocarbia with venoarterial admixture (Ayres et al., 1964). As this becomes more severe, some cyanosis is observed, hyperventilation is

more marked, and hypocarbia is more profound. The respiratory situation now becomes much more worrisome, not only because of these physiologic findings but because of increasingly widespread rales and rhonchi (sometimes with marked evidence of bronchospasm) on auscultation and an increasingly widespread spotty or flecky soft infiltrate visualized by x-ray.

PROGRESSIVE PULMONARY INSUFFICIENCY. As the pulmonary problem begins to predominate in the clinical picture, the patient enters the third phase, that of progressive post-traumatic pulmonary insufficiency. Before its recognition and during the free interval many patients have been transferred to other parts of the hospital. In some instances this syndrome is doubtless recognized for the first time when fully developed, during its third phase; greater vigilance for the early subtle signs would disclose that the problem had already been present for several days.

Difficulty in oxygenation now becomes the predominant clinical feature. Under no circumstances should tracheostomy be carried out for anoxia alone until a suitable trial of endotracheal intubation has indicated that direct access to the lower airway will yield an improvement that justifies its hazard. If the difficulty is purely that of venoarterial admixture (i.e., passage of venous blood through the lungs without ventilation), then great increases in oxygen tension in the airway yield a disappointing increase in arterial oxygen tension. One must be satisfied with an arterial oxygen tension that is achieved with "safe" airway oxygen levels in the vicinity of 60 to 75 per cent, and usually yielding arterial oxygen tensions in the general neighborhood of 70 mm. Hg.

The relation of inhaled oxygen concentration to achieved arterial oxygen tension is the basis of the "oxygen tolerance test," which we first used as a rough quantification of venoarterial admixture in patients at this stage. This test, repeated daily, or more often as needed, enables one to tailor the oxygen therapy to the patient's needs; changes in its response over the course of time are a guide to prognosis.

Tracheostomy can often be avoided. Endotracheal intubation is far preferable and is tolerated for periods of a week or more;

withdrawal of the tube restores to the lower airway its normal anatomic relationship, a restoration that is never easily or quickly done with a tracheostomy. When endotracheal suction is necessary, it can safely be done through the endotracheal tube.

Survival of patients who have reached the severe anoxia of Phase III can still occur if the airway is managed with restraint and if certain of the promoting or maintaining factors in systemic therapy, which further hazard the lungs, are avoided. In many cases, even with the most elaborate measures to avoid damage to the lungs and airway, the lesion becomes progressive; there are progressive and diffuse infiltrates and widespread pulmonary infection. This is manifested both by a change in the x-ray appearances and by a febrile course. The aspiration of purulent material from the lower airway discloses very large numbers of a single organism, in many cases an organism that has previously been identified in cultures of wounds, septic surgical incisions, or the blood.

TERMINAL PHASE. Oxygenation now be-

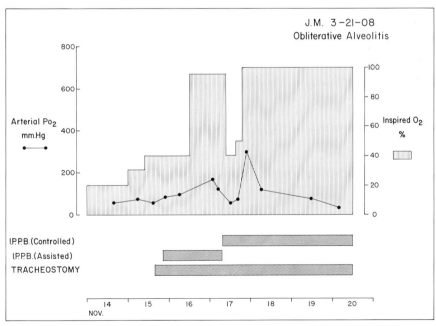

Figure 1-3. Increasing alveolar-arterial oxygen gradient in a patient with severe abdominal injury. Initial stepwise increase of oxygen concentration in inspired air was associated with only a moderate increase in arterial oxygen content. When, on November 17th, the inspired gas mixture oxygen concentration was reduced to 40 per cent, the arterial oxygen tension fell to approximately 62 mm. Hg. Thereafter, oxygen concentration in the inspired air was again increased to 100 per cent with some increase in arterial oxygen tension to about 300 mm. Hg, indicating venoarterial admixture of about 25 per cent. Thereafter, on continuous administration of 100 per cent oxygen, the patient's blood oxygenation failed progressively and he died. This course is reminiscent of that seen in animals maintained on prolonged inhalation of 100 per cent oxygen.

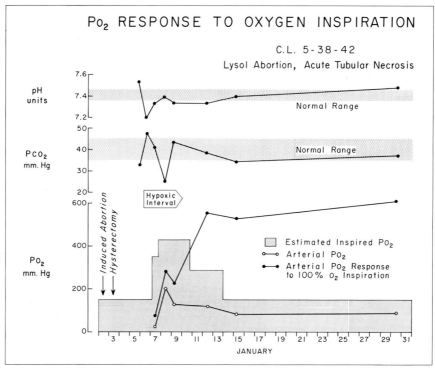

Figure 1-4.   Data from a patient with gram-negative bacteremia following a self-induced abortion. The patient was initially hypoxic on room air. A test inhalation of 100 per cent oxygen showed only a modest response (closed circles), indicating a very large shunt fraction. The inspired oxygen fraction was increased to a level of about 60 per cent on January 7th. There was a modest increase in arterial oxygen concentration (open circles) sufficient to satisfy peripheral oxygen needs. Successive improvement in performance on test periods of 100 per cent oxygen inhalation is shown by the closed circles; levels finally rose to approximately normal. Therefore, on January 13th and 14th, it was possible to return the patient to room air, and on this inspired oxygen concentration she maintained arterial oxygen tensions that were satisfactory for the tissues. In this patient, by successive tests of the response to 100 per cent oxygen inhalation for short periods, it was possible to avoid the prolonged use of high oxygen tensions in the inspired air. This course is to be contrasted with that of the patient shown in Figure 1-3.

comes progressively more refractory to any increase in airway oxygen tension, as the shunting defect increases in severity. Finally, as ventilation-perfusion abnormalities in the lung become more widespread, with some areas perfused but not ventilated at all, and others evidently ventilated but poorly perfused, there is an increase in dead space and a rise in the carbon dioxide tension of the blood from its chronically hypocarbic levels. This presages death. It is often accompanied by other evidences of deterioration, particularly a return of circulatory failure with hypotension, oliguria, and the resumption of a severe low-flow state with mounting lacticacidosis. During the last day or two of this disease the auscultatory and roentgen findings in the lungs change but little and are of remarkably little assistance to the therapist. Pulmonary infection is severe; bloodstream infection is commonplace. A few warning changes in the electrocardio-

gram may suggest subendocardial ischemia; slowing to asystole may be abrupt and with no prior warning.

The combination of metabolic and respiratory acidosis with severe anoxia produces this final event: asystole refractory to any form of cardiac resuscitation.

CHEMICAL BEHAVIOR

With the foregoing as a summary of the clinical syndrome, it is now appropriate to examine the physiologic events in greater detail.

As already indicated, hypocarbia (the biochemical reflection of hyperventilation) is characteristic of the first three phases of this disease. The carbon dioxide tension varies from 25 to 35 mm. Hg. At the very outset this hyperventilation seems clearly related either to a prolonged anesthesia (and the tendency to hyperventilate patients during prolonged general anesthesia) or to such factors as pain, apprehension, or motion of injured limbs. If assisted ventilation is instituted, using some sort of mechanical respiratory support, hypocarbia is apt to become even more marked, as there is a pernicious tendency to hyperventilate patients with shunt-induced anoxia. The therapist considers that a higher minute volume and increased alveolar ventilation should result in better oxygenation. In some cases this can be demonstrated to be true owing either to higher airway pressure or to the expansion of collapsed peripheral alveolar segments. More frequently, the induced hyperventilation merely promotes respiratory alkalosis without improving oxygenation.

Severe hypocarbia is dangerous to these patients because of cerebral vasoconstriction and myocardial irritability (Lyons and Moore, 1966). Every effort should be made to avoid it. If the arterial carbon dioxide tension is below 32 mm. Hg, active steps should be taken to restore it to normal. This is usually done by introducing additional dead space into the ventilatory tubing. The progression of the pulmonary lesion to the point at which the arterial carbon dioxide tension returns to normal and then rapidly progresses to high levels is a characteristic preterminal event.

Lacticacidosis is commonplace in the early phase. The initial low-flow state produces a rise in arterial blood lactate to levels generally in the range of 2 to 5 mM per liter. The metabolic acidosis observed is almost wholly due to lactate accumulation; the lactate is almost wholly present as excess lactate (i.e., as lactate over and above that accounted for by any increase in pyruvate). During the free interval, most of this excess lactate is oxidized or excreted, and the lactate value returns toward normal. Just as prolonged spontaneous hyperventilation presages further pulmonary trouble, so also a long-continued slight elevation of blood lactate is an indication of continued anoxic or vasoconstricted areas in muscle — evidence that the circulation is not as normal as one might be led to believe by superficial appearances. The rapid or massive infusion of lactated Ringer's solution or other forms of sodium lactate can produce mild transient elevations of total blood lactate, particularly in individuals whose renal function is abnormal. The interpretation of slight elevations of lactate

level must be tempered by analysis of the infusion therapy. During the terminal phase, lactate again rises abruptly to levels that are far higher than any that were observed in the first phase; levels of 10 to 20 mM per liter are not uncommon, and at the time of death, lactate levels may be 30 mM per liter or higher, a load of metabolic acid that is apparently incompatible with survival.

Blood pH changes are wholly accountable on the basis of a balance between the carbon dioxide tension and the lactic acid load. While other factors may enter transiently into the acid-base balance (such as the infusion of buffers, the removal of gastric juice, or the presence of small amounts of renal acids), the pH of the blood is the net vector of carbon dioxide removal and lactate accumulation.

Other chemical features of these patients are determined by the rest of the clinical picture. These include renal failure with its attendant acidosis and azotemia, liver injury (either direct or resulting from prolonged hypoperfusion), further elevation of blood bilirubin due to the metabolism of heme pigments arising from the breakdown of poorly preserved blood, and disorders of electrolyte equilibrium.

PATHOPHYSIOLOGY

Venoarterial admixture is so characteristic a cause of anoxemia in post-traumatic pulmonary insufficiency, that it has become the biochemical trademark of the disease. The pathophysiology of pulmonary shunting deserves special consideration.

In normal individuals, some venous blood with oxygen saturation below 70 per cent, passes to the left heart output without full oxygenation. This is the normal or physiologic shunt and includes blood passing through small areas of unventilated lung tissue, bronchial artery return, and probably some components of coronary flow. The total is less than 8 per cent of normal cardiac output, and it manifests itself as a minor alveolar-arterial oxygen difference on test inhalation of 100 per cent oxygen for 30 minutes. The gradient thus observed is considered to be due to shunt rather than to diffusion defects, and in a normal person the achieved arterial oxygen tension ranges between 450 and 550 mm. Hg rather than the theoretical maximum at 1 atmosphere of 100 per cent oxygen (760

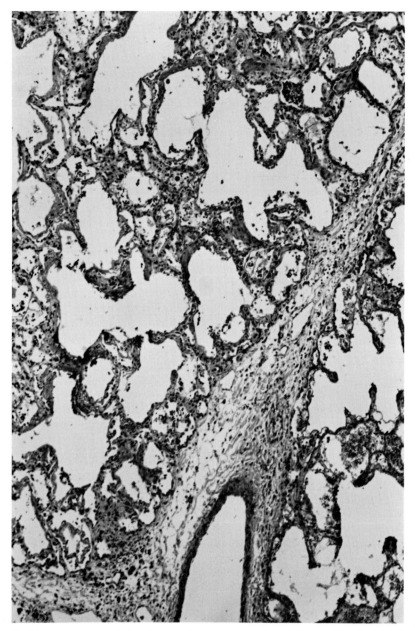

Figure 1-5. Postmortem findings in post-traumatic pulmonary insufficiency. The interlobular septum which traverses the field is prominent because of interstitial edema and fibroblastic proliferation. The alveolar septa are moderately widened, and many of the alveoli are lined with dark-staining hyaline membrane deposits.

mm. Hg corrected for water vapor and carbon dioxide) of about 680 mm. Hg.

What, then, are the pathophysiologic mechanisms that, in patients with post-traumatic pulmonary insufficiency, cause as much as 50 per cent or 70 per cent of the cardiac output to pass through the lungs without being oxygenated?

Atelectasis has always been considered the principal cause of increased pulmonary shunting. The word "atelectasis" means "collapsed airlessness." The condition is shown in the x-ray as streaky or plate-shaped shadows containing essentially no gas at all. Blood perfusing such alveoli will return to the left heart with the same oxygen tension, concentration, and content with which it entered the lungs. This venous blood, mixing with the normal arteriolized blood, lowers its average or observed oxygen tension.

In the post-traumatic lung, other forms of airlessness are just as important as atelectasis in producing shunting. Alveolar edema or interstitial edema due to retained secretion or inflammatory exudate will do precisely the same thing so long as air is exchanged and perfusion maintained.

It is fundamental to the understanding of pulmonary shunt that the airless lung, if not perfused, will not show shunting. The classic experiment here was done by Nilsson et al., using a Carlens tube, and consisted in producing an airless lung by occluding a bronchus without altering its blood supply (Nilsson et al., 1956). All the blood passing through that lobe entered the arterial tree without being oxygenated. The subject became anoxic with a low arterial oxygen tension unresponsive to an increased oxygen fraction in the inspired gas mixture, i.e., shunting. Then the lobe was removed, or the blood supply occluded. Here the anatomic damage had obviously increased (ischemia or absence of a whole lobe). Nonetheless, because the airless lung was now no longer perfused (and therefore no reduced hemoglobin returned from it to the arterial circulation) the arterial oxygen tension paradoxically returned to normal and the subject superficially appeared to be improved. *Airless lung must be perfused in order to demonstrate the phenomenon of shunting, and if perfusion stops, the shunt ceases.*

Occasionally the clinical counterpart of this "Carlens phenomenon" is observed if it is carefully sought out. If a patient has the changes of pulmonary edema plus atelectasis in one lobe, he will show shunting as manifested by a low arterial oxygen tension on room air and a greatly increased alveolar-arterial oxygen difference on 100 per cent oxygen inhalation. If, now, the pathologic process progresses to the point of full consolidation with reduced perfusion of that lobe (or if a pulmonary embolus were to lodge in that branch of the pulmonary artery), the blood supply would be shut off and the patient's arterial oxygen values would paradoxically improve even though he was becoming much sicker, as evidenced by a gross increase in the severity of the lobar change while shunting decreased.

Other possible causes of increased pulmonary shunting in post-traumatic pulmonary insufficiency include several mecha-nisms whose importance has never been proven in man. The first of these is decreased passage time of the erythrocyte. The resuscitated patient who has been in a low-flow state characteristically has a very high cardiac output; values as high as twice normal have frequently been observed. If this output is being accommodated through the same or a decreased number of pulmonary capillaries, then the mean transit time of the erythrocyte must be shortened. It is conceivable that under some circumstances this could result in incomplete oxygenation and add to the appearances of shunting.

Blood entering the lung in a severely acidotic state is oxygenated less readily because of the shift of the oxyhemoglobin dissociation curve. This would show itself as shunting. Any abnormality of hemoglobin itself would manifest itself as venoarterial admixture.

Most important, and of unknown significance in this syndrome, are those components of pulmonary disease that interfere with the diffusion of oxygen from the alveolus to the capillary. Most notable of these in post-traumatic pulmonary insufficiency are interstitial edema, alveolar cell hypertrophy, and hyaline membrane formation. We may clump these three together as anatomic changes that increase the distance and the tissue barrier between alveolar gas and hemoglobin molecules in the erythrocyte passing through the pulmonary capillary. It has long been assumed that this type of diffusion barrier is no longer significant when tested on 100 per cent oxygen inhalation for a significant period of time (i.e., over 20 minutes). The assumption is that all the nitrogen in body fluids and tissues has been "washed out" so that the only gases present in the alveolus and in the tissues and blood are water, carbon dioxide, and oxygen. It is, therefore, held that barriers to diffusion, such as thickening of the tissues at the blood-gas interface, would no longer impair oxygenation. It remains to be proven whether or not this is the case with such extensive pulmonary changes as are seen in post-traumatic pulmonary insufficiency. The barrier to oxygen diffusion is evident under the microscope; whether this is reflected physiologically in an alveolar-arterial gradient on 100 per cent oxygen inhalation remains to be established.

In addition to pulmonary shunting, the role of peripheral shunting must be considered at least briefly. If any large number of peri-

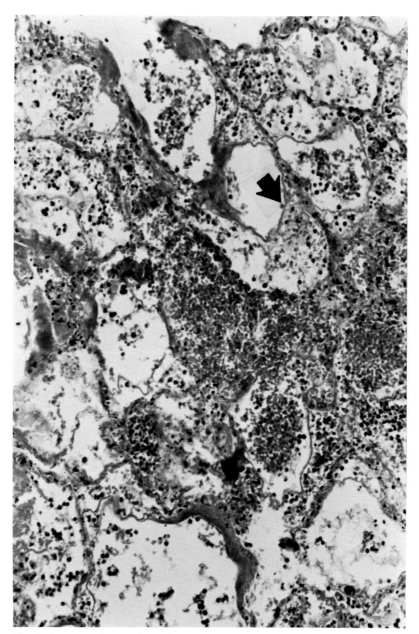

Figure 1-6.   This higher magnification from the same case illustrated in Figure 1-5, illustrates the uniformity of hyaline membrane deposition with alveolar and interstitial hemorrhage. The membranous deposits vary in width, and it appears that some were formed before fluid and cellular extravasation separated them from the alveolar wall (arrow).

pheral arteriovenous shunts open up, then peripheral resistance is lowered and the maintenance of blood pressure requires a considerable increase in cardiac output, as is so commonly observed. At the same time areas of peripheral tissue, presumably skeletal muscle, would be shunted out of the circulation and would be the source of a constant trickle of lactic acid into the veins. This sequence could be established by find-

ing anomalous high venous oxygen tensions in the right atrium, or in veins draining some localized anatomic area, with a rising lactate level. Such findings have been reported (Siegel et al., 1967), but we have observed them only terminally. It is noteworthy that, with any given arterial oxygen tension, the higher the mixed venous oxygen content, the higher will be the calculated figure for shunt fraction at any given cardiac output; the darker the venous blood, the less it takes to darken arterial blood.

The terminal hypercarbia seen in these patients is due to the ventilation of pulmonary parenchyma that is not perfused (the opposite of the ventilation-perfusion anomaly of shunting). When the ventilatory gas mixture fails to meet a blood interface because of an increase in alveolar dead space, the end-expiratory carbon dioxide tension falls below that of arterial blood and hypercarbia results. This lung finally becomes one in which the normal 1:1 relationship of ventilation to perfusion has been so distorted that many areas are perfused but not ventilated, and the remainder ventilated but not perfused, with a huge increase in the ratio of dead space to tidal volume. The result is a lethal anoxia with a rising carbon dioxide tension. When to this is added the infiltration of large segments of lung by a pneumonic process that prevents both ventilation and perfusion, pulmonary artery pressure rises, and the terminal events become inevitable.

PATHOLOGY

The term "bronchopneumonia" has been used for many years to describe the consolidated, heavy, wet, airless, and infected lung found at autopsy. The term has come to include any sort of mixed infectious pulmonary lesion other than lobar pneumonia, pulmonary edema, or pulmonary embolism. In late-stage post-traumatic pulmonary insufficiency, if the patient's life has been maintained for several days on assisted respiration, very large areas of the lung are occupied by a bronchopneumonic process. The case can all too often be dismissed as one of bronchopneumonia. Looking more closely, one finds underlying other more subtle changes. There are parts of the lung that demonstrate these earlier and more subtle changes unobliterated by supervening infection. In those patients in whom death has occurred earlier, the pure pulmonary lesion may be seen with little or no infection.

The outstanding features of the uninfected lesion are interstitial edema with widening of the interalveolar septa, hypertrophy of the alveolar lining cells, and the formation of hyaline membrane. By electron microscopy, the characteristic inclusion bodies in the alveolar lining cells, probably the synthetic organelles for surfactant, are pathologically distributed or lacking entirely.

Hyaline membrane is a nonspecific change in the lung found in many disease states. If the fluid of alveolar edema, containing some protein, were to be dehydrated by opening up those alveoli with positive pressure ventilation, leaving behind a residual strip of desiccated protein, it should lie against the alveolar lining and show itself under the microscope as hyaline membrane. It appears to us that desiccation of proteinaceous alveolar edema induced by prolonged mechanical ventilation is the most important source of hyaline membrane in these lungs; whether specific pulmonary injury such as oxygen toxicity will, in and of itself, produce hyaline membrane, remains unproven. The importance of hyaline membrane lies in the fact that it denotes a pulmonary injury long antedating the supervening infection carelessly referred to as "bronchopneumonia." If the hyaline membrane is relatively impervious to the passage of oxygen, it could contribute to venoarterial admixture, particularly under circumstances in which the inhaled gas mixture contained some nitrogen.

Other pathologic changes in the lung, including interstitial hemorrhage, aspiration pneumonitis, and multiple small pulmonary emboli, are evident in many cases. The finding of lipid material in the pulmonary circulation always leads to the conclusion that fat embolism has been an important component of pulmonary damage. In some patients with peripheral skeletal trauma, gross evidence of marrow-globular pulmonary fat embolism is easily gathered during life or after death. The florid picture of severe marrow-globular pulmonary fat embolism is quite different in its evolution from post-traumatic pulmonary insufficiency, although minor degrees of marrow-globular fat embolism would contribute to the embarrassment of pulmonary function.

A source of controversy that remains unsettled has to do with the production of fat emboli by some mechanism other than outright venous embolization. This type of fat embolism might be called "biochemical fat embolization" to differentiate it from "marrow-globular embolism." Carlsson has shown, and our laboratories have confirmed that prolonged injection of catecholamines in the dog will produce very high levels of free fatty acids in the blood with widespread

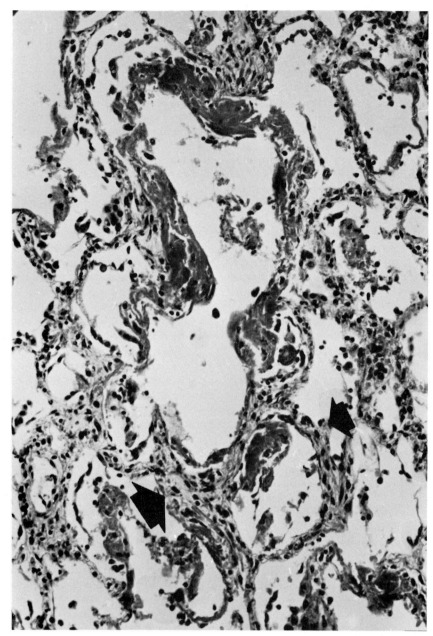

Figure 1-7.   Same case as Figures 1-5 and 1-6. There are hyperplasia of alveolar lining cells and massive deposits of hyaline membrane in many of the alveoli. Most of the alveolar walls are abnormally wide and some show beginning fibrosis.

evidence of re-esterification of fatty acids to neutral triglycerides in peripheral tissues, particularly muscle, liver, kidneys, and heart (Carlsson, 1966; Eltringham et al., 1969). This gives the appearance of fat embolization. In our animals the lungs were spared. The production of very high levels of free fatty acids after trauma has been documented, but the relationship of this to lipid clearing

factors such as heparin has never been elucidated for the uncomplicated traumatic state. When triglycerides are injected intravenously, the administration of heparin greatly hastens the clearing of the triglycerides and thus adds immensely to the level of free fatty acids in the blood, the lipoprotein lipase activity of heparin evidently acting to clear triglycerides by hydrolysis of fatty acids, the clearance of which is limited by peripheral tissue requirements (Coran and Nesbakken, 1969). Disorders of this sequence can produce widespread fatty deposits in tissues; whether or not such deposits occur in the lung is still uncertain.

Blood platelets, once aggregated to form white thrombi, later degenerate histologically into globules of material that stain with Sudan III. A final possible explanation for some of the fat observed in the lungs of traumatized patients is, therefore, that it is the end stage of multiple small platelet thrombi.

The role of multiple small thromboemboli in the production of post-traumatic pulmonary insufficiency remains important in some cases. If transfusion blood is poorly filtered, or if multiple small emboli are forming in traumatized tissue and pass to the lungs, poor perfusion of pulmonary segments, with transient pulmonary hypertension, will be an inevitable result. Granting the importance of such a mechanism, it remains very difficult to prove in any given patient. Pulmonary artery catheterization has been carried out in these patients; for the most part pulmonary hypertension is not a prominent feature in those without pulmonary embolization, until the terminal few hours. At that time pulmonary artery hypertension may be a manifestation of left heart failure as well as pulmonary arterial vasospasm or embolization (Dollery and Glazier, 1966).

ETIOLOGY AND PREVENTION

Within the limitations of this chapter, the causes, prevention, and management of post-traumatic pulmonary insufficiency can best be listed under general headings, with a brief comment after each.

DIRECT TRAUMA TO THE LUNGS; INHALATION INJURY; ASPIRATION

Sudden compression of the thorax or the abdominal cavity or explosive compression communicated to the airway damage the lung directly and increase its vulnerability to the formation of edema. Traumatic wet lung is merely an extreme form of direct trauma in which normal capillary permeability is altered with the production of interstitial and alveolar edema regardless of fluid overload.

The pulmonary injury of burns is another example wherein a variety of chemical substances, usually the products of incomplete combustion of organic substances, damage the lining layer so that alveolar edema is produced. The importance of lesser degrees of pulmonary trauma cannot be overemphasized in evaluating infusion therapy. An otherwise healthy young person whose circulation and renal function could support a considerable overdose of sodium salts at isotonic concentrations will, when his lung is injured, develop interstitial and alveolar pulmonary edema as a result of the hypoproteinemia induced by the infusion. The fluid overload and hypoproteinemia, combined with minor increases of capillary permeability due to trauma to the pulmonary parenchyma, result in edema even if left atrial pressure and pulmonary artery diastolic pressure are normal.

The elevated diaphragm that regularly follows abdominal operations can scarcely be regarded as a cause of pulmonary capillary permeability changes analogous to traumatic wet lung. In contrast, however, the direct handling of the lung in any sort of transthoracic operation and the prolonged use of mechanical ventilation or careless application of positive pressures during inhalation anesthesia must be regarded as forms of pulmonary trauma that render the lung sensitive to fluid overloads. This is the elective counterpart of the lesser degrees of traumatic wet lung so often seen after extrathoracic injury. Injury to the lung by aspiration of gastric contents is easily preventable in most circumstances by the insertion of a nasogastric tube. This should be routine in any seriously injured or freshly postoperative patient.

There are two components in the care of the traumatized patient that make aspiration of gastric juice difficult to control. First is malfunction of the nasogastric tube. This is commonplace and is due to a whole variety of common-sense factors too numerous to be listed here. It is preventable only by detailed attention to the function of bedside apparatus. A nasogastric tube should never be trusted unless it is checked frequently for total function from gut to suction. Under no circumstances should the patient be given any significant oral intake until peristalsis and the expulsion of flatus indicate normal ability to empty the intestinal tract.

Despite this meticulous attention to detail, there still remain patients in whom some degree of aspiration from the gastrointestinal tract into the pulmonary system seems to be inevitable and virtually continuous. These are patients who have severe trauma to the brain or throat, or who have varying degrees of diminished consciousness with motor and sensory paralysis of the hypopharynx. If some aspiration appears to persist despite a well functioning nasogastric tube, this is an indication for an indwelling nasotracheal tube or, in rare cases, tracheostomy.

If aspiration of gastric contents has been sudden and massive, bronchoscopy should be performed and the bronchial tree lavaged with saline solution or cortisone. There may be some advantage in administering cortisone in high dosage for 24 hours.

INFUSION IN RESUSCITATION

Given a severe injury to both legs occurring without percussive violence, one might be challenged to explain how this could result in any sort of pulmonary difficulty. If the trauma is viewed alone as a local anatomic event, pulmonary damage would most likely result from multiple small emboli coming from platelet thrombi in the damaged extremity, from gross pulmonary emboli arising from major venous thrombosis many days after the trauma, or from marrow-globular embolism, should there be long bone fractures.

Turning from the trauma itself to the treatment of that trauma, many factors emerge that are of a systemic character that profoundly affects the lungs. Most important of these are intravenous infusion and the positional management of the patient. The commonest cause of interstitial pulmonary edema (which sets the stage for post-traumatic pulmonary insufficiency) is fluid overload in the course of initial resuscitation. This usually takes one of two forms: blood or noncolloid solutions. Fluid overload from blood transfusion occasionally results when high-volume transfusion is continued after circulatory needs have been met or in the face of some central lesion producing myocardial damage. The best way to prevent this obvious cause of pulmonary edema is to match the patient's transfusion program to his needs. The keys to this match are central venous pressure, blood pressure, urine output, and a clinical estimate of circulatory stability. If needs cannot be met by transfusion, or if an elevation of central venous pressure is unaccompanied by restoration of peripheral pressure and flow relationships, one may safely assume that other central lesions are involved. These could be pulmonary components such as pneumothorax, mediastinal emphysema, chest wall instability, or direct cardiac components such as myocardial ischemia and heart failure.

When the infusion is of non-colloid-containing solution (usually some modification of saline solution such as lactated Ringer's) there are several points worthy of emphasis. First, that severe degrees of hypoproteinemia going on to frank pulmonary edema can occur with a perfectly normal central venous pressure. Second, that left heart failure reflected in an elevation of the left atrial pressure, the pulmonary venous pressure, and the pulmonary arterial diastolic pressure can coexist with a normal right ventricular end-diastolic pressure (and normal right atrial and central venous pressures) for periods up to several hours or even days so long as the pulmonary valve is competent and the right ventricle not in failure. Third, that if hypoproteinemia results from external losses plus excessive infusion of salt-containing colloid-free solutions, then frank fluid overloading with pulmonary edema can occur long before there is any alteration in these central pressures.

There are several warning signs that such overload might have occurred. First, it is found in a quantitative review of the actual fluids administered to the patient. The dose of crystalloid or electrolyte solution given must be adapted to the observed need for such fluids in terms of traumatic edema, the need for blood replacement, the patient's body weight and previous state of hydration. To these should be added measurements of the hematocrit (or other indices of the peripheral concentration of erythrocytes) and the hourly urine output. In previously healthy young individuals the hourly urine output will be the most sensitive index of fluid overload, and any maintained urine volume higher than 80 to 100 ml. per hour should warn the therapist that he is crowding the extracellular fluid with excess volume unless a rising blood urea level after the second day indicates polyuric renal failure.

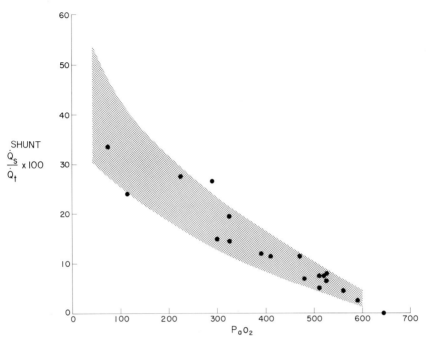

SHUNT FRACTION VERSUS OXYGENATION ON 100% O_2

Figure 1-8. Shunt fraction as a function of alveolar-arterial gradient on test inhalation of 100 per cent oxygen. The points are taken from a number of patients and studies carried out in these laboratories. Although the relationship is a loose one, and can only be quantified accurately with mixed venous oxygen data, it is evident that arterial oxygen tensions of 100 mm. Hg or lower, while on short test periods of 100 per cent oxygen inhalation, indicate that 30 to 50 per cent of the cardiac output is passing through the lungs without oxygenation.

The importance of moderation in intravenous infusion in the prevention of pulmonary insufficiency arises not only from its obvious causative relationship, but from the extreme difficulty of correcting errors. If a patient has been seriously overcrowded with crystalloid or electrolyte solutions, and is developing rales and some elevation of central pressures, this is not a matter that is easily or readily repaired merely by the administration of a very active diuretic agent such as ethacrynic acid or a drug such as digitalis. The massive diuresis that results from ethacrynic acid therapy can be associated with cardiac arrhythmias, especially in older persons who are already digitalized, and it is often disappointing to note that a large diuresis has not rectified the damage done in the lungs.

POSITION

Positional management of the patient is a matter of nursing care so obvious that often it escapes the attention of the surgeon who

may be devoting most of his thinking to other more subtle matters. The fact remains that the supine position held for many hours, or even days, will produce a ventilation-perfusion imbalance in the lungs that is a normal response to a new posture; it represents the same sort of blood-air distribution described for the sitting or standing human being, in which perfusion is devoted largely to the lower pulmonary segments. It will result in dorsal segment shunting and ventral segment dead space. Changing of position, deep breathing, and exercise are all significant in maintaining normal ventilation-perfusion relationships in the lung. The squirm is as important as the sigh.

Although the experiment has never to our knowledge been performed, it is conceivable that a perfectly normal person, placed in bed, rigidly immobilized in the supine position, bled a few units, given several transfusions and a large load of electrolyte, heavily sedated, and treated with multiple broad-spectrum antibiotics, would ultimately become very ill and possibly succumb to a

EFFECT OF MIXED VENOUS OXYGEN TENSION ON SHUNT
FRACTION AT CONSTANT P_aO_2 (OXYGEN BREATHING)

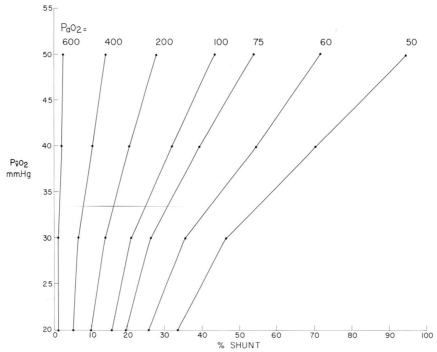

Figure 1-9. Effect of mixed venous oxygen tension on shunt fraction at constant arterial oxygen tensions during test inhalation of 100 per cent oxygen. It is evident that the higher the oxygen tension of mixed venous blood entering the right heart, as shown in the vertical coordinate, the larger will be the calculated shunt for any given arterial tension, as indicated by the isopleths. It is also noteworthy that this effect is most marked when arterial oxygen tensions are very low. Stated otherwise, it takes only a small amount of venous blood to darken the arterial blood if the venous blood is very desaturated to begin with. As the oxygen saturation of venous blood rises, for any given value of arterial oxygen tension achieved on a test inhalation of 100 per cent oxygen, the larger is the shunt fraction indicated thereby.

sequence of events bearing a close resemblance to post-traumatic pulmonary insufficiency. It is important not to add these difficult burdens to the problems of a patient who has, in addition, been severely injured before admission.

MEASURES IN PULMONARY CARE

Once the downward spiral has commenced, as manifested by some increasing shunt, some anoxia with concomitant hypocarbia, measures are instituted for the improvement of pulmonary function. It was formerly commonplace to do a tracheostomy before there had been any demonstration that access to the lower airway would improve the patient's ventilation or blood gas findings. The hazards of tracheostomy are too well known at this time to bear repetition here save to emphasize that all tracheostomy incisions become infected, that the organism

is usually *Pseudomonas aeruginosa* or one of the *Proteus* species, that this organism is later recovered from the lungs, that tracheobronchial ciliary action is inhibited at the site of the tracheostomy tube, that secretions are dried, and that the patient can no longer communicate with his attendants. A high price has been paid for direct access to the lower airway, the benefits of which must be clearly demonstrated by preliminary nasotracheal intubation before tracheostomy is justified. In the stage of acute injury, particularly with trauma around the neck and the face, the function of tracheostomy is entirely different, and immediate tracheostomy must often be done to establish an airway. It is in the later phases, after one to five days and with anoxia due to beginning shunt, that one must question most actively the advisability of a tracheostomy. In most instances a tracheostomy does little for shunt-induced anoxia.

There are three other steps often taken in pulmonary care that can also be damaging to the lungs and that have been a part of the fatal progression in post-traumatic pulmonary insufficiency. They must be done perfectly to avoid injury. These steps are: endotracheal suction, mechanical assistance to ventilation, and elevated oxygen tensions in the airway.

First, as to endotracheal suction. This is unquestionably a useful step if carefully done. In performing suction in a patient whose lower airway has never previously been contaminated and in whom the only problem is the removal of secretions, the surgeon must bear in mind that as he passes his catheter through the nasopharynx and into the lower airway he is carrying with it all the organisms that are present in the pa-

tient's nose, mouth, and pharynx; many of these are organisms that the patient has recently picked up in the hospital and to which he has little immunity. The procedure, no matter how many sterile precautions are taken, will thus inevitably contaminate the lower airway with these organisms. One must question whether it should be done or whether other methods (particularly non-invasive assistance to coughing and ventilation) are superior. When properly indicated and well done, endotracheal suction is important; for early post-trauma cases it is unquestionably hazardous.

Second, as to mechanical assistance to ventilation. The proper handling of mechanical ventilatory apparatus, particularly with respect to the norms to be met and the detailed management procedures, form the

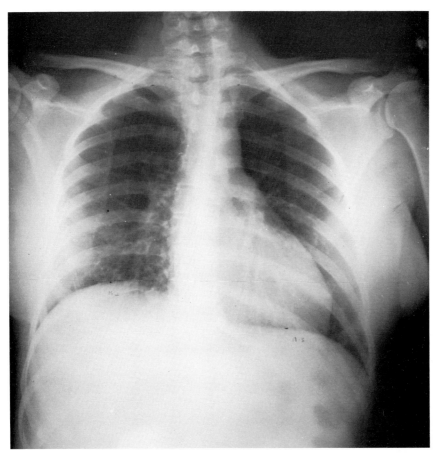

Figure 1-10. This and the subsequent three figures are x-rays of the same patient whose course is documented in Figure 1-4. This was a patient with gram-negative bacteremia, a severe low-flow state, and pulmonary insufficiency due to a septic self-induced abortion. This first film shows the diaphragm at a rather high level. There is some blurring of the vascular markings. The transverse diameter of the heart is normal for a film taken with portable equipment. This film was taken shortly after admission and indicates early interstitial edema especially at the right base.

subject of separate chapters in the monograph previously published from these laboratories (Moore et al., 1969). If mechanical ventilation is used, on an assist basis, with the patient's own diaphragmatic descent initiating the inspiratory cycle, there is some semblance of normal respiratory activity. Once the patient is heavily sedated and put on completely controlled respiration, he will show at least transient spectacular improvement as prolonged deep respirations with high inspiratory pressures and very large tidal volumes are imposed. The problem is to release the patient from this form of therapy and wean him back upward to his own control and finally to room air on spontaneous respiration. The farther the patient descends down this ladder, the more difficult the upward reascent becomes. One should be tolerant of some respiratory inadequacies,

particularly spotty atelectasis. Anoxemia, down to oxygen tensions in the range of 55 to 70 mm. Hg, are tolerable if hematocrit and pH are normal. One should beware of moving on to the deep and fully controlled respiration that initially looks so effective, but that brings in its wake extremely difficult problems two to five days later.

Finally, as to oxygen toxicity. The guidelines seem to be clear. Although it is very difficult to demonstrate damage to the normal human lung during a 12-hour continuous exposure to 100 per cent oxygen there seems little question from animal evidence that prolonged oxygen exposure is damaging, and there may be factors in the traumatized state that make the lung particularly vulnerable to oxygen-induced damage (Van De Water et al., in press).

The pathophysiology of increased veno-

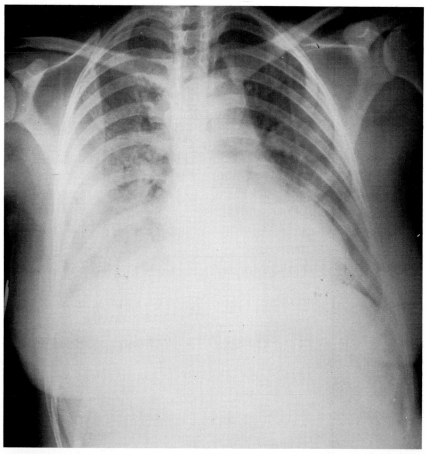

Figure 1-11. There has been a slight increase in the size of the heart in this film taken one day after that shown in Figure 1-10. There is now gross evidence of interstitial and alveolar edema with complete opacification of the lower two-thirds of the right lung with an air bronchogram. These are the appearances of acute combined alveolar and interstitial edema of very sudden onset. At this time the patient's oxygenation was failing and she was becoming acidotic.

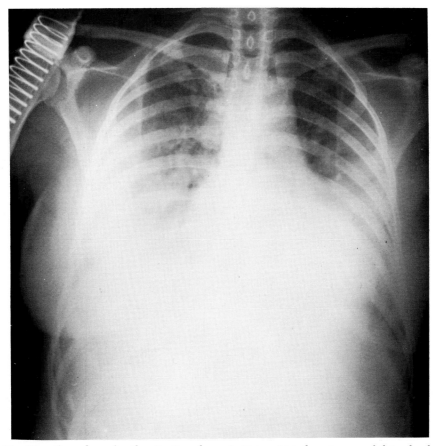

Figure 1-12. Now, three days after the situation shown in Figure 1-11, there is severe bilateral pulmonary edema sparing only the apices. There is engorgement of the primary pulmonary process rather than cardiac failure. At this time the patient's arterial oxygen tension on room air was less than 40 mm. Hg, and on a test period of 100 per cent oxygen inhalation, rose only to 90 mm. Hg, indicating a physiologic shunt of at least 30 per cent of cardiac output.

arterial admixture indicates both the futility of prolonged high oxygen tensions in the airway and the importance of making compromises.

When the alveolar-arterial gradient is severe, the inhalation of 100 per cent oxygen may suffice only to bring the arterial oxygen tension from a level of 30 or 40 mm. Hg on room air to 100 mm. Hg. The use of 75 per cent oxygen under these circumstances would suffice to bring the arterial oxygen tension to an acceptable level (about 70 mm. Hg) without at the same time threatening the lungs with the downward spiral that follows prolonged inhalation of 100 per cent oxygen by mechanical ventilation.

The gradual widespread realization of this fact has tempered the view so long held by anesthetists and respiratory therapists that all caution must be thrown to the winds and all other conditions subjugated merely to obtain the highest possible oxygen tension in arterial blood. Many patients have unfortunately suffered from such a dictum when a more sophisticated view would have let them inhale 60 or 75 per cent oxygen, remain somewhat deoxygenated, but save their lungs. Many persons who are heavy smokers or who have chronic lung disease from other causes (asthma, emphysema, bronchiectasis) live out useful lives with oxygen tensions between 60 and 75 mm. Hg. There is no use jeopardizing the sanctity of the alveolar membrane to achieve air oxygen tension over 100 mm. Hg. If one examines respiratory care records, one will find that over the years patients have been repeatedly superoxygenated, exposing their lungs to 100 per cent oxygen in order to achieve oxygen tensions in the arterial blood of about 250 to 400 mm. Hg. In persons who have normal acid-base balance and normal

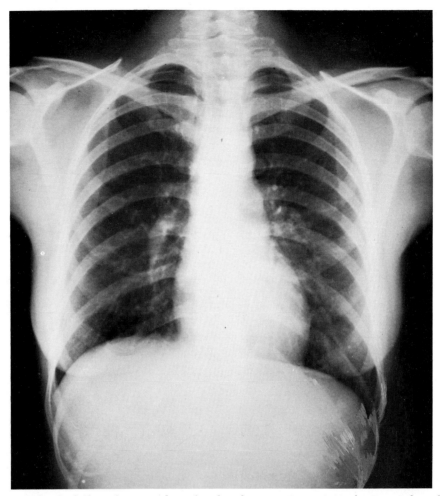

Figure 1-13. This final film, taken nine days after that shown in Figure 1-12, shows complete clearing of the pulmonary edema, with heart size and configuration well within normal bounds. At this time the lungs were normal to percussion and auscultation. There was no longer any physiologic shunt, and the respiratory situation had returned essentially to normal. These four films demonstrate the development and then the clearing of a form of post-traumatic pulmonary insufficiency due either to gram-negative bacteremia, endotoxemia, or the local effects on the lungs of microemboli from the uterine circulation, including the possibility that some of the Lysol soap is itself appearing in the pulmonary circulation.

hemoglobin, there is nothing to be gained by moving their arterial oxygen tension higher than 125 mm. Hg. At that level the hemoglobin is completely saturated and the oxygen content close to maximal. Any further small increase in oxygen content (for example, 3 to 5 per cent) achieved by increasing the oxygen tension in arterial blood to 250 mm. Hg is only done by extreme hazard to the alveolar membrane. As in most other things in medicine, restraint is essential to success.

In order to achieve oxygen tensions in the airway of fixed and known value, it is essen-tial to have respiratory devices that deliver oxygen mixtures of known composition to the airway equipment. A new oxygen mixing valve recently perfected by Drinker makes this possible, with delivery of fixed and known percentages of oxygen regardless of the pressures of flow rates on either side of the valve (Drinker et al., 1967). This is im-portant because certain types of demand-operated respiratory assist devices achieve humidification by entrainment of oxygen. At high flow rates or under certain conditions of adjustment, an oxygen concentration over 90 per cent can be delivered for many days at a time, despite a setting on "air mix" that indicates a presumed concentration around 40 per cent.

BACTERIOLOGY

Lobar pneumonia, empyema, lung abscess, and multiple septic pulmonary emboli may all occur after trauma and lead to severe illness or death from pulmonary infection. The infection is usually the primary event.

In post-traumatic pulmonary insufficiency the bacterial process is secondary; if the patient lives long enough it is inevitable. This bacterial colonization of the already damaged lung occurs by three predominant routes: the bloodstream, the airway, and tracheostomy.

The first is of primary importance in those patients in whom the source is a septic peripheral injury such as an infected wound or fracture, or peritonitis. In such patients, with high swinging fever and intermittent colonization of the bloodstream, the lungs are found a few days later to harbor the same organism cultured from the peripheral injury and the blood. The process seems clear enough although the precise pathogenetic mechanism may be poorly understood; organisms in the periphery have invaded the bloodstream and passed from there to the lungs.

The second predominant pathway is infection of the lungs from the upper airway of the patient, usually with organisms that are common in the hospital ambience. If the patient has had repeated endotracheal catheterization for suction, direct trauma to the airway or lungs, or repeated or prolonged nasotracheal intubation, then it is not difficult to understand how these hospital flora from the upper airway arrive in the lower airway. Once there, they find a friendly soil for growth in the edematous pulmonary interstitium and in poorly expelled mucus and bronchial fluid accumulation, characteristic of the severely injured patient.

The third route of pulmonary colonization is from the tracheostomy site itself. All tracheostomy incisions become colonized and most become infected. The predominant infecting organisms are bacilli of *Proteus* or *Pseudomonas* species. Once these organisms are present around the tracheostomy site itself, then despite aseptic precautions taken in suction or manipulation, such organisms

will be passed to the lower airway. The normal lung can withstand these hazards of tracheostomy as indicated by the prolonged tracheostomy management of patients with carcinoma of the larynx. The lung of the severely injured patient is less able to withstand such a challenge, and infection regularly results. The lower airway in man is normally sterile. Once it is infected it cannot become sterile again until its anatomic and ciliary integrity have been restored.

The restriction of antibiotics is essential in the treatment of post-traumatic pulmonary insufficiency, once infection has supervened. The antibiotic should be chosen according to the organism present in tracheal suction. It is remarkable how frequently this will be a single organism that far predominates over any others. It is also quite characteristic for an injured patient with multiple infected sites (a burn, for example) finally to show colonization by some one organism in virtually pure culture throughout the body. This is a preterminal event.

Once having started treatment with an appropriate antibiotic, and then making repeated cultures from the lower airway, one finds himself in the familiar dilemma of naming his bacteriologic objective. Does one expect this antibiotic to sterilize the lower airway? With the continued presence of a tracheostomy or repeated tracheal suction, this is impossible. If the objective is to protect the lung tissue from invasion, the organism that is sensitive to the antibiotic will be obliterated and replaced by another. Oftentimes the organism that finally colonizes the lower airway (when the initial infecting organism has been controlled) is either *Monilia* or *Pseudomonas*. Finding a change in organism on culture after three to seven days of antibiotic treatment, the therapist is then placed in the impossible position of changing antibiotics to suit that organism. He should again ask the question—what is the bacteriologic objective now? Since sterility of the lower airway cannot be attained so long as there is continued access to it by instrumentation, suction, or endotracheal invasion, the bacteriologic objective—avoidance of alveolar or interstitial invasion—obviously results in alteration of strain until one wholly resistant strain survives.

This all-too-familiar series of events makes it essential to use antibiotics sparingly and only with a precise clinical objective. It is best to use antibiotics in short courses at high dosage and then withdraw them. The normal human body carries a variety of bacteria in several sites. Prominent among these are the upper airway, the colon, the vagina, the ear canal, and the skin-hair-nails. There is a normal balance of flora in these sites including organisms that exhibit some degree of reciprocal growth inhibition by substrate competition or metabolite antibiosis. When multiple broad-spectrum antibiotics are used, this normal healthy polyglot flora is changed to a dangerous monocolonization. This colonization with a single organism throughout the body is a hazardous deterioration that presages a fatal pulmonary or bloodstream infection. The finding of the same organism in all sites is an ominous development in the traumatized patient, particularly one with pulmonary insufficiency.

The bacteriologic aspects of post-traumatic pulmonary insufficiency thus epitomize all the problems so prominent in surgical bacteriology: the hazards of unbalancing the normal flora, monocolonization with a single resistant strain, yeast infection, the impossibility of sterilizing certain areas of the human body, the passage of hospital organisms to a vulnerable tissue, and the difficulty of achieving any worthwhile bacteriologic objective so long as normal anatomic barriers are destroyed or bypassed.

It is for this reason that the initial management of the severely injured patient, particularly one who shows persistent hyperventilation or other evidences of pulmonary injury, must be accomplished with the strictest attention to asepsis right from the start. If it is possible to avoid extensive colonization of the patient with hospital organisms, if antibiotics can be restricted in their range and duration, and if violation of the lower airway can be avoided, then, and only then, can one hope that a fatal infection will be avoided in patients with post-traumatic pulmonary insufficiency.

REFERENCES

Ayres, S. M., Criscitello, A., and Grabovsky, E.: Components of alveolar-arterial O_2 difference in normal man. J. Appl. Physiol., *19*:43, 1964.

Carlsson, L. A.: Lipid mobilization in trauma—friend and foe. *In* Morgan, A. O. (ed.): *Proceedings of Conference on Energy Metabolism and Body Fuel Utilization.* Cambridge, Harvard University Printing Office, 1966, p. 50.

Coran, A. G., and Nesbakken, R.: The metabolism of intravenously administered fat in adult and newborn dogs. Surgery, *66*:922, 1969.

Dollery, C. T., and Glazier, J. E.: Pharmacological effects of drugs on the pulmonary circulation in man. Clin. Pharmacol. Ther., *7*:807, 1966.

Drinker, P. A., Carter, J. W., Howard, J. F., Kelley, T. L., and Peterson, R. S.: A constant ratio air-oxygen mixer. JAMA, *202*:531, 1967.

Eltringham, W. K., Hester, W. J., and Morgan, A. P.: Fat mobilization and fat infiltration from prolonged catecholamine infusion. Postgrad. Med. J., *45*:545, 1969.

Lyons, J. H., Jr., and Moore, F. D.: Posttraumatic alkalosis: incidence and pathophysiology of alkalosis in surgery. Surgery, *60*:93, 1966.

MacLean, L. D., Mulligan, W. G., McLean, A. P. H., and Duff, J. H.: Patterns of septic shock in man—a detailed study of 56 patients. Ann. Surg., *166*:543, 1967.

Moore, F. D., Lyons, J. H., Jr., Pierce, E. C., Jr., Morgan, A. P., Jr., Drinker, P. A., MacArthur, J. D., and Dammin, G. J.: Post-traumatic Pulmonary Insufficiency. Philadelphia, W. B. Saunders Company, 1969.

Nilsson, E., Slater, E. M., and Greenberg, J.: The cost of the quiet lung: Fluctuations in PaO_2 when the Carlens tube is used in pulmonary surgery. Acta Anaesth. Scandinav., *9*:49, 1956.

Proceedings of Conference Feb. 29-March 2, 1968 on Pulmonary Effects of Nonthoracic Trauma. Conducted by Committee on Trauma, Division of Medical Sciences, National Academy of Sciences-National Research Council. J. Trauma, *8*:666, 797, 865, 930, 952, 1968.

Shoemaker, W. C.: Personal communication.

Siegel, J. H., Greenspan, M., and Del Guercio, L. R. M.: Abnormal vascular tone, defective oxygen transport and myocardial failure in human septic shock. Ann. Surg., *165*:504, 1967.

Van De Water, J. M., Kagey, K. S., Miller, I. T., Parker, D. A., O'Connor, N. E., Sheh, J-M., MacArthur, J. D., Zollinger, R. M., Jr., and Moore, F. D.: Oxygen toxicity: a study in normal man. In press.

Weil, M. H., and Shubin, H.: Diagnosis and Treatment of Shock. Baltimore, The Williams & Wilkins Co., 1967.

CHAPTER 2

SHOCK AND CARDIAC ARREST

by JAMES D. HARDY, M.D.

*Department of Surgery, University of Mississippi Medical Center,
Jackson, Mississippi*

SHOCK

The management of shock constitutes a major segment of surgical endeavor. The operation performed may have produced the shocklike state, or, in turn, an operation may be required to reverse the shock. In other circumstances, the patient may not yet have had an operation and, in fact, operation may be contraindicated until treatment has been effective in controlling the hypotension. Thus the possibility of shock with its potential complications is ever present on any large surgical service.

The word "shock" means different things to different observers. To the laboratory investigator and, indeed, to many clinicians the term denotes a metabolic state caused by a prolonged reduction in arterial blood pressure. However, the writer prefers to consider the patient to be in shock as soon as his systemic arterial blood pressure is substantially below his normal value. If this hypotension is allowed to persist for a long enough period of time, the metabolic alterations produced will become sufficiently gross to be measured. When these metabolic changes are at an advanced state, virtually everyone would concede the existence of "shock." But again, we prefer to treat significant arterial hypotension at once, before serious biochemical changes have had time to develop. The simple or moderate hypotension produced by a dose of analgesic or a tranquilizer drug may not be significant, but it still represents a deviation from the normal physiologic state.

The level of the blood pressure per se does not establish or exclude the diagnosis of shock. For example, the blood pressure of a patient in profound shock can often be elevated temporarily to a normal level with an intravenous drip of norepinephrine, but it would not be concluded that the patient whose blood pressure was thus artificially elevated with a drug was no longer in shock. Conversely, a "normal" blood pressure level may actually represent a shocklike state in a patient who was previously severely hypertensive.

THE HAZARDS OF HYPOTENSION

The basic metabolic changes in shock, due primarily to cellular hypoxia and acidosis, affect all organs, but the heart is our primary concern. All other organs are dependent upon its pumping action, and hypotension permits inadequate coronary artery perfusion, which may lead to cardiac arrest. This is a particularly serious hazard in elderly patients, in whom coronary atherosclerosis may have already reduced myocardial blood flow to a critical level. Even if cardiac arrest does not occur, definite renal damage may develop in the presence of severe hypovolemia, even when marked vasoconstriction prevents a profound fall in blood pressure. In fact, any organ that is already diseased or has a reduced blood flow because of vascular disease may be further damaged by hypotension (Fig. 2-1). Brain damage may be evidenced by coma, liver damage by jaundice, and renal damage by oliguria and azotemia. When profound hypotension persists long enough, a state of cellular damage develops that precludes recovery and is termed "irreversible shock." However, the surgeon should ever be on guard lest the "irreversibility" simply represent inadequate diagnosis or inadequate treatment.

The orientation of this chapter is a clinical one, and an orderly approach to the diagnosis and management of shock in surgical patients

23

MECHANISMS OF HYPOXIA

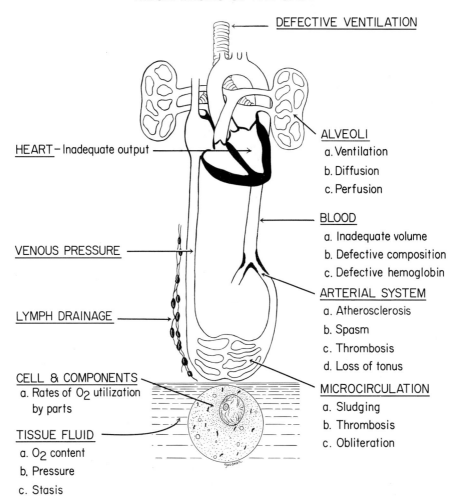

DEFECTIVE VENTILATION

HEART – Inadequate output

ALVEOLI
a. Ventilation
b. Diffusion
c. Perfusion

BLOOD
a. Inadequate volume
b. Defective composition
c. Defective hemoglobin

VENOUS PRESSURE

ARTERIAL SYSTEM
a. Atherosclerosis
b. Spasm
c. Thrombosis
d. Loss of tonus

LYMPH DRAINAGE

CELL & COMPONENTS
a. Rates of O_2 utilization
   by parts

MICROCIRCULATION
a. Sludging
b. Thrombosis
c. Obliteration

TISSUE FLUID
a. O_2 content
b. Pressure
c. Stasis

Figure 2-1. The amount of oxygen supplied to the individual cell may be influenced by many factors. (From Hardy, J. D.: Tissue hypoxia in surgical practice. Amer. J. Surg., 106:476, 1962)

will be emphasized. After consideration of causes and a general discussion about the patient in an undiagnosed state of shock, the management of shock in specific disease states will be considered. The management of shock ranges from simple blood replacement in the patient with a bleeding peptic ulcer to tracheostomy for laryngeal obstruction, and to all the measures available for the patient with massive blunt trauma, flail chest, sepsis, or acute heart failure.

FACTORS THAT MAINTAIN NORMAL BLOOD PRESSURE

The factors that maintain a normal blood pressure in healthy patients are known to all physicians. These are the blood volume, the peripheral resistance, and the heart. Yet it is surprising how often this knowledge is not applied in the diagnosis and management of shock. If one can but identify which of the three factors is or are deficient, the appropriate therapy will usually be apparent.

BLOOD VOLUME

The blood volume of the person of average obesity represents approximately 80 ml. per kilogram of body weight. Since fat contains little blood (or water) as compared with lean tissue, the blood volume of the fat person may be only 75 ml. or less per kilogram (Hardy et al., 1951). Furthermore, it has been estimated that the arteries contain approximately one-fourth of the blood volume, the veins one-half, and the heart and lungs one-fourth. This emphasizes the large role played by venous constriction or dilatation in the prompt adjustment to variations in the total blood volume. The blood volume of a 70-kilogram man of average obesity should be approximately 5 liters, but the figure varies somewhat from person to person, and it may vary in the same person, according to his state of physical conditioning. The blood volume is composed of the plasma volume and the red cell mass. The plasma volume can be measured with dye or isotope (RISA) and the red cell mass with the venous hematocrit or with Cr^{51}-tagged red cells. The error in these methods is approximately 10 per cent. The previously healthy adult can lose a large amount of blood without evidence of shock, as long as compensatory reflexes are not interfered with. By the time clinical shock is evident, the patient may have lost one-fourth to one-third of his blood volume.

Notwithstanding the normal blood volume and the methods for its measurement, the surgeon is primarily concerned with the "effective" blood volume. That is, regardless of what the blood volume may be in liters, is it adequately filling the right atrium to permit an effective cardiac output? For example, in certain disease states the blood volume may be normal or actually increased, but the return to the right heart may be inadequate because of vasodilatation and venous pooling in the splanchnic area or in the muscles. A similar situation could be produced by giving ganglionic blocking drugs. Therefore, it is necessary to think in terms of the effective or functional blood volume, one which at the moment in question is producing an adequate but not excessive flow into the right atrium. At times an augmented blood volume is advantageous in permitting a needed increase in cardiac output, but in other circumstances a diseased heart cannot accept even a moderate increase in venous return. This dynamic relationship is reflected in variations in the central venous pressure, a measurement commonly monitored in the treatment of shocklike states. If the heart cannot accept the venous return without a significant rise in central venous pressure, and if the systemic blood pressure remains low, digitalization and perhaps isoproterenol to improve myocardial contractile strength may be in order.

The composition of the total blood volume, comparing red cell volume or mass with plasma volume, may vary considerably in disease states. In general, the red cell mass remains rather stable over brief periods, in the absence of gross hemorrhage. In contrast, plasma volume may increase in cases of heart failure or decrease in the case of dehydration due to vomiting or to peritonitis (Fig. 2-2) or to plasma loss beneath burn

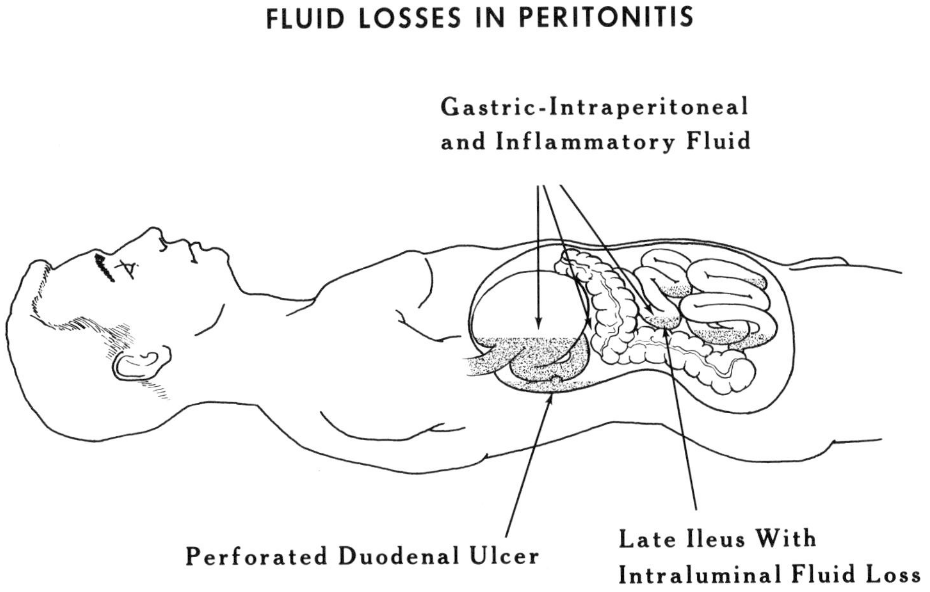

FLUID LOSSES IN PERITONITIS

Gastric-Intraperitoneal and Inflammatory Fluid

Perforated Duodenal Ulcer

Late Ileus With Intraluminal Fluid Loss

Figure 2-2. The massive fluid losses that can occur in peritonitis may result from fluid sequestration in the gastrointestinal tract, the peritoneal cavity, and the retroperitoneal space, as well as from diarrhea and nasogastric suction or vomiting.

wounds, for example. Plasma loss results in hemoconcentration with an elevation of the blood hematocrit level (normal, 45 per cent). Hemoconcentration usually also reflects a reduction in the interstitial fluid volume, which constitutes the supporting reservoir for the plasma volume. For effective support of the plasma volume the interstitial fluid must be adequate not only in amount but also in its ionic composition. The sodium ion in particular is very important in maintaining the extracellular volume, from which, in turn, the intracellular fluid volume replenishes itself (Fig. 2-3). A striking example of the importance of the sodium ion may be seen in the patient undergoing hemodialysis on the artificial kidney. If hypotension develops, it is often corrected by giving 100 ml. of isotonic sodium chloride intravenously. Other solutions containing no sodium do not have an equal effect.

A low plasma sodium level may indicate an absolute sodium deficit or a relative or absolute excess of water. An elevated sodium level may reflect inappropriate renal excretion of this ion or it may reflect a relative or absolute water deficit. In addition to an adequate volume of extracellular fluid, there must also be an adequate concentration of plasma proteins to preserve the normal colloid osmotic pressure to hold the appropriate volume of water in the vascular bed.

It has been seen that plasma is a component of the extracellular fluid, and that when the volume of one is diminished, that of the other is usually diminished. Likewise, it has become increasingly apparent that similar interrelationships exist between the extracellular fluid and the intracellular fluid. Even in simple hemorrhage, significant fluid shifts may occur (Shires et al., 1961). For example, a sudden significant hemorrhage is followed by hemodilution, effected by the movement of fluid from the interstitial space and probably from the intracellular space into the vascular compartment. This hemodilution occurs in several hours in the dog but requires from 18 to 24 hours in man. A normal well-hydrated person can thus compensate for the loss of a liter of blood by fluid shifts within 24 hours, with a resultant hemodilution that will reduce the hematocrit by 10 per cent. However, since this hemodilution occurs slowly, the hematocrit is a poor guide to blood replacement immediately after significant blood loss has occurred. The advantages and disadvantages of massive Ringer's lactate therapy in various clinical disease states are discussed in Chapter 3.

PERIPHERAL RESISTANCE

A normal blood volume will permit a normal cardiac output, which will produce a normal systemic arterial blood pressure, so long as there exists an adequate degree of resistance at appropriate sites in the vascular tree. However, sudden and massive vasodilatation, as may occur in certain drug responses or hypersensitivity states, can result in a marked fall in blood pressure. The viscosity of the blood, particularly due to red cell content, also assists in the maintenance of normal peripheral resistance. For example, studies have suggested that the hypotension often seen immediately after the initiation of cardiopulmonary bypass using hemodilution may be due to decreased peripheral resistance, despite a normal flow into the arterial tree (Hardesty et al., 1969). A significant increase in blood viscosity, as in marked polycythemia, can lead to a reduced rate of peripheral flow, sludging, and even thrombosis in small vessels.

A decrease in peripheral resistance is often seen in endotoxin shock, and stasis and pooling in the splanchnic area is a prominent feature of this condition, especially when it occurs in the laboratory, where it can be measured. While the logical treat-

BODY COMPOSITION OF A NORMAL MALE OF AVERAGE OBESITY

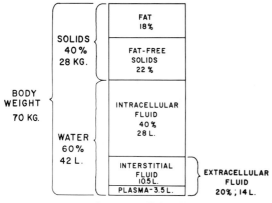

Figure 2-3. The intracellular fluid is dependent for its volume and constituents upon water and ions that must traverse the extracellular fluid. Evidence increasingly documents a continuous dynamic exchange between the two compartments. (From Hardy, J. D.: Fluid Therapy. Philadelphia: Lea and Febiger, 1954)

ment under such circumstances would appear to be the use of a vasopressor drug, in actual practice these agents have frequently been disappointing. They almost invariably raise the blood pressure, but actual tissue perfusion may remain defective and the recovery rate is often not clearly improved.

Excessive and clearly abnormal vasoconstriction occurs in some patients, as in endotoxin shock or following cessation of cardiopulmonary bypass in the presence of continuing hypovolemia. In general, it is preferable to transfuse such patients steadily, using the central venous pressure as a guide, as the vasoconstriction recedes and normal vascular tone returns. Some clinicians have recommended the use of phenoxy-benzamine (Dibenzyline) to dissipate severe vasoconstriction, coupled with adequate blood transfusion, as will be described subsequently. We ourselves have witnessed remarkable improvement produced by intravenously administered Thorazine (25 mgm.) in a few patients who had pathologically intense vasoconstriction: skin perfusion improved, respiration became more quiet and effective, the CVP declined, systemic arterial blood pressure stabilized, urine output increased, and the sensorium cleared.

Much remains to be learned regarding the factors that regulate vascular tone, but endogenous vasoactive substances such as epinephrine and norepinephrine surely have important roles.

CARDIAC OUTPUT

The importance of the heart in maintaining a normal blood pressure level can hardly be exaggerated. Given an adequate blood volume, inadequate heart action is a most common cause of hypotension in surgical patients. This reduced strength of myocardial contractions may be due to pre-existing heart disease, but it is often due to defective respiration leading to hypoxia and acidosis. Electrolyte imbalance, especially with regard to potassium and calcium but probably sodium also, can have a markedly deleterious effect on heart action.

The immediate danger of severe hypoxia or hypotension due to hypovolemia is cardiac arrest, either in asystole or ventricular fibrillation. This precipitates a crisis of stark proportions, one that might have been avoided if the blood pressure had been maintained at an adequate level by arterialization of the blood, if normal blood volume had been maintained or if a vasopressor drug had been used temporarily to support the blood pressure while the precise diagnosis and appropriate therapy were being developed.

The normal cardiac output is usually expressed as the "cardiac index," and it represents the cardiac output in liters per minute per square meter of body surface area. This value is from 4 to 6 liters in an adult of average size, for a cardiac index of 3 to 4 liters, since the surface area of the average adult is approximately 1.5 sq. meters. The value of using the "cardiac index," as contrasted with the cardiac output in liters, is that it permits comparison between individuals of varying sizes.

Unfortunately, the correlation between cardiac output and blood pressure often exhibits a very inexact relationship, for severe vasoconstriction may temporarily prevent a fall in blood pressure even when the cardiac output is seriously reduced secondary to hypovolemia or to cardiac disease per se. Furthermore, in the shock patient the pre-injury cardiac output is rarely known and, since even in health there is a considerable variation in the cardiac output between individuals of equal size or in the same person at different times, the actual determination of the cardiac output in the shock patient is often of limited therapeutic assistance unless the value is grossly abnormal. Therefore, the overwhelming majority of patients in shock are treated, usually successfully, without dependence upon measurement of the cardiac output, though its use is increasing.

Actually, a diminished cardiac output may be virtually assumed if there is a reduced urine output reflecting reduced renal perfusion and body surface evidence of low output, such as vasoconstriction, clammy skin, cyanosis, and a sluggish capillary refill. The patient may also exhibit restlessness due to cerebral hypoxia and thirst due to oligemia. However, in septicemia significant shock and oliguria may at times occur in the presence of a high cardiac output. While clinical evidence of a reduced cardiac output does not disclose whether it is due to defective heart action, to inadequate blood volume, or to a combination of the two, the measurement of the central venous pressure is helpful. If the central venous pressure is high, the blood volume is at least adequate for the pumping action that the heart can effect at that given time. Once the heart action has been rendered more effective by digitalis, isoproterenol, better lung function, or necessary electrolyte adjustment, the total blood volume may prove actually to be diminished and transfusion may be required. This illustrates the intimate interrelationships that exist among the heart, the lungs, and blood volume. Again, defective peripheral resistance, with inappropriate arterial-capillary-venous function, is not a major problem in most surgical patients early in shock. Such defects may be found in endotoxin shock and in the terminal phases of other types of unsuccessfully treated shock.

DIFFERENTIAL DIAGNOSIS OF SHOCK

The precise, expeditious, and successful treatment of shock depends upon an orderly approach to diagnosis, with recognition of physiologic priorities.

The *history*, abbreviated to meet the immediate clinical circumstances, is essential even in the extreme emergency. Has there been obvious blood loss, or fluid loss by vomiting, diarrhea, or sequestration in the gut, in wounds or elsewhere? Is there evidence of respiratory insufficiency of whatever type, from whatever cause? Is the patient febrile? Has he sustained trauma? Has he experienced chest or abdominal pain that might suggest myocardial infarction, pulmonary embolus, or aneurysm?

Other items of history can be gleaned as emergency measures are initiated at once to prevent cardiac arrest while the total clinical situation is being further evaluated.

The physical examination will also be directed to the requirements at hand. Repeated blood pressure measurements reflect the diagnosis and progress of the shocklike state. Is there an adequate airway and is pulmonary ventilation effective, as indicated by chest expansion and auscultation? Is the patient cyanotic? Has he vomited, with possible pulmonary aspiration of gastric contents? Is blood loss visible, or do severe pallor and vasoconstriction suggest internal bleeding, as from duodenal ulcer or ruptured aneurysm? Are the neck veins distended, which would suggest an adequate blood volume but defective heart action secondary to valvular or myocardial disease, to hypoxia from defective lung function or coronary atherosclerosis, or to pulmonary

embolism or pericardial tamponade? What is the character of the pulse? Does it suggest an inadequate blood volume or arrhythmia? A rapid pulse, or one that taps the finger and then falls quickly away, or the pulse that diminishes in volume on inspiration suggests inadequate venous return to the heart with reduced cardiac output. Dyspnea may reflect respiratory difficulty, but it also may reflect hypovolemia. In a postoperative patient, hypovolemia may be reflected in excessive cyanosis and pallor of a leg with arterial occlusive disease long before the blood pressure has fallen.

The *clinical* and *laboratory measurements* that are readily available and useful are the blood pressure, respiratory rate, pulse rate, urine output, central venous pressure (CVP), electrocardiogram, hematocrit, plasma electrolytes, portable chest x-ray, and BUN. Moreover, measurements of the arterial blood pH, P_{O_2}, and P_{CO_2} should be available in every general hospital of significant size, on a 24-hour basis. Blood volume and cardiac output determinations are frequently available in the larger hospitals, but they are not commonly used in clinical practice unless a research project is underway.

Once a tentative diagnosis of the probable defect or combination of defects—heart, blood volume, or peripheral resistance—has been made, emergency measures are instituted at once, to be followed by more orderly and precise therapy on a continuing basis.

A check list of the usual causes of hypotension is presented in Table 2-1. Failure of therapy to raise the blood pressure and to improve the metabolic state may reflect inadequate therapy or an incorrect or incomplete diagnosis of the cause or causes of shock. Unfortunately, in the most advanced shock state, so-called "irreversible shock"—a conclusion which, again, often reflects erroneous diagnosis and inadequate or inappropriate treatment—it may be impossible to demonstrate which of the factors that normally preserve an adequate blood pressure level is most at fault.

In concluding these remarks regarding diagnosis, one must emphasize the great importance of continued observation of the patient by an experienced clinician. He may detect early or delayed clues to diagnosis and proper therapy that often escape the less experienced observer. Furthermore, since the shocklike metabolic state is an everchanging continuum in the given pa-

TABLE 1.　Causes of Hypotension*

1. Volume deficits 　Whole blood loss 　Plasma loss 　Interstitial fluid loss or shift 　Water deficit 2. Electrolyte deficits or excesses 　Na, K, Cl, Ca, Mg 3. Acid-base imbalance 　Respiratory acidosis 　Metabolic acidosis 　Respiratory alkalosis 　Hypokalemic alkalosis 4. Sepsis 　Septicemia 　Infection with fluid shift (peritonitis) 5. Respiratory insufficiency 　Hypoxia 　Hypercapnia 　Right-to-left pulmonary shunts (atelectasis, 　　pneumonia, lung contusion) 　Pneumothorax 　Mechanical disturbances due to trauma (flail 　　chest, tracheolaryngeal injury) 　Pulmonary embolism 6. Cardiac causes 　Cardiac arrest or fibrillation 　Coronary occlusion 　Pericardial tamponade 　Cardiac arrhythmia 　Myocardial failure 　Cardiac contusion 7. Central nervous system causes 　Brain injury 　Increased intracranial pressure 　Reflex vagal stimuli 　Psychic stimuli 　Brain-stem and spinal cord injury	8. Endocrine causes 　Adrenocortical insufficiency 　Adrenomedullary dysfunction (e.g., shock before 　　and following resection of pheochromocytoma) 　Thyroid crisis 　Hyperinsulinism 　Diabetic coma 9. Shock during operation 　Hypovolemia (from anesthetic vasodilatation and 　　pre-existing blood-volume deficit, or acute 　　blood loss) 　Heart failure 　Hypoxia 　Hypercarbia 　Myocardial ischemia 　Arrhythmia 　Miscellaneous other causes 10. Shock in recovery room 　Hypovolemia 　Cardiac failure 　Hypoxia 　Hypercarbia (due to inadequate ventilation) 　Coronary insufficiency 　Arrhythmia 　Electrolyte imbalance 　Endotoxin shock 　Pulmonary embolus 　Excessive medication 11. Miscellaneous 　Drug reactions 　Transfusion reactions 　Fat embolism 　Hepatic failure 　Anaphylaxis

*From Gurd, with modifications and additions.

tient, a single initial decision regarding treatment is usually inadequate, and it must be followed up by reassessment and redirected therapy at frequent intervals. The ability to manage shock successfully is essential to good surgical results.

MANAGEMENT OF THE PATIENT IN SHOCK

BASIC PROCEDURE AND ORGANIZATION OF SHOCK THERAPY

This discussion will begin with consideration of the most imminently fatal clinical shock circumstances and will then expand outward to less exacting physiologic requirements. The essential features of immediate therapy are presented in Figure 2-4.

CASE ANALYSIS: SHOCK FOLLOWING ABDOMINAL OPERATION. As an example, take the 70-year-old obese female in the Recovery Ward whose blood pressure is found to be 60/40 mm. Hg one hour following completion of an abdominoperineal resection for carcinoma of the rectum. A fat-soluble inhalation anesthetic agent (most inhalation anesthetic agents are fat soluble) was used, and 30 minutes after operation the patient was given 10 mg. of morphine sulfate intramuscularly for pain.

Clearly the coronary artery perfusion at such a low pressure, especially in an elderly patient who surely has a degree of coronary atherosclerosis, will not long support the myocardium, and arrhythmia and cardiac arrest threaten. It is far simpler to treat shock prior to cardiac arrest than after arrest has occurred. When cardiac arrest occurs because of the prolonged hypoxic effects of inadequate pulmonary ventilation or hypovolemia, these defects must be corrected concurrently with heart resuscitation or the resuscitative efforts cannot be successful. Furthermore, the heart that arrests after a brief period of hypoxia is usually more easily

MANAGEMENT OF SHOCK

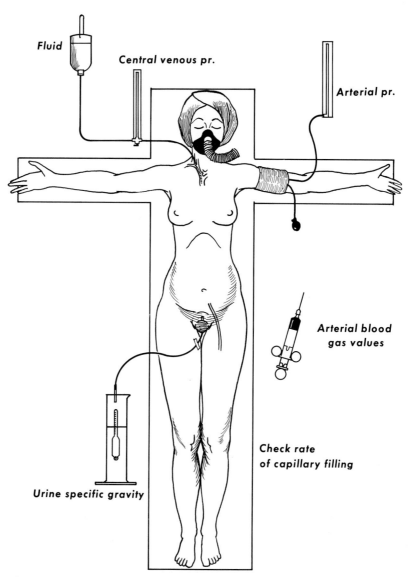

Fluid

Central venous pr.

Arterial pr.

Arterial blood gas values

Check rate of capillary filling

Urine specific gravity

Figure 2-4. The systemic arterial blood pressure, the effectiveness of pulmonary ventilation as reflected in arterial gas values, the central venous pressure as a gauge of effective blood volume, the rate of urine formation, and the rate of capillary re-fill are all important considerations in the management of shock.

resuscitated than one that has failed after prolonged hypoxia, usually due to defective pulmonary ventilation or to hypovolemia.

The patient in this case is an obese and elderly woman who was given a fat-soluble anesthetic agent, which will be slowly mobilized from the fat depots, and on whom an operation was performed that leaves a large raw surface and that usually involves significant blood loss. In addition, she received morphine for pain.

The most urgent consideration, and fortunately the most quickly correctable problem

if it exists, is the possibility of inadequate pulmonary ventilation. This may have developed because of continued effects of the anesthetic agent, respiratory depressant effects of the morphine, advanced age, or a diaphragm elevated by fat within the peritoneal cavity. Incidentally, we have found that more energy is necessary for adequate pulmonary ventilation in fat patients than in lean patients (Neely et al., 1970). Thus the physician immediately checks the adequacy of pulmonary ventilation by inspection, manual palpation at the nares, the expansions of the thorax, and auscultation. Even if ventilation appears to be reasonably adequate, one should draw an arterial sample for blood-gas analyses. Hypoventilation is usually reflected in a reduced PO_2 (normal, 90 to 100 mm. Hg) and an increased PCO_2 (normal, 40 mm. Hg). However, even with good ventilation the arterial PO_2 may be reduced and the PCO_2 increased if a diffusion defect across the alveolar membrane exists, such as might develop following excessive fluid administration, after pulmonary aspiration of gastric contents, or in congestive heart failure.

But assuming that inadequate pulmonary ventilation does not exist or is quickly corrected by positive pressure face mask assistance, or by insertion of a nasotracheal or oral endotracheal tube and airway, or even by tracheostomy in unusual circumstances, the next consideration is the possibility of an inadequate blood volume. Before leaving the problem of pulmonary ventilation, however, it should be noted that we and many other surgeons and anesthesiologists often leave the endotracheal tube in place postoperatively for hours or even several days, with assisted positive pressure ventilation, using a respirator when indicated. However, if the endotracheal tube is to be left for a prolonged period, it is well to replace the orally inserted tube with a nasotracheal tube, since the latter is better tolerated and produces less salivation owing to lessened oral stimulation. The advantage of the endotracheal tube over the nasotracheal tube is that it is more difficult to suction the tracheobronchial tree through the latter. If assisted ventilation is to be continued for more than 48 to 72 hours, a tracheostomy will usually be required.

Gross evaluation of lung function requires but a few moments, and it takes priority because severe hypoxia from hypoventilation will produce cardiac arrest much more quickly than will a reduced blood pressure level with good pulmonary ventilation.

Next, attention is turned to the adequacy of the blood volume. If pulmonary ventilation is satisfactory, the hypotension is probably caused by an inadequate effective blood volume. This inadequacy may be caused by a relative vasodilatation from the remaining effects of anesthesia or the morphine, but it is more likely caused by a chronically reduced blood volume in a patient who had rectal malignancy, by unreplaced blood loss

at operation, or by continuing blood loss into the operative area. Actually, the precise explanation for the relative hypovolemia is not essential for appropriate corrective action. If the neck veins are not distended, as they might after a myocardial infarction or pulmonary embolus, a pint of blood should be infused briskly to determine the effect on the blood pressure. Meanwhile, a catheter for measuring the central venous pressure (CVP) should be inserted, if one has not been introduced prior to operation. As long as the CVP remains below 100 mm. of saline and the patient remains hypotensive, blood should be infused at a rather rapid rate (500 ml. every 10 to 15 minutes). When the CVP has risen to 100 to 150 mm. of saline, further blood should be given with caution. If blood for transfusion is not immediately at hand, an electrolyte solution, plasma volume expander, or a vasopressor drug should be infused as a temporary expedient. In general, transfusion will restore the blood pressure to normal, reduce the pulse rate, diminish the sympathomimetic signs of cold sweat and vasoconstriction, and increase the urine output, as measured with an indwelling catheter. The perineal wound should be inspected for excessive oozing or for frank hemorrhage, which should be corrected by surgical means. The general objective should be to stop hemorrhage promptly and to minimize the amount of blood transfusion required, for the transfusion of homologous blood involves certain hazards itself and ultimately the patient becomes more and more refractory to transfusion.

If lung function is good and if the CVP is satisfactory or elevated, but arterial hypotension persists, the adequacy of heart action must be questioned. An electrocardiogram should usually be performed and digitalization should usually be effected. An isoproterenol drip may be helpful.

Respiratory acidosis due to hypercarbia should be corrected by adequate respiratory function, and metabolic acidosis is corrected with sodium bicarbonate infusion. The risk of pulmonary aspiration should be minimized by nasogastric suction to keep the stomach empty and to relieve respiratory embarrassment from gastric distention.

These several measures will correct arterial hypotension in the vast majority of patients in the Recovery Ward, but additional possible causes of hypotension are presented in Table 2-1.

Intra-arterial blood pressure monitoring can be extremely valuable in many critically ill patients, and it should be used much more often. In the presence of intense vasoconstriction the intra-arterial measurement (taken in a femoral artery) may reveal actual hypertension at a time when the brachial arterial pressure is not obtainable with the blood pressure cuff. In addition, continuous monitoring by intra-arterial catheter gives a minute-by-minute index of the state of cardiovascular function, and thus permits prompt and rapid adjustments in the many facets of effective therapy.

FURTHER COMMENTS ON SHOCK THERAPY IN GENERAL

VOLUME REPLACEMENT

The question is often asked, How much blood replacement does the patient in hemorrhagic shock need? The answer is, Enough. For example, it may be assumed that the average adult in profound shock has lost perhaps 2000 ml. of blood, or almost one-third of his blood volume. Furthermore, blood loss may be continuing, internally or externally, at an indeterminate rate. Blood loss into the abdomen is hard to diagnose or to estimate, even if drains were inserted at operation: clotted blood may have blocked the drainage tract while fresh hemorrhage continues. Blood loss into the chest can usually be detected with roentgenograms, but even here the films can be misleading. Factors such as lung and heart status as well as peripheral resistance and individual patient variations come into play, and it is not only impossible but even hazardous to replace blood rapidly by any pre-set formula. The first several pints may be given rapidly, if hemorrhage is continuing and the situation is urgent. In general, though, it is well to follow the CVP, arterial blood pressure, pulse rate, and urine output as guides to blood replacement. Massive and rapid loss must be rapidly replaced, and to do this successfully at least two large bore needles or catheters should be placed in good peripheral veins. Blood is given until the CVP rises or the arterial blood pressure rises, after which further blood is often needed but should be given more slowly and more cautiously.

Serial measurements of the hemoglobin and hematocrit levels are useful guides to blood replacement for slow but continuing bleeding, but, again, these measurements are useless and even misleading guides to blood replacement in massive and rapid hemorrhage. They are useless because almost six hours are required for the hematocrit to change significantly following a hemorrhage in man, and by that time the patient might well have exsanguinated. Blood volume measurements are occasionally helpful for the detection of major blood deficits or overloads, but in clinical practice they are used infrequently.

Adequately crossmatched blood should be used in most patients, but in a dire emergency it may be necessary to use low-titer O-negative blood initially, followed by proper typing and crossmatching as quickly as possible. For example, the occasional patient with a ruptured abdominal aortic aneurysm may survive only minutes unless blood is infused. If typed and crossmatched blood cannot be made available within minutes, O-negative blood should be used. Some temporary assistance can be gained from electrolyte solution, serum albumin, or other plasma expander, but these do not provide red cells to carry oxygen. Furthermore, if the patient fails to secrete urine promptly, excessive electrolyte solution can ultimately produce hypoxia due to pulmonary edema.

Before leaving the subject of whole blood replacement, we should consider the prevention of hypovolemia. Blood transfusion is rarely required for certain operations such as simple cholecystectomy or simple thyroidectomy. However, the patient who is to undergo radical neck dissection or abdominoperineal resection will almost always require transfusion, and this should be initiated before substantial blood loss has so stained the compensatory mechanisms that hypotension, tissue hypoxia, and an oxygen debt occur.

WATER AND ELECTROLYTE REPLACEMENT

Blood loss and its replacement have been emphasized because of the urgent emergency created by such loss. However, the red cell mass may remain satisfactory in some types of shock that are due to body water and salt loss. Such circumstances may occur in prolonged vomiting, diarrhea, mechanical intestinal obstruction, ileus, gastrointestinal fistula, massive thermal burns and peritonitis secondary to perforated peptic ulcer, pancreatitis, or intestinal leakage. Massive external or internal fluid loss results in a diminished plasma volume and an elevated hematocrit level, and appropriate fluid replacement will promptly increase the cardiac output (Fig. 2-5). In massive trauma with multiple fractures, both red cells and plasma (extracellular fluid) are lost. The surgeon expects substantial fluid losses

through a high-output small bowel fistula, but the relatively huge functional losses that occur in small bowel ileus, with or without peritonitis, are not always appreciated.

Such fluid losses should be replaced with electrolyte solutions. (See Chapter 3.) Relatively large volumes may be required, for example, following perforation of a duodenal ulcer and peritonitis (Fig. 2-2). However, whereas serial measurements of the central venous pressure are helpful in preventing excessive transfusion of whole blood, these measurements do not provide an adequate safeguard against excessive

SOME CAUSES OF SHOCK IN TRAUMA

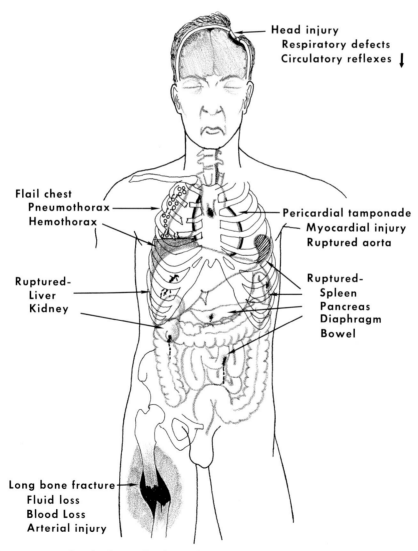

Head injury
Respiratory defects
Circulatory reflexes ↓

Flail chest
Pneumothorax
Hemothorax

Pericardial tamponade
Myocardial injury
Ruptured aorta

Ruptured-
Liver
Kidney

Ruptured-
Spleen
Pancreas
Diaphragm
Bowel

Long bone fracture
Fluid loss
Blood Loss
Arterial injury

Figure 2-5. In trauma, the shock may be due to hypovolemia, respiratory insufficiency, sepsis, pump failure, vasomotor collapse, or mixed causes. Continuous observation of the patient is essential.

noncolloid fluid administration: pulmonary edema may develop before a significant rise in the CVP is produced by electrolyte solutions, which promptly leave the bloodstream. For rule of thumb, body fluid losses should be replaced with solutions containing electrolytes. A modest volume of 5 per cent dextrose in water is given to provide for losses through urine and sweat, for which the body can control the electrolyte loss to some extent. Perhaps the commonest "low sodium" syndrome seen in otherwise stable postoperative patients is that produced by the intravenous infusion of large volumes of dextrose in water when a solution containing electrolytes is what is needed. Isotonic sodium chloride solution is often preferable for the replacement of gastric fluid losses with chloride depletion, since this salt solution contains a physiologic excess of chloride ions; potassium supplementation will also be required in most instances. For replacement of balanced losses with little change in the plasma electrolyte levels, Ringer's lactate solution is frequently used.

The adequacy of water and salt replacement is reflected in the vital signs, especially in the urine output, the appearance of the tongue and the skin turgor, the plasma electrolyte values, and the red cell hematocrit.

RESPIRATORY FUNCTION

This subject deserves additional comment. Few advances in recent years have so improved surgical care as has the realization that a substantial segment of surgical morbidity and mortality is a result of defective respiration. This realization has come about largely through the widespread and routine use of arterial blood gas determinations and pH. These measurements permit early detection of impending respiratory insufficiency, which is frequently relieved by vigorous measures to mobilize pulmonary secretions. Prolonged use of the endotracheal tube and assisted positive pressure ventilation have markedly reduced the incidence of postoperative hypoxemia and resulting shock from myocardial depression. Incidentally, it is not always realized that hypertension characterizes the initial stages of hypoxia and hypercarbia, but that this hypertension is eventually followed by severe hypotension due to myocardial failure. If doubt exists

regarding the probable adequacy of pulmonary ventilation in the obtunded postoperative patient, who was perhaps already debilitated and elderly, the closest supervision is mandatory. Hypoventilation is usually preventable, but it still constitutes a prominent cause of surgical morbidity and mortality.

Again, the hazard of pulmonary aspiration of gastric contents before, during, and following operation should be minimized by nasogastric suction to empty the upper reaches of the alimentary tract. A cuffed endotracheal tube offers good ventilation and considerable protection from pulmonary aspiration once it is in place, but the patient often vomits and aspirates before the cuff has been inflated.

CARDIOGENIC SHOCK

The well-oxygenated normal heart has a tremendous functional capacity, but hypoxia is poorly tolerated. Hypoxia may develop in many ways, including defective respiration, hypovolemia with reduced cardiac output and hypotension, and localized hypoxia as a result of coronary artery occlusive disease. Each of these should be anticipated and prevented to the extent possible (Fig. 2-1). In addition, the heart may have pre-existing valvular, conduction, or myocardial disease. Digitalization is usually indicated when heart failure is a definite possibility. Careful attention to achieving normal plasma electrolyte concentrations will reduce arrhythmias.

VASOPRESSOR DRUGS

Much has been written regarding the use of vasopressor drugs in the treatment of shocklike states. In the writer's experience, these drugs are clearly valuable if used for specific purposes and discontinued as soon as possible. First, a vasopressor drug such as Neo-synephrine is often useful in supporting the blood pressure for brief periods, until blood is available for transfusion. Secondly, an isoproterenol or even norepinephrine drip often permits the heart to gain needed vigor following cardiopulmonary bypass. Thirdly, the occasional patient may require vasopressor support, when blood volume and respiration are adequate, and then eventually stabilize and go on to recover. Again, vasopressor drugs should theoretically be useful in endotoxin shock, but here their value has been difficult to confirm and, in fact, some workers prefer to use vasodilator drugs to treat this condition. If cardiac support is the primary requirement, isoproterenol is preferable to norepinephrine if it will suffice, since the former strengthens myocardial contractions and rate without the peripheral vasoconstriction produced by norepinephrine. Moreover, a slow drip of isoproterenol (Isuprel) is well tolerated without tissue damage for many hours or even days, whereas norepinephrine may result in such severe arteriolar constriction that organ damage results. However, norepinephrine may be required when isoproterenol is ineffective.

The vasopressor drug should be administered continuously in a slow drip in sufficient concentration and low volume to avoid overloading the oliguric patient with excess fluid. Once a satisfactory blood pressure level has been achieved (90 to 110 mm. Hg), it should be sustained with the minimal amount of drug possible. The use of "doses" of drugs, injected in a single slug, is to be discouraged, since the marked swings in blood pressure levels that result are best avoided.

VASODILATOR DRUGS

Considerable laboratory and clinical experience has now been accumulated with the use of the adrenergic blocking agent, phenoxybenzamine hydrochloride (Dibenzyline) in the treatment of shock, especially endotoxin shock. Gurd and his associates found beneficial effects in certain patients who were already transfused to the point of an elevated central venous pressure and pulmonary edema and whose blood pressure remained low. The blood pressure and cardiac output values indicated a high peripheral resistance, supported by clinical evidence of intense adrenergic activity in the form of cold, moist, and cyanotic extremities. Despite all efforts to improve ventilation and oxygenation, such patients showed a low arterial PO_2 and a falling blood pH. After the administration of 1 mg. of Dibenzyline per kilogram of body weight, vasodilation and a reduction of CVP were often seen, at which time further blood transfusion almost always became necessary. These effects of Dibenzyline, which appeared in

approximately 10 minutes and lasted approximately 24 hours, frequently permitted the extremities to become warm, dry, and pink. Pulmonary edema was found to clear, and arterial PO_2 values improved.

The writer has had limited clinical experience with adrenergic blocking agents in apparently "irreversible shock" due to sepsis, but the results thus far have not been dramatically encouraging. However, as noted earlier, we have observed very gratifying improvement after intravenous injection of Thorazine for severe vasoconstriction following cardiopulmonary bypass and in certain other circumstances. In animal experiments with induced endotoxin shock, we were unable to demonstrate a significant reduction in mortality rates with norepinephrine, isoproterenol, or Dibenzyline, but isoproterenol did prolong survival (Anas et al., 1969).

STEROID THERAPY

Much has been written about the value or lack of value of massive doses (e.g., 1000 to 1500 mg.) of hydrocortisone in the management of shock, especially septic shock. Here again, few if any patients have been saved by this drug in our experience, but we do use it when all other therapy has proved inadequate. It has often been used instead of Dibenzyline, since it also has an adrenergic blocking effect. Of course, if the shock is a result of adrenocortical insufficiency, the steroid therapy will be beneficial.

HYPOTHERMIA

Hypothermia has been advocated in the management of shocklike states associated with fever. We have preferred to maintain the body temperature at an essentially normal level, avoiding either marked hyperthermia or hypothermia.

SEPTIC SHOCK

Septic shock occurs frequently following instrumentation of the urinary tract, as well as in association with biliary tract infection, peritonitis, septic burn wounds and pulmonary infection. The mechanisms by which bacteria produce profound shock are far from clear, though extensive investigations have added much to the information available (Ebert and Stead, 1941; Lillehei et al., 1964; MacLean et al., 1967; Udhoji and Weil, 1965).

Peripheral pooling of blood occurs regularly in the dog and probably in many patients, and thus blood transfusion is usually indicated, guided by central venous pressure measurements. The peripheral resistance may be high, for which Gurd and his associates use Dibenzyline therapy, or it may be low. A markedly increased cardiac output has been found in some cases of septic shock by ourselves and by others and, since the heart is able to produce this output with the substantial amount of blood returning to the right atrium, it has been concluded that peripheral resistance is deficient in at least some cases of endotoxin shock. The strength of myocardial contraction is rather well preserved until late in the course of irreversible endotoxin shock (Alican et al., 1962), but Clowes and associates have reported an apparent benefit of empirical digitalization in shock due to severe infection.

Endotoxin shock is best treated with saline and blood transfusion as guided by the CVP, drainage of pus where possible, massive antibiotic therapy, and digitalization when indicated. Many patients in septic shock exhibit alkalosis, but when metabolic acidosis exists it should be treated with sodium bicarbonate. Hemodialysis may be required for renal failure, and to reduce fluid overload when necessary. Respiratory function should be made as effective as possible. We use isoproterenol in an intravenous drip when other measures appear to be failing. This drug produces both ionotropic and chronotropic effects upon the heart, and at the same time it decreases resistance at the tissue level by stimulating the beta receptors. It has appeared to offer assistance in the management of a few cases of septic shock that had proved refractory to other measures. Nevertheless, isoproterenol is as yet not fully established as an effective agent in the management of clinical endotoxin shock. It should not be forgotten that endotoxin shock represents an assault that the body must first limit and then gradually overcome. If the patient can be kept alive by whatever means available, his own defenses may gradually triumph.

Massive steroid therapy in doses of 1000 to 1500 mg. of hydrocortisone, given intravenously, has frequently been employed by us and by others. However, the effects achieved have been less than impressive, and fluid replacement remains a primary therapeutic measure in endotoxin shock.

Arterial blood lactate measurements are useful in following the effectiveness of therapy, and a progressive rise in the lactate level indicates a poor prognosis. However, lactate levels are not usually necessary to assess the efficacy of treatment.

SPECIAL SITUATIONS IN CLINICAL SHOCK

IRREVERSIBLE SHOCK

In some patients the shocklike state is so profound and so prolonged, refractory to all therapy, that it is termed "irreversible shock." However, we have found that in many patients the shock has not responded to treatment because the diagnosis of the cause of the shock was either incorrect or incomplete, or the treatment inappropriate or inadequate. The presence of a Shock Study Team in our hospital has resulted in a more orderly and precise approach to diagnosis and management of shock states.

SHOCK IN COMPLEX BLUNT TRAUMA

The patient who has sustained severe blunt trauma, as from an automobile injury, may be in shock from internal hemorrhage, inadequate respiration, cardiac contusion, brain injury, fat embolism, body fluid translocation and sequestration, or other causes (Fig. 2-6). Frequently, a decision to explore the abdomen for possible rupture of spleen, liver, kidney, or gut must be made in a patient comatose from head injury, with a flail chest and lung contusion and with multiple long-bone fractures. To render matters worse, he may be in renal shutdown, and fluid overload must be avoided to the extent possible. Judicious blood and fluid replacement, and perhaps assisted ventilation through a cuffed endotracheal tube, may be required to preserve life until the various diagnostic possibilities have been eliminated or dealt with effectively.

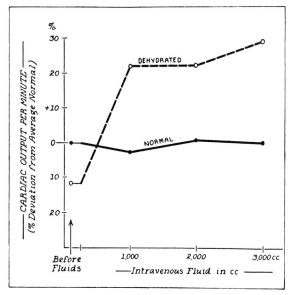

Figure 2-6. The administration of fluid to dehydrated patients promptly increased the previously reduced cardiac output. The same volume of fluid produced little change in normal volunteers. (From Hardy, J. D., and Godfrey, L., Jr.: Effect of intravenous fluids on dehydrated patients and on normal subjects. JAMA, 126:23, 1944)

should be discontinued temporarily and blood should be infused, unless the CVP is elevated already.

The shock that follows prolonged clamping and then release of the abdominal aorta is a result of both abrupt filling of the distal vascular bed and the return of acid metabolites to the heart from the previously ischemic portion of the body. The clamp should be released somewhat slowly, and sodium bicarbonate should be given intravenously to combat the acidosis. An initial dose of one or perhaps two ampules, 44.5 mEq. each, is appropriate in the adult, to be repeated if indicated by arterial blood pH measurements.

The hypotension that often follows the initiation of cardiopulmonary bypass, using hemodilution, may be caused by diminished peripheral resistance as a result of dilution of the blood and reduced blood viscosity. It has been shown that the "cardiac" output (by the pump oxygenator) and blood volume may be normal under these hypotensive circumstances (Hardesty et al., 1969).

SHOCK DURING OPERATION

The commonest cause of shock during operation is a functionally inadequate circulating blood volume. This may have developed through vasodilatation as a result of the anesthetic agent, preoperative blood volume deficit, or blood loss at operation. In any case, blood transfusion is required. The second most common cause of sustained hypotension is defective anesthetic management. This may be reflected in hypoxia, hypercarbia, or excess anesthetic agent with a toxic effect on the heart. Traction on the abdominal viscera or compression of the vena cava may produce hypotension temporarily, but this is usually a fleeting phenomenon. Other causes of shock during operation are transfusion reaction, heart failure from heart disease, a fresh myocardial infarction, pulmonary embolism, aspiration of material into the lungs, or some metabolic state such as adrenocortical crisis, pheochromocytoma, or thyroid crisis.

When the blood pressure falls sharply during operation, the patient should usually be ventilated with pure oxygen and with minimal or no anesthetic agent. Retraction

SHOCK IN POSTOPERATIVE PERIOD

Shock in the Recovery Ward was considered previously. Suffice it to re-emphasize here that inadequate blood volume, residual anesthetic effect, and inadequate pulmonary ventilation are the most common causes of hypotension in the immediate postoperative period. This is also true of patients who have had open-heart surgery, in which case, however, failure of the heart itself must be given serious consideration. If the operation involved the heart, cardiac tamponade must be considered. A roentgenogram is helpful in excluding abnormal collections of blood, fluid, or air within the thorax, but relatively huge amounts of blood may be lost into the abdomen without producing changes detectable on roentgenogram or by physical examination. If serious question exists, the abdomen should be explored. A negative peritoneal tap does not exclude the diagnosis of intraperitoneal hemorrhage.

To re-emphasize, the monitoring of blood pressure, pulse rate, CVP, respirations, urine output, and arterial blood gases will afford most of the data required to prevent shock in the postoperative patient.

HYPOTENSION DURING ENDOSCOPY

A severe fall in blood pressure, often associated with convulsions, may occur during bronchoscopy or esophagoscopy. This may be due to hypoxia, but it may also be a result of overdosage or allergic reaction to the topical anesthetic agents. These drugs are absorbed rapidly through the mucous membranes and toxic blood levels can easily be produced. If such a severe reaction occurs, along with bronchospasm, positive pressure ventilation with a face mask or endotracheal tube and intravenous injection of a barbiturate are indicated. The most serious possible immediate complication is cardiac arrest from hypoxia.

ACUTE HEART FAILURE

The management of acute heart failure, which can have a variety of causes, ranging from excessive blood transfusion to myocardial infarction, cannot be discussed in detail here. Suffice it to note that rapid digitalization, positive pressure pulmonary ventilation with oxygen, aminophylline, effective diuretics, and perhaps phlebotomy in special circumstances are all useful measures upon occasion.

CARDIAC ARRHYTHMIAS

Shock due to cardiac arrhythmias embraces a specialized field, which need not be considered in detail here. (See Chapter 27.) Suffice it to note that an excessive ventricular rate due to atrial fibrillation can be controlled with digitalization. Rapid atrial tachycardia can be slowed with quinidine. Premature ventricular ectopic beats and ventricular irritability may be controlled with an intravenous drip of Xylocaine, or lidocaine, or Pronestyl. Finally, every effort must be made to render the plasma electrolytes normal and respiration optimal. If ventricular fibrillation appears to threaten on the basis of excessive cardiac irritability, the cardiac defibrillator should be kept at the bedside and the electrocardiograph should be monitored continuously in an Intensive Care Unit.

SHOCK FOLLOWING ENDOCRINE OPERATIONS

Certain endocrine tumors are often associated with shocklike states, especially upon their removal. The pheochromocytoma may be associated with profound hypotension preoperatively and following its excision. The preoperative shock usually follows a hypertensive crisis as a result of the abrupt release of large amounts of epinephrine or norepinephrine or both into the bloodstream. If the patient does not die from acute left ventricular strain, pulmonary edema, or intracranial hemorrhage, spontaneous recovery ensues. This same train of events may follow manipulation of the tumor at operation, but, being forewarned, the anesthetist should have prepared a drip of Regitine (phentolamine), a sympatholytic agent that neutralizes the effects of the catecholamines. Recently, phenoxybenzamine (Dibenzyline) has been advocated for preoperative preparation to minimize cardiac arrhythmias and to permit blood volume augmentation and adjustments prior to surgery (Sjoerdsma et al., 1966).

The hypotension that may follow removal of the functioning tumor is largely a result of a blood volume inadequate to fill the vascular tree, which is no longer constricted. If transfusion to a CVP level of 100 to 150 mm. saline does not overcome the hypotension, a slow drip of a vasopressor agent may be required temporarily. A relative adrenocortical insufficiency has been suggested as a contributing cause of the hypotension, but the writer has not been convinced that adrenal insufficiency plays a significant role. Nonetheless, there is little or no contraindication to the administration of 100 mg. of hydrocortisone every 6 hours in a drip for 24 hours, and it should be used if blood volume augmentation and, if needed, a vasconstrictor drip are not sufficient to raise the blood pressure. Digitalization should be considered.

Thyroid crisis represents a complex metabolic state, the pathogenesis of which has never yet been fully explained. It may occur spontaneously in hyperthyroid patients, and it may develop following subtotal thyroidectomy for thyrotoxicosis. The crisis or "storm" is possibly caused by the release of excessive amounts of thyroid hormone into the bloodstream, but even this has been difficult to document. In any case, the condition is characterized by irritability, disorientation, fever, tachycardia, and, at times, pulmonary edema. The treatment begins with prevention, for a patient who cannot be rendered euthyroid should not be operated upon, regardless of the risks of radioiodine. Once crisis has developed, it should be treated with sedation, reserpine, digitalization, mild hypothermia, and an oxygen tent. Intravenous hydrocortisone therapy has occasionally seemed helpful. Even so, the mortality rate of full-blown thyroid crisis is still significant.

Adrenocortical crisis and shock, following adrenal surgery or operations upon other organs where adrenocortical function was inadequate, are also diffuse metabolic phenomena. However, it has now been shown that the hypotension is at least partly cardiac in origin, reduced peripheral resistance being perhaps an additional factor. The myocardium requires an adequate amount of adrenocortical hormone to function properly (Webb et al., 1965). The treatment of adrenocortical insufficiency consists primarily of the infusion of hydrocortisone or related adrenocortical substance, supplemented with transfusion and other supportive measures. A dosage of 100 mg. of hydrocortisone every 6 hours, given in an intravenous drip beginning at operation, is almost always sufficient. Incidentally, in acute adrenocortical insufficiency there will not have been time for plasma electrolyte changes to occur, and treatment must be instituted on presumptive clinical evidence. The presence of a normal number of eosinophiles in the peripheral blood following a major operation suggests reduced adrenocortical activity. In our experience, adrenocortical insufficiency has been rare, and it has usually occurred when least expected, as in the cancer patient with adrenal metastases.

CARDIAC ARREST

Cardiac arrest occurs on all busy surgical services. The causes are multiple, but the major cause in patients without serious pre-existing heart disease is hypoxia. This hypoxia usually results from inadequate pulmonary ventilation, hypotension due to hypovolemia or other causes. The patient with pre-existing heart disease, especially coronary atherosclerosis, is especially predisposed to cardiac arrest. The physician should be forever alert to correct quickly any condition that might lead to myocardial

irritability or depression. Basically, hypotension and hypoxia should be avoided.

Cardiac arrest may be considered to exist when the heart can no longer eject properly the blood that returns to the right atrium. The "arrest" may consist of regular contractions so weak as to be ineffectual, complete standstill, or ventricular fibrillation. In either situation, remedial measures must be instituted at once.

DIAGNOSIS

The diagnosis of circulatory arrest is usually simple but can be somewhat difficult. At operation it is usually discovered by the anesthetist when he cannot feel the carotid pulse or get a blood pressure reading. The surgeon should quickly palpate the aorta, if the abdomen is open, or observe the heart, if the chest is open. Otherwise, the femoral artery should be palpated. If an effective pulse cannot be detected, the patient should be treated as if he had sustained cardiac arrest, whether or not a weak beat may still be present. The suspicion of arrest can be further verified with the electrocardiogram, but treatment should not be postponed while the electrocardiograph machine is being fetched.

MANAGEMENT

Speed is of the essence. Closed-chest cardiac massage should be instituted immediately (Fig. 2-7) and the lungs should be ventilated with pure oxygen if the patient has been intubated for operation. A useful synchronization is for the surgeon to give three brisk compressions of the chest over the heart, then pause briefly to permit the lungs to be inflated, and then give three more cardiac compressions. Two ampules of sodium bicarbonate (44 mEq. each) should be given intravenously to combat the metabolic acidosis caused by hypoxic metabolism.

After effective circulation has been restored, as reflected in a palpable femoral pulse with each cardiac "massage" or chest compression, the leads for the electrocardiogram should be applied to determine whether the heart is beating, is in standstill, or is in ventricular fibrillation.

MANAGEMENT OF CARDIAC ARREST

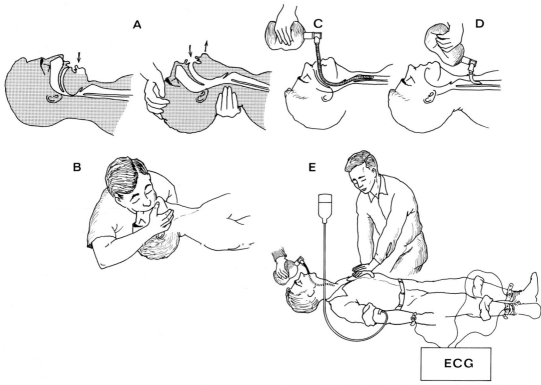

Figure 2-7. In the management of cardiac arrest, mouth-to-mouth breathing should be replaced with an airway and face mask and endotracheal tube. This procedure is supplemented by closed-chest massage and the ECG should be determined.

FURTHER MANAGEMENT

The initial steps of external cardiac massage and pulmonary ventilation have been mentioned. Mouth-to-mouth breathing may be necessary initially, but it should be replaced with an airway and face mask, followed by an endotracheal tube as soon as possible. Pulmonary aspiration of vomitus is always a hazard until a cuff has been inflated within the trachea. If massive pulmonary aspiration of gastric contents occurs, the patient who has sustained cardiac arrest will not often recover.

It has been estimated that about one-half the normal cardiac output can be achieved by external compression of the chest (Jude, 1967). If the heart is still beating weakly or is in standstill, external massage and pulmonary ventilation should be continued until a good femoral pulse and a systolic blood pressure of 90 to 100 mm. Hg are present.

As soon as effective pulmonary ventilation and closed-chest massage (palpable femoral pulse) have been achieved, the electrocardiogram should be employed to detect the presence or absence of ventricular fibrillation. If fibrillation exists, it must be abolished with the electrical defibrillator. One gram of calcium chloride may be given intravenously, and blood volume deficits should be quickly corrected with transfusion. An intravenous drip of isoproterenol or norepinephrine may be required to support the circulation temporarily.

If the heart has not sustained a coronary thrombosis or if it was not subjected to severe and prolonged hypoxia before it arrested, resumption of cardiac activity is the rule. Again, if ventricular fibrillation exists, the external defibrillator should be used to convert the organ to arrest, following which it will commonly assume a regular beat. The pulse or direct current defibrillator is preferred. The more difficult the defibrillation, the worse the prognosis, by and large. Failure of the heart to maintain a regular rhythm, that is, if it reverts back repeatedly to ventricular fibrillation, is often a bad sign.

If defibrillation cannot be accomplished through the closed chest wall, the chest should be opened and the defibrillator electrodes applied directly to the heart through the opened pericardium. However, efforts should not be made to defibrillate the heart until it has been well oxygenated by ventilation of the lungs and cardiac massage.

REASSESSMENT

Once an effective heart beat has been re-established, the following minutes, hours, and days are critical ones. The heart should be supported with continued massage until a good femoral pulse can be palpated and a brachial blood pressure obtained. The drip of vasopressor drug may be slowed to a level that will support the blood pressure above 90 mm. Hg, and this drip should be discontinued altogether as soon as possible. If the resuscitated heart cannot sustain an adequate blood pressure level without drug support, the prognosis is uncertain. The arterial blood pH should now be checked and additional sodium bicarbonate given intravenously if needed. Next, if indicated, either an endotracheal tube, preferably passed through the nose, or a tracheostomy tube should provide a secure means for assisted pulmonary ventilation during the next 48 hours. The cardiac defibrillator should be at the bedside, and the heartbeat should be monitored continuously. The patient who has sustained one cardiac arrest, regardless of the cause, is often predisposed to further arrests. It is often impossible to exclude, initially, the possibility that a myocardial infarction precipitated the cardiac arrest. However, if prompt action is taken each time the heart arrests, the patient will often survive repeated arrests and resuscitations and be restored to normal life. The presence of a dependable airway, either endotracheal tube or tracheostomy, vastly improves the possibility of successful (cardiac) resuscitation. The previously intubated patient may and often does survive many episodes of cardiac arrest.

ADDITIONAL MEASURES

Digitalization should be instituted on the basis of the merits of the given case, and appropriate drug therapy should be used to reduce ventricular irritability. The patient may be rendered hypothermic, to minimize cerebral edema and brain compressions, but we elect simply to prevent hyperthermia.

The neurologic condition should be assessed as soon as the situation has stabilized. If the pupils are widely dilated and fixed to light, irreversible brain damage may have occurred, though not always. If the patient exhibits spontaneous respirations, has nondilated pupils that react to light, and moves all four extremities, the prognosis for neurologic recovery is probably good.

PROGNOSIS

The prognosis depends upon numerous factors such as the age of the patient, the duration of hypoxia prior to cardiac arrest, the time required for resuscitation, whether or not organic heart disease existed prior to arrest, whether myocardial infarction occurred, whether severe hypovolemia existed at the time of arrest, whether or not the patient has aspirated gastric contents and thus made pulmonary gas exchange defective, the location of the patient in the hospital at the time of arrest, whether significant brain or renal damage has occurred and, last but not least, the experience of the team providing the cardiac resuscitation.

The cardiac arrest that occurs at thoracotomy, with the heart exposed, is usually detected quickly and readily corrected. In contrast, the arrest that occurs on one of the hospital floors distant from the operating rooms is often associated with delayed resuscitation and pulmonary aspiration of vomitus. Furthermore, the physicians and nurses at hand may not be sufficiently experienced to cope quickly and effectively with the situation, and the salvage rate under such circumstances is poor. Finally, if the arrest was primarily due to pre-existing heart disease, the resuscitative efforts may be unsuccessful, though occasionally success is achieved.

In conclusion, it is stressed that all physicians must expect to encounter patients who have sustained unexpected cardiac arrest. Prevention yields substantial returns, but prompt and effective management of actual arrest can provide successful resuscitation in a gratifying percentage of cases.

REFERENCES

Alican, F., Dalton, M. L., Jr., and Hardy, J. D.: Experimental endotoxin shock; circulatory changes with emphasis upon cardiac function. Amer. J. Surg., *103*:702, 1962.

Altemeier, W. A., and Cole, W. R.: Septic shock. Ann. Surg., *143*:600, 1965.

Anas, P., Neely, W. A., and Hardy, J. D.: The effect of vasoactive drugs on oxygen consumption in endotoxin shock. Arch. Surg., *98*:189, 1969.

Baue, A. E.: Recent developments in the study and treatment of shock. Surg. Gynec. Obstet., *127*:849, 1968.

Baue, A. E., and McClerkin, W. W.: A study of shock: acidosis and the declamping phenomenon. Ann. Surg., *161*:41, 1965.

Clowes, G. H. A., Jr., Farrington, G. H., Zuschneid, W., Crossette, G. R., and Saravis, C.: Circulating factors in the etiology of pulmonary insufficiency and right heart failure accompanying severe peritonitis. Ann. Surg. (In press.)

Crenshaw, C. A., Canizaro, P. C., Shires, G. T., and Allsman, A.: Changes in extracellular fluid during acute hemorrhagic shock in man. Surg. Forum, *13*:6, 1962.

Dietzman, R. H., and Lillehei, R. C.: The treatment of cardiogenic shock. V. The use of corticosteroids in the treatment of cardiogenic shock. Amer. Heart J., *75*:274, 1968.

Ebert, R. V., and Stead, E. A., Jr.: Circulatory failure in acute infections. J. Clin. Invest., *20*:671, 1941.

Gurd, F. N.: Shock as a Complication in the Surgical Patient. *In* Artz, C. P., and Hardy, J. D. (eds.): Complications In Surgery and Their Management. 2nd ed. Philadelphia, W. B. Saunders Company, 1967.

Hardesty, R. L., Baker, L. D., Gall, D. A., and Bahnson, H. T.: Systemic resistance during cardiopulmonary bypass. Surg. Forum, *20*:185, 1969.

Hardy, J. D.: Cardiac arrest. *In* American College of Surgeons' Manual of Preoperative and Postoperative Care. Philadelphia, W. B. Saunders Company, 1967.

Hardy, J. D., and Godfrey, L., Jr.: Effect of intravenous fluids on dehydrated patients and on normal subjects; cardiac output, stroke volume, pulse rate and blood pressure. JAMA, *126*:23, 1944.

Hardy, J. D., Sen, P. K., and Drabkin, D. L.: The relation of body fluid compartments to body fat. Surg. Gynec. Obstet., *93*:103, 1951.

Hardy, J. D., Neely, W. A., Wilson, F. C., Jr., Milnor, E. P., and Wilson, H.: Fluid kinetics following thermal burns in man. Surgery, *34*:457, 1953.

Jude, J. R.: Cardiac Arrest and Resuscitation. *In* Artz, C. P., and Hardy, J. D. (eds.): Complications In Surgery and Their Management. 2nd ed. Philadelphia, W. B. Saunders Company, 1967.

Kinney, J. M., and Wells, R. E.: Problems of ventilation after injury and shock. *In* Symposium on Shock. J. Trauma, *2*:370, 1962.

Lillehei, R. C., Longerbeam, J. K., Block, J. H., and Manax, W. G.: The nature of irreversible shock: experimental and clinical observations. Ann. Surg., *160*:682, 1964.

MacLean, L. D., Mulligan, W. G., McLean, A. P. H., and Duff, J. H.: Patterns of septic shock in man—a detailed study of 56 patients. Ann. Surg., *166*:543, 1967.

Martin, A. M., Soloway, H. B., and Simmons, R. L.: Pathologic anatomy of the lungs following shock and trauma. J. Trauma, *8*:687, 1968.

Moore, F. D., Lyons, J. H., Jr., Pierce, E. C., Jr., Morgan, A. P., Jr., Drinker, P. A., MacArthur, J. D., and Dammin, G. J.: Post-Traumatic Pulmonary Insufficiency. Philadelphia, W. B. Saunders Company, 1969.

Moyer, C. A., Margraf, H. W., and Monafo, W. W., Jr.: Burn shock and extravascular sodium deficiency—treatment with Ringer's solution and lactate. Arch. Surg. (Chicago), *91*:92, 1965.

Neely, W. A., Martin, H., McMullan, M. H., Bobo, W. O., Meadows, D. L., and Hardy, J. D.: Postoperative respiratory insufficiency. Ann. Surg., *171*:679, 1970.

Nickerson, M., and Gourzis, J. T.: Blockade of sympathetic vasoconstriction in the treatment of shock. *In* Symposium on Shock. J. Trauma, *2*:399, 1962.

Shenkin, H. A., Cheney, R. H., Govons, S. R., Hardy, J. D., and Fletcher, A. G., Jr.: On the diagnosis of hemorrhage in man. A study of volunteers bled large amounts. Amer. J. Med. Sci., *208*:421, 1944.

Shires, G. T., Williams, J., and Brown, F.: Acute change in extracellular fluids associated with major surgical procedures. Ann. Surg., *154*:803, 1961.

Siegel, J. H., and Del Guercio, L.: Peripheral and central factors influencing the pulmonary complications of nonthoracic trauma in man. J. Trauma, *8*:742, 1968.

Sjoerdsma, A., Engelman, K., Waldmann, T. A., Cooperman, L. H., and Hammond, W. G.: Pheochromocytoma: current concepts of diagnosis and treatment. Ann. Intern. Med., *65*:1302, 1966.

Thal, A. P., and Wilson, R. P.: Shock. *In* Current Problems in Surgery. Chicago: Year Book Medical Publishers, Inc., 1965.

Trinkle, J. K., Rush, B. F., and Eiseman, B.: Metabolism of lactate following major blood loss. Surgery, *63*:782, 1968.

Udhoji, V. N., and Weil, M. H.: Hemodynamic and metabolic studies on shock associated with bacteremia. Ann. Intern. Med., *62*:966, 1965.

Webb, W. R., Degerli, I. U., Hardy, J. D., and Unal, M.: Cardiovascular response in adrenal insufficiency. Surgery, *58*:273, 1965.

Weil, M. H., and Shubin, H.: Shock following acute myocardial infarction. Current understanding of hemodynamic mechanisms. Progr. Cardiov. Dis., *11*:1, 1968.

Wilson, J. N., Grow, J. B., Demong, C. V., Prenedel, A. E., and Owens, J. C.: Central venous pressure in optimal blood volume maintenance. Arch. Surg., *91*:121, 1965.

Wilson, R. F., Chiscano, A. D., and Quadros, E.: Some observations on 58 patients with cardiac shock. Anesth. Analg. (Cleveland), *46*:764, 1967.

Wilson, R. F., Chiscano, A. D., Quadros, E., and Tarver, M.: Some observations on 132 patients with septic shock. Anesth. Analg. (Cleveland), *46*:751, 1967.

CHAPTER 3

POSTOPERATIVE OLIGURIA, ACID-BASE IMBALANCE, AND FLUID DISEQUILIBRIUM*

by H. T. RANDALL

Henry Thomas Randall was born in New York City and received his education at Princeton University and Columbia University College of Physicians and Surgeons. Always an outstanding scholar, he developed an abiding interest in shock and fluid balance while still in training at Columbia-Presbyterian Hospital. He was appointed Clinical Director, Memorial Hospital for Cancer and Allied Diseases, and Associate Professor of Surgery at Cornell University only two years after completion of his residency. There he later served as Vice President of Medical Affairs, Memorial Hospital, and full Professor of Surgery. He is now Surgeon-in-Chief of Rhode Island Hospital and Professor of Medical Science, Brown University. Dr. Randall has been a vigorous national and international leader in the investigation, writing, and teaching of the pathophysiology and treatment of body fluid disequilibrium in surgical patients.

The purpose of this chapter is to discuss the etiology, diagnosis, and management of several major disorders of body fluid distribution and of acid-base balance in critically ill patients.

Since the kidneys are active regulators of the volume, concentration, and pH of body fluids, as well as the organs effecting excretion of nonvolatile end products of metabolism, adequate renal function is an important part of prevention and correction of fluid and acid-base abnormalities. Alterations in renal function play a major role in the development and maintenance of serious disequilibria in the critically ill patient. Early and proper treatment can prevent or attenuate the severity of postoperative renal insufficiency.

POSTOPERATIVE OLIGURIA

Postoperative oliguria may be defined as an hourly urine volume of 17 ml. or less in the average adult male (70 kg.) and of 15 ml. per hour or less in the average adult female (60 kg.). These rates of flow represent 24-hour urine volumes of 408 ml. and 360 ml., which, even with maximum urine concentration, are below the minimum volumes necessary to excrete the daily solute load of urea, creatinine, uric acid, and electrolytes of normal, inactive, semistarving adults. Such volumes are completely inadequate for excretion of the increased solute load of urea, phosphate, sulfate, and potassium that follows major surgery, trauma, or invasive infection.

Severe oliguria is present when urine volume is 10 ml. per hour or less and 24-hour urine volume is below 200 ml.

Anuria, or failure of urine production (< 50 ml. per day), is usually due to obstruction of the postrenal urinary tract or to

*This work was supported in part by a grant from the United States Public Health Service, #5501RR-05644.

Appreciation is expressed to Dr. Charles W. Cashman, Jr., for permission to use the case report of patient S. K., and to the resident and nursing staff of the Surgical Intensive Care Unit of the Rhode Island Hospital for their skills and detailed care, which made possible both the patient's survival and a very complete record of his case.

The author thankfully acknowledges Dr. Robert V. Stephens for permission to publish Figure 3-4. A paper describing the derivation and clinical application of this nomogram is in preparation.

43

cardiovascular collapse with marked hypotension. Rarely it may be due to occlusion of renal blood flow by thrombosis or embolus, or to renal cortical necrosis.

ETIOLOGY

Postoperative oliguria is an indication of renal insufficiency existing at the time the observation is made. The commonest cause of postoperative oliguria is inadequate perfusion of the kidneys with well-oxygenated blood of normal pH and electrolyte content and therefore is prerenal in its origin.

Prolonged inadequate perfusion of the kidneys, or their perfusion with blood containing bacterial, chemical, or other toxins, results in degenerative and obstructive changes within the kidney, usually most obvious in renal tubular cells under a light microscope. Intrinsic renal failure is then present.

Obstruction of the urinary tract distal to

TABLE 3-1. Etiology of Postoperative Oliguria
(Functional Renal Insufficiency)

I. *Prenal causes: Renal ischemia, pigments, toxins*
  1. Hemorrhage—acute depletion of circulating volume.
  2. Dehydration—volume depletion of blood and ECF from external losses unreplaced—particularly acute desalting dehydration.
  3. Internal dehydration—third space formation as seen in burns, large wounds, sepsis—with plasma loss and ECF shift into the area of injury.
  4. Cardiogenic hypotension—primary pump failure, with water and salt retention if subacute.
  5. Increased pulmonary resistance, emboli, fat emboli, lung infection—may produce right heart failure.
  6. Hemolytic transfusion reaction—hemoglobinemia and red-cell debris, sometimes with hypotension as well. May be masked under anesthesia.
  7. Extensive trauma—a combination of hemorrhage, myoglobin release from injured muscle, extensive third space formation, pain, and hypotension.
  8. Vasoconstriction—initiated by volume reduction, potentiated by vasoconstricting drugs—results in renal cortical ischemia, initiates renal failure.
  9. Shock—in the sense of prolonged inadequate perfusion of the kidneys, usually with hypotension < 80 mm. Hg systolic for some time, but not necessarily so.
  10. Sepsis—usually affects cardiac output and vascular tone, as well as renal blood flow.
  11. Metabolic disturbance—hypercalcemia, severe hypokalemia, hyponatremia, acidosis with severe volume depletion, hypoxia, metabolic alkalosis, or respiratory alkalosis.
II. *Intrarenal causes: Tubular injury or obstruction*
  1. Acute tubular necrosis with acute renal failure.
    A. Ischemic type—prolonged inadequate perfusion with cellular injury and breakdown.
    B. Pigment type—Heme or myoglobin—tubular obstruction.
    C. Mixed type—seen in burns, crush injury, hemolysis.
  2. Nephrotoxins
    A. Chemical nephrotoxins present incidentally to surgery.
    B. Nephrotoxic antibiotics.
    C. Endotoxins of septicemia.
    D. Cortical necrosis of obstetrical hemorrhage.
  3. Drugs
    A. Morphine and meperidine (Demerol)—reduce GFR.
    B. Vasopressin (ADH)—increases distal tubular water permeability.
    C. Vasoconstricting drugs (Aramine, L-norepinephrine)—reduce glomerular filtration by afferent renal arteriolar vasoconstriction.
  4. Vascular accidents
    A. Renal arterial or venous thrombosis or obstruction.
    B. Emboli to renal artery.
  5. Pre-existing renal diseases—may be exacerbated by hypoperfusion, hypotension, or hypoxia; renal reserve is often severely reduced. Glomerulonephritis, pyelonephritis, and arteriosclerosis with decreased blood flow are common causes.
III. *Postrenal causes: Obstruction*
  1. Failure to void—incontinence—obstructed catheter—stricture.
  2. Prostatism.
  3. Surgical accidents to ureters or urethra.
  4. Renal pelvic, ureteral, or bladder calculi, with dislodgment.
  5. Tumors of the bladder or pelvis.
  6. Drugs (sulfa)—hyperuricemia following chemotherapy of cancer.
  7. Infection—acute pyelonephritis.

the collecting ducts results in *postrenal* obstructive oliguria or anuria, sometimes interrupted by periods of high-volume excretion. Prolonged obstruction will produce secondary intrinsic renal injury.

Pre-existing renal disease, whether vascular, glomerular, tubular, or due to chronic infection, diminishes renal reserve and increases the probability of development of postoperative renal insufficiency, either oliguria or high-volume output in type. History of previous organic renal disease, hypertension, or diabetes is of great importance in assessing the contribution of pre-existing renal disease to an acute problem postoperatively.

Table 3-1 lists the common causes of postoperative oliguria.

DIFFERENTIAL DIAGNOSIS OF POSTOPERATIVE OLIGURIA

Postoperative oliguria must be established as a true observation. Failure to void; failure to empty the bladder completely, particularly in older men with prostatic hypertrophy; failure to measure and record the urinary output completely; incontinence, a poorly placed or obstructed urinary catheter, or a kinked or excessively long and looped outflow tube may singly or in combination result in an apparent, but not necessarily real, decrease in urine production.

A carefully and aseptically placed, self-retaining *bladder catheter* of a sufficient size to minimize obstruction by mucoid secretions or small blood clots should be used in most critically ill surgical patients. A catheter carries with it some risk of infection, but is essential to monitor urinary output adequately in the critically ill. In patients suffering from major trauma and in those who are to undergo major surgery in which blood loss is likely to be substantial or in which extensive dissection is required, it is wise to insert a bladder catheter early during initial resuscitation or preoperatively to permit intraoperative as well as postoperative recording of urine flow. The catheter should be connected by means of an adaptor of the same bore and of sufficient length to permit ease of disconnection without contamination. Straight gravity drainage, avoiding an uphill course over siderails or pillows and pinching or kinking of the tubing, is effective

except in patients with markedly atonic bladders. One of several varieties of commercially available, disposable graduated cylinders may be attached for ease in determination of hourly volumes. A plastic bag may be incorporated as a reservoir for collecting total output over a longer period of time, but samples of hourly output should be easily available for a variety of important tests.

In the critically ill patient, urine output should be determined at one- or two-hour intervals and the amount and time recorded in an orderly, sequential fashion. Such records are often a part of the vital signs or input and output sheet and should be retained as a part of the permanent record.

When oliguria has been clearly demonstrated in a patient, it is necessary to determine whether it is pre-renal, renal, or postrenal in origin. Time is of great importance because functional renal insufficiency of pre-renal, renal, or postrenal origin requires vigorous treatment that can often prevent acute organic renal failure.

The following check list will be found useful in establishing a differential diagnosis of oliguria:

1. What is the status of the patient's circulating blood volume? Has the patient lost significant amounts of blood either externally, into the gastrointestinal tract, or into an area of massive trauma? Has this been adequately replaced? In hemorrhagic shock, has at least one transfusion, and preferably two, been given beyond the amount necessary to bring the systolic blood pressure above 100 mm. in the average-size adult? Has the pulse rate slowed significantly with therapy? What is the central venous pressure, and what is its response to a test load of blood, plasma, or dextran? Does the patient have peripheral vasoconstriction? Does the patient have septicemia? Septic shock? (See Chapter 2 on Shock.)

2. What is the status of the extracellular fluid? Was the patient dehydrated prior to surgery or trauma? Has he had abnormal external losses of fluid and electrolytes that have not been adequately replaced? What has happened to hematocrit values, to plasma protein concentration, to plasma osmolality? Does the patient have a large wound, burn, or area of crush injury or infection into which significant amounts of extracellular fluid and plasma have been sequestered? Does he have an ileus with substantial transcellular fluid in the gut? What changes have occurred in the patient's body weight, and can they be accounted for? Has sufficient saline or balanced salt solution been given to replace adequately both abnormal external losses and internal fluid shifts? What is the effect on hourly urine flow and on central venous pressure of 500 to 1000 ml. of a balanced salt solution without glucose administered at 20 ml. per minute?

3. What is the status of plasma electrolytes and of blood gases? Are plasma sodium, potassium, chloride,

and total bicarbonate concentrations within normal limits? If not, are corrective measures under way that are compatible with the patient's volume tolerance? Is the patient acidotic or alkalotic? Why? What are values of arterial PO_2, PCO_2, and hemoglobin saturation? Have corrective measures been instituted if these values are abnormal?

4. Does the patient have clinical signs and symptoms of cardiac failure? Is there a history of previous cardiac disease? Is the patient elderly, extensively arteriosclerotic? Has he been on digitalis or diuretics? Is the patient on a respirator with positive pressure ventilation that interferes with venous return to the heart? Does the patient require digitalis or other cardiotonic drugs?

TABLE 3-2. Laboratory Tests in Differential Diagnosis of Postoperative Oliguria

Urine	Prerenal	Renal	Postrenal
Urine volume (see text)	Oliguria	Oliguria (or high volume) (see text)	Anuria; may show high volume if partial obstruction is present. (1.018–1.014 if urine excreted.)
Specific gravity*	>1.018 (1.014–1.018 if low solute load)	<1.018 (1.008–1.014)	History and surgical procedure are significant. Drip pyelography sometimes helpful.
Creatinine concentration (mgm./100 ml.)	>100 U/P ratio > 30 often > 100	<70 U/P ratio < 20	Early retrograde evaluation is very important.
Urea concentration (mgm./100 ml.)	>2000 U/P ratio > 14	300± U/P ratio< 10	Angiography may reveal rare vascular occlusion if distal urinary tract is normal and anuria present.
Osmolality (mOsm.)	>600 U/P ratio > 1.3	300–350 U/P ratio < 1.1	
Na^+ (mEq./l.)**	<20	>30	
K^+ (mEq./l.)	30–70	<20–40	
Na/K ratio**	<1.0 usually < 0.2	0.8 to > 1.0	
Microscopic	Hyaline and fine granular casts. WBC if infection present (RBC from catheter trauma)	Tubular cells, cell casts, coarse granular casts, RBC	
Protein	Negative or trace, unless pre-existing	Often positive when previously negative	
Plasma Creatinine (mgm./100 ml.)	0.6–2.0	>2.0 Daily rise of 1–2 mgm./100 ml.	
Blood Urea Nitrogen (mgm./100 ml. plasma)	Depends on prerenal catabolic load; may be 40–80 + mgm./100 ml.	Daily rise of 10–40 mgm./100 ml., depending on catabolism and protein intake	

Note: U/P ratios compare urine and plasma concentration or value expressed in the same term for each, i.e., mgm./100 ml., mEq./liter, or milliosmols.

*Urine specific gravity will be increased, often substantially, by glucose, proteins, mannitol, dextran, and Keflin, and by organic iodides used for angiography and intravenous pyelography. Osmolality may be increased by glucose, mannitol, and contrast media, but is affected much less by larger molecules.

**Urine sodium may be increased in patients receiving large volumes of sodium-containing solutions, particularly Ringer's lactate or other balanced salt solutions, and by mannitol, furosemide, ethacrinic acid, or other diuretics.

5. Is the patient diabetic? What are urine and blood glucose and acetone levels? Has he been on steroids previously and does he need them now?

Table 3-2 summarizes laboratory findings which are of help in the diagnosis and treatment of postoperative oliguria.

The *urine specific gravity* may be helpful, if substances such as glucose, mannitol, dextran, Keflin, and x-ray contrast media are excluded. A high specific gravity and low-volume urine in the absence of these substances and of protein and hemoglobin is indicative of good renal function in a dehydrated or hypovolemic patient.

Renal function, both glomerular filtration and tubular function, can be *approximated* from knowledge of the urine and plasma concentration of urea and creatinine, measurement of urine and plasma osmolality, and determination of urine electrolyte content.

U/P UREA RATIO

Forland (1966), Lindsay (1965), Luke (1965), and Shires (1970) are among many who suggest using the ratio of urine to plasma urea concentrations as a measure of renal function and to differentiate renal from prerenal failure.

$\dfrac{U \text{ urea}}{P \text{ urea}}$ values of greater than 14 indicate a prerenal cause of oliguria, while U/P ratios of less than 10 and particularly those less than 5 are likely to be due to intrinsic renal failure. The problem involved with using urea as an index under these circumstances, as pointed out by Pitts (1968), is that urea clearance is urine-flow dependent, and at low-flow rates, a high percentage of the urea filtered is reabsorbed by the renal tubules.

U/P CREATININE RATIO

A somewhat better approximation of glomerular filtration can be obtained by comparing the ratio of urine creatinine to plasma creatinine. The ratio Ucr/Pcr is normally greater than 50 and may be 100 or more with mild dehydration. Pitts (1968) described two problems in the use of creatinine to measure filtration: the chemical problem of accurate measurement of low plasma creatinine levels, and the fact that at high plasma levels there is some tubular secretion of creatinine. Nevertheless, creatinine is concentrated by the kidney, is not reabsorbed at low flow rates, as is urea, and is easy to measure by modern, automated laboratory procedures. Values can be obtained in one hour on an emergency basis.

In oliguric patients, a Ucr/Pcr ratio of 30 or more indicates good renal function and a probable prerenal cause of the oliguria. A Ucr/Pcr of less than 20 is suggestive of intrinsic renal failure. Stokes (1968) believes that a Ucr/Pcr ratio of less than 7 is diagnostic of acute tubular necrosis. He differentiates among three types of oliguria—hypovolemic oliguria, catabolic urea loading with hypovolemia, and acute tubular necrosis as follows:

Hypovolemic oliguria: Normal plasma creatinine, modest elevation of BUN, high Ucr/Pcr ratio, oliguria.

Catabolic urea loading with hypovolemia: Rapid rise in BUN, modest rise in plasma creatinine, high Ucr/Pcr ratio, reduced urine volume.

Acute tubular necrosis (ATN): Elevated BUN, elevated plasma creatinine, low Ucr/Pcr ratio, oliguria.

On the Surgical Service at Rhode Island Hospital, the Ucr/Pcr ratio and urine volume are used together to approximate renal efficiency (RE). A simple formula provides an estimate of glomerular filtration rate (GFR).

$$RE = \frac{Ucr \cdot Volume}{Pcr \cdot 1000} \times \frac{24}{\substack{Number \ of \ hours \\ urine \ collected}}$$

Ucr and Pcr are expressed in milligrams per 100 ml. and urine volume in milliliters. The time correction factor—24 ÷ hours of collection—permits evaluation of urine collected over a short period of time, with some sacrifice in accuracy. Plasma creatinine is measured on blood drawn at the midpoint of the urine collection.

Normal renal function is assumed to be present if $\dfrac{Ucr \cdot Vol.}{Pcr \cdot 1000} \times \dfrac{24}{\substack{Collection \\ time}} = 100$ or more. Values less than 100 are an approximation of renal efficiency based on 100. The formula permits the plotting of hour-by-hour changes in glomerular filtration, with treatment in acute situations, and the day-by-day observation of the progress of patients with renal failure. Since both urine volume and concentration are considered, the formula is useful in patients with high-output renal failure, in the diuretic phase of recovery from ATN, and in assisting in decision-making about dialysis.

For example, patient S. K. (Table 3-3) had a urine creatinine value of 24 mgm. per 100 ml. on the seventh postoperative day and a plasma creatinine of 5.1 mgm. per 100 ml. His urine volume was 1321 ml. with Na^+33 and K^+68 mEq./l.

$$RE = \frac{24 \cdot 1321}{5.1 \cdot 1000} = 6.6$$

On the following day urine volume was 1345 ml. and plasma creatinine had risen to 5.6 mgm. per 100 ml. However, urine creatinine had risen to 74 mgm. per 100 ml. and urine sodium had dropped to 10 mEq./l. with no real change in urine potassium.

$$RE = \frac{74 \cdot 1345}{5.6 \cdot 1000} = 17.7$$

This is a distinct improvement. Had the values been continued, which unfortunately they were not, the creatinine in the plasma would have begun to fall at an RE value of about 25, which corresponds to a GFR of 18 to 20 per cent of normal.

Delayed oliguria may develop after a latent period of one or two days following an episode of hypotension. While urine volumes may be "adequate" during the interval, a progressive fall in renal efficiency will be seen if Ucr/Pcr ratios are obtained. Particular attention should be paid to the maintenance of fluid balance and normal electrolyte and acid-base values in this situation to prevent, if possible, the onset of intrarenal oliguria. A high-volume urine flow may prevent oliguric ATN, as pointed out by Shires (1966, 1970).

U/P OSMOLALITY RATIO

Determination of the osmolality of biological fluids is easily accomplished by determining freezing-point depression, and osmolality can be an important diagnostic aid in the differential diagnosis of the etiology of oliguria. Normal urine osmolality is from 400 to 800 mOsm., and depends greatly on water intake and the amount of protein and salt ingested. A patient whose urine volume is diminished because of dehydration will excrete a higher concentration of solutes in a smaller volume, and urine osmolality will be high, the upper limit being about 1200 mOsm., or four times the plasma osmolality.

Eliahou (1965) differentiated functional renal insufficiency from acute tubular necrosis, noting that oliguric patients who responded to mannitol had average Uosm/Posm ratios of 1.35, while the average ratio in patients with ATN was 1.035. Forland (1966) reported urine osmolality greater than 800 mOsm. and Uosm/Posm ratios of about 3.0 with prerenal oliguria, while urine osmolality was 300 to 350 mOsm., and Uosm/Posm ratios about 1.0 in patients with intrinsic renal failure. Rosenbaum (1967) used a Uosm/Posm ratio of less than 1.1 as diagnostic of intrinsic renal failure when oliguria was present. Merrill (1970) states that if Uosm/Posm is greater than 1.5, it may be assumed that the kidney has retained function and oliguria is reversible. In Table 3-2 urine osmolality of greater than 400 mOsm. and a Uosm/Posm ratio of greater than 1.3 have been chosen as levels representing prerenal oliguria.

URINE ELECTROLYTES: THE NA/K RATIO

Urine electrolytes, particularly the concentration of sodium in urine, may be of some value in the differential diagnosis of oliguria. With decreased kidney perfusion due to vasoconstriction, glomerular filtration is decreased and proximal tubular sodium and water absorption is increased. Urine flow through the loop of Henle and the distal convoluted tubule is decreased. Sodium exchange for potassium is enhanced by high aldosterone levels. Water diffusion is increased by the action of ADH on the distal tubule and collecting ducts. The result is a low volume of urine with a high solute concentration containing low sodium and high potassium concentrations. However, treatment of patients with large volumes of electrolyte solutions, particularly Ringer's lactate or other balanced salt solutions; the use of osmotic diuretics, such as mannitol; or the use of diuretics such as furosemide or ethacrinic acid that inhibit proximal tubular water and sodium transfer will result in higher levels of sodium in the urine.

If urine sodium is less than 20 mEq. per liter in an oliguric patient, and renal tubular function is good, the oliguria is probably prerenal in origin. However, urine sodium values in excess of 30 mEq. per liter may be due to a variety of causes and are not necessarily due to ATN.

The ratio Na/K in the urine is of some value in predicting a prerenal etiology of oliguria if the value is 0.5 or less. Values of 0.2 indicate both active sodium conservation and potassium secretion and, therefore, good renal function in handling these electrolytes under the stimulus of hypovolemia.

PRE-RENAL CAUSES OF POSTOPERATIVE OLIGURIA

HYPOVOLEMIA

The commonest cause of postoperative oliguria is *hypovolemia* due to blood loss, dehydration, or blood, plasma, or ECF translocation into areas of tissue injury or sepsis. Often two or more of these factors exist simultaneously. In the treatment of shock (see Chapter 2), monitoring of central venous pressure and, when possible, mean central arterial pressure produces information of great value in judging the rate and adequacy of volume replacement. Values of central venous pressure of less than 3 to 4 cm. of saline almost always indicate hypovolemia. Above this value, the response of the central venous pressure to a test load of blood, plasma, or electrolyte solution given fairly rapidly is more important than the absolute CVP, which may be misleading as an isolated observation. A rise of several centimeters in pressure, with a slow return toward the starting pressure, suggests caution in rate and volume of intravenous therapy and consideration of digitalis or Isuprel. No response or a small and transient rise encourages further volume expansion if lungs remain clear and urinary findings are compatible with hypovolemia (see Table 3-2). Such information permits the clinician to titrate blood, plasma, and electrolyte solutions needed by the patient in quantities beyond the amounts needed simply to restore blood pressure and somewhat to reduce pulse rate. Its importance lies in the fact that renal ischemia *appears early* and *disappears late* in the cycle of volume reduction and restoration, and that persistent renal ischemia over a period of a few hours to one or two days, even with a normal blood pressure, can result in acute renal insufficiency (acute tubular necrosis), just as does 60 to 120 minutes of virtually no perfusion at normal body temperature.

ELECTROLYTE DISORDERS

Electrolyte disorders influence renal function, and their correction is important in the treatment of postoperative oliguria. Schwartz and Relman (1967) have defined the effects of changes in sodium and potassium metabolism on renal function.

Sodium Depletion

Sodium depletion is defined as the net loss of substantial amounts of sodium from the body or its sequestration in a third space of injury or sepsis. Sodium loss exerts an effect on renal function that depends on the absolute amount of sodium lost and on the relative water balance that co-exists with sodium depletion. If net water balance is proportional to sodium loss, then there is no significant change in plasma sodium concentration, and the major effect is reduction of functional extracellular fluid space and plasma volume. With reduced circulatory volume there are the usual effects of reduced cardiac output, increased peripheral resistance, and renal vascular vasoconstriction, with reduced glomerular filtration rate and renal blood flow.

Sodium depletion affects tubular handling of sodium. The fraction of filtered sodium reabsorbed is increased, probably by a combination of increased proximal tubular reabsorption of sodium and water and by distal tubular sodium reabsorption resulting from production of increased aldosterone through the renin-angiotensin pathway.

Renal tubular secretion of potassium is affected by sodium depletion. Inability to handle an increased potassium load may result in hyperkalemia. Severe hypoperfusion of any cause produces a similar defect in renal tubular secretion of potassium, and hyperkalemia is a threat in functional hypovolemic states such as congestive heart failure and cirrhosis, as well as in postoperative catabolic states.

Sodium depletion influences renal tubular handling of water. One of the first effects is the inhibition of dilution of the urine and the prevention of free-water diuresis. Sodium depletion also reduces maximum free-water clearance during solute loading—a situation often seen in the critically ill postoperative patient because of heightened catabolic response. Even when they are hyponatremic, salt-depleted patients tend to excrete an iso-osmotic or slightly hypertonic urine, the volume of which is solute-dependent. As a result they tend to retain water loads and are vulnerable to water intoxication.

Patients with chronic debilitating diseases, such as cancer, chronic congestive heart failure, malnutrition, chronic infection, and cirrhosis, are particularly vulnerable to postoperative water overloading and severe hyponatremia.

Sodium depletion also affects renal tubular mechanisms that control acid-base balance. Augmented proximal tubular sodium absorption interferes with excretion of bicarbonate in the urine, as does depletion of potassium and chloride ions. Regulation of pH by renal excretion of bicarbonate in respiratory alkalosis is inhibited, a common problem in critically ill patients. On the other hand, excretion of titratable acid is not usually interfered with, since excretion of phosphate and ammonium is relatively unimpaired.

Sodium depletion may produce the clinical picture of acute or chronic renal insufficiency. According to Schwartz and Relman (1967) a loss of 4 to 5 mEq. of sodium per kilogram significantly impairs glomerular filtration and renal blood flow. Urea clearance is decreased more than filtration rate, probably owing to back diffusion of urea with low tubular urine flow, and blood urea nitrogen and creatinine levels rise. Sodium depletion may be severe enough to produce vascular collapse with severe oliguria, leading to acute tubular necrosis.

In moderate salt depletion, urine volume is low, urine osmolality is equal to or greater than that of plasma, depending on hydration. Urine sodium concentration is low, and the urine Na/K ratio is considerably reduced. In patients with pre-existing renal disease that interferes with sodium conservation, sodium depletion accompanying abnormal external losses such as vomiting, diarrhea, intestinal intubation, or bowel fistulas is likely to be more rapid and deterioration of renal function is likely to occur earlier than in patients with previously normal renal function.

Potassium Depletion

Potassium depletion produces clinical problems in renal function that are of immediate concern in care of the critically ill patient. The ability both to concentrate urine and to dilute it is impaired, as reported by Schwartz and Relman (1967). Inability to concentrate urine is caused by interference with water reabsorption in the distal convoluted tubules and collecting system. In severe cases, urine becomes increasingly hypotonic with solute loading and remains hypotonic even with vasopressin (ADH) administration. Low potassium levels decrease renal tubular capacity to handle sodium, so that *neither very low nor very high levels of sodium* are found in urine, and both excretion and conservation of sodium are impaired.

Potassium depletion also results in increased renal tubular absorption of bicarbonate, producing a metabolic alkalosis refractory to the administration of NaCl. Chloride as well as potassium levels in the plasma are usually below normal, and both potassium and chloride, usually as KCl, must be administered.

Potassium deficiency may be an important contributing factor, with volume and sodium imbalance or pre-existing renal disease, in the development of severe renal failure.

CARDIAC FAILURE

Cardiac failure may produce oliguria in the critically ill patient. The mechanism is that of functional hypovolemia, with renal vasoconstriction and markedly diminished renal blood flow. Forland (1966) has stated that when cardiac output is reduced by 50 per cent because of failure, renal plasma flow in man is 25 per cent of normal. The ratio of glomerular filtration to renal plasma flow is increased, and renal arterial perfusion pressure falls.

Renal effects are essentially the same as those seen with hypovolemia due to dehydration or hemorrhage, and urine findings are the same (Table 3-2). The differential diagnosis between oliguria due to cardiac failure and that due to hypovolemia must depend on the history, particularly of pre-existing heart disease, and on clinical observations, the appearance of chest x-rays, electrocardiographic evidence, and the central venous pressure, both initially and in response to a volume load. A high initial venous pressure or a rapid rise with the administration of a small test volume intravenously are suggestive of cardiac insufficiency. Phlebotomy for reduction of circulating volume may result in improved cardiac output, reduction in pulmonary edema, and, indirectly, in improvement in renal function. Diuretics that decrease renal tubular reabsorption of sodium and water are useful both in treatment of congestive heart failure and in solving the problems of oliguria.

PROTEIN AND PIGMENT LOADS

Incompatible blood transfusion will result in rapid lysis of transfused cells and occasionally of recipient cells as well. The result is flooding of the plasma with hemoglobin and the membranes of lysed cells. Some hemoglobin is filtered through glomeruli and may be precipitated in the tubules and collecting ducts as water and sodium are withdrawn. Initially, the urine will have a distinct red color and, at the same time, will be clear, unlike urine containing whole red blood cells, which make the urine turbid. Plasma will show the presence of free hemoglobin and should be checked for this at once while blood compatibility is being rechecked. Incompatible blood may be lysed under anesthesia without any sign other than transient hypotension, often attributed to blood loss during operation.

Onesti (1967) reported that renal blood flow need not fall significantly in dog or man to produce acute renal failure as the result of a hemoglobin load. He observed, however, that experimental reduction of perfusion pressure by 15 to 20 mm. Hg in one kidney in the dog, followed by an intravascular load of hemoglobin, consistently produced renal shutdown of that kidney despite minimal or no reduction in blood flow or GFR. He attributed the effect to a significant reduction in urine flow due to increased tubular reabsorption of water and precipitation of hemoglobin in the tubules.

Similar protein loads may be presented to patients' kidneys when there is hemolysis due to burns or myoglobin release with extensive injury to muscle. Early recognition and early treatment is essential. The objective is to maintain a high rate of urine flow

to prevent tubular deposition of protein until the excess load has been cleared. Compatible blood must be transfused if needed, and it often is. Electrolyte solutions of saline or balanced salt solution such as Ringer's lactate must be given in sufficient volume to assure hydration and provide for a urine volume of ±100 ml. per hour.

Austen (1968), Mueller (1967), and Powers (1970) advocate the use of mannitol as an osmotic diuretic under conditions of abnormal globin loading. All point out the importance of *volume restoration* as the initial and vital step. Mannitol, 12.5 to 25 gm. in 500 ml. of isotonic saline, given fairly rapidly intravenously should then produce a prompt osmotic diuretic effect. Additional small doses of mannitol may be required to maintain a high urine volume, but the total dose should probably not exceed 50 gm. Rapid urine flow will interfere with concentration and produce an obligatory loss of electrolyte, particularly sodium. Urine specific gravity and Na/K ratios are significantly altered by mannitol diuresis.

INTRARENAL CAUSES OF RENAL INSUFFICIENCY

The pathology of acute renal insufficiency (tubular necrosis) has been excellently reviewed by Teplitz (1969). He points out that the light-microscope picture of the kidneys of patients dying of acute renal failure is remarkably variable. In some instances, only minimal tubular cloudy swelling can be seen; in other cases, heme casts, damaged distal convoluted tubules, and tubular epithelial thinning and degeneration are present, but usually in focal areas only. He postulates that the basic lesion of so-called acute tubular necrosis may be at the ultrastructural or enzymatic level and thus not visible to the light microscope.

The etiology of intrinsic renal failure also remains controversial, although the relationship of hypovolemia, vasoconstriction, electrolyte imbalance, toxins, and, in specific instances, globin loads has long been recognized. Recent reports by Hollenberg (1968, 1970) bring renal insufficiency of varied etiology into a common pathway of acute, persistent renal cortical ischemia. Using ^{133}Xe clearance and selective angiography to evaluate renal blood flow and with a control of 36 patients being evaluated as potential kidney donors, he and his associates reported 20 patients with acute oliguric renal insufficiency (1968) and seven with nephrotoxin-induced renal failure (1970). Identical abnormalities were found in both groups of ill patients, consisting of absence of identifiable cortical arterial vessels, absence of a cortical nephrogram, delayed transit of the contrast material through the kidney, and the absence of the rapid, cortical phase of washout of ^{133}Xe. Blood flow was reduced to about one-third of normal, a level comparable to patients with chronic renal failure who retained some renal function. He concluded that there exists a common pathogenic final pathway involving undefined mediators that induce severe, sustained preglomerular vasoconstriction.

HIGH-OUTPUT RENAL FAILURE

The critically ill patient may have a "good" urinary output of 1000 ml. or more of urine in 24 hours and usually will not have had an hourly urine volume of less than 20 ml., and yet may have a progressive rise in BUN and creatinine.

Patient S. K., the illustrative case in this chapter, demonstrates this phenomenon (see Table 3-3). Although oliguric (345 ml.) on the sixth postoperative day due to dehydration, the patient thereafter had urine volumes of 1300 ml. or more per day, while the BUN rose to 177 mgm. per 100 ml. on the tenth day, and the plasma creatinine increased from 2.5 mgm. to 6.3 mgm. per 100 ml. This was followed by a gradual fall in BUN and creatinine, the creatinine level falling earlier and more rapidly and the BUN level being maintained, in part because of some bleeding into the gastrointestinal tract, with a resulting protein overload. Note that *urine* creatinine levels were 24 mgm. per 100 ml. on the seventh day and 71 mgm. per 100 ml. on the eighth day, with plasma creatinine values of 5.1 and 5.6 mgm. per 100 ml. These values give urine/plasma creatinine values of 4.7/1. and 12.7/1., which contrast with normal values of > 50/1. and usually > 100/1. (Table 3-2). The patient obviously had a markedly diminished glomerular filtration rate despite a "good" urine volume, much of which was probably the result of the osmotic diuretic effect of his glycosuria.

Shires (1966, 1970) observed that uremia without oliguria was the most common form of renal insufficiency observed in his series of trauma patients. He reported the incidence of high-output failure as five to ten times the incidence of classic oliguric renal failure. He felt that high-output renal insufficiency was a milder form of renal disease and noted that none of 26 patients died of renal failure, although one-third of the group died because of complications of their injuries. Urine volumes of 3 to 5 liters a day were observed while the BUN continued to rise for 8 to 12 days before a downward trend occurred. Urine/blood urea ratios were about 10/1., and GFR was less than 20 per cent of normal in the acute phase. Attempts at volume restriction resulted in hypernatremia without a volume fall. These patients were refractory to Pitressin administration during the acute phase and for several weeks thereafter.

It is probable that the procedure advocated by Shires, that is, the administration of substantial volumes of Ringer's lactate solution in addition to whole blood in the treatment of patients in shock due to trauma, altered the picture by providing rapid and substantial expansion of the extracellular fluid space and a considerable solute load as sodium salts. Oliguria was avoided, but renal efficiency was nevertheless markedly reduced in these patients. Urine volume roughly paralleled blood urea concentration, indicating a solute-dependent urine volume.

Merrill (1965) stated that acute tubular necrosis may occur without periods of detectable oliguria. He indicated that the course of events is identical with that seen in the diuresis phase following a prolonged period of urinary suppression. Merrill also reported a series of patients with "high-output failure" in which cardiac failure also was present. The use of digitalis in this setting was less than satisfactory in treating the heart failure. Hemodialysis resulted in marked improvement, suggesting a metabolic component affecting the heart. He cautioned that digitalis should be used in patients with renal insufficiency only to treat frank cardiac failure and that these patients require less digitalis because of reduction of renal excretion of the drug and because of increased sensitivity due to the metabolic acidosis present.

Schreiner (1967) defined high-output renal failure as a loss of concentrating ability of the renal medulla accompanied by a high pre-renal load of urea, and he notes that severe renal failure may be present with an output of 1 to 2 liters of urine a day.

POSTRENAL OLIGURIA OR ANURIA

The key word here is *obstruction*. The important clinical criterion is a very low urine volume, less than 50 ml. a day, occurring immediately after operation or injury or occurring *suddenly* at any time during the course of illness. Partial obstruction of the distal urinary tract is likely to result in a high-volume output of dilute urine, resembling that of high-output renal failure. Anuria may alternate with episodes of polyuria if intermittent obstruction occurs because of blocking of the catheter or movement of a stone or tumor.

Table 3-1 lists the common causes of postrenal obstruction. Prompt investigation is indicated because most causes of postrenal obstruction are remediable.

If the distal urinary tract is clear and anuria or marked oliguria with considerable bleeding exists, angiography may reveal renal vascular thrombosis or embolus.

MANAGEMENT OF OLIGURIA PERSISTENT AFTER VOLUME REPLACEMENT: USE OF DIURETICS

Luke (1965) reported 35 patients who, after an episode of hypotension treated with blood and electrolyte replacement, demonstrated oliguria and severely diminished urea clearance. These patients were treated with mannitol and 25 of the 35 responded with increased volume of urine. Of the 10 who did not respond, treatment was instituted *50 hours or more after the insult in eight* and two had glomerular lesions. These observations lend additional support to the importance of early diagnosis and treatment of oliguria based on hypovolemia or depleted extracellular fluid volume before acute renal failure becomes fully established.

Powers (1970) has observed that the factors which seem to be associated with prevention of acute renal failure are the presence of a high urine flow and the reversal of vasoconstriction. Prompt restoration to normal of blood volume and extracellular fluid space

following trauma usually results in restoration of renal function. With delay, he feels that an osmotic diuretic and possibly a ganglionic blocking agent should be employed. Powers postulates that renin released by low renal blood flow has both an intrarenal and a systemic effect—the intrarenal effect is control of blood flow via the afferent arteriole, and the systemic effect is increasing aldosterone production via angiotensin and shunting blood away from the renal medulla. Mannitol increases urine PO_2 and increases renal blood flow, offering indirect evidence of improved renal medullary circulation. He recommends its use when volume restoration fails to result in an adequate urine output.

Merrill (1970) recommends the use of mannitol, 12.5 to 25 gm., dissolved in no more than 200 ml. of isotonic fluid and infused in 10 to 15 minutes, in situations in which oliguria persists *after adequate restoration of volume deficit*. He also notes that the intravenous administration of ethacrinic acid or furosemide has recently been shown to be a simpler, and perhaps more effective, method of determining the kidney's ability to increase urine volume. Substantial doses—150 to 200 mgm.—of ethacrinic acid (or 80 to 120 mgm. of furosemide) are suggested. It should be remembered that very substantial sodium losses occur with both ethacrinic acid and furosemide, both of which block renal tubular sodium reabsorption, probably in the proximal tubules. These losses may have to be replaced to avoid dehydration and hyponatremia. They also may be beneficial in patients who are fluid overloaded or in congestive heart failure.

MANAGEMENT OF OLIGURIA: SUMMARY OUTLINE

1. Is the oliguria real? What is the hourly urine volume? A bladder catheter is required. Start laboratory evaluation of urine and plasma. (See Table 3-2.)

2. Be certain that the patient's circulating blood volume and extracellular fluid space are at *functionally* normal levels. Blood pressure (preferably by a central arterial catheter) and central venous pressure are essential for adequate monitoring. What is the effect of additional blood, plasma, or dextran on CVP? On urine flow? If hemato-

crit is adequate, and peripheral vasoconstriction not great, what is the effect of 500 to 1000 ml. of Ringer's lactate at 20 ml. per minute on urine flow?

3. Institute correction of abnormalities of plasma electrolyte values early, as a part of volume restoration. Check pH and blood gases; take appropriate measures to correct abnormalities.

4. If oliguria persists after volume restoration is completed, or at once if the patient has had a high globin load from hemolysis or from crushing injury to muscle, administer mannitol, 12.5 to 25 gm. in 500 ml. or less of saline. Repeat doses may be necessary, but do not exceed 50 gm. in most instances.

Ethacrinic acid or furosemide may be useful in initiating a high level of urine flow in persistent oliguria. This type of diuretic is particularly suggested if the CVP is elevated, or rises rapidly with a small fluid load, and in the presence of heart failure.

5. If all measures fail, *do not persist* with fluid loading. Accept the fact that the patient has intrinsic renal insufficiency, and institute a conservative regimen of management, being prepared for dialysis if indicated. See articles by Merrill (1965, 1970), Johnson (1967), and Teschan (1967) for examples.

CASE STUDY

S.K., a 75-year-old retired salesman, was admitted to Rhode Island Hospital in January, 1970, with a chief complaint of a "spot" in his right lung. Eight months previously his chest x-ray was normal. Two months prior to admission a round shadow, 2 cm. in diameter, was observed in the right upper lobe. The patient was completely asymptomatic as far as this lesion was concerned.

Significant past history included documented myocardial infarctions in 1937 and in 1958 and anginal attacks with myocardial ischemia in 1961 and 1962. The patient smoked one package of cigarettes daily for 40 years, doubling this in the past four years. Previous surgical history included cholecystectomy in 1951, choledochoplasty in 1952, left inguinal hernia repair in 1957, hemorrhoidectomy in 1958, and tendon graft in the right hand in 1958. His previous history and hospital records were negative for evidence of diabetes and tuberculosis.

The patient was a wiry, alert individual who appeared to be about his stated age. Blood pressure was 160/70, an electrocardiogram showed that a right bundle branch block, present in 1962, had disappeared and demonstrated only some flattening of T waves in lead 1 and AVL with generalized low voltage. Laboratory tests showed the following: fasting blood sugar = 164 mgm. per 100 ml., BUN = 12 mgm. per 100 ml., plasma cre-

atinine = 0.9 mgm. per 100 ml., sodium = 136 mEq./l., potassium = 3.7 mEq./l., chloride = 102 mEq./l., and total CO_2 = 25 mEq./l. Repeat fasting blood sugar test was 92 mgm. per 100 ml., hemoglobin was 13.9 gm., and hematocrit was 43 per cent. Plasma protein was 7.2 gm. per 100 ml., and albumin was 4.7 gm. per 100 ml. Alkaline phosphatase, transaminase, and LDH were within normal limits. Urinalysis was negative for protein, glucose, and acetone; pH = 5.0; specific gravity = 1.016. Ventilation studies revealed moderate constrictive pulmonary disease, improved by bronchodilators.

Because of marked stiffness of the lung, noted at thoracotomy, a segmental resection of a very small bronchogenic carcinoma was performed.

Immediately postoperative, blood gases showed pH = 7.41, Po_2 = 55 mm. with 88 per cent oxygen saturation, Pco_2 = 37 mm. with 40 per cent oxygen delivered through a face mask; hemoglobin was 13.1 gm.; hematocrit was 44 per cent. The following day he was doing well; Po_2 had risen to 62 mm. with oxygen saturation 92 per cent, Pco_2 = 39 mm., and pH = 7.45. The patient exhibited a moderate tachycardia. He was alert and cooperative. Hemoglobin was 13.3 gm.; hematocrit was 41 per cent.

On the second postoperative day his temperature rose to 101°, blood gases were as follows: pH = 7.54, Po_2 = 52 mm. with 90 per cent oxygen saturation, TCO_2 = 27 mEq./l. and Pco_2 = 32 mm. with 100 per cent oxygen from a Puritron face mask. X-ray showed a moderate infiltrate of the left lower lobe. Keflin was started. Hemoglobin was 12.8 gm.; hematocrit was 41 per cent. A Levin tube, placed on the night of the first postoperative day because of some gastric distention, began to drain increasingly large volumes of fluid, and during the next three days this volume rose to a peak of 4140 ml. in 24 hours (see Table 3-3). Partly as the result of this, by the third postoperative day the arterial blood pH had risen to 7.54 and TCO_2 had increased from 27 to 33 mEq./l. Plasma sodium was 134, potassium was 4.0, chloride was 87 mEq./l., hemoglobin was 11.7 gm., and hematocrit was 37 per cent. The evening of the third postoperative day, the TCO_2 was 37 mEq./l., with a pH of 7.55, Po_2 was 59 mm. with 93 per cent saturation, and Pco_2 was 36 mm. The patient was febrile and restless. Because of the large volume of gastric drainage, and persistent ileus, the patient was treated with an intravenous administration of 0.9 per cent NaCl with 5 per cent dextrose in water, with 40 mEq. KCl as baseline. Twenty grams of L-Arginine monohydrochloride (90 mEq. HCl) was given on the third postoperative day to provide additional chloride.

By the fourth day the patient's temperature had risen to 104° F. and he was restless, disoriented, and hypoxic. On the fourth postoperative day a CVP catheter was placed and CVP was less than 3 cm., nasogastric tube drainage was 4140 ml., and urinary output was 1205 ml. The gastric drainage contained 83 mEq./l. sodium, 9 mEq./l. potassium, and 124 mEq./l. chloride and had a pH of 2.0. Fluid replacement was kept about 2000 ml. less than needed on this day, partially in the hope of decreasing the large volume of gastric drainage.

On the fifth postoperative day the BUN had risen to 59 mgm. per 100 ml., creatinine to 2.5 mgm. per 100 ml. and CVP was less than 3 cm. Urine specific gravity was 1.020 and 1.032 during that day. Urinary output was 1150 ml.

It was recognized that the patient's total fluid replacement had been inadequate to replace the very large volume of nasogastric tube drainage and that additional fluid was needed. Because a prolonged period of parenteral therapy was anticipated, 1000 ml. of 5 per cent Amigen 10 per cent fructose and 1000 ml. of 20 per cent dextrose were given in addition to 5 per cent dextrose in saline, thus increasing the carbohydrate load substantially. A central venous pressure catheter was replaced and CVP was less than 3 cm. of saline.

On the sixth postoperative day it was found that the patient's blood glucose level was 320 mgm. per 100 ml., despite the fact that his urine was negative for both glucose and acetone. Urine showed hyaline and occasional granular casts, 1 to 3 RBC. This day the patient's urinary output fell to 345 ml. CVP was 4.5 cm. Because of severe tachypnea and inability to clear secretions, a tracheostomy was done and the patient was placed on assisted respirations at 15 cm. positive pressure. Arginine HCL, 20 gm., was given because of low chloride and high pH; hemoglobin was 10.4; hematocrit was 35.

The seventh postoperative day blood glucose was 160 mgm. per 100 ml., BUN was 117 mgm. per 100 ml., creatinine was 5.1 mgm. per 100 ml., plasma sodium was 138, potassium, 4.2, chloride, 83, PCO_2 was 37 mEq./l., hemoglobin was 10.0, and hematocrit 35. Urine electrolyte determination showed urine sodium = 33 mEq./l., potassium = 64 mEq./l., and chloride = 21 mEq./l. Urinary output this day was 1321 ml. and was repeatedly negative for both glucose and acetone. The nasogastric tube drainage was 3985 ml. Urinary creatinine was 24 mgm. per 100 ml., creatinine clearance was 6.42 liters. A mixed metabolic and respiratory alkalosis persisted (Table 3-3). High caloric parenteral fluids were stopped and the patient was treated with 5 per cent glucose with 0.9 per cent and 0.45 per cent saline. Twenty grams arginine HCl was given again; hematocrit was 35.

On the eighth postoperative day blood glucose was 300 mgm. per 100 ml., urinary glucose was +3 to +4, urine volume was 1345 ml., gastric tube volume was 2500 ml., urinary creatinine was 71 mgm. per 100 ml., BUN was 150 mgm. per 100 ml., plasma creatinine was 5.6 mgm. per 100 ml., and creatinine clearance was calculated to be 17 liters. Urine sodium was 10; potassium was 62 mEq./l. On this day a lumbar puncture was performed, revealing clear fluid, no cells, pH = 7.40, TCO_2 = 22 mEq./l., PCO_2 = 38 mm., and glucose = 248 mgm. per 100 ml. CVP was again less than 3 cm. saline, and 3560 ml. was given parenterally, with a total carbohydrate load of 375 gm. Urine ketones were absent.

On the ninth postoperative day BUN was 168 mgm. per 100 ml., creatinine was 6.3 mgm. per 100 ml., urine volume this day was 2540 ml. and showed occasional 1+ glucose, 0 acetone; tube drainage was 1840 ml. Urine sodium was 8 mEq./l. and potassium was 51 mEq./l., plasma TCO_2 was 24 mEq./l., pH = 7.47, PO_2 = 155 mm. with 99 per cent oxygen saturation, and PCO_2 = 34 mm. The patient remained febrile with temperature ranging between 100.6° and 102.0° F. He was disoriented and restless despite the much improved PO_2. Oxygen was reduced from 70 to 40 per cent.

On the tenth postoperative day urine volume rose to 2795 ml., tube drainage decreased to 1015 ml., plasma electrolyte determination showed sodium = 145, potassium = 4.4, chloride = 106, and TCO_2 = 30 mEq./l. A severe alkalosis, now largely respiratory, persisted. Hemoglobin was 8.8, and hematocrit was 28, after some bleeding from the Levin tube.

On the eleventh postoperative day urine volume rose to 3210 ml., Levin tube drainage decreased to 835 ml., plasma sodium was now 153, potassium = 4.1, chloride = 113, total CO_2 = 29 mEq./l., urine sodium was 6 and urine potassium was 25 mEq./l. The patient was confused and uncooperative. Temperature was 101° F, hemoglobin was 9.7, and hematocrit was 30.

On the twelfth postoperative day the plasma sodium was again 153, potassium = 4.2, chloride = 114, TCO_2 = 23 mEq./l. Urine volume was 2870 ml. The nasogastric tube had stopped draining and was removed. Plasma pH was 7.55, PO_2 = 133 mm., and PCO_2 = 31 mm. The patient was judged to have a respiratory alkalosis. He became progressively unresponsive, reacting only to painful stimuli.

The rate of infusion was slowed to 150 ml./hour. Plasma glucose was in the range of 240 to 300 mEq./l., with a total of 70 units of regular insulin administered. Urine sodium was 1, 2, and 3 mEq./l. in three separate specimens, potassium = 29, and chloride = 8 mEq./l. Urine sodium rose to 10, potassium to 42, and chloride to 10 mEq./l. after the administration of 80 mgm. of furosemide intravenously. Long-acting insulin, 15 units a day, was added to help control blood-glucose levels, with regular insulin supplementation based on blood-glucose determinations taken every six hours. After the twenty-first day there was no further glycosuria, and regular insulin was omitted after the twenty-second day.

On the thirteenth postoperative day the patient remained deeply obtunded. Urine volume rose to 4730 ml. with specific gravity of 1.018 to 1.030, BUN was 67 mgm. per 100 ml., creatinine was 2.3 mgm. per 100 ml., serum sodium was 162 mEq./l., potassium = 4.0, chloride = 118, TCO_2 = 29 mEq./l., hemoglobin was 10.7, and hematocrit was 38. A total of 4755 ml. dextrose in water with KCl was given parenterally.

On the fourteenth postoperative day the A.M. blood glucose was 260 mgm. per 100 ml., blood acetone was negative, urine volume was 3110 ml., and showed +4 glucose on three of four determinations. Plasma sodium was 166, potassium = 4.1, chloride = 123, and total CO_2 = 26 mEq./l. The plasma osmolality was 378 mOsm. and urine osmolality was 508 mOsm. Urine sodium was 3, potassium = 10, chloride = 9 mEq./l., and CO_2 = 26 mEq./l. The patient was treated this day with 300 ml./hour of 5 per cent dextrose in water, a total of 5690 ml., and the +4 glucose in the urine was covered with 20 units of regular insulin every four hours. Hypertonic nonketotic coma was present. A water deficit of 7 liters was estimated from weight and plasma sodium concentration.

In the early morning of the fifteenth day the patient became cyanotic and his blood pressure fell to 120/90 with a pulse of 150. CVP was 5 cm. saline. He was given 4.0 gm. of dihydrocortisone in a single dose intravenously, followed by 750 ml. of plasma. CVP rose to 11 cm. with marked clinical improvement in perfusion and blood pressure. Blood cultures taken at this time failed to grow any organisms and the episode was later considered to have been cardiogenic shock. Hemoglobin was 9.0; hematocrit was 28.

On the fifteenth postoperative day the patient continued to receive large volumes of 5 per cent dextrose in water intravenously. Total urine volume was 2550 ml. with sodium = 1 mEq./l. and potassium = 11 mEq./l.; blood glucose was 720 mgm. per 100 ml. at 3 A.M., 326 mgm. per 100 ml. at 8 A.M., 575 at noon, 630 at 6 P.M., and 920 at 10 P.M. All urine sugars were +4 for glucose

TABLE 3-3. Segmental Resection of Right Lung
(Patient S.K., Age 75)

Days	I.V. Volume	CVP (cm H_2O)	Urine Vol. (ml.)	Urine Sp.G.	Urine Electrolytes	N.G. Vol. (ml.)	N.G. Electrolytes	Na	K	Cl	CO_2	pH	Po_2	% Saturation	Pco_2	Blood Glucose	Urine Glucose	Ketones	BUN	Creatinine Plasma	Creatinine Urine	Weight Kg	Notes (see text)
Preop				1018				136	3.7	102	25					164/92	0	0	12	0.9		76.5	
OR 1	2600/3200		860/650	1026/1026		675/1950		139	3.9	101	22/26	7.41/7.45	55/62 (40%)	88/92	37/39				16	1.0	1.0		Mild ileus
2	2460		770	1025		2200					27	7.54	52 (100%)	90	32								Somewhat confused and restless; LLL infiltrate
3	3070		1015	1026		4000		140	4.5	97	33	7.54	59 (100%)	93	36				24	1.0			Behind on fluids; gastric pH = 2.0
4	3100	<3	1205	1024	Na 69 / K 93 / Cl 8	4140		131	H.	89	37	7.58	53	92	39				30	0.9			T = 104°, hydrocortisone and Keflin started
5	2860	<3	1150	1023		2910		144	3.5	95	37	7.54	56	92	38								Marked tachypnea; further dehydration
6	3070	4.5	345	1016		4865	Na 83 / K 9 / Cl 124	134	4.2	89	31	7.57	85 (V-25)	97 (V-53)	31 (V-38)	320	0	0	59	2.5			Lactic acid 9 mEq./l.; tracheostomy
7	4840	6.0	1321	1022	Na 33 / K 68 / Cl 21	3985		138	4.0	83	37	7.56	59	93	37	160	+++	0	117	5.1	24		T = 104°, CVP = 37 cm. Tachypnea
8	3560	<3	1345	1015	Na 10 / K 62 / Cl 76	2500		141	4.4	87	33	7.57	80 (70%)	97	36	300	++++/+++	0	150	5.6	71	71.0	Digitalized, (?) congestive failure
9	2810	5.6	2540	1010/1015	Na 8 / K 51	1840		135	5.1	103	24	7.47	155 (70%)	99	34		+		168	6.3		70.7	Low urine Na in increased volume
10	3020	8.0	2795	1010		1015		145	4.4	106	30	7.58	105 (40%)	99	36				177	5.4		68.5	High-output renal failure
11	4045	10.5	3210	1015		835		153	4.1	113	29	7.56	85	97	24				155	3.8			Confused, T = 101°; diuresis
12	2710	—	2870	1015		0		153	4.2	114	33	7.55	133	99	31				126	2.7			Progressively unresponsive
13	4755	—	4730	1018/1030		25		162	4.0	118	29	7.54	61	93	35				67	2.3			Renal function improving; obtunded
14	5690	5	2250	1030	Na 13 / K 10 / Cl 9	25		166	3.0	123	27	7.61	132	99	27	260	++++	0	73	2.7	67.0	Urine osmol = 508; blood osmol = 378; blood acetone negative

No.						Na	K	Cl	CO₂	pH	pO₂	O₂%	pCO₂	Sugar	Acetone				Wt.	Clinical notes
15	6990	11	2250	1033	Na 1 / K 11 Out	166	3.7	122	25	7.50	155 (V-40)	99 (V-77)	28 (V-35)	720 326 260 / 920	++++	0	64	2.6	69.5	Blood acetone negative; dihydrocortisone 4.0 gm. at 2 A.M. for hypotension
16	3935	10	2940	1013	Na 1 / K 29	151	4.5	111	26	7.58	106	99	26	230	++++	0	72	1.3		Insulin by blood sugars begun; blood cultures negative
17	2650	7	3660	1027	Na 23 D / Na 5	144	4.7	110	28	7.59	85	98	25	184	++++ +00	0	46	1.0	70.5	Still comatose; diuretic to unload Na
18	2750	7	2525	1025	Na 47 / K 60 D	148	3.8	109	28	7.60	73	97	26	190 +++	+++	0	42	1.2	69.1	Hyperpnea with tachypnea
19	3975	9	1960	1024		154	3.4	111	30	7.59		93	86	480 / 300 +++ / ++++			30	1.0	67.5	Insulin changed to NPH 15 U; narcotics and Valium for tachypnea and alkalosis; redigitalized
20	2450	18 / 24	1600	1025		150	4.2	114	30	7.58	92	98	27	266 225	++++ 0	0	37	0.9		
21	2600	14	1750	1024	Na 118 / K 5	141	4.0	106	28					318	+++++	0	32	1.0	67.8	Insulin 20 U+; NPH 15 U; still comatose
22	2100	–	1225	1025		139	3.9	104	26	7.68	110 (40%)	99	21	180	+	0				Marked respiratory alkalosis persists despite Valium
23	2500	–	1350	1020	Na 148 / K 48 / Cl 168	No	3.9	103	23	7.66	68 (Air)	96	21	116	0	0	11	1.0	68.2	Responding; off respirator several hours
24	1750	–	1195	1015										146	0	0				Talking with tracheal tube corked
25	1280	– / P.O. 700	1760	1015		No	3.8	108	23	7.53	69 (Air)	85	27	142	0	0	10	0.5		Eating soft food
26	1440		1300	1020	Na 41 / K 26 / Cl 30	137	4.3	106	23	7.52	81 (Air)	97	25	121	0	0	12	0.9		Eating moderately well, quite alert; discharged from ICU
27	1885	600	1185	1016																

Blood and packed red cells were given in two preoperative transfusions, plus 1/23 P.C. (10), 1/25 P.C. (12), 2/4 P.C. (22), 2/13 W.B. (31), 1/24 P.C. (11), 1/30 W.B. (17), 2/8 P.C. (26). A total of 2000 ml. Plasmanate was used.

and negative for acetone. The morning electrolyte determination showed sodium = 166, potassium = 3.7, chloride = 122, and TCO$_2$ = 25 mEq./l. A total of 6990 ml. of 5 per cent dextrose in water was given by infusion. Eighty milliequivalents of furosemide was given as a diuretic in an attempt to get his kidneys to release sodium. Regular insulin was given in accordance with blood sugars taken every four hours, with doses limited to 20 units to avoid hypersensitivity.

On the sixteenth postoperative day the patient remained deeply obtunded. The serum sodium had fallen to 151 mEq./l., then to 147 and 143 during this day. Urine volume was 2940 ml. average with, +2 glucose.

On the seventeenth postoperative day the patient had six loose stools, and a persistent ileus began to abate. The presence of ileus was the contraindication to the administration of substantial volumes of water into the gastrointestinal tract on days 13 through 16, as would have been desirable, and necessitated the use of large volumes of parenteral 5 per cent dextrose in water with the resultant high blood-sugar levels.

The seventeenth day plasma sodium was 144 mEq./l., urine volume was 3600 ml. with +2 to +3 glucose. Blood glucose was at the level of 200 to 300 mg. per 100 ml. with insulin. The urine sodium, following furosemide, rose to 23 mEq./l. but dropped back to 5 mEq./l. in six hours.

The major problem from the eighteenth to the twenty-fourth postoperative day was a severe respiratory alkalosis. The patient remained hyperpneic and tachypneic despite the administration of Valium and Dilaudid or morphine in order to attempt to slow his respiratory rate. At this time the advisability of paralyzing the patient to take over ventilation was considered, but this was not done. His CVP rose to 24 cm. on the twentieth day and fell with re-digitalization. The patient began to respond more actively to motion or painful stimuli by the twenty-third postoperative day, and suddenly, on the morning of the twenty-fourth postoperative day, he woke up, recognized members of his family, and seemed quite cooperative. The following day he was able to talk with his tracheal tube corked temporarily, and on the twenty-sixth postoperative day he began eating a soft diet and tolerated being off the respirator for prolonged periods of time, Po$_2$ being maintained in the range of 69 to 81 mm. on room air. On the twenty-seventh postoperative day he was eating moderately well, was quite alert and capable of conversing, and was discharged from the Intensive Care Unit to a ward. His convalescence following this was slow with difficulty in regaining his ability to walk, and a pronounced instability of balance for some time, but with physiotherapy this gradually improved. On the sixty-fourth postoperative day he was discharged to his home, walking with the assistance of a cane.

COMMENT

As is true of so many critically ill patients, this patient had a variety of complications, both simultaneous and sequential. Initially he presented with a ventilation perfusion defect, with low Po$_2$ despite relatively normal pH and Pco$_2$. This was, at first, fairly easily corrected with 40 per cent oxygen by face mask, but by the second postoperative day, Po$_2$ was 52, with the patient on 100 per cent oxygen via face mask, probably representing an inspired oxygen concentration in the range of 50 per cent. His arterial pH gradually rose, reaching a high of 7.58 on the fourth postoperative day, despite a Pco$_2$ of 39 mm. The elevation of the pH was largely the result of extraordinarily high levels of hydrochloric acid loss from his stomach and a resultant metabolic alkalosis.

By the sixth postoperative day, respiratory function began to play a larger role; pH was 7.57, TCO$_2$ = 31 mEq./l., Pco$_2$ = 31 mm., and a mixed metabolic and respiratory alkalosis was present. At this point the patient's respiratory rate was 36 to 40 per minute, and his tidal volume was ± 500 ml., so that he was breathing approximately 20 liters a minute. The work of breathing was considered to be excessive and likely to be lethal to the patient. In addition, the patient's restlessness and confusion made it very difficult to perform tracheal suction. Therefore, on the sixth postoperative day, a tracheostomy was done, both to clear pulmonary secretion and because of the extraordinary work of respiration. Tracheostomy and assisted respiration, however, did not rectify his acid-base imbalance, although with sedation it was possible to slow his respiration sufficiently to raise the Pco$_2$ to 37 mm. It was not until after the tenth postoperative day, when the drainage from the Levin tube diminished below 1000 ml. a day, that it was possible to correct the chloride loss and to reduce and then eliminate the element of metabolic alkalosis.

High volume losses from his nasogastric tube which were under-replaced not only resulted in a metabolic alkalosis but also in hypovolemia and a drop in urine output on the sixth day; this was followed by climbing creatinine and BUN, while the patient became further dehydrated with urine volumes in the range of 2500 to 3000 ml. per day (see Table 3-3, Figure 3-1).

Serum sodium began to climb during the tenth postoperative day and by the fourteenth postoperative day reached 166 mEq./l. Despite the intravenous administration of 5690 ml. this day, the patient became cyanotic and hypotensive late at night, with blood pressure falling to 120/90 and pulse rising to 160. Since it was thought that he was possibly in septic shock, the patient was given 4.0 gm. of dihydrocortisone intravenously in a single push, followed by 750 ml. of plasma. He responded by becoming better perfused and his blood pressure slowly rose back to his normal level of 160/95. It is probably significant that urine volume did not fall except very transiently during the period of hypotension, although the BUN and creatinine (see Figure 3-2), which had been rapidly falling at this point, reached a plateau for a period of three to four days, suggesting that there had been some decrease in renal function.

When, on the thirteenth day, the patient's serum sodium rose to 162 mEq./l., he became comatose, having previously been confused and restless. He remained in a comatose state from the fourteenth postoperative day until he began to respond on the twenty-third postoperative day, following which he cleared mentally very rapidly. The coma persisted despite the fact that the osmolality had been reduced to normal and his diabetes was believed to be under relatively good control (see Table 3-3, Figure 3-3). An electroencephalogram suggested diffuse brain injury at the peak of the coma.

It is of interest that urinary sodium excretion during the period of severe hypertonicity was 3 mEq./l. of sodium prior to the administration of hydrocortisone and was 1 mEq./l. on two consecutive days following this. Administration of a diuretic yielded only a urine

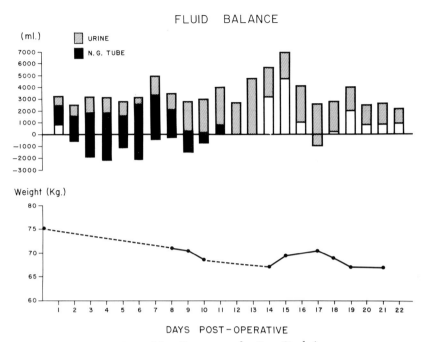

Figure 3-1. (See text under Case Study.)

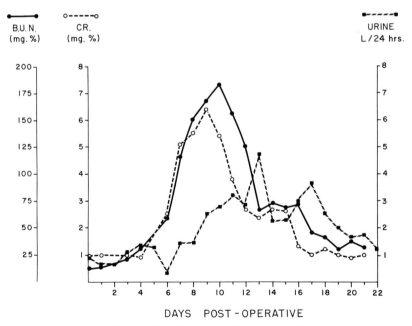

Figure 3-2. (See text under Case Study.)

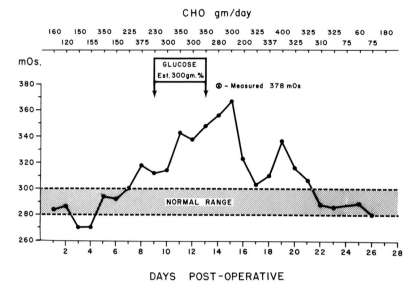

Figure 3-3. *(See text under Case Study.)*

sodium of 23 mEq./l. on the seventeenth postoperative day and 47 mEq./l. on the nineteenth postoperative day. It was not until the twenty-first postoperative day, that, following re-digitalization and without a diuretic, the urine sodium rose to 118 mEq./l. and to 148 mEq./l. on the twenty-third postoperative day. By the twenty-sixth postoperative day the urine sodium had reached levels normal for his dietary intake at that time.

The sequence of events can be summarized as follows:

1. Preoperatively: Age 75, cancer of the lung, cigarette smoker, constrictive pulmonary disease, two or more old myocardial infarctions, one of two blood-sugar determinations abnormal. Normal renal and hepatic tests.

2. Intraoperatively and immediately postoperatively: Stiff lungs, infiltration of LLL, ventilation perfusion defect with shunting, improved with elevation of Po₂. High-volume gastric secretion loss, with metabolic alkalosis developing by the second day (see Table 3-3).

3. Progressive dehydration, with metabolic alkalosis increasing as a result of highly excessive gastric drainage. Acute renal insufficiency with oliguria on the sixth day; then progressive azotemia despite increasing urine volumes, followed by rising serum sodium (see Table 3-3, Figures 3-1 and 3-2).

4. Improving renal function, with falling BUN and creatinine in the face of a serum sodium of 166 mEq./l. and blood glucose levels of 260 mgm. per 100 ml. Coma, with measured plasma osmolality of 378 mOsm., urine osmolality 508 mOsm., and now +4 glucose. Blood and urine acetone negative (see Table 3-3, Figures 3-1 and 3-2).

5. Resolution of hypertonic nonketotic coma complicated by necessity of giving glucose in water intravenously and by a very large dose of dihydrocortisone given for peripheral and central circulatory collapse. Renal conservation of sodium to extreme degree (see Table 3-3, Figure 3-3).

6. Persistent respiratory alkalosis and coma, despite return to normal of osmolality, plasma electrolytes, and renal function. Followed by dramatic recovery of mental

faculties with decrease, but not total resolution, of respiratory alkalosis (see Table 3-3).

ACID-BASE IMBALANCE AND FLUID DISEQUILIBRIUM

HYPEROSMOLAR AND OTHER TYPES OF NONKETO-ACIDOTIC COMA IN PATIENTS WITH KNOWN OR UNSUSPECTED DIABETES

Classic diabetic coma with dehydration, hydroxybutyric acid, has long been recogduced by the presence of excessive amounts of keto acids, aceto-acetic acid and beta-hydroxybutyric acid, has long been recognized. Critically ill patients of all types who are either known diabetics or potentially diabetic, whose glucose intolerance is made evident or intensified by severe illness, may develop diabetic ketoacidosis and progress to the stage of diabetic coma unless the condition is recognized and the patient appropriately treated. Much is known and is available in the literature about the management of this condition as a complication of surgery. Hypoglycemic coma in the patient either on insulin therapy or on a variety of drugs that interfere with glucose mobilization is also well-recognized. A review by Steinke (1970) summarizes the essential points of management of diabetes in surgical patients.

However, two types of coma are less common but equally important in the management of patients who may develop them. They are hyperosmolar nonketotic diabetic coma and nonketotic lactic acidosis with coma.

Nonketotic diabetic coma is characterized by severe dehydration, with a marked elevation of the blood glucose or plasma sodium or both. The result is a marked increase in the plasma osmolality, accompanied by lethargy, stupor, and usually coma. Schwartz and Apfelbaum (1966) have reported 63 cases, collected from the literature and through their own experience, of patients with hyperglycemic hyperosmolar coma. Forty-one of these are pure, in the sense that there was no change toward acidosis in the blood pH. Of particular significance is the fact that 43 patients were *not* known to be diabetic prior to the onset of the coma. Blood glucose in these patients ranged from 400 to 2200 mgm. per 100 ml. Serum sodium was almost always in excess of 150 mEq./l. Serum osmolality, when measured, ranged from 362 to 462 mOsm.

All patients suffered from *severe* dehydration from polyuria, vomiting, or diarrhea. All had fever, tachycardia, and usually tachypnea. Blood pressure was normal to low. Abdominal tenderness was frequently present. The patients did *not* demonstrate Kussmaul respiration. Areflexia was common in severe cases. Danowski and Nabarro (1965) noted that most patients with hyperosmolar coma were in the older age group, that they had diabetes of recent onset or undiagnosed diabetes, and that all were dehydrated and had some other acute illness. They observed that nonketotic patients had normal bicarbonate levels in the blood and were not acidotic.

A mild initial ketosis was observed in a few patients but disappeared with infusions in the cases discussed by Daughaday (1967). He feels that all these patients had uncontrolled diabetes and, at the same time, inadequate renal sodium excretion.

Schwartz (1966) observed that the condition may develop following hemodialysis, presumably with a high glucose level in the dialysate, and in patients with burns. Rosenberg (1965) reported a well-documented case of a 36-year-old male with 45 per cent third-degree burns who, 22 days after the burns, while on a high-caloric, high-carbohydrate diet, became comatose, with hyperglycemia; plasma sodium was 160, chloride was 120, potassium was 4.6, and CO_2 was 20.2 mEq./l. Urine glucose was +4 with negative ketones. Plasma pH was 7.38; hematocrit was 40 per cent. Plasma osmolality was 459 mOsm. and urine osmolality was 478 mOsm. The patient had experienced four days of a high urine output and high urine glucose prior to the development of coma. The coma lasted five days. Urinary steroids were high, 30 mgm. 17-OH in urine per day, and dropped to 15 mgm. per day on recovery. The patient was treated with intravenous fluids and insulin.

Recently, high-caloric parenteral feeding has been implicated in producing hyperosmolar coma. Rea et al. (1970) included two cases of hyperosmolar coma in their study of hyperosmolar intravenous feeding, and another is mentioned in discussion of the paper. The patient, S.K., presented as an illustrative case in this chapter, developed hyperglycemic, hypernatremic, and hyperosmolar coma on the twelfth postoperative day following a thoracotomy. He had both excessive drainage of gastric juice from a Levin tube and a diuresis following acute renal insufficiency to provide excessive water loss. There was marked urinary retention of sodium, glycosuria developed five days prior to coma, and his high-caloric parenteral fluid regimen provided an average of 300 gm. of glucose per day for several days prior to onset. Of interest also is the effect of 4 gm. of dihydrocortisone in increasing the severity of the hyperglycemia. At no time was this patient ketotic, arterial pH determinations were always alkalotic, and TCO_2 values were normal to somewhat elevated.

The etiology of the syndrome would seem to be:

1. Severe dehydration, whether due to polyuria, GI-tract losses, burn surface evaporation, or some combination of these factors.

2. A high-level intake of carbohydrate, either in diet or by infusion.

3. An unrecognized diabetes, often developing several days after the onset of a severe illness. This is a nonketotic hyperglycemia, with relatively normal blood pH and TCO_2.

4. Pancreatic "fatigue," as suggested by Rosenberg (1965).

5. Perhaps related to endogenous steroid

excess with stressful prolonged illness and apparently exacerbated by steroid administration.

6. The lack of ketosis may be the result of dehydration, excessively high glucose, and increased adrenocortical steroid production, all of which are antiketogenic.

TREATMENT

Primary attention must be focused on the severe hyperosmolality. Large volumes of water appear to be required and, when possible, the gastrointestinal tract should be used to avoid further glucose or sodium load. Usually 5 per cent glucose (or fructose) in water by infusion is required with insulin administration based on frequently determined blood glucose levels. The dosage of insulin should be kept small, since sensitivity to insulin seems to be greater in these patients. The rate of fall of plasma osmolality should not be too rapid, for fear of sudden fluid shifts, particularly into the central nervous system. Plasma potassium may fall abruptly, and large amounts of KCl (100 to 200 mEq.) may be required per day to keep the plasma level near normal.

PROGNOSIS

In the series of patients reported by Schwartz and Apfelbaum (1966), 41 per cent of 63 patients died. Prompt recognition and early treatment, together with reduction of high carbohydrate intake in patients with persistent glycosuria or blood glucose levels consistently above 180 mgm. per 100 ml. in nondiabetics, should reduce the mortality to that of the serious illness which underlies the development of the syndrome. Several days of deep coma do not preclude recovery.

LACTIC ACIDOSIS WITH COMA

Danowski (1964) and Schwartz (1966) have pointed out the occurrence of marked elevation of blood lactate without ketosis in some diabetic patients with hyperosmolarity and coma or stupor. Normal levels of lactic acid (lactate) in the blood are from 6 to 16 mgm. per 100 ml., or 0.6 to 1.8 mEq./l. A high level of lactate is to be expected in patients in

shock, in those with severe anemia, after vigorous muscular exercise (shivering), and in patients with severe hyperventilation or hypoventilation. In each instance, lack of oxygen at the cellular level results in anaerobic metabolism of glucose through the Embden-Meyerhof pathway to produce both an absolute excess of lactate and an increase of the normal ratio of blood lactate to pyruvate. Blood pH is decreased, indicating a metabolic acidosis.

Elevated blood lactate can be suspected in any patient in whom there is an anion gap not accounted for by either renal insufficiency or keto acids. The sum of CO_2 plus Cl plus 10 mEq. in the plasma should equal the plasma sodium in milliequivalents within about ± 3 mEq. As discussed by Randall (1969), plasma CO_2 plus Cl plus 10 is less than plasma sodium by more than 3 mEq. when there is excessive retention of either $SO_4^=$ and $HPO_4^=$, as in renal failure, or an abnormal increase of organic anions, such as aceto-acetate and beta-hydroxybutyrate in ketoacidosis, or of lactate in hypoxia and lactate diabetic acidosis. Schwartz (1966) pointed out that diabetics treated with phenformin seem particularly susceptible to lactic acidosis and coma.

Treatment of lactic acidosis is treatment of the underlying cause of cellular hypoxia. The use of sodium bicarbonate-containing solutions partially to correct a severe acidosis is indicated, but the use of sodium lactate in the treatment of metabolic acidosis characterized by lactic acid excess is illogical, at least until the underlying cause of tissue hypoxia has been corrected and lactate can be metabolized normally.

In patients with hyperglycemia and hyperosmolality with elevated blood-lactate levels, the prognosis is usually grave, according to Schwartz.

HYPERTONIC AND HYPOTONIC STATES

Normal osmolality of the plasma in man is 285 milliosmoles (mOsm.), ± 10 mOsm. Cells, extracellular fluid, and plasma are in osmotic equilibrium, and any change in osmotic pressure of any compartment is immediately adjusted by a transfer of water from or to the others to restore equilibrium.

Only the central nervous system, because of the unique permeability characteristics of the blood-brain barrier, responds somewhat differently in adjusting to alterations in extracellular fluid and plasma solute concentration changes.

Determining osmolality of plasma and other biological fluids is a relatively simple laboratory procedure, based on the fact that one gram molecular weight of any substance, dissolved in a liter of water, will depress the freezing point of that solution 1.86° C.

The osmolality of plasma, and thus of most of the body, can be approximated quite accurately if the sodium concentration of the plasma in milliequivalents is doubled and 6 is added. Thus, 2 Na + 6 = milliosmoles. This approximation is accurate only if there is no significant elevation of plasma glucose or urea. (See articles by Randall [1967, 1969] for further discussion of the principles involved.)

A patient is hypertonic when plasma osmolality exceeds 300 mOsm. and hypotonic when plasma osmolality is less than 270 mOsm. Both conditions can exist with dehydration, with a normal complement of water, or with an excess of water, although usually hypertonicity is seen with dehydration and hypotonicity with fluid overloading.

A serious form of hypertonicity—hypertonic nonketotic diabetic coma—is separately discussed, and is illustrated in the case report of patient S.K. in this chapter.

HYPERTONICITY DUE TO SOLUTE LOADING

The mechanism is that of excessive loading of solutes, both salt and protein, in the absence of sufficient water to permit renal excretion of the total solute load. Common clinical settings involve patients being tube-fed a formula following head and neck surgery or for forced feeding, unconscious patients who are being given tube feedings, and patients with brain-stem injuries or brain tumors. Occasional patients on high-caloric, high-glucose parenteral feedings have been reported to have developed this syndrome (Rea, 1970). The patient usually does not appear clinically dehydrated and may be relatively asymptomatic until severe hypertonicity is present. The urine volume is normal or even high because of an osmotic diuresis created by the solute load.

LABORATORY FINDINGS

An increased concentration of plasma solutes, both electrolytes and crystalloids, in concentrations out of all proportion to a change in hematocrit is found. An elevated plasma sodium in the presence of a substantial urine volume is the key to diagnosis. The urine volume is normal or polyuria may be present; the specific gravity is often elevated but not to maximal levels. This is in contrast to the desiccated patient, who is oliguric and hypertonic with an elevated hematocrit.

TREATMENT

The basic problem is that of a water intake inadequate to permit urinary excretion of a large solute load and the inability to drink water to provide more solvent. Treatment consists of the administration of large volumes of water orally, or parenterally as 5 per cent glucose in water, while withholding or at least reducing the amount of tube feeding or parenteral feeding. A remarkably high output of urine may persist for some time as the hypertonicity gradually falls.

In patients who excrete large volumes of dilute urine while becoming dehydrated and hypertonic, a response to Pitressin tannate is both diagnostic of diabetes insipidus and therapeutic in restoring water balance.

WATER LOADING, HYPOTONICITY, AND WATER INTOXICATION

The direct opposite of solute loading hypertonicity is excessive water intake in the presence of antidiuresis. The mechanism is the administration of an excess of water beyond baseline requirements and the replacement of abnormal losses, in a patient who is incapable of excreting the water during antidiuresis due to illness, trauma, or renal failure.

The source of water may be oral intake but more often is ill-advised excessive parenteral therapy with glucose and water. Colonic irrigations, particularly those designed to reduce postoperative distention, may result in the retention of substantial volumes of water, as much as 4 liters in two days in one case in our records.

Patients with chronic wasting illness, cancer, congestive heart failure, or hepatic or renal disease are likely to have an expanded ECF and some degree of hypotonicity before they come to surgery or suffer accidental trauma. These patients are particularly prone to hold excess water postoperatively and to expand and further dilute their ECF.

Drowsiness, weakness, and a fall in urine volume are early symptoms, followed by convulsions and coma. A rapid weight gain will always occur; peripheral and pulmonary edema may be noted. Laboratory findings include a rapid fall in the serum sodium concentration and in plasma osmolality. The urine may contain substantial amounts of sodium, which, in the presence of a low plasma concentration, indicates an inappropriate sodium release due to excess ECF volume, if renal tubular disease and adrenal insufficiency are ruled out.

The rate of fall of the plasma sodium appears to be of greater importance than the absolute sodium value. Brain edema is the cause of the coma and convulsions. Plasma sodium values of 120 mEq. or less will usually be found in water intoxication.

Treatment

Stopping the intake of water is the first step in treatment. Either no intake at all for a while or very small volumes of slowly administered hypertonic glucose solution are indicated.

If pulmonary edema and increased central venous pressure are not present, the administration of a small volume of hypertonic salt, 300 ml. of 3 per cent NaCl, will begin restoration of osmotic equilibrium and promote the renal excretion of water. No attempt should be made to give a "calculated replacement of sodium deficit" based on ECF volume and unit sodium deficiency, for severe overloading would result. Time, with the loss of insensible water via the lungs and skin, together with urine output, will gradually restore the patient to normal. Hemodialysis with plasma ultrafiltration has been used successfully in treating severely ill patients with water intoxication.

DEHYDRATION

The type of dehydration and its effect on the patient depend on the *rate* and the *route* of water loss. Rapid dehydration by external fluid loss is initially almost entirely an extracellular fluid loss. Replacement should be rapid and should contain the electrolyte components of extracellular fluid. Slow dehydration, extending over a period of several days, permits renal retention of water and salt and involves the loss of substantial amounts of intracellular water and potassium. Repletion must be slower, the total volumes required are larger, and once reasonable renal function is assured, substantial amounts of potassium chloride are required.

There are three types of dehydration: desiccation, acute dehydration, and chronic dehydration. Each presents a different problem in management.

DEHYDRATION BY PRIMARY WATER LOSS: DESICCATION

The mechanism is that of excessive loss of water vapor or of very hypotonic solutions. The common clinical settings are those involving excessive evaporation of water from the lungs, as is seen with fever, dyspnea, tracheostomy, and dry oxygen administration by nasal or tracheal catheter. A high-volume output of dilute urine in diabetes insipidus and excessive sweating also produce excess water loss, as does the evaporation of water from injured body surface, as occurs in the open treatment of burns. Fever, disorientation, oliguria, azotemia, coma, convulsions, and death will follow. Hypotension is not a major feature in development of hypertonicity.

Laboratory Findings

There is an increase in all the solutes in the plasma, with a rise in the plasma osmolality. The plasma sodium is the key and may reach levels of 160 mEq. or more in a patient with oliguria. The hematocrit rises in proportion to the loss of total body water and thus more slowly than in a fresh burn or in peritonitis, when major plasma losses accentuate the hematocrit increase. The urine volume is small and the urine is concentrated.

Treatment

Water is administered orally or as a 5 per cent dextrose solution intravenously in sufficient volume to restore renal function and hematocrit to normal and gradually to decrease the plasma sodium to about 140 mEq./l. The rate of administration will depend on the rapidity of dehydration: the faster it occurred, the more rapid can be the administration rate. Some salt will be required in later stages of repair if sweating has contributed significantly to the water loss. The total volume of water required is large and can be estimated from the total body water reduction necessary to raise the plasma osmolality from normal to the concentration found.

ACUTE DEHYDRATION WITH LOSS OF ECF

The mechanism is that of the rapid loss of body fluid containing nearly isotonic concentrations of extracellular fluid electrolytes. Clinically this usually occurs as loss from the gastrointestinal tract. The volume loss is so rapid that there is little initial change in tonicity. Pyloric obstruction, acute bacterial dysentery, small bowel fistulas, pseudomembranous colitis, ulcerative colitis, and infantile diarrhea are examples. Acute small bowel obstruction produces the same pattern. If the obstruction is high, there is usually vomiting, but lower small bowel obstruction may exhibit little external loss, with an equally shocking loss of fluid into a distended bowel.

The patient appears clinically dehydrated and initially may be thirsty but rapidly passes into a state of apathy with tachycardia, a low-grade fever, oliguria progressing to anuria, hypotension, and shock.

Laboratory Findings

There is a diminished plasma volume, with a sharp increase in the hematocrit, an increase in plasma protein concentration, and perhaps some elevation of the plasma potassium. If the loss has been primarily that of gastric juices, there will be a fall in plasma chloride concentration, with a compensatory elevation of the plasma bicarbonate, resulting in a metabolic alkalosis. Usually there is little change in plasma electrolyte concentration. If there is hypotension, there may be a metabolic acidosis due to excess lactic acid. There will be an acute fall in body weight if the loss is external. An acute loss of 4 per cent of body weight (20 per cent of ECF) is sufficient to produce major symptoms and a loss of 6 per cent is sufficient to produce shock.

Treatment

The loss is almost entirely that of interstitial fluid and plasma. Replacement should be rapid and consist of extracellular electrolytes in isotonic solution. If vomiting has been a predominant feature and the CO_2 content of the plasma is high, isotonic sodium chloride is the ideal replacement fluid for the deficit of interstitial fluid, while some plasma will be needed to replace lost plasma protein. If the loss has been from diarrhea, small bowel fistula, or retained small bowel content, the plasma CO_2 content will be low, and replacement should be with two-thirds the calculated volume as 0.9 per cent NaCl and one-third as one-sixth molar $NaHCO_3$. Ringer's lactate solution may be used for total replacement if plasma potassium and lactate levels are not elevated. Potassium chloride should be added to replacement fluid as soon as renal output increases to normal volume but should be avoided initially in the oliguric patient. Baseline fluids containing glucose must be added to the replacement regimen at the rate of about 500 ml. every six hours, and any continuing abnormal loss must be replaced.

A "rule-of-thumb" estimate of initial requirements in *acute* dehydration can be obtained from the following formula:

$$\text{Deficit in liters} = \left(1 - \frac{40}{\genfrac{}{}{0pt}{}{\text{hematocrit}}{\text{of patient}}}\right) \times 20 \text{ per}$$

cent of body weight in kg.

In a 70-kg. man with a hematocrit of 55 this becomes:

$$\left(1 - \frac{40}{55}\right) \times 14, \text{ or } \frac{3}{11} \times 14 = 3.8 \text{ liters}$$

Four-fifths of this should be given as non-colloid-containing electrolyte solution and one-fifth as plasma albumin solution.

Chronic dehydration with electrolyte loss: Chronic salt loss

The mechanism is a slower version of acute dehydration with extracellular fluid loss. It is more common than acute shocking ECF loss. Dilutional hypotonicity develops as abnormal losses of electrolytes continue and are under-replaced and as water is retained by the kidneys to defend volume. The loss of electrolyte is usually from the gastrointestinal tract, either by diarrhea or by a fistula or its medical equivalent, a tube in the stomach or small bowel. The patient is usually oliguric and weak and frequently has fever but is not usually thirsty.

Laboratory Findings

The serum sodium is low without a significantly elevated hematocrit. Serum potassium is likely to be low, particularly with protracted loss of fluid from the gastrointestinal tract. If there has been loss of HCl from gastric suction or vomiting, the plasma CO_2 content and pH are likely to be elevated, the plasma chloride quite low, and the plasma potassium strikingly low—the typical picture of hypokalemic alkalosis. Some degree of azotemia may be present along with the oliguria.

If loss of base has been dominant, as in small bowel loss and particularly a biliary or pancreatic fistula, the plasma potassium may be normal or slightly elevated, the CO_2 content and pH of the plasma tend to be reduced, and a metabolic acidosis is present. The plasma protein concentration is usually low, particularly if bowel losses have been replaced over several days with only electrolyte solutions and water. Urine volume is related to solute load and may have a fixed specific gravity because of hyponatremia.

Treatment

The major problem is that of extracellular electrolyte deficiency with additional hypotonicity. Extracellular volume is much less reduced than in acute dehydration. Initial treatment with hypertonic salt solution or a hypertonic mixture of NaCl and $NaHCO_3$ is indicated. Additional water should be restricted to minimal baseline and to quantitative isotonic replacement of external abnormal loss. There is little point in giving a hypertonic solution and then giving enough water so that the total retained load is hypotonic!

A test of 300 ml. of 3 per cent NaCl should begin osmotic restitution. Sodium bicarbonate should constitute one-third of this load if acidosis is present. Potassium will be needed as osmolality is increased, to provide potassium for intracellular depletion. It is particularly important in the presence of a metabolic alkalosis. Further addition of concentrated electrolyte should depend on observation of the effect of the initial dose after several hours of equilibration. Often an increased urine volume will further assist in repair, since free-water clearance becomes possible with increased sodium concentration. Intracellular potassium losses will be large if the process has gone on for some time, and substantial amounts of KCl will be needed in the later state of repair. Since dehydration occurred *slowly*, replacement will, of necessity, be *slow* and will take several days.

USE AND LIMITATIONS OF RINGER'S LACTATE AND OTHER BALANCED SALT SOLUTIONS IN TREATMENT OF CRITICALLY ILL PATIENTS

USE OF RINGER'S LACTATE SOLUTION

In recent years there has been great interest in the use of large volumes of buffered salt solution, particularly Ringer's lactate solution, in the treatment of patients with shock due to trauma and burns. Discussion of the use of Ringer's lactate in the treatment of shock will be found in Chapter 2. Extension of the use of large volumes of buffered salt solution to the other types of surgical patients requires careful consideration.

There is no doubt that healthy, vigorous young patients can tolerate a massive load of acute infusions of buffered salt solutions after injury and that most will respond to such treatment with an immediate and extensive diuresis while tolerating quite well the marked overhydration, decreased plasma oncotic pressure, and hemodilution that are involved. An increase in cardiac output of considerable amount apparently accompanies massive fluid loading, and the key to tolerance seems to be the ability to raise cardiac output and to institute and maintain massive diuresis of urine containing not only urea, sulfates, phosphates, and potassium but much of the administered electrolytes as well.

The virtues of infusion of large volumes of buffered salt solutions resembling extracellular fluid are described as production of a large volume of urine, reduced viscosity of blood, with increased perfusion of peripheral tissues, and a decreased need for blood transfusions.

The risks of administration of large volumes of saline or buffered salt solutions include overloading patients who are unable to raise cardiac output sufficiently to handle the load or who have inadequate renal function to dispose of a substantial volume, and overloading patients who for some endocrinological reason do not suppress secretion of antidiuretic hormone and aldosterone and, therefore, cannot release either the water or the salt components of the infusion. In such patients both plasma volume and interstitial fluid become grossly overexpanded; circulatory failure, usually manifested by pulmonary edema, is not an infrequent consequence, and major disruption of normal fluid equilibrium results in distorted equilibrium within the brain, compromised pulmonary function with atelectasis and local pulmonary infection, decrease in oxygenation of the blood, anastomotic edema, and generalized peripheral edema.

The rationale for the administration of large volumes of Ringer's lactate solution or other solution containing sodium, chloride, and lactate or bicarbonate is derived from many observations on the temporary effect of saline solution in large volumes in treatment of shock.

Shires and associates (1964, 1966) reported a reduction in the space of distribution of $^{35}SO_4$ in the functional extracellular fluid space of as much as 40 per cent in hemorrhagic shock in dogs and similar apparent deficits in human patients. Infusion of Ringer's lactate solution, 5 per cent of body weight, in addition to transfusion, markedly reduced the mortality of the experimental shock preparation in dogs and restored the distribution of $^{35}SO_4$ to normal.

Subsequent reports by Dillon (1966), Rush (1967), Moss (1969), and Gilder (1970) support the effectiveness of salt solution containing sodium, chloride, and bicarbonate or lactate in treatment of hemorrhagic hypotension in otherwise healthy dogs. At least one-half the volume of blood lost had to be replaced in order to avoid a severe drop in hematocrit, and volumes of Ringer's lactate or similar solutions that were used varied from 5 per cent of body weight, as reported by Shires et al., to 12 per cent or more, according to Dillon and associates.

Recently, however, doubt has been expressed concerning the interpretation of the volume measured by early diffusion of $^{35}SO_4$ and of ^{22}Na and ^{24}Na in shock as representing a true loss of extracellular fluid of the magnitude suggested. The time required for equilibration of isotopic anions or cations of small size is prolonged in hemorrhagic shock and following surgical operations, but ultimate volumes of distribution do not appear to be reduced more than would be expected from measured blood loss. Multiple sampling of blood during isotope dilution and prolongation of the observation period beyond 20 or 30 minutes to an hour or more has been shown to be important to avoid errors in interpretation.

Anderson (1969) studied 60 patients immediately after their evacuation from the battlefield to a surgical hospital in Vietnam. Using ^{125}I-tagged serum albumin and $^{35}SO_4$ to measure plasma volume and extracellular fluid, they were unable to demonstrate any interstitial fluid deficits that were not due to dehydration (also seen in all field controls) or to transcapillary refilling of the plasma volume. They found no evidence for isotonic intracellular redistribution of extracellular fluid in patients with major trauma and hemorrhage who were in various degrees of shock.

Roth (1969) reported studies of extracellular fluid space in dogs and in patients undergoing both general surgical and open-heart procedures. A mean decrease in extracellular fluid volume of 5.7 per cent was found in dogs after one and a half hours of severe hemorrhagic shock, much of it due to blood sampling and respiratory loss. In patients undergoing open-heart surgery and general surgery, increases in extracellular fluid volume and interstitial fluid volume were found, all of which could be accounted for by postoperative fluid balance. Increases of 9 and 15.5 per cent of extracellular fluid volume which Roth reported are compatible with the formation of areas of sequestered fluids in wounds and within the gastro-intestinal tract.

Moore and Shires (1967) and Randall (1969) have emphasized that the purpose of administering balanced salt solutions during and after surgical procedures is to provide for extracellular fluid sequestration in areas of surgical or traumatic injury and to replace pre-existing deficits, if they are present. They emphasize that the volume of salt solution used must be related to the extent of injury and that excessive use is ill-advised and potentially dangerous.

INDICATIONS

The use of Ringer's lactate or other balanced salt solutions during surgical treatment and in the treatment of trauma in previously healthy adults is indicated in the following situations:

1. During major surgical procedures and during the first 24 to 48 hours postoperatively, to provide for sequestration of extracellular fluid in the wound and in viscera subject to manipulation. The volume administered should be *proportional* to the extent of the surgical procedures and probably should not exceed 3000 to 3500 ml. *total for the most major operations,* with *much less for most routine cases.*

Studies of the rate of formation of wound edema suggest that in a clean, incised wound, about one-half the total excess fluid accumulates in the first five hours, more than three-fourths in 24 hours, and the process of wound edema formation is complete in 36 to 48 hours in the absence of infection. As in treating a patient with a burn, salt solutions given for major operations should be proportionate to the extent of injury. Half the solution or more should be given intra-operatively and in the first six hours postoperatively, and the remaining half given over the next 24 hours or so. After this, the use of balanced salt solutions should stop, except to replace abnormal external losses or to provide additional ECF if there is advancing sepsis, such as peritonitis.

2. In severe cases of trauma in volumes determined by hourly urine volume and central venous pressure (in addition to the administration of whole blood). In the most major injury the total volume should not exceed 10 per cent of ideal body weight in 48 hours and in most cases should be retricted to 5 *per cent or less of body weight.*

3. In patients with extensive plasma-losing diseases, such as diffuse peritonitis, pancreatitis, or perforated hollow viscus. Solution should be given in addition to plasma, albumin, or plasma substitute and in volumes guided by central venous pressure and hourly urinary output. Volumes should rarely exceed 5 per cent of body weight.

4. In patients with pre-existing deficits due to dehydration or fluid loss who do not have a metabolic alkalosis due to hypochloremia or potassium deficit. Isotonic sodium chloride is indicated for volume expansion in the presence of a metabolic alkalosis.

5. In patients with sudden major venous obstruction, solution used with whole blood or plasma to treat a functional blood-volume deficit.

CONTRAINDICATIONS AND RESTRICTIONS

Situations in which the use of Ringer's lactate and other extracellular fluid volume-expanding solutions is contraindicated or restricted include the following:

1. In elderly patients, particularly if they fail to respond with an increase in urine volume or have a significant rise in central venous pressure.

2. In patients with an already overexpanded extracellular fluid volume, as with valvular heart disease, heart failure, liver disease, chronic infection, starvation, renal insufficiency, and recent previous surgical treatment or major trauma. These patients require careful control of circulatory volume and efforts to increase cardiac output through digitalization, but further expansion of the extracellular fluid may be highly dangerous in many, although necessary in some.

3. In patients with elevated venous pressure, particularly if a small volume of fluid added parenterally results in a sharp rise. A sudden increase in venous pressure, even within normal limits, is an indication for slowing or stopping of further parenteral therapy temporarily. Accurate measurement of central venous pressure is essential.

4. To replace blood loss in excess of 15 to

20 per cent of the estimated total blood volume. Anemia and hypoproteinemia are limiting factors.

5. In patients with established acute renal failure, unless severe dehydration and extracellular fluid electrolyte deficits are clearly established.

6. In lieu of baseline provision of glucose in water or glucose and saline solution, with potassium when indicated. Ringer's lactate and most other balanced salt solutions contain virtually no calories and far too much sodium for maintenance therapy. Potassium content is inadequate as well.

7. During the phase of diuresis with resolution of sequestered fluid in an area of injury or infection. The danger of serious overload and pulmonary edema is great at this time.

8. As a routine replacement fluid for gastrointestinal tract fluid losses, particularly gastric juice.

DIFFERENTIAL DIAGNOSIS OF METABOLIC AND RESPIRATORY ACID–BASE IMBALANCE

The hydrogen-ion concentration of the blood is normally held within very narrow limits at a level which keeps the blood in a slightly alkaline state, with a pH between 7.38 and 7.42. Close control is accomplished by a series of buffers, of which, in the blood, the bicarbonate-carbonic acid system and hemoglobin are the most important.

The Henderson-Hasselbalch equation for the bicarbonate-carbonic acid buffer system states that the ratio of base (largely sodium) bicarbonate to carbonic acid at pH 7.4 is 20:1.

$$pH = pK + \log \frac{(BHCO_3)}{(H_2CO_3)}$$

$$7.4 = 6.1 + \log \frac{20}{1}$$

where   pK = dissociation constant of (H_2CO_3) = 6.1

$(BHCO_3)$ = bicarbonate associated with cations (other than hydrogen ion), mEq./l.

(H_2CO_3) = carbonic acid, mEq./l.

Since the amount of dissolved CO_2 which is hydrated to form (H_2CO_3) is proportionate to total dissolved CO_2, both the denominator of the ratio $(BHCO_3/H_2CO_3)$ and pH depend on PCO_2 and are functions of CO_2 production and respiratory excretion.

Inorganic acidic radicals, such as Cl^-, $HPO_4^=$, and $SO_4^=$, and organic acid radicals, such as lactate, pyruvate, and the keto acids, combine with $(BHCO_3)$, yielding the sodium salt of the acid and (H_2CO_3), which is then excreted as CO_2. $HAc + NaHCO_3 \rightarrow NaAc + (H_2CO_3)$; pH is defended, since a neutral salt and CO_2 are formed at the expense of bicarbonate reserve.

Inorganic acid anions are selectively excreted by the kidneys, together with hydrogen ion or as ammonium salts, to maintain the normal bicarbonate concentration of the plasma and pH of the blood. Organic anion excesses are usually metabolized as the underlying defect that has caused accumulation is corrected, but in the presence of excessive levels, some renal excretion occurs as well and may be a guide to diagnosis and therapy.

Since it is the ratio of $(BHCO_3)$ to (H_2CO_3) that determines pH and not the absolute amounts present, it is apparent that the acid-base status of a patient's blood can be determined only if at least two of the three values of CO_2 content, PCO_2, and pH are determined. Since all three are interdependent, any one can be calculated from the other two.

Inspection of the Henderson-Hasselbalch equation indicates that the ratio of $(BHCO_3)$ to (H_2CO_3) can be disturbed either by a change in the bicarbonate concentration or by a change in the (H_2CO_3) concentration, as well as by disproportionate changes in both. These changes can result from primary disturbances in pulmonary regulation of PCO_2, by changes in concentration of bicarbonate and other buffer ions produced by metabolic disturbances, or by some combination of these factors.

Blood determinations, which involve measuring pH, PCO_2, total CO_2 and PO_2 of *arterial* blood, are easily accomplished and are essential for evaluation of acid-base balance as well as pulmonary function.

Table 3-4 describes the primary changes which represent acidosis or alkalosis.

Note that respiratory acidosis and respiratory alkalosis involve a change in PCO_2 and pH. Acute respiratory acidosis or alkalosis

TABLE 3-4. Primary Changes in $BHCO_3$ and H_2CO_3 Leading to Acid-Base Disturbances

CO_2 content $\downarrow$ pH $\downarrow$	Metabolic acidosis
CO_2 content $\uparrow$ pH $\uparrow$	Metabolic alkalosis
$P_{CO_2} \uparrow$ pH $\downarrow$	Respiratory acidosis
$P_{CO_2} \downarrow$ pH $\uparrow$	Respiratory alkalosis

frequently exists without any significant change in the CO_2 content of plasma and can be determined only by measurement of pH and CO_2 content, or pH and P_{CO_2}.

Unfortunately, these simple changes are not sufficient for complete evaluation of the acid-base status of patients, for primary changes induce secondary compensations which must be taken into consideration as well. It is widely recognized that respiratory disturbances result in secondary changes in plasma bicarbonate concentration, and that metabolic disturbances produce compensatory changes in respiration and in P_{CO_2}. Thus a complete evaluation of the acid-base status of a patient requires knowledge of pH, P_{CO_2} and total CO_2 (T_{CO_2}), and at least two of these must be measured. Fortunately, laboratory apparatus has now been developed which makes it easy to determine pH and P_{CO_2} directly, to add to the determination of CO_2 content which has been in use for many years. Usually P_{O_2} is also determined and the percentage of O_2 saturation is calculated, determinations that are of great value in assessment of pulmonary function. (See Chapter 1.)

METABOLIC ACIDOSIS

This is an excess of hydrogen ion with a fall in pH of the blood, accompanied by a decrease in plasma bicarbonate concentration, as bicarbonate is used up in buffering or is lost externally. Bicarbonate is less than 24 mEq./l. and pH is less than 7.38. (See Figure 3-4.)

The common causes of metabolic acidosis are:

1. Acute and chronic renal failure, with retention of $SO_4^=$ and $HPO_4^=$ ions.

2. Dehydration due to loss of small bowel content, bile, or pancreatic fistulas, with loss of bicarbonate and sodium.

3. Hypoxia, with the production of an excess of lactic acid.

4. Diabetes mellitus and starvation acido-

sis, with the production of an excess of keto acids.

5. Ureterosigmoidostomy with chloride reabsorption and hyperchloremia.

6. Adrenal insufficiency.

COMPENSATION

Compensation for metabolic acidosis is both respiratory and renal. Respiration is increased in rate and particularly in depth, with a lowering of P_{CO_2}, and a partial return of pH toward normal. Renal adjustment, if renal function permits, is a slower process involving an increase in both ammonia and titratable acidity, with increased hydrogen-ion excretion and conservation of base to restore plasma bicarbonate toward normal.

TREATMENT

Treatment of metabolic acidosis is directed toward the cause of the acidosis. In addition, therapy must be planned to reinforce the diminished bicarbonate reserve and combat the hyperkalemia which may become a serious threat. Efforts should be made to keep the CO_2 content of the plasma at or above 15 mEq./l., and the best drug for this purpose is sodium bicarbonate.

Experience has demonstrated that it takes 2 mEq. of $NaHCO_3$ per liter of ECF to raise the plasma CO_2 by 1 mEq. Thus a patient with a CO_2 content of 10 mEq. and who weighs 70 kg. will require 140 mEq. of $NaHCO_3$ to restore the CO_2 to 15 mEq./l. ($70 \times 0.2 \times 5 \times 2 = 140$).

This may be administered as an isotonic solution (1.2 per cent) or in critically ill patients as a 5 per cent solution given intravenously very slowly. A sharp fall in the serum potassium must be watched for, and potassium must be administered if this occurs. It is seldom necessary to give sodium bicarbonate sufficient to bring the plasma CO_2 to normal levels, and the amount of sodium required to do so may be excessive. Titration of the patient to maintain a CO_2 above 15 mEq./l. is usually adequate.

RESPIRATORY ACIDOSIS

This is an increase of hydrogen ion and a decrease in pH of the blood caused by an increase in PCO_2 and in $HHCO_3$. The pH of blood is less than 7.38 and the PCO_2 more than 45 and usually more than 50 mm. Hg. The CO_2 content of the plasma is not altered in the acute phase but rises with compensation. (See Figure 3-4.)

Common causes of respiratory acidosis are:

1. Hypoventilation. Mechanical hypoventilation may be due to airway obstruction, pneumothorax, pleural effusion, atelectasis, pneumonitis, thoracotomy, upper abdominal incisions, or skeletal-muscle weakness. Carbon dioxide retention often may occur in chronic pulmonary disease—emphysema, asthma, chronic bronchitis, or radiation fibrosis of the lung—or acutely as the result of medications, such as anesthesia, narcotics, barbiturates, or muscle relaxants.

2. Venous-arterial shunting in poorly ventilated segments of the lungs due to atelectasis or pneumonitis. This may result in elevation of arterial PCO_2.

COMPENSATION

Compensation for respiratory acidosis is renal, with increased tubular reabsorption of sodium and bicarbonate and increased excretion of chloride and hydrogen ion. The result is a rise in plasma bicarbonate, which partially or completely restores pH to normal.

TREATMENT

Treatment of acute respiratory acidosis is an emergency, the success of which rests on recognition of inadequate ventilation long prior to the development of cyanosis. Restlessness and a rise in blood pressure and pulse rate may be the first signs of hypercapnea and hypoxia. Hypotension follows. The use of narcotics only increases the problem through suppression of the respiratory center. Making certain that the airway is clear, administering oxygen cautiously, and assisting respiration are indicated. Problems in ventilation are discussed in detail in Chapter 1, to which the reader is referred.

METABOLIC ALKALOSIS

Metabolic alkalosis is a deficit of hydrogen ion, reflected as a rise in blood pH. The pH is in excess of 7.42, and the CO_2 content of the plasma is more than 29 mEq./l. Usually the plasma potassium level and the plasma chloride level are low. The common causes of metabolic alkalosis are:

1. Loss of hydrochloric acid due to vomiting or gastric drainage.

2. Antidiuresis and sodium retention in excess of chloride following trauma or in wasting disease, potentiated by pre-existing potassium deficit.

3. The administration of diuretics, particularly the chlorothiazides, with renal loss of potassium and chloride.

4. Combined hypochloremic, hypokalemic alkalosis, with an acid urine—a very common finding in the post-traumatic state in patients with gastrointestinal drainage.

5. The administration of adrenal steroids.

COMPENSATION

Compensation for metabolic alkalosis is also respiratory and renal. In some patients there is diminished ventilation with some increase in PCO_2, particularly when the CO_2 content of the plasma rises above 35 mEq./l. However, respiratory compensation is small and is limited by oxygen demand.

Renal compensation initially is by excretion of sodium bicarbonate in an alkaline urine. Unless adequate amounts of sodium, potassium, chloride, and water are available, however, this soon leads to dehydration and to hyponatremia. Metabolic alkalosis increases renal excretion of potassium and, as depletion develops, renal tubular absorption of bicarbonate increases, leading to the paradox of an acid urine in an alkalotic patient and helping to perpetuate the alkalosis.

TREATMENT

Treatment of metabolic alkalosis is directed to correction of the cause. Alkalosis caused by sodium retention (steroids, exogenous sodium bicarbonate administration) will correct itself on cessation of therapy. Alkalosis caused by chloride and potassium loss responds to the administration of chloride and potassium. Both ions are required; the potassium chloride is the drug of choice.

RESPIRATORY ALKALOSIS

Respiratory alkalosis is a primary decrease in PCO_2 and in $HHCO_3$ and is reflected in an increase in pH of the blood above 7.42. The cause is increased ventilation, both in rate and depth, with a reduction of the normal alveolar PCO_2 below 35 mm. Hg. Initially there is no change in the CO_2 content of the plasma.

The causes of hyperventilation and respiratory alkalosis are multiple and include:

1. Apprehension and pain.
2. Fever, particularly if associated with some lung infection or atelectasis.
3. Hepatic failure with elevated blood ammonia.
4. Central nervous system injury.
5. Respirators.
6. Septicemia, particularly gram-negative sepsis.
7. Salicylate intoxication.

A *mild* degree of respiratory alkalosis is a common finding in a high percentage of postoperative patients and is often associated with some degree of metabolic alkalosis as well (Lyons, 1966).

Severe respiratory alkalosis produces hypocapneic vasoconstriction, which reduces cerebral circulation, and hypoxia, by decreasing the release of oxygen from hemoglobin and decreasing arterial PO_2, with the production of excess lactic acid. In addition, depression of the ionization of calcium leads to tetany, and the fall in plasma potassium leads to cardiac arrhythmias and digitalis intoxication. With circulatory failure, there is rapid conversion to a severe and often lethal metabolic acidosis.

COMPENSATION

The compensation for respiratory alkalosis is renal, with the excretion of sodium bicarbonate in the urine. However, sodium retention and antidiuresis following trauma substantially or completely block this compensation and, as a result, an alkaline urine is seldom seen.

TREATMENT

Treatment of respiratory alkalosis depends on its severity. A mild degree of alkalosis, partially respiratory in origin, is seen in a large percentage of postoperative patients upon whom blood-gas analysis is performed.

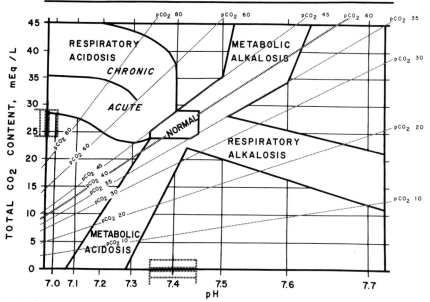

···ACID-BASE PATTERN-ANALYSIS DIAGRAM···

Figure 3-4. Acid-base pattern—Analysis diagram, useful both for diagnosis of acid-base imbalance and for following the course of a patient and the effectiveness of treatment. Arterial blood analysis (blood gases) gives values for pH, total CO_2, and PCO_2. All three should be determined as an internal check on accuracy and should result in a single plot point on the diagram. Combinations of metabolic and respiratory derangements are common and will fall between the areas that represent "pure" disturbances. The upward turn of the arm designated metabolic alkalosis beyond TCO_2 of 35 mEq/l. allows for respiratory compensation. Shaded areas on the abscissa and ordinate represent normal ranges. (Developed by and reproduced with permission of Dr. Robert V. Stephens, senior resident in Surgery at Rhode Island Hospital.)

In general, these patients have good cardiac, pulmonary, and renal function and will recover without treatment.

Severe respiratory alkalosis has a poor prognosis owing to the underlying causes of the hyperventilation. Within the limits imposed by oxygen demand, narcotics have proved effective in reducing ventilation. Theoretically, the inhalation of an oxygen-carbon dioxide mixture, with sufficient CO_2 to raise the PCO_2 to normal, should be effective. In the few instances tried, patients have tolerated this procedure poorly.

COMBINED ALTERATIONS

Combinations of metabolic and respiratory changes in acid-base balance are often seen, not only as compensation for the initial derangement, but also because of two or more co-existing causes. The importance of measurement of arterial pH, CO_2 content, and PCO_2 cannot be overemphasized in the accurate determination of the cause of acid-base imbalance in a seriously ill patient.

A nomogram that visually demonstrates normal and abnormal values of pH, total CO_2, and PCO_2 and the relationships which must exist among these three is of great value in clinical evaluation and patient treatment. Such a nomogram is shown in Figure 3-4. The pH scale is logarithmic (pH is $\frac{1}{\log [H]^+}$) and this permits the PCO_2 isobars to be shown as straight lines.

Relatively "pure" metabolic and respiratory acidosis and alkalosis are shown as areas within the four arms radiating from the very small zone representing normal values. Often blood-gas data will plot as a point lying between two of the arms, indicating a combination of respiratory and metabolic derangements. Such a diagram, as an insert for the patient's chart, not only assists in diagnosis, but can be used to follow the patient's course and the effectiveness of treatment.

REFERENCES

Anderson, R. W., Simmons, R. L., Collins, J. A., Bredenberg, C. E., James, P. M., and Levitsky, S.: Plasma volume and sulfate space in acute combat casualties. Surg. Gynec. Obstet., *128*:719, 1969.

Arney, G. K., Pearson, E., and Sutherland, A. B.: Burn stress and pseudodiabetes. Ann. Surg., *152*:77, 1960.

Austen, G., Jr.: Management of postoperative acute renal failure. Amer. J. Surg., *116*:346, 1968.

Danowski, T. S., and Nabarro, J. D. N.: Hyperosmolar and other types of non-ketoacidotic coma in diabetes. Diabetes, *14*:162, 1965.

Daughaday, W. H.: Acidosis and coma. Chapter XXVI. In Diabetes Mellitus: Diagnosis and Treatment. New York, American Diabetes Association, Inc., 1967.

Dillon, J., Lynch, L. J., Myers, R., Butcher, H. R., Jr., and Moyer, C. A.: A bio-assay of treatment of hemorrhagic shock, Part I. Arch. Surg., *93*:537, 1966.

Eliahou, H. E., and Bata, A.: The diagnosis of acute renal failure. Nephron, *2*:287, 1965.

Forland, M., and Pullman, T. N.: Renal aspects of cardiac disease. Med. Clin. N. Amer., *50*:255, 1966.

Gilder, H., Cortese, A. F., Loehr, W. J., Moore, H. V., and deLeon, V.: Dilution studies in experimental hemorrhagic shock: a critical look at the excessive deficits of extracellular space in shocked dogs. Ann. Surg., *171*:42, 1970.

Hollenberg, N. K., Adams, D. F., Oken, D. E., Abrams, H. L., and Merrill, J. P.: Acute renal failure due to nephrotoxins: renal hemodynamic and angiographic studies in man. New Eng. J. Med., *282*:1329, 1970.

Hollenberg, N. K., Epstein, M., Rosen, S. M., Basch, R. I., and Merrill, J. P.: Oliguric renal failure in man: evidence for preferential renal cortical ischemia. Medicine (Balt.), *47*:455, 1968.

Johnson, W. J.: Principles of management of acute renal failure. Chapter 33. *In* Brest, A. N., and Moyer, J. H. (eds.): Renal Failure. Philadelphia, J. P. Lippincott Company, 1967, pp. 273–280.

Lindsay, R. M., Linton, A. L., and Longland, C. J.: Assessment of postoperative renal function. Lancet, *1*:978, 1965.

Luke, R. G., Linton, A. L., Briggs, J. D., and Kennedy, A. C.: Mannitol therapy in acute renal failure. Lancet, *1*:980, 1965.

Lyons, J. H., Jr., and Moore, F. D.: Post-traumatic alkalosis: incidence and pathophysiology of alkalosis in surgery. Surgery, *60*:93, 1966.

McClelland, R. N., Shires, G. T., Baxter, C. R., Coln, G. D., and Carrico, J.: Balanced salt solutions in the treatment of hemorrhagic shock. JAMA, *199*:166, 1967.

Merrill, J. P.: Acute renal failure. JAMA, *211*:289, 1970.

Merrill, J. P.: The Treatment of Renal Failure. New York, Grune and Stratton, 1965.

Moore, F. D., and Shires, G. T.: Moderation. Ann. Surg., *166*:300, 1967.

Moss, G.: Fluid distribution in prevention of hypovolemic shock. Arch. Surg., *98*:281, 1969.

Mueller, C. B.: Use of solute diuresis in the prevention of acute renal failure. Amer. J. Surg., *114*:695, 1967.

Onesti, G.: Renal hemodynamic alterations in renal disease and renal failure. Chapter 8. In Brest, A. N., and Moyer, J. H. (eds.): Renal Failure. Philadelphia, J. P. Lippincott Company, 1967, pp. 85–93.

Pitts, R. F.: Physiology of the Kidney and Body Fluids, 2nd ed. Chicago, Year Book Medical Publishers, Inc., 1968.

Powers, S. R.: Renal response to systemic trauma. Amer. J. Surg., *119*:603, 1970.

Randall, H. T.: Fluid and electrolyte therapy. Chapter 3.

In Randall, H. T. (ed.): Manual of Preoperative and Postoperative Care, By The Committee on Pre and Postoperative Care, American College of Surgeons. Philadelphia, W. B. Saunders Company, 1967, pp. 15–51.

Randall, H. T.: Fluid and electrolyte therapy in surgery. Chapter 2. In Schwartz, S. I. (ed.): Principles of Surgery. New York, McGraw Hill Book Company, 1969, pp. 46–81.

Rea, W. J., Wyrick, W. J., McClelland, R. N., and Webb, W. R.: Intravenous hyperosmolar alimentation. Arch. Surg., *100*:393, 1970.

Rosenbaum, J. L.: Differential diagnosis of acute renal failure. Chapter 31. In Brest, A. N., and Moyer, J. H. (eds.): Renal Failure. Philadelphia, J. P. Lippincott Company, 1967, pp. 253–258.

Rosenberg, S. A., Brief, D. K., Kinney, J. M., Herrera, M. G., Wilson, R. E., and Moore, F. D.: The syndrome of dehydration, coma and severe hyperglycemia without ketosis in patients convalescing from burns. New Eng. J. Med., *272*:931, 1965.

Roth, E., Lax, L. C., and Maloney, J. V.: Ringer's lactate solution and extracellular fluid volume in the surgical patient: a critical analysis. Ann. Surg., *169*:149, 1969.

Rush, B. F., Jr., and Morehouse, R.: Volume replacement following acute bleeding compared to replacement after hemorrhagic shock: effectiveness of dextran and buffered saline. Surgery, *62*:88, 1967.

Schreiner, G. E.: Acute renal failure. Chapter 12. In Black, D. A. K. (ed.): Renal Diseases. 2nd ed. Philadelphia, F. A. Davis Company, 1967, pp. 309–326.

Schwartz, T. B., and Apfelbaum, R. I.: Nonketotic diabetic coma. In: Yearbook of Endocrinology, 1965–1966 Series, Chicago, Year Book Medical Publishers, Inc., 1966, pp. 165–181.

Schwartz, W. B., and Relman, A. S.: Effects of electrolyte disorders on renal structure and function. New Eng. J. Med., *276*:383–389, 452–458, 1967.

Shires, G. T. (ed.): Care of the Trauma Patient. New York, The Blakiston Division, McGraw Hill Book Company, 1966.

Shires, G. T., Coln, D., Carrico, J., and Lightfoot, S.: Fluid therapy in hemorrhagic shock. Arch. Surg., *88*:688, 1964.

Shires, G. T., Carrico, C. J., Baxter, C. R., Gieseeke, A. H., Jr., and Jenkins, M. T.: Principles in the treatment of severely injured patients. In Welch, C. E. (ed.): Advances in Surgery. vol. 4, Chicago, Year Book Medical Publishers, Inc., 1970, pp. 255–324.

Steinke, J.: Management of diabetes mellitus and surgery. New Eng. J. Med., *282*:1472, 1970.

Stokes, J. M.: Diagnostic indices and postoperative renal failure. Arch. Surg., *97*:291, 1968.

Stremple, J. F., Ellison, E. H., and Carey, L. C.: Osmolar diuresis: success and/or failure: a collective review. Surgery, *60*:924, 1966.

Teplitz, C.: Pathology of burns. In Artz, C., and Moncrief, J. (eds.): Treatment of Burns. 2nd ed. Philadelphia, W. B. Saunders Company, 1969, pp. 22–88.

Teschan, P. E.: Indications for dialysis. Chapter 34. In Brest, A. N., and Moyer, J. H. (eds.): Renal Failure. Philadelphia, J. P. Lippincott Company, 1967, pp. 281–283.

CHAPTER 4

POSTOPERATIVE FEVER

by FRED ALLISON, Jr., M.D.

Fred Allison, Jr., received his college education at Auburn University where his father was Chairman of the Department of Physics and an internationally recognized scientist. A member of Alpha Omega Alpha at Vanderbilt Medical School, he served his medical residency there and at the Peter Bent Brigham Hospital. Following two years as instructor in microbiology and medicine at Louisiana State University and a fellowship in infectious diseases at Washington University, he joined the faculty of the University of Mississippi Medical Center where he rose to the rank of full professor. There he established a solid reputation as an inspiring teacher, clinician, and investigator. Following a sabbatical year as Guest Investigator at the Rockefeller University in 1966–67, he returned to Louisiana State University as Head of the Department of Medicine. His rich clinical experience permits him to bring the investigative approach to the solution of problem infections in the surgical patient.

No clinical or laboratory measurement approaches the usefulness or the reliability of accurately recorded body temperature as a means for documenting the state of a patient's health. This fact has been a well-worn cornerstone of clinical medicine for centuries, long before sophisticated devices were available for recording temperatures objectively. Precise ways for documenting body temperature, i.e., thermometry, now provide a dependable means for following the progress of postoperative patients. When an elevated body temperature is found, therefore, it must be regarded as a warning sign and as an indication that all is not well. Under these circumstances all patients in a postoperative state must be evaluated completely for evidence of complications that may jeopardize or protract recovery.

Prior to the introduction of surgical aseptic techniques and before the idea that infectious agents caused disease had gained acceptance, almost all wounds, regardless of their cause, were associated with an elevation of body temperature. In these instances, infection was the cause of fever and the finding of "laudable pus" in a wound was regarded as an acceptable or expected step in the healing process. At present, however, when it is possible to control wound infections with far greater effectiveness, the finding of fever often indicates that factors other than infection of the surgical site may be at fault in the postoperative patient. As a result, the physician must not only be alerted to but must also look for the many possible mechanisms that may produce fever in patients.

PHYSIOLOGY OF TEMPERATURE CONTROL

Before considering specific aspects of the febrile patient, it will be useful to consider briefly certain simple yet important aspects of heat regulation by the human body. To begin, it is important to remember that the accepted oral temperature for healthy adults is 98.6° F. with a variation of 0.5° F. above or below this range. Axillary temperatures may be somewhat lower, whereas values found by rectal measurement may be somewhat higher.

Neurophysiologic studies have clearly established that thermostatic centers located within the hypothalamic region of the brain are responsible for limiting the variations of body temperature to remarkably narrow ranges. Sensory endings, located nearby in viscera and more distantly in the skin, are responsible for the input of signals that assist the body in maintaining a reasonably stable level of heat balance despite wide fluctuations of environmental temperature (Atkins,

1960). Compromise of function of these hypothalamic centers, usually the result of injury, may seriously derange the regulation of body temperature and lead to major fluctuations that are expressed most often as hyperpyrexia (above 106° F.) or hypothermia (below 94° F.).

Exposure to extremes of environmental temperature may activate appropriate mechanisms for either the conservation or the dissipation of body heat. For example, when very high environmental temperatures are encountered, man will bring into action measures that hasten loss of excessive body heat. These include an increased rate and depth of respiration, dilatation of blood vessels within the skin, and an increased production of sweat. This last mechanism, the loss of heat carried in body water, is the most efficient device we have to remove heat from the body. Very high ambient temperatures compromise the effectiveness of heat loss mechanisms by convection and radiation so that the only reliable means left to the body is in the loss of body water by sweating. Quite the opposite type of compensation develops when extreme environmental cold prevails; i.e., the depth and rate of respiration are reduced, there is a reduction in the rate and volume of cutaneous blood flow caused by vasoconstriction, and the loss of body water by sweating is minimized. In addition, if chilling of the body occurs, extra heat may be produced by increased muscular activity in the form of shivering or a shaking chill.

Protracted exposures to high environmental temperatures may in time overwhelm body homeostatic mechanisms and lead to unchecked rises of body heat (above 106° F.) with the eventual emergence of the "heat stroke" syndrome that may be attended by serious and often fatal neurologic, hepatic, and renal injury. By the same token, undue exposure to cold may cause a gradual reduction of the body temperature to such low levels (below 94° F.) that general anesthesia occurs accompanied by dangerous cardiac arrhythmias. Neither hyperthermia nor hypothermia of advanced degree is compatible with sustained life. The presence of either should be recognized promptly so that vigorous corrective measures may be used to bring the body temperature back to within normal ranges.

From a practical point of view it should be kept in mind that children under the age of two years lack sufficiently stable homeostatic mechanisms to prevent wide fluctuations of body temperature when they are subjected to extreme temperature ranges encountered in the environment. Likewise, there is reason to believe that the elderly, i.e., persons over the age of 70 years, may be less able to compensate cardiovascularly for unusual ranges of temperature encountered in the environment. As a consequence, it is not unusual to find that both of these age groups often respond in an exaggerated fashion to the challenge of infection by developing very high levels of body temperature.

It is also always worth keeping in mind that body heat regulation normally varies in a diurnal pattern, with lowest temperatures usually recorded in the early morning hours just before awakening and with highest values found in the late afternoon. Presumably, this peak reflects the culmination of physical and metabolic activity while one is awake. This rhythm may be reversed simply by changing one's sleeping and working hours (Bennett, 1966).

MECHANISMS OF FEVER PRODUCTION

For many years it has been recognized that elevated body temperatures are found to be associated most often with inflammatory lesions (Atkins and Snell, 1965). In connection with this fact it is important to know that injury with destruction of tissue per se is an event that leads to inflammation and, as a result, may be responsible for causing fever even in the absence of infection. The search for pyrogenic substances responsible for causing fever by altering the set of thermostatic centers in the hypothalamus is a problem that has attracted the attention of investigators for a number of years. Since experiments on the pathogenesis of fever in man are not done easily, most of the work bearing on this subject has been conducted with laboratory animals.

It is known that some bacteria produce large amounts of pyrogenic material (endotoxin) in the form of complex lipopolysaccharide molecules that may be identified and distinctly separated from the organism. The widespread occurrence of endotoxin throughout nature suggested originally that it was responsible for fever production in man in most clinical conditions. However, about 20 years ago Beeson first showed that leukocytes collected from sterile exudates free of bacterial endotoxin were capable of inducing fever (Beeson, 1948). Within a few more years, after intensive investigation by a number of workers, it was found by Atkins and Wood that the pyrogenic substance derived from polymorphonuclear leukocytes was distinctly different both chemically and biologically from bacterial endotoxin (Atkins and Wood, 1955). Since then, it has been proved conclusively that bacterial endotoxin evokes a febrile response from experimental animals and probably also from man by activating phagocytic cells. These "turned on" cells then release a leukocytic or *endogenous pyrogen* which in turn acts directly to reset hypothalamic temperature conservation centers. Very recently it has been found that granulocytes are not the only cells that produce this type of endogenous pyrogenic material—circulating monocytes also have the same capability (Atkins et al., 1967; Hahn et al., 1967). The fever produced by autolized tissue may thus actually stem from endogenous pyrogen released from white blood cells trapped within the damaged tissue. This system, therefore, must explain why trauma to tissue after extensive surgical manipulation can cause fever.

CLINICAL ASPECTS OF POSTOPERATIVE FEVER

As a rule of thumb, patients facing elective surgery should never be operated upon when found to be febrile. Rather, surgery should be delayed until the cause for fever has been identified and appropriate corrective measures have been initiated; or, at least until after the fever has abated and the patient is proved to be afebrile for at least seven days. Otherwise, the presence of disease of sufficient severity to produce fever preoperatively may seriously jeopardize not only surgical procedures but also the postoperative course.

When the cause for fever is relatively benign and the course of the process is of limited duration, as in the case of most viral infections, a febrile postoperative course will confuse clinical management. As a result, patients with intercurrent viral infections unrelated to surgery may be unwittingly subjected to unnecessary and potentially dangerous diagnostic and therapeutic measures. Thus, common sense dictates that elective surgery for febrile patients should be postponed until recovery has been established.

On the other hand, pyrexia in the postoperative period may be an obvious and predictable event in patients with illnesses that require surgical intervention and in whom fever is a part of the disease. In this case, surgery often represents a crucial diagnostic maneuver needed to establish clearly the nature of the process causing the fever. Of even greater importance, operative intervention may be essential for treatment of closed tissue infections or of undrained abscesses. Correction of mechanical or obstructive lesions and release of pus under pressure by incision and drainage are classic examples of basic surgical therapy that may greatly ameliorate the course of fever in patients. Under these specific conditions, operative intervention becomes the treatment of choice in patients with fever.

After putting aside obvious situations that result in postoperative fevers as just described, there are patients to whom fever represents an unexpected, unwanted, and generally alarming complication of surgery. A body temperature of 100° F. taken orally in the immediate postoperative period or fever that persists for more than six hours must cause the physician to consider certain specific problems that often complicate recovery.

IATROGENIC CAUSES OF POSTOPERATIVE FEVER

Early in the postoperative period overheating may cause fever as a result of interference with the patient's heat loss mechanisms. This may be caused by high environmental temperatures that lead to dehydration and inadequate heat loss by way of sweat. Likewise, excessive body cover used to keep patients warm may prevent heat loss by way of convection and radiation. These problems arise particularly in the very young and in the elderly in whom heat loss adaptation may be compromised easily. Injudicious use of atropine or other parasympathomimetic drugs that interfere with sweating and that dry mucous membranes may enhance heat conservation and thereby lead to the development of high body temperature in postoperative patients when little else is wrong.

A more important and often more dangerous cause of fever may result from true drug idiosyncrasy (hypersensitivity). Under circumstances where such a possibility may exist, the patient should be carefully questioned regarding past allergic events. Preoperatively, a good rule to follow should include documentation of all recognized instances of hypersensitivity to pharmacologic agents. Unfortunately, even an accurate allergic history may fail to help in pointing out potential reactions to drugs. For this reason, the physician must use his powers of deduction in attempting to connect an unexplained febrile course to drug usage. It is not uncommon to find, however, that drug hypersensitivity may emerge late in the postoperative period and, as a consequence, may be fairly easily related etiologically to fever since elapse of at least five to seven days may be necessary before symptoms become apparent. Peripheral eosinophilia associated with pruritic skin eruptions and joint pain often accompany drug reactions and may help hasten the diagnosis in febrile patients.

WOUND INFECTIONS

The operative wound should always be considered first as the most obvious source for fever. Frequent inspection with meticulous care of wounds will lead the surgeon to an early decision regarding wound infection as the cause of postoperative fever. When wounds are traumatic in origin, delayed in primary closure or otherwise grossly contaminated, i.e., known to contain bowel contents, or already clearly infected, fever due to infection may occur even though prompt and vigorous treatment has been initiated (see Chapter 8). On the other hand, the presence of stitch abscesses, purulent drainage, failure to obtain prompt primary healing with dehiscence, unexplained discoloration of wound edges, obvious cellulitis or suppuration should suggest strongly that the wound is infected and, therefore, is a likely cause for postoperative fever. Appropriately stained smears of exudate should reveal pus cells along with the responsible bacterium. Systemic or local prophylaxis with

antimicrobial agents for elective surgical procedures known to be free of contamination is not regarded as justifiable, since drug usage in itself may enhance the likelihood of other complications. As discussed in Chapter 8, however, antimicrobial agents should be used for treatment of wounds known to be either contaminated or infected, and therapy may best be guided by smears and cultures.

ANTI-INFLAMMATORY AGENTS AND FEVER

The physician must always be aware that antipyretic agents may dampen or block the febrile response of patients with mild to moderate inflammatory lesions. In particular, when aspirin is used on a continuing or around-the-clock basis as an analgesic, fever may be reduced materially. Salicylates, however, do not eliminate fever completely when the inflammatory process is widespread or vigorous.

Much greater confusion occurs, however, when patients are operated upon after an established course of treatment with glucocorticoids. Two interesting situations may occur. The dosage of glucocorticoid may be of sufficient size to block completely the capacity of the host to respond with fever to infectious or inflammatory lesions. This dampened reactivity may be beneficial and desirable when diseases of hypersensitivity require treatment with glucocorticoids. On the other hand, the antipyretic effect can be of serious consequence when patients develop complicating bacterial infections as a direct result of glucocorticoid suppression of cellular and humoral defense mechanisms. When this happens, serious and even fatal infections may become far advanced before fever appears, to provide a clinical clue that trouble is afoot.

Another mechanism may be operative to cause fever after glucocorticoid therapy. It is seen after glucocorticoids have been given for an extended time, i.e., for weeks or months. Inevitably, chronic administration of glucocorticoids leads to suppression of endogenous hormone production. Sudden cessation or reduction of glucocorticoid therapy, as may occur inadvertently during surgery, leaves the patient inadequately supported by an exogenous hormone; adrenal hypofunction then becomes apparent. The certain result is clinical hypoadrenalism. Under these circumstances, a striking febrile response may serve as a prominent and pressing clue that glucocorticoid replacement is needed for survival. This complication can be avoided or prevented when patients are well known to their physician and a complete documentation of all drug therapy is at hand.

PULMONARY COMPLICATIONS AS A CAUSE OF POSTOPERATIVE FEVER

As a result of unconsciousness during general anesthesia, the cough reflex is suppressed, and aspiration of mouth contents into the lungs is a common postoperative event. Furthermore, the thickened mucus produced by atropine or other agents to reduce the volume of secretions during general anesthesia is almost always aspirated into the lower reaches of the respiratory tract. These viscous plugs of mucus and other aspirated material obstruct small bronchi and cause patches of atelectasis. It is not unusual, therefore, for viable bacteria from the mouth to reach the lower respiratory tract. Under these circumstances, in which the cleansing movements of respiratory tract cilia are seriously compromised, conditions are ideal for the development of infection. Thus, the combination of lower respiratory tract obstruction with contamination by mouth organisms leads to development of atelectasis and infection in the form of bronchopneumonia. This complication is usually not encountered within the first six hours after surgery but is seen 18 to 24 hours after recovery from general anesthesia.

It should be noted that, unless infection is present, atelectasis in itself is probably not sufficient to cause fever. Consequently, those measures that are effective in preventing, correcting, or, at least, minimizing development of atelectasis will assist in preventing the complication of postoperative pneumonitis. Under these circumstances, it is usually possible to detect radiographically small disc-like areas of infiltration at the lung bases; over these areas one may hear an accentuation of breath sounds as evidence of partial consolidation with both crepitant and moist sibilant rales. These findings, plus modest to moderate increases in the peripheral white blood cell count, predominantly polymorphonuclears, indicate that a complicating bacterial infection has developed.

A rigorous program of deep breathing with forced coughing early in the postoperative period is often successful in minimizing the extent of atelectasis and pneumonitis. Unfortunately, surgical procedures involving either the thoracic cage or abdomen produce enough pain to discourage forced breathing or coughing exercises, a turn that will surely minimize effectiveness of these prophylactic maneuvers. When this occurs, the proper use of appropriate analgesics during the immediate postoperative period should assist the patient in performing suitable prophylactic measures.

It is worth remembering that the prophylactic use of antimicrobial agents to prevent this complication may not be completely successful, since material aspirated into the lower respiratory tract will usually contain resistant bacteria. For this reason, it is felt that prophylactic antibiotics are not indicated as a routine measure. Rather, once infection and fever appear with atelectasis, appropriate smears of sputum should be taken, and, from this preliminary information, a reasonable selection of antimicrobial agents can be made. Confirmatory cultures should establish precisely within the next 24 or 36 hours the bacterium responsible for infection and thus confirm the choice of antimicrobial agent. Such simple diagnostic measures are predicated upon procurement of a true specimen of sputum. Care should be taken to ensure proper collection, utilizing either tracheal or transtracheal aspiration if the patient is unable to cough adequately. Under hospital conditions, a careful watch must always be maintained for pulmonary staphylococcal or gram-negative infections (coliform or Pseudomonas species), since these two groups of bacteria are more resistant to antimicrobials and are acquired after the normal upper airway flora have been eliminated.

PULMONARY EMBOLISM

Sterile or chemical thrombophlebitis involving superficial veins is a common postoperative event. This is particularly so with increased usage of intravenous catheters for uninterrupted administration of fluids, medications, and blood during the postoperative care period. It is worth noting that a sterile inflammatory process within veins, but without embolism, may be sufficient to provoke a febrile response in patients. Fever, however, in association with thrombophlebitis should suggest that pulmonary embolism has occurred. The risk of venous inflammatory lesions produced by plastic catheters is now well established and, for this reason, they should be moved to a new location every 72 hours. The risk of bacterial infection with indwelling venous catheters is lessened when peripheral body sites are used, since infusions administered by routes nearer the trunk of the body are more apt to become infected by fecal or airway bacteria. Once thrombophlebitis becomes clinically obvious, the risk of pulmonary embolization increases substantially.

The postoperative patient is an ideal subject for the formation of intravascular thrombi with subsequent embolization, since hypovolemia with increased viscosity of blood is often present. Likewise, in inactive patients a sharp reduction in venous return may contribute to the formation of thrombi. Finally, hypercoagulability of blood may be present in the immediate postoperative period when wound healing and the response of the body to stress are at peak levels. Under these circumstances, it is likely that pulmonary embolization is even more common than realized and may be attended by a febrile response.

Classically, pulmonary embolization becomes apparent in patients in one of two ways. It may be of catastrophic proportions ending in sudden death when a large embolus is dislodged from a distant site with passage through the chambers of the right side of the heart to occlude major portions of the pulmonary arterial supply. Under these circumstances, the embolus may lead to acute pulmonary hypertension associated with dilatation of the right ventricle. This may be further complicated by the sudden appearance of fatal cardiac arrhythmias. Few, if any, premonitory symptoms may precede the event. Once it has developed, the patient acutely experiences the sensation of breathlessness, a sense of impending doom, chest discomfort, confusion, syncope, peripheral evidence of vasomotor insufficiency, and eventually death. Heroic measures may succeed in salvaging the patient, and within a relatively short period of time, i.e., within hours, recovery may occur.

Another type of presentation results when smaller emboli are discharged into the pulmonary circulation to produce a clinical picture that is more confusing. In this case, fever associated with coughing, occasionally blood-tinged sputum, repeated bouts of breathlessness, sibilant rales, chest pains, varying electrocardiographic evidence of right ventricularity with transient arrhythmias, and, finally, changing radiographic findings should suggest the occurrence of recurrent pulmonary embolism. It is recognized that pulmonary embolism may occur commonly after fractures, especially those that involve the lower extremities, and after prolonged immobilization of an extremity with venous stasis caused by a cast. Even though fever and tachycardia are found under these circumstances, there may be little or no evidence of thrombophlebitis from which thrombi propagate before becoming emboli.

A high index of suspicion coupled with careful surveillance of the clinical course and the appropriate use of diagnostic measures, such as serial enzyme determinations, isotopic lung scans, and pulmonary angiography, will lead to an early diagnosis of pulmonary embolism. Treatment with appropriate anticoagulation is usually indicated unless there is significant risk of blood loss from a wound or from some other site such as a peptic duodenal ulcer. In most instances, anticoagulation with either heparin or Coumadin will control the process satisfactorily. Unfortunately, failure to prevent additional embolism may dictate more aggressive therapy with ligation of either the inferior vena cava or the peripheral veins in order to achieve control.

As a word of warning, it should be emphasized that recurrent pulmonary embolism is often confused with either atelectasis or bouts of pneumonia. Because fever attending embolism may be transient, it may seem that pulmonary infiltrates have responded to antimicrobial therapy. Such an association tends to cloud the issue and delay the arrival at the correct diagnosis until it eventually becomes clear that the pneumonic process is not responding at all to antimicrobial therapy.

URINARY TRACT INFECTIONS AS A CAUSE OF POSTOPERATIVE FEVER

Infection of the lower urinary tract, i.e., the urethra and bladder, rarely develops *de novo* unless there has been preexisting disease or unless obstruction requires urinary catheterization for relief. In almost every instance, infection is accompanied by the classic symptoms of inflammation with frequency, urgency, dysuria, and pain on voiding (stranguria). Examination of the urine will reveal many leukocytes, often in clumps, a variable number of red blood cells, and almost always it is possible to detect both intracellular and extracellular bacteria. Thus, the febrile postoperative patient with such a history and findings should present no great diagnostic problem.

Extension of infection to the upper urinary tract leads to a more complex situation therapeutically, although from a diagnostic point of view the problem is usually clear. This is so because involvement of the upper urinary tract, particularly of the renal pelvis, medullary portions of the kidney, and renal cortices, causes pain and tenderness in the flanks and costovertebral angles. In addition, chill with fever, vomiting, and hypotension may accompany infection of the kidney. Unless there has been an operative procedure in the area, the clinical impression of upper urinary tract infection as a cause of fever is easily established. The finding of white cell casts in the urine with bacteria helps clinch the diagnosis. With a careful study of the appropriate smears taken from the urinary sediment, an early selection of the right antimicrobial therapy may be made.

Under less typical conditions it is also possible for urinary tract infections to cause fever. For example, pyuria may be the only clue to implicate this area as the cause for trouble. Thus, the urine should *always* be examined carefully when evaluating postoperative patients with fever.

MANAGEMENT OF POSTOPERATIVE FEVERS

Presented with the problem of a postoperative patient with fever, in which there is little doubt that it has developed *de novo* in the postoperative period, certain meaningful and useful procedures should be immediately undertaken in order to arrive at a prompt diagnosis.

1. A careful and thoughtful appraisal of the patient's entire clinical status should be undertaken with particular attention directed to the state of hydration of the patient, the relationship of medications employed to the febrile course, and a careful reevaluation of the possibility of hypersensitivity phenomena in the patient's past.

2. Wounds should be examined and cultured if there is suggestive evidence of infection.

3. The lungs and urinary tract should be evaluated clinically and appropriate studies made of the sputum and urine for evidence of infection. Whenever in doubt, cultures employed under these circumstances may be of specific help. Smears of material from any of the sites should be examined with the Gram stain and with other appropriate techniques, such as methylene blue stains.

4. Blood cultures should be obtained whenever there is the slightest suggestion of sepsis, bacteremia, or peripheral vascular collapse of unexplained etiology.

5. X-rays of the chest and other radiographic measures should be utilized to determine if infection or pulmonary embolization has occurred.

6. An electrocardiogram is often helpful both pre- and postoperatively in evaluating the possibility of a pulmonary embolus.

From these measures, which are attainable in a short time, the alert physician can find the cause for postoperative fever most of the time. Since the wound often represents a prime source for spreading infection, an early decision regarding antimicrobial drugs must be made. In general, in those instances in which the wound is known to be contaminated or dirty preoperatively, wound management should include a drug with a broad antibacterial spectrum. In those instances of postoperative fever in which the wound has been considered clean, the contents should be carefully examined for bacteria; therapy should be largely couched upon results of preliminary smears and stains. In most instances, it is possible to make a rational and intelligent selection of drugs.

REFERENCES

Atkins, E.: Pathogenesis of fever. Physiol. Rev., *40*:580, 1960.

Atkins, E., and Snell, E. S.: Fever. *In* Zweifach, B. W., Grant, L., and McCluskey, R. T. (eds.): The Inflammatory Process. New York, Academic Press, 1965.

Atkins, E., and Wood, W. B. Jr.: Studies on the pathogenesis of fever. II. Identification of an endogenous pyrogen in the blood stream following the injection of typhoid vaccine. J. Exp. Med., 102:499, 1955.

Atkins, E., Bodel, P., and Francis, L.: Release of endogenous pyrogen in vitro from rabbit mononuclear cells. J. Exp. Med., 126:357, 1967.

Beeson, P. B.: Temperature-elevating effect of a substance obtained from polymorphonuclear leucocytes. J. Clin. Invest., 27:524, 1948.

Bennett, I. L., Jr.: Alterations in body temperature. *In* Harrison, T. R., Adams, R. D., Bennett, I. L., Jr., Resnik, W. H., Thorn, G. W., and Wintrobe, M. M. (eds.): Principles of Internal Medicine. 5th ed., Blakiston Div. New York, McGraw-Hill Book Co., 1966.

Hahn, H. H., Char, D. C., Postel, W. B., and Wood, W. B., Jr.: Studies on pathogenesis of fever. XV. The production of endogenous fever by peritoneal macrophages. J. Exp. Med., 126:385, 1967.

CHAPTER 5

POSTOPERATIVE DISORDERS OF CONSCIOUSNESS

by HILARY H. TIMMIS, M.D.

Hilary H. Timmis was born in Detroit and received his degrees from the University of Detroit and Wayne State University College of Medicine, where he was elected to Alpha Omega Alpha. Following his residencies in general and thoracic surgery at the University of Pennsylvania, he joined the National Naval Medical Center, where he was a member of the heart team for two years. In 1964 he joined the faculty of the University of Mississippi Medical Center, where he holds the rank of Associate Professor of Surgery and is executive officer of the heart surgery service. Dr. Timmis is an accomplished surgical academician, and this is reflected in the perceptive and penetrating discussion which follows.

Even such a man, so faint, so spiritless, so dull, so dead in look, so woe-begone, . . .

———Shakespeare
King Henry IV, Part II

In hospital areas set aside for the delivery of intensive care, there is usually a paucity of patients who are obviously wide awake and active. Although most are simply sleeping as a natural response to serious illness or recent operation, there are invariably some whose state of reduced awareness is beyond that of normal repose. A spectrum of pathologically reduced levels of consciousness is commonly seen in the postoperative period, ranging from somnolence and confusion through delirium and stupor to frank coma. In each instance, the capacity for arousal is progressively lower until the comatose state is met, at which point no intelligible response can be evoked even with vigorous stimulation.

Seriously ill patients, especially the elderly, will often pass through a period of reduced awareness characterized by confusion and disorientation, that is difficult to delineate, partly because of the myriad etiology and partly because of obscure metabolic changes not measured by the usual studies. One fact is certain: every patient manifesting central nervous system depression does so for definite and ultimately definable anatomic or biochemical reasons or both. If these can be identified, care can be planned intelligently and delivered more effectively.

This chapter is not intended to be an exhaustive review of all the causes of coma, since it is restricted to the surgical patient. Rather, it has as its goal a concise and orderly description of the etiology of coma commonly or occasionally seen in the postoperative period, an evaluation of central nervous system depression in terms of diagnosis and extent, the emergency and long-term care of the comatose patient, and the prevention and management of complications.

DEFINITION. Coma is commonly defined as a negative quantity, the antithesis of consciousness, and there is virtually no information regarding its subjective implications (Schaefer, 1966). The intellectual response to afferent stimuli is apparently depressed in a manner comparable to sensory and motor depression. Moreover, the construction of mental images, the readiness to react, and the association of present and past experiences with their emotional implications all appear to be absent (Locke, 1968). The lack of response alone must not be confused with coma, since certain psychotic states (catatonia) may mimic coma, and psychogenic coma is a well-documented entity (Hill, 1965; Thomas, 1964). Several dramatic instances have also been reported of total and complete immobilization due to midbrain lesions that simulate coma but do not alter the state of awareness (Nathanson and Bergman, 1966).

Investigation has failed to delineate within the brain a site exclusively occupied with the maintenance of consciousness. However, the ascending midbrain reticular formation is anatomically and functionally integrated with the diffuse thalamic projection system, the cerebral hemispheres, and the hypothalamus and is currently thought to be the most probable location for the collection and integration of information and its transmission for storage or action (Moruzzi, 1963; Scheibel and Scheibel, 1967). Although lesions of the cortex alter perceptual response and associative functions, it is well established clinically that diffuse alteration of the cerebral hemispheres is necessary to produce a state resembling coma (Chapman and Wolff, 1959). Conversely, certain focal lesions of the brain stem, particularly in the region of the reticular formation, characteristically produce coma (Brain, 1958; French, 1952).

BIOCHEMICAL BACKGROUND. The energy expended by the brain is derived almost exclusively from the oxidation of glucose, through the Embden-Meyerhof and Krebs-Hensleit cycles at a respiratory quotient that approaches unity (Dixon, 1965). Since only 6 per cent of its energy requirement is available through anaerobic metabolism, the brain experiences irreversible cellular damage quickly in the absence of sufficient oxygen. To meet this limitation, the brain receives approximately 20 per cent of the total cardiac output, similar to the percentage of total oxygen consumption (Gardner, 1968), although the organ constitutes only 2 per cent of the total body weight. Normal cerebral O_2 consumption averages 50 cc. per minute or 3.3 cc. per 100 gm. per minute with no appreciable change during sleep (Kety, 1950; Mangold et al., 1955). In the absence of sufficient oxygen, the brain literally metabolizes itself to meet its energy demand. In the comatose patient, however, oxygen consumption of the brain is invariably reduced (Ingvar et al., 1964). With normal cerebral blood flow, cerebral hypoxia is likely to occur if the arterial PO_2 falls below 40 mm. Hg. In this situation, cerebral vasodilatation resulting from the low oxygen tension and

the commonly associated hypercarbia may produce a modest increase of blood flow (Kety and Schmidt, 1948).

The complete oxidation of glucose produces high energy pyrophosphate compounds (30 mols ATP per mol of glucose) to drive cerebral neurons. A lack of sufficient glucose, in turn, is manifested rapidly by cerebral dysfunction and, if uncorrected, will also result in irreversible cellular damage. Hypoglycemia always becomes symptomatic

TABLE 5-1.   Etiology of Postoperative Disorders of Consciousness

Cerebral Hypoxia
  Systemic hypoxemia
    Restricted oxygen supply
    Respiratory insufficiency
    Reduced O_2-carrying capacity
  Diminished cerebral perfusion
    Reduced cardiac output
      Arrhythmia
      Primary or secondary cardiomyopathy
      Structural changes of heart or great vessels
    Peripheral vascular collapse
      Neurogenic reaction
      Hypovolemia
      Vasomotor paralysis
    Aortocranial vascular occlusion
      Embolism
      Thrombosis
      Positional compromise
      Reflex vasoconstriction
    Intracranial hemorrhage

Disturbances of Cerebral Metabolism
  Deficiency of substrate and cofactors
    Hypoglycemia
  Abnormalities of ionic or acid-base environment
    Water (Hyperosmolarity and water intoxication)
    Sodium (Hypernatremia and hyponatremia)
    Potassium (Hyperkalemia and hypokalemia)
    Magnesium (Hypermagnesemia and hypomagnesemia)
    Acidosis (Respiratory and metabolic)
    Alkalosis (Respiratory and metabolic)
  Hyperfunction and hypofunction of endocrine organs
    Thyroid
    Parathyroid
    Adrenal
    Pancreas
  Enzymatic alterations
    Hepatic failure
    Renal failure
    Drug intoxication
    Thermal extremes

Infection
  Primary brain abscess
  Meningitis
  Remote septicemia
  Endotoxemia

when the blood glucose falls below 30 mg. per 100 ml., although there is still adequate glucose to meet the metabolic demand (Fazekas and Alman, 1962). A further reduction of glucose results in a well-defined, stepwise deterioration of CNS function. Various cofactors in the Krebs "citric acid" cycle such as thiamine pyrophosphate, nicotinic acid, pyridoxine, and cyanocobalamin are also essential for normal cellular function, and their absence produces well-defined deficiency states (Plum and Posner, 1966). It has been suggested that cerebral fat and amino acids may also make a minor contribution to the energy pool by entry into the Krebs cycle as acetyl CoA (Gardner, 1968). However, the energy derived from this source is insignificant even during hypoxic stimulation. The aerobic oxidation of glucose is absolutely essential to maintain functional capability and normal physiochemical characteristics of cerebral cells. All central nervous system dysfunction, whether or not it is of sufficient severity to express itself as coma, results from or is associated with an alteration of biochemical integrity so that the oxidation of glucose to carbon dioxide and water is unable to proceed normally. Therefore, a physical or chemical block to substrate utilization is a feature common to the causes of coma listed in Table 5-1. The loss of energy to drive CNS function in terms of synthesis of neurohumoral transmitters, maintenance of membrane potential, and transmission of impulses is proportionately impaired, and consciousness is lost.

ETIOLOGY

CEREBRAL HYPOXIA. In view of the strict oxygen requirement that exists for normal CNS function, it is not surprising that hypoxia is one of the major causes of postoperative coma. One or both of the two primary factors determining the delivery of oxygen to the brain, namely, the oxygen content and cerebral flow rate, are altered by a variety of mechanisms. Normally, the brain receives 15 to 20 per cent of the total cardiac output, and this can be reduced as much as 60 per cent before cerebral dysfunction occurs (Finnerty et al., 1954). On the other hand, the effect of reducing the arterial oxygen content is more difficult to evaluate because of the compensatory in-

crease of cerebral flow. Below an ambient oxygen tension of 80 mm. Hg, which is about 50 per cent of that found at sea level, changes in cerebral function will appear (Fazekas and Alman, 1962). At this partial pressure of oxygen and a normal hemoglobin level, the oxygen content is reduced to about 10 vols.%. Expressed in terms of the amount of oxygen available to the brain per unit time, then, cerebral hypoxia can result from arterial desaturation or reduced oxygen-carrying capacity of arterial blood (hypoxemic hypoxia); generalized reduction of peripheral blood flow (pump failure, systemic hypotension); and local reduction of cerebral blood flow (alteration of aortocranial vascular tone or patency).

HYPOXEMIC HYPOXIA. Postoperative hypoxemic hypoxia most commonly results from respiratory insufficiency, which, in turn, follows upper- and lower-airway obstruction, depression of the respiratory center due to drug idiosyncrasy, atelectasis, pneumonitis, and, now with increasing frequency, the alveolar-capillary block of interstitial pulmonary edema caused by overly aggressive fluid therapy. Patients with pre-existing parenchymal disease and hypercarbia are especially prone to respiratory depression following injudicious administration of narcotics, barbiturates, and other depressants. An additional hazard is incurred if the non-ionic buffer, Tham, is used to reverse a reduced pH due to respiratory acidosis. This agent can paralyze the respiratory center and thus cause respiratory arrest and should be used only when mechanical ventilation is available. Hypoxemia may also occur during operation as a result of unrecognized airway obstruction, malpositioning of the endotracheal tube, or inadequate oxygen concentration in the anesthetic gas mixture (particularly when nitrous oxide is used). Reduced oxygen-carrying capacity due to anemia or acquired hemoglobinopathies of sufficient severity to produce postoperative cerebral depression is rarely met. On the one hand, reduction of the red cell mass to a point producing hypoxemia tends to be compensated by increased flow resulting from a lowered blood viscosity; on the other hand, drugs causing methemoglobinopathies and sulhemoglobinopathies are now used infrequently.

REDUCED FLOW—GENERALIZED. Cerebral hypoxia secondary to reduced cardiac output and an over-all reduction of peripheral blood flow, including the brain, causes a spectrum of neurologic changes depending upon its severity and duration. Intermittent complete heart block (Stokes-Adams syndrome) with transient cardiac arrest or severe bradycardia is a classic and frequent example. However, any cardiac arrhythmia that seriously interferes with ventricular filling or emptying, such as second-degree heart block, atrial flutter, or recurrent ectopic ventricular activity, may critically reduce cerebral blood flow.

Postoperative cardiomyopathies leading to a critical fall in cardiac output and cerebral depression are usually metabolic in origin and are, therefore, potentially reversible. In some instances, though, neurologic depression that progresses to coma is seen, or there is no recovery from anesthesia in patients succumbing to the low-output syndrome following cardiopulmonary bypass. The heart and brain may share a common lesion here, such as platelet thrombosis, air embolism, or interstitial edema. However, since the cardiac output is below a level necessary for adequate peripheral perfusion, cerebral depression may result from cerebral ischemia alone.

Aortic stenosis is characterized by loss of consciousness that is usually limited to syncopal episodes and probably results from functional or electric cardiac standstill. In most instances, circulatory arrest is transient and complete neurologic recovery is usual. Absence of cardiac response results in the sudden-death syndrome. Cardiac output may also be critically reduced by massive pulmonary embolism that severely obstructs right ventricular output and produces right ventricular heart failure. Immediate loss of consciousness results from the acute fall of peripheral perfusion that includes the brain. The gradual onset of coma with this lesion may be a result of hypoxemia from impaired gas exchange, cerebral edema secondary to brachiocephalic venous hypertension, and cerebral ischemia occurring from progressive cardiac failure.

Systemic hypotension, whether reflex and transient, as in the vasovagal response, or prolonged because of toxin-induced vasodilatation (gram-negative shock), can produce an immediate fall in cerebral blood supply and cerebral depression ranging from dulling of the sensorium to loss of consciousness. A number of pharmacologic agents that produce hypotension by decreasing vasomotor tone also exert a direct depressing effect on the brain (barbiturates, phenothiazine derivatives). It should be emphasized here that arterial pressure per se is not critical for normal cerebral function provided that the delivery of O_2 per unit time to the brain is within normal limits. (Eckenhoff et al., 1963). Induced hypotension is used clinically without untoward central nervous system effects because of the maintenance of adequate cerebral flow in the face of reduced peripheral vascular resistance (Larson, 1964). Regardless of the factors decreasing cerebral flow, the critical level below which consciousness occurs is approximately 30 cc. per 100 gm. brain per minute, about 60 per cent of normal flow (McHenry et al., 1961).

REDUCED FLOW—LOCALIZED: ARTERIAL OCCLUSION. Localized cerebral hypoxia results from partial or complete occlusion of the carotid and vertebral arteries or their intracranial ramifications. Here, as elsewhere, atherosclerotic segmental lesions tend to occur at sites where flow is altered by acute angulation or bifurcation of vessels resulting in plaque formation, intramural degenerative changes, ectasia, and stenosis. Subclinical narrowing of aortocranial branches may seriously compromise flow before a measurable fall of pressure can be elicited at the point of stenosis. Perivascular and vascular inflammatory changes such as those seen in periarteritis and Takayasu's disease may also produce asymptomatic narrowing or occlusion (Hardy, 1960). Hypotension during or after operation predisposes to thrombosis in these areas and it is imperative that marked fluctuations of pressure and flow be avoided, since thrombogenesis may be enhanced further by the hypercoagulable states associated with trauma (surgical or otherwise), certain neoplasms (kidney, pancreas), blood dyscrasias, and collagen disease.

EMBOLISM. The incidence of postoperative ischemic brain damage as a result of the introduction of air, clot, fat, or calcium, in that order of frequency, into the cerebral circulation is still significant. Arterial air embolism is most common in those patients undergoing cardiac surgery with cardiopulmonary bypass, but also occurs as a result of other mechanisms. Large volumes of air can be introduced into the right atrium and across the pulmonary vascular bed by the misuse of air pressure for rapid transfusion (Ruesch et al., 1960; Yeakel, 1968), during the insertion of large-bore central venous pressure catheters (Levinsky, 1969), at neurosurgical procedures carried out in the sitting position, particularly those in the posterior fossa (Michenfelder et al., 1969), and during operative procedures such as radical mastectomy in which the transected veins are subject to negative intrathoracic pressure. Air may enter the pulmonary venous tree directly during thoracentesis (Diamond et al., 1964) and following pulmonary rupture by positive pressure ventilation (Lenaghan et al., 1969). The cerebral manifestations of air embolism can be extremely variable, ranging from mild obtundation to a state of decorticate or decerebrate rigidity. Although neurologic dysfunction is usually diffuse, localizing findings may be present. We have seen two instances of paralysis of lateral gaze beyond the midline toward the side of transient left-sided hemiparesis in patients undergoing open mitral valvulotomy with the right side elevated. Fortunately, the degree of damage is often limited and temporary, and the level of cerebral depression is relatively superficial, so that with time, substantial recovery is possible.

Cerebral embolism resulting from the migration of clot is usually secondary to acquired or congenital cardiovascular disease (Fisher et al., 1966). Atrial fibrillation is a frequent finding and is thought to predispose to intra-atrial thrombosis because of the absence of coordinated atrial systole and stasis within this chamber (Marshall, 1968). This arrhythmia is especially common in the elderly patient with minor postoperative pulmonary complications. Myocardial infarction is complicated by the disruption of fragments of intraventricular laminated clot at the site of myocardial damage. Since clot here is usually adherent, the incidence of cerebral embolism following myocardial infarction is quite low. The formation of clots on and adjacent to prosthetic heart valves has been a major cause of late morbidity and mortality in patients undergoing valve replacement and is still an unsolved problem despite the use of long-term anticoagulation at therapeutic levels (Sanders, 1969; Matloff et al., 1969). Cloth-covered prostheses and homograft valves exhibit less thrombogenesis and may eventually provide a solution. Other sources of arterial emboli include venous thrombi that gain access to the systemic arterial tree through a patent foramen ovale and the migration of clot distally from areas of intimal damage in the aortocranial branches. We have seen several instances of aneurysms of the internal carotid artery filled with the characteristic friable, crumbling, partially organized clot, and it is always a wonder that embolization does not occur more frequently.

Fat embolism is probably infrequently recognized, since most cases diagnosed clinically fail to survive (Hamilton, 1964). It usually follows major trauma with multiple fractures, especially of the long bones (Derian, 1965), and was also seen occasionally in the early days of open-heart surgery when relatively crude filters allowed particulate matter, including fat, to pass through the pump oxygenator and back into the patient's arterial circulation (Wright et al., 1963). Rarely, it occurs with pancreatitis, osteomyelitis, and other infections (Tedeschi et al., 1968). The cerebral manifestations of fat embolism are similar to those of air embolism (Murley, 1964). The classic clinical sequence consists of the sudden onset of diffuse nonspecific central nervous system alterations as well as evidence of acute respiratory insufficiency 30 minutes to several days following skeletal injury (Linscheid and Dines, 1969). Crops of petechial hemorrhages characteristically appear over the chest and flanks (Garner and Peltier, 1967). Fat embolism is suggested by the presence of fat globules in the urine and sputum (Evarts, 1965; Peltier, 1965) and by elevated serum lipase and tributyrinase levels several days later, but may be distinguishable only by postmortem histologic examination with special strains.

Calcific embolization, on the other hand, is almost exclusively a result of manipulation of calcified mitral and aortic valves. When closed-mitral commissurotomy was popular, morbidity and mortality were largely caused by cerebral occlusion by calcium fragments. Although open techniques of valve repair have largely replaced these "blind" techniques and reduced the incidence of embolization in general, unrecognized dislocation and gravitation of calcium particles, particularly during valve excision, is still a problem and is continuously stimulating the development of new "trapping" devices (Ibarra-Perez et al., 1969).

Intracranial hemorrhage. Postoperative intracranial bleeding is an infrequent clinical occurrence that may complicate cerebral vascular occlusion, blood dyscrasias, and marked transient elevations of systemic arterial pressure regardless of etiology (Fisher et al., 1966). Pre-existing cerebral atherosclerosis or congenital anomalies of cerebral vessels are often present. In our experience, an early postoperative transient elevation of the systemic arterial pressure is commonly seen during recovery from anesthesia, especially in those patients with a history of hypertension, and in instances of hypoventilation with carbon dioxide retention. Arterial hypertension may be pronounced and persistent incident to obstruction of venous drainage from the head and after the onset of cerebral edema due to other causes. We have never seen cerebral hemorrhage resulting from serious postoperative bleeding diatheses, such as those complicating cardiac and genitourinary surgery, after massive transfusion, and during anticoagulation with coumarin or derivatives.

POSITIONAL COMPROMISE. Rotation of the head to the opposite side consistently results in a decrease of ipsilateral internal carotid arterial flow (Hardesty et al., 1961). When coupled with contralateral aortocranial disease, the potential is present for significant cerebral ischemia during rotational extremes that are used for some operative procedures of the head and neck. In the anesthetized, unconscious patient, there are no symptoms of cerebral hypoxia to forestall irreversible neurologic damage.

HYPERTENSION. Pre-existing hypertension occasionally undergoes an accelerated phase resulting in hypertensive encephalopathy characterized by severe headache, vomiting, rising blood urea nitrogen, convulsions, and progressive cerebral depression (Leavitt and Polansky, 1968). Cerebral vascular resistance rises disproportionately at higher levels of arterial pressure, so that cerebral blood flow is reduced to the point at which ischemia occurs. Secondary factors also contribute to cerebral depression and retard recovery, such as cerebral and vascular-wall edema, perivascular hemorrhages, and microinfarction (Fazekas and Alman, 1962). Hypertensive encephalopathy may be difficult to differentiate from that due to uremia, since the systemic arterial pressure and blood urea nitrogen are commonly elevated in both, and each condition causes seizures, delirium, stupor, and increased intracranial pressure. However, papilledema, cortical blindness, and aphasia are rare in uremia and common in hypertensive encephalopathy (Plum and Posner, 1966).

SUBSTRATE DEFICIENCY. In some instances, cerebral changes are only temporary, regardless of the duration of severity of the inciting cause, since only neuronal function is disturbed. In others, intracellular protein denaturation eventually occurs, producing irreversible structural changes, death of neurons, and permanent central nervous system damage.

HYPOGLYCEMIA. While oxygen deprivation is the specific deficit causing postoperative coma by a variety of mechanisms, a host of other entities with obvious metabolic implications can also interfere with aerobic energy production and the formation of high-energy phosphate bonds, the basic intermediary for normal neurologic function. The most common of these is hypoglycemia due to exogenous insulin or oral hypoglycemic agents, severe liver disease, or the secretion of an insulin-like factor by certain tumors, i.e., sarcomas, hepatoma, and the like (Hurwitz, 1968; Unger, 1966). There is now ample experimental data that glucose is the only substrate that the brain can utilize in vivo to maintain metabolic and functional integrity, and then only by aerobic degradation, which necessitates a continuous adequate supply of oxygen (Dixon, 1965). The average adult brain metabolizes 70 mg. glucose per minute, an amount slightly in excess of the quantity required to account for the total cerebral oxygen consumption (Sokoloff, 1960). Since the brain removes oxygen and produces carbon dioxide in equivalent quantities, its respiratory quotient is almost unity, indicating complete dependence on glucose for energy production. The discrepancy between glucose and oxygen consumption can be attributed to the synthesis of glycogen and, to a lesser extent, to the anaerobic degradation of minute quantities of glucose (Fazekas and Alman, 1962).

Clinically, hypoglycemia is manifested by tremor, anxiety, diaphoresis, diplopia, giddiness, confusion, convulsions, and progressive central nervous system depression. The serial progression of neurologic decompensation originating from uncorrected hypoglycemia is well documented and summarized in Table 5-2. It is not generally appreciated that irreversible cen-

Table 5-2. Symptoms of Hypoglycemia

Order of Appearance	Symptoms	Localization
First	Muscular relaxation (hypotonia) Fine tremor Somnolence Excitement	Depression of activities of cerebral hemispheres and cerebellum
Second	Loss of environmental contact	Release of subcorticodiencephalon

	Motor phenomena
	  Myoclonic twitching
	  Clonic spasms
	  Motor restlessness
		1. Subcortical motor nuclei

	Sensory changes Increased sensitivity to stimulation	2. Thalamus

	Changes in the autonomic nervous system
	  Increased sympathetic activity
	  Periodic exophthalmos
	  Dilatation of pupils; still react to light
		3. Hypothalamus

Third	Diminished sensitivity Tonic spasms Independent movement of the eyes Babinski reflex	Release of midbrain
Fourth	Extensor spasms	Release of medulla 1. Upper 2. Lower
Fifth	Pin-point pupils No light reaction Depressed respiration Muscular flaccidity Depressed reflexes Loss of corneal reflex	

Modified from Himwich, H. E.: Brain Metabolism and Cerebral Disorders. Williams & Wilkins Company, 1951

tral nervous system damage may result from insufficiency of glucose as well as oxygen. This may follow a single severe episode of hypoglycemia or repeated milder episodes that occur not infrequently in poorly controlled diabetics.

COFACTOR DEFICIENCY. The absence of essential cofactors that participate in the complete degradation of glucose is usually found with chronic malnutrition and produces recognizable syndromes. Whereas these states are unlikely in the postoperative period characterized by prolonged lack of oral intake, the absence of essential cofactors and crucial trace elements such as magnesium from parenteral supplements may contribute to the obtundation that is commonly seen. As a cocarboxylase, thiamine is necessary for the oxidative decarboxylation of pyruvic, lactic, and ketoglutamic acids. Thiamine deficiency results in Wernicke's disease owing to vascular and neuronal

damage in the diencephalic and periaqueductal gray matter. Patients are obtunded and confused and exhibit dysarthria and ataxia. However, diagnosis is questionable without ophthalmoplegia and nystagmus (Buckle, 1967).

Nicotinic acid is a major component of di- and triphosphopyridine nucleotides, which are concerned with a number of cerebral oxidation and reduction reactions. Niacin deficiency causes a diffuse chronic encephalopathy with muscle rigidity, prominent sucking and grasping reflexes, and delirium that progresses to coma (Plum and Posner, 1966). Pyridoxine (B_6) deficiency is most common in those patients receiving pyridoxine antagonists such as isoniazid or hydralazine and is manifested by polyneuropathy and generalized convulsions (Minard, 1967; DeJong, 1967). Cyanocobalamin (B_{12}) deficiency occurs most frequently beyond middle age and all but the cerebral signs of the disease, including anemia, may be absent. Neurologic symptoms consist of progressive apathy, lethargy, and confusion leading to chronic delirium. Like the other deficiency states, symptoms can be halted promptly in most instances by the administration of appropriate vitamins (Shulman, 1967).

PHYSIOCHEMICAL ABNORMALITIES

HYPONATREMIA. The end products of normal cerebral metabolism are water and carbon dioxide, and the accumulation of either substance in the brain results in progressive cerebral dysfunction. A sudden or severe reduction of serum sodium may result in the syndrome of water intoxication, which is characterized initially by headache, nausea, vomiting, cramps, myoclonus, asterixis, hyperactive reflexes, convulsions, and delirium, followed by central nervous system depression and coma. Almost invariably, water is of exogenous origin and the excess usually results from the injudicious administration of hypotonic fluids either orally or intravenously. In some instances, there may also be an element of inappropriate ADH secretion (Goldberg and Reivich, 1962). All constituents of both the intra- and extracellular compartments are diluted and the resulting hypoosmolarity and dilution of electrolytes, rather than cerebral edema per se, are thought to produce the functional alterations of this syndrome (Plum and Posner, 1966). A serum sodium concentration below 120 mEq./liter in a symptomatic patient is suggestive of water intoxication, whereas a serum osmolarity measured directly or calculated by the formula, Osmolarity (mOsm.) $= 2 \times Na + (mEq./l.) + \dfrac{glucose\ (mg\%)}{18}$, which is less than 260 mOsm./l., is diagnostic of this condition.

HYPEROSMOLARITY. Hyperosmolar states are complicated by neurologic dysfunction and cerebral depression when the serum osmolarity reaches 325 to 350 milliosmols (Johnson, 1969). Hypernatremia resulting from unrecognized, heavy, insensible gastrointestinal or renal losses, or both, with excessive salt replacement is foremost among these causes. Neurologic symptoms consist of restlessness, delirium, hypertonicity, hyperactive reflexes, myoclonus, convulsions, and coma. Irreversible dysfunction may follow focal hemorrhages. Cerebral

depression resulting from uncontrolled diabetes mellitus probably has a multifaceted etiology but dehydration of the brain is the only consistent gross pathologic finding. Hyperglycemic, nonketotic coma presents similar neurologic changes along with focal seizures in about 20 per cent of patients (Schwartz and Apfelbaum, 1966). The metabolic and osmotic derangements are usually more severe than those of diabetic coma, resulting in a mortality of over 40 per cent of patients. This syndrome is characterized by failure of ketogenesis, absence of ketoacidosis, hyperglycemia ranging from 400 to 2000 mg. per 100 ml., and, in some instances, lactic acidosis (Goldberg, M. E., 1969). The inappropriate secretion of antidiuretic hormone that occurs with some tumors, such as bronchiogenic carcinoma, occasionally produces pathologic sodium retention and encephalopathy (Claxton et al., 1966). Hyperosmolarity can also be induced with postoperative tube feedings containing a proportionately small quantity of free water and a high concentration of solute. Prerenal azotemia and diarrhea are commonly present and contribute further to the serum hyperosmolarity.

OTHER ELECTROLYTE DISTURBANCES

While abnormal levels of the sodium cation account for the bulk of neurologic disorders attributed to electrolyte imbalance, the roles played by other cations in promoting or maintaining neurologic function are frequently overlooked. Severe shifts away from the normal range can either precipitate central nervous system dysfunction in the postoperative patient or potentiate encephalopathy primarily due to other causes (Table 5-3).

HYPERCALCEMIA. Primary hyperparathyroidism rarely manifests itself initially in the postoperative period, and the onset of hypercalcemia here should direct one to seek other causes. Immobilization alone may result in calcific deposits of the kidneys and elsewhere, without an elevation of the serum calcium. Severe postoperative hypercalcemia occurs most often in patients with malignant neoplasms or metastatic bone disease (Miller, 1968). We have seen two instances of calcemic crises caused by a parathyroid-like activity of nonresectable tumors. The first was a poorly differentiated

TABLE 5-3. Major Neurologic Manifestations of Electrolyte Disturbances

	Coma, Delirium, or Dementia	Seizures	Paralysis or Weakness	Asterixis	Myoclonus	Tetany
Extracellular Fluid						
Volume Depletion	O					
Excess	R					
Hyponatremia	C	C	W	O	C	
Hypernatremia	C	C			C	
Hypokalemia	D		C			R
Hyperkalemia			C			
Metabolic acidosis	C			O	O	
Respiratory acidosis	C	O		C	O	
Metabolic alkalosis	O	R	W		O	O
Respiratory alkalosis	O	O	W	O	O	O
Hypocalcemia	D	C				C
Hypercalcemia	C	R	W			
Hypomagnesemia	R	C	W		O	C
Hypermagnesemia	O		C		O	

C (common), O (occasional), R (rare) refer to the frequency with which the neurologic disorder is observed in patients with the indicated electrolyte disturbance and do not necessarily imply that the electrolyte disturbance is of the stated frequency in the indicated neurologic disorder.

D refers to dementia or delirium only, not coma.

W refers to severe weakness only, not paralysis.

From Miller.: Surg. Clin. N. Amer., 48:383, 1968.

bronchiogenic carcinoma and the second, a squamous cell carcinoma of the bladder. Regardless of etiology, mild hypercalcemia can be precipitously elevated to a critical level by the action of thiazide diuretics. Neurologic symptoms tend to parallel the rise of serum calcium and consist of headache, delusions, change of affect, muscle weakness, hallucinations, and cerebral depression ranging from delirium to coma.

HYPOCALCEMIA. Operative compromise of the parathyroid glands or their blood supply is the most common cause of an absolute decrease of serum calcium, whereas a transient fall of the ionized fraction often occurs with hyperventilation and respiratory alkalosis. In either case, tetany is the cardinal manifestation and is characterized by nausea, vomiting, abdominal cramps, paresthesias, laryngeal and carpopedal spasm, and marked apprehension. More severe hypocalcemia produces delirium, psychotic behavior, seizures, and occasionally papilledema (Katzman, 1966). Coma rarely occurs except as a postictal state.

Potassium has a pronounced neuromuscular effect and antagonizes the action of calcium. Consequently, the relative levels of either cation may potentiate or lessen neurologic changes due to the other.

HYPOMAGNESEMIA AND HYPERMAGNESEMIA. Postoperative hypomagnesemia is rarely indicated as a cause of disordered consciousness because magnesium is universally present in food far in excess of the daily maintenance requirement. However, in some instances of prolonged nutritional deprivation, the serum magnesium may fall below a critical level (1.5 mEq./l.) and cause symptoms (Barnes, 1962). Tetany, extreme weakness, coarse tremors, tremulousness, muscle cramps, hyperreflexia, personality changes, delirium, and stupor have all been attributed to a specific magnesium deficit (Katzman, 1966).

An elevated serum magnesium is rarely seen without renal failure, to which its symptoms may be falsely ascribed. Occasionally, hypermagnesemia may be induced by magnesium salt enemas or by the therapeutic administration of magnesium sulfate. Symptoms are mainly neurologic and cardiovascular and result in progressive central nervous system depression, a curare-like effect on the neuromuscular function and hypotension (Randall et al., 1964).

RESPIRATORY ACIDOSIS (HYPERCAPNIA, CO_2 NARCOSIS)

Carbon dioxide retention is most commonly seen in patients with primary pulmonary insufficiency (alveolar hypoventilation, alveolar-capillary block) and is occasionally met in some instances of general anesthesia (closed-circle) and after cardiopulmonary bypass, when there has been inadequate removal of carbon dioxide. The association of marked obesity, plethora, cor pulmonale, hypercapnia, and progressive cerebral depression constitutes the "Pickwickian syndrome" (Robin, 1966). Whereas carbon dioxide retention usually occurs together with hypoxia and acidosis, neurologic changes correlate most closely with the carbon dioxide tension (Sieker and Hickman, 1956). Experimental acidosis without hypercarbia is tolerated to pH 6.5, a level seldom reached clinically without cardiac arrest (Swanson et al., 1958). On the other hand, severe central nervous system depression is consistently seen only when marked elevations of PCO_2 (above 130 mm. Hg) are combined with profound acidosis. Since cerebral depression occurs clinically at much lower carbon dioxide tensions, the association of hypoxemia and other factors must be significant (Dulfano and Ishikawa, 1965). Hypercapnia causes symptoms of diffuse headache, inattentiveness, and drowsiness, which may progress to stupor and coma as carbon dioxide accumulates. Tremors, myoclonus, and asterixis are common, and evidence of increased intracranial pressure with papilledema is present in about 10 per cent of patients (MacDonald, 1965). In the absence of hypoxic brain damage, neurologic symptoms are usually completely reversible, although recovery is often not synchronous with reduction of arterial PCO_2. Rapid correction by artificial ventilation can induce severe alkalosis and serious secondary neurologic symptoms (Miller, 1968).

OTHER ACID-BASE DISTURBANCES

Less frequently, other disturbances of acid-base balance produce metabolic encephalopathy, although the direct influence of the inciting cause itself on neurologic function is often difficult to separate, i.e., uremia, hepatic failure, circulatory collapse. While changes of spinal fluid pH correlate best with central nervous system manifestations, neurologic dysfunction occurs most readily with respiratory acidosis and is least likely with metabolic acidosis (Posner and Plum, 1967). Encephalopathy due to metabolic acidosis is regularly seen when the spinal fluid pH falls below 7.25 (Posner et al., 1965), and it consists of headache,

asterixis, hyperventilation, hyperactive reflexes, and cerebral depression. However, there is poor correlation between the pH of blood or spinal fluid and neurologic symptoms of metabolic and respiratory alkalosis. Both may cause confusion, myoclonus, tetany, convulsions, obtundations, or coma. In general, therapy should be directed at the underlying disease and only secondarily (very cautiously) at the acid-base imbalance, needless to say, with the guidance of serial blood pH measurements.

ENDOCRINE DISEASE

A number of endocrinopathies can be manifested in part by encephalopathies and central nervous system depression. In the postoperative period, they are often associated with less esoteric conditions that are also characterized by neurologic changes. Here, as in few other areas, the prompt institution of correct therapy is followed by rapid improvement. Consequently, it is essential that these diagnostic possibilities, while uncommon, be kept in mind.

HYPOTHYROIDISM. Since the onset of hypothyroidism is spontaneous in over 40 per cent of patients (Watanakumakorn et al., 1965), it may remain unrecognized prior to the increased metabolic demands of operation or surgical sequelae. The brain, like other tissues, is dependent upon thyroid hormone for normal oxidative metabolism, and deficiency results in central nervous system depression (Rosenberg, 1968). Coma can be precipitated by a variety of stresses, including surgery and infection. More severe states of deficiency are characterized by a reduction of body temperature, hypotension, hypoventilation, and hypercapnia (Hyams, 1963). Neurologic signs of moderate CO_2 retention coupled with hyponatremia and hypothermia should suggest this disease. Mortality in myxedema coma is still above 60 per cent, despite the use of thyroactive agents, corticoids, appropriate fluid and electrolyte replacement, and respiratory support (Forester, 1963).

HYPERTHYROIDISM. Occasionally, a fulminating increase of thyroid function will be precipitated by surgery or sepsis in the postoperative period. The syndrome is characterized by extreme restlessness, irritability, tachycardia, hypotension, vomiting, diarrhea, delirium or coma, and elevation of body temperature to 106° F. or more.

Rarely, the clinical picture may be more subtle, with apathy, severe prostration, coma, and only mild pyrexia (Selenkow and Ingbar, 1966). In addition to the overwhelming circulatory load that threatens the patient, temporary or irreversible brain damage can result from the sustained high fever. Emergency measures must be directed toward reversing the severe pyrexia, since thermal-induced neuronal changes of membrane permeability, enzymatic activity, and protein configuration will produce neurologic signs that mimic cerebral ischemia.

Adrenal insufficiency. Improper mineral and corticoid replacement therapy following surgical ablation of the adrenal glands, unrecognized adrenal cortical atrophy due to antecedent infection, and prolonged use of corticoids may be complicated by postoperative adrenal insufficiency (Edgahl, 1968). Neurologic symptoms include apathy, muscular weakness, lassitude, convulsions, and somnolence to mild delirium. Stupor and coma usually appear only during addisonian crises (Plum and Posner, 1966). Unlike other causes of metabolic coma, flaccid weakness and reduced or absent deep tendon reflexes are usual and may be due to hyperkalemia. Hyponatremia, hypocalcemia, and hypoglycemia are also present. Hypotension alone may be severe enough to produce symptoms by the reduction of cerebral blood flow. Absent deep tendon reflexes combined with papilledema and the characteristic electrolyte changes should be diagnostic.

There is probably a far more frequent and subtle manifestation of adrenal insufficiency in the postoperative patient burdened with the stress of one complication after another. Although usually unproved or unprovable, it is reasonable to suppose that some degree of adrenal exhaustion is reached that, along with other deficiencies, contributes to the obtunded state that is commonly present.

Diabetes mellitus. Infrequently, ketoacidosis and coma will complicate a postoperative diabetic state made brittle and unmanageable by sepsis or other untoward sequelae. In addition to the grossly disordered metabolic events characterizing the disease, the combination of hemoconcentration and hypotension further predisposes to neurologic complications by intravascular obstruction of cerebral blood flow. Hemorrhagic infarcts are occasionally seen in those succumbing with diabetic coma and may produce focal neurologic changes. Lesser levels of cerebral depression may be manifested by various neurologic abnormalities such as areflexia, reflex asymmetry, hemiparesis, hemianopsia, and aphasia. The Kussmaul pattern of hyperventilation is characteristically present due to severe metabolic acidosis. The exact cause of cerebral dysfunction is unknown. However, it does not result from an absolute or relative lack of insulin, since the brain does not require insulin for utilization of glucose (Elliott and Wolfe, 1962). At the same time, the usual levels of hyperglycemia, electrolyte imbalance, ketoacidosis, and dehydration that accompany diabetic coma do not cause coma independently in the experimental animal (Fazekas and Alman, 1962). The cerebral manifestations correlate better with the level of ketonemia than with the degree of acidosis and tend to improve with clearing of ketosis (Hurwitz, 1968).

Drug intoxication

Accidental drug overdosage and idiosyncratic responses are rarely of sufficient severity to cause significant postoperative disturbances of consciousness. On the other hand, widespread administration of the ever-expanding pharmacopeia of neurotrophic drugs, singly or in combination, to treat mild mental aberrations with metabolic roots can precipitate major neurologic disturbances. Drugs may be selective or nonselective central nervous system depressants or may initially stimulate and later depress neurologic function. Regardless of their mode of action, they have several features in common. Permanent neuronal damage is uncommon in the absence of hypoxia, and prompt treatment invariably results in recovery (Plum and Swanson, 1957). Unlike other metabolic encephalopathies, brain-stem depression parallels cortical depression, so that the patient is threatened with respiratory or circulatory failure, or both, at a relatively early stage of intoxication. Premonitory signs of vestibular and cerebellar dysfunction may precede the onset of coma after which the oculocephalic response is often lost and the vestibulo-ocular responses markedly reduced (Plum and Posner, 1966). Muscle tone and tendon reflexes are usually diminished, giving a picture of generalized flaccidity. Barbiturates, glutethimide (Doriden), chloral hydrate, methyprylon (Noludar), the phenothiazine derivatives, meprobamate, chlordiazepoxide (Librium), diazepam (Valium), reserpine, and narcotics may all produce these changes (Henderson et al., 1966; Maddock and Bloomer, 1967; McKown et al., 1963; Maher et al., 1962; Quastel, 1962). The pupils are usually small and reactive except in the case of glutethimide, atropine, and similar drugs. The phenothiazines and reserpine may produce tremors, dyskinesia, and parkinsonian-like signs because of their action on extrapyramidal centers (DeJong, 1967), and their interference with catecholamine metabolism may result in severe refractory hypotension (Adriani et al., 1962). Xylocaine, like other local anesthetics, initially produces symptoms of central nervous system stimulation followed by neurologic depression, particularly of the respiratory center. Consequently, it must be used with care in high doses (3 to 4 mg. per min.) for the treatment of refractory ventricular arrhythmias. Certain antibiotics have a myoneural blocking action and can potentiate the effect of muscle relaxants, thereby producing prolonged apnea. Neomycin is most potent in this regard, and since it can be actively absorbed by serosal surfaces (Benz et al., 1961; Corrado et al., 1959), it should not be used intraoperatively. A similar action has also been ascribed to streptomycin, bacitracin and Coly-mycin (Bennetts, 1964; Ream, 1963; Small, 1964; Ryan et al., 1969).

VISCERAL DECOMPENSATION

HEPATIC COMA. Hepatic coma is the ultimate expression of liver failure and is seen in the postoperative period following drug-induced or toxic hepatitis (Ritt et al., 1969), after operative complications directly interfering with hepatic blood supply or biliary drainage, and incident to challenge of a compromised hepatic reserve by the stress of surgery, sepsis, multiple transfusions, or ischemia (McDermott, 1967). The frequent association of remote infection, fluid and electrolyte imbalance, and subacute malnutrition makes liver failure a common terminal event along with varying degrees of cardiorespiratory and renal dysfunction. The exact cause of hepatic coma is unknown, although it may also be triggered by the presence of a large nitrogenous content in the gastrointestinal tract, derived from dietary intake and intestinal bleeding in the face of pre-

existing liver damage or a previously constructed portacaval shunt (McDermott, 1968). There is abundant experimental and clinical evidence that aerobic glycosis is impaired by ammonia and/or other nitrogenous substances to which the neuronal cell membranes are freely permeable (Chalmers, 1968). However, poor correlation exists between the extent of neurologic findings and the blood ammonia level, although coma can be precipitated clinically with ammonia-releasing drugs, such as ammonia ion exchange resins (Gabuzda et al., 1952) and the thiazide derivatives (Sherlock et al., 1958), and, experimentally, by the administration of glycine, which is metabolized by ammonia and urea. Sedatives, analgesics, and other drugs detoxified by the liver may also result in coma when hepatic reserve is marginal (Norcross, 1962). Hepatic encephalopathy is characterized by a spectrum of neurologic signs ranging from personality changes to a quiet or sometimes maniacal delirium to coma. Liver flap (asterixis) is common in the precoma period and can be brought out by dorsiflexing the hands and spreading the fingers. This sign is also seen in encephalopathies associated with cor pulmonale, congestive heart failure, polycythemia, uremia, and bromism. At deeper levels of cerebral depression, muscle spasticity, extensor reflexes, and decerebrate rigidity may appear. Focal signs such as hemiparesis alternating between sides are seen occasionally. Hyperventilation is a characteristic finding and causes respiratory alkalosis in most patients.

UREMIC COMA. The incidence of postoperative renal insufficiency appears to be on the upswing and is commanding increasing attention with respect to earlier recognition and more aggressive treatment (Hollenberg, 1969; Merrill, 1969; Goldberg, 1969; Maffly, 1969). The distressing frequency with which it emerges to complicate an already difficult clinical situation may be related to the widespread use of potentially nephrotoxic drugs, the practice of massive fluid administration for shock, and the increased subacute survival after overwhelming sepsis, circulatory collapse, and postoperative cardiac arrest. Failure to adjust fluid intake to accommodate declining renal function or, in some cases, a conscious effort to force the production of urine by loading commonly results in the accumulation of sodium and water. Interstitial fluid overload is a major problem in these patients and supersedes hyperkalemia and azotemia as the primary indication for postoperative hemodialysis. When dialysis cannot be supplied by the peritoneal or circulatory routes, the uremic syndrome quickly emerges and, if progressive, produces cerebral depression and coma by a mechanism that is still unknown. Whereas electrolyte and fluid imbalances, metabolic acidosis, and hypertension each may contribute to neurologic dysfunction, uremic encephalopathy also occurs in their absence (Plum and Posner, 1966). Furthermore, there is poor correlation between the level of cerebral depression and the blood urea nitrogen or other serum constituents. The clinical picture is characterized by dull delirium with inappropriate behavior, stupor, coma, convulsions, and focal neurologic changes such as asterixis, asymmetrical stretch reflexes, and, occasionally, hemiparesis. These signs are completely reversible by hemodialysis, although several days may be necessary for complete resolution.

THERMAL ABNORMALITIES

Completely normal activity of the central nervous system necessitates the maintenance of body temperature within a narrow range. This demand is supplied by the thermal regulating centers of the hypothalamus, which direct heat conservation and dissipation mechanisms. Temperature changes alone can affect cerebral function by altering intracellular constituents, cell membrane characteristics, and the rate of enzymatic reactions and interactions (Brown, 1956). However, deviations of body temperature capable of producing central nervous system depression are rarely seen in the postoperative period. Here cerebral depression is usually secondary to inciting agents causing temperature shifts, i.e., hypoglycemia, depressant drug intoxication, and brain-stem infarcts, rather than to the thermal abnormalities. With the exception of myxedema coma, postoperative reduction of body temperature below 95° F. invariably requires the agency of exogenous cooling measures (Ivy, 1965), and hypothermia at this level is used mainly to protect the brain after a known insult, usually of a hypoxic nature. Coma due to hypothermia alone is seen experimentally below 27° C. (McQueen, 1956). Mild hypothermia (down to 95° F.) is common in infants as a result of excessive heat loss and is occasionally seen in adults with overwhelming sepsis, endocrine deficiency, accidental exogenous cooling, and as a terminal sign indicating imminent dissimilation.

Hyperthermia is a far more frequent postoperative phenomenon, which reaches its highest levels with pyrogenic reactions, sepsis, thyroid crisis, atropine overdosage, and hypothalamic dysfunction (Modell, 1966). General anesthesia may also be complicated by a dramatic and often fatal rise of body temperature (Hogg and Renwick, 1966; Saidman et al., 1964) apparently caused by a disturbance of oxidative phosphorylation (Wilson et al., 1966). Tolerance to pyrexia declines steadily with age, and the elderly are often obtunded from temperature elevations in the range of 101 to 102° F. (Haerer, 1969). In general, delirium appears around 104° F., with progressively greater cerebral depression at higher levels of body temperature. At 107 to 110° F., the metabolic rate is almost doubled and the heat dissipating mechanisms are overcome (Guyton, 1966). Despite the uninterrupted delivery of oxygenated blood, irreversible brain damage intervenes due in part to relative hypoxia, protein denaturation, and altered cell membrane and capillary permeability. A variable neurologic picture emerges that resembles postanoxic encephalopathy but from which recovery is less likely.

SUBARACHNOID HEMORRHAGE

While subarachnoid hemorrhage may follow intracranial occlusive disease and massive intracerebral hemorrhage, it usually results from rupture of a congenital, mycotic, or leutic aneurysm, bleeding from a cerebral neoplasm, blood dyscrasia, or hypertensive and/or arteriosclerotic arteriopathy (Grinker and Sahs, 1966). In children, ruptured intracerebral angiomas and arteriovenous anomalies are the most common cause of recurrent subarachnoid hemorrhage (DeJong, 1967). Neurologic signs depend upon the rapidity, magnitude, and persistence of bleeding and may be precipitous and catastrophic or relatively gradual in evolution. Coma is commonly preceded by sudden severe occipital headache, vertigo, vomiting, lethargy, and convulsions. The signs are those of focal neurologic changes, ocular palsies, nuchal rigidity, retinal hemorrhages, papilledema, and other evidence of increased intracranial pressure (Gardner, 1968). Cerebral spinal fluid obtained by lumbar puncture is grossly bloody or at least xanthochromic.

INFECTION

Coma in the postoperative period may be secondary to remote sepsis, such as pneumonitis, peritonitis, or extensive burns, or may result from primary intracranial infection, usually either meningitis or brain abscess. In the former, cerebral depression is caused by the infectious process itself or from endogenous toxic substances released into the circulation (Procter, 1966). Postoperative intracranial infection is usually a result of metastatic sepsis, contiguous infection of the middle ear or the paranasal sinuses, or a contaminated craniotomy or spinal puncture. The cardinal signs of meningitis are fever, nuchal rigidity, spasm of the paraspinous musculature, cerebral depression, evidence of increased intracranial pressure, and, occasionally, focal neurologic changes and convulsions. The Kernig* and Brudzinski** signs are commonly present owing to stretching of and tension on irritated nerve roots and meninges. Brain abscess is more likely to cause focal neurologic signs that depend upon the location of the lesion. The systemic manifestations of infection are often absent. Coma here results from necrosis of brain tissue, pressure on adjacent structures, and from increased intracranial pressure (DeJong, 1967). Premonitory signs and symptoms are common and include stupor, vomiting, headache, papilledema and bradycardia, and changes in the pattern of respiration. In general, the onset of brain abscess is more subtle than that of meningitis, which tends to delay detection. The diagnosis is supported in either case by lumbar puncture that shows increased pressure, elevated protein and cellular content, and reduced glucose and chloride levels.

EMERGENCY MEASURES

IMMEDIATE SUPPORT OF VENTILATION. Coma is commonly associated with an altered response of the respiratory center to the

---

*Involuntary flexion of the knee occurs during flexion of the thigh with the leg extended.

**Passive flexion of the head is followed by flexion of both thighs and legs.

extent that ventilation is seriously compromised. With a fluctuating level of consciousness, what appears to be a satisfactory respiratory drive one moment may be totally inadequate the next. Furthermore, relaxation of the pharyngeal and glottic musculature in deep coma allows the tongue to fall posteriorly and partially obstruct the airway. Slight flexion of the neck or at least the absence of extension in many instances will complete the obstruction. Along with these changes, both saliva and nasopharyngeal secretions collect in the posterior oral and nasal pharynx and are likely to be aspirated into the tracheobronchial tree. Consequently, it is essential to evaluate ventilation immediately from the standpoint of airway patency as well as the pattern, frequency, and depth of the respiratory effort. An airway obstructed by a collapsed tongue usually can be effectively managed with an oral airway, supplemented in some instances by extending the neck to straighten out the hypopharynx. The posterior pharynx should be inspected and secretions removed by suction. The lateral decubitus position prevents further pooling and affords drainage in the event of vomiting (Rosomoff and Safar, 1965). If the tendency for airway obstruction persists or function of the respiratory center is erratic, tracheal intubation is indicated, with a balloon-cuffed tube to seal the trachea as well as to permit positive pressure ventilation. Since a balloon pressure of 10 to 15 mm. Hg is required for an air-tight system, the balloon should be deflated periodically to permit capillary perfusion at the site of mucosal contact. Considerable experience has been accrued with the long-term use of both endotracheal and nasotracheal intubation, and it is evident that these adjuncts are well tolerated for periods as long as two weeks when adequate care is given to avoid pressure necrosis with an overinflated or persistently inflated intratracheal balloon cuff (Kuner and Goldman, 1967). Nasotracheal tubes are particularly useful when one wishes to avoid tracheostomy. However, in our experience, the caliber of the tube is limited by the size of the nasal orifices, and kinking of the tube at the point at which it crosses the roof of the mouth tends to impede the passage of a suction catheter into the trachea. If and when tracheostomy is performed, the old metal, 90-degree angle tube should be avoided, mainly because of the danger of erosion of the anterior tracheal wall. A 60-degree angle tube, which conforms to the angle that the trachea makes as it passes postero-inferiorly, is now widely available. Trauma may be reduced further by the use of tracheostomy tubes made of Silastic* or polyvinyl chloride.**

Tracheostomy is indicated when the advantages afforded by endotracheal intubation are required for a long period or when intubation fails to provide the protection for which it was intended, namely, to support ventilation and to facilitate tracheobronchial toilet. In a medium of adequate observation, it seldom has to be done as an emergency procedure. Since the procedure can be fraught with hazard, it should be performed in the operating room with adequate lighting, proper positioning (shoulders elevated and neck extended), sufficient instruments, and adjuncts to control bleeding, and by an operator who is skilled and familiar with the technique. The preliminary use of an endotracheal tube permits a relatively safe, unhurried procedure through a cosmetic, transverse incision. It is essential that the endotracheal tube not be completely removed from the larynx until the cuffed tracheostomy tube is securely inserted and its position checked by the passage of a suction catheter through the tracheostomy tube into the tracheobronchial tree. I prefer a cruciate incision through the second tracheal ring without the removal of tracheal tissue. To our knowledge, this has never resulted in tracheal stenosis.

Comatose patients commonly have ileus and retention of gastric contents early in the course of neurologic depression. The danger of aspiration should be foremost in mind and any suggestion of distention of the stomach must be checked immediately by nasogastric intubation. A suction machine must be at hand in the event of vomiting. If gastric residuum is more than 150 cc., intermittent evacuation of gastric contents is indicated until return of satisfactory gastrointestinal motility.

In order to provide an optimal environment for neurologic recovery, it is essential to have the best possible peripheral arterial oxygen saturation and to avoid the retention of carbon dioxide which may increase intracranial pressure by vasodilatation (Rosomoff and Safar, 1965). Ventilation should, therefore, be assessed at regular intervals by inspection of the rate and depth of respiration and the color of the capillary beds of the nails and mucous membranes as well as by periodic auscultation of the breath sounds supplemented with roentgenologic examination. There is no substitute for direct appraisal of the end product of the total respiratory effort by measurement of the arterial pH, PO_2, and PCO_2. If, for any reason, these studies are less than optimal, pulmonary function must be reappraised and, if necessary, assisted ventilation instituted without delay.

When function of the respiratory center is uncertain because of an active neurologic process, mechanical ventilation should be immediately available. In most instances of progressive neurologic deterioration, respiratory arrest occurs long before peripheral vascular collapse. When long-term assisted ventilation is anticipated, compressed air should be used to avoid the high arterial oxygen concentration that is obtained with high inspiratory pressures. The currently available oxygen-air mix systems provide concentrations as high as 90 per cent that produce very high arterial PO_2 early in the course of therapy, and a progressive fall with prolonged use because of parenchymal changes of patchy intra-alveolar edema, pneumonitis, and hemorrhage, and perivascular interstitial emphysema, edema, infiltration, and hemorrhage (Pautler et al., 1966). A commonly unrecognized problem that attends the use of pressure-controlled respiration is inadequate tidal volume. For this reason, it is helpful to measure periodically the inspiratory volume and adjust the inspiratory pressure control accordingly to deliver an adequate intake with each respiratory cycle.

It is absolutely necessary that adequate humidification be used continuously to avoid the marked drying effect that can complicate positive pressure breathing. Humidifiers must be capable of reducing the droplet size to the region of 1 to 3 microns in order to permeate to the entire tracheobronchial tree (Holder, 1969). On several occasions, we have seen a syndrome of terminal bronchiolitis that follows positive pressure breathing without adequate wetting

---

* "Moore," Dow Corning
** Hardy-Shiley, Shiley Laboratories

and that is simply a result of inspissated secretions in the terminal bronchioles adjacent to the alveoli.

Certain procedures are necessary to facilitate the evacuation of pulmonary secretions, promote full expansion, and prevent atelectasis and pulmonary vascular shunting. Tracheal aspiration should be carried out at regular intervals with a soft sterile catheter and sterile glove technique to avoid "seeding" the tracheobronchial tree with pathogenic organisms. Along with the use of adequate humidification, it is helpful to irrigate periodically the tracheobronchial tree with small increments of saline to wash out the upper-air passages and assist the removal of plugs, crusts, and mucous casts. In proper dilution (1:3) the mucolytic enzyme acetyl cysteine is also of considerable benefit in liquefying secretions and may be instilled by way of the intratracheal tube or through a small (PE 90), percutaneously inserted indwelling catheter. Bronchoconstriction sometimes complicates its use, particularly in higher concentration, and caution should, therefore, be exercised when asthma, severe emphysema, or other obstructive pathological conditions are present. When the expiratory phase of respiration is prolonged and accompanied by wheezing or whistling rales, bronchodilators are indicated. We prefer a 0.5 per cent solution of isoproterenol given by nebulization along with the systemic administration of aminophylline. Since the benefits derived by coughing are drastically reduced by the presence of a tracheostomy or intratracheal tube, it is helpful to use the respirator for periodic instantaneous hyperinflation to fully expand the lungs and deter the build up of patchy atelectasis. Fastidious pulmonary hygiene and attention to the proper application of pulmonary adjuncts will permit the use of positive pressure ventilation in patients with inadequate pulmonary reserve for remarkedly long periods without permanent injury to the respiratory system.

IMMEDIATE SUPPORT OF CIRCULATION. It is imperative that normal circulatory dynamics be maintained to provide or restore adequate cerebral flow. An integral aspect of intensive care today consists of continuous monitoring of circulatory parameters (Dammann et al., 1969). Frequent measurement of arterial pressure in the critically ill is expedited by the use of an indwelling Teflon catheter in the radial or brachial artery and a recording system that provides information both at the bedside and in a central nursing area. When the catheter is inserted with operating room precautions and maintained in the manner prescribed for prolonged use, morbidity due to sepsis is very low (Dudrick et al., 1968). A continuous infusion technique will avoid the problem of clotting despite the absence of anticoagulation. The pulse rate can be recorded directly with an electronic counter or as a by-product of the electrocardiogram. The latter suffices admirably and replaces the need for manual measurement every 15 minutes. The information provided by monitoring the central venous pressure also has been emphasized recently (Langerbeam, 1965; Maier et al., 1969). To obtain reliable measurements, a large vein must be cannulated proximal to the extremities, and either the external jugular or the subclavian vein can be used safely and effectively. In the face of incipient circulatory collapse, the continuous recording of venous pressure permits an appraisal of cardiac performance, the ability of the heart to handle that circulatory load, and, to a lesser extent, blood volume. However, it is a poor index of the state of hydration and, consequently, should not be relied upon as a guide for the administration of noncolloid fluids.

Hourly measurements of urine production are helpful to appraise volume replacement, cardiac performance, and the process of rehydration, but require the use of an indwelling catheter. These measurements are also a reliable index of the quality of tissue perfusion in general, since reduction of cardiac output is almost immediately reflected by a proportionate decline of urine production. In many instances, particularly when the integrity of the kidneys themselves is in question, the measurement of urinary electrolytes, blood urea nitrogen, creatinine, and osmolarity are helpful. When the serum sodium is near normal, a low urinary sodium (below 40 mEq./liter) and a high osmolarity (specific gravity above 1020) indicate adequate tubular function despite a reduced output.

Circulatory failure tends to compound itself by virtue of the effect of reduced coronary flow on myocardial contractility. Consequently, the temporary use of vasopressors is not only permissible but advocated to increase myocardial perfusion and to increase the strength of myocardial contractions. However, if vasoconstriction is undesirable, beta-stimulating drugs such as isoproterenol, mephentermine, or glucagon should be employed. In an environment of adequate oxygen, the heart will rapidly adjust its disturbed enzyme systems and restore its content of ATP. Myocardial performance is acutely augmented by the use of agents such as epinephrine, phenylephrine, and norepinephrine, which increase coronary perfusion. Not only is the circulatory load handled more effectively, but with cardiac function restored, volume loading to enhance diastolic filling and myocardial contractility is possible. When volume replacement is indicated to restore and stabilize circulatory function, it is best carried out with whole blood or, if necessary, blood substitutes. Noncolloid fluids are rapidly lost from the vascular tree, reaching an equilibrium between the intravascular and extravascular-extracellular compartments in about two hours. The rise of interstitial fluid volume is uniform throughout the body including the lungs and brain. The sequestration of fluid in the interstices of the lungs can deter diffusion of gases across the alveolar-capillary membrane and eventually result in hypoxemia.

A rise of water content in a brain that is already the site of cerebral edema obviously should be avoided. In the face of fluid overload, which potentiates or is the primary cause of cerebral depression, the administration of a diuretic agent is indicated along with electrolyte replacement. In our experience, mannitol has been useful to promote an active osmotic diuresis while simultaneously reducing brain volume. At least 25 gm. should be given as a primary dose over a period of 30 minutes to test the ability of the kidney to respond to osmotic diuresis. Ethacrynic acid and furosemide stimulate massive diuresis by another mechanism and, although of recent vintage, they are widely used because of their safety and effectiveness even when renal function is depressed (Goldberg, 1969). In all instances, care should be exercised to prevent electrolyte imbalance mainly by the loss of serum potassium. The diuretic response can be augmented by the administration of human albumin, which remains for the most part within the intravascular compartment while mobilizing water from the extravascular space. It is commonly prepared in increments of 25 gm., which have the osmotic equivalence of 500 cc. whole blood. As such, it is a potent volume expander and should be used with caution.

REGULATION OF BODY TEMPERATURE. There is uniform agreement that hyperthermia, which commonly complicates brain damage because of dysfunction of hypothalamic thermoregulating centers, should be avoided. Consequently, attention must be directed to reduction of an elevated body temperature and prevention of recurrent pyrexia. A rectal or pharyngeal thermocouple is necessary to monitor adequately the body temperature and the response to antipyretic therapy. Whenever primary causes are identifiable, such as sepsis or pyrogenic reaction, they should be managed with specific measures. At the same time, the use of external cooling with ice packs, alcohol and ice sponging, or more commonly, a hypothermia blanket, is indicated. Supplemental oxygen helps offset the hypermetabolic state and increased oxygen consumption imposed by fever. There is now solid experimental and clinical evidence that the reduction of body temperature to the range of 30° C. prior to or following a neurologic insult exerts a protective effect on the brain by suppressing the reactive cerebral edema that occurs with most neurologic injury (Blair, 1964), as well as by reducing the metabolic requirement to about 50 per cent without altering normal cerebral metabolic pathways (Michenfelder and Theye, 1968). Therapeutic hypothermia is usually induced with a hypothermia blanket that carries a circulating coolant. The temperature of the blanket should not be less than 40° F. because of the danger of cold injury to pressure areas. Antishivering agents, such as chlorpromazine, greatly augment the cooling process. When a therapeutic level of hypothermia is reached, neurologic function itself is depressed, as are all other vegetative processes including the blood pressure, pulse rate, respiratory rate, and the like. Despite these changes, hypothermia has been continued for periods of several days without untoward effects (Rosomoff and Safar, 1965).

Spontaneous hypothermia is usually undesirable, particularly in the very young in whom it is prone to occur. Consequently, continuous external warming is necessary to avoid the fall in cardiac output and tendency toward anaerobic metabolism that occurs with hypothermia in this age-group. In adults, the necessity for active warming in the postoperative period is uncommon and the external application of heat usually suffices. However, hyperthermia by internal perfusion has been reported for the treatment of accidental hypothermia (Davies et al., 1967).

SUPPRESSION OF SEIZURE ACTIVITY

Whereas cerebral oxygen consumption is reduced in quiet coma, there is a sharp rise above normal during seizure activity (Gottstein, 1965). When cerebral oxygenation is borderline, the implication is obvious; convulsions themselves may precipitate further brain damage or at least prolonged postictal coma (Plum and Posner, 1966).

Primary reliance is still placed upon the intravenous administration of Sodium Amytal occasionally coupled with supplements of diazepam (Valium). The tongue and extremities must be protected from injury and precautions taken to prevent aspiration of gastric contents and airway obstruction. The infusion of a short-acting muscle relaxant such as succinylcholine may be necessary for cases of continuous, refractory seizure activity (Evanson, 1959; Robinson, 1963).

Once convulsions are halted, control can be maintained with phenobarbital and diphenylhydantoin (Dilantin). Dosage is titrated until a response is obtained, and very high levels may be required, depending upon the magnitude of cerebral irritability.

DIAGNOSIS

For practical purposes, postoperative patients in coma can be divided into two groups, namely, those in whom unconsciousness is a sudden, abrupt, and unexpected deviation from the anticipated hospital course and those who have gradually and relentlessly passed through the clinical stages of progressive cerebral depression to finally become frankly comatose. In general, the former demands immediate evaluation and the application of emergency measures to support vital functions while diagnosis is being obtained, whereas the latter requires the use of conventional supportive therapy during re-examination and scrutiny of the hospital course preceding the gradual deterioration of central nervous system function. The historical aspects of every case

should be carefully investigated through available records, family members, and acquaintances to expose potential causes of coma, such as antecedent trauma and Stokes-Adams episodes or conditions predisposing to cerebral dysfunction that occur with many chronic diseases, i.e., diabetes mellitus, hypertension, and chronic renal insufficiency. Historical inquiry should determine the chronic use of drugs (depressants, analgesics, ataractics, and anticoagulants), the possibility of mental disorder (memory loss, insomnia, depression, agitation, emotional lability), and previous head injury or neurologic disease (seizures, dizziness, syncopal episodes) (Nathanson and Bergman, 1966).

Physical examination with emphasis on the character and extent of neurologic changes is then in order. Cyanosis, pallor, jaundice, petechiae, diaphoresis, dehydration, and the stigmata of weight loss may suggest the presence of acute or chronic systemic illness. Certain postures in bed may also be informative, such as the opisthotonos of meningitis, the characteristic attitudes of decorticate and decerebrate rigidity, and the unnatural and uncomfortable positions of the extremities with paralysis. Spontaneous normal movements suggest an intact motor system, whereas marked restlessness and flocciLation (tugging and picking at the bed clothes), and asterixis (flapping tremor) are common in precoma states (DeJong, 1967). The degree of urinary and fecal continence and the response to loud noises and spoken commands are a guide to the status of vegetative functions. An elevated pulse rate is seen with sepsis, toxemia, fever, congestive heart failure, and other hypermetabolic states, whereas bradycardia is characteristic of heart-block, increased intracranial pressure, and, occasionally, acute blood loss. The systemic arterial pressure, in turn, is altered by a host of conditions affecting cardiac output, blood and fluid volume, and peripheral vascular tone; and whereas the direction of response is usually downward, a marked elevation of pressure is met in hypertensive crisis and uremia. Fever can result from damage to the thermoregulatory center but is far more commonly a response to sepsis, pyrogens, or dehydration. Examinations of the neck and extremities should include the arterial pulses and lymphatic structures, which may point to cerebral arteriopathy or metastatic disease. Primary neoplasms, foci of infection, and circulatory disorders may also be discovered during appraisal of the chest and abdomen.

Frequently, the cerebral insult is well defined and the primary diagnostic interest is directed to the extent of neurologic damage rather than to etiology as is usually the case with postanoxic encephalopathy. Whereas there is some tendency to shift the responsibility to a consulting neurologist, it is helpful, if not imperative, for the attending physician to be equipped to carry out a basic neurologic examination. This includes an evaluation of the state of consciousness, pupillary response, ocular movements, respiration, deep tendon reflexes, and motor function.

Metabolic coma, unlike some structural lesions causing cerebral depression, is almost invariably preceded by disorders of cerebration and is manifested by variable alterations of awareness, cognition, memory, perception, association, and attitude (Plum and Posner, 1966). Reduced alertness is a characteristic incipient sign of postoperative metabolic encephalopathy which imperceptibly progresses to drowsiness and then stupor. Simultaneously, there is a more or less orderly regression of orientation—first to time, then to distance, and finally to persons and places. Associative and abstract cognitive processes are replaced with monosyllabic responses and there is a progressive decline of memory, especially for recent events. Affect and attitude are also altered and, although usually marked by apathy and indifference, the onset of encephalopathy following sensory and nutritional deprivation, as in the "recovery room syndrome," is frequently associated with anxiety and hostility. The magnitude of altered mentation is thought to parallel the extent of diffuse neuronal dysfunction with specific areas affected more severely than others in some cases.

RESPIRATION. Both metabolic coma and structural brain lesions commonly produce changes in rhythm, rate, and depth of ventilation. In some instances, the respiratory center is specifically involved as a discrete part of the pathologic process, whereas in others, ventilatory alterations are simply a manifestation of diffuse brain stem dysfunction. Several nonspecific patterns of breathing have been described. Posthyperventilation apnea and Cheyne-Stokes respiration are seen with diffuse metabolic or structural lesions of the cerebral hemispheres, whereas neurogenic hyperventilation indicates more profound brain-stem dysfunction. Apneustic breathing is characterized by prolonged inspiratory pauses and occurs with basilar artery occlusion and less commonly with hypoglycemia. Structural lesions of the respiratory center that interfere with reciprocal inspiratory and expiratory relationships produce the totally irregular respiratory pattern of ataxic breathing. Areas of the brain stem controlling ventilation are especially sensitive to hypoglycemia, hypoxia, drug intoxication, and intracranial pressure. Consequently, apnea usually precedes the onset of vascular collapse and the cessation of other vital activities.

In the absence of altered gas exchange owing to pulmonary parenchymal changes, the dominant pattern of breathing is of diagnostic importance. Chemoreceptors in the aortic and carotid bodies as well as chemosensitive areas in the medulla itself influence the rate and depth of ventilation by responding to changes of hydrogen-ion concentration, PO_2, and PCO_2 (Mitchell et al., 1963).

HYPOVENTILATION. Depression of the respiratory center and the compensatory reduction of respiration that accompanies a rising blood pH are the two principal causes of hypoventilation in the comatose patient. The former is the result of metabolic or structural alteration of the central and/or peripheral neuromuscular respiratory apparatus that leads to respiratory insufficiency and carbon dioxide retention. The blood pH is usually less than 7.35 and the CO_2 combining power is seldom below 20 mEq./liter. However, the PCO_2 is characteristically elevated above 50 mm. Hg. Differentiation between central and peripheral respiratory insufficiency is made mainly by physical examination supplemented by simple x-ray examination. Metabolic alkalosis, in turn, is seen after prolonged use of corticoids and diuretic agents but is most severe because of persistent gastric losses through heavy nasogastric drainage. The pH is elevated above 7.5 and the CO_2 combining power above 30 mEq./liter while the PCO_2 is usually below 50 mm. Hg. Accurate measurement of the blood gases coupled with the serum carbon dioxide combining power pinpoint the specific acid-base imbalance and facilitate reaching a specific diagnosis.

HYPERVENTILATION. Sustained hyperventilation may represent the normal response of the respiratory center to the accumulation of acid metabolites that is seen with diabetes mellitus, uremia, or severe lactic acidemia secondary to peripheral vascular insufficiency. Simple laboratory studies will suffice to establish the cause in the first two instances, whereas circulatory collapse of sufficient severity to cause widespread tissue hypoxia should be easily recognizable on physical examination.

Hepatic coma, irritative stimulation of the respiratory center by noxious agents, and structural lesions of the reticular formation in the low midbrain and the pons can all produce hyperventilation, which eventually results in respiratory alkalosis. The pH is usually above 7.5 and the PCO_2 below 30 mm. Hg. The administration of oxygen may elevate the PO_2 but will not slow the respiratory rate. When bronchopulmonary disease is also present, hypoxemia may be superimposed on CO_2 retention. Here, hyperventilation may reflect hypercarbia or reduced arterial oxygen saturation or both. In any event, blood-gas studies are essential to clarify the issue.

PUPILS.   In the absence of drugs that alter the size and activity of the pupils, the pupillary responses to light and to painful cutaneous stimuli[*] are of great diagnostic significance, particularly if coma is profound. Extensive structural damage of the cortex and many metabolic encephalopathies produce small pupils. The pupils become dilated and fixed with diffuse lesions of the cortex and brain stem secondary to hypoxia, air and fat embolism, encephalomyelitis, and markedly increased intracranial pressure. Inequality of size or response strongly suggests the presence of a structural lesion, whereas the pupils will almost always show some activity when coma is purely metabolic in character (Hill, 1965).

Optic-nerve lesions produce ipsilateral dilatation, absent reaction to light, and consensual constriction during stimulation of the opposite eye. The pupils remain in the midposition or slightly dilated with lesions of the optic tracts, and the response to light is present with ipsilateral and absent with contralateral stimulation. Lesions of the upper brain stem are associated with small, equal pupils that react to light over a small arc. The ciliospinal reflex is intact. Damage

in the region of the midbrain nuclei causes irregular and sometimes unequal pupils that tend to be fixed to light and painful stimuli. Structural lesions of the pons that interrupt sympathetic pathways initially produce pinpoint pupils. With extension of damage, they later become dilated and fixed, and involvement of the autonomic pathways in the lateral medulla and cervical cord is likely to produce a mild Horner's syndrome. Space-occupying lesions that compress the oculomotor nerve against the cerebral tentorium result in dilatation of the ipsilateral pupil, followed by a sluggish or absent response to light by direct and contralateral stimulation (Smith, 1965). If the pupillary reaction is equivocal, magnification should be used along with a high-intensity light source to facilitate the examination.

The funduscopic examination is likely to be useful in instances other than metabolic coma. Papilledema indicates the presence of significant cerebral edema or a space-occupying lesion such as free or clotted blood or hematoma. Extensive retinal hemorrhage is seen with subarachnoid bleeding, and small retinal hemorrhages and exudates are characteristic of diabetes mellitus, hypertensive crises, and blood dyscrasias.

EXTRAOCULAR MOVEMENTS.   An appraisal of spontaneous and reflex eye movements will often contribute additional significant information concerning the etiology, depth, and course of cerebral depression. In general, asymmetric motion, dysconjugate gaze, and fixed conjugate lateral deviation are more characteristic of structural lesions. Random conjugate or dysconjugate movements similar to those seen in sleep occur with mild metabolic encephalopathy. At deeper levels of unconsciousness the eyes become fixed in a neutral position. Abnormalities of lateral gaze may be produced by extensive hemispheral lesions, brain-stem damage involving the ocular nuclei, or extraocular nerve injury. Lateral conjugate deviation due to a hemispheral lesion can be overcome during testing of the reflex extraocular movements to be described later. Destructive lesions of supranuclear cerebral pathways result in ipsilateral conjugate deviation, whereas damage in the region of supranuclear oculomotor fibers of the pons produces conjugate deviation to the opposite side or paralysis of horizontal movement beyond the midposition to the ipsilateral side. Resting dysconjugate lateral gaze and

---

[*]The ciliospinal reflex consists of homolateral, and to a lesser extent, contralateral mydriasis in response to painful stimuli of the head, neck, and trunk. Its presence indicates an intact brain stem.

homolateral mydriasis indicate damage to the oculomotor nuclei or peripheral pathways, whereas lesions of the abducens nucleus or nerve cause dysconjugate medial deviation.

Abnormalities of vertical gaze are usually associated with structural injury to the brain stem. Damage involving the pretectal area of the midbrain or the tracts connecting the oculomotor, trochlear, and abducens nuclei (medial longitudinal fasciculi) causes upward conjugate deviation. Downward deviation is usually the result of severe metabolic or structural alterations in the brain stem. Resting dysconjugate vertical gaze or skew deviation results from damage to internuclear fibers of the medial longitudinal fasciculus (Plum and Posner, 1966).

Reflex extraocular movements can be elicited by passive movement of the head or during caloric (cold) stimulation of the vestibular apparatus. With some exceptions, the responses coincide and, at all but profound degrees of metabolic encephalopathy, are usually intact, with the vestibular reflex being the stronger of the two. When cortical influence on an intact brain stem is lost, the reflexes are active. The oculocephalogyric reflex is elicited by rotating the head rapidly from side to side and coming to rest at one of the extremes. If the eyes deviate to the opposite side, the response is positive (normal). Vertical motion can be tested by rapidly flexing and extending the neck. The oculovestibular reflex follows stimulation of the intact tympanic membrane with cold water injected into the auditory canal. Nystagmus is produced in the awake normal patient with the rapid component toward the opposite side. The comatose patient with an intact brain stem will exhibit conjugate deviation of the eye to the side of stimulation.

The reflexes are most useful in providing information concerning brain-stem function. Lesions in the midbrain or pons that produce paralysis of lateral or vertical gaze cause the ocular reflexes to be absent in one direction or the other. Dysconjugate responses usually result from lesions of the medial longitudinal fasciculus (Nathanson and Bergman, 1966). The oculovestibular reflex can also differentiate psychogenic coma in which, despite the absence of sensory reaction, the wakeful response is intact. Both ocular reflexes disappear with deep coma from any cause. Roving conjugate or dysconjugate eye movements occur with light coma (Aserinsky and Kleitman, 1955) and are, consequently, an encouraging prognostic sign. The oculocephalogyric reflex is usually positive when these movements are present, and both disappear when the brain stem is depressed.

SENSORY AND MOTOR ACTIVITY. Evaluation of sensory and motor activity in the comatose patient is hampered by the inability to communicate perceptual interpretations. Since sensation is diminished to absent at a relatively mild level of coma, those parts of the brain involved with sensory function may be difficult to appraise. As in other areas of the neurologic examination, a comparison of response in the two halves of the body can provide information that is essential for accurate diagnosis.

When muscular activity is impaired due to a contralateral cerebral lesion, sensation is usually retained partially; although the response to noxious stimuli is absent on that side, an expression of pain may be manifested by grimacing or withdrawal elsewhere. A total absence of response occurs with bilateral interruption of the corticospinal pathways, with pontomedullary lesions, or with deep coma from any cause. The superficial reflexes, i.e., abdominal, cremasteric, and the like, have a cortical pathway as well as a spinal reflex arc and these too are altered by processes affecting cerebral function. Consequently, they are diminished or disappear with pyramidal tract lesions and may be increased in psychogenic disorders and disease of the extrapyramidal system, possibly as a result of the loss of inhibitory impulses. However, the activity of superficial and deep reflexes is a poor index of the level of cerebral depression, since it may be altered without a commensurate change in the state of consciousness. The deep reflexes persist beyond the superficial reflexes but also may be lost in deep coma.

The examination of motor activity should include an appraisal of muscular tone and function and the presence of abnormal movements such as twitches, tremors, and focal seizures. Palpation of the muscle masses and the response to passive movement give information regarding tonicity. Motor function, in turn, is evaluated in the unconscious patient by inspection of the facies and the response of the extremities to attitudes other than the resting position. Unilateral facial movements, blowing out of one cheek in breathing and lack of closure of the ipsilateral eye indicate a facial palsy (Thomas and Klass, 1964). When the arms are elevated and released, an extremity that is paralyzed will descend as dead weight, whereas the functionally unimpaired extremity tends to float down. Similarly, when the legs are flexed and supported on the heels, the functionally intact side tends to maintain this position, whereas the paralyzed extremity immediately flops into the resting position. Although asymmetric motor abnormalities are much more likely with structural brain lesions, there are several instances of metabolic encephalopathy, such as hepatic coma and hypoglycemia, with at least transient localization of neurologic signs, i.e., hemiplegia.

Disease of the pyramidal system, resulting from lesions of the motor cortex, its projection fibers, and the descending corticospinal tracts, manifests itself by impaired motor activity on the contralateral side plus diminished to absent superficial reflexes, exaggerated deep tendon reflexes, and muscular hypertonicity. Clonus of the ankles, wrists, and petellae is common due to hyperactive stretch reflexes. A host of pyramidal tract signs have been described, the most important of which is the Babinski phenomenon.* This pathologic reflex is present with both suppressive as well as destructive neurologic disease from the motor cortex through the descending corticospinal pathways. Intact basal ganglia are necessary for its presence, and if they are damaged, the Babinski sign disappears (DeJong, 1967). Since the pyramidal system is involved by most processes affecting the state of consciousness, the Babinski sign is also present. However, a spurious response, a pseudo-Babinski sign, can result from involuntary withdrawal in overly sensitive individuals, from plantar hyperesthesia, and from too strong a plantar stimulation.

Extrapyramidal structures may be involved alone or, more commonly, along with the pyramidal tracts. This area of the brain is phylogenetically the primitive motor system and its chief components, the basal ganglia, are the oldest part of the cerebrum. Its primary function appears to be the mainte-

nance of a fluidity of motion on voluntary muscular action mediated through the pyramidal system, although many voluntary or automatic movements related mainly to posture are initiated in extrapyramidal centers. Postoperative encephalopathy commonly involves the extrapyramidal tracts producing hypertonicity, tremors, and dyskinetic movement. Paratonia is a form of extrapyramidal hyperactivity, variously described as a plastic, waxy, or lead-pipe type of resistance to passive movement, that is present from any position and is most common with metabolic and diffuse vascular brain disease and mass lesions of the frontal lobe (Plum and Posner, 1966).

Fixed patterns of inappropriate response are observed with specific levels of brain damage. Decorticate rigidity follows extensive destructive lesions of the internal capsule or cerebral hemisphere with or without injury to the adjacent basal ganglia and thalamus. A characteristic habitus is met consisting of flexion of the arms, wrists, and fingers, adduction of the upper extremities, and internal rotation, extension, and plantar flexion of the lower extremities. Decerebrate rigidity, in turn, occurs with both structural and metabolic encephalopathy and is characterized by extension of the back, arms, and legs, adduction and pronation of the upper extremities, plantar flexion of the feet, and clenching of the teeth. This phenomenon results from release of the vestibular nuclei from extrapyramidal control. Depression of the brain stem by anoxia, hypoglycemia, depressant drugs, and endogenous or exogenous toxins, as well as extensive structural injury to the midbrain and pons, can produce these changes.

Needless to say, both decorticate and decerebrate rigidity are grave neurologic signs even when they are brought out only by noxious stimuli. However, they do not necessarily indicate irreversible neurologic damage (Haerer, 1969). The likelihood of recovery is proportional to the duration of these patterns of response and is rare after one week.

Spasticity follows pyramidal tract lesions that result in an imbalance between inhibitory and facilitatory centers of the midbrain and brain-stem reticular formation. In contrast to the responses discussed earlier, spasticity consists of sustained contraction of a muscle when it is passively stretched. At one extreme, slow passive movement may

---

*The Babinski sign is present when stimulation of either side of the plantar surface of the foot beginning from the heel forward to the metatarsophalangeal joints is followed by dorsiflexion of the great toe and fanning of the remainder of the toes.

permit a relative freedom of motion, whereas at the other, spastic muscles may be continuously hard and unyielding so that they cannot be moved. In the presence of spasticity, the deep tendon reflexes are exaggerated and pathologic reflexes, such as the Babinski sign, are usually present.

Convulsive disorders complicating postoperative cerebral depression are usually secondary to metabolic disturbances, systemic toxicity, acute hypoxia, or focal cerebral disease. It has been the author's impression, perhaps because of some neurologic naïveté, that those patients with postanoxic encephalopathy who exhibit grand mal or focal convulsive activity carry a more optimistic prognosis for ultimate recovery. At any rate, it does suggest that the cortex is irritable and, hence, viable.

LABORATORY STUDIES. Laboratory examinations of blood, serum, and urine may both facilitate diagnosis and assist in evaluating the therapeutic response. In each instance, the spectrum of studies must be tailored to the clinical findings. However, the blood count is informative in the presence of acute and chronic infection, polycythemia, and recent blood loss. Blood cultures may also be indicated. Measurement of the arterial blood pH, PO_2, and PCO_2 permits appraisal of the quality of tissue perfusion as well as the effectiveness of ventilation. Hypoglycemia must always be ruled out and the blood ammonia should be measured when hepatic insufficiency is suspected. Serum studies should evaluate the electrolyte profile and the status of hepatic and renal function. The serum calcium, phosphorus, and proteins may also be useful in evaluation. The urine should be examined for glucose, acetone, and protein, and in borderline perfusion states such as congestive heart failure and circulatory collapse, hourly measurements of output are indicated.

AUXILIARY DIAGNOSTIC STUDIES. In some instances, supplemental studies are necessary and are usually embarked upon in conjunction with and at the discretion of the consulting neurologist. Among the more common diagnostic adjuncts that can be applied with minimal manipulation or movement of the patient are electroencephalography and spinal puncture.

The electroencephalogram records electrical activity of cortical neurons adjacent to the skull, which, in turn, depend partly upon stimuli from deeper brain structures for normal function. Consequently, it follows that the EEG can be altered by both cortical and brain-stem abnormalities. The predominant changes consist of slow waves that are to some extent proportional to the severity of the disturbance of the brain. Supratentorial or cortical lesions tend to produce focal or unilateral changes, whereas bilateral slow activity appears when the deeper brain structures with bilateral projection fibers to the cortex are involved. However, when coma results from caudal lesions sparing the midbrain reticular formation, the EEG may be normal. Alpha rhythms, usually the most prominent feature of the recording of a normal, waking patient, are also present with hysterical states that simulate organic coma (Thomas and Klass, 1964). Coma due to diffuse encephalopathy results in bilateral slowing that parallels the depth of cerebral depression. Electric cortical activity begins to wane early in the course of metabolic brain disease, and bursts of very slow, high-voltage waves are seen in the precoma period of hepatic, uremic, and other metabolic encephalopathies.

Spinal puncture is often an essential part of the neurologic examination and may supply chemical, cytologic, and bacteriologic information concerning the etiology of postoperative coma as well as the level of intracranial pressure. However, the study should never be embarked upon across a contaminated field and probably should be avoided in the presence of generalized systemic infection or contiguous infections of the head, such as mastoiditis. It should be used only with extreme caution in the presence of increased intracranial pressure because of the danger of fatal herniation of the cerebellar tonsils and medulla into the foramen magnum or of the hippocampal gyrus through the incisura of the cerebellar tentorium, with subsequent brain-stem compression.

The spinal fluid pressure is elevated with increased formation or decreased absorption. The former occurs with encephalitis, meningitis, and other infections, and during periods of increased systemic venous pressure regardless of cause. Absorption is reduced by the presence of blood, pus, or a high-protein content within the cerebral spinal fluid, as well as by inflammatory changes of the arachnoid villi. Cerebral edema and space-occupying lesions can produce or augment an elevation of spinal fluid pressure.

A low spinal fluid pressure probably has little significance per se and is due most commonly to systemic arterial hypotension, dehydration, and hypovolemia. Drugs that increase the serum osmolarity cause the pressure to fall because of the reduced formation of spinal fluid. The agents most effective in producing a sustained elevation of the serum osmolarity are a 30 per cent solution of urea in 10 per cent fructose or a 25 per cent solution of mannitol.

The cerebral spinal fluid is normally crystal clear and colorless and contains less than 5 cells per cubic centimeter. The total protein ranges from 15 to 40 mg. per 100 ml., although higher levels than normal are a ubiquitous finding in a host of neurologic disorders, including the metabolic encephalopathies of myxedema and hyperparathyroidism. The protein may be fractionated to provide further information concerning certain neuropathies such as multiple sclerosis. The glucose content is also significant in that it is characteristically altered in some instances. The cerebral spinal fluid glucose rises above the normal range of 50 to 65 mg. per 100 ml. in clinical conditions when the blood glucose is also elevated. Hypoglycorrhachia, on the other hand, is most common in bacterial, tuberculous, mycotic, and neoplastic meningitides. The chloride content is commonly reduced in these instances and also tends to parallel the blood level when the protein content of spinal fluid is normal. Otherwise, the chloride decreases as the spinal fluid protein rises.

Postoperative disorders of consciousness are occasionally evaluated by other methods. In some instances of pre-existing intracranial disease, *skull roentgenography* can be helpful. Unsuspected fracture lines, punched-out lesions of the cranium, and shifts of the calcified pineal gland may be defined. Views in the coronal and sagittal planes are useful for demonstrating erosion of the intracranial processes by primary or metastatic neoplasms and intracranial calcification resulting from chronic foci of infection, certain benign tumors, and vascular anomalies. Additional information and localization may be obtained by *cerebral angiography* when a space-occupying lesion, vascular anomaly, or occlusive disease is suspected (Pevehouse and Brown, 1962). Even a single bedside film may be informative, as in a recent case in which there was a sudden onset of coma in a patient recovering from a neck wound. A primary or metastatic neoplasm may exhibit the characteristic tumor "stain" as well as displacement of adjacent vascular structures. *Ophthalmodynamometry*, which is an indirect method of measuring retinal artery pressure, is also useful for the diagnosis of unilateral occlusive disease. A difference of 20 per cent or more between pressures of the retinal arteries indicates definite and significant reduction in blood flow in the ipsilateral carotid system (Calderon and Eisenbrey, 1965). However, it correlates poorly with angiographic appraisal in the presence of bilateral lesions. *Echoencephalography*, a developing study, measures the distance of midline structures by ultrasonic scanning and has been used to outline intracranial neoplasms, demonstrate ventricular size, and record intracranial pulsations (Kurze et al., 1965). Biplane examination gives additional localization. *Brain scanning* following the administration of radioactive isotopes that have a propensity for nervous tissue, especially in the cerebral hemispheres, is useful for the diagnosis of cerebral neoplasms, abscesses, infarcts, and hematomas. Although many isotopes have been employed, Technetium[99] is currently popular, and the use of recently available scintillation cameras shortens a single study from 30 to about 3 minutes (Handa, 1969).

DEFINITIVE MANAGEMENT

When acute metabolic aberrations that express themselves in part by disorders of consciousness are correctly identified and reversed, recovery from neurologic alterations follows in most instances. On the other hand, failure to institute correct therapy promptly can lead to irreversible brain damage or death. The foregoing section deals in a general manner with specific measures that are essential or at least useful in handling the more common causes of postoperative coma. Additional details can be obtained from the designated reference material.

Hypoxemic hypoxia.   In the absence of

chronic pulmonary disease, hypoxemia of sufficient severity to cause central nervous system symptoms usually results from catastrophic pulmonary accidents, such as massive atelectasis, tension pneumothorax, or aspiration of gastric contents. The success of therapy depends largely upon prompt diagnosis and the use of specific measures to evacuate the tracheobronchial tree and to re-expand the pulmonary parenchyma. The injudicious administration of drugs that depress the respiratory center can also precipitate hypoxemic crises. To avoid cardiac catastrophes, alveolar hypoventilation must be corrected immediately by measures that increase the depth of respiration and the transfer of oxygen, mainly by assisted ventilation with a respirator.

Recently, there has been a growing incidence of pulmonary diffusion abnormalities in the seriously ill who are overtreated with balanced electrolyte solutions to expand blood volume. Noncolloid fluids begin to "leak" from the intravascular compartment almost immediately, reaching an equilibrium in the extracellular space in about two hours. The rising level of pulmonary interstitial water both decreases the lung compliance and directly interferes with gas exchange. As the arterial oxygen tension falls, the circulatory status deteriorates, removing any likelihood of effective renal compensation. Poor tissue perfusion produces lactic acidosis, completing a vicious and often fatal cycle. In our experience, a dramatic improvement of arterial oxygen saturation can follow a vigorous diuresis induced by ethacrynic acid. If diuresis is ineffective or contraindicated, aggressive dialysis by the peritoneal or circulatory routes may be the only satisfactory way to manage this difficult problem.

VASCULAR OCCLUSIVE DISEASE. The medical management of cerebrovascular disease, whether occlusive or hemorrhagic, is similar in that it is primarily supportive in nature. In both instances, a cardiopulmonary status must be achieved or maintained that will provide optimal tissue perfusion and oxygenation while avoiding extremes of blood pressure. At the onset of the stroke syndrome due to thrombosis or embolic occlusion of major vessels, accurate diagnosis by aortocranial or carotid angiography may reveal an obstructing lesion that is amenable to repair, particularly with the advent of the Fogarty balloon catheter. With the possibility of spontaneous recovery or at least partial return of function on one hand and the danger of additional brain damage due to vascular manipulation on the other, one is naturally hesitant to suggest surgical intervention. However, there have been several instances of reversal of neurologic symptoms following aggressive operative therapy (Hardy, 1963). During the period of recovery, the supine position is recommended for one week or more, since postural hypotension can precipitate cerebral ischemia. The role of anticoagulant therapy is still being contested. It appears to have some effect in checking the progression of an evolving stroke and in reducing the early mortality of cerebral embolus. Anticoagulants are contraindicated in patients with cerebral hemorrhage and are of questionable benefit after completed strokes due to cerebral thrombosis. However, many will institute anticoagulation with heparin or coumarin derivatives (Dicumarol, Coumadin) if the cerebrospinal fluid is free of blood or xanthochromia after thrombotic infarction (Marshall, 1968).

Because of the diffuse nature of the insult, embolization of fat or air to the brain can compromise function at all levels. Reactive cerebral edema is often severe and is the primary cause of early mortality. If involvement of precapillary vessels is patchy and the effects of increased intracranial pressure can be avoided, partial or complete recovery is possible even from a state of prolonged coma. Measures to decrease cerebral edema are not indicated for all patients but should be used when cerebral depression is progressive or is already profound. The inflammatory reaction is reduced by (1) hypothermia to 90° by external cooling with increments of chlorpromazine to prevent shivering (Rosomoff and Safar, 1965), (2) intravenous hyperosmolar solutions such as 25 per cent mannitol in a dose of 1.5 gm. per kilogram of body weight at 12-hour intervals to promote sustained dehydration of the brain, and (3) intravenous dexamethasone (Decadron) in pharmacologic doses, i.e., 4 mg. at 6-hour intervals (French, 1966). The efficacy of treatment is inversely proportional to the interval from neurologic injury. Administration of heparin at less than anticoagulant doses may be useful for its fat clearing effect while the infusion of 5 per cent alcohol solution, 500 to 1000 cc. daily, appears to accelerate resolution of pulmonary infiltrates due to fat emboli (Tedeschi et al. 1968).

The effect of low molecular weight dextran on cerebral capillary flow under these circumstances requires further evaluation.

Recently, an extracellular surface active agent, Pluronic F-68, has come into limited clinical use following experimental demonstration of the dramatic protection it provides against air embolism. Its role in future therapy for cerebral fat and air embolism remains to be determined (Hymes et al. 1968).

Coma resulting from malignant hypertension is an emergent problem requiring immediate therapy. Methyldopa and reserpine are the antihypertensive agents of choice and initially should be given parenterally (Leavitt and Polansky, 1968). Both drugs are titrated at prescribed intervals until the blood pressure begins to fall. Maintenance therapy is then instituted once the blood pressure reaches a satisfactory level.

HYPOGLYCEMIA. When postoperative patients receiving insulin exhibit bizarre neurologic signs or cerebral depression, the likelihood of a hypoglycemic reaction is so great that intravenous glucose solution should be given empirically, immediately after a sample is drawn for blood glucose. Following the administration of 50 cc. of 50 per cent glucose solution, an infusion of isotonic glucose is given until the clinical picture is clarified. The speed and quality of response depend upon the duration and severity of hypoglycemia. Sufficient glucose can also be mobilized to reverse hypoglycemic coma by the intramuscular administration of 1 mg. of glucagon. If inappropriate administration of exogenous insulin is at fault, care must be taken to err on the conservative side when altering the total insulin dosage or adjusting a combination of rapid and long-acting insulin preparations. Mild to moderate glycosuria (2 or 3+) is preferable to avoid this very problem. Hypoglycemia secondary to hepatic insufficiency should be readily apparent from liver function studies, whereas that caused by excessive circulating endogenous insulin or insulin-like factor may be identified only by special diagnostic techniques. Whatever the case, every effort must be made to provide a continuous supply of glucose until the underlying cause is corrected. It is generally not appreciated that lack of substrate over a sufficient period can cause widespread brain damage similar to cerebral ischemia. Fortunately, recovery from hypoglycemic coma is usually rapid and complete with prompt and adequate therapy.

WATER INTOXICATION (HYPONATREMIA). When confronted with a reduced sensorium, cortical hyperactivity, and a fluid balance tally that is consistent with the possibility of water intoxication, the serum electrolytes (sodium) and osmolarity should be measured without delay. If both are significantly reduced, the best management is to dissipate the relative or absolute positive balance of water by sharply restricting intake well below that level of insensible and urinary loss. When more aggressive measures are indicated and renal function is adequate, solute diuresis can be promoted by the administration of mannitol or urea solutions. Since incipient congestive heart failure is often present due to the fluid overload, these volume expanders must be used with great caution. Hypertonic saline should be administered only when the patient is severely threatened with irreversible damage by the hyponatremia per se. The dose required to elevate the serum sodium can be calculated from the formula: Na+ increase × 60% body wgt. (kg) = Na+ mEq. required. In these instances the removal of extra water by hemodialysis or peritoneal dialysis may be the safer course.

HYPERNATREMIA. Hypernatremic encephalopathy due to osmoregulatory defects (inappropriate ADH) should be treated by correcting fluid deficits and establishing a positive water balance (Wolfman et al., 1968). This is best accomplished by giving solute-free water orally or isotonic glucose solution intravenously. When hypernatremia is the result of excessive salt replacement rather than water loss, the total body water is also usually increased. Dialysis may be necessary to avoid further loading and congestive heart failure (Miller, 1968).

HYPERGLYCEMIC NONKETOTIC COMA. About two-thirds of the patients with this syndrome lack an antecedent history of hyperglycemia. Consequently, unlike diabetic coma, failure of early recognition in the postoperative period may be justified to some extent. Emphasis must be placed on aggressive fluid therapy, which is absolutely essential to avoid the high mortality that threatens this state. Hypotonic solutions of saline (0.45 per cent) and glucose (2.5 per cent) should be used in place of the usual isotonic fluids that may actually worsen the hyperosmolarity (Ashworth et al., 1968).

Ten to 15 liters of fluid may be required in the first 24 hours, with the use of repeated determinations of the serum and osmolarity, the hourly urinary output, and an estimate of the total body water as guides. The serum potassium level must be carefully monitored and this cation replaced as required. The insulin dose should be tailored to the individual demand but in general it is less than that required for diabetic coma. In fact, when the acute crisis is passed, satisfactory control of hyperglycemia is often possible with oral hypoglycemic agents or diet (Goldberg, 1969).

HYPERCALCEMIA. The therapy of hypercalcemic crisis may be almost as dramatic as that of hypoglycemic coma when mental symptoms are present. A number of agents are available but the most effective appear to be the sodium salts of phosphate and sulphate, which can be given by infusion of isotonic solutions (Goldsmith et al., 1967). Sodium or potassium phosphate is effective for 6 to 15 days after the intravenous administration of 100 mM. When sodium sulphate is used in equivalent amounts (122 mM.), the drug has to be repeated within 48 to 72 hours (Kahil et al., 1967). Reports concerning metastatic calcification are conflicting but all agree that the calcium level should not be lowered too rapidly (Shackney and Hasson, 1967; Breuer and LeBauer, 1967). Consequently, the prescribed doses must be given over a period of 8 to 12 hours. The simultaneous administration of corticoids may be helpful (Cavagnini et al., 1968). Thyrocalcitonin is ineffective for calcemic crisis because of its relatively mild and slow action in reducing the serum calcium (Munson and Hirsch, 1967). Edetic acid (EDTA) which is a chelating agent of calcium, is both nephrotoxic and calcium depleting and should also be avoided. Recently, both hemodialysis and peritoneal dialysis have been advocated as the most effective method for safely reducing markedly elevated calcium levels.

HYPOCALCEMIA. When hypocalcemia is accompanied by hypoproteinemia or mild metabolic acidosis, it is rarely symptomatic. Measures to augment the serum calcium level become necessary with the onset of tetany. Immediate improvement can be obtained by the intravenous infusion of 10 per cent calcium gluconate solution in 1-gram increments. Adequate long-term support is provided in most cases by the use of oral calcium salts. Calcium chloride in doses of 300 mg. three times per day is most effective, since it forms an acid solution that favors calcium absorption and also contains a higher percentage of available calcium (Bernstein and Thorn, 1966). Occasionally, vitamin D is also required to enhance the plasma calcium levels and may be given as calciferol, 50,000 to 150,000 units daily. Interval therapy with parathyroid hormone or dihydrotachysterol is rarely necessary.

CO_2 NARCOSIS. The role of arterial carbon dioxide tension in precipitating the syndrome of CO_2 narcosis is unknown. As alluded to previously, the absolute level of hypercarbia appears less significant than its relationship with the arterial oxygen tension. When high concentrations of oxygen are administered in the presence of chronic hypercapnia and hypoxemia, progressive nervous system depression occasionally is met. The loss of respiratory drive by the peripheral chemoreceptors that are primarily responsive to hypoxemia results in progressive hypoventilation and further carbon dioxide retention. Consequently, although oxygen administration is fraught with hazard, the severe hypoxia must be relieved. Intubation and controlled ventilation with 40 per cent oxygen or compressed air is probably the safest therapeutic recourse, although occasionally supplemental oxygen can be titrated by mask or catheter without ensuing apnea until the patient can tolerate oxygen continuously. When the hypoxemic dependent respiratory drive is reduced by the administration of oxygen, respiratory stimulants such as nikethamide (Coramine), diethylaminovanillic acid (Ethamivan), and methamphetamine may be beneficial (Tyler, 1969).

Ordinarily, alkalizing agents, such as bicarbonate and THAM, should not be used since they may either worsen encephalopathy by further reducing ventilation and the cerebral spinal fluid pH (Posner and Plum, 1967) or produce fatal convulsions as a result of the rapid development of alkalosis (Ratherham et al., 1964). If assisted ventilation fails to elevate a pH below 7.2 or metabolic acidosis is present, bicarbonate therapy may be given cautiously (Ferguson and Gaensler, 1968). Hypokalemic hypochloremia, which is present in a high percentage (Dulfano and Ishikawa, 1965; Robin, 1963), is corrected by the addition of potassium chloride supplements to the fluid intake, and the over-all response to therapy should be charted by blood-gas studies and electrolyte determinations.

HYPERTHYROIDISM. Thyroid crisis is rarely met as an incidental postoperative complication or with proper preoperative preparation for thyroid surgery. Prompt recognition and effective control of hyperthermia and the hypercirculatory status are paramount for a successful outcome. External cooling should be coupled with the administration of corticoids, reserpine, and thyroid suppressive drugs to reverse the hypermetabolic state. Supplemental oxygen by mask, tent, or nasal catheter and the infusion of isotonic glucose solution containing vitamin-B complex supplements are used to cover the marked rise of oxygen and glucose consumption. Digitalis may be necessary to control high-output congestive heart failure, and supraventricular tachyarrhythmias.

HYPOTHYROIDISM. The combination of severe carbon dioxide retention and hypoxia, hypothermia, electrolyte imbalance, and altered cardiovascular responses resulting from thyroid and often adrenal insufficiency make the successful management of postoperative coma due to hypothyroidism (myxedema coma) a major therapeutic challenge (Cline et al., 1969). Thyroid replacement therapy must be carefully titrated according to response, mainly in terms of recovery from hypothermia, hypotension, and hypoventilation. Thyroprotein, thyroid extract, L-thyroxin, L-triiodothyronine, and L-triiodothyroacetic acid (Triac) have all been used, but the latter two are recommended because of their rapid onset of action and controllability when used intravenously (Hyams, 1963; Perlmutter and Cohn, 1964). Corticoids are indicated primarily because of the associated adrenal insufficiency and the danger of adrenal crisis during recovery from the hypothyroid state (Dillinger, 1963). However, they also potentiate the impaired vascular response to endogenous catecholamines, improve cardiovascular stability, and may augment the rewarming process. Severe hypoventilation alone can depress both the sensorium and vascular reactivity (Forester, 1963). It is best corrected with a respirator and the response to pulmonary support monitored with blood-gas studies. Fluid and electrolyte replacement must be controlled by attention to the net fluid balance and the serum electrolytes to prevent

further hyponatremia on one hand and cardiac decompensation on the other. Since the oxygen and, hence, circulatory demands are greatly reduced by hypothermia, the reduced body temperature is a protective response. External rewarming should, therefore, certainly be avoided until reversal of the endocrine deficiency state has begun and should be used advisedly thereafter (Hyams, 1963).

ADRENAL INSUFFICIENCY. When unexplained hypotension occurs with hyperkalemia and/or a low serum sodium in the absence of oligemia or myocardial failure, adrenal insufficiency should always be suspected. The lethal character of this deficiency in the face of major surgical or postoperative stress warrants aggressive management, particularly with the low morbidity attending the use of brief corticoid replacement therapy. The use of steroids with some mineralocorticoid activity, such as hydrocortisone sodium succinate, is preferred along with the restoration of blood volume and electrolyte replacement. Initial adjunctive therapy is best given by the parenteral route to ensure an adequate level of circulating steroids and should begin with the immediate intravenous administration of 100 mg. of hydrocortisone. Additional 100-mg. increments can be given by continuous perfusion at 8-hour intervals until the acute episode has passed (Nelson, 1964). A reduced daily maintenance dose may then be instituted or corticoids discontinued to permit evaluation of adrenal function (Adams et al., 1966).

DIABETIC COMA. Rarely, the stress of surgery or its sequelae make unrecognized demands on the known or unknown diabetic, with the result that hyperglycemic ketoacidosis emerges, which, if not reversed with exogenous insulin, may rapidly progress to coma. This is a true medical emergency in which treatment must be prompt and vigorous and, if possible, directed by someone skilled in the management of these patients. Crystalline insulin is administered both intravenously and subcutaneously in conjunction with rehydration with hypotonic solutions (Cohen et al., 1960) and the replacement of electrolytes, especially sodium, potassium, and bicarbonate. Whereas an initial response is often obtained with an insulin dose of 200 to 300 units, there is no hard and fast rule concerning total dosage. A lag period of 1 to 3 hours is common in severe acidosis before insulin effects appear (Goodner, 1965). Therapy is guided by repeated measurements of blood and urine glucose and acetone levels at frequent intervals as well as by periodic determination of the serum electrolytes. Circulatory decompensation from severe dehydration is best managed by judicious fluid replacement guided by the vital signs and the hourly urine output. The precipitating cause of uncontrolled diabetes must then be corrected.

DRUG INTOXICATION. Postoperative coma due to accidental overdosage, drug idiosyncrasy, or unsuspected potentiation and synergistic action by other agents or metabolic disturbances is treated in a manner similar to that for malicious drug intoxication, namely, by support of ventilation and circulatory function and maintenance of a state of hydration that promotes diuresis (Bunn and Lubash, 1965). In some instances, analeptics can effectively antagonize cerebral depression (Table 5-4) and, although their use is controversial, ethimivan (Emivan) and methylphenidate (Ritalin) appear to hold some promise (Hoagland and McCarty, 1963; Powell, 1960). When the latter is administered in pharmacologic doses beginning with 100 to 200 mg. by intravenous injection, it reverses the effect of chlorpromazine, reserpine, barbiturates, and Compazine, and shortens the recovery after general anesthesia (Adriani et al., 1962). The total dose is response-dependent and must be titrated accordingly (Hoagland, 1964). In addition to reversing the induced drug depression of arterial pressure, methylphenidate has the unique quality of restoring consciousness.

Central nervous system depression can also be reversed with the use of specific inhibitors, which compete for receptor sites on the cell membrane. Both nalorphine (Nalline) and levallorphan (Lorfan) are competitive inhibitors of morphine and other narcotic drugs and are themselves weak depressants. Unfortunately, there is no such agent to compete with barbiturates, although bemegride, a potent analeptic, was mistakenly thought to fill this role. This drug is even more effective than methylphenidate in causing arousal. It is given intravenously in increments of at least 50 mg., according to the response. Hemodialysis is another tool to acutely lower toxic drug levels but it probably should be reserved for phenobarbital intoxication and that caused by other long-acting depressants (Setter et al., 1966). The relative effect of analeptics in reversing drug depression is shown in Table 5-4.

HEPATIC COMA. While there is no clearcut optimal or proven therapy for the encephalopathy of liver failure, clinical experience indicates that measures must be taken to reduce the blood level of one or more potentially toxic metabolites that are ordinarily removed by the liver. Elevation of the blood ammonia derived mainly from the digestion and bacterial degradation of protein in the bowel has often been indicted as the immediate cause of hepatic coma, although there is poor correlation between the magnitude of neurologic dysfunction and the ammonia level. Signs of encephalopathy are usually present when the arterial ammonia is above 4 μg. per milliliter (normal less than 1 μg. per milliliter). However, measures to reduce ammonia selectively, such as with the ion exchange resins, have only limited effectiveness in reversing neurologic changes.

The keystone of treatment consists of restriction of dietary protein, mechanical cleansing of the bowel, and reduction of the

TABLE 5-4. Comparative Potency and Effectiveness of Analeptics

Number of Patients	Drug	Average Dose (Mg.)	Recovery Time (Min.)*
32	Bemegride	50	2 to 5
33	Methylphenidate	30	10 to 50
15	Ethamivan	50	15 to 25
14	Picrotoxin	3	20 to 25
15	Pentamethylenetetrazol	100	20 to 35
12	Nikethamide	250	30 to 35
12	Caffeine	1000	30 to 35

*Arousal times when the analeptic was given 40 minutes after 150 to 200 mg. secobarbital intravenously. Average sleeping time in control receiving same dose 3 to 5 days previously was 73 minutes.

From Adriani et al.: JAMA, 179:756, 1962.

intestinal bacterial population by bacteriocidal antibiotics such as neomycin. Once encephalopathy is established, exchange transfusion with blood or plasma (Berger et al., 1967; Burnell et al., 1967; Jones et al., 1967), coupled in some instances with large doses of corticoids, has been most effective in restoring consciousness. The efficacy of dialysis (Ritt et al., 1969), cross-perfusion with a normal volunteer (Burnell, 1965), and porcine liver perfusion (Eiseman et al., 1965) have all been disappointing and there is no substantial evidence to support the usefulness of arginine-glutamate preparations.

UREMIC COMA. Clouding of the sensorium, confusion, and progressive cerebral depression are the rule in advanced uremia and their onset appears to parallel the rate of rise of azotemia. The absence of central nervous system changes with a blood urea nitrogen level between 250 to 300 mg. per 100 ml. is not uncommon in chronic uremia, whereas much lower levels are complicated by convulsions and coma in the postoperative patient with previously normal renal function. Hyponatremia, acidosis, and dehydration may precipitate cerebral depression in the azotemic patient, along with the retention of depressant drugs ordinarily excreted by the kidneys.

When the cause of renal insufficiency is unknown, upper- and lower-tract obstructive uropathy, renal arterial or venous occlusive disease, and any other mechanical impediment to renal function must be ruled out by appropriate studies. Serial measurements of the blood urea nitrogen, creatinine, creatinine clearance, urine electrolytes, and Addis count also assist in appraising the renal status.

A number of "stop-gap" measures can and should be instituted to tide the patient over an episode of acute renal insufficiency. Most important of these are exemplary management of fluid and electrolyte balance, usually in the direction of restriction and reversal of hyperkalemia by the oral and rectal administration of ion exchange resins, such as sodium polystyrene sulfonate (Kayexalate) (Flinn et al., 1960), by correction of anoxia, acidosis, and dehydration, which all potentiate hyperkalemia, and by the infusion of hypertonic glucose solutions with or without insulin. All medications that are wholly or in part removed by the kidneys must be sharply reduced or discontinued to prevent drug intoxication. Since sepsis is a common cause

of death in renal failure, particularly from foci of infection in the lungs and urinary tract, prophylactic therapy or active definitive treatment with appropriate antibiotics is imperative. However, particular caution must be exercised with the use of streptomycin, kanamycin, colymycin, and polymyxin B during renal insufficiency.

Neuromuscular irritability can result from either hyponatremia or hypocalcemia and is controlled by replacement of the appropriate cations in hypertonic solutions. If alkalizing agents are used to correct metabolic acidosis, supplemental calcium should also be given to prevent the onset of tetany, which may be confused with uremic seizures (Earley, 1968). When progressive cerebral depression is manifested, dialysis becomes mandatory (Epstein, 1966). Hemodialysis is strongly preferred because of the rapidity of its effectiveness as well as the relative ineffectiveness of peritoneal dialysis following abdominal surgery. If repeated dialysis is likely, the insertion of an arteriovenous shunt (Scribner) will expedite the procedure and eliminate the necessity for repeated cutdowns. There is no question in our experience that an aggressive hemodialysis team will salvage many postoperative patients who would otherwise succumb to the complications of renal failure.

GENERAL CARE OF THE COMATOSE PATIENT

Since many neurologic disorders producing cerebral depression defy definitive therapeutic measures, the successful management of coma often resides in personally supervised, conscientiously delivered, day to day medical and nursing care, along with an unrelenting effort to reduce morbidity while awaiting neurologic recovery. Meanwhile, one is confronted with an imposing array of potential complications that can emerge suddenly and reverse an optimistic course. Respiratory and urinary tract infections, thrombophlebitis, parotitis and glossitis, corneal ulceration, tracheitis and tracheal bleeding, cutaneous pressure necrosis, upper-G.I. bleeding, obstipation and contractures, to mention a few, all threaten the comatose patient. Treatment must be directed to avoiding these pitfalls while maintaining the integrity of all body systems.

RESPIRATORY TRACT. Following the elimination of possible inciting causes of neurologic dysfunction and the correction of conditions predisposing to cerebral depression, therapeutic measures must initially be directed to the maintenance of adequate cardiopulmonary function, as outlined under "Emergency Measures." Satisfactory oxygenation presupposes an intact bellows system, patent airways, and unimpaired gas transfer. Measures to promote effective tracheobronchial toilet are the first line of defense against atelectasis and pneumonitis. Pulmonary care must be prophylactic as well as therapeutic and should begin with intermittent positive pressure breathing at regular intervals, complemented by periodic tracheal aspiration to stimulate coughing and assist in the removal of secretions. Needless to say, tracheal instrumentation should be avoided when the stomach is full. Standard nasal hygiene and the use of a sterile catheter and sterile glove technique will reduce the risk of contamination of the bronchial tree with pathogenic organisms. The removal of viscid secretions can be expedited by heated steam inhalation therapy, which both humidifies the air passages and produces a bronchorrhea. Periodic bronchial lavage with small increments of saline and the percutaneous intratracheal instillation of acetyl cysteine to hydrolyze the mucus component will also assist in liquefying secretions. Dilution of acetyl cysteine with saline to produce a 1:3 solution will almost eliminate the incidence of bronchospasm seen occasionally. When peripheral oxygen desaturation is suspected, serial arterial blood-gas studies should be obtained until levels are normal. If tracheostomy has been necessary, a change of tracheobronchial flora is almost inevitable. However, clinical infection can be kept to a minimum by regular cleansing of both the inner cannula and the cutaneous stoma and by use of the prescribed technique of tracheal aspiration.

CIRCULATORY SYSTEM. Cardiac decompensation is best managed by promoting an optimal environment for cardiac activity in terms of adequate oxygenation and the maintenance of fluid, electrolyte, and acid-base balance. The administration of a short-acting digitalis preparation, such as digoxin, to control heart failure provides some therapeutic malleability. When the response to the organomercurials, chlorothiazides, and other conventional diuretics is poor, potent agents such as ethacrynic acid and furosemide will often vigorously stimulate the excretion of retained fluid. Cation replacement, especially potassium, may be necessary to cover the loss of electrolytes.

Circulatory failure secondary to cardiac dysfunction is best treated with agents that do not further decrease cerebral perfusion. An isoproterenol infusion is recommended because of its lack of alpha-stimulating properties as well as its inotropic effect on the heart. Cardiac arrhythmias are usually controlled by digitalis when they are supraventricular in origin, i.e., atrial flutter-fibrillation, or by quinidine or Pronestyl, and potassium supplements when they arise from ventricular foci. In some instances, cardiac pacing or direct current cardioversion can be used effectively.

GASTROINTESTINAL TRACT. Until adequate G.I. tract function is established by the presence of bowel sounds and the passage of stools, nutritional supplements should be given intravenously to avoid vomiting and aspiration or possible bleeding from an overloaded, atonic stomach. If reflex ileus is present, as is often the case in the critically ill, intermittent suction may be necessary to both prevent the onset of abdominal distention owing to the passage of swallowed air into the small bowel as well as to keep the stomach empty. In some instances, however, the use of a nasogastric tube may be complicated by gastric irritation or superficial erosion, which manifests itself in the inevitable appearance of "coffee-ground" gastric drainage. To obviate this problem the author has found that the periodic instillation of a solution containing porcine gastric mucin is extremely useful. A commercial preparation combined with antacids and dispensed under the trade name Mucotin* is available, which, when administered in a warm aqueous solution at four- to six-hour intervals, seems to exert a protective effect that is absent with antacids alone.

Fluid replacement must be based upon the combined daily output from the urinary and G.I. tracts as well as from the estimation of the insensible loss and the daily weight. Initially, determination of serum electrolytes and carbon dioxide combining power may be necessary to guide replacement

---

*Warner-Chilcott Laboratories

therapy with exceptional losses from the gastrointestinal or urinary tract. Intake should be instituted by way of a gastric feeding tube as soon as possible to supply adequate calories, protein, and tract elements that are almost always lacking in parenteral fluids. At first, feedings should be small and given at frequent intervals to evaluate the assimilating capacity of the intestinal tract and to avoid the danger of vomiting and aspiration. When G.I. tract function is established, maintenance therapy is greatly simplified. Adequate water must be given with gastrostomy feedings containing a high-solute and high-protein concentration to avoid serum hyperosmolarity and prerenal azotemia. For the long haul, the administration of a regular house diet passed through a Waring blender probably provides the most balanced nutritional intake. Comatose patients receiving tube feedings seem predisposed to fecal impactions, as a result in part of immobilization and the lack of body tone, as well as the constituents of their nutritional supplements. Consequently, it is necessary to perform rectal examination at regular intervals and to use stool softeners such as the various liquid preparations of dioctyl sodium sulfosuccinate (Colace). One of the most common manifestations of fecal impactions is the onset of watery stools and this type of diarrhea must be distinguished from that related to the use of feedings with a high concentration of solutes. Fecal incontinence quickly results in the development of perianal excoriations and the continuously damp, contaminated, macerated presacral area becomes even more susceptible to pressure necrosis and infection. There is also a considerable danger of introducing organisms into the urinary tract from a continuously unclean perineum.

URINARY TRACT. The major prerequisite for preserving functional integrity of the urinary tract is the maintenance of sufficient hydration to provide a urinary output of at least 2000 cc. per day. An indwelling catheter is often necessary in these patients and should be inserted under surgically sterile conditions. Since hardened mucosal secretions and cellular detritus tend to build up rapidly at the urethral meatus, the catheter should be cleansed daily with a germicidal soap. This decreases the necessity for catheter replacement at intervals more frequent than every two weeks and reduces the danger of instrumental contamination of the bladder. Urinalysis and cultures should be obtained at regular intervals to detect pyuria and to define the types of bacteria that are inevitably present. Several adjuncts are advocated to suppress the urinary bacterial population and prevent the onset of clinical infection. Among these are acidification of the urine with Mandelamine, the prophylactic administration of Furadantin or a water-soluble sulfa drug, and the use of triple irrigation with or without nonabsorbable antibiotics to mechanically "flush" the bladder. If clinical urinary tract infection does not appear, appropriate systemic antibiotic therapy should be instituted.

INTEGUMENT, TRUNK, AND EXTREMITIES. The musculoskeletal system often is directly compromised by virtue of the postoperative neurologic disorder, and supportive care here must be actively carried out to prevent or delay the development of lasting deformities. In all instances, positional extremes must be avoided and the posture should be one of normal repose. Since the skin over bony prominences that are subjected to pressure may show discoloration and inflammation almost within hours, an immediate effort must be made to properly pad and protect these areas. The position of both the trunk and extremities should be changed at frequent intervals to permit unhindered circulatory perfusion of dependent parts. The skin overlying pressure areas must be carefully examined, massaged, and kept meticulously clean to prevent defects that can rapidly become ulcerated. Devices such as the "Total Flotation Therapy"* mattress or the new Silastic "Gel-Fom"** pad may provide remarkable protection. The alternating pressure "Air Mattress APP"*** is also useful. Muscle tone will be augmented by the use of passive exercises and galvanic stimulation, and early mobilization will take advantage of the effect of gravitational forces on muscle activity. The development of proprioceptive, neuromuscular facilitation exercises, which utilize all stretch and proprioceptive reflexes to restore and maintain muscle tone, is a major physiotherapeutic breakthrough (Knott and Voss, 1969). The patterned diagonal and rotary exercises that characterize this technique simulate physiologic movements and have largely replaced

---

*DePuy Manufacturing Co.
**Stryker Corp.
***Grant Airmass Corp.

the straight up and down range of motion exercises. When spasticity is present, some relief may be obtained by passive motion, hydrotherapy, and the administration of spasmolytic agents such as Valium. Well-padded splints should be used prophylactically to prevent the development of contractures, and nonforceful movements of joints will allay the development of ankylosis. In brief, physiotherapy has much to offer, particularly when it is used before deformities are established.

With the impaired ability to perceive noxious visceral sensations on one hand and the inability to communicate symptomatic impressions on the other, the comatose patient is defenseless by his own devices. He is, therefore, completely dependent on the perspicacity, fastidiousness, and perseverance of those providing care to prevent morbidity and effectively treat unavoidable complications.

There are few clinical instances that convey the rewards of an unrelenting therapeutic effort more dramatically than does the management of the patient in prolonged coma who eventually awakens. The author first recognized this fact as a medical student when he became acquainted with the nursing supervisor of a large city hospital. She had recently recovered without disability from a seven-month period of coma due to a ruptured cerebral aneurysm. Complete rehabilitation, therefore, is possible following a prolonged state of coma when medical and nursing support is intelligently organized, conscientiously directed, and sympathetically applied.

GLOSSARY

Asterixis — An intermittent, involuntary relaxation and sudden restoration of posture that is characteristic of metabolic encephalopathy.

Coma — A state of complete or almost complete loss of consciousness with no arousal by ordinary stimuli.

Delirium — A state of disordered perception, loss of attention, disorientation, and motor and sensory irritability.

Dementia — A state of mental deterioration characterized by emotional lability, abnormal affect, decreased memory, and variable loss of contact with reality.

Floccillation — An involuntary tugging at the sheets and picking of imaginary objects from the bed clothes.

Myoclonus — Abrupt, brief, lightning-like arrhythmic, involuntary contractions involving portions of muscles, entire muscles or groups of muscles regardless of their functional association.

Paratonia — A plastic-like increase of muscle tonus, present from all positions and common with diffuse metabolic and vascular brain lesions.

Stupor — A state of partial unresponsiveness to the environment, in which consciousness is impaired in varying degrees.

REFERENCES

Adams, D. A., Gold, E. M., Ganick, H. H., and Maxwell, M. H.: Adrenocortical function during intermittent corticosteroid therapy. Ann. Intern. Med., 64:542, 1966.

Adriani, J., Drake, P., and Arens, J.: Use of antagonists in drug-induced coma. JAMA, 179:752, 1962.

Aserinsky, E., and Kleitman, N.: Two types of ocular motility occurring in sleep. J. Appl. Physiol., 8:1, 1955.

Ashworth, C. J., Sacks, Y., Williams, L. F., and Byrne, J. J.: Hyperosmolar hyperglycemic non-ketotic coma: Its importance in surgical problems. Ann. Surg., 167:556, 1968.

Barnes, B. A.: Current concepts relating magnesium and surgical disease. Amer. J. Surg., 103:309, 1962.

Bennetts, F. E.: Muscular paralysis due to streptomycin following inhalation anesthesia. Anesthesia, 19:93, 1964.

Benz, H. G., Lunn, J. H., and Foldes, F. F.: Recurization by intraperitoneal antibiotics. Brit. Med. J., 2:241, 1961.

Berger, R. L., Stanton, J. R., Liversage, R. M., McGoldrick, D. M., Graham, J. H., and Stohlman, F.: Blood exchange in the treatment of hepatic coma. JAMA, 202:119, 1967.

Bernstein, D. S., and Thorn, G. W.: Diseases of the parathyroid. In Harrison, T. R., Adams, R. D., Bennett, I. L., Resnik, W. H., Thorn, G. W., and Wintrobe, M. M.: Principles of Internal Medicine. New York, McGraw-Hill Book Co., 1966, pp. 438–448.

Blair, E.: Clinical Hypothermia. New York, McGraw-Hill Book Co., 1964.

Brain, R.: The physiological basis of consciousness. Brain, 81:426, 1958.

Breuer, R. I., and LeBauer, J.: Caution in the use of phosphates in the treatment of severe hypercalcemia. J. Clin. Endocr., 27:695, 1967.

Brown, D. E.: Some considerations of physiochemical factors in hypothermia. In The Physiology of Induced Hypothermia. Publication 451, National Academy of Science, National Research Council, Washington, D.C., 1956.

Buckle, R. M.: Wernicke's encephalopathy. Studies on blood pyruvic acid and aketoglutaric acids. Acta. Neurol. Scand., 43:149, 1967.

Bunn, H. F., and Lubash, G. D.: A controlled study of induced diuresis in barbiturate intoxication. Ann. Intern. Med., 62:246, 1965.

Burnell, J. M.: Observations on cross-circulation in man. Amer. J. Med., 38:832, 1965.

Burnell, J. M., Dawborn, J. D., Epstein, R. B., Gurman, R. A., Leinvoch, G. E., Thomas, E. D., and Volwiler, W.: Acute hepatic coma treated by cross-circulation of exchange transfusion. New Eng. J. Med., 276:935, 1967.

Calderon, R., and Eisenbrey, A.: Postural ophthalmodynamometry in the surgical management of occlusive aortocranial disease. J. Neurosurg., 22:30, 1965.

Cavagnini, F., Cortellaro, M., and Praga, C.: Treatment of hypercalcemia. Lancet, 1:750, 1968.

Chalmers, T. C.: The management of hepatic coma. A continuing problem. Med. Clin. N. Amer., 52:1475, 1968.

Chapman, L. F., and Wolff, H. G.: The cerebral hemispheres and the highest integrative functions of man. Arch. Neurol., 1:357, 1959.

Claxton, C. P., McPherson, H. T., Sealy, W. C., and Young, W. G.: Hyponatremia from inappropriate antidiuretic hormone elaboration in carcinoma of the lung. J. Thorac. Cardiov. Surg., 52:331, 1966.

Cline, M. J., Williams, H. E., and Smith, L. H.: Coma in myxedema. Calif. Med., 110:61, 1969.

Cohen, A. S., Vance, V. K., Runyan, J. W., and Hurwitz, D.: Diabetic acidosis: An evaluation of the cause, course, and therapy of 73 cases. Ann. Intern. Med., 52:55, 1960.

Corrado, A. P., Ramos, A. O., and DeEscobar, C. T.: Neuro-muscular blockade by neomycin, potentiation by ether anesthesia and d-tubocurarine and antagonism by calcium and prostigmine. Arch. Int. Pharmacodyn., 121:380, 1959.

Dammann, J. F., Updike, D. J., Updike, O. L., and Bowers, D. L.: Assessment of continuous monitoring in the critically ill patient. Dis. Chest, 55:240, 1969.

Davies, D. M., Millar, E. J., and Miller, I. A.: Accidental hypothermia treated by extracorporeal blood-warming. Lancet, 1:1036, 1967.

DeJong, R. N.: The Neurologic Examination. New York, Harper & Row, 1967.

Derian, P. S.: Fat embolization — current status. J. Trauma, 5:580, 1965.

Diamond, S., Kaplitz, S., and Novick, O.: Cerebral air embolism as a complication of thoracentesis. Gen. Pract., 30:87, 1964.

Dillinger, G. R.: Myxedema and coma. J. Med. Assoc. Georgia, 52:8, 1963.

Dixon, K. C.: Ischaemia and the neurone. In Adams, C. W. M.: Neurohistochemistry. New York, Elsevier, 1965, pp. 558–598.

Dudrick, S. J., Wilmore, D. W., and Wars, H. M.: Long-term parenteral nutrition with growth, development, and positive nitrogen balance. Surgery, 64:134, 1968.

Dulfano, M. J., and Ishikawa, S.: Hypercapnia: Mental changes and extrapulmonary complications. An expanded concept of the "CO_2 intoxication" syndrome. Ann. Intern. Med., 63:829, 1965.

Earley, L. E.: Effects of uremia on the cardiovascular and central nervous system. Surg. Clin. N. Amer., 48:371, 1968.

Eckenhoff, J. E., Enderby, G. E., Larson, A., Davies, R., and Judevine, D. E.: Human cerebral circulation during deliberate hypotension and head up tilt. J. Appl. Physiol., 18:1130, 1963.

Edgahl, R. H.: Shock and the adrenal. Surg. Clin. N. Amer., 48:287, 1968.

Eiseman, B., Leim, D. S., and Raffucci, F.: Heterologous liver perfusion in treatment of hepatic failure. Ann. Surg., 162:329, 1965.

Elliott, A. C., and Wolfe, L. S.: Brain tissue respiration and glycolysis. In Elliott, D. A., Page, I., and Quastel, J. E.: Neurochemistry: The Chemistry of Brain and Nerve. Springfield, Ill., Charles C Thomas, 1962.

Epstein, F. H.: Chronic renal failure, clinical features of renal insufficiency. In Harrison, T. R., Adams, R. D., Bennett, I. L., Resnik, W. H., Thorn, G. W., and Wintrobe, M. M.: Principles of Internal Medicine. New York, McGraw-Hill Book Co., 1966, pp. 858–864.

Evanson, J. M.: Treatment of status epilepticus by muscle relaxants and artificial respiration. Lancet, 2:72, 1959.

Evarts, C. M.: Diagnosis and treatment of fat embolism. JAMA, 194:899, 1965.

Fazekas, J. F., and Alman, R. W.: Coma. Springfield, Ill., Charles C Thomas, 1962.

Ferguson, A., and Gaensler, E.: Respiratory failure and unconsciousness. Surg. Clin. N. Amer., 48:293, 1968.

Finnerty, F. A., Jr., Wilkin, L., and Fazekas, J. F.: Cerebral hemodynamics during ischemia induced by acute hypotension. J. Clin. Invest., 33:1227, 1954.

Fisher, C. M., Dalal, P. M., and Adams, R. D.: Cerebrovascular diseases. In Harrison, T. R., Adams, R. D., Bennett, I. L., Resnik, W. H., Thorn, G. W., and Wintrobe, M. M.: Principles of Internal Medicine. New York, McGraw-Hill Book Co., 1966, pp. 1146–1184.

Flinn, R. B., Merrill, J. P., and Welzant, W. R.: Treatment of the oliguric patient with a new sodium-exchange resin and sorbitol: A preliminary report. New Eng. J. Med., 264:111, 1960.

Forester, C. F.: Coma in myxedema. Arch. Intern. Med., 111:734, 1963.

French, J. D.: Brain lesions associated with prolonged unconsciousness. Arch. Neurol. Psychiat., 68:727, 1952.

French, L. A.: The use of steroids in the treatment of cerebral edema. Bull. N. Y. Acad. Med., 42:301, 1966.

Gardner, E.: Fundamentals of Neurology. 5th ed. Philadelphia, W. B. Saunders, 1968.

Garner, J. H., and Peltier, L. F.: Fat embolism: The significance of provoked petechiae. JAMA, 200:556, 1967.

Gabuzda, G. J., Phillips, G. B., and Davidson, C. S.: Reversible toxic manifestations in patients with cirrhosis of the liver given cation-exchange resins. New Eng. J. Med., 246:124, 1952.

Goldberg, M. E.: Hyperglycemic hyperosmolar nonketotic coma. Current Med. Dig., 36:302, 1969.

Goldberg, M.: Is post-surgical acute renal failure preventable? Presented at American Heart Association Postgraduate Seminar, Dallas, Texas, November, 1969.

Goldberg, M., and Reivich, M.: Studies on the mechanism of hyponatremia and impaired water excretion in myxedema. Ann. Intern. Med., 56:120, 1962.

Goldsmith, R. S., and Ingbar, S. H.: Phosphate, sulfate, and hypercalcemia. Ann. Intern. Med., 67:463, 1967.

Goodner, C. J.: Newer concepts in diabetes mellitus, including management. Disease-a-Month. Chicago, Year Book Medical Publishers, September, 1965.

Gottstein, U.: Physiologie und pathophysiologie des Hirnkruslaufs. Med. Welt., 15:715, 1965.

Grinker, R. R., and Sahs, A. L.: Neurology. Springfield, Ill., Charles C Thomas, 1966.

Guyton, A.: Textbook of Medical Physiology. 3rd ed. Philadelphia, W. B. Saunders, 1966.

Haerer, A. F.: Personal communication, 1969.

Hamilton, U. H.: Coma due to fat-embolism treated with hypothermia and dehydration. Lancet, 2:994, 1964.

Handa, J.: Serial brain scanning with technetium 99 M and scintillation camera. Amer. J. Roentgen., 106:708, 1969.

Hardesty, W. H., Roberts, B., Toole, J. F., and Royster, H. P.: Studies on carotid artery flow. Surgery, 49:251, 1961.

Hardy, J. D.: On the reversibility of strokes. Case of carotid artery repair with prompt recovery after hemiplegia and coma for two days. Ann. Surg., 158:1035, 1963.

Hardy, J. D.: Surgery of the Aorta and Its Branches. Philadelphia, J. B. Lippincott, 1960.

Henderson, L. W., and Merrill, J. P.: Treatment of barbiturate intoxication. Ann. Intern. Med., 64:876, 1966.

Hill, F. C.: Evaluation of the unconscious patient. Rocky Mountain Med. J., 62:54, 1965.

Hoagland, R. J.: Analeptic treatment of coma. Hawaii Med. J., 23:103, 1964.

Hoagland, R. J., and McCarty, R. J.: Treatment of drug-induced coma: Effectiveness of methylphenidate. Amer. J. Med. Sci., 245:189, 1963.

Hogg, S., and Renwick, W.: Hyperpyrexia during anesthesia. Canad. Anaesth. Soc. J., 13:429, 1966.

Holder, T. M.: Thoracic surgery in infants. In Gibbon, J. H., Sabiston, D. C., and Spencer, F. C.: Surgery of the Chest. Philadelphia, W. B. Saunders, 1969, pp. 108–119.

Hollenberg, N. K.: The renal response to surgery. Presented at American Heart Association, Postgraduate Seminar, Dallas, Texas, November, 1969.

Hurwitz, D.: Hypoglycemia and hyperglycemic coma. Surg. Clin. N.Amer., 48:361, 1968.

Hyams, D. E.: Hypothermic myxedema coma. Brit. J. Clin. Pract., 17:1, 1963.

Hymes, A. C., Safavian, M. H., Arbulu, A., and Baute, P.: A comparison of Pluronic F-68 low molecular weight dextran, mannitol, and saline as priming agents in the heart-lung apparatus. J. Thorac. Cardiov. Surg., 56:16, 1968.

Ibarra-Perez, C., Ersek, R. A., and Lillehei, C. W.: A trapping device to prevent calcium embolism during the removal and replacement of heart valves. J. Cardiov. Surg., 10:155, 1969.

Ingvar, D. H., Haggendal, E., Nillson, N. J., Sourander, P., Wickbom, I., and Lassen, N. A.: Cerebral circulation and metabolism in a comatose patient. Arch. Neurol., 11:13, 1964.

Ivy, H. K.: Myxedema precoma: Complications and therapy. Mayo Clin. Proc., 40:403, 1965.

Johnson, B. B.: Personal communication, 1969.

Jones, E. A., Clair, D., Clink, H. M., MacGillivary, M., and Sherlock, S.: Hepatic coma due to acute necrosis treated by exchange blood transfusion. Lancet, 2:169, 1967.

Kahil, M., Orman, B., Gyorkey, F., and Brown, H.: Hypercalcemia; experience with phosphate and sulfate therapy. JAMA, 201:721, 1967.

Katzman, R.: Effect of electrolyte disturbance on the central nervous system. Ann. Rev. Med., 17:197, 1966.

Kety, S. S.: Circulation and metabolism of the human brain in health and disease. Amer. J. Med., 8:205, 1950.

Kety, S. S., and Schmidt, C. F.: The effects of altered arterial tensions of carbon dioxide and oxygen on cerebral blood flow and cerebral oxygen consumption of normal young men. J. Clin. Invest., 27:484, 1948.

Knott, M., and Voss, D.: Proprioceptive Neuromuscular Facilitation. New York, Harper & Row, 1969.

Kuner, J., and Goldman, A.: Prolonged nasotracheal intubation in adults. Dis. Chest, 31:270, 1967.

Kurze, T., Dyck, P., and Barrows, H.: Neurosurgical evaluation of ultrasonic encephalograph. J. Neurosurg., 22:437, 1965.

Langerbeam, J. K.: Central venous pressure monitoring. Amer. J. Surg., 110:220, 1965.

Larson, A. G.: Deliberate hypotension. Anesthesiology, 25:682, 1964.

Leavitt, M. A., and Polansky, B. J.: Cardiogenic aspects of shock and coma. Surg. Clin. N. Amer., 48:273, 1968.

Lenaghan, R., Silva, Y. J., and Walt, A. J.: Hemodynamic alterations associated with expansion rupture of the lung. Arch. Surg., 99:339, 1969.

Levinsky, W. J.: Fatal air embolism during insertion of CVP monitoring apparatus. JAMA, 209:1721, 1969.

Linscheid, R., and Dines, D.: The fat-embolism syndrome. Surg. Clin. N. Amer., 49:1137, 1969.

Locke, S.: The neurological aspects of coma. Surg. Clin. N. Amer., 48:251, 1968.

Macdonald, F. M.: Respiratory acidosis. Arch. Intern. Med., 116:689, 1965.

Maddock, R. K., and Bloomer, H. A.: Meprobamate overdosage. JAMA, 201:123, 1967.

Maffly, R. H.: The management of the oliguric postoperative patient with cardiac insufficiency. Presented at American Heart Association Postgraduate Seminar, Dallas, Texas, November, 1969.

Maher, J. F., Schreiner, G. E., and Westervett, F. B.: Acute glutethimide intoxication. Amer. J. Med., 33:70, 1962.

Maier, W. P., Goldman, L. I., and Rosemond, G. P.: Central venous pressure monitoring. Penn. Med. J., 72:58, 1969.

Mangold, R.: Effects of sleep and lack of sleep on cerebral circulation and metabolism of normal young men. J. Clin. Invest., 34:1092, 1955.

Marshall, J.: The Management of Cerebrovascular Disease. Boston, Little, Brown and Co., 1968.

Matloff, J. M., Collins, J. J., Jr., and Sullivan, J. M.: Control of thromboembolism from prosthetic heart valves. Ann. Thorac. Surg., 8:133, 1969.

McDermott, W. V., Jr.: Liver disease in the differential diagnosis of coma. Surg. Clin. N. Amer., 48:327, 1968.

McDermott, W. V., Jr.: Postoperative liver failure and complications of shunt surgery. In Artz, C. P., and Hardy, J. D.: Complications in Surgery and Their Management. 2nd. ed., Philadelphia, W. B. Saunders, 1967, pp. 196–203.

McHenry, L. C., Fazekas, J. F., and Sullivan, J. F.:

Cerebral hemodynamics of syncope. Amer. J. Med. Sci., 241:173, 1961.

McKown, C. H., Verhulst, H. L., and Crotty, J. J.: Overdosage effects and danger from tranquilizer drugs. JAMA, 185:425, 1963.

McQueen, J. D.: Effects of cold on the nervous system. In The Physiology of Induced Hypothermia. Publication 451, National Academy of Sciences, National Research Council, Washington, D.C., 1956.

Merrill, J. P.: Differential diagnosis of post-operative oliguria. Presented at American Heart Association Postgraduate Seminar, Dallas, Texas, November, 1969.

Michenfelder, J. D., and Theye, R. A.: Hypothermia. Effect on canine brain and whole body metabolism. Anesthesiology, 29:1107, 1968.

Michenfelder, J. D., Martin, J. T., Altenburg, B. M., and Rehder, K.: Air embolism during neurosurgery. JAMA, 208:1353, 1969.

Miller, R. B.: Central nervous system manifestations of fluid and electrolyte disturbances. Surg. Clin. N. Amer., 48:381, 1968.

Miller, R. B.: Fluid and electrolyte disturbances. In Packman, R. C.: Manual of Medical Therapeutics. Boston, Little, Brown and Co., 1966.

Minard, F. N.: Relationships among pyridoxal phosphate, vitamin B_6-deficiency and convulsions induced by 1,1-dimethylhydrazine. J. Neurochem., 14:681, 1967.

Mitchell, R. A., Loeschke, H. H., and Severinghaus, J. W.: Respiratory responses mediated through superficial chemosensitive areas of the medulla. J. Appl. Physiol., 18:523, 1963.

Modell, J. H.: Septicemia as a cause of immediate postoperative hyperthermia. Anesthesiology, 27:329, 1966.

Moruzzi, G., Fessard, A., and Jasper, H. H.: Brain Mechanisms. Amsterdam, Progress in Brain Research, 1963, p. 493.

Munson, P. L., and Hirsch, P. F.: Discovery and pharmacologic evaluation of thyrocalcitonin. Amer. J. Med., 43:678, 1967.

Murley, A. H. G.: Coma due to fat-embolism. Lancet, 2:1120, 1964.

Nathanson, M., and Bergman, P.: The evaluation of the unconscious patient. Including oculocephalic and vestibulo-ocular testing. J. Mount Sinai Hosp., 33:252, 1966.

Nelson, D. H.: Treatment of adrenal insufficiency. Gen. Pract., 29:135, 1964.

Norcross, J. W.: The management of hepatic coma. Med. Clin. N.Amer., 46:1313, 1962.

Pautler, S., Cimons, I., Cauna, D., Totten, R., and Safar, P.: Pulmonary oxygen toxicity at one ATA. Acta. Anaesth. Scand. (Supplement 24), 10:51, 1966.

Peltier, L. F.: The diagnosis of fat embolism. Surg. Gynec. Obstet., 121:371, 1965.

Perlmutter, M., and Cohn, H.: Myxedema crisis of pituitary or thyroid origin. Amer. J. Med., 36:883, 1964.

Pevehouse, B., and Brown, B.: Cerebral angiography. Its use in acute head injuries and undiagnosed coma. Calif. Med., 97:268, 1962.

Plum, F., and Posner, J. B.: Diagnosis of Stupor and Coma. Philadelphia, F. A. Davis, 1966.

Plum, F., and Swanson, A. G.: Barbiturate poisoning treated by physiological methods. JAMA, 163:827, 1957.

Posner, J. B., and Plum, F.: Spinal-fluid pH and neuro-logic symptoms in systemic acidosis. New Eng. J. Med., 227:605, 1967.

Posner, J. B., Swanson, A. G., and Plum, F.: Acid-base balance in cerebrospinal fluid. Arch. Neurol., 12:479, 1965.

Powell, J. R.: Treating the comatosed patient. Value of methylphenidate. Texas J. Med., 56:363, 1960.

Procter, D. S. C.: Coma in burns—the cause traced to dressings. S. Amer. Med. J., 40:1116, 1966.

Quastel, J. H.: Effects of anesthetics, depressants, and tranquilizers on brain metabolism. In Elliott, D. A., Page, I., and Quastel, J. E.: Neurochemistry: The Chemistry of Brain and Nerve, Springfield, Ill., Charles C Thomas, 1962.

Randall, R. E., Jr., Cohen, M. D., Spray, C. C., Jr., and Rossmeisl, E. G.: Hypermagnesemia in renal failure: Etiology and toxic manifestations. Ann. Intern. Med., 61:73, 1964.

Ream, C. R.: Respiratory and cardiac arrest after intravenous administration of kanamycin with reversal of toxic effects of neostigmine. Ann. Intern. Med., 59:384, 1963.

Ritt, D. J., Whelan, G., Werner, D. J., Eigenbrodt, E. H., Shenker, S., and Combes, B.: Acute hepatic necrosis with stupor or coma. Medicine, 48:151, 1969.

Robin, E. D.: Abnormalities of acid-base regulation in chronic pulmonary disease. With special reference to hypercapnia and extracellular alkalosis. New Eng. J. Med., 268:917, 1963.

Robin, E. D.: Restrictive and diffusional pulmonary disorders. In Harrison, T. R., Adams, R. D., Bennett, I. L., Resnik, W. H., Thorn, G. W., and Wintrobe, M. M.: Principles of Internal Medicine. New York, McGraw-Hill Book Co., 1966, pp. 910–925.

Robinson, J. S.: Therapeutic use of the muscle relaxants. Brit. J. Anaesth., 35:570, 1963.

Rosenberg, I. N.: Hypothyroidism and coma. Surg. Clin. N. Amer., 48:353, 1968.

Rosomoff, H. L., and Safar, R.: Pathophysiology and general patient care. Clin. Anesth., 1:244, 1965.

Rotheram, E. B., Jr., Safar, P., and Robin, E. D.: CNS disorder during mechanical ventilation in chronic pulmonary disease. JAMA, 189:993, 1964.

Ruesch, M., Miyatake, S., and Ballinger, C. M.: Continuing hazard of air embolism during pressure transfusions. JAMA, 172:1476, 1960.

Ryan, K. J., Schaenuck, L. I., Hickman, R. O., and Striker, G. E.: Colistimethate toxicity. JAMA, 207:2099, 1969.

Saidman, L. J., Haraad, E. S., and Enger, E. I.: Hyperthermia during anesthesia. JAMA, 190:1029, 1964.

Sanders, C. A.: Prosthetic problems. New Eng. J. Med., 281:501, 1969.

Schaefer, H.: Psychosomatic problems in vegetative regulatory function. In Eccles, J. C.: Brain and Conscious Experience, New York, Springer-Verlag, 1966.

Scheibel, M. E., and Scheibel, A. B.: Anatomical basis of attention mechanisms in vertebrate brains. In Quarton, G. C., Melnechuk, T., and Schmitt, F. O.: The Neurosciences. New York, The Rockefeller University Press, 1967.

Schwartz, T. B., and Apfelbaum, R. I.: Yearbook of Endocrinology, Chicago, Year Book Medical Publishers, 1965–66.

Selenkow, H. A., and Ingbar, S. H.: Diseases of the thyroid. In Harrison, T. R., Adams, R. D., Bennett, I. L., Resnik, W. H., Thorn, G. W., and Wintrobe, M. M.: Principles of Internal Medicine. New York, McGraw-Hill Book Co., 1966, pp. 421–438.

Setter, J. G., Maher, J. F., and Schreiner, G. E.: Barbiturate intoxication. Arch. Intern. Med., *117:*224, 1966.

Shackney, S., and Hasson, J.: Precipitous fall in serum calcium, hypotension and acute renal failure after intravenous phosphate therapy for hypercalcemia. Ann. Intern. Med., *66:*906, 1967.

Sherlock, S., Read, A. E., Laidlaw, J., and Haslam, F.: Chlorothiazide in hepatic cirrhosis. Ann. N. Y. Acad. Sci., *71:*430, 1958.

Shulman, R.: A survey of vitamin B_{12} deficiency in an elderly psychiatric population. Brit. J. Psychiat., *113:*241, 1967.

Sieker, H. O., and Hickman, J. B.: Carbon dioxide intoxication: The clinical syndrome, its etiology and management with particular reference to the use of mechanical respirators. Medicine, *35:*389, 1956.

Small, G. A.: Respiratory paralysis after large dose of intraperitoneal polymyxin B and bacitracin. Anesth. Analg., *43:*137, 1964.

Smith, B. H.: Principles of Clinical Neurology. Chicago, Year Book Medical Publishers, 1965.

Sokoloff, L.: *In* Field, J., Magoun, H. W., and Hall, V. E.: Handbook of Physiology, Section I. Neurophysiology, Vol. III, Washington, D.C., American Physiological Society, 1960, p. 1849.

Swanson, A. G., Stavney, L. S., and Plum, F.: Effects of blood pH and carbon dioxide on cerebral electrical activity. Neurology, *8:*787, 1958.

Tedeschi, C. G., Walter, C. E., and Tedeschi, L. G.: Shock and fat embolism: An appraisal. Surg. Clin. N. Amer., *48:*431, 1968.

Thomas, J. E., and Klass, D. W.: Evaluation of the comatose patient. Postgrad. Med., *36:*207, 1964.

Tyler, M. D.: Personal communication, 1969.

Unger, R. H.: The riddle of tumor hypoglycemia. Amer. J. Med., *40:*325, 1966. (Editorial).

Watanakumakorn, C., Hodges, R. E., and Evans, T. C.: Myxedema. Arch. Intern. Med., *116:*183, 1965.

Wilson, R. D., Nichols, R. J., Dent, T. E., and Allen, C. R.: Disturbances of oxidative phosphorylation mechanism as a possible etiology factor in sudden unexplained hyperthermia occurring during anesthesia. Anesthesiology, *27:*231, 1966.

Wolfman, E. F., Coon, W. W., and Kahn, E. A.: The recognition and management of severe hypertonicity of the extracellular fluid associated with cerebral lesions. Surgery, *47:*410, 1968.

Wright, E. S., Sarkozy, E., Dobell, A. R. C., and Murphy, D. R.: Fat globulinemia in extracorporeal circulation. Surgery, *53:*500, 1963.

Yeakel, A. E.: Lethal air embolism from plastic blood-storage container. JAMA, *204:*267, 1968.

CHAPTER 6

MASSIVE ABDOMINAL INJURY IN CIVILIAN PRACTICE

by J. D. MARTIN, Jr., M.D.

John Daniel Martin, Jr., is a distinguished Georgian who was elected to both Phi Beta Kappa and Alpha Omega Alpha at Emory University and Medical School. Following his residency there, he had special training in Vienna before joining the Emory faculty where he was ultimately made Joseph B. Whitehead Professor and Chairman of the Department in 1957. Although heavily involved in teaching at all levels and in administration and clinical surgery, he has continuously pursued his investigations in the field of trauma and burns to become an outstanding authority in this field. He has served with the Grady Memorial Hospital since 1930, becoming Chief of Surgery in 1961. It is from this extensive experience that the following discussion is derived.

There is no condition the surgeon may be called upon to treat that is more critical than trauma to the abdomen. In this era of high-speed transportation, with the desire to get to our destinations scarcely before we start, it is inevitable that massive trauma can be expected. Not only speed, but the inability to control the vehicle both on busy super-highways and on remote roads less geared to modern transportation, is responsible for many accidents.

A factor that compounds the problem is that these injuries often occur in the less-populated regions some distance from medical centers. This frequently overburdens the already taxed medical profession and facilities. Whether they desire it or not, all hospitals must be equipped to receive, evaluate, and manage those conditions that require immediate treatment. An appreciation of this responsibility is mandatory for those who treat such conditions.

The evaluation of the bluntly traumatized abdomen is the most important consideration in the early management of these critical injuries. The decision as to whether or not there is intra-abdominal involvement is an extremely difficult one and requires the utilization of every known method of evaluation. If a wound of entrance is present, there is little doubt, in most cases, that an exploration should be made; however, occasionally ob-

scure evidence may require a delay, perhaps for the manifestation of more obvious symptoms, before proceeding. There are few clues that are absolutely infallible. Experience in management is necessary to evaluate the clinical appearance, which may be influenced by other injuries, particularly those involving the chest and head.

The prognosis for patients with associated intracranial and pulmonary trauma is adversely affected by an unnecessary exploratory abdominal operation. On the other hand, these patients cannot tolerate a delay in the correction of intra-abdominal injury. Thus, after the assessment of the patient with multiple injuries, the first consideration should be: Is there an associated abdominal injury that may complicate the entire problem? No doubt, in some instances, a delay may be necessary for some change in the patient's general condition to specifically dictate surgical intervention. The mechanism of the injury may determine certain expected forms of trauma. For example, when the driver of an automobile sustains a steering-wheel injury, one can suspect trauma to the upper abdomen or chest wall, as well as accompanying cardiac, pancreatic, duodenal, and mesenteric injuries as a result of the localized force exerted on this area. If there is a resulting fracture of the lower rib cage, the liver and spleen must be suspected. Crush-

120

ing injuries to the lower pelvis, resulting in massive fractures, should always be suspected of producing damaged viscera in the lower abdomen, particularly the urinary bladder and the urethra, with a frequent loss of a large quantity of blood in the retroperitoneal area.

EVALUATION OF THE TRAUMATIZED ABDOMEN

In the evaluation of the abdomen, there are specific findings that must be considered indicative of intra-abdominal trauma. After an over-all assessment of the degree of shock and associated injuries, the immediate vital signs upon inspection of the abdomen should reveal noteworthy evidence of abdominal involvement (Martin and Adams, 1958). The pulse and blood pressure are of considerable value in estimating the massiveness of intra-abdominal hemorrhage. Repeated observation will determine whether the bleeding continues and whether fluid replacement, particularly of blood, is adequate. It has been suggested that when vital signs are affected by an increase in the pulse rate to more than 100, a 10 per cent reduction in blood volume has occurred; whereas, with the pulse over 120 or a blood pressure of 90/60 in a previously normal individual, this is evidence of at least a 20 per cent blood-volume reduction (Stone and Martin, 1969).

Careful inspection of the abdomen may confirm the occurrence of such an injury. Increased respiratory movements are commonly encountered in massive abdominal trauma. If marked distention occurs immediately after the injury, intra-abdominal trauma is indicated. This carries with it a serious prognosis and signifies the rupture of a hollow viscus or massive bleeding. Any local evidence of associated contusion, bruises, or ecchymosis offers further confirmation. On palpation, the muscle spasm is dependent upon the contusion to the abdominal wall and also the severity of the injury within the abdomen and subsequent irritation of the peritoneum. A rigid abdomen indicates either chemical or bacterial contamination, while a mild accompaniment of muscle spasm may be the only indication of hemoperitoneum. Rebound tenderness associated with muscle spasm is usually evidence of intra-abdominal trauma. A mass is not found except in the late stages when a localized hematoma has occurred. Peristalsis may be diminished or absent; however, intra-abdominal trauma can also exist with peristalsis present.

Rectal examination may be significant. Extreme tenderness, the presence of blood on the examining finger, or a palpable mass from a localized hematoma, particularly one associated with pelvic fracture, may be found. Following injuries to the bladder or the urethra, an anterior mass of collected blood and urine may be felt.

The introduction of a nasogastric tube into the stomach may be useful in the aspiration of the stomach contents, which may reveal blood and further indicate intra-abdominal trauma. The tube may also be of considerable value in lessening distention in preparing for further diagnosis. The insertion of an indwelling catheter into the bladder assists in determining urinary tract injuries to either the bladder or kidney, and it also serves as an important aid in determining the function of these organs if the patient is in a state of shock.

RADIOLOGIC EXAMINATIONS

In most instances sufficient time is afforded to obtain radiologic examination, which may be helpful in the diagnosis. In rare instances, however, as in the presence of uncontrolled shock, the time spent in the x-ray department may be critical to the patient's life unless immediate control of the massive bleeding has been achieved. Perhaps the most useful radiologic examination in determining the intra-abdominal trauma is the flat, upright, and lateral decubitus abdominal film. The visualization of the individual loops of intestine, space in the upper lumbar regions, and the depths of the pelvis should be studied closely for the presence of extraluminal gas, particularly following duodenal and rectal perforations. Free fluid may separate one segment of intestine from another and from the lateral wall of the peritoneal cavity. Lower rib fractures are frequently associated with kidney, spleen, and liver injuries. If the pelvis is fractured, particularly the pubic bones, rupture of the bladder or urethra should be considered. When vertebral fractures have occurred, injuries to the pancreas and liver should be suspected.

Following splenic injuries, a displacement of the air pattern in the upper abdomen may be seen. Introducing air into the nasogastric tube can help the physician to note the displacement of the stomach and the characteristically serrated edges of the greater curvature in the attachment of the short gastric arterial branches to the spleen. Introduction of Gastrografin or thin barium likewise may be helpful. The examination of the chest may show the presence or absence of fluid and air within the pleural space, and also the presence or absence of rib fractures and evidence of injuries to the mediastinum and great vessels in the thorax. These conditions may require attention before suspected intra-abdominal injuries. In a situation in which the diaphragm has been ruptured, the presence of the intestines above the diaphragm may be seen without difficulty.

The evaluation of the urinary tract for injuries is mandatory both for diagnostic purposes and also to avoid difficulties during the operation. Intravenous pyelogram can be helpful for determining the presence or absence of injuries and, in addition, evidence of kidney function. However, it must be remembered that an individual in shock may have kidney function impaired to such a degree that an intravenous pyelogram would not be valid.

Cystograms and urethrograms are extremely helpful when properly carried out. These should always be done when injuries to the pelvis have occurred or when there is evidence of bleeding or other trauma in the liver, bladder, or urethra.

ABDOMINAL ASPIRATIONS

Much has been written about paracentesis as a diagnostic aid in recognizing and determining the presence or absence of intra-abdominal trauma. A negative, four-quadrant aspiration is worthless for confirmation of intra-abdominal injury. When the examination is made, it is extremely important that it be carried out under adequate circumstances to obtain complete information. With the patient lying supine, an 18-gauge needle is introduced with an attached 10 ml. syringe. While this is being done, the patient is requested to hold his breath to reduce the likelihood of lacerating an abdominal viscus. Dilute blood that fails to clot has probably been obtained from the peritoneal cavity; however, blood that clots is most often indicative of a false positive result. Cloudy fluid may suggest a pre-existing intra-abdominal inflammatory process or chemical peritonitis, which occurred when aspiration was done some hours after the injury. In some instances, the intestine may be entered and the contents aspirated, but this does not usually cause a very serious problem.

The second method of abdominal paracentesis may be accomplished by inserting a small trocar in the lower quadrant of the abdomen and placing a small catheter through the lumen of the trocar. With the trocar in place, normal saline can be infused into the peritoneal cavity and then aspirated. Blood obtained in moderate quantities is significant, but a negative aspiration may be more significant.

LABORATORY FINDINGS

Laboratory evaluations have limited value except in cases in which there are sudden variations from the normal or initial hemoglobin and hematocrit determinations, taken upon admission of the patient. The initial hematocrit and hemoglobin may show evidence of pre-existing anemia and may be useful for comparison with later determinations and in estimating blood volume loss and adequacy of blood replacement. Initial specific blood volume determinations, and also those of patients in shock, are notoriously inadequate and sometimes confusing.

A significant elevation of the white blood count within a few hours following injury denotes massive contamination of the peritoneal cavity from bowel contents or other irritating substances. Liver or splenic injuries are likewise suspected in the presence of a large quantity of bile or blood.

There are certain chemical analyses that may be significant within the first 24 hours. In the presence of injury to the pancreas, there is a rise in the value of the serum amylase. Trauma to the pancreas may show a brief elevation or a rising amylase but later may become more marked if a pseudocyst develops.

An elevation of the serum bilirubin may be variously interpreted by noting the absorption of blood and the breakdown products of the blood. These products are reduced within serous-lined cavities and hematomas associated with injuries, such as fractures of the pelvis or liver injury, particularly in patients with pre-existing liver diseases. It must be remembered that the administration of large quantities of blood to the trauma patient may lead to liver damage subsequent to mismatched blood.

Proctoscopic examination may afford some value, particularly for injuries to the rectum and rectosigmoid. Such an examination should be done with precaution in view of difficulties encountered from patients unable to cooperate. Frequently this cannot be done except under anesthesia, but the risks involved may outweigh the benefits for the critically ill patient.

Cystoscopic examination, however, may be more beneficial and sometimes offers practical assistance in determining the presence or absence of injury to the bladder. A definitive and thorough evaluation of the kidney and its ability to function is obtained by means of a retrograde pyelogram; it is more complete than that obtained by an intravenous pyelogram. Occasionally, a selective angiography may be helpful in determining the site where the retroperitoneal hemorrhage has occurred. This is particularly noteworthy following pelvic fractures because at the time of operation one cannot be certain of the presence or absence of injury to the hypogastric artery, and knowledge before laparotomy is considerably helpful.

ABDOMINAL WALL

The abdominal wall may be injured without associated involvement of the peritoneal cavity. The major concern on examination is whether or not penetration of the abdominal wall has taken place. There are a number of surgeons who have emphasized that differentiation should be made between these injuries and that an exploratory laparotomy can be avoided.

It has been recommended that radiographic examination of the abdominal wall following the introduction of sodium diatrizoate (Hypaque) through a previously placed catheter into the wound of entrance be done (Tobias et al., 1967). A pursetring suture should be placed around the catheter to secure it (Fig. 6-1). The results obtained following the injection of this material may aid in differentiation. However, a carefully performed laparotomy should prove most satisfactory.

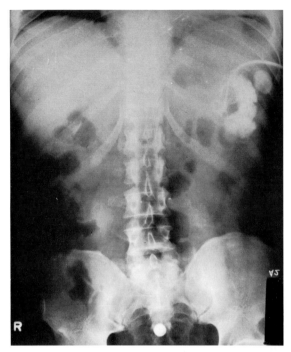

Figure 6-1. Roentgenogram after the introduction into the stab tract of Hypaque, showing that the material does not penetrate the abdominal cavity.

Recently, much enthusiasm has been expressed for refraining from exploring stab wounds until obvious signs of peritoneal irritation exist. Under carefully controlled circumstances when one person is observing these patients, the results may be satisfactory (Cohn). In an adequately performed exploration of the abdomen, there is minimal or no risk. In a recent review of 100 patients (Grady Memorial Hospital) explored for stab wounds, there was only one death (Woodhams). This was associated with a massive injury to a major vessel which resulted in exsanguination.

HEMATOMAS

The rectus abdominis muscle is divided by a series of transverse inscriptions. When an episode of severe, sudden stress occurs along the long axis of this muscle, a vessel may be torn, with a resultant hemorrhage into one of the segments of this muscle, confining the hematoma to this section. This may occur during pregnancy or when a paratrooper lands following a jump, producing a stretching of the rectus muscle. Martin and Thompson in 1957 reported an elderly patient who had a rupture of the transversalis fascia below the semicircular fold of Douglas, resulting in an accumulation of a large quantity of blood beneath the muscle.

Recognition of this condition is essential to avoid an unnecessary exploratory laparotomy. Bouchacourt's sign aids in the differentiation between a mass in the abdominal wall and within the abdominal cavity. When the trunk and the shoulders are raised from the examining table, a mass within the abdominal cavity may no longer be palpable. However, a mass localized to the abdominal wall usually becomes more prominent.

When one is certain that the mass is within the abdominal wall, aspiration of the hematoma may result in rapid resolution. When one is not certain, an exploratory laparotomy is in order.

Crushing trauma, particularly when the force is of a compressing character, may be limited to the abdominal wall, although involvement of the structures in the abdominal cavity frequently occurs. When destruction or loss of soft tissue of the abdominal wall occurs, an assessment must be made and utilization of all structures available must be carried out to correct this defect either with or without intra-abdominal involvement. When intra-abdominal involvement occurs, this becomes paramount and correction of this injury must be instituted immediately. The devitalized skin and fascia should be excised to avoid consequent infections, which should be limited as much as possible.

Wound infections may be manifested under many circumstances but more frequently when there has been an associated penetration of the abdominal cavity and perforation of a viscus. Protection of the wound, adequate irrigation with normal saline, careful closure and the utilization of the basic surgical principles assist in lessening these difficulties. Dehiscence of the wound occurs very infrequently unless there is an associated infection or marked debility, as in individuals who develop fistulas from the gastrointestinal tract. If adequate care has not been exercised, and there has not been sufficient restoration of blood, healing may be delayed and evisceration through these weakened wounds may be the consequence.

EXPLORATION

Once the decision has been made for exploration, certain factors are important: the general health status of the patient; the availability of proper anesthesia; the likelihood of associated injuries outside the abdomen; attention to factors that would interfere with a safe abdominal exploration, such as comatose head injuries, a flail chest injury, and massive unstabilized fractures of the extremities. Only after a thorough evaluation of all problems may one safely proceed with the exploratory laparotomy.

One should not proceed with extensive examination or treatment, except in the most severe emergency, without having access to an adequate amount of blood. The value of properly administered anesthesia should not be underestimated in the final outcome of critical intra-abdominal trauma. If administration of anesthesia is of the highest quality, one can safely proceed with an orderly and satisfactory exploration. Thorough preliminary planning for anesthesia is imperative to avoid considerable waste of time, needless unproductive effort, and iatrogenic difficulties.

The incision should be extensive enough to allow thorough, adequate evaluation and control of any situation that may be encountered within the abdominal cavity. For this reason, vertical incisions serve most advantageously, although there are certain disadvantages with this type of incision. The benefit, however, is obvious in that the incision can be extended in either direction to allow for a complete evaluation of all the injuries that might have occurred within the abdominal cavity. When the diaphragm and the upper abdomen are involved as well as the lower thoracic injuries, a planned thoracoabdominal incision may be made either on the right or left side, as the case may be, in order to approach the abdominal and thoracic cavities and to manage combined problems. This is particularly true when subtotal resections of the liver may be encountered or a particularly difficult injury to the upper stomach or to the spleen has occurred with an associated diaphragmatic rupture or perforation.

An orderly exploration of the abdomen should be made beginning with an evaluation of the contents in situ. The presence or absence of blood, bile, or gastrointestinal contents can be immediately determined. These substances, found separately or in conjunction with others, indicate in which direction one should proceed. In the presence of continued bleeding, immediate control of the site of bleeding is required in order to avoid unnecessary blood loss and exsanguination of the patient. Compression of the aorta by means of digital compression or with aortic clamps may be extremely beneficial. On the other hand, it must be remembered that in instances in which the bleeding is of a venous nature, particularly from torn venae cavae, exsanguination may occur in spite of total compression of the aorta. Under those circumstances, adequate incision and a rapid evaluation of the site of bleeding are in order to digitally compress and control venous as well as arterial bleeding.

After control of bleeding, carefully detailed and thorough exploration of the abdomen should be made: starting first in the upper quadrant, evaluate the spleen and liver and their attachments and blood supply; then explore the stomach, the pancreas, the kidneys, and the retroperitoneal areas in which a hidden loss of blood can take place. Then one can proceed with the complete evaluation of the small and large intestines; most often this necessitates visualizing every segment of these structures. Only in this way can one determine the exact location of the significant injury and proceed with the major problem without undue attention to those of lesser degree.

STOMACH AND DUODENUM

Following the evaluation and exploration of the entire intestinal tract, attention to the specific organs must be given and especially injuries to the stomach. Since it occupies such a large part of the upper abdomen, it requires an immediate consideration. These wounds may be divided according to the site and type of injury: (1) the esophagogastric junction, (2) the body of the stomach, and (3) the pyloric area (Thoroughman and Haynes, 1969). The esophagogastric junction is the first to be overlooked and certainly is the most difficult to manage. A thoracoabdominal incision affords the very best exposure and should be utilized when there is any doubt. Small perforations from stab wounds or bullets can be closed without difficulty and

usually most successfully by the two-layer method, followed by the maintenance of nasogastric suction for a short period postoperatively. With shotgun blasts or extensive trauma, esophagogastrectomy may be required. When these injuries are involved with other structures, particularly the liver and the great vessels, attention must be given to them before the stomach is repaired. The massive injuries to the esophagogastric area should be thoroughly debrided, and a closure of the proximal end of the stomach and reimplantation of the esophagus into the fundus instituted. Following such a procedure, the performance of pyloroplasty is mandatory for adequate postoperative function.

More frequently, the main body of the stomach may be involved and it is well to evaluate both the anterior and posterior walls of the stomach before proceeding, to determine if a primary closure will be adequate and to be certain that there are no perforations on the posterior wall. It is essential that blood supply be adequate on completion of either the closure of the perforation or resection of a segment of the pylorus. When the pylorus is involved, restorative procedures can be totally satisfactory without resection. In rare instances a pyloroplasty may be done when viability is unquestioned. In some instances a jejunal patch may be utilized.

In most injuries to the stomach, the performance of a vagotomy is contraindicated to avoid late stasis. Gastric dilatation can be lessened by the nasogastric tube, but in some instances a tube gastrostomy may serve more effectively as a means of decompression. Once you are committed to such a means, it is essential that the tube be kept in place in order to effectively perform its function.

DUODENAL INJURIES

Management of either penetrating or blunt trauma to the duodenum presents some of the most difficult problems encountered in trauma to the abdomen. Following nonpenetrating injuries, delay in exploration may produce contamination of the peritoneal cavity with duodenal contents which may cause additional prolongation of morbidity and an increase in mortality. (Burrus et al., 1961). The majority of duodenal injuries are of the penetrating variety, and for this reason early exploration should be carried out. Following blunt trauma, however, retroperitoneal perforation of the second portion of the duodenum may result in extravasation of air and bile-stained duodenal contents in this area without involving the general peritoneal cavity.

Injuries in this location may be overlooked during the exploration. Following blunt trauma, the second and third portions of the duodenum are most frequently involved, as a result of compression against the second and third lumbar vertebrae. Either a partial or complete division of the bowel may result. Extensive hemorrhage may occur into the wall of the duodenum without perforation of the bowel, and a characteristic appearance of intraluminal hematoma can be found on radiographic examination (Stone and Garoni, 1966). This is described as multiple fingerprint appearances on either side of the duodenum. When the abdominal paracentesis is done, the presence of bile or intestinal contents should be highly suggestive of duodenal involvement. There is an elevation in the white blood cell count, and it is not unusual for counts of 20,000/cu mm. to be obtained in the first 24 hours (Cleveland and Waddell, 1966). The serum amylase may be elevated and leukocytosis can be expected. This evidence should be quite significant and confirm the involvement of either the duodenum, pancreas, or biliary tract. An exploration and orderly evaluation of all portions of the duodenum should be made, beginning first with the portion that is most easily approached and examined.

The management of injuries in this location, like those at the end of the stomach, can be made by closure. When extensive damage has occurred and resection is not feasible, and when closure of the lateral wall cannot be accomplished, a jejunal patch to the injured area may be utilized (Barnett and Tucker, 1964). It is impossible to thoroughly evaluate the second and third portions of the duodenum without first mobilizing the duodenum by the Kocher maneuver. This is most satisfactorily accomplished by dividing the hepatocolic ligament and exposing both the posterior and anterior walls of the second portion of the duodenum as well as dividing the omentum and its attachments to the transverse mesocolon and the third portion of the duodenum (Stone, 1969b). The relationship with the superior mesenteric vessels must be visualized in order to avoid damage to these structures.

Injuries in the region of the ligament of Treitz are rare except by penetration, and when such an injury does occur, exposure may be difficult unless the duodenojejunal junction has been fully mobilized.

Control of bleeding and debridement must be completed before any attempt is made at repair of the anatomical defects. Many of the perforations of the duodenum may be closed with two-layer closure, but when extensive destruction has occurred, a jejunal patch and anastomosis of the proximal end or a *Roux-en-Y*-segment of the jejunum may be successful.

In many instances it is essential that adequate proximal decompression be maintained as is done in the stomach. This can be accomplished in most instances with gastrostomy; retrograde duodenal decompression with jejunostomy may also be considered. It is essential that drainage be accomplished by gravity rather than by the use of suction to avoid some of the late sequelae that may occur. When utilized, a Witzel-type jejunostomy is essential in order to avoid leaks or later complications.

INTRAMURAL HEMATOMA

The relief of intramural hematoma can in some instances be accomplished by simple evacuation of the collected blood by longitudinal incision through the serosa and muscularis of the bowel. On the other hand this may be difficult and not entirely satisfactory, since late stenosis can occur. This obstruction can be corrected through a gastrojejunostomy, bypassing the duodenum. Drains should be used cautiously in the region of the duodenum except when the pancreas is involved.

A fistula at the anastomotic site can be a most serious complication. This can and does occur in spite of all efforts, and under these circumstances, a sump drain becomes mandatory. A duodenal fistula should not be allowed to remain for a long period of time and should be closed as soon as possible by one of the usually acceptable methods — either with the establishment of a *Roux-en-Y* closure or a side-to-end jejunal patch.

JEJUNUM AND ILEUM

There has been a gradual decrease in the mortality rate for both penetrating and non penetrating injuries to the small intestine (McGarity, 1969). This, in part, has been brought about by an appreciation of the significance of these injuries, and of the necessity for adequate preoperative preparation and immediate exploration and repair (Thorlakson, 1960).

Blunt traumas are more difficult to evaluate. A wide variety of forms of violence may produce these changes within the bowel (Baxter and Williams, 1961). They may be caused by direct blows on the anterior abdominal wall, compressing the bowel across the vertebrae and resulting in various degrees of tears or total division.

Another mechanism is that related to tearing at fixed points, such as at the duodenojejunal junction, in the region of the ileocecal valve, and also at the attachments of the mesentery to the posterior abdominal wall. A rapid increase of intraluminal pressure may also result in a disruption of the wall of the bowel (Williams and Sargeant, 1963).

Recently, injuries related to the use of seat belts have been seen. When improperly used, this safety measure may be just as devastating and significant in producing injuries within the abdominal cavity as it has been protective. These are brought about by forces directed against the abdomen, in which tearing of the small bowel or hemorrhaging within the mesentery may occur as a result of this violent compression (Fish and Wright, 1965). Usually this type of injury may be suspected when there are bruises and contusions on the skin over that area and obvious peritoneal irritation.

The presence or absence of shock, infection, or signs of hemorrhage should create a suspicion of intra-abdominal injury. When seen early in minor trauma, evidence may be unclear, whereas, a few hours later, when signs of peritonitis appear, intraperitoneal damage is obvious. Diagnosis should be made before this period to avoid many of the late complications.

Radiographic examinations may or may not be useful. The demonstration of free air in the peritoneal cavity beneath the diaphragm, obliteration of psoas shadow, or associated fractures of the lower and upper framework may confirm damage when all other signs are only suggestive. In any event, when there is doubt, an immediate exploration is in order (Wilder et al., 1967).

A complete exploration of the abdominal cavity is essential. This may require an adequate incision so that a thorough exploration may be made to prevent overlooking a perforation. This requires a careful evaluation and caution in protecting the bowel with moist packs to avoid unnecessary exposure and injury. Rapid control of the retroperitoneal or mesenteric bleeding is required. Attention should be given to the blood supply in mesenteric injuries, and caution should be exercised to avoid leaving devitalized bowel (Zollinger and Sirak, 1953).

The manner of control of small bowel injuries depends on the type of involvement. With a single perforation or with minimal perforations, closure may be accomplished by purse-string sutures of nonabsorbable material, provided there is no compromise of the lumen of the bowel (Maingot, 1963). However, a careful end-to-end anastomosis following resection of the devitalized portion with proper debridement may be required when there is irregular damage to the surface.

The basic principles of surgical repair of the bowel must of necessity be exercised. In the treatment of both the devitalized bowel and mesentery, resection of both the bowel and the mesentery may be required. An end-to-end anastomosis should be accomplished in preference to a side-to-side. The late difficulties of unexplained bleeding, possible intussusception, or an associated anemia may be avoided.

An avulsion of the mesentery from the posterior abdominal wall requires careful attention in order to prevent ischemia in larger segments of the small bowel (McCune et al., 1952). In some instances, this may not be appreciated unless, after careful control of bleeding, one determines the presence or absence of blood flow to the segment before final closure of the abdomen.

COMPLICATIONS

When extensive crushing or thrombosis occurs, resection of large segments of small bowel may be required; this may result in severe malnutrition and can be incompatible with life. All perforations must be closed to avoid the development of peritonitis. A localized abscess may result when there has been extensive contamination of the peritoneal cavity. This begins to be evident either immediately after the injury or after the patient has apparently withstood a difficult postoperative course. Diagnosis of the abscess and determining its location are not always easy, but after carefully observing the patient, such a complication can be recognized and adequate drainage established. One of the most dreaded complications is leakage following the closure of a perforation. With careful technique and adequate attention to the basic surgical principles this can be minimized.

The development of spontaneous fistulas may occur as a catastrophic event after a few days of apparently varying degrees of normal convalescence of the patient. Obviously, the management of the patient with multiple intestinal fistulas becomes very serious and requires an immediate diversion and drainage of the area, maintenance of proper alimentation, and the early re-establishment of bowel continuity before extreme anemia or malnutrition develops. The more recent use of the method of hyperalimentation through continuous infusion, as described by Dudrick and others (1969), may permit many of these patients to be saved who otherwise would not survive.

Late thrombosis and occlusion of either the superior mesenteric artery or vein should be suspected, particularly in those patients who suddenly become quite ill and who experience unusual distention and abdominal pain. Associated and marked leukocytosis may be the clue for such an occurrence. As soon as a diagnosis has been made, an immediate exploration should be considered, and when the bowel is found to be necrotic, resection is required.

As has been noted in the experiences of many, the development of intestinal obstruction, either during the immediate postoperative period or as a late complication, should always be considered following injury to the small bowel. Obstruction may occur as a result of adhesions after peritoneal contamination and injury; such adhesions cause various types of fibrosis and stricture formations (Giddings et al., 1955). They may present as closed-loop lesions or single bands that compress the lumen of the bowel and interfere with normal continuity. An intraluminal stricture may be manifested in the late period as a result of fibrosis within the lumen.

The prognosis of injuries to the small intestine is directly related to the extent of the involvement and the associated injuries to other organ systems (Geoghegan et al., 1955). If patients with stab wounds alone are properly treated, a near-zero mortality rate can be expected (Mason, 1964).

COLON

There has been marked improvement in the treatment of traumatic wounds of the colon in the past few years. A progressive decrease in mortality has been noted in each of the periods in which studies have been made in this country. During the Civil War, wounds of this variety carried a mortality of 90 per cent (Colcock, 1952); in World War I, a mortality of 59.6 per cent was recorded (Elkin et al., 1943); and in World War II, the percentage was 31.4 (Graham, 1958). The improvement has been continuous, as is shown in a recent report of cases at Grady Memorial Hospital in which the mortality is 14.6 per cent (Haynes, 1969).

This marked improvement, both in time of war and also in civilian practice, can be attributed to many factors: the shorter delay in reaching a center where definitive therapy can be administered; the availability of blood and plasma in the preoperative period, assuring a safer operation; the proper evaluation and administration of the necessary antibiotic therapy; the availability of safe anesthesia; and the performance of exteriorization of the damaged area to the colon without attempting a closure of the primary perforation. The method of decompression by colostomy, in the opinion of most authorities, has contributed most in the reduction of morbidity and mortality in colon injuries (Sanders, 1963). There are rare incidences in which primary closure should be considered (Woodhall and Ochsner, 1951). One example is a simple stab wound by a clean ice pick or other small missile in those individuals who are seen early and have minimal peritoneal soiling. It must be admitted that there are certain risks even with this variety of injury. The development of distention of the bowel can be followed by a breakdown of the suture line, with fatal peritonitis following contamination of the peritoneal cavity.

There are a variety of methods of management by decompression either approximate to or at the site of the injury. In a rare group, the closure of the perforated bowel by a loop or transverse colostomy, particularly in the region of the midtransverse colon, may be indicated. A safer method, however, when feasible, would be the exteriorization of the entire colon wound. The transverse colon and the sigmoid flexure of the descending colon are areas that lend themselves more easily to treatment. Mobilization of the other regions can be carried out in most instances, although it is not as easily done. The perforation can be closed and left on the outside. Another method is to insert a mushroom catheter into the opening and fasten it securely with a purse-string suture. The open bowel may be left open and exposed to the outside, along with an adequate segment of the adjacent proximal and distal areas. The colostomy may function from two to three months before being closed by resection and an end-to-end anastomosis or by extraperitoneal closure of the stoma ends when a loop type of procedure is used.

It is essential that the colostomy be performed as simply as possible. There are four basic types of operation applicable to trauma to the large bowel — the loop colostomy, the diverting colostomy, the venting colostomy, and the cecostomy. These are done to protect questionable anastomosis when the wound is closed, to decompress the bowel in acute traumatic obstruction, to divert the fecal stream away from the questionable potential inflammatory processes, and to exteriorize the injured segment of the bowel.

COMPLICATIONS

Unless properly done, the colostomy may be equally damaging and result in difficulties as great as the original injury. Some complications that may be encountered are: retraction of the stoma, prolapse of the colon, herniation at the stoma site, small bowel obstruction, perforation of the colon, bleeding from the colonic mucosa, or stenosis of the colostomy either at the skin or fascial level (Haynes, 1969). Results have been gratifying following adherence to the basic principles just described.

SPLEEN

The spleen, of all the solid organs in the abdomen, is one of the most frequently injured by blunt trauma. This is particularly true in children who are more active and subject to falls (Martin and Cooper, 1950;

Stone, 1969a). Direct blows to the spleen can cause serious damage, since the spleen is vulnerable and sometimes unprotected, especially if it is enlarged. In left chest injuries associated with fractures of the lower ribs, trauma to the spleen should always be suspected. There are essentially two varieties that may be seen — one in which there is an immediate parenchymal rupture, and a subcapsular hematoma, which occurs in the body or hilum of the spleen. When the former is encountered, there is usually a massive escape of blood into the peritoneal cavity; immediate evidence depends on the blood lost and the degree of peritoneal contamination. In the case of a subcapsular hematoma, immediate evidence may not be quite so obvious. In injuries of this particular variety, however, a delayed rupture may occur, sometimes up to a week or ten days following the injury. This can be catastrophic, with massive loss of blood into the peritoneal cavity.

In both adults and children splenic injury should be suspected in all forms of abdominal trauma. When massive hemorrhage occurs, the signs are obvious; but in the presence of multiple injuries, they may be more difficult to evaluate. Depending on the amount of blood in the peritoneal cavity, the patient may experience left upper quadrant pain and difficulty in breathing, particularly when a positive Kerr's sign is present. This can be demonstrated by putting the patient in the Trendelenburg position, which allows the blood to gravitate to beneath the diaphragm, thereby becoming an irritant to this part, and resulting in difficulty in breathing and referred pain to the left shoulder through the path of the phrenic nerve.

Roentgenograms of the chest may be of great value in determining the fracture of ribs, fluid above the diaphragm, enlargement of the spleen, or elevation of the diaphragm. As has been mentioned before, the characteristic picture of irregularity along the greater curvature of the stomach may suggest hemorrhage into the hilum of the spleen along the course of the short gastric arterial branches from the stomach (Fig. 6-2). This irregularity can be demonstrated by the insertion of air through a nasogastric tube, if such has been placed, by permitting the swallowing of a carbonate drink (Stone, 1969c), or, finally, by the introduction of Gastrografin or barium into the stomach. Specific laboratory tests may be helpful: leukocytosis or a drop in the

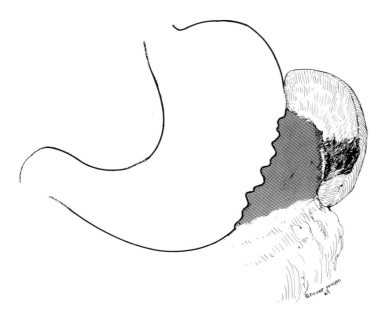

Figure 6-2. Injury to the spleen with extravasation of blood into the gastrosplenic ligament, producing irregular defects on the greater curvature of the stomach. (Changes can be seen on the radiograph.)

hemoglobin and hematocrit, and evidence of hypovolemia may thereby be revealed.

Final confirmation may be made by four-quadrant aspiration. Once the decision has been made that a possible ruptured spleen exists, laparotomy should be performed without further delay in order to lessen the likelihood of massive exsanguination. If multiple injuries have occurred in the left upper abdomen or lower chest, a thoracoabdominal incision may be made. On the other hand, in most instances a long, left subcostal incision may afford adequate exposure, which is most essential. The entrance into the lesser peritoneal sac by dividing the short gastric vessels and exposing the hilum and the tail of the pancreas affords a more careful dissection of the spleen. This approach is preferable if time and the condition of the patient permit it. The ligation of the individual vessel allows a dry operating field; on the other hand, this is not always feasible when bleeding is severe.

On exposure of the spleen, it is essential to carefully ligate the splenocolic ligament, divide the attachments to the under surface of the diaphragm, and avoid injury to the tail of the pancreas. The other approach is the immediate removal of the spleen; it involves bringing the spleen into view and controlling the hilum of the spleen with mass ligatures. However, this may not as safely control the bleeding nor avoid possible injuries to the adjacent structures, particularly the greater curvature of the stomach, the tail of the pan-

creas, and the splenic flexure of the transverse colon (Fig. 6-3).

COMPLICATIONS

The three basic complications following splenectomy for trauma are delayed bleeding, thrombosis, and infection. It is felt that in all injuries to the spleen the area should be drained because of the likelihood of recurrent bleeding and also because the bed of the spleen may have exposed surfaces with the potential for continued oozing of blood. There is also the possibility that bleeding or infection may develop, particularly in the presence of associated injuries to the intestinal tract, especially the colon. It has been pointed out that infections occur in approximately 4 per cent of all traumatic splenectomies. Immediate and delayed bleeding may occur in approximately 2.8 per cent (Martin and Cooper, 1950).

Much has been written regarding thrombosis and pulmonary embolism as a further complication, and concern for these is encountered in approximately 3.7 per cent. They have variously been ascribed to the ligation of large blocks of tissue when the crash type of splenectomy has been performed. Also, the elevation in the platelet count, in some instances as high as 1 million, may be significant in hastening and contributing to the development of thrombosis and subsequent embolization. It should be remembered that when the spleen alone is injured there are available large quantities of blood that can be utilized for autotransfusion, and plans should be carried out for recovering the blood for immediate replacement in each patient.

THE LIVER

The liver is often involved in severe direct blunt trauma to the upper abdomen. This is because of its size, position, and character. It is impossible for it to escape penetrating wounds within this area. Up until recent times, it was expected that massive trauma would be associated with a comparably high morbidity and mortality (Martin, 1947). If the patient did not immediately bleed to death, delayed hemorrhage and sepsis were the primary problems encountered. With a better appreciation of pathophysiology and with the knowledge of the more recently described segmental anatomy and physiology, a new era has been reached in the treatment of injuries to this organ. The mortality rate, therefore, has correspondingly decreased, but there are many associated problems, the manner of treatment has become more complex, requiring exceptional skill, more attention to the details of preoperative management, and, to be sure, better surgical technique and postoperative care.

It is essential to remember the three varieties of injuries encountered. The first, and by far the most common, is rupture of the capsule with an escape of bile and blood into the peritoneal cavity. The second variety is subcapsular hemorrhage with an accumulation of blood within the substance of the liver without a disruption of Glisson's capsule. One feature of this type of injury is that it may spontaneously rupture several days after the injury and be associated with a massive blood loss into the peritoneal cavity, and may result in exsanguination. The third variety is associated with extensive destruction of the central portion of the liver, resulting in devitalization, delayed sloughing, hematoma formation, accumulation of bile within an encapsulated area, and possible development of an intrahepatic abscess. This is frequently seen in individuals who apparently withstand the immediate trauma only to develop an abscess that may erode a large vessel and massively bleed into a major bile duct, with blood escaping into the intestinal tract. This condition is known as hemobilia (Amerson and Blair, 1959).

In those individuals with extensive injury to the liver, immediate recognition is not difficult, but in those with a subcapsular hematoma or a minor injury, an early diagnosis is obviously difficult. The question of exploration depends to a very great extent on the severity of the symptoms, early diagnosis, and the availability of facilities for management of this type of injury. The initial step in the exploration is through the peritoneal route. A full assessment of the findings and visualization of the associated injuries should be accomplished before proceeding with specific management of the liver wounds, except to control bleeding by compression. In a number of wounds of this variety, the bleeding has stopped in some cases, even though there may be a large quantity of blood within the peritoneal cavity (Madding, 1955).

In those individuals with lacerations of a minor degree, drainage alone may be adequate, provided that there is no associated devitalization from fragmentation of the liver substance (Mikal et al., 1950). However, continued bleeding can be controlled by

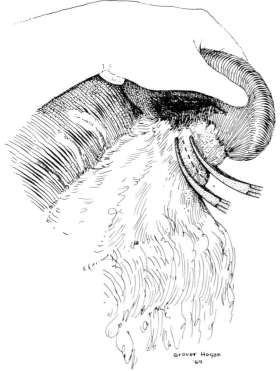

Figure 6-3. Control and resection of the spleen by the crash method (recommended only in emergency situations).

suturing the lacerations, using blunt needles provided for this purpose. This procedure, in many instances, is satisfactory. The use of gelatin foam or Surgicel for assistance in bringing about hemostasis may be satisfactory if small lacerations have occurred. Muscle, omentum. and peritoneum have been sutured into this type of wound with fair to satisfactory results.

When deep laceration or large linear tears occur, one should be thoroughly aware of the degree of involvement before closing superficial lacerations with destroyed liver beneath. This would be followed by necrosis or central accumulation of blood, and secondary rupture could occur a few days after injury. If the surface liver wounds are closed and have been well protected or sealed by the omentum, the bleeding can occur into the biliary tract. The first manifestation may be that of massive bleeding through the common duct into the duodenum, producing hemobilia, which has been previously described.

If extensive destruction has occurred and the patient is rapidly bleeding from the liver site at the time of the operation, control of the blood flow through the portal vein and hepatic artery can be accomplished by means of compression through the foramen of Winslow. This allows for further assessment of the degree of injury and for the consideration of resection of the involved area of the liver.

Recently, the knowledge of the segmental anatomy, as described by Goldsmith and Woodburne (1951), has made possible resections that were heretofore impossible. Essentially, these divisions permit a partial resection or hepatectomy to the right of the gallbladder and, secondly, to the inner side of the gallbladder; the major portion of the right hepatic lobe is removed. The left lobe can be more easily identified and safely resected by utilizing the falciform ligament as the division marking. The technical procedure permits effective division of the liver by means of a knife (Quattlebaum, 1953). Hemostasis can then be accomplished by ligation of the individual ducts and vessels encountered as they are exposed.

During World War II experience with this type of injury emphasized the inability to control bleeding with applications of large gauze packs to the area of destruction (Martin, 1947). When the process of further necrosis and bleeding occur behind the packs, second-

ary bleeding and peritonitis may follow and prove fatal.

Postoperative hemorrhage from the site of injury is usually minimal, provided there has not been central damage. On the other hand, if infection and necrosis develop, a large variety of subsequent difficulties can be expected. Subphrenic hematoma, abscess, or peritonitis, as has been mentioned, can be serious accompaniments.

It should be mentioned that an indwelling, common duct T-tube should be inserted in most liver injuries. This is particularly true when a segmental or partial resection of the liver is done. It should be stated that under no circumstance should resection of the liver be done unless adequate preparation has been made. This includes the availability of safe anesthesia, a sufficient amount of blood, and able assistance in undertaking the management of liver injuries both during and following the operation.

Once the decision has been made, the original exploratory abdominal incision through the midline should be extended through the right diaphragm to afford adequate exposure of all of the ligamentous attachments of the liver (Amerson, 1969). Resection of the liver can then be carefully performed. The control of all individual vessels by ligation is absolutely necessary. Certainly the operation must be undertaken with great concern; the magnitude and implications must be fully understood and appreciated. This approach has saved the lives of many patients but it must be emphasized that, even under the most ideal circumstances, the high mortality rate continues to exist.

EXTRAHEPATIC BILIARY TRACT

Fortunately, extrahepatic biliary tract injuries are not frequently encountered (Barnes and Diamonon, 1963; Cattell and Braasch, 1960; Hinshaw et al., 1952; Shires, 1966; Stewart, 1961; Stewart and Silen, 1961; Sturmer and Wilt, 1963). When they are recognized, there are certain requirements that should be met in order to avoid many later difficulties and allow patients to recover who otherwise would not survive.

Penetrating wounds affect the extrahepatic biliary tract more frequently than do blunt wounds. There are three locations to be considered: deep within the hilum of the liver, at or near the entrance of the hepatic duct into the common duct, and the common duct below this level (Fletcher et al., 1961). The most frequent location, however, for penetrating injuries is that of the gallbladder. Fortunately for these patients, cholecystectomy for injuries to the cystic duct and gallbladder is sufficient. In most instances, it is not necessary to leave the gallbladder in unless there is a very minor injury.

When the patient has had extensive damage to the hepatic duct and there is nonviable liver tissue, the situation may be incompatible with life. However, with minor injuries of the ductal system, reconstruction over a T-tube stent may be effective if an adequate amount of duct remains and can be mobilized. The primary concern in this variety of injury is the associated involvement of the vena cava, the portal vein or, perhaps, the hepatic artery. When present, these must be safely controlled and repaired before proceeding with repair of the bile ducts (Haynes and Martin, 1969). When the ducts are extensively involved and anastomosis cannot be done, the *Roux-en-Y* loop of jejunum can be attached to the proximal end of the duct.

When injury to the liver is also present, it may be necessary to subsequently resect the destroyed area. Bile duct injuries are frequently accompanied by a variety of complications. Leaks at the anastomotic site are the first concern. Peritonitis can ensue with collection of bile and possible subphrenic abscesses with the associated metabolic and nutritional problems.

Delayed hemorrhage, intestinal fistulas, or other complications may be demonstrated if the individual is fortunate enough to survive the initial trauma. Delayed stricture may occur and, if uncorrected, the development of jaundice, chills, fever, and biliary cirrhosis can be anticipated. The latter will depend on the degree and duration of obstruction. Management of the strictures should be accomplished under the most ideal circumstances after thorough preparation of the patient for re-exploration. The use of vitamin K to prevent a bleeding problem when jaundice exists and the administration of broad-spectrum antibiotics before and after repair are essential. The correction of electrolyte and nutritional deficiencies is absolutely necessary.

Complete exploration and assessment of the remaining biliary tract and the establishment of communication with the gastrointestinal tract may be required. One should determine whether a suitable proximal duct is available, which may be anastomosed to the intestinal tract by utilizing again, preferably, the *Roux-en-Y* jejunum loop. As has been previously stated, injury to the biliary tract is not common, but when it occurs it taxes the ingenuity of the surgeon.

PANCREAS

Pancreatic trauma may be easily overlooked, particularly when it does not involve penetration of the abdomen. Initially, the vital signs may be stable and the findings indefinite. A delay in manifestations occurs frequently unless there has been severe trauma and escape of pancreatic enzymes. Late signs become apparent after delayed hemorrhage and peritonitis are evident. Fortunately trauma to the pancreas is mainly of the penetrating variety except when it is massive, such as following compression against an object like a steering wheel.

During the operation for penetrating wounds, attention may be focused on other organs in the upper abdomen, and the lesser peritoneal sac may not be explored. Therefore, in all penetrating trauma, it is necessary that the pancreas be completely visualized. Due to the close proximity of large major vessels, accompanying injuries to these structures should be expected. They are primarily the inferior vena cava, superior mesenteric artery and vein, and the portal vein. An accompanying wound to the duodenum may likewise be suspected, particularly when the object is penetrating. The presence of crepitation, bile-stained tissue, and evidence of massive retroperitoneal bleeding further add to the suspicion that the pancreas has been damaged.

The anatomical divisions of the pancreas (the head and neck, the body, and the tail) should be considered in association with certain injuries. The head and neck are usually associated with major vessel and duodenal injuries; the body is involved when the pancreas is severely compressed against the vertebrae and the force anteriorly; the tail of the pancreas is frequently involved in injuries to the spleen. When the hilum of the spleen is injured, a certain degree of pancreatic damage can be expected; this may be manifested early or late.

The prognosis in injuries to the pancreas alone can be related to injuries to the other organs involved. Suffice it to say that a reasonably high mortality rate is around 23 per cent, whereas with injuries associated with other organs it may be as high as 60 per cent (Stone et al., 1952).

Diagnosis

The earlier the operation for pancreatic injury the less the mortality; therefore, it is imperative that early definitive treatment be rendered. After the usual preliminary preparations essential for all abdominal trauma have been made, the operation should proceed without delay (Stone and Walker, 1969). In order not to overlook the presence of pancreatic wounds, a careful and detailed exploration and dissection of the three separate divisions are essential. The first procedure is to expose the body and tail of the pancreas through an opening in the lesser sac made by dividing the gastrocolic omentum. A division of the gastroepiploic vessels may be required. In this manner the anterior surface of the neck, body, tail, and, to some degree, the head of the pancreas can be visualized. The inferior margin can be seen by reflecting the transverse colon and omentum superiorly and the under surface can be demonstrated by going through the avascular area of the mesocolon, exercising extreme care to avoid the middle colic artery and its lateral branches.

The pancreatic head can best be demonstrated by taking down the hepatic flexure of the colon, dividing the superior attachments to the liver and dissecting the angle at the base of the superior aspect of the transverse mesocolon. This is followed by an extended Kocher maneuver, allowing further visualization of the head and the posterior wall.

There are three principles of management of pancreatic injuries: (1) assessment of the extent of injury, (2) conservative debridement of devitalized tissue, and (3) control of the pancreatic secretion. Hemostasis can be safely achieved only when one determines the full extent of injury to the vessels involved. The application of instruments to control bleeding within this area may result in changes more destructive than beneficial.

Some injuries of the pancreas may be safely sutured by transfixation, after the bleeding from major vessels has first been controlled. In injuries to the superior aspect of the pancreas, it should be remembered that the main blood supply to the spleen may be compromised and a splenectomy may be required.

The escape of pancreatic secretions must be controlled where the pancreatic duct is divided. The proximal and distal divisions of the duct must be ligated. If separation of the pancreas has occurred, a resection of the distal end of the pancreas may be necessary. The essential concern in the management of postoperative secretion is that preparation be made for leakage from the devitalized pancreatic tissue or exposed pancreatic ducts. This can be accomplished satisfactorily by means of an effective sump drainage.

A negative pressure must be accomplished in order to maintain continuous and uninterrupted suction. A pressure of approximately 100 mm. of mercury is required to keep this area reasonably free of the accumulated pancreatic enzymes. A sump suction should be maintained for at least a week or until drainage has become negligible (Fig. 6-4).

Complications

In a review of some 20 patients, four developed fistulas, two had chemical peritonitis, and two had hemorrhage. There was an overall mortality within this group of 30 per cent (Stone et al., 1952). A less vital but distressing complication that may occur is a pseudocyst. This occurs in traumatic injury to the pancreas when there has been inadequate drainage of the pancreatic secretions or a major duct has been injured. There is always the possibility that with damage to the pancreas, either with or without resection, exocrine function may be insufficient. This would result in abnormal pancreatic function and may require the administration of pancreatic enzymes. Diabetes mellitus rarely occurs as a result of these injuries.

THE RECTUM

The rectum is not as frequently injured as other parts of the gastrointestinal tract, and

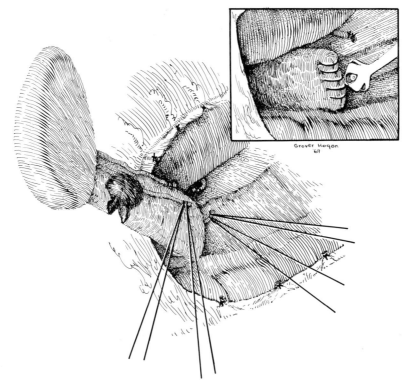

Grover Hogan
'69

Figure 6-4. Mobilization of the traumatized pancreas with partial transection. The damaged area is completely resected along with the spleen.

for this reason it may easily be overlooked. The types of rectal injuries are generally the same as those encountered elsewhere. The method of wounding, the anatomical location, and the delay in treatment account for the differences. Injuries above the peritoneal fold are distinctive and should be considered individually.

Massive trauma is associated with crushing injuries. Penetrating wounds from objects such as missiles and knives are frequently associated with the involvement of other organs. An increase in iatrogenic injuries, occurring during diagnostic studies and operative procedures, has been noted (Andresen, 1947).

The relationship of rectal injuries to other associated organs is a serious problem, particularly when seen in the patient in profound shock or in a comatose state. In the presence of extensive intra- or extra-abdominal injury, the rectum is often overlooked.

With abdominal trauma the early systemic signs and symptoms may be absent, although they become quite severe as infection and other late sequelae develop. In injuries to the rectum above the reflection of the peritoneum, the initial findings may be either

mild peritoneal irritation or overt signs of intra-abdominal trauma (Bailey, 1958). The extent, type, and location of the rectal wound should be determined for proper primary treatment.

Because of its location and size, the rectum is seldom missed by penetrating objects in this area. Insignificant stab wounds around the buttocks demand thorough investigation to exclude the presence of rectal penetration. Digital examination alone can be conclusive in some instances. Anoscopic and proctoscopic examinations, although very important, may be negative because of extreme discomfort and associated pain, making the examination unsatisfactory.

A barium enema may be helpful, but it also involves risk. The introduction of barium into a perforated rectum or rectosigmoid colon should be avoided. When a barium enema is indicated, a small quantity of contrast medium is instilled under low pressure in order to limit the amount of extravasation.

TREATMENT

Once the lost blood has been replaced, a decision must be made as to the need for operation. Insertion of an indwelling urethral catheter is helpful, not only in making the diagnosis of a urinary tract injury but also in its management. The first considerations in the case of rectal perforations are a primary colostomy and determining whether or not the local injury can be repaired.

In extensive losses of the rectal wall, primary reconstruction should be deferred. A preliminary colostomy necessitates the thorough debridement of the perineal wound and provision for drainage (Laufman, 1946). The site of injury must be exposed even if it necessitates resecting the coccyx or dividing the levator ani muscle.

If primary closure is not selected initially, it can be performed within six weeks to three months after the injury when the risk of infection is minimal and after other major problems have been resolved. Antibiotics are usually administered but are not always required. Widespread infection may occur, but can be controlled by adequate drainage and the arrest of hemorrhage.

Following an operative repair or a complicating infection, distortion of the normal perianal anatomy may result in functional impairment. There may be scarring, prolapse of rectal mucosa, loss of continence, and the inability to maintain normal cleanliness because of constant soiling.

Blunt trauma occurs rarely because the rectum is surrounded by a muscle sling and is supported in the hollow of the sacrum by the bony framework of the pelvis. It is attached by folds of the peritoneum to the presacral fascia and may extend as high as the promontory of the sacrum and into the rectosigmoid. With this degree of fixation, blunt trauma seldom occurs except in crushing wounds of the pelvis. Suspicion of such an injury and a thorough investigation from below by proctoscopic visualization will facilitate early recognition. In combined lesions, exploratory laparotomy may be necessary to ascertain the extent of injury into the pelvis and allow immediate visualization and repair of the injury.

The bladder rather than the rectum is more frequently injured in blunt trauma. Attention should therefore be directed to this organ by the introduction of an indwelling catheter, by cystograms, and direct visualization through the cystoscope. When trauma is primarily to the bladder and urethra, proper treatment is first given to these organs.

An unusual injury, known as *impalement*, is caused when an individual falls and the rectal area is pierced by a sharp object. A fall onto a spike can be expected to tear, penetrate, or invade any portion of the perineum (Mathieson and Mann, 1965). In such an accident, immediate careful assessment, debridement, and repair of the perineal structures are required (Berry and Wylie, 1953). In most instances a decompressing colostomy should be performed. In extensive injuries a delayed repair may be advisable, but if a puncture wound alone has occurred, repair can be done immediately.

Stab wounds in and around the buttocks should lead to suspected involvement of the rectum. These wounds are difficult to assess and may require a period of observation. In the deep penetrations involving the ischiorectal space, hemorrhage, secondary infection, and delayed abscess formations may follow unless such wounds are recognized earlier and effectively treated.

Penetrating wounds of the buttocks may produce considerable bleeding into the perineum and pelvis. When such a condition is anticipated, a direct approach to the site of injury from below should be avoided, since it may be impossible to control the proximal blood supply. It is safer to open the abdomen first and then to expose the hypogastric artery for control of the bleeding before proceeding to explore the perineal injury.

Trauma to the rectum caused by the insertion of foreign bodies is common among mental patients. The articles vary from small fragments that do no appreciable harm to large objects that produce major damage. The consequences are tears of the sphincter, disruption of the mucosa, and perforation of the wall into the perirectal tissues even beyond the reflection of the peritoneum.

Recognition and immediate treatment of iatrogenic trauma are essential if deleterious effects are to be avoided. During the administration of a barium enema, particularly if there is a proximal obstructive lesion, perforation of the rectosigmoid can occur and permit the escape of barium into the peritoneal cavity (Zheutlin et al., 1952). In such cases very high morbidity and mortality can be expected.

Radiation is so commonly used in treating cancer of the pelvic organs that the rectum and the small intestine are often secondarily affected. The injuries produced may be considerable and are noted first as simple inflammatory changes that progress to chronic cellulitis and fibrosis. The end result may be necrosis with fistula formation. The possibility of such injury is becoming more significant with the extensive use of radiation therapy.

THE ABDOMINAL GREAT VESSELS

The most distressing abdominal injury is one that involves the major intra-abdominal vessels. Until recently, the results of management of such injuries have been poor. It was only during World War II and the Korean conflict that a more aggressive approach was attempted in an effort to salvage the victims of such injuries. The availability of rapid evacuation, particularly by means of helicopters, has made possible the survival of individuals with this type of trauma.

The present status of management of these civilian injuries has been presented by Perdue and Smith in a study in which treatment of 90 patients resulted in 55 survivors with a 61 per cent survival rate (Perdue and Smith, 1969).

A large number of retroperitoneal vascular injuries, both penetrating and nonpenetrating, are associated with intra-abdominal involvement. The nonpenetrating variety occur in crushing injuries associated with pelvic fractures and in which the vessels in the lower abdomen may be involved. More frequently injuries in the upper abdomen are produced by penetration involving the aorta and vena cava and their tributaries. The retroperitoneal area is protected to some extent by the limiting boundary of the peritoneum, which may prevent a sudden escape of a large quantity of blood into the peritoneal cavity. The diagnosis of injuries of the penetrating variety is much more easily made than that following blunt trauma. With extravasation of large quantities of blood into the retroperitoneal area, arterial thrombosis, and signs of ischemia to the lower extremity may become apparent.

Asymmetric pulses in the legs may be significant as well as the development of a bruit, which may become readily audible on auscultation. In those rare situations in which the injuries may be located at the level of the kidneys, thrombosis of the renal vessels may become apparent, denoted by

oliguria followed by anuria. In management of the acute phase, roentgenograms may not be possible, since it is important to get the patient into the operating room immediately. Abdominal films can be obtained and may prove helpful when the patient is more stable.

The x-ray findings may include hazy abdominal contents, and psoas outlines may indicate a large amount of intra-abdominal blood. The obliteration of the psoas shadow and the displacement of gas patterns in a large retroperitoneal hematoma are significant. Intravenous pyelogram indicates renal function of one or both of the kidneys. Angiography may be helpful, if time permits, in indicating thrombosis of a visceral artery or vein.

There are certain basic principles that are essential for treatment in such cases. First, two or more large-bore polyethylene catheters should be introduced into the veins of the upper extremity, remote from the site of possible venous injury. The urinary catheter must be placed in order to monitor urine output and to determine injury to this system. A central venous catheter is more advantageous in determining blood volume replacement. The introduction of crystalloid solutions and plasma expanders is necessary while an adequate amount of cross-matched blood is being obtained. The use of dextran should be restricted to 1000 ml. in order to avoid the bleeding diathesis that may result from excessive administration of this substance (Perdue and Smith, 1969).

As soon as the patient can be taken into the operating room, anesthesia must be induced with a minimal amount of agent, using controlled ventilation in all instances. A midline incision from the xiphoid to the pubis should be made to afford maximal approach for controlling and repairing damaged vessels. The first step is the rapid assessment and exposure of the aorta and the accurate identification of the bleeding point, which can be controlled by the use of a sponge stick quickly applied to the aorta beneath the diaphragm; the vessel should be occluded after the point of injury has been determined.

Next, bleeding from the vena cava must be controlled. This can best be done by utilizing the three segments of this structure — that above the renal portion, that below the renal vessels, and that behind the liver in the retrohepatic area. The infrarenal cava is made up, of course, by the iliac vessels entering to the right of the aorta. The exposure of this portion of the cava can be accomplished by releasing the lateral peritoneal reflections of the cecum and ascending colon, and mobilizing the intestines anteriorly and medially. Care must be taken to avoid injury to the ureter and duodenum. On visualization of this portion, compression of the vena cava, above and below, can be accomplished by the application of proximal and distal spongestick compression, usually from the level of the renal veins to the common iliac veins.

The suprarenal portion of the cava can best be visualized by the Kocher maneuver once the hepatocolic ligament has been released. When the vena cava has been divided, the exposure can be increased from the caudate lobe of the liver to a point below the tributaries of the renal vein. It is essential to avoid injuries to the tributaries, particularly those of the adrenals.

Access to the retrohepatic portion of the vena cava can best be obtained through a thoracoabdominal approach with an incision of the diaphragm, exposing the vena cava by rotation of the liver into the right chest. Control of the vena cava can be established by placing umbilical tapes both above and below the liver. At this time precaution must be taken not to injure the vena cava, since air embolism may be a threat, which in most instances can be lethal. Temporary venous bleeding from the liver can be controlled by inflow occlusion through compression of the hepatoduodenal ligament. This can be safely accomplished up to a maximum of 15 to 20 minutes without damage to the liver.

THE ABDOMINAL AORTA

The abdominal aorta can best be exposed by dividing it into its three portions: above the pancreas, behind the pancreas, and below the pancreas. The portion above the pancreas can be visualized by entering between the stomach and liver; the portion behind the pancreas can be approached both above and between the stomach and liver, and alternately by incising the posterior parietal peritoneum along the base of the transverse mesocolon along the superior mesenteric vessels. The infrapancreatic aorta can be exposed in the same manner as the infrarenal vena cava.

In the operative repair of injuries to the aorta, the utilization of the sound principles of control of arterial bleeding is necessary. In the high injuries, control can only be ac-

complished by going above the diaphragm in the left hemithorax to place a tape from above. On the other hand, injuries below this area may safely be controlled by placing tapes both below and above the injury within the abdominal cavity. After the immediate control of the bleeding vessels, attention to the normal blood flow may be required for adequate resuscitation.

Restoration of normal blood flow must be accomplished as rapidly and completely as possible, preserving continuity when possible. Clean lacerations may be successfully repaired without too much difficulty. On the other hand, when disruption of larger areas has occurred, replacement of damaged segments by the use of a prosthesis may be required.

There may be a tendency toward clotting in the distal segments after the application of vascular occluding instruments. When absolute hemostasis is assured, systemic administration of heparin in the dosage of 75 units per kilogram of body weight is recommended to prevent intravascular coagulation during repair (Perdue and Smith, 1969). However, when massive trauma has occurred, systemic heparinization may be dangerous and only local anticoagulation can be obtained by injecting a solution of 1000 units of heparin in 50 ml. saline into the artery proximally and distally. One should be cautioned that before final completion of the repair, the presence or absence of clots should be determined by introducing a Fogarty balloon catheter to clear this area.

In the postoperative period, the continued use of broad-spectrum antibiotics is recommended to control the late development of infection. This is particularly advantageous in those individuals in whom injury to the small or large bowel may have been present. Vigorous treatment of acidosis, which accompanies shock and prolonged muscle ischemia, may be required during this period. The judicious use of an osmotic diuretic, such as 20 per cent mannitol, is helpful to maintain adequate postoperative urine flow in individuals in whom clamps may have been placed on the aorta. The development of thrombophlebitis in the postoperative period may prove to be significant, particularly when treatment of major vessels consisted of ligation. Postoperative use of dextran or heparin at a safe time may prove of value. The use of support stockings worn by individuals for a long period of time may also prove to be beneficial.

REFERENCES

Amerson, J. R.: The liver. *In* Trauma to the Thorax and Abdomen. Springfield, Ill., Charles C Thomas, 1969.

Amerson, J. R., and Blair, H. D.: Traumatic liver injuries. Amer. Surg., 25:648, 1959.

Andresen, A. F. R.: Perforations from proctoscopy. Gastroenterology, 9:32, 1947.

Bailey, H.: Emergency Surgery. 7th ed., Bristol, Wright, 1968, p. 538.

Barnes, J. P., and Diamonon, J. S.: Traumatic rupture of the gallbladder due to nonpenetrating injury. Texas State J. Med., 49:785, 1963.

Barnett, W. O., and Tucker, F. H., Jr.: Management of the difficult duodenal stump. Ann. Surg., 159:794, 1964.

Baxter, C. F., and Williams, R. D.: Blunt abdominal trauma. J. Trauma, 1:241, 1961.

Berry, F. B., and Wylie, R. H.: Wounds of perineum, rectum and buttocks. *In* Bowers, W. F. (ed.): *Surgery of Trauma.* Philadelphia, J. B. Lippincott Company, 1953, p. 251.

Burrus, G. R., Howell, J. F., and Jordan, G. L., Jr.: Traumatic duodenal injuries: An analysis of 86 cases. J. Trauma, 1:96, 1961.

Cattell, R. B., and Braasch, J. W.: Repair of benign strictures of the bile duct involving both or single hepatic ducts. Surg. Gynec. Obstet., 110:55, 1960.

Cleveland, H. C., and Waddell, W. R.: Retroperitoneal rupture of the duodenum due to nonpenetrating trauma. Surg. Clin. N. Amer., 43:413, 1963.

Cohn, I., Jr.: Personal communication.

Colcock, B. P.: Colostomy: historical role in the surgery of the colon and rectum. Surgery, 31:794, 1952.

Dudrick, S. J., Wilmore, D. W., Vars, H. M., and Rhoads, J. A.: Can intravenous feeding as the sole means of nutrition support growth in the child and restore weight loss in an adult? Ann. Surg., 169:974, 1969.

Elkin, D. C., and Ward, W. C.: Gunshot wounds of the abdomen. A survey of 238 cases. Ann. Surg., 118:780, 1943.

Fish, J., and Wright, R. H.: The seat belt syndrome— does it exist? J. Trauma, 5:746, 1965.

Fletcher, W. S., Mahnke, D. E., and Dunphy, J. E.: Complete division of the common bile duct due to blunt trauma. J. Trauma, 1:87, 1961.

Geoghegan, T., Gordon, S. J., and Brush, B. E.: Small intestinal rupture from nonpenetrating abdominal trauma. J. Mich. Med. Soc., 54:1223, 1955.

Giddings, W. P., and McDaniel, J. R.: Wounds of jejunum and ileum. In *Surgery in World War II.* Washington, D.C., Surgeons General Office, Department of the Army, 1955, chapter 19.

Goldsmith, N. A., and Woodburne, R. T.: The surgical anatomy pertaining to liver resection. Surg. Gynec. Obstet., 105:310, 1957.

Graham, A. S.: Penetrating wounds of the colon. Surg. Clin. N. Amer., 38:1639, 1958.

Haynes, C. D.: The colon. *In* Trauma to the Thorax and Abdomen. Springfield, Ill., Charles C Thomas, 1969.

Haynes, C. D., and Martin, J. D., Jr.: The extrahepatic biliary tree. *In* Trauma to the Thorax and Abdomen. Springfield, Ill., Charles C Thomas, 1969.

Haynes, C. D., Gunn, C. H., and Martin, J. D., Jr.: Colon injuries. Arch. Surg., 96:944, 1968.

Hinshaw, D. B., Turner, G. R., and Carter, R.: Transection of the common bile duct caused by nonpenetrating trauma. Amer. J. Surg., 104:104, 1962.

Laufman, H.: The initial surgical treatment of penetrating wounds of the rectum. Surg. Gynec. Obstet., 82:210, 1946.

Madding, G. F.: Injuries of the liver. Arch. Surg., 70:748, 1955.

Maingot, R.: Abdominal injuries. *In* Mathews, D. N. (ed.): Recent Advances in Surgery of Trauma. Boston, Little, Brown & Company, 1963.

Martin, J. D., Jr.: Wounds of the liver. Ann. Surg., 125:756, 1947.

Martin, J. D., Jr., and Adams, C. P.: Multiple nonpenetrating wounds of the abdomen. Southern Med. J., 51:62, 1958.

Martin, J. D., Jr., and Cooper, M. N.: Complications of splenectomy. Southern Surg., 16:1047, 1950.

Martin, J. D., Jr., and Thompson, E. B., III: Spontaneous hemorrhage into the rectus muscle: Two case reports and a review of the literature. Amer. Surg., 23:309, 1957.

Mason, J. H.: The expectant management of abdominal stab wounds. J. Trauma, 4:210, 1964.

Mathieson, A. J., and Mann, T. S.: Rupture of the posterior urethra and avulsion of the rectum and anus as a complication of fracture of the pelvis. Brit. J. Surg., 52:309, 1965.

McCune, W. S., Keshishian, J. M., and Blades, B. B.: Mesenteric thrombosis following blunt abdominal trauma. Ann. Surg., 135:606, 1952.

McGarity, W. C.: The jejunum and ileum. *In* Trauma to the Thorax and Abdomen. Springfield, Ill., Charles C Thomas, 1969.

Mikal, S., and Papen, G. W.: Morbidity and mortality in ruptured liver. Surgery, 27:520, 1950.

Perdue, G. D., Jr., and Smith, R. B., III: Abdominal great vessels and the retroperitoneal space. *In* Trauma to the Thorax and Abdomen. Springfield, Ill., Charles C Thomas, 1969.

Quattlebaum, J. K.: Massive resection of the liver. Ann. Surg., 137:787, 1953.

Sanders, J. J.: The management of colon injuries. Surg. Clin. N. Amer., 43:457, 1963.

Shires, G. T. (ed.): Care of the Trauma Patient. New York, McGraw-Hill Book Company, 1966, p. 392.

Sparkman, R. S., and Fogelman, M. J.: Wounds of the liver. Ann. Surg., 139:690, 1954.

Stewart, J. H.: Severance of the common bile duct due to external blunt trauma. J. Louisiana Med. Soc., 113:377, 1961.

Stewart, R., and Silen, W.: Traumatic rupture of the common bile duct. Arch. Surg., 82:387, 1961.

Stone, H. H.: The duodenum. *In* Trauma to the Thorax and Abdomen. Springfield, Ill., Charles C Thomas, 1969b.

Stone, H. H.: The spleen. *In* Trauma to the Thorax and Abdomen. Springfield, Ill., Charles C Thomas, 1969a.

Stone, H. H., and Garoni, W. J.: Experiences in the management of duodenal wounds. Southern Med. J., 59:864, 1966.

Stone, H. H., and Martin, J. D., Jr.: Evaluation of the bluntly traumatized abdomen. *In* Trauma to the Thorax and Abdomen. Springfield, Ill., Charles C Thomas, 1969.

Stone, H. H., and Walker, L. G., Jr.: The pancreas. *In* Trauma to the Thorax and Abdomen. Springfield, Ill., Charles C Thomas, 1969.

Stone, H. H., Stowers, K. B., and Shippey, S. H.: Injuries to the pancreas. Arch. Surg., 85:525, 1952.

Sturmer, F. C., Jr., and Wilt, K. E.: Complete division

of the common duct from external blunt trauma. Amer. J. Surg., *105*:781, 1963.

Thorlakson, R. H.: Rupture of the small intestine due to nonpenetrating abdominal injuries. Canad. Med. Assoc. J., *82*:989, 1960.

Thoroughman, J. C., and Haynes, C. D.: The stomach. *In* Trauma to the Thorax and Abdomen. Springfield, Ill., Charles C Thomas, 1969.

Tobias, S., DeClement, F. A., and Cleveland, J. C.: Management of abdominal stab wounds; roentgenographic technique for diagnosis for peritoneal penetration. Arch. Surg., *95*:27, 1967.

Wilder, J. R., Habermann, E. T., and Schaner, S. J.: Selective surgical intervention for stab wounds within the abdomen. Surgery, *61*:231, 1967.

Williams, R. D., and Sargeant, F. T.: Mechanism of intestinal injury in trauma. J. Trauma, *3*:288, 1963.

Woodhall, J. P., and Ochsner, A.: Management of perforating injuries of the colon and rectum in civilian practice. Surgery, *29*:305, 1951.

Woodhams, J. A.: Personal communication.

Zheutlin, N., Lasser, E. C., and Rigler, L. G.: Clinical studies on effect of barium in the peritoneal cavity following rupture of the colon. Surgery, *32*:967, 1952.

Zollinger, R. M., and Sirak, H. D.: Abdominal wounds. *In* Bowers, W. F. (ed.): Surgery of Trauma. Philadelphia, J. B. Lippincott Company, 1953, chapter 13.

CHAPTER 7

CHEST TRAUMA

by EMIL BLAIR, M.D., CEMALETTIN TOPUZLU, M.D., and
ROBERT S. DEANE, M.B., B. Ch.*

Emil Blair graduated from the Medical College of Georgia and served residencies in both general and thoracic surgery at the University of Maryland and the City Hospitals in Baltimore. Depth in thoracic physiology was gained as a Fellow in Cardiopulmonary Physiology at Duke University Medical Center in 1952–54, as a Halsted Fellow in Experimental Surgery at the University of Colorado in 1954–55, and as a USPHS Fellow in Cardiovascular Surgery at Colorado in 1955–56. He received the Career Research Development Award from the USPHS National Heart Institute. After serving as associate director of the famed shock-trauma program at the University of Maryland, he became Professor of Surgery, Chief of Thoracic and Cardiovascular Surgery, and Director of Surgical Research at the University of Vermont. In 1969 he was appointed Professor of Surgery at the University of Colorado.

Cemalettin Topuzlu received his medical education at the University of Istanbul with high distinction. He served his surgical residency at the University of Vermont College of Medicine and was appointed Assistant Professor of Surgery in 1968. Chest trauma constitutes his field of special interest.

Robert S. Deane was born in England and graduated from medical school at the University of Witwatersrand in South Africa. After taking his residency in anesthesiology at the University of Vermont College of Medicine, he joined the staff and is presently Director of the Respiratory Therapy Department, Division of Anesthesiology.

THE PROBLEM

Annually there is a magnitude of over 13,000,000 traffic accidents with a death every 10 minutes and a serious injury every 10 seconds (Stapp et al., 1967). Accidents rank third, next to cardiovascular diseases and cancer, as major causes of death in the United States. Since 1966 automobile accidents have accounted for over 50,000 deaths annually and are responsible for almost half of all accidental fatalities (Table 7-1). Most victims are in the young and productive age group between 20 and 40 years of age. Of 50,000 deaths, 25 per cent were due entirely to thoracic injuries, while in another 50 per cent chest involvement was a major factor. Thus, major chest injury occurs in about 75 per cent of traffic deaths. Traffic mishaps are the cause of 40 to 73 per cent of hospitalizations for chest trauma (Ashbaugh et al.,

1967; Bassett et al., 1968; Blair et al., 1968).

The next most common cause is falls (15 to 25 per cent), followed in turn by blunt missiles, industrial crush injuries, contact sports, and other miscellaneous forms of violence. Overall accidental death rates have increased progressively during the past 20 years. Deaths caused by motor vehicles rose from 38 per cent of accidental deaths in 1950 to 46 per cent in 1965, while falls, as a cause of death, declined from 23 to 19 per cent.

The type of chest injury (flail, for example), and accompanying complications (lung contusion, major vascular) or subsequently developing complications (pneumonia, tension pneumothorax), exert significant influence on morbidity and mortality. Limited to serious problems of the chest alone, mortality varies from 4 to 12 per cent (Ashbaugh et al., 1967; Blair et al., 1968; Howell et al., 1963). If another organ system is involved, the death rate increases to 13 to 15 per cent, and with two or more systems, accelerates to 30 to 35 per cent. Significant multiple injuries occur in over half of the patients, with fractures

*Supported by U.S.P.H.S. Grant No. HE 11493, the Surgical Associates Fund, and the Herman Blair Research Fund.

141

TABLE 7-1A. Motor Vehicle Accidents*

	1950	1955	1960	1965	1966
Deaths	34,763	38,426	38,137	49,000	52,500
Injuries (millions)	1799	2400	3078	4100	4400

TABLE 7-1B. Comparative Accidental Death Rates*

	1950		1955		1960		1965	
	Number	(Per cent)	Number	(Per cent)	Number	(Per cent)	Number	(Per cent)
All	91,249	(−)	93,443	(−)	93,806	(−)	108,004	(−)
Motor vehicle	34,763	(38.2)	38,426	(41.3)	38,137	(40.6)	49,163	(45.5)
Falls	20,783	(22.9)	20,192	(21.6)	19,023	(20.3)	19,984	(18.5)
Firearms	174	(2.4)	2120	(2.3)	2334	(2.5)	2344	(2.2)

*(From Statistical Abstract of the United States, U.S. Bureau of the Census, Washington, D.C., 1967.)

predominating, followed by head injuries, and, to a smaller extent, intra-abdominal (D'Abreu et al., 1964; Howell et al., 1963; Hughes, 1965).

The injury rate is estimated at 16 per 1000 population, amounting to over 4 million in 1966. About 10 per cent of hospital admissions are for accidents. Over 65,000 hospital beds are needed at present to treat injuries. Over 2 million working years of life are lost through disability from accidents (Table 7-2).

Death and disability, caused by firearms and stabbing, create a dramatic public reaction. They are commonly identified with occasional melodramatic forays of organized youth gangs, or multiple murders by a demented individual, due to the emphasis imposed by news media. The cold fact is that more Americans are killed or wounded annually in "private" forays than in the politically volatile Vietnam conflict. Statistics on violence have once again become as imposing as they were during the "sensational" crime orgies of the depression (Table 7-3). Accidental deaths from firearms have per-

sisted at a consistent rate during the past 15 years. As in motor vehicle accidents, the predominant victim is the young male (15 to 35 years).

Stab wounds are the leading cause of civilian penetrating chest injuries (69 to 79 per cent) in contrast to the predominance of gunshot wounds in battlefield casualties (Beall et al., 1966; Conn et al., 1963; Gray et al., 1960; Sherman, 1966). Mortality from penetrating chest wounds is directly related to the extent of intrathoracic and remote organ involvement, as in blunt trauma. All factors considered, death rates from stabbing are significantly lower (2 to 3 per cent) than those from firearms (14 to 20 per cent). Combined stab and gunshot mortality vary from 3 to 10 per cent.

The injuries in a seriously traumatized patient transfer themselves exponentially into a vector, which can lead to death. The avowed purpose of resuscitation and of treatment is directed at reversal of this vector. Of cardinal importance is the elimination of delay, error, and therapeutic impropriety, which often serve as positive feedbacks, pushing the vector forward at a more rapid rate.

The problems with respect to the resolution of the overall difficulties include clarification of pathoanatomy and pathophysiology, correct emergency care, and proper subsequent management. Pathophysiology is based on anatomic abnormalities. Critical features often may not be manifest as direct correlates of clinical signs and symptoms. Nevertheless, the basis for logical decision

TABLE 7-2. Etiology of Trauma

Cause	Number	Per cent
Automobile	48	68
Falls	14	20
Miscellaneous*	8	12
Total	70	100

*Industrial, sports, fights.

TABLE 7-3. Death Rates from Firearms and Stabbing*

	1930	1940	1950	1960	1965
Homicide					
Firearms	6,995	4,655	4,179	4,627	6,158
Stabbing	1,553	2,064	1,879	1,836	2,292
Totals	8,548	6,719	6,058	6,463	8,450
Suicide					
Firearms	7,735	3,554	3,592	3,366	3,197

*From Statistical Abstract of the United States, U.S. Bureau of the Census, Washington, D.C., 1967.

and execution rests in a good grasp of clinical fundamentals.

Care at the scene is very incomplete and frequently amounts to nothing other than inappropriate movement and handling of the traumatized individual. Patients are frequently transferred without proper care or attention in ambulances inadequately equipped and staffed. Often the victim is admitted to the Emergency Room in a much more serious state than that which existed initially. Figures showing the number of patients who potentially might have been saved have not been documented, but may be anywhere from 10 to 25 per cent for blunt chest trauma. A similar probability exists with knife penetrating chest injuries. On the other hand, the potential in gunshot wounds, particularly with injury to the heart, is considerably less.

In the Emergency Room the lack of the development and enforcement of a programmed protocol for ascertaining the immediate critical problems remains a predominant factor in delayed or missed diagnoses (DOMD). Flirtations with disaster are all too common. The obvious injuries—head and facial injury, lower extremity fractures, deceptive skin wounds that appear innocuous—continue to come under attention. Too often the first call for help rings out to the neurosurgeon or the orthopedist. Awareness of intrathoracic injury, of airway obstruction, or of major vascular involvement lingers somewhere in the stream of the subconscious. The penchant for lab results and the time spent waiting for x-rays compound delays and may accelerate the pathophysiologic vector.

After the initial evaluation and resuscitation, the third phase is entered. The patient is in the Intensive Care Unit, plugged into monitors, on the respirator, fluids pouring in, and under an umbrella of attentive, devoted nurses. There follows a period of emotional and mental relaxation. But the gratification of immediate rescue may dissolve with rupture of an aortic transection, a major blowout of a contused lung, creeping pneumonia, or a "sudden second" tamponade. A high level of tense, programmed pursuit is essential to avoid such consequences.

PATHODYNAMICS

Blunt chest trauma is defined as injury to the chest in which there is no communication with the outside environment by virtue of the primary impact. This is distinguished from penetrating chest injury, such as from missile or knife wounds. In a strict sense, there should be no communication in blunt trauma, but secondary forces occasionally come into play and create communication by virtue of avulsions or rib penetrations.

BLUNT TRAUMA

The destructive nature of forces in chest trauma can be both direct and indirect. The direct collisive impact produces injuries primarily to the chest wall by the forces of the steering wheel or dashboard barrier, blunt missile, crushing load, or flying tackle. Indirect forces are principally responsible for injuries to intrathoracic contents. These mechanical phenomena include positive acceleration, negative acceleration (deceleration), shearing, torsion, compression, and decompression (Table 7-4).

DIRECT IMPACT. The extent of injury produced by direct impact is related to (1) the magnitude and direction of the force applied, (2) the area of application, and (3) the rate of onset and decay of the force (Stapp, 1967). Over 50 per cent of automobile in-

TABLE 7-4. Pathodynamics in Blunt Chest Trauma

Structure	Damage	Mechanism		Incidence
		Primary	Secondary	
A. Thorax				
Soft tissue	Tear, avulsion, penetration	Rib fragment	"Burst" phenomena	Common
Intercostal vessel	Laceration	Rib fragment	–	Fairly common
Ribs	Fracture	Direct impact	"Shock" wave	Common
Sternum	Fracture; dislocation	Direct impact	–	Uncommon
B. Pleura	Tear	Rib fragment	"Burst" phenomena	Common
C. Lung	Tear	Rib fragment	–	Common
	Rupture	Closed system compression	–	Common
	Hematoma	Rib fragment	Closed system compression	Common
	Contusion	Compression/decompression	Rapid deceleration	Common
D. Tracheobronchus	Rupture	Shearing, compression	Rib fragment	Uncommon
E. Mediastinum	Hematoma (primary)	"Burst" phenomena	Shearing	Common
F. Pericardium	Tamponade	Pericardial vessel rupture	Heart, aorta rupture	Uncommon
G. Heart				
Myocardium	Contusion	Direct impact	Compression	Fairly common
Atria, vena cava	Laceration	Rib fragment	Rupture	Rare
Valves, chordae, septa	Rupture	Compression	Rib fragment	Rare
H. Great vessels				
Aorta	Transection	Deceleration, shearing	–	Uncommon
Subclavian	Transection	Deceleration, shearing	–	Rare
Great veins	Tear	Direct impact	Shearing	Rare
Pulmonary	Transection	Direct impact	Shearing	Rare
I. Diaphragm	Rupture	Compression	Shearing	Uncommon
J. Esophagus	Rupture	Compression	Shearing	Rare

juries occur at speeds below 40 mph. with a decelerating force of 20 G. At 60 mph. the force rises to 60 G. At 36 mph., at the instant of impact, the unrestrained occupant continues in a forward motion, but exponentially decelerating so that the chest strikes the steering wheel or instrument panel (the impact barrier) at less than half the original velocity (Kulowski, 1960). Fortunately impact time is brief, only 1 to 20 milliseconds. The thorax can withstand a load in excess of 1000 pounds for 10 milliseconds. Impact tolerance is highest for force applied in the chest-to-back direction or vertical to the long axis of the body, as in steering wheel injuries (Stapp, 1967). In contrast, tolerance is lowest horizontal to the long axis, as in falls and landing on the feet. The mass (weight) of the object (occupant), the distance to the steering wheel, and the velocity are significant factors in the actual impact force sustained. Estimates of impact force are highly variable, ranging anywhere from 300 to 3000 pounds or more (Blair et al., 1969; Kulowski, 1960).

The energy of direct impact is partially dissipated as heat. Vascular damage and bleeding may occur from compression with a sudden rise in intravascular pressure (above 150 mm. Hg) resulting in bursting (Clark, 1967). Clothes provide effective cushioning for the skin so that often the extent of underlying soft tissue damage and the severity of intrathoracic injury is concealed. Muscle avulsion may result from shearing phenomena, but most often from rib fractures. The extent and wide distribution of rib fractures are due in part to the dissemination of force, in turn influenced by tissue structure (bone, cartilage, muscle), and in part to secondary compressive force (Fig. 7-1). The sharp rib fragment may tear muscle, pleura, and vessels (intercostal and internal thoracic). Experimental studies have demonstrated that the force of impact can actually shove the sternum almost against the spinal column (Border et al., 1968).

COMPRESSION AND DECOMPRESSION. A second action of the direct impact is compression with a sudden increase of pressure within a closed system (Blair et al., 1969). Ordinarily the airway is open. At the moment of or just prior to impact, the open system is converted into a closed box by closure of the glottis. The increase in pressure may result in bursting phenomena; and mediastinal pleural, tracheobronchial, or intrapulmonary damage. When the force is removed (occupant is thrown backward), the distorted thorax springs back creating an instant of increased negative (decompressive) intrathoracic pressure. One possible mechanism for lung contusion may lie in these compressive-decompressive phenomena. At the moment of impact a subsegmental bronchus is suddenly pinched off. The pressure within the alveoli, served by this segmental bronchus, is suddenly elevated. The limits of intra-alveolar pressure are exceeded. The alveoli burst and capillaries rupture. Along with this disruption of alveoli, blood extravasates within the enclosed area. Just as suddenly the compressive force is released. There is an explosive decompression with abrupt, negative intra-alveolar pressures leading to alveolar collapse; hence, the morphologic picture of patchy, disseminated congestive and hemorrhagic atelectasis.

Shock waves, from blast phenomena or secondary to an impact, with a velocity of 66 feet per second and a duration of 0.5 milli-seconds or less can produce lung injury. Experimentally, abrupt deceleration from a terminal velocity of 100 feet per second or higher resulted in diffuse pulmonary hemorrhage, at 75 to 104 feet per second, more localized lesions, and at 66 to 75 feet per second, multiple scattered foci. The characteristics of lung pathology are likely related to combinations of these secondary forces. Similar events may explain the dynamics of injury with respect to the diaphragm, the trachea or bronchus, and the esophagus. The sudden increase in pressure causes, not a laceration, but a rupture, and secondary shearing tangential forces may also contribute to the injury.

The compressive force in automobile injuries is of split-second duration. In industrial accidents, such as mine cave-ins, landslides, or other sustaining, crushing loads, the direct compressive force is responsible for most of the injuries.

OTHER SECONDARY FORCES. Mediastinal injuries rarely result from direct impact, since the lungs (momentarily at positive pressure) presumably serve as protective cushions, somewhat like plastic air splints (Border et al., 1968). The damaging forces are compressive, decelerative, shearing, and torsional. At chest barrier impact, the sternum is shoved posteriorly. The heart is swung to the left and twisted. The forward motion of

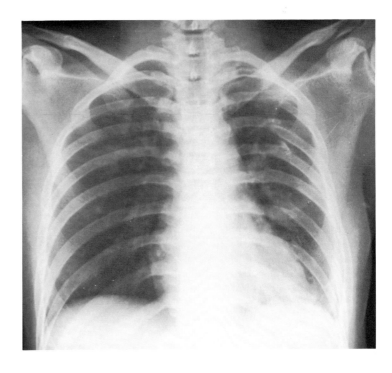

Figure 7-1. Admission x-ray following an automobile accident. Flail was not apparent in Emergency Room. Fractures involve ribs 3 to 9 on left. The infiltrate in midlung proved to be a contusion.

the thorax suddenly is arrested while mediastinal contents continue to decelerate.* The deceleration is arrested sharply at points of attachment, such as the ligamentum arteriosum of the aorta. This action alone, however, cannot account for transection, which is more common than "tears." Torsion stress is more critical at the base of the heart, with shearing stress at the ligamentum (Carmack et al., 1959). Force per se does not cause the injuries, but an imbalance of forces of acceleration and restraint (Clark, 1967). Similar stresses may account for the rare avulsion of a major pulmonary vessel or lobe. In falls, where loads are not as well tolerated and vertical deceleration is the primary factor in aortic tears, all which occur are at the ligamentum. The sudden deceleration in a relatively closed system can cause bursting of smaller vessels in the mediastinum and therefore may well account for the development of hematomas. The mechanisms for myocardial contusion probably include the combination of direct impact as well as shearing force (Parmley et al., 1958).

PENETRATING TRAUMA

MISSILES.   Direct impact is the more important factor in penetrating injuries, particularly in civilian casualties, since missiles usually are of low to medium velocities. Secondary effects include negative (suction) pressure, the formation of a temporary cavity, and tangential stresses related to trajectory — all significantly greater in high velocity missiles. Wound capability is directly proportional to bullet type, weight, velocity, and flight characteristics (yaw and spinning or tumbling) (French et al., 1962).

Bullets are characterized by weight, composition, and whether or not they expand upon impact. Most bullets are of the nonexpansive type except in hunting, in which the bullet explodes on impact, producing a wound tract that may be 30 to 40 times greater than that of the nonexplosive type. Velocity is considered in terms of kinetic energy imparted. It is classified as low (1200 fps.†), medium (1200 to 2500 fps.), and high (greater than 2500 fps.). Civilian weapons most commonly utilized are of low to medium velocity. Low velocities usually produce clean

wounds; medium velocities, more extensive wounds with some explosive effects; and high velocities, extreme explosive effects with maximum tissue destruction. An impact velocity of 125 to 170 fps. is required to penetrate the skin. If there is no exit of the bullet, there is no residual velocity, indicating that all of the energy was expended in wound production. Other factors influencing wound production include yaw, which is the deviation from the longitudinal axis in the line of flight. This increases with tissue density to as much as 800 times that experienced in air. The net result of yaw is to increase kinetic energy, which in turn increases tissue destruction. The retardation factor represents distance to the line of flight of the missile and varies with the density of the tissue. Generally there is an increase in kinetic energy, which is magnified in tissue. Spin is the rotation of the bullet and may vary from 100,000 to 200,000 revolutions per minute. The higher the spin, the more tissue is destroyed (Table 7-5A and B).

A 150-grain, .30 caliber bullet with an initial velocity of 2400 fps. strikes the skin, and, as it proceeds through the tissue, produces a permanent cavity termed the bullet tract. This is the direct impact effect. Beyond the skin, there is a negative suction pressure effect, which pulls in clothing, debris, and dirt. As the missile continues to traverse tissue, shock waves are produced, resulting in vascular rupture and extravasation beyond the tract. With further progression a temporary cavity is produced that is directly related to the velocity characteristics of the missile. The volume of the temporary cavity may be as much as 27 times that of the permanent cavity (wound tract). The extent of the cavities produced by various types of missiles is noted in Table 7-5. The higher the velocity (hence the kinetic energy imparted in tissue), the larger the cavity, with greater tissue destruction. The effects may be experienced two to three inches beyond the normal wound tract.

Another secondary effect is the tangential nonpenetrating trajectory, producing a force that will result in injury some distance from the wound tract itself. This may account for lung contusions, vascular and nerve injury, myocardial contusion, and bone fractures.

Immediately after penetration by a bullet, the skin, because it is elastic, tends to close and is therefore no index of the extent of injury. Muscle is the site of tremendous

---

*Negative acceleration — Newton's second law of motion.

†Feet per second.

TABLE 7-5A. Missile Ballistics Classification

	Low		Medium		High	
Velocity (fps)°	Kinetic energy (ft. lb.)°	Velocity (fps)	Kinetic energy (ft. lb.)	Velocity (fps)	Kinetic energy (ft. lb.)
500	55	2000	887	4000	3549
1000	222	3000	1996	5000	5545

TABLE 7-5B. Wound Characteristics of Low-medium Velocity (Civilian) Missiles

Velocity (fps)	Wound tract (in³)°	Adjacent zone (in³)°	Temporary cavity (in³)°
500	1.27	15.05	33.13
1000	2.55	30.11	66.25
2000	5.09	60.21	132.49

°*fps* = feet per second; *ft. lb.* =foot pound; *in³* = cubic inches. *Wound tract* is the visible permanent tissue defect. *Adjacent zone* refers to extent of tissue damage beyond the wound tract. *Temporary cavity* refers to the magnitude of tissue defect at the instant of missile flight through tissue. (Adapted from French and Callender: Wound Ballistics, 1962).

damage because it is the tissue in which the temporary cavity is most expansive. Ribs are usually fractured by direct impact, although occasionally this results from the explosive effect of a temporary cavity or the force from a tangential trajectory. Direct penetration of the lungs results in intra-alveolar hemorrhage and collapse. Frequently the extent of injury is remote from the wound tract. The mechanism for this is that the temporary cavity opens perpendicular to the line of flight of the missile. There is first a negative pressure followed by a much higher positive pressure. The sudden compressive and decompressive pressure changes result in alveolar-capillary ruptures. Most cardiovascular injuries are due to impact (Fig. 7-2). Occasionally contusions are due to secondary tangential forces or shock waves.

STAB WOUNDS. Approximately 75 per cent of stab wounds are inflicted with a knife and the remainder with ice picks. In the United States the most frequently used knife is a switchblade, which is six to eight inches long. Wound potential is directly related to the characteristics of the knife blade and the strength and angle of the thrust. All stab

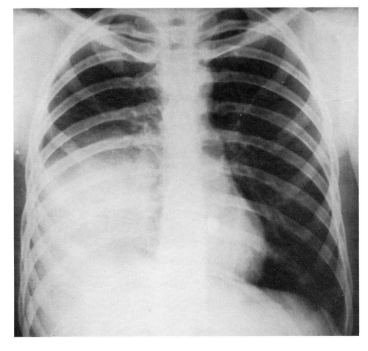

Figure 7-2. Admission x-ray following .32 caliber gunshot. Bullet entered on right and at surgery was found to be in the right atrium.

wounds tend to look more innocuous than they actually are, since the elasticity of skin tends to reduce the apparent size of the wound injury. Some protection is afforded by the victim's garments. As with bullet wounds, the anterior projection of the trunk is the most vulnerable, except for the sternum. This is due to the larger posterior thoracic muscle mass, which increases the traverse tract required for the blade to reach intrathoracic structures and be potentially lethal.

Muscle damage is limited to the wound tract entirely. Occasionally parts of garments or external debris are carried within the tract, but as a rule, knife wounds are considered "clean." Ribs are rarely fractured by a knife wound although occasionally costal cartilage may be severed. Of particular importance is the severance of intercostal vessels, a major source of hemothorax in knife wound victims. Pulmonary structures per se are rarely lacerated to a severe degree, the wound usually being a peripheral laceration. Direct penetration of a heart chamber or a major mediastinal vessel is the leading cause of early death, either from exsanguination or tamponade.

CHEST ANATOMY

RIB CAGE

The thorax is designed structurally to resist atmospheric pressure, so that the necessary differentials of negative dynamic intrapleural pressure may develop, and to permit normal flow of air into the lungs and minimal impediment to venous return. In addition, the thorax also serves as protection against possible injury, not only to intrathoracic contents but also to those in the upper abdomen. In accordance with orthopedic principles, fragments of long bones resulting from fractures are influenced by the force of impact and muscle pull. The rib is characterized essentially as flat, long bone. In rib fractures the force of impact is far more important than that of muscle pull. On the other hand, the musculature of the chest wall, by splinting, does exercise an influence over a flail segment, albeit temporary, because of reactive spasm secondary to trauma. The pectoralis major and minor splint primarily potential anterior or anterolateral flail segments, while the posterolateral segments

also include action of the anterior and posterior serratus muscles. Posteriorly, the back muscles, including the trapezius and the spinalis group, which are extremely strong, account for the fact that posterior flail chests rarely present any problem with respect to chest instability. On the inner surface of the chest wall, the subcostal muscles contribute to the splinting of posterior rib fractures in ribs 8 to 10. Anteriorly, the transthoracic muscles may contribute to splinting, but these are rather delicate slips and probably have no significant effect. Because it is quite small and protected by the shoulder girdle, the first rib is rarely fractured. When it is fractured, it is almost always accompanied by a fracture of the clavicle and also indicates that the force of the impact must have been tremendous. To produce a flail chest, double fractures of several ribs must occur. As the spasm wears off, the relatively minor effect of the intercostals, the subcostals, and the transverse thoracic muscles is easily overcome by forces in the opposite direction (flail segment and gravity). The plane of the posterior (proximal) rib fractures may remain unchanged or may be elevated slightly (more so in the upper three to six ribs), while the floating segment retains a position below (Blair et al., 1968). An associated fractured clavicle may accentuate the downward displacement of the flail portion. Ribs 3 to 8 are most commonly involved in fractures. These are more exposed and have the least protection from muscles. The lower ribs are not fractured as frequently primarily because of an increased degree of mobility and elasticity even at an older age. In the younger group of patients fractures are seen rather infrequently even if they sustain a relatively large force of impact.

PLEURAL SPACE

This is only a potential space. Visceral and parietal pleura usually separate easily by virtue of air or blood or both, incident to trauma. Once the space is created (whether open or closed) the relatively negative intrapleural pressure is converted into either a positive pressure or neutralized to zero, inhibiting lung expansion.

THE LUNGS

The lungs functionally may be classed as open-ended, elastic cushions, containing air and surrounded by a vacuum. The air sacs are in a constant state of imminent collapse, due to elastic force. A surfactant in conjunction with the negative pull (force) keeps the alveoli open. Thus, a balance exists between forces to maintain the intra-alveolar norm. Disruption of this balance often results in alveolar collapse. The alveoli are interlaced by capillary networks resting on a delicate stroma. The air sacs are connected to ducts, which are devoid of cartilage, and to respiratory (terminal) bronchioles, with some, but scanty, cartilage. Both structures are richly embossed in elastic fibrils. The communications continue progressively to more rigidly supportive segmental lobar and stem bronchi. The peripheral (lateral) surfaces abut the inner chest wall right against the ribs. The bases sit astride the diaphragmatic leaves and the apices crowd into the narrow, but solid, upper thorax. The medial surfaces wrap about the mediastinal contents, serving as protective cushions, particularly effectively under increased transpulmonary pressure. The hila are fairly rigid, but relatively pliable in children. These vital regions are also protected by the pulmonary umbrella.

TRACHEOBRONCHIAL TREE

This structure is fairly well protected by its anatomic location and relative resistance to force imbalance. The most common site of injury in blunt trauma is at the main stem bronchus, just distal to the trachea. The lung is most mobile at this region.

MEDIASTINUM

The upper third of the mediastinum is encased in a fatty areolar pad, through which course many small blood vessels. Generally, these are well protected by the relatively rigid upper thorax so that direct "crush" rarely produces serious damage. On the other hand, sudden decelerative phenomena may result in bursting of these vessels, causing hematomas.

HEART

The heart, relatively speaking, dangles freely in the mediastinum, suspended from the aortic root. It is encased in a rather stiff envelope, the pericardium. As noted previously, at the moment of impact the sternum moves backward, shoving the heart to one side and producing shearing and tangential forces. The point of suspension to the aortic root is a critical area of injury. Sudden deceleration may result in damage to high volume-low pressure regions, possibly accounting for most of the injuries to the right side (atrial and vena caval). On the other hand, anterior "crush," involving particularly the costal cartilages by direct injury, per se may produce cardiac tears. Sudden decelerative or compressive phenomena account most likely for bursting lacerations of the valves. Direct impact has some bearing on myocardial contusion, but decelerative and shear phenomena or trajectory shock waves, resulting in capillary rupture and diffuse hematomas, may be as significant. In blunt trauma, the left ventricle is rarely ruptured, the right ventricle very occasionally, whereas direct penetration by missiles is common. The pericardium contains many blood vessels, the rupture of which probably accounts for tamponade in the absence of direct injury to the heart or a coronary vessel. The pericardium is rather firmly fixed at the superior end around the aortic root and the pulmonary vessels. It is a closed type of sac and accounts for the rather drastic events should an acute effusion occur. It is somewhat grudgingly elastic and can accommodate fairly large-sized effusions, if they develop slowly. On the other hand, the sudden ingress of a relatively small amount (200 to 300 ml.) may result in tamponade of sufficient magnitude to cause cardiac arrest. The pericardium itself is rarely burst by decelerative phenomena, although it may be torn by sharp rib fragments, missiles, or knives.

LARGE VESSELS

The aorta is attached anteriorly to the heart at the root, superiorly by the three major aortic divisions, and posteriorly by the ligamentum arteriosum. Inferiorly, it is encased firmly in pleura, the point of maximal fixation in the thorax. These are, therefore, critical points of stress. The nature of damage is a transection and not a "tear," as popularly conjectured. The reasons are (1) the ligamentum is the last fixed point parallel to the long axis of the body, and (2) the attachment is stronger (more rigid) than those at the root or at the arch branches. The secondary forces are therefore more effective at this site. The proximity of the subclavian artery to the ligamentum accounts for this vessel's occasional involvement. Other major systemic arteries of significance are the intercostals and the internal thoracic. Because of their proximity to ribs, damage consists of laceration caused by rib fragments. The major systemic veins are concentrated in the superior mediastinum, huddling beneath the firm, protective roof of the clavicle and the first two ribs. An unusually enormous direct impact force is required to produce damage. Even when the first rib is fractured, underlying vascular injury is rare. The clavicle gets the brunt of the impact. In penetrating trauma the damage is always by direct force.

Pulmonary hilar vessels are protected by the lung air cushion and, in contrast to the bronchi, by their own elasticity. Direct impact or shearing and torsion phenomena can cause injury only if of enormous energy. Damage is unusual, but when it occurs it is usually lethal.

DIAPHRAGM

The extreme degree of mobility of the diaphragm generally permits a position of wide latitude. At the moment of impact there is a sudden positive intrathoracic pressure, which appears to be well met by a positive intra-abdominal pressure. This neutralization of pressures apparently accounts for the fact that diaphragmatic injuries are fairly uncommon as burst phenomena. The diaphragm is tensed and susceptible to "burst" forces. Injury is almost always on the left, which is the more mobile leaf. The subdiaphragmatic immediately adjacent structures are important to bear in mind, since injury can occur to the spleen or liver. This is particularly pertinent in penetrating trauma.

PHYSIOLOGY

From a functional standpoint the lungs serve to maintain normal oxygen and carbon dioxide tensions. This is accomplished by the mass movement of air in and out of the lungs by virtue of alternating pressures intrathoracically, with the chest wall serving as a buffer against the relatively positive atmospheric pressure. Uniform action of the thoracic muscles and of the diaphragm results in geometric enlargement of the intrathoracic volume. At the same time there is an increase in the relative negativity of the intrapleural pressure, creating a gradient between it and the atmosphere. Air flows (or is pushed) into the lungs. Conversely, by virtue of recoil of the lungs and the upward movement of the diaphragm, the intrapleural pressure becomes less negative. The intrapulmonary pressure becomes somewhat positive in relation to the atmosphere, and the air is thence expelled. Mechanical

TABLE 7-6.   Terminology and Normal Values in Respiratory Physiology

Term	Meaning	Normal Values
P_AO_2	alveolar O_2 tension in mm. Hg	100–104
P_aO_2	arterial O_2 tension in mm. Hg	90–100
A-aDO$_2$	alveolar-arterial O_2 gradient	5–60° (100% O_2 = max. 60)
P_ACO_2	alveolar CO_2 tension in mm. Hg	38–42
P_ECO_2	fraction of expired CO_2	28–30
$PaCO_2$	arterial CO_2 tension	Same as P_AO_2
$CaCO_2$	arterial CO_2 content in Vol %	55–60
VT	tidal volume in cc.	500†
$\dot{V}_T$	minute ventilation (total) in cc.	6000†
$\dot{V}_A$	alveolar ventilation in cc.	4200†
VD	"physiological" dead space in cc.	100% O_2 = max. 60
P_B	barometric pressure in mm. Hg	760 (sea level)
P_{H_2O}	water vapor pressure in mm. Hg	47
$^FIO_2$	fraction of inspired O_2	—
$\dot{V}/\dot{Q}$	ventilation-perfusion ratio	0.7–0.8

°Varies with $^FIO_2$.
†Young male, recumbent, BTPS. (Body temperature, pressure, saturated with water vapor).
Calculations:
$P_AO_2 = (P_B \times {}^FIO_2) - (P_{H_2O} + PaCO_2)$
$A\text{-}aDO_2 = P_AO_2 - PaO_2$
$$VD/VT = \frac{PaCO_2 - P_ECO_2}{PaCO_2} \qquad (normal = 0.3 - 0.4)$$

(resistance) and elastic (compliance) factors are involved in the mass movement of air in and out of the lungs, since the system is visco-elastic (Table 7-6).

In order to maintain a normal P_aO_2 and a normal P_aCO_2, inspired air must be dispersed throughout the lungs. The mixture of intrapulmonary gas under normal circumstances, is considered uneven; that is, certain portions of the lungs are not ventilated at equivalent rates. The lung, physiologically, is compartmentalized, so that ventilation rates and volumes vary considerably. In order to assure the transport of oxygen and carbon dioxide, perfusion is required, also with varying distribution. Ventilation/perfusion ($\dot{V}_A/\dot{Q}$) ratios vary in different parts of the lungs, and average out at approximately 0.8. This $\dot{V}_A/\dot{Q}$ may be altered when areas with adequate perfusion are inadequately ventilated. This has been termed physiological shunting. Diffusion across the alveolocapillary membrane is proportional to gas pressure gradients and to the physical state of the membrane itself.

PATHOPHYSIOLOGY

PULMONARY EFFECTS

The physiological manifestations of chest trauma derive from cumulative effects of loss of integrity of the chest wall, intrapleural accumulations, airway obstruction, and pulmonary parenchymal damage. The bellows action of the muscles of the chest wall is reduced (Avery et al., 1956). On inspiration, the loose segment (flail) is pushed inward due to the loss of the quality of thoracic resistance. On expiration the gradient is reversed, so that the intrathoracic pressure exceeds atmospheric pressure. The flail segment is shoved outward. It has been speculated that a segment of air pendulates (moves) back and forth between two lungs, resulting in increased dead space ventilation. The magnitude of the "pendelluft" is not as significant as was formerly believed (Blair et al., 1969).

The open chest wound also causes an alteration in pressure dynamics, but in a different fashion. Communication with the atmosphere neutralizes the intrapleural pressure to zero at rest. On inspiration, the induced negative pressure is greater than on the contralateral, unaffected side. There is, therefore, a larger gradient. Air rushes in at a greater rate than into the normal hemithorax. The intrapleural pressure rises rapidly to atmospheric. To push the air out of the pleural space on expiration requires positive effort, since there is no potential energy build-up (elastic recoil) during inspiration, as occurs within the lungs. A tissue flap or blood clot may produce a ball-valve effect, causing tension pneumothorax. The resultant bobbing back and forth of the flail or sucking open wound, together with airway obstruction from secretions, causes increased resistance and decreased compliance (Garzon et al., 1966). Gas distribution is impaired causing a net reduction in alveolar ventilation; with a continued perfusion, this results in disproportion in the $\dot{V}_A/\dot{Q}$ relationship (Bassett et al., 1968; Blair et al., 1969).

In an attempt to overcome the impairment, there is an increase in respiratory work. The accumulation of air or blood, or both, in the pleural space reduces the ventilative lung volume, producing a restrictive pulmonary insufficiency. Parenchymal damage, in the form of pulmonary contusions or intrapulmonary hematomas, results in a decrease in compliance and an increase in elastic work. The P_aO_2 is decreased with reduction in net diffusion across the alveolocapillary membrane. Assuming that perfusion is relatively adequate, and that the hemoglobin is also within normal limits, the reduced gas oxygen transport culminates in a decreased arterial oxygen tension.

Positive identification of the defect is obtained by analysis of the P_aO_2, a mandatory procedure in evaluation (Blair et al., 1969; Wise et al., 1968). The reduction in oxygen tension produces hypoxia, which in turn causes a reflex hyperventilation, lowering the carbon dioxide level. The pH rises. Respiratory alkalosis is present. The initial ventilatory insufficiency is for oxygen. If this disarray is allowed to persist, or secondary complications, such as airway obstruction from secretions or aspirate, are permitted to intervene, the insufficiency spreads to include carbon dioxide. Respiratory acidosis ensues. Continued hypoxia eventually causes increased anaerobic cellular metabolism with the accumulation of fixed acids, or metabolic acidosis (Fig. 7-3).

The degree of pulmonary dysfunction existing in a patient upon initial observation in an Emergency Room is often compounded significantly by the development of complications of a secondary nature during the interval before admission. These usually are

PULMONARY UNITS

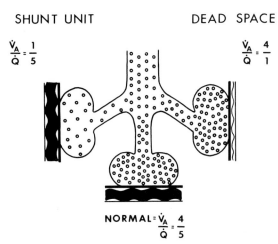

SHUNT UNIT   DEAD SPACE

$$\frac{\dot{V}_A}{\dot{Q}} = \frac{1}{5}$$ $$\frac{\dot{V}_A}{\dot{Q}} = \frac{4}{1}$$

$$NORMAL = \frac{\dot{V}_A}{\dot{Q}} = \frac{4}{5}$$

Figure 7-3. A pulmonary unit consists of the terminal airway (alveolus) and circulation (capillary), separated by a membrane. Lung dysfunction in chest trauma is attributed to the "shunt" unit. $\dot{V}_A$ = alveolar minute ventilation; $\dot{Q}$ = minute blood flow.

related to airway obstruction, further ventilatory restriction of an iatrogenic nature, and shock. Retained secretions or aspiration of vomitus or blood from facial injuries lead to airway obstruction, increasing alveolar hypoventilation, airway resistance, and work of breathing. Strapping the chest with different devices to diminish the flail movement often inhibits contralateral mechanical ventilation. Immense acute gastric dilatation is very common in trauma and causes restriction of diaphragmatic motion and vomiting.

Pulmonary dysfunction is often further staggered because of improprieties of management, lack of intensity of vigil and follow-up, and pneumonia. Retained secretions with persistent or recurring atelectasis lead to a further decrease in compliance and elevation of airway resistance, with concomitant worsening in alveolar hypoventilation. Over-zealous fluid therapy may produce "wet lungs." Pneumonitis, a common complication of lung contusion, and occasionally "blowouts" during respiratory therapy also contribute to impairment.

CARDIOVASCULAR EFFECTS

As early as 1889 Cohnheim demonstrated that the injection of oil into the pericardium caused elevation in peripheral venous pressure and a drop in the arterial pressure. A recent investigation of experimental techniques included raising the intrapericardial pressure by introducing saline, whole blood, or air. Change in peripheral arterial pressure occurred only when the intrapericardial pressure was increased above 50 mm. Hg, at which point there was a precipitous drop in arterial pressure. As the intrapericardial pressure approached the resting venous pressure, this began to increase. There was also an elevation in right atrial pressure. In the pulmonary system, the venous and capillary pressure also increased. Pulmonary arterial pressure subsequently also rose. The cardiac output demonstrated a progressive decline with an elevation in peripheral resistance. Arterial pressure fell only when the intrapericardial pressure reached 50 mm. Hg.

The dynamics producing diminished cardiac output are unsettled. One possible mechanism is diminished ventricular filling pressure, which can limit diastolic fiber length, with a subsequent reduction in stroke volume and ventricular stroke work. Obstruction to venous return into the right atrium per se was not considered a significant factor. Another mechanism is concerned with the gradient between the pulmonary arterial and venous pressures; diminished pressure results in insufficient force for forward propulsion of blood through the lungs. A third factor is the increased intrapericardial pressure producing some obstruction to coronary flow. A report of patients has demonstrated the diminished effects of pressure in the right ventricle with reduction in central blood volume and cardiac output. The experimentally demonstrated compensatory mechanisms of increased peripheral resistance, increased heart rate, and increased intravenous pressure were confirmed. Also, in these clinical studies it was noted that arterial pressure remained within a reasonably normal level until very late, at which time there was a precipitous fall. The maintenance of a gradient between the pulmonary artery and the left atrium was considered to be the most important factor in maintaining cardiac output.

Waterpump tamponade, blood loss, or a cardiac arrhythmia causes a critical low perfusion state. The net effect is reduced oxygen transport to tissue, compounding the effect of pulmonary dysfunction and accelerating hypoxia (Fig. 7-4).

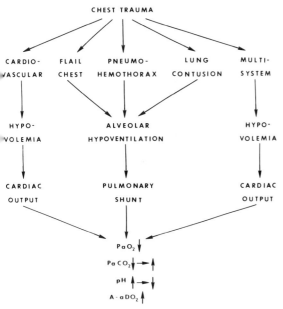

Figure 7-4. In blunt chest trauma the primary deficit is in ventilation (alveolar), resulting in hypoxia and "shunting" within the lung. Because of reflex (hypoxic) ventilation, carbon dioxide retention is not seen initially. Respiratory alkalosis is present, and acidosis supervenes later if correct therapy has not been effected. Hypovolemia is a secondary problem. On the other hand, in penetrating chest trauma hypovolemia is often the primary problem. This leads to reduced cardiac output and subsequent reduced oxygen transport. If any lung impairment is also present, the resultant hypoxia is further aggravated.

DIAGNOSIS

Prompt assessment of the nature and magnitude of chest trauma is necessary to save the patient's life or to reduce morbidity. Since injuries often are of a highly complex, multiple-organ nature, the examination of the patient must include a survey of all systems possibly involved. While the pulmonary-cardiovascular complex is the most crucial with respect to life-saving procedures (thereby dictating the initial direction of resuscitation), ascertainment of danger elsewhere is of equal importance.

In the majority of instances, diagnosis and evaluation can be made by accurate history and by the four fundamentals of physical diagnosis: inspection, palpation, percussion, and auscultation, based on a knowledge of biodynamics, anatomy, and physiology. Information relative to the intensity of the incident may be obtained from the police or ambulance attendants.

In every automobile accident, the possibility of blunt chest trauma should be considered. The burden of ruling this out rests upon the physician. Accident victims sitting in the driver's seat, or in the front seat, are more prone to chest injury because of sudden impact against the steering wheel or dashboard. The patient's past history is of importance, particularly as related to his pulmonary status. Pre-existing chronic lung disease heralds poor tolerance to injury. In penetrating injury, relevant information includes the weapon, range or assailant stance, and amount of blood lost at the scene.

CLINICAL ASPECTS

INSPECTION. Careful systematic inspection provides valuable information, noting blood loss (clothes), wound entry and exit, a pulsating knife handle, ventilatory pattern, skin color, mental status, collapse or dilatation of peripheral veins, and, if present, a flailing chest segment. Approximately 35 per cent of patients with crushed chest fail to show any thoracic wall abnormality when initially seen, but develop a flail chest subsequently (Bassett et al., 1968; Blair et al., 1968). Repeat examinations are therefore essential. Missing the flail effect may result in "hidden" hypoxia. Absence of motion in a hemithorax is usually the result of a sizeable pneumothorax or hemothorax. Extreme distress in ventilation, together with cyanosis and deviation of the trachea from the midline, frequently is due to tension pneumothorax, massive hemothorax, or massive atelectasis. In the first two instances, the trachea deviates contralaterally and in the last to the ipsilateral side. Stridor points to obstruction in a major airway. Pale skin and flat peripheral veins may be the result of major hemorrhage, suggesting hypovolemia with possible shock. Dilated peripheral veins, especially in the neck, should suggest the presence of a cardiac tamponade or impaired myocardial function.

PALPATION. The presence of subcutaneous emphysema indicates an air leak, secondary to pneumothorax or a tracheobronchial rupture or perforation. Absence of tactile fremitus is usually the result of pneumothorax. In the majority of instances wherein the flail segment cannot be noted by visual perception, careful palpation will usually denote its presence. Most sternal injuries (fractures or separations) can be accurately diagnosed by careful palpation. Manual examination of the larynx and trachea leads to early diagnosis of fractures or contusions in these areas. Localization of the site of the rib fractures may point to possible underlying organ damage in the upper abdomen. Wound entry and exit should create a mental picture of the trajectory.

AUSCULTATION. Absence of breath sounds is suggestive of a pneumothorax, a hemothorax, or atelectasis. The presence of bowel sounds in the chest is secondary to diaphragmatic rupture. Auscultation of the heart should be performed meticulously; however, the distress of the patient frequently renders physical examination difficult. Distant or absent heart sounds should signal the presence of a cardiac tamponade. Abnormal murmurs may be secondary to the development of intracardiac shunt. Friction rubs, particularly if synchronous with the heart sounds, should suggest pericardial involvement.

PERCUSSION. The loss of normal sonority of the chest is usually the result of an abnormal collection of air or fluid. Dullness should raise the question of hemothorax, hyperresonance, and pneumothorax. Percussion is rarely helpful in distinguishing enlargement of the mediastinum.

RADIOLOGY

Too often in the routine of the Emergency Room, the staff is admonished to take the blood pressure, start I.V., and take an x-ray. While there is no question that x-rays are of great value, most of the patient's emergent problems can be discerned by careful physical examination. X-rays are a supplementary procedure and should be kept in the proper perspective as a confirmation of initial impressions. In particular, tension pneumothorax, massive hemothorax, and cardiac tamponade should be established on a clinical basis and proper therapy instituted prior to x-ray examination. The ascertainment of a patent airway and stabilization of ventilation and of hemodynamics are urgent requirements prior to moving a patient about. The delay in getting films, poor quality, and the difficulties in interpretation contribute to missed or delayed diagnoses of serious complications, secondary to the chest injury. Simple posteroanterior (PA) projections of the chest will supply most of the information required in blunt chest trauma. Most of the anteroposterior (AP) films are taken because

of patient problems. Mediastinal shadows tend to be prominent. The eye trained to read PA projections must be alert for a different pattern. Most of the rib fractures can be seen readily, but in certain instances lateral fractures cannot be viewed. Costal cartilage involvement will not show up. Immediate delineation of the rib fractures is superfluous, delaying therapy. Identification of retained missiles is extremely important, especially if the missile lies outside of the projected horizontal axis of entry.

PNEUMOTHORAX. Most sizable pneumothoraces are readily visible. If the volume of pneumothorax is small, physical signs will be absent and undetectable by routine x-rays. These then would indicate that no immediate serious problem is present, but since collections may be somewhat delayed, repeated subsequent examinations are of importance. Should the ascertainment of pneumothorax be significant, additional films of a supine projection with expiration may demonstrate small pneumothorax not observable in the standard film.

HEMOTHORAX. The blood that enters the pleural cavity rapidly coagulates, but presumably because of physical agitation of the heart and lungs, the clot is defibrinated and the blood is usually in liquid form. In most instances the blood moves with gravity and therefore is in a dependent position. An upright film is of importance in order to establish whether or not the magnitude of hemothorax is of significance. At times the lateral decubitus position may demonstrate a very small hemothorax, although this information rarely is of practical value. When blood and air are present in the pleural space, the resulting air-fluid level will permit easy detection in the standard upright film.

LUNG DAMAGE. Parenchymal infiltrates in the lung most often are due to contusion, although they may result from hematomas and lacerations. Contusions may be focal or disseminating and range from mild linear to nodular infiltrates, and finally to rather massive spread with some degree of consolidation. X-ray recognition of pulmonary contusion is rather poorly defined and initially it is frequently difficult to differentiate from other types of infiltrates. The contusion usually appears after the injury but may be delayed as long as 48 to 72 hours after injury. The radiologic criteria for diagnosis of pulmonary contusion are as follows: (1) isolated or confluent regular nodular densities with peribronchial and perivascular infiltrates; (2) homogeneous opacification resulting from intra-alveolar hemorrhage and traumatic rupture of the alveoli; (3) a combination of the preceding with and without pulmonary effusion. Frank consolidation occurs rarely, but when present, the pattern does not conform to the shape of any lung segment. An intrapulmonary missile that is peripheral and close to the site of entry indicates problems of small magnitude compared to one in the mediastinum or imbedded in soft tissue across the thorax.

LACERATED TRACHEA OR BRONCHUS. In the majority of instances, patients with tracheobronchial rupture will demonstrate pneumomediastinum and subcutaneous emphysema extending up into the neck. Ipsilateral rib fractures are often present. Fractures of the first and second ribs, which are relatively unusual, should raise a question of bronchial injury, since these indicate an unusual magnitude of impact. Occasionally, only a pneumothorax and very little in the way of a pneumomediastinum may be present. Suspicion should escalate when there is continued escape of air through a thoracotomy tube. Definition of a rupture may be obtained through laminography and bronchoscopy. Bronchograms are rarely required.

ESOPHAGUS. Damage to the esophagus is extremely rare. Rupture of the upper segment causes mediastinal and cervical emphysema. Injury in the lower esophagus is accompanied by hydropneumothorax in about 50 per cent of instances. The effusion may be bilateral. Should any question exist, a Gastrografin swallow is of value.

AORTA AND LARGE VESSELS. It has been estimated that only 20 per cent of patients with blunt traumatic rupture of the aorta live long enough to arrive at an Emergency Room. The figure is even lower in missile perforations. In an injury predominantly of the chest existence of shock should lead to suspicion of a major vascular injury. The initial x-ray is of importance, particularly if there is a massive hemothorax on the left side. The sign most often searched for is widening of the mediastinum. Unfortunately, this is not a very accurate guide in the absence of left side effusion. Widening of the mediastinum may result from many factors, the most common of which are inadequate films, which falsely enlarge the mediastinal area, and mediastinal hematomas. Repeat films are often necessary. Most often a questionably wide mediastinum, "present" upon the admission, will "resolve" within 24 hours with properly obtained chest films.

CARDIAC TAMPONADE. The rapid effusion of blood may be sufficient to induce a cardiac arrest, but at the same time may not demonstrate radiologic enlargement of the heart. The diagnosis should be made initially on clinical grounds, and if any question exists, repeat films and pericardiocentesis should be performed.

DIAPHRAGM. Most blunt traumatic ruptures occur in the left hemidiaphragm, posteriorly at the dome. Pathognomonic evidence includes gas-filled viscus above the level of the diaphragm. Suggestive findings include an abnormally high diaphragm, fluoroscopic evidence of decreased or absent movement, or disc-like atelectasis above an elevated diaphragm. A thoracic entry wound with the missile in the abdomen is pathognomonic for diaphragmatic perforation and intra-abdominal injury. The injection of contrast media into the upper or lower G.I. tract may be of assistance, should any question exist.

LABORATORY

Important initial laboratory examinations include a hematocrit, urine samples, and arterial blood gases. Studies in our institution have demonstrated that 80 per cent of patients who arrive in the Emergency Room with major blunt chest trauma are hypoxic. Estimation of the alveolar-arterial oxygen gradient (A-aDO$_2$) provides important information about pulmonary function, particularly shunting (Blair et al., 1969; Wise et al., 1968). This can be obtained by having the patient breathe 100 per cent oxygen for 30 minutes through an endotracheal tube or a well-fitted mask. Normal A-aDO$_2$ values range from 8 to 60 mm. Hg, depending on the concentration of inspired oxygen.

SPECIAL PROCEDURES

Special procedures are designed primarily for confirmation of suspicion of critical lesions, such as tension pneumothorax, aortic tear, or bronchial laceration. Diagnostic thoracentesis is an extremely useful procedure should any question exist as to the presence of a sizable pneumothorax, particularly if under tension. In the latter situation, the insertion of a large bore needle may prove lifesaving. The suspicion of a cardiac tamponade should immediately lead to pericardiocentesis. Aortography is essential in a suspected rupture. Facilities and a trained staff must be available on a 24-hour basis. Double venous injection has been used, but visualization is not nearly so satisfactory. Tracheal or bronchial tears, if present, will frequently be revealed through bronchoscopy or laminography. Emergency exploratory thoracotomy may be required for penetrating injuries, but is rarely indicated in blunt trauma.

DELAYED OR MISSED DIAGNOSES (DOMD)

Delay in detecting a serious injury or missing it completely is the primary cause of early post-admission deaths, practically all of which are preventable. The "sudden" deluge of an Emergency Room by several seriously injured victims; the turbulence of ambulance attendants, police officers, orderlies, nurses, doctors, students, and technicians; the delay in getting back lab reports; the poor x ray; the puzzle of whom the patient "belongs" to—all serve only as weak excuses. The development of and strict adherence to a simple, logical routine is almost foolproof.

Tension pneumothorax and severe heart contusion were the most common DOMD and were fatal in most instances. Aortic rupture, when missed, is almost uniformly disastrous. Diaphragmatic ruptures and tracheobronchial tears are frequently missed, but not as fatal. In our experience, flail chest was missed in the early period (3 to 6 hours), and was detected on the next morning's rounds. The time of delay is of interest; in the vast majority of blunt trauma cases there was adequate time afforded to have made the necessary detection: tension pneumothorax—10 hours to 2 days. DOMD is due to the failure to exercise clinical acumen and to adhere to established and proven protocol. Victims dead on arrival are common in penetrating injuries, especially gunshot. Death shortly after admission to the Emergency Room also occurs with

agonizing frequency as a result of hemorrhage, tamponade, or tension pneumothorax. Youth and an "insignificant" skin wound lead to paralyzing deceptions. Hemodynamic compensatory mechanisms, sustaining arterial pressure, may collapse precipitously (Tables 7-7 and 7-8).

MANAGEMENT

PRINCIPLES

THORACIC. The fundamental principle in therapy of chest trauma is to reverse the pathophysiologic vector by correcting (1) the anatomic defects (flail, open-wound, pneumohemothorax, atelectasis) and (2) ventilatory ($\dot{V}_A$ and $\dot{V}/\dot{Q}$) and perfusion deficits (hypovolemia, tamponade) (Fig. 7-5). The rationale for the anatomic correction is based upon the physiologic changes. Both problems are treated at the same time. In serious blunt trauma, the most ideal and practical solution is utilization of intermittent positive pressure ventilation (IPPV) (Avery et al., 1956; Blair et al., 1968). Stabilization of the thorax and restoration of thoracic and ventilative lung volume are the anatomic goals. Continued clearance of airway obstructions and assurance of restoration of lung volume by rapid removal of intrapleural air or fluid or both by intrathoracic catheter are similarly important (Tables 7-9 and 7-10).

A patient, since he is already hypoxic, should not be permitted to work excessively. The initial and vital factor with respect to use of IPPV is the elimination of the pressure differential phenomena responsible for flail effects and its replacement by a controlled, positive-zero pressure system. With IPPV the pressure differential is abolished. The loose, bobbing segment is pushed and kept outward by the lungs, which serve as internal pneumatic splints. By the constant and steady push of the lungs against the fragments, reduction similar to that in long bone fracture takes place. The free, displaced, and rotated segment falls back into usually satisfactory realignment. The position is then maintained by the lungs under positive-zero pressures for the period of time required for adequate fixation, as in any fracture.

Physiologically, IPPV serves as the only

TABLE 7-7. Delayed or Missed Diagnoses (DOMD) in Chest
Trauma—Anatomic Aspects

Lesion	Reason for DOMD	Diagnostic aids	Time interval
A. Thorax			
1. Flail	Muscular splinting; double fractures not visualized by x-ray (costal cartilages)	Careful, thorough palpation; Repeat examination	1-6 hours
2. Fractured (dislocated) sternum	Same	Same	Same
B. Lungs and pleura			
1. Contusion	Develops in 2-24 hours; x-ray evidence nonspecific early	Arterial blood gases; calculation of A-aDO$_2$; serial x-rays	4-48 hours
2. Tension pneumothorax	Inadequate awareness and examination	Initial—dyspnea, cyanosis Later—increased leak; subcutaneous emphysema; x-ray	10-48 hours
C. Heart			
1. Hemopericardium	Not considered—physical findings nonspecific	High index of suspicion, elevated CVP; distended neck veins; fluoroscopy; pericardiocentesis	4-24 hours
2. Contusion	Physical findings nonspecific Initial ECG normal or nonspecific	High index of suspicion; repeat ECG; precordial pain; acute failure	2-10 days Some never
3. Tear, perforation	Not suspected	Continued bleeding from thoracotomy tube; shock; missile	12-48 hours
4. Valve rupture	Not suspected	Murmur of insufficiency, heart	Days-months
D. Great vessels			
1. Aortic rupture	Findings nonspecific in two-thirds	Widening mediastinum; hypertension; loss of femoral pulses; hemothorax (left); shock; aortogram	4 hours-16 days Months-years
2. Aortic penetration	Rapid exsanguination	Profound shock	None
3. Lung vessel laceration	Not suspected	Continued brisk bleeding from thoracotomy tube; shock; missile in mediastinum	4-12 hours
E. Miscellaneous			
1. Tracheobronchial rupture, wound	Not suspected	Continued and pronounced air leak from thoracotomy tube; tension pneumothorax; subcutaneous emphysema	4-72 hours Months-years
2. Diaphragmatic	No specific signs	Bowel in chest (auscultation and x-ray); missile in abdomen	48-72 hours
3. Esophageal rupture	Not suspected	Subcutaneous emphysema; hydrothorax	Years 24-72 hours

TABLE 7-8.   Delayed or Missed Diagnoses (DOMD) of Chest
Trauma—Physiologic Aspects

Deficit	Reason for DOMD	Causes	Diagnostic aids
A. Hypoxia	Clinical signs (dyspnea, cyanosis) absent. Restlessness attributed to head injury	Airway obstruction Flail chest Lung contusion Tension pneumothorax Massive atelectasis	Airway aspiration Blood gases; A-aDO$_2$ Diagnostic thoracentesis X-rays Oxygen administration
B. Hypovolemia	Arterial pressure and pulse may be misleading Bleeding not obvious Underestimate due to lack of appraisal	Nonthoracic injury Laceration of intercostal vessel Aortic rupture Pulmonary vessel tear	Careful examination (abdomen, fractures) Thoracentesis High index of suspicion Aortography
C. Cardiac dysfunction	Not suspected initially	Tamponade Contusion Lacerations Arrhythmias	Distended neck veins; elevated CVP; low output syndrome; diagnostic pericardiocentesis Serial ECG Persistent bleeding Auscultation; ECG

consistently effective means of overcoming the insidious effects on ventilation resulting from (1) diminished chest expansion due to initial muscular spasm, (2) the flail condition, and (3) disturbance secondary to atelectasis, pulmonary contusion, and aspiration pneumonitis. IPPV is rarely re-

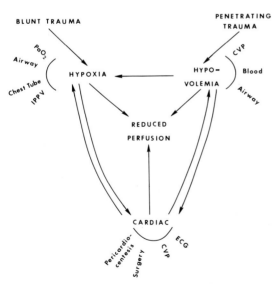

Figure 7-5. The primary pathophysiologic features are indicated and reduced perfusion is the preterminal event (due to hypovolemia, direct cardiac injury, or myocardial ischemia). Principal positive feedback develops which hastens cardiac dysfunction and decreases blood flow. Resuscitation is directed to relieve hypoxia and hypovolemia.

quired in penetrating chest trauma unless severe pre-existing chronic lung disease is present or a severe pulmonary complication develops. Plugging the open chest wound with concomitant catheter drainage restores integrity. It is emphasized that the impact of the dysfunction causing hypoxia can be assessed early and accurately only by arterial gas tension analysis. The increased dead space ventilation may be reduced by tracheostomy, but initially nasotracheal intubation is most satisfactory.

CARDIOVASCULAR. Assessment of myocardial states in blunt trauma is critical, especially if general anesthesia and surgery are contemplated. Severe contusions are the likely cause of acute failure or of cardiac arrest. Significant hypovolemia requires whole blood transfusion. Estimates based on hematocrit values coupled with dilutional modifications of rapid fluid administration lead to serious errors. Reliance solely on solute is as grave a mistake as overtransfusion. The best indices are (1) overt loss of blood from hemothorax, or other obvious active major bleeding, and multiple lower extremity fractures with or without pelvic fractures; (2) urinary output; (3) central venous pressure changes with test loads; and (4) clinical evaluation Penetrating cardiovascular wounds are catastrophic. Blood transfusion races to balance active and huge losses are usually futile. Early surgical intervention is re

TABLE 7-9. Emergency Management of Blunt Chest Trauma

Place	Problem	Procedure
A. On site	Crushed chest	External splint (strap-type)
		Oropharyngeal tube
		Oronasopharyngeal suction
		Oxygen by mask
		IPPV by hand-bag
	Bleeding	Compresses (no tourniquets!)
		I. V. with Ringer's solution
	Fractures	Splint (cushion type)
	Cardiac arrest	External massage
	Head injury	Dress open wound
B. In transit	Crushed chest	Continue A
	Bleeding	" "
	Fractures	" "
	Cardiac arrest	" "
C. Emergency Room	Crushed chest	Nasotracheal intubation
		IPPV (respirator or hand-bag)
		Intratracheal suction
		Oxygen at 100%
		Remove external splints, clothes
		Chest tube
		Chest x-ray
		ECG
	Bleeding	Continue Ringer's; blood, if indicated
		Insert CVP catheter
		Hematocrit
		Search for site
	Fractures	In splint. (Postpone treatment of fracture unless there is vascular involvement)
	Head injury	Stabilize cardiopulmonary, then attend
	Abdomen	Careful and repeated exam
		Catheter lavage
		X-ray
		Careful and repeated exam
		Urinalysis
	Renal	IVP

Table 7-10.   Emergency Management of Penetrating Chest Trauma

Place	Problem	Procedure
A. On site	Open wound	External compress
		Oropharyngeal tube
		Oronasopharyngeal suction
		Oxygen by mask
		IPPV by hand-bag
	Bleeding	External compresses
		I. V. with Ringer's solution
	Cardiac arrest	External massage
B. In transit	Open wound	Continue A
	Bleeding	" "
	Cardiac arrest	" "
C. Emergency Room	Open wound	Vaseline compress
		Nasotracheal intubation, if
		indicated
		Intratracheal suction
		Oxygen at 100%
		Remove clothes
		Chest tube
		Chest x-ray
		ECG
	Bleeding	Continue Ringer's; whole blood
		Insert CVP catheter
		Hematocrit
		Urinary catheter
		Search for site
		If massive, thoracotomy
	Cardiac	Pericardiocentesis
	tamponade	Rapid recurrence, thoracotomy
	Cardiac arrest	Thoracotomy, open massage
		(*Never* closed massage!)

quired. Relief of pericardial tension by aspiration is the prime step in tamponade; rapid recurrence would indicate the need for surgery. Imminent or actual cardiac arrest demands open thoracotomy massage. Local massage is ineffectual and potentially dangerous.

Clinical state. A third and important factor is the clinical state of the patient. Dyspnea, pain, anxiety, and restlessness are common features of the critically injured victim. The proper use of IPPV in crushed chests eliminates the first three symptoms and, by producing distraction of the rib fragments, relieves pain. Prudent use of narcotics and of sedatives may be required. Occasionally, automatic control ventilation will necessitate heavier sedation and curare-like drugs.

BLUNT TRAUMA

CHEST WALL. The most striking and critical injury is a flail chest due to fractures of many ribs, including double fractures of several individual ribs. In addition, there is considerable damage to chest wall musculature, causing reactive spasm. Occasionally there may be a laceration through the chest wall musculature and a penetrating wound.

Minor Trauma. Minor trauma usually encompasses one or more rib fractures with or without pneumothorax. There is no flail effect and no significant parenchymal injury. The dominant problem is pain. Ventilatory movements and cough are inhibited. There is one, and only one, proper technique in treatment—intercostal nerve block. This should include one interspace above and one below the rib fracture(s) and should be performed either in the posterior midline or the posterior axillary line. Topical anesthetics in a water base, not oil, is advised. If this simple and excellent method fails, it is for one reason— neglect in performance of repeat blocks. As many as four may be required in the first 24 to 48 hours. There are two measures to avoid: External binding of any type is contraindicated. The idea of therapy is to free-up mobility of the thorax, not to inhibit it further. Narcotics relieve pain and anxiety, but the positive benefit of a quiet immobile patient accrues only to the nurse and the intern. Depression of the respiratory center reflexes, cilia motility, and cough are serious hazards. If urgently required, tranquilizers (antihistamines for the elderly) or very small dosages of Demerol (25 mg. intravenously) may be used. The patient should be up and about the next morning, unless other injuries are prohibitive.

The second important problem is retention of secretions. There is considerable, and unfortunate, reluctance in the performance of nasotracheal catheter suctioning by staff members. This is the only effective means of assisting the victim in clearing his airway immediately and in the first 24 to 48 hours after injury. If the patient complains bitterly, then the intercostal block was not performed effectually or needs to be repeated. Administration of 100 per cent humidity in the form of a mist by face-tent is useful. Occasionally in the elderly or in the presence of chronic lung disease nasal oxygen may be indicated. Respirator therapy may be required.

Major Trauma. Flail chest constitutes the major problem. Approximately one-third of patients in our series did not demonstrate this abnormality in the Emergency Room due to the marked degree of muscular spasm. Flail is apparent in most of the patients within three hours and in all within 12 hours after the accident. Bilateral chest injury was present in 25 per cent of the patients (Table 7-11). The flail was on the right side in 45 per cent and on the left in 55 per cent. In the majority of instances six ribs or fewer were involved in the flail segment. This included patients with bilateral thoracic cage rib fractures. The number of fractured ribs was higher in immediate fatalities. The flail segments were mostly lateral or posterolateral with anterior or anterolateral

locations next in rate of frequency. Estimation of the degree of displacement of the rib fractures demonstrated this to be minimal in 21 per cent, moderate in 68 per cent, and marked in 11 per cent. The sternum was involved in about 7 to 15 per cent of patients, with either a fracture or a dislocation. These were associated with anterior rib fractures.

RESPIRATOR MANAGEMENT

Management may fall into two broad categories: I, the chest injured patient requiring only IPPV/I (intermittent or noncontinuous) and II, patients requiring IPPV (continuous) (Table 7-12).

CATEGORY I — IPPV/I THERAPY. This includes patients with the following criteria: (a) blunt chest trauma with usually fewer than five fractured ribs; (b) a minimal degree of splinting or flailing; (c) the ability to maintain satisfactory PaO_2 and $PaCO_2$ with nasal oxygen only, (d) ability to maintain a normal or somewhat alkalotic pH; (e) little or no lung contusion; (f) mental alertness without head injuries; (g) no pre-existing lung disease; and (h) a ventilatory rate under 30 per minute.

Arterial blood gases, drawn on admission, usually reveal some hypoxia, hypocarbia with a $PaCO_2$ of less than 40 mm. Hg, and a pH which is normal or slightly elevated. Additional oxygen is given via a nasal catheter sufficient to raise the PaO_2 to acceptable levels. Flows of over 5 liters per minute are not used owing to the complication of intragastric distention, which results in added impairment to ventilation. Following the administration of nasal oxygen for about 15 to 30 minutes, blood gases are checked again.

Vital signs are monitored at frequent intervals. Those indicating hypoxia include a rise or fall in pulse rate or arterial pressure, usually a rise in both; cyanosis, which is a late sign; an increase in respiratory

TABLE 7-11. Time Interval in Appearance of Flail (70 Patients)

Hours Prior to Admission	<3	<6	<12	>24	Total
Splint (per cent)	29	3	0	0	32
Flail (per cent)	16	1	1	13	31
None (per cent)	6	1	1	1	9
No record (per cent)	19	4	4	1	28

TABLE 7-12. Management of Blunt Chest Trauma

Criteria	Essential features
A. Conservative—IPPV/I (Category I)	
Usually less than 5 fractures	Vital signs
Minimal to no flail, minimal splinting	Serial blood gases
Adequate coughing possible, ability to raise secretions not impaired	Intercostal block
	Minimal doses of narcotics
Small to no chest contusion present	Nasal O_2, if indicated
Mentally alert—no associated head injury	Humidity via humidifier and half-face tent
	Chest physical therapy and IPPV/I
No pre-existing lung disease	Adequate hydration and blood volume
Cooperative, able to take IPPV/I	Chest x-ray
Satisfactory PaO_2 with or without nasal O_2	
B. Active—IPPV (Category II)	
Patients who show deterioration from conservative group	Vital signs
	Serial blood gases
Usually more than 5 fractures	Serial x-ray, chest
Flailing or splinting	Nasotracheal intubation
Inadequate cough with retained secretions	Controlled ventilation
Large lung contusions, costochondral separations	Inspired O_2 concentration, enough to ensure adequate PaO_2 (70 to 80 mm. Hg)
Pre-existing lung disease	$PaCO_2$ (32 to 36 mm. Hg)
Non-cooperative, unable to take IPPV/I	pH (7.40 to 7.46)
Associated head injury with stupor or coma	Hydration and blood, if required
Hypoxia with added nasal O_2	Chest physical therapy, suction, etc.
A rising $PaCO_2$	Nasogastric tube
Respiratory rate of 35+ per minute	Adequate doses of narcotics
Associated injuries requiring laparotomy	Tracheostomy when convenient

rate over 30 per minute; and a change in the level of consciousness. In terms of mechanical work, the rate of lung oxygen utilization in breathing for a normal person is approximately 0.5 to 1.0 ml. per liter of ventilation. The oxygen requirement rises dramatically in patients with severe chest injury. Physical signs are often unreliable and may lead to a false sense of security. Therefore, serial blood gases are absolutely essential and should be recorded on an acid-base nomogram. This has proved to be the only effective means to evaluate a patient's progress.

Intercostal nerve block is performed as noted under Minor Trauma. Elimination of secretions is extremely vital. Since the mucus often is thick and viscid and difficult to remove, it is essential to keep the secretions as thin as possible. This can be achieved in two ways: one is by maintaining adequate hydration of the patient and the other by administering well-humidified, oxygen-enriched air to the patient. A suitable humidifier with a plastic hose attached to a half-faced tent is preferable to placing the patient in an oxygen tent. In the latter

situation oxygen concentration cannot be controlled. The patient cannot be attended to adequately by either the nursing or the professional staff.

IPPV/I in this group of patients is administered at intervals as required, depending upon the clinical status. Generally it is administered every 4 to 6 hours and a bronchodilator medication is utilized, since a nebulizer itself may give rise to bronchospasm. Micronephrin, 5 drops in 5 cc. of sterile distilled water, is recommended. If bronchospasm is severe, 5 cc. of aminophylline with 5 drops of Micronephrin in a nebulizer has proved to be highly effective. Isuprel is not recommended because of possible deleterious side effects.

Narcotics may be utilized, but with caution. The agents depress ventilation, particularly in large dosages. Small dosages given intravenously relieve pain dramatically, with minimal respiratory depression. The intravenous administration is essential because in this way the correct dosage can be given. The effects of the drug take place in a very short period of time. Phenothiazines generally are not desirable because they have a tendency to produce thick secretions.

Measurement of lung volumes is extremely helpful in assessing progress. Vital capacity of a single breath of less than twice the normal tidal volume of the patient, or a vital capacity of 15 cc. per kg. body weight or less, would indicate that progress is not being maintained adequately and that active treatment (Category II) should be given.

It is preferable, if at all possible, to monitor these patients in the Intensive Care Unit where they can receive appropriate attention 24 hours a day. Patients with a few fractured ribs and minimal flail and small contusions usually respond well to this conservative regimen of therapy. On the other hand, some of these individuals do become fatigued and demonstrate progressive deterioration of function, which is evidenced by physical signs and, in particular, by blood gases. Daily x-rays are important to determine the presence or absence of pneumothorax or the development of complications such as atelectasis and/or pneumonitis. Lung contusions are best diagnosed by calculating the A-aDO$_2$ gradient, which often precedes x-ray appearance of change by at least 12 to 24 hours.

CATEGORY II—CONTINUOUS IPPV THERAPY. This includes patients with critical chest injury (disease) and consists of the following: (1) those in Category I whose respiratory status has deteriorated; (2) a significant flail effect with multiple fractured ribs and lung contusion; (3) entirely ineffective coughing; (4) ventilatory rate greater than 30 per minute; (5) hypoxia unresponsive to increased oxygen by half-face tent or nasal oxygen catheter; (6) elevated PaCO$_2$; (7) neurologic signs such as depressed sensorium or coma; (8) undue fatigue.

Maintenance. The following points are vital: (1) A *nasotracheal tube*, firmly fixed to the patient with a marker, enables the nursing staff to ascertain any change from its original position. (2) *Gastric decompression*—plastic nasogastric intubation through the other nostril vents the stomach of swallowed air, a condition that always occurs with IPPV. The tube is attached to a plastic enema bag held about two feet above the level of the patient's head to permit escape of air and collection of gastric juice, which

is returned to the patient. Tube patency must be ascertained hourly. (3) *Removal of secretions*—suctioning is carried out under sterile conditions, including disposable gloves and 22-inch long plastic catheters (#10 or #14 French) with a side arm. The catheters are used for one suction period only. Sterile normal saline is supplied in 100 cc. plastic water bottles, which are used for a period of 8 hours only and replaced with fresh bottles at the end of this time. Nurse instruction in suction techniques and constant checks are critical. One hand is kept sterile, the other being used to undo the plastic cap at the back of the swivel, handle the wash bottle, and so on. Suctioning should always be as brief as possible. The catheter can partially obstruct the tube. Suctioning precipitously reduces P$_a$O$_2$ and induces acute hypoxia. The actual suctioning period is limited to 5 seconds. The catheter is removed from the nasotracheal tube and the patient is adequately reventilated before suctioning is repeated. There is no set timetable. The procedure is done at least every hour but, more important, as frequently as necessary. (4) *Cuff inflation*—the cuff is inflated with air at a pressure just sufficient to obtain the seal with a small leak, at end-inspiration. It is preferable to make respirator adjustments than to permit excessive cuff pressure on tracheal mucosa. Deflation is not done regularly, but only once or twice a day. Strict attention to the proper degree of inflation of the cuff is in professional hands. Hourly deflation and inflation by different sets of hands increases the risk of improper cuff pressures.

Initial control: Emergency Room. These patients are usually hypoxic with rapid, shallow, ineffective ventilation and a small tidal volume. Furthermore, they are restless, in pain, and emotionally distraught. Assisted ventilation generally is introduced first. The Mark 7 Bird respirator, with flow and mixing cartridges and maximum inspired oxygen concentration, is used. High inspiratory flow rates and usually pressures of 25 cm. to 35 cm. water are established. More may be necessary. Narcotics are given intravenously as noted previously. Once intubation and IPPV have been instituted, it is essential to check regularly for possible pneumothorax. A closed tube thoracotomy on the injured side should be performed, whether or not a pneumothorax is present, to serve as a vent. Not infrequently the patient reacts to nasotracheal intubation by bucking and coughing. This can be handled by instillation of 2 to 3 cc. of 4 per cent Xylocaine through the nasotracheal tube or by a nebulizer. With these procedures, it has been noted that the patient's tidal volume can be stepped up. By opening the expiratory time for apnea on the Bird respirator, ventilation can be controlled within a relatively short period of time. Control of ventilation is absolutely essential in order to stop the flail effect and to stabilize the chest wall. Rarely does a patient require a muscle relaxant.

Blood gases constitute the single most important tool for the management of a patient on the respirator. These are repeated within 15 minutes after the institution of IPPV. When the patient's evaluation has been completed and he is considered to be in a relatively stabilized state, he is moved to the Intensive Care Unit or to the Operating Room, if indicated. Emphasis is placed strongly upon establishing control of the patient's ventilatory status before he is moved from the Emergency Room.

Intensive Care Unit. It is desirable to maintain a large tidal volume and to use the lungs as pneumatic splints. The volume delivered is generally 1200 cc. to 1500 cc. with a respiratory control set at 6 to 8 breaths per minute. The Bird Mark 7, powered by oxygen with the flow cartridge in the fully open position, delivers an oxygen concentration to the patient of approximately 93 per cent. The nasogastric tube is checked for patency with frequent aspiration of air. Gastric contents are returned to the stomach, unless there is an indication for continuous gastric suction. After several days it may be removed, if the patient is conscious. Repeated checks are required in the event of recurrent gastric distention.

Analgesics, as indicated previously, are continued. One of the great advantages of utilizing respirator therapy, rather than fixed stabilization equipment, is that the patient can be turned frequently, as indeed they do require. Turning the patient on the flail side, however, is avoided owing to the presence of the double fractures, which may prove injurious. The technique of vibration and percussion of the chest, together with suctioning, is carried out on an hourly basis. Great care must be exercised

in suctioning, particularly in patients who are extremely hypoxic so that they are not off the respirator for an undue period of time.

Blood gases are repeated as often as indicated during inspiration of a known oxygen concentration. It is not uncommon to find that the $PaCO_2$ is quite low. It is not desirable to permit alkalosis for a long period of time, because of shifting of the oxygen dissociation curve to the left with possible impairment in cardiac contractility with reduced output. Furthermore, a marked degree of respiratory alkalosis renders weaning off the ventilator difficult. To correct for this, dead space is placed into the system between the expiratory valve and the patient. Initially, the dead space is increased by approximately 100 cc. and blood gases repeated after 15 minutes. The dead space then is altered so that the $PaCO_2$ is maintained at a level of 34 mm. to 36 mm. Hg. A nomogram is available for predicting the dead space required to bring the $PaCO_2$ to a desired level. In general, PaO_2 is maintained at 70 mm. to 90 mm. Hg and the pH at 7.40 to 7.46.

Since infections are so common, Luken's tube specimens of intratracheal tube secretions are taken under sterile conditions and sent for cultures and sensitivity every 48 hours. Bronchodilators are administered four times daily or more often, as dictated by the degree of bronchospasm. The procedures, including adjustments, patient care, and gas analysis, are carried out as frequently as required in order to ensure that the adjustments are correct.

The effective lung compliance is determined along with adjustments for necessary input of volume of air. This, in addition to blood gases, is the most valuable indicator of the state of the lung. A progressively decreasing compliance is indicative of a worsening situation and is common with contusion, pneumonia, secretions, atelectasis, and other disorders.

Initially, feeding is carried out by intravenous therapy. Fluids, subsequently, are given by nasogastric tube. Once the tube has been removed, fluids can be given by mouth and may include anything that is suitable in a liquid state, avoiding fruit juices. It must be borne in mind that an inflated cuff is no guarantee against aspiration.

WEANING THE PATIENT OFF THE RESPIRATOR. This is a most critical step and should be executed only by trained, experienced professionals. Readiness is based upon the patient's physiologic and clinical state. The criteria in general are as follows: (1) a PaO_2 of greater than 250 mm. Hg on 100 per cent oxygen, (2) a $PaCO_2$ of less than 55 mm. Hg on the respirator, (3) a tidal volume of 10 cc. per kg. of body weight, (4) reasonable stability of the chest wall, (5) resolution of pulmonary contusion, and (6) reduction in $A\text{-}aDO_2$. In flail injuries, as a rule, at least a 10-day period is required before weaning is begun (Table 7-13).

The first and most vital step is to explain to the patient in detail what is to be done and what he can expect. Most patients have become quite accustomed to the respirator. A tremendous amount of anxiety can occur when the patient is taken off. Loss of this very important support upon which he has become so dependent may be a terrifying experience. All essentials should be prepared and readily at hand—a suitable humidifier able to supply varying oxygen concentrations, plastic hosing, and a Briggs adaptor with reservoir tubing. The inspired oxygen concentration delivered to the patient is somewhat higher than that received on the respirator. The flow also is about twice the patient's estimated minute volume on the respirator to prevent rebreathing. The dead space is limited to tubing from the adaptor to the nasotracheal tube, about 10 cc. to 20 cc.

When the patient is removed from the respirator, the initial period of spontaneous breathing is carefully observed for indications of mild respiratory distress, which always develops. The other sign carefully looked for is recurrence of the flail effect. If the latter does occur, the patient is reattached to the respirator and weaning is deferred for another period of at least a week. If the flail effect does not recur, the length of time for development of signs and symptoms of respiratory difficulty is noted.

Blood gases are drawn at this period. If the blood gases are within acceptable limits

Table 7-13. Weaning Patient off Respirator

A. Patient Orientation
(Single most important step)
Explain in detail: the equipment
the changeover
what to expect
Reassure often—before, during, and after

B. Indications		C. Preparations
On respirator:		Equipment for inhalation (see text)
PaO_2 250+ mm. Hg on 100% O_2		High humidity source
$PaCO_2$ 50 mm. Hg		O_2 higher than that on respirator
VD/VT 0.6		Thorough clearance of airway
Thorax reasonably stable		Thorough clearance of pharynx
Stable vital signs		Deflate cuff (if no excess secretions)

D. Monitoring

Pulse rate or	Hypoxia	Back on respirator
Arterial pressure or	Hypoxia	Back on respirator
Sweating	Anxiety; hypoxia	Reassure; respirator
Respirations	Hypoxia, anxiety	Respirator; reassure
Dyspnea	Hypoxia	Back on respirator
Flail recurrence	Instability	Back on respirator

E. Period off Respirator
Determinants: 1. Length of time to first sign of respirator distress—
disphoresis; dyspnea; flail; tachypnea
2. Evidence of physiological respiratory status—
PaO_2 80 mm. Hg; $PaCO_2$ 45 mm. Hg; pH 7.36
3. Time off respirator in the hour—
half of (1) if (2) OK

F. Progression	G. Extubation
Reduce inspired O_2	PaO_2 OK on 40% O_2
Extend time off respirator	$PaCO_2$ 45 mm. Hg
When 45 mins./hr., extend	pH 7.36
to a few hours with IPPB/I	

(no hypoxia and little or no hypercarbia), a period of about half the length of time it took for the distress to develop is selected as the initial period of time off the respirator. For example, if the patient was able to remain off for 30 minutes, then the initial weaning period for institution of the program would be 15 minutes off the respirator at hourly intervals. The weaning process is performed only during the time the full complement of staff is available. Patients are kept on the respirator during the night.

Based upon blood gases and clinical signs, the time off the respirator is extended, and the oxygen concentration is reduced as rapidly as can be tolerated by the patient. When 45 minutes of spontaneous breathing on 40 per cent oxygen or less is possible, a further period of spontaneous breathing is allowed for a number of hours with IPPV/I treatments via the tracheostomy or nasotracheal tube for 15 minutes every 4 hours. If the patient progresses well, then the period is extended from 4 to 24 hours. If the patient's status and blood gases are satisfactory, extubation is carried out.

It is emphasized that extubation should not be performed at night or over the weekend when there is only a minimal staff present. Following extubation, high humidity is administered via ultrasonic or some other suitable humidifier via a face tent for 48 to 72 hours with sufficient nasal oxygen to maintain an acceptable PaO_2. Periodic IPPV/I treatments, together with chest physiotherapy, are given as indicated, to raise secretions and to encourage coughing in order to prevent atelectasis.

The overall period required for successful weaning of a patient with a flail chest varies considerably. The shortest time is about 7 to 10 days. The longest has been as much as 4 to 5 weeks. The average time required is after 2 to 3 weeks of continuous ventilatory support. There has been no difficulty encountered in not being able to wean a patient off the respirator in our series of 70 patients.

Results of Respirator Management. The duration of IPPV varies considerably depending upon the patient's response and degree of lung dysfunction (Table 7-14). Approximately 30 per cent of our patients did not receive prolonged IPPV therapy, since the flail segment proved to be rather small. In most other individuals IPPV therapy was continued from 1 to 3 weeks (Table 7-14). There appeared to be no relationship of external thoracic cage injury to the duration of the time required for IPPV therapy, except for those individuals with anterior and anterolateral injuries, which generally required treatment for longer periods of time. The presence of other complications, such as lung contusion, necessitated prolonged therapy. Administration of IPPV was almost 100 per cent effective in stabilizing the thoracic cage. Early restoration of thoracic volume was not as consistent (Blair et al., 1968). In 28 per cent of patients there was no improvement, and in 5 per cent the thoracic volume actually decreased somewhat more. Flails of the lateral rib cage were less prone to early reconstruction.

In patients free of significant parenchymal disease, the PaO_2 prior to institution of therapy was uniformly low, varying from 25 mm. to 65 mm. Hg, with the majority of patients at 50 mm. Hg (Fig. 7-6). In only about one-third of the patients in whom initial blood gases were obtained was the flail effect obvious. Following the institution of IPPV, arterial blood gases improved progressively, so that it was possible to reduce the oxygen input into the respirator. Delay of therapy usually occurred because the flail effect was not clinically evident. In situations such as this, the patients appear to do fairly well as determined by clinical signs, but eventually a severe degree of hypercarbia develops (Blair et al., 1968). In the literature it is stated that patients with posterior flail segments generally are not in very serious condition

TABLE 7-14. Duration of (Continuous) Intermittent Positive Pressure Ventilation (IPPV)

Days	*0-2*	*3-7*	*8-12*	*13-17*	*18-21*	*22-25*	*No. IPPV*
Number	0	12	16	13	16	6	7
Per cent	0	16	23	19	23	9	10

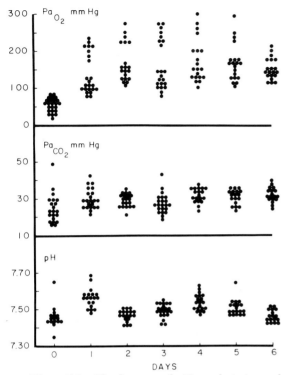

Figure 7-6. Blood gases and pH on admission and after institution of IPPV.

(Hughes, 1965). This is generally true, but in our study some of these showed reduction in PaO_2 and, therefore, were managed with IPPV therapy.

NASOTRACHEAL INTUBATION

Endotracheal intubation was introduced by Sir William McEwen in 1881. Over the years sentiment has fluctuated for and against this procedure, which initially was limited to anesthesia and, for very brief times, in the immediate post-anesthetic period. Rather significant complications have been reported (Tonkin et al., 1966). We have recently reviewed a series of 225 of our own patients (Deane et al., accepted for publication). The incidence of laryngeal complications was severe in 2.4 per cent and moderate in 4.6 per cent.* In 93 per cent there were none. There were no instances of perforation or of stenosis. Intubations were maintained from a few hours to over 300 hours, with the majority in the 48- to 200-hour period.

---

*Severe—mucosal ulcerations and pronounced edema; Moderate—minor erosions and edema.

The advantages of nasotracheal intubation as an initial procedure are (1) the institution of rapid and effective ventilation, (2) the enhanced use of time available for patient evaluation and the initiation of resuscitative procedures, (3) adequate suctioning and (4) avoidance of untoward experiences with emergency tracheostomy. The safe duration of intubation is somewhat in dispute, but we have noted very minimal or no laryngeal damage with intubation for as long as six days. On the other hand, in severe chest trauma in which it is quite likely that assisted ventilation may be prolonged, elective tracheostomy, usually within 48 to 72 hours, is recommended. Nasotracheal intubation is preferred to endotracheal, since the latter is much more uncomfortable for the patient and further gives rise to a higher incidence of laryngeal complications.

TECHNIQUE. The larger nostril is selected and 5 per cent cocaine is applied with cotton sticks. This helps to reduce the incidence of epistaxis on passing the tube. A well-lubricated tube is pushed through the nose without force into the nasopharynx. The tube size selected for an adult usually is 7.5 mm. or 8.0 mm. The pharynx is cleared of any foreign material (mucus, blood) by suction. Oxygen is administered through the adjacent nostril via a catheter. The neck is extended at the atlanto-occipital joint, providing that associated trauma does not contraindicate this positioning. A small pillow is placed under the shoulders; the head is held in midline position. At this point, while listening to the breath sounds, the tube is introduced further into the nasopharynx and, as the patient inspires, it is introduced into the trachea.

In the vast majority of instances, blind nasotracheal intubation is successful at the first attempt with minimal discomfort. The presence of a tube in the trachea is confirmed by cough and breath sounds through the tube. If the first attempt is not successful, the head is rotated to the side of the nostril being used, and the procedure is tried again. In 90 per cent of instances blind intubation can be carried out. In the rest the glottis is visualized with a laryngoscope and sprayed with local anesthetic. Under direct vision then, intubation is carried out. It is better to avoid the use of intravenous barbiturates and muscle relaxants to achieve intubation and these are only rarely necessary. After the patient is connected to the respirator, the cuff is inflated. Enough air is introduced to obtain an air-tight seal in the inspiratory phase of ventilation. A high oxygen concentration is delivered to the patient following a few cycles of ventilation. The position of the tube is checked carefully by means of auscultation to ensure that it is not down the right main stem bronchus. X-ray confirmation is a must and is taken as soon after intubation as conditions permit.

Complications (Table 7-15)

MANAGEMENT. (1) *Accidental extubation.* The chief deterrent to extubation is (a) constant vigilance to prevent or correct loosening and movement and (b) control of patient restlessness, which, if due to reasons other than hypoxia, indicates judicious use of analgesics, sedatives, or hand restraints. (2) *Sore throat.* Xylocaine viscopaste, or some other local anesthetic drug, given orally and held in the pharynx for a few minutes before swallowing, has worked

very well. (3) *Epistaxis.* This has occurred very infrequently and has never been a serious problem. (4) *Excoriation of the nostrils.* If the nasal mucous membrane or the skin adjacent to the tube becomes edematous or infected, cultures are taken and a suitable local antibiotic applied to the area. This also has been a very rare occurrence. (5) *Suctioning.* Inability to introduce the suction catheter all the way down the nasotracheal tube indicates trouble, which may be due to (a) too large a suction tube, (b) inadequate lubrication of the suction tube (wetting with sterile saline solves this), or (c) obstruction due to secretions. (6) *Overinflation of the cuff.*

EXTUBATION. This would apply only to those cases in which the flail segment is minimal and when extubation is possible without tracheostomy.

Loss of Voice and Laryngitis. This occurs in 100 per cent of patients and is treated by administering high humidity, usually with an ultrasonic or heated humidifier, for a period of 48 to 72 hours and constant vigi-

TABLE 7-15.   Common Problems and Hazards Associated with Intubation

Problem	Remedy
A. Nasotracheal	
During Intubation	
1. Obstruction	Adequate hydration, humidity and suction
Secretions	Replace tube
Kinking of tube	Inflate pilot balloon with just enough air to obtain
Overinflation of cuff	a seal during inspiratory phase
Intubation right main stem bronchus	Auscultation and x-ray to assess tube position
2. Accidental extubation	Vigilance, correct taping of tube, prevention of restlessness
3. Sore throat	Local anesthetics
4. Aspiration	Feed via nasogastric tube; nothing orally except water, ice chips
Following Intubation	
1. Laryngitis	High humidity via nebulizer or ultrasonic and half-face tent for 48–72 hours
2. Hoarse voice	As above; if persists for 24 hours, indirect or direct laryngoscopy
3. Subglottic	Early: as above plus steroids; vigilance Worse: Reintubate; tracheostomy
4. Aspiration	Initial oral fluids – water only (If cough occurs feed via nasogastric tube until laryngeal competence intact)
B. Tracheostomy	
During Intubation	
1. Obstruction	Same as for nasotracheal tubes
2. Hemorrhage	Change tube; regain hemostasis; check coagulation status
3. Dislodgment	Firm fixation; vigilance
4. Infection	Smear and culture; antibiotics
5. Dilation of trachea	Use longer tube
6. Tracheoesophageal, tracheopleural fistula	Minimal air in cuff; strict aseptic suction techniques; surgery
After Extubation	
Tracheostenosis	Reintubate, if required; surgery

lance. Indirect laryngoscopy is indicated if hoarseness persists for longer than 24 hours.

Subglottic Edema and Obstruction. We have had three instances in the past 315 nasotracheal intubations in which acute obstruction, usually 48 to 200 hours following extubation, has occurred, necessitating tracheostomy. In all cases, obstruction was due to a thickened membrane situated superior to the level of the cuff on the nasotracheal tube. Following tracheostomy in all cases, it was possible to remove the tracheostomy tube within a period of 5 to 7 days and no further complications occurred in a follow-up period of longer than six months.

TRACHEOSTOMY

Tracheostomy is never performed as an emergency. Nasotracheal intubation is carried out and then tracheostomy is done on an elective basis in the Operating Room under sterile conditions. Furthermore, the performance of the tracheostomy is always done under complete control of the patient's ventilation and with a patent airway via the nasotracheal tube. Suitable premedication is generally ordered. A general anesthetic is avoided, if possible, although there is no hesitancy in its use when required. A superficial cervical block is executed by injecting 10 cc. of 1 per cent Xylocaine along the posterior border of each sternocleidomastoid muscle. Additional local infiltration with 1 per cent Xylocaine is carried out when needed.

During performance of the tracheostomy, the patient is ventilated by the respirator, which was brought with him either from the Emergency Room or from the Intensive Care Unit. The surgical procedure is routine. The dissection is carried out under a calm, relaxed atmosphere. Large vessels are avoided, and hemostasis is effectively maintained. Following mobilization of the trachea, a segment of at least two rings is removed in an ellipse in order to permit ease of introduction of the tracheostomy tube and to insure against undue necrosis. At the time the incision is made into the trachea, the cuff of the nasotracheal tube is usually ruptured and this can then be withdrawn. The tracheostomy tube is connected to a 15 cm. Mörch swivel. It is extremely important to maintain active suction through-

out the procedure when required. Instillation of a few cc. of 1 per cent Xylocaine can be utilized if there is any coughing.

Maintenance

The basic respiratory management of the patient with a tracheostomy is exactly that of the patient on a nasotracheal tube. An ordinary, sterilized, red rubber catheter may be used for suction purposes. Provided the level of consciousness is adequate and no paralytic ileus exists, oral feedings may be instituted with a fluid or a soft diet. It is important to keep the tracheostomy tube in the midline at all times. Lateral displacement may cause erosion of the tracheal wall with perforation or tracheoesophageal erosions of arteries and the like. Fixation is achieved by placing two or three layers of Reston self-adhesive plastic material on skin prepared with tincture of benzoin. Two pieces of tracheostomy tape approximately 10 inches long are placed underneath and then tied over the short piece of green plastic Bird tubing running from the exhalation valve or the Y of the respirator to the Mörch swivel.

Complications

INTUBATION. (1) *Obstruction of the tracheostomy tube due to inspissated secretions.* This should never occur and is caused by inadequate humidity from the respirator. (2) *Hemorrhage.* Small amounts may be initiated by frequent and rough suctioning. Large amounts should be viewed with alarm because this indicates a possible erosion of a large vessel or a sign of disseminated intravascular thrombosis. (3) *Tube dislodgement,* either to the exterior or into the neck tissues. This can be prevented by attention to the tension of the tracheostomy tape. When it occurs during the first 24 hours of tracheostomy, it is a potentially dangerous situation. A spare sterile tracheostomy tube should be available at the patient's bedside for instant use. All the necessary equipment for reintubation should be available in the Intensive Care Unit. (4) *Infection.* (5) *Dilation of the trachea.* It is not uncommon to find that progressive amounts of air are necessary to obtain an air-tight seal. If this occurs, it is probably preferable to change over to a different kind of tracheostomy tube, or to use a double cuffed tube with alternating filling. (6) *Tracheoesophageal and tracheopleural fistulas.* (7) The tube may be inappropriate—too long, too short, or the wrong kind of tube.

EXTUBATION. Tracheostenosis is an ever increasing problem following the prolonged tracheostomy with positive pressure ventilation. The site of the stenosis may be at the stoma itself or at the site of the cuff. Difficulties in extubation due to tracheostomy complications and to respirator problems have been noted.

PLEURAL CAVITY (FIG. 7-7)

The development of a pneumothorax usually is due to a pulmonary tear, caused by rib fragment in blunt trauma, or penetration by a missile or knife blade. The incidence varies from 12 per cent to 33 per cent and bilaterally 6 per cent to 19 per cent. The most serious is a tension pneumothorax, which may occur because of a tremendous loss of air through a defect in a large-sized bronchial segment. Hemothoraces derive from lung tears, a severed vessel, or a heart wound, and occur in from 21 to 36 per cent (Blair et al., 1969; Conn et al., 1963; Malm et al., 1965; Sherman, 1966). In both situations, it is urgent to eliminate the existing dead space or any restriction of the ventilable lung by promptly evacuating all the air. Multiple and delayed aspirations of blood are poor and improper substitutes. A large-sized chest tube (#26 to #28) should be placed into the thorax by the clamp technique. Trocars limit catheter size and are hazardous. The ancient adage about blood in the intrapleural space tamponading a bleeding vessel is misleading and potentially dangerous. Should the vessel be of significant magnitude, most likely it will bleed again and will require operative intervention.

The chest tube constitutes a very important mechanism with respect to management of the patient, not only in the evacuation of air and blood, but also in the detection of continued bleeding from a major source. If continued blood loss is massive or rebleeding occurs, then the principle of operative intervention, utilized in other problems (e.g., gastrointestinal) is invoked. The probability of involvement of a major pulmonary or systemic vessel should become strikingly clear. A catheter has another important function as a source of decompression if a patient is on IPPV. If a hemothorax persists, early delayed surgery is recommended in order to avoid the higher morbidity and mortality rates associated with decortication of fibrothoraces. The problem arises most frequently in gunshot wounds.

LUNGS

Damage to the lungs consists of pulmonary contusion, parenchymal tears or wounds, intrapulmonary hematomas, aspiration pneu-

BLUNT   PENETRATING

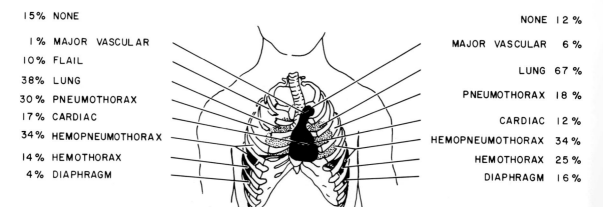

BLUNT		PENETRATING
15% NONE		NONE 12%
1% MAJOR VASCULAR		MAJOR VASCULAR 6%
10% FLAIL		
38% LUNG		LUNG 67%
30% PNEUMOTHORAX		PNEUMOTHORAX 18%
17% CARDIAC		CARDIAC 12%
34% HEMOPNEUMOTHORAX		HEMOPNEUMOTHORAX 34%
14% HEMOTHORAX		HEMOTHORAX 25%
4% DIAPHRAGM		DIAPHRAGM 16%

Figure 7-7. Injuries commonly accompanying chest trauma.

monitis, and atelectasis. In the late stage, the development of pneumonia, particularly as a sequel to contusion, is a serious matter.

Contusions

Pulmonary contusion constitutes one of the most serious complications in chest trauma. Pathogenesis is poorly understood. It is the most frequent pulmonary complication with an overall incidence as high as 70 to 75 per cent (Reynolds et al., 1966). Flail injuries are complicated by contusion in about 57 per cent (Blair et al., 1969). Contusions occur when there are no rib fractures, particularly in the younger individual. Clinically, the patient may not appear at all incapacitated soon after the accident. Further deception by indecisive x-rays may delay proper treatment. The PaO_2 and especially the $A\text{-}aDO_2$ correctly identify the serious degree of involvement. Oxygen gradients may be increased enormously. We have found the $A\text{-}aDO_2$ to be the most reliable means of assessing patient status, progress, and prognosis. Changes in $A\text{-}aDO_2$ often precede x-ray evidence of progression and of resolution (Fig. 7-8).

The essentials of therapy include a patent airway, continuous IPPV, 100 per cent humidity, and scrupulous antibacterial measures. The contused lung hosts the most serious complications in blunt chest trauma—pneumonia and blowouts with tension pneumothorax. It is absolutely vital that a decompressing thoracotomy tube be inserted and retained, whether or not a pneumothorax is present. Suctioning must be performed only under aseptic conditions, utilizing a sterile, disposable catheter each time. Lukens tube aspirates are cultured at least every 48 hours with antibiotic manipulations as indicated. The critical period is five to seven days (Blair et al., 1969; Reynolds et al., 1966). Decreasing PaO_2 and widening $A\text{-}aDO_2$ herald spreading infirmity and pneumonia. Constant nursing attention and frequent status review are urgent. Respirator adjustments are crucial in order to maintain an adequate PaO_2 at the minimal oxygen input. (Fig. 7-9).

HEMATOMAS. Lung hematomas are the result of severe localized trauma in the region of the actual injury (Reynolds et al., 1966). These are associated with significant destruction of lung parenchyma and hemor-

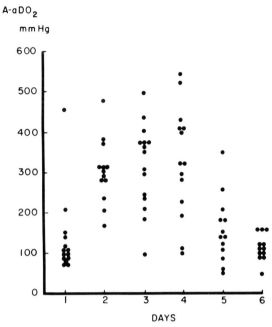

Figure 7-8. Alveolar-arterial oxygen gradients ($A\text{-}aDO_2$) in lung contusion Peak gradients developed within several days, declining as the contusion resolved. All patients were on IPPV.

rhage. Shearing and crushing of lung parenchyma against the chest wall or laceration of the lung by a rib fragment are the probable reasons for the development of pulmonary hematoma in blunt trauma, just as is the missile in penetrating injuries. Hematomas may be central or peripheral. Central hematomas are located in the central portions of the lung and appear shortly after the injury or several days later. They are poorly defined densities and become more circumscribed approximately three days to two weeks after injury. Several months may be required for total resolution. Cystic cavities may develop when the damage has been extensive. Slowly resolving hematomas tend to develop characteristics suggestive of a solitary coin lesion, and at times patients have been explored. At exploration the findings consisted of a cystic cavity containing blood surrounded by dense, injured lung tissue.

Peripheral hematomas consist of subpleural accumulations and are probably more common. Radiologically, they appear as extensive, lateral densities, very difficult to distinguish from organized hemothorax

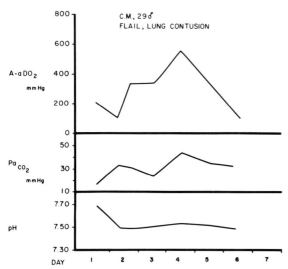

Figure 7-9. Blood gases and pH in a patient with flail chest and lung contusion. Peak A-aDO$_2$ was reached on the fourth day after the accident. Initially with IPPV, the PaCO$_2$ was low and the pH was alkalotic, but they returned to normal by means of respirator adjustments and resolution of lung dysfunction.

in the pleural space. The treatment of pulmonary hematomas is expectant; most hematomas tend to clear up completely. A small number resolve as cysts and a few heal by scarring.

LACERATION. Lung tears are due to direct injury from a fractured rib. Occasionally a shearing effect may cause a tear. The severity of the laceration is variable, but usually is superficial and produces relatively little bleeding or air leak. On the other hand, the laceration may involve pulmonary vessels and bronchial segments. These lead to major hemothorax and pneumothorax. In the absence of significant hemothorax or pneumothorax, the diagnosis of the lung tear may be difficult, until there is some clearance of the infiltrates in the lacerated area. The majority of lacerations may be treated conservatively with tube thoracotomy in the presence of pneumothorax or hemothorax.

In stab injuries lung laceration is generally of no serious consequence. Prompt evacuation of intrapleural air or blood by closed tube thoracotomy is followed by re-expansion of the lung. The laceration is sealed by apposition to the inner chest wall. The same is true for the majority of gunshot wounds. Intraparenchymal retention of the

missile has proved of no consequence. Surgical intervention is never indicated for missile retrieval alone, but only for an emergency, such as large vessel or tracheobronchial perforation.

WET LUNG SYNDROME. The wet lung syndrome was described as an entity, deriving from experiences in World War II casualties. Most of these individuals suffered blast injuries of a nonthoracic type. The syndrome was characterized by large amounts of fluid accumulated in the tracheobronchial tree causing considerable respiratory difficulty and hypoxia. It was believed that the mechanisms included pulmonary trauma, increased respiratory effort, tracheal obstruction, and anoxia. The "wet lung" syndrome is most likely quite different from true pulmonary contusion. Experiences in Korea and, more recently, in Vietnam suggest another "wet lung" syndrome, probably due to overly enthusiastic fluid replacement with resulting congestion and edema. The treatment of wet lung syndrome is essentially that of pulmonary contusion. If it is severe, nasotracheal intubation and IPPV are necessary. Great care must be exercised in the administration of fluids. In some instances, it may be necessary to use diuretics, such as ethacrynic acid and Mercuhydrin, in order to assure removal of fluid.

LUNG HERNIATION. Although occasionally a complication of thoracotomy, herniation is rarely observed after blunt chest injury. Repair is not required, since the hernias are quite small, as a rule.

TORSION. Torsion of a lobe is a bizarre occurrence, quite rare and occurring in children (Selmonsky et al., 1967). Middle-lobe clockwise and left-lung counterclockwise torsions may occur. The involved structure is infarcted and requires surgical removal.

CARDIOVASCULAR INJURY

PRINCIPLES. Cardiac injury means crippling of the central pump mechanism. The problems may be classed as major dramatic (exsanguination or arrest) or major undramatic (tamponade or contusion). There are no minor cardiac injuries. There is no such thing as emergency surgery, but there is emergency resuscitation, including open-chest massage. The fundamental principle is restoration of cardiodynamics in order to maintain an adequate blood flow. The vehicles are surgical and nonsurgical. (*Conservative* treatment is a misleading and dangerous state of mind. There is nothing conservative about acute trauma.)

The prime indication for surgical management is an impending or actual threat to life (for example, exsanguination or massive tamponade with arrest), and requires early major operative intervention. The next category is early delayed surgery and includes problems of continued major hemorrhage or unsuccessful cardiocenteses. The third category is delayed surgery for such cases as unresolved hemothorax or empyema. The fourth is "elective" surgery for late complications or missed diagnoses, including traumatic aortic or ventricular aneurysm, traumatic valvular insufficiency, and so on.

Nonsurgical management includes pericardiocentesis (surgery, but distinguished from major operation), closed tube thoracotomy, and vigilant patient care.

Blunt Trauma

The circumstances of accidents considered along with the dynamics of impact and the subsequent forces that develop would suggest that injuries to the heart would be very common. Reports, however, fail to confirm this (Howell et al., 1963; Hughes, 1965; Reynolds et al., 1966). Patients who died immediately, or very shortly after automobile accidents, do indeed demonstrate high incidences of heart injury at autopsy (Parmley et al., 1958).

On the other hand, in patients who survive, or who die some days or weeks after the injury, involvement seems to be unusually infrequent. Studies of immediate fatalities have demonstrated that there is a 65 per cent incidence of rupture of one or more chambers of the heart, a 12 per cent incidence of contusion, and 46 per cent pericardial lacerations. In practically all of these there was a hemopericardium. Reports from immediate survivals have indicated that myocardial contusions occur at the rate of approximately 7 to 8 per cent. On the basis of electrocardiographic change, the incidence might have been construed as being anywhere between 17 and 40 per cent (Blair et al., 1969).

The actual incidence in survivals is not yet established. The problem is much more than an academic one. Myocardial contusion, upon which is superimposed hypoxia from the chest injury or secondary perfusion deficits from hypovolemia, readily leads to cerebral anoxia and to cardiac arrest. The occurrence is probably much more common than it is reported or suspected.

Hemopericardium is difficult to diagnose unless there is a massive effusion. Admission x-rays often are "equivocal," since technique may be unsatisfactory. Portable films are deceptive, tending to exaggerate the mediastinal shadows. Should any suspicion exist (and it should often), a pericardiocentesis is required. Intrapericardial blood of large magnitude usually signals a catastrophic injury, such as aortic rupture. On the other hand, there have been a number of instances of hemopericardium without rupture of the large vessels, probably due to tear of pericardial vessels (Blair et al., 1969; Reynolds et al., 1966). The diagnosis too often is established at the moment of circulatory collapse.

Contusions predominate in the right rather than the left ventricle (38 per cent as opposed to 18 per cent) and have been noted to be bilateral in 23 per cent of instances (Parmley et al., 1958). The contusions may be from a few millimeters to more than 3 cm. in diameter. They may resemble an early infarct with interstitial hemorrhage and subendocardial or epicardial hematoma. Progressive changes have demonstrated that they behave very much like an infarct during the healing process (Demuth et al., 1965). Very occasionally the septum may also show hemorrhagic necrotic changes. Ruptures are observed very infrequently in the Emergency Room because few patients survive the accident. The few who do reach a hospital are DOMD, so that the reports are based on autopsies, with an occasional one from surgery. Eight per cent of patients with these critical cardiac injuries do reach a hospital and could be saved. In autopsy studies, the ruptures were noted as follows: right ventricle, 19 per cent; left ventricle, 17 per cent; right atrium, 12 per cent; left atrium, 7 per cent; and multiple chambers, 30 per cent. The interventricular septum was ruptured in 9 per cent and the interatrial septum in 7 per cent of cases. There was a 23 per cent incidence of rupture of the aorta in these fatal injuries. The coronary vessel was lacerated in approximately 3 per cent and there was a tear of papillary muscle in 7 per cent. A few patients able to survive the initial acute episode were successfully treated. Most of these had leaflet ruptures, detected subsequently by signs of aortic tricuspid insufficiency. An occasional right atrial or vena caval tear has been suspected by virtue of continued bleeding via the chest tube, with diagnosis established at thoracotomy. This and the lack of programmed protocol and lack of pursuit are the main factors in DOMD.

Definitive signs and symptoms often are masked because of the nature of extensive trauma. In the early stages, friction rubs, chest pain, tachycardia, or a murmur are often attributed to problems other than those occurring in the heart. When the initial crisis has become stabilized, the persistence of precordial pain, of tachycardia, the presence of a systolic murmur and of a friction rub should signal the possibility of myocardial injury.

The ECG constitutes the single most useful aid. There are many loopholes, however. The very signs that would indicate myocardial damage unfortunately are nonspecific RS-T and T-wave changes. In hypoxic patients these abnormalities may be present in the absence of myocardial damage. Nevertheless, the ECG remains valuable and should be one of the very first procedures in the Emergency Room evaluation. This is often done, but the "error" lies in the failure of repetition, since the initial ECG may appear normal. The subsequent development of flat and inverted T-waves in AV_f and in V_1 leads is significant. ECG changes may persist anywhere from 5 to 20 days and most often are picked up several days after the injury, emphasizing the need for pursuit. In a small number of patients the injury is obvious by virtue of atrial fibrillation or flutter or pulsus paradoxus or both.

Continued brisk bleeding from a thoracotomy tube in the right hemithorax must lead one to suspect a major vascular source. Probably an intercostal or internal thoracic artery is responsible, but it may be the right atrium, superior vena cava, or a pulmonary vessel. The rate of bleeding is an important index and should be recorded. The precise diagnosis is established at thoracotomy.

The management of myocardial contusion is precisely that of an acute myocardial infarction (Demuth et al., 1965). It is obvious that a diagnosis or a strong suspicion of a laceration of a chamber requires immediate surgery. Hemopericardium, as a rule, is adequately treated by pericardiocentesis. Although an initial pericardiocentesis, perhaps followed by a second one, may be successful, the persistence of a significant amount of blood in the pericardial sac would necessitate surgical intervention. Usually, a major vascular rupture is the cause, but rarely tears of pericardial vessels are responsible. Evacuation of the blood and suitable drainage is all that is required.

Long-term follow-up in patients has yielded left ventricular aneurysms in occasional instances. If the problem is not appreciated immediately, the course may be as follows: the patient seems to be progressing

TABLE 7-16.   Management of Cardiac Injuries in Chest Trauma

Trauma	Problem	Management
Pericardial	Hemopericardium	Pericardiocentesis; surgery
	Tamponade with arrest	Open chest massage
		Pericardiotomy and repair of cardiac wound
	Tamponade, no arrest, but shock	Whole blood; crystalloids
		Pericardiocentesis (If recurs, surgery)
	Tamponade, no arrest, no shock	Pericardiocentesis (If recurs, repeat pericardiocentesis; if recurs again, surgery)
Cardiac	Contusion	Treat as acute myocardial infarct
	Laceration; rupture	Pericardial tamponade or major hemorrhage; surgery
		Otherwise, as in hemopericardium
	Valve rupture	Elective surgery
	Traumatic aneurysm	Elective surgery

well, when suddenly he develops ventricular fibrillation, acute myocardial failure, or acute collapse due to rupture, usually of a left ventricular aneurysm secondary to the contused area. Most patients with left ventricular aneurysms rupture from 2 to 90 days after trauma (Blair et al., 1969). Patients with myocardial contusion usually show an uneventful recovery with follow-up to 16 years (Lidstrom et al., 1968). Tricuspid insufficiency has been observed anywhere from 3 months to 24 years later. Aortic incompetence is usually detected much earlier, within two months or so (Table 7-16).

Penetrating Trauma

In 1819 Baron Larrey, surgeon to Napoleon, decompressed a wound of the heart for the first time by draining the pericardial sac. The first direct suturing of a heart wound was performed by Cappelen in 1895 but the patient died. In 1897 Rhen sutured an acutely bleeding wound of the right ventricle with subsequent recovery. In 1929, the great French surgeon, Tuffier, published 305 cases of heart injuries with a 50 per cent recovery rate. Considerable controversy exists as to the approach and management of penetrating cardiac wounds (Beall et al., 1966; Hardy et al., 1967; Sugg et al., 1968; Yao et al., 1968). A number of factors are responsible for this: (1) the lack of consistent classification of heart wounds; (2) increasing skill and experience as reflected by improvement in statistics of management; (3) delayed or missed diagnosis; and (4) the influence of military experiences. The two approaches consist of either immediate exploration of all heart wounds or initial pericardiocentesis with observation followed by surgery, if indicated on the basis of signs and symptoms.

Since the nature of wounds produced by knives and by bullets differs, it would be reasonable to develop a protocol accordingly. Stab wounds tend to produce cardiac tamponade more frequently than gunshot wounds, since in the latter situation there is a possibility for egress of blood, whereas with stab wounds the pericardium often remains a closed space. Secondly, gunshot wounds produce more extensive wounds, with massive bleeding extending to the mediastinum and to one of the pleural cavities. Therefore, hemothorax is more frequently seen in gunshot wounds and cardiac tamponade in stab wounds. Gunshot wounds produce hemothorax in all victims and tamponade in only 22 per cent, whereas 92 per cent of stab wounds cause hemopericardium only.

A singular problem with regard to pericardiocentesis is that the blood clots, consequently making complete evacuation impossible. Clots are present in about 50 to 60 per cent of patients with hemopericardium. Yao and associates noted that in 15 per cent of pericardiocenteses in 71 patients a positive aspirate was not obtained, while blood was present at surgery (Yao et al., 1968). On the other hand, blood can be obtained as a false positive. Most of the clots are over the right ventricle and since pericardiocentesis is usually done in the area of the left ventricle, it is very possible to miss blood. Pericardiocentesis may be adequate therapy for tamponade. The issue as to management is decided by the patient. A victim with a penetrating chest wound (especially gunshot) with massive bleeding, as evidenced by blood pouring from the wound in conjunction with a large hemothorax, is a candidate for prompt, major surgery. On the other hand, the patient whose hemodynamics are somewhat depressed, but who is not in shock, with minimal or no hemothorax and a somewhat enlarged cardiac shadow by x-ray, will be approached initially by pericardiocentesis.

Pericardiocentesis is carried out usually by the paraxiphoid route, using a thin-walled, spinal needle, #16 or #18. The evacuation of 100 ml. of blood, or less, often proves to be dramatic. As much blood as possible should be removed. The patient is then observed very carefully with all vital signs monitored. Should there be recurrence, pericardial aspiration is repeated. If the amount removed again is in excess of 100 ml. or if there is no improvement, then preparation for open thoracotomy should be seriously considered. Not infrequently tamponade will occur once more in these individuals and the third time is a signal for major surgery. Over-transfusion has been recommended in the therapy of pericardial tamponade in order to ensure an adequate filling pressure. This should not be carried to extremes, however, since the logical maneuver is not to pour fluids in, but rather to relieve the pressure and allow for ventricular filling.

The staff of an Emergency Room is occasionally struck by the sight of a patient brought in on a stretcher, or even occasionally walking in, with a pulsating knife protruding from his chest. Although the situation demands a cool and calm consortium, bedlam often breaks out. The patient is handled in the same manner as an individual with severe trauma when prepared for surgery. The knife is untouched until the patient is in the Operating Room, wherein control can be achieved, and the mediastinum has been approached by means of a remote incision.

The vast majority of cardiac wounds can be treated without resort to supplementary devices, such as bypass or hypothermia. Most wounds can be compressed temporarily with the finger and closed by direct suturing. The heart is a sponge-like mass of muscle and, it must be recalled, the extent of the injury is far greater than that presented by the bullet hole or wound tract. The sutures, therefore, must be placed widely. Furthermore, since they tear through very easily, Teflon buttresses are extremely important to assure the retention of sutures. As a rule, a single layer of interrupted sutures is all that is required. Occasionally, a small coronary vessel may have been lacerated. This requires ligation or oversewing with a #5-0 suture.

The mortality rate from cardiac wounds is the highest of all problems in open wounds of the chest. In one large series the overall rate was 25 per cent (Beall et al., 1966). From 33 to 50 per cent of the patients who expired did so immediately upon arrival in the Emergency Room, before therapy could be instituted adequately. Mortality was insignificant among patients who were treated by pericardiocentesis, whereas those who were operated on showed a mortality rate of about 15 per cent. It is quite apparent that the figures do not necessarily represent the technique, but rather the severity of injury. Combined pericardiocentesis and surgery yielded a mortality of only 7 per cent (Yao et al., 1968). In this particular study it was noted that 4 of 10 patients who died could have been saved if exploration had been done earlier.

In summary, gunshot wounds suggest early surgery whereas this is less true of stab wounds. A patient in profound shock with obvious massive bleeding will require early surgery after resuscitation measures have been taken and once his hemodynamic status

shows some degree of stabilization. In the absence of profound shock, a pericardial infusion with tamponade should be approached initially with nonsurgical measures, including pericardiocentesis. If the shock state or imminent circulatory collapse exists after two taps, then surgery is required.

One of the objections to pericardiocentesis alone, particularly if clots exist in the pericardial space, is the development of chronic constrictive pericarditis. This, however, appears to be relatively infrequent in survivals, since blood is pretty well absorbed from the space. Post-traumatic murmurs suggest intracardiac lesions, which generally require surgery at an elective date utilizing cardiopulmonary bypass.

Major Vessels

The diagnosis of injury to major vessels, particularly the aorta, from blunt trauma continues to be elusive despite its increasing emphasis. This is due to the fact that the mechanisms leading to injury are not fully appreciated. Especially in young people, very often there does not appear to be any obvious thoracic or superficial external evidence of serious trauma. It has been estimated that in 36 per cent of aortic ruptures there is minimal external evidence of thoracic injury (Parmley et al., 1958; Spencer et al., 1961).

In former years, falls usually were the mechanism leading to rupture. At the present time, 67 per cent are due to automobile accidents. Rupture of the aorta is a catastrophic event with approximately 20 per cent surviving the initial injury, but only 10 to 15 per cent surviving long enough to reach the hospital. This means that of 100 individuals with a ruptured aorta, at least 20 survive and are available for cure. Five to 10 are lost en route to a hospital. Approximately 10 to 15 then arrive at a major hospital, but because of delays in diagnosis, the majority of these individuals also succumb.

Complete transections are far more common than tears (Jahnke et al., 1964; Spencer et al., 1961). About 56 per cent are at the ligamentum arteriosum, 16 per cent are in the descending thoracic aorta, and 10 per cent are in the ascending thoracic aorta. Occasionally, other major vessels may be involved, such as the subclavian or the innominate artery.

It is distressing that for patients who *do*

survive long enough to get to a major hospital there is still time for diagnosis. It has been estimated that such patients, arriving at an Emergency Room of a large hospital, have a 50:50 chance of surviving for at least 48 hours. Some have survived as long as 21 days before catastrophe intervened (Jahnke et al., 1964). Survival is due to the fact that the transection begins in the tissues of least resistance to impact and decelerative forces, the endothelium and intima. The adventitial tissue is extremely strong and will sustain for a while. There have been reports of survivals anywhere from 4 months to 37 years with diagnoses established as post-traumatic aneurysms (Hughes, 1965; Spencer et al., 1961). The survivals for this period of time have been limited entirely to injuries at the ligamentum arteriosum.

In diagnosis, the problems once again are the multiple nature of the injury, the more obvious problems taking precedence, the lack of the classic signs and, most important of all, the lack of a high index of suspicion on the part of the physician. The expected signs of massive left hemothorax occur in only about 33 per cent (Hughes, 1965). A wide mediastinum is very frequent, reported in one series to be up to 100 per cent. But a wide mediastinum may be difficult to ascertain. Indeed, there have been instances of complete transections where the mediastinum is not very greatly increased.

It is important to bear in mind that in only 17 per cent of instances there are accompanying rib fractures. Two very important signs are present and should aid in setting into motion the machinery for establishing diagnosis. These are the presence of a systolic murmur and hypertension in a young individual (Hughes, 1965). Both occur in 66 per cent of instances. On admission, such hypertension is not detectable because these individuals may be hypotensive as a result of blood loss. However, the next day the blood pressure may rise to above 180 mm. to 200 mm. Hg (Laforet, 1965).

Reduced arterial pressure in the lower extremities as compared to the upper is a singularly suspicious sign. But unfortunately differential pressures are rarely done. Reduced or suddenly disappearing femoral pulses are practically pathognomonic. The diagnosis should be confirmed by aortography in order to avoid needless exploration, particularly in patients who have other serious injury, such as myocardial contusion. Facilities for performing emergency aortography should be available. These procedures, in themselves, present minimal risks.

There have been an encouraging number of successful repairs. In general, resection with grafting of the defect is the best procedure.

As in blunt trauma, few patients with penetrating injuries to major intrathoracic vessels reach the Emergency Room alive, especially in the case of a gunshot wound. The incidence of aortic (or major branch) perforation is about 6 per cent. In contrast to aortic ruptures from blunt trauma, profound shock is uniformly present in perforations (Steichen, 1967 [Aug.]). Hemothorax is massive. Often other injuries are present—pulmonary and cardiac, depending on the trajectory. As a result of exsanguination or arrest in the Emergency Room or en route to the Operating Room, even fewer patients reach surgery.

Establishing a diagnosis is urgent, but is often done for the first time at the operating table. Most repairs can be effected by finger tamponade or partial occlusion. In some instances partial cardiopulmonary bypass is often required. Occasionally, simple tube bypass from the subclavian to the distal thoracic aorta may be sufficient. In civilian injuries, primary repair with direct suture or a patch graft is sufficient (Table 7-17).

MEDIASTINUM

Mediastinal hematomas are a common occurrence (Reynolds et al., 1966). They are small, diffuse, and insignificant in the vast majority of instances. The most dramatic are those due to aortic rupture. Other sources for gross hematomas include rupture of small vessels from the aorta and veins from fractures of thoracic vertebrae. The significance of large hematomas is in the critical differential diagnosis of an aortic transection or perforation.

TRACHEOBRONCHIAL TRAUMA

Tracheobronchial involvement occurs in 2 to 6 per cent of blunt chest trauma (Blair et al., 1969; Howell et al., 1963). The incidence of burst trachea or bronchus in immediate traffic fatalities is somewhat higher. The injuries in survivors who reached hos-

TABLE 7-17. Indications for Major Surgery in Chest Trauma

Problem	Source	Type of Wound Blunt	Type of Wound Penetrating	Indication for Surgery Immediate	Indication for Surgery Early	Indication for Surgery Early elective
Major hemorrhage	Intercostal artery	✓	✓	—	✓	—
	Cardiac	○	✓	✓	✓	—
	Aorta	✓	✓	—	✓	—
	Pulmonary artery	○	○	✓	✓	—
Cardiac tamponade	Unresolved hemopericardium	○	✓	—	✓	—
Constrictive pericarditis	Persistent clot	○	○	—	—	✓
Major air leak	Trachea/bronchus	✓	○	—	✓	—
	Lung rupture	○	—	—	✓	—
Lung collapse	Unresolved hemothorax	○	○	—	—	
Bowel in chest	Diaphragm tear	○	○	—	✓	—

✓ = frequent
○ = infrequent
— = not applicable

pitals fall into two categories. The first is early and directly from the trauma episode itself, and most often involves a main-stem bronchus. The second is a relatively recent complication of IPPV therapy, the rupture of a necrotic area of contused lung or of a residual cyst. Both complications can lead to potentially disastrous tension pneumothorax. Otherwise, the two are quite dissimilar, anatomically and mechanistically.

The presence of severe subcutaneous emphysema and pneumomediastinum with pneumothorax (especially tension) marks the provisional diagnosis of the rupture of a major-sized segment of the airway. In this infrequent injury, these signs are not so obvious, however. Suspicion usually derives from continued massive leakage through a thoracotomy tube with persistent pneumomediastinum and subcutaneous emphysema. Detection is usually 24 to 48 hours late and the rupture sometimes missed completely. Complete transections produce dramatic distress and are easily detected. Most injuries, however, are only partial. The smaller ones may seal up, either to be popped open later by IPPV, or go on to heal with varying degrees of stenosis. Laminography and bronchoscopy will convert suspicion into documentation. In rare instances bronchography may be required.

The complete type of rupture is more dramatic and constitutes the second most common cause of death during therapy

(Blair et al., 1969). The first indication is a composite of signs and symptoms of tension pneumothorax, the earliest being subcutaneous emphysema. But tragically these often fail to impress the attending staff. Crises can be averted by an indwelling thoracotomy tube in all respirator patients.

Management of transections or perforations from gunshot is operative as an emergency. These patients are too ill not to be operated on. Conservative therapy of partial tears is given out of ignorance. Primary repair is uniformly possible and successful. The secondary ruptures are treated as a rule by tube thoracotomy and negative suction with underwater seal. An occasional case will require surgery to close the leak or for resection, since continued IPPV will not permit sealing. Surgical intervention of this nature has much to recommend it and is more desirable than keeping a patient chained to a respirator continuously and needlessly.

The true incidence of initial ruptures is not known, since most seem to be partial and proceed to heal. Subsequent bronchostenosis is apparently unusual, judging from the paucity of reports.

ESOPHAGUS

Traffic accidents are the least common cause of trauma to the esophagus, which is even more rare in penetrating injuries (Conn et al., 1963; Hughes, 1965). The damage in blunt trauma consists of vertical tears, usually at the tracheal bifurcation, suggesting a bursting type of mechanism. A tear in the upper segment is manifested by cervical subcutaneous emphysema; lower tears are accompanied by hydrothorax. Urgent treatment consists of exploration and primary repair, as with any esophageal perforation or tear. Unusual complications such as traumatic tracheoesophageal fistulae may occur.

DIAPHRAGM

Injuries to the diaphragm in blunt trauma are uncommon, about 3 per cent in survivors and 7 per cent in immediate fatalities (Bassett et al., 1968; Demuth et al., 1966). Left-dome rupture predominates 25 to 1 (Ebert et al., 1967). The incidence is higher in penetrating trauma (8 to 16 per cent) and mostly originates from gunshot wounds.

The magnitude of initial injury (blunt or penetrating) does not influence the probability of diaphragmatic involvement, since external evidence often is trivial. Multiple rib fractures were present in over 50 per cent of victims in automobile accidents. The possibility of ipsilateral, as well as contralateral, intra-abdominal injury exists in missile wounds. A posterocentral tear with medial extension is the most common injury in blunt trauma, followed by avulsion from the anterolateral rib cage and finally rupture of the dome. The tear is usually quite large, permitting intrathoracic migration of abdominal contents.

Diagnosis in the Emergency Room is difficult and almost always missed. Transient paralytic ileus removes the important physical sign of bowel sounds in the chest. At times bowel migration occurs later. Dyspnea and restlessness are attributed to the oft accompanying and more obvious thoracic trauma. The initial x-rays may fail to give a clue (particularly if the technician neglected to include the diaphragm and costophrenic sinus). However, follow-up films usually are conclusive. A barium swallow is rarely indicated. DOMD is mostly a result of the failure to suspect this unusual event. Except for a rare bowel infarction, no catastrophe derives from the rupture. Detection is usually made after 24 hours; sometimes it is made many years later. An early incidental diagnosis is often made at the time of a laparotomy for an accompanying suspected intra-abdominal injury, particularly in penetrating trauma.

Early operative repair is advised. It is best to first stabilize the cardiovascular-pulmonary system complex. Most interventions are transthoracic, but those which are transperitoneal are just as satisfactory. Simple closure by suture is all that is needed in early repairs. Older, post-traumatic hernia may require some material (Marlex, fascia lata) to bridge a wide defect. Also, a transthoracic approach in these patients is preferred, since they often retain intrapleural adhesions or partial obliteration of the pleural space. Decortication should be done, if required.

URGENT PROBLEMS

During the course of management, urgent problems often erupt, requiring prompt detection and resolution (Table 7-18). These crises are almost always due to (1) failure to diagnose the injury or its severity, or (2) complications arising from therapy.

The respirator and the patient are not natural partners. Constant supervision for proper cycling and hook-up are required. Furthermore, the use of the respirator may cause abnormalities to be masked. Atelectasis or unresolved pneumothorax, or both, may be present, despite the apparently satisfactory recovery of the patient. "Blowouts" from contused lungs are abrupt and serious. The chest tube is the hapless patient's lifeline and the doctor's sure-fire indicator of tension pneumothorax or of major bleeding. Pulmonary edema may appear "suddenly," caused by heart failure due to hypoxia, contusion, excessive fluids, alone or in combination.

Tachycardia, after management has been established, usually means hypoxia. Hypovolemia, sepsis, or apprehension are also factors or causes. Bradycardia is much more serious and always means severe myocardial ischemia. The heart is warning the physician or the nurse of impending calamity. Arrhythmias are common in the elderly and not infrequent in the young. The cause is not esoteric—hypoxia, insufficiency. Hypotension usually means hypovolemia but may be caused by hypoxia or acute heart failure. Every sick patient is constantly feeding

TABLE 7-18.   Urgent Problems During Management of Chest Trauma

Problem	Cause	What to do
A. Thoracic		
Flail	Segment not stabilized	Adjust respirator pressure
	Patient not in cycle	Narcotic or muscle relaxant
	Patient is hypoxic	Check for cause (atelectasis, respirator function, worsening A-aDO$_2$).
		Increase O$_2$ input
Lag	Atelectasis	Suction; x-ray confirmation
	Pneumothorax	X-ray; check chest tube
Subcutaneous	"Blowout" with tension pneumothorax	Trocar relief; x-ray; chest tube
	Missed tracheobronchial rupture	X-ray; bronchoscopy; planigrams; surgery
	Missed esophageal tear	Gastrografin swallow; surgery
	Chest tube bottle mix-up	Check and correct
Increased air leak (chest tube)	Tension pneumothorax	See above
	Missed tracheobronchial rupture	See above
Bleeding (chest tube)	Major vessel	X-ray; transfusion; aortogram; surgery
Pulmonary edema	Acute myocardial failure	X-ray; ECG; adjust respirator; digitalis; diuretics
	Overhydration	
B. Cardiovascular		
Tachycardia	Hypoxia	X-ray; adjust respirator;
	Hypovolemia; sepsis	CVP and test fluid load;
	Apprehension	x-ray; sedation
Bradycardia	Ischemia	Check and correct
	Tamponade	hypoxia; hypovolemia; ECG; x-ray; Isuprel
Arrhythmias	Contusion; ischemia; failure	As above; digitalis
Hypotension, shock	Hypovolemia; hypoxia	Fluids and whole blood; check
	Myocardial contusion	pulmonary status; x-ray;
	Delayed aortic rupture	ECG; aortogram

back vital information. It is incumbent upon the staff to be alert to this information — to look for it, interpret it, and act upon it.

COMPLICATIONS AND DEATHS

PULMONARY

Complications following initial resuscitation and institution of therapy in blunt chest trauma are usually pulmonary (Ashbaugh et al., 1967; Blair et al., 1969). These include pneumonia, empyema, fibrothorax, tension pneumothorax, atelectasis, aspiration, acute anoxia, respiratory failure, and oxygen toxicity. Pneumonias frequently become superimposed on lung contusions (Wise et al., 1968). They were the single most common cause of complications (35 per cent) in our patients. The hemorrhagic necrotic beds are not only vulnerable to infection, but serve as culture media. The previous dominance of *Staphylococcus aureus* has now given way to gram-negative microorganisms —*Escherichia coli, Pseudomonas aeruginosa* and Aerobacter (*Klebsiella*). Initial "wide spectrum" antibiotic coverage suppresses gram-positives preferentially. Emerging resistant strains also are a problem. (See Tables 7-19A and B.)

Contusions that fail to show some indication of resolution within five to seven days are interlaced with infections. Spreading infiltrates (including to the opposite lung and temperature elevation mark the subsequent course. Consolidation is unusual and is a late, terminal sign. We have found the A-aDO$_2$ to be of inestimable value in anticipating pneumonia prior to x-ray evidence. Pneumonia precedes the appearance of acute respiratory failure. In uncomplicated flail injuries, pneumonia is less frequent and more readily resolves (Fig. 7-10).

TABLE 7-19A. Complications in Chest Trauma

Complication	Number	Per cent	Died
Pneumonitis	21	30	4
Empyema	1	1	0
Atelectasis°	36	46	0
Tension pneumothorax†	4	6	1
Suction hypoxia	1	1	1
Septicemia	3	4	‡
Disseminated intravascular thrombosis	10	14	‡
Respiratory failure	10	14	‡

° Major (segmental or lobar)
† Secondary to "blowout" (respirator)
‡ Included in pneumonitis

TABLE 7-19B. Mortality Rate

Category	Number	Per cent	Total	Per cent
Thoracic			8	11
Immediate	1	1		
Late	7	10		
Nonthoracic			12	17
All			20	28

The sequence of events before terminus has become classic. The patient with a moderate contusion is in a stabilized, presumably controlled state on the respirator, with a reduced input of 40 to 50 per cent oxygen. Consternation envelops the staff as the infiltrate, instead of resolving, begins to spread. The temperature rises. The patient "doesn't look as well." The PaO_2 drops and the $A\text{-}aDO_2$, which had declined, rises again. The oxygen input is cranked up. Cultures and sensitivities are rechecked,

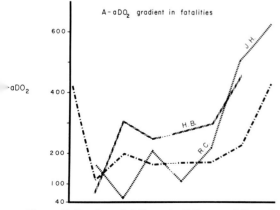

Figure 7-10. Initial fall in $A\text{-}aDO_2$ was followed by a secondary and greater rise due to the development of pneumonia.

and antibiotics are manipulated. The infiltrate spreads first throughout the lobe, then the lung, and finally spills over into the contralateral lung (which had been "supporting" the patient). The intensity magnifies. Intratracheal suction yields are scanty. The oxygen input is 100 per cent; the PaO_2 drops to 70, 60, 50, 40 mm. Hg; the $A\text{-}aDO_2$ levels out at 500 to 600 mm. Hg. Acute respiratory failure exists. Days go by. Oxygen toxicity gradually envelops the system (Soloway et al., 1968). The lungs are consolidated into a rubbery, stiff mass. Respiratory, then mixed, metabolic acidosis supervenes. The heart slows down and stops (Fig. 7-11).

Tension pneumothorax occurs with alarming frequency in lung contusion patients. Two factors are significant—pneumonia and the respirator. The lung responds to contusion and pneumonia by developing weak spots caused by cystic, necrotic changes. The resistive intra-alveolar tension is lost. Normally impervious to reasonable positive pressure blasts from the respirator, these weak areas rupture. A quiescent thoracotomy tube suddenly erupts into frantic bubbling. This patient is fortunate. If the tube had been removed (as it often is), acute respiratory, followed by circulatory, collapse would occur. We have lost one patient this way.

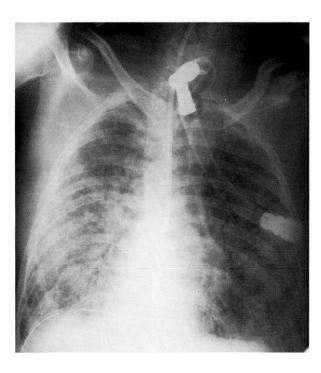

Figure 7-11. Appearance of the lungs the day before death. Contusion was complicated by pneumonia and oxygen toxicity.

Atelectasis is a constantly recurring problem, resulting from inefficient clearance of the airway, and it is a greater problem in blunt trauma than in penetrating trauma. The mechanism is in a large part also due to the tendency of damaged parenchyma to collapse, probably because of the loss of surfactant. Patchy atelectases are constant cohabitants of the damaged lung. Without vigilant, frequent suction, segmental and lobar collapse occurs. Usually a dilated, paralytic stomach must be aspirated because it has not been carefully watched. In a marginal patient acute anoxia from prolonged suctioning is a constant threat. The nurse must be adept, decisive, and strictly timed in this procedure. The critical patient can only tolerate interruption from the "mother" respirator for a brief period. The negative pressure sucks air more easily than it sucks secretions. In a few seconds the precariously maintained PaO_2 can be precipitously depleted.

Acute respiratory failure is generally associated with advanced emphysema or the neonatal respiratory disease syndrome. More recently the problem has been espoused as a leading complication in other crises, such as shock or nonthoracic trauma. Oxygen toxicity from prolonged administration of high concentrates has been implicated. This problem has emerged as a relatively new syndrome in the young chest trauma patient. The indictments include pneumonitis, superimposed on lung contusion, and prolonged respirator therapy with high oxygen input. The inevitable pattern emerges whenever the patient cannot be taken off the respirator, much less endure reduced oxygen concentration.

There is no objective evidence for or against "prophylactic" antibiotic therapy in severe blunt chest trauma. Contamination is a reality by the time the patient arrives in the hospital, especially with a gunshot wound. To be sure, infections per se have not developed, but the conditions are ideal. The principle of a specific, lab-documented antibiotic for a specific microorganism is most pertinent in trauma. Early methicillin, 12 gm./day, (or another penicillinase synthetic drug) is advised, until culture and sensitivities are available. In the hustle and bustle of the Emergency Room, sputum for cultures is often forgotten. It is even more important to get Lukens tube cultures of intratracheal secretions with aseptic precautions. Whenever possible partial isolation should be imposed to protect the trauma patient from those in the Intensive Care Unit with clinical infections. Airborne and cross contamination (personnel carriers) and unsterile equipment are principal sources of infection. Emergence of gram-negative bacteria secondary to suppression of gram-positives is another.

Empyemas are relatively unusual in major thoracic trauma, being somewhat more common after gunshot wounds. These are secondary to pneumonia and to infection of hemothoraces. Therapy consists of the control of pneumonitis and prompt evacuation of intrapleural fluid with complete re-expansion of the collapsed lung. Repeat thoracentesis invites infection. Tube thoracotomy is the only sure, safe, and effective method. Chronic empyema, often with loculation, requires rib resection and drainage.

Fibrothorax is relatively unusual. Early decortication is recommended, preferably during the same hospital stay. The procedure is simpler, less traumatic to the lungs, and far more effective than a delayed procedure. Tension pneumothorax is best treated by anticipation and a decompression thoracotomy tube. In chronic cases with repeat blowouts, more than one tube is required. It should be borne in mind that a tension pneumothorax may be due to a respirator blowout of a previously sealed tracheobronchial laceration. The failure of prompt re-expansion and seal heralds the need for operative intervention—either for the primary tracheobronchial tear or the secondary blowout. In either situation a tight seal is urgent, either by primary closure or lobectomy. Segmental resection is ill-advised. Since the patient will continue to be on the respirator, he would only continue to leak air profusely.

Death from aspiration is a tragic climax to an otherwise brilliant program of resuscitation. Nasogastric decompression and vigilant nursing care are the mainstays of prevention.

Acute anoxia is prevented by strict adherence to suction techniques, as outlined previously. Acute respiratory failure can only be treated effectively by not permitting it to develop. The important factors include suppression of pneumonitis, avoidance of excessive oxygen concentrations, and meticulous respirator handling.

Subcutaneous emphysema is a dramatic and distressing development. It is almost always due to an air leak under tension—a pleural tear or tracheobronchial injury. Treatment is directed at the source. Patients on the respirator often will not show pneumothorax. Insertion of a chest tube into the affected side, nevertheless, is mandatory.

Pneumomediastinum is not infrequently present with tension pneumothorax. If the pericardium is lacerated, pneumopericardium may also occur. Again, therapy is directed at the source through effective, closed-tube thoracotomy and negative suction.

CARDIOVASCULAR

The early complications are due to DOMD and, in blunt trauma, they include acute failure, arrhythmias, and cardiac arrest or rupture secondary to cardiac injury. In penetrating injuries, the problem is lengthy "delay" of surgery and arrest due to tamponade or exsanguination from the "blowout" of a precarious clot when the arterial pressure is restored.

Later hospital complications include acute failure from myocardial contusion or traumatic valvular insufficiency. Patients who, days after the injury, require digitalization, more likely suffered a contusion rather than some nebulous, mysterious, myocardial assault. Inappropriate fluid therapy may cause overload, especially in older patients. Again, some pre-existing fault most likely exists, such as contusion or ischemia from other sources.

Problems months or years later include post-traumatic aneurysms, valvular insufficiency, and chronic constrictive pericarditis, most of which require surgical correction. These are relatively uncommon.

HYPOVOLEMIA

Hypovolemia and shock are early complications and most often are due to non-thoracic injuries in blunt trauma. On the other hand, in penetrating injuries the source is thoracic and is the greatest cause of death. A falling hematocrit, later on in the course of recovery, may be due to dilutional fluid therapy, continued blood loss, a fresh source (stress ulcer), or intrathoracic crises (delayed vascular rupture, intercostal vessel). Renal shutdown secondary to hypovolemia is not uncommon. Hemodialysis is recommended.

DISSEMINATED INTRAVASCULAR THROMBOSIS

Trauma is presumed to be accompanied by intravascular phenomena. Documentation is scanty since, as a rule, a search is not made. We have observed this problem in three patients (Blair et al., 1969). The syndrome is due to inappropriate activation of clotting mechanisms with subsequent intravascular fibrin deposits and depletion of coagulation precursors. Bleeding of unexplained origin is the primary overt clinical manifestation—at the tracheostomy site, petechial hemorrhages, undue bleeding from a venous puncture. The late signs result from organ failure, secondary to major vascular thrombosis. The patient may demonstrate a falling hematocrit for no discernible reason. A platelet count provides a simple and ready clue. Prothrombin time is reduced and fibrinogen is depleted. As lysis takes place, plasminogen levels may decline. Our patients had pneumonias and the infection may well have been a contributing factor. A survey of 10 other patients with chest trauma revealed thrombocytopenia and decreases in clottable protein. The diagnosis can be established before an advanced stage is reached or prior to intervening sepsis by simple laboratory tests, including hematocrit, platelet count, prothrombin time, and estimate of clottable protein.

Since the problem is one of intravascular thrombosis, initial therapy requires full heparinization. Caution and careful observation is essential, since the patient may have a potential, latent bleeding problem from an injury site.

SUMMARY

Major chest trauma is a multifaceted, complex problem—its rising incidence, deficiencies in emergency care, inadequate comprehension of dynamics and of pathophysiology, inordinately delayed or missed diagnoses, controversies in and complications deriving from management all add to the difficulties. The major problem in blunt trauma is the flail chest, which may be further complicated by an accompanying lung contusion. Thoracic pathoanatomy causes interference with the mechanical components of lung function—such as occurs with flail, intrapleural collections, loss of ventilable lung tissue, and parenchymal damage, culminating in disturbances in effective alveolar ventilation. Impairment of the many components of lung function boils down to abnormalities in V_A/Q manifested by low PaO_2 and increased $A\text{-}aDO_2$. Current research indicates the fundamental defect is increase in venoarterial admixture. In contrast, the major problem of penetrating trauma stems from cardiovascular involvement—massive hemorrhage and pericardial tamponade, with the thoracic component secondary.

Pathodynamics in blunt trauma are poorly understood and have been inadequately studied. Thoracic cage injury appears to be due primarily to the force of direct impact, whereas pulmonary and mediastinal involvement result from secondary phenomena, derived from the direct force and the dynamic environment of the accident. Because of military interest in ballistics, the mechanics of wounding is better understood. Civilian casualties are primarily due to low to medium-velocity missiles. The extent of tissue damage is far greater than that indicated by the actual wound tract, but in the main these are comparatively "clean" wounds. In contrast to blunt trauma, the significant injuries are mediastinal, especially cardiovascular. The force from direct impact and penetration is responsible for most damage. Secondary "shock" waves and shearing effects can cause lung or myocardial contusion. Stab wounds are more common and less lethal.

Clinical perception stands as the sole sure way of rapid, accurate assessment of life-threatening components of thoracic injury and of patient progress during therapy. Radiology and laboratory tests are supplemental and confirmatory, except in special situations. Delayed or missed diagnoses are due to lack of, or faulty, perception. The singular laboratory aid is the PaO_2 and calculation of $A\text{-}aDO_2$. Shock is due to a thoracic-oriented injury primarily in penetrating trauma. Significant hypovolemia in blunt injury heralds a complicating nonthoracic problem, such as long bone or pelvic fracture, or an intra-abdominal catastrophe. The emergency dictum is resuscitation, not surgery. Cardiac massage is performed as an "open" procedure only. Surgery, however, may be urgent (aortic transection or perforation).

A step-by-step protocol, executed with deliberate, programmed tension by team effort, will ensure immediate action and will save lives. A clear airway is achieved by prompt eradication of secretions and blood and by *nasotracheal intubation*. Tracheostomy in the hospital is an *elective* procedure and never performed as an emergency. Until the extent of chest pathology can be discerned, respirator support with 100 per cent oxygen should be instituted. Respirator management should be in the hands of skilled, experienced professionals, functioning as members of a team. The respirator does *not* reconstitute normal ventilation. A flail segment is stabilized and alveolar ventilation improved. Arterial blood gases and the estimated A-aDO$_2$ are the best guides for respirator and other technical adjustments. For patient adjustments the best guide unequivocally is clinical judgment, which in turn is sharpened by relentless pursuit and tenacity. Evacuation of air or blood or both by large tube thoracotomy is vital. External stabilization of the flail segment should be limited to on-the-site and in-transit operations. IPPV with the lungs as pneumatic splints is the preferred in-hospital procedure. Flail injuries, uncomplicated by lung contusion, are uniformly controlled. Not all flail injuries require respirator support. It is wise to institute IPPV, however, until the magnitude of the instability can be ascertained.

Lung contusions are the problem in blunt trauma, giving rise to the majority of complications, particularly pneumonia. Relatively new problems related to gram-negative pneumonias and to the respirator have emerged. If not arrested, progressively increasing oxygen concentrations are required over long periods of time. The spreading pneumonitis culminates in acute respiratory failure. Coupled with prolonged oxygen therapy, the lungs may become converted into a rubbery, functionless mass. In a well-organized and well-run trauma service, lives may be saved only to be lost because of acute respiratory failure and respirator-generated complications, such as O$_2$ toxicity and lung rupture. Since these complications are iatrogenic, they can be prevented.

Lung damage with intrapleural accumulations, due to penetrating injury, is treated as it is for blunt trauma. The singular problem is mediastinal involvement, especially cardiac. Pericardiocentesis is the preferred initial procedure for hemopericardium. Surgery is reserved for unsuccessful aspirations, but should not be unduly delayed.

REFERENCES

Ashbaugh, D. C., Peters, G. N., Halgrimson, C. G., Owens, C., and Waddell, W.: Chest trauma. Analysis of 685 patients. Arch. Surg., 95:546, 1967.

Avery, A. E., Mörch, E. T., and Benson, S. W.: Critically crushed chest. J. Thorac. Surg., 32:291, 1956.

Bassett, J. S., Gibson, R. D., and Wilson, R. F.: Blunt injuries to the chest. J. Trauma, 8:418, 1968.

Beall, A. C., Jr., Bricker, D., Crawford, H. W., and DeBakey, M. E.: Surgical management of penetrating thoracic trauma. Dis. Chest, 49:568-77, 1966.

Beall, A. C., Jr., Diethrich, E. B., Crawford, W., Cooley, D. A., and DeBakey, M. E.: Surgical management of penetrating cardiac injuries. Amer. J. Surg., 112:686-692, 1966.

Blair, E., and Mills, E.: Rationale of stabilization of the flail chest with intermittent positive pressure breathing. Am. Surgeon, 34:860, 1968.

Blair, E., Topuzlu, C., and Deane, R.: Major blunt chest trauma. Curr. Prob. Surg., May, 1969.

Border, J. R., Brian, R., Hopkinson, M. B., and Schenk, W. G.: Mechanisms of pulmonary trauma. An experimental study. J. Trauma, 8:47, 1968.

Carmack, K., Rapport, R. Z., Paul, J., and Baird, W. C.: Deceleration injuries of the thoracic aorta. Arch. Surg., 79:244, 1959.

Clark, C. C.: Airbag Restraints and Air Systems for the Alleviation of Highway Injury. In *Prevention of Highway Injury*. Highway Safety Res. Inst., Ann Arbor, Mich., pp. 221-237, 1967.

Conn, J. H., Hardy, J. D., Fain, W. R., and Netterville, R. E.: Thoracic trauma: Analysis of 1072 cases. J. Trauma, 3:22, 1963.

D'Abreu, A. L.: Thoracic injuries. J. Bone Surg., 46:581, 1964.

Deane, R. S., and Mills, E.: Prolonged nasotracheal intubation in adults—a successor and adjunct to tracheostomy. To be published, Anesth. Analg.

Demuth, W. E., Jr., and Fallah-Mejad, M.: Delayed recognition of serious thoracic injury. Amer. J. Surg., 111:587, 1966.

Demuth, W. E., Jr., and Zinsser, H. F., Jr.: Myocardial contusion. Arch. Intern. Med., 115:434, 1965.

Ebert, P. A., Gaertner, R. A., and Zuidema, G. D.: Traumatic diaphragmatic hernia. Surg., Gynec., Obstet., 125:59, 1967.

French, R. W., and Callender, G. R.: Ballistics Characteristics of Wounding Agents. In *Wound Ballistics*. Office of the Surgeon General, Washington, D.C., pp. 91-2, 1962.

Garzon, A. A., Gourin, A., Seltzer, B., Chiu, C. J., and Karlson, K. E.: Severe blunt chest trauma. Studies of pulmonary mechanics and blood gases. Ann. Thorac. Surg., 2:629, 1966.

Gray, A. R., Harrison, W. H., Couves, C., and Howard, J.: Penetrating injuries to the chest—clinical results in the management of 769 patients. Amer. J. Surg., 100:709, 1960.

Hardy, J. D., and Williams, R. D.: Penetrating heart wounds: Analysis of 12 consecutive cases individualized without mortality. Ann. Surg., 166:228-231, 1967.

Howell, J. F., Crawford, E. S., and Jordan, G. S.: The flail chest: An analysis of 100 patients. Amer. J. Surg., 106:628, 1963.

Hughes, R. K.: Thoracic trauma. Ann. Thorac. Surg., 1:778, 1965.

Jahnke, E. J., Fisher, G. W., and Jones, B. C.: Acute traumatic rupture of the thoracic aorta. Report of six consecutive cases of successful early repair. J. Thorac. Cardiov. Surg., 48:63, 1964.

Kulowski, J.: Crash Injuries. Springfield, Ill., Charles C Thomas, 1960.

Laforet, E. O.: Acute hypertension as a diagnostic clue in traumatic rupture of the thoracic aorta. Amer. J. Surg., 110:948, 1965.

Lidstrom, P., Lindholmer, C., and Orinius, E.: The late cardiac prognosis after nonpenetrating chest trauma. Acta Med. Scand., 183:243, 1968.

Malm, A., Svanberg, L., Holen, O., and Bäckstrom, C. G.: Chest injuries and their treatment. Acta Chir. Scand. (Suppl.), 332:7, 1965.

Parmley, L. F., Manion, W. C., and Mattingly, T. W.: Nonpenetrating traumatic injury of the heart. Circulation, 18:377, 1958.

Parmley, L. F., Mattingly, T. W., Manion, W. C., and Jahnke, E. J.: Nonpenetrating injury of the aorta. Circulation, 17:1086, 1958.

Reynolds, J., and Davis, J. T.: Injuries of the chest wall, pleura, pericardium, lungs, bronchi, and esophagus. Radiol. Clin. N. Amer., 4:383, 1966.

Selmonosky, C. A., and Ehrenhaft, J. L.: Torsion of lobe of the lung due to blunt thoracic trauma. Ann. Thorac. Surg., 4:166, 1967.

Sherman, R. T.: Experiences with 472 civilian penetrating wounds of the chest. Milit. Med., 131:63, 1966.

Soloway, H. B., Castillo, Y., and Martin, A. M.: Adult hyaline membrane disease: Relationship to oxygen therapy. Ann. Surg., 168:937, 1968.

Spencer, F. C., Green, P. F., Blake, H. H., and Bahnson, H. T.: A report of 15 patients with traumatic rupture of the thoracic aorta. J. Thorac. Cardiov. Surg., 41:1, 1961.

Stapp, J. P.: The Problem: Biomechanics of Injury. In The Prevention of Highway Injury. Ann Arbor, Mich., Highway Safety Res. Inst., pp. 159–164, 1967.

Steichen, F. M.: Penetrating Wounds of the Chest and the Abdomen. Current Problems in Surgery. Chicago, Year Book Medical Publishers, Inc., August, 1967.

Sugg, W. L., Rea, W. J., Ecker, R. R., Webb, W. R., Rose, E. F., and Shaw, R. R.: Penetrating wounds of the heart. An analysis of 459 cases. J. Thorac. Cardiov. Surg., 56:531–545, 1968.

Tonkin, J. P., and Harrison, G. S.: The effect on the larynx of prolonged endotracheal intubation. Med. J. Australia, 2581:587, 1966.

Wise, A., Topuzlu, C., Mills, E. L., Page, H. G., and Blair, E.: The importance of serial blood gas determinations in blunt chest trauma. J. Thorac. Cardiov. Surg., 56:520, 1968.

Yao, S. T., Vanecko, R. M., Printen, K., and Shoemaker, W. C.: Penetrating wounds of the heart: A review of 80 cases. Ann. Surg., 168:67–68, 1968.

CHAPTER 8

WOUND SEPSIS AND DEHISCENCE*

by W. A. ALTEMEIER, M.D., and EDWARD BERKICH, M.D.

William A. Altemeier was born in Cincinnati and received his baccalaureate and medical degrees at the University of Cincinnati, where he graduated with high distinction. As a medical student and later during residency training at Henry Ford Hospital he developed his profound interest and research in bacteriology and surgical infections. In 1952 he was appointed the Christian R. Holmes Professor of Surgery and Chairman of the Department at Cincinnati and Chief of the Surgical Services of Cincinnati General Hospital. His honors have been many and outstanding, including being elected President of the American Surgical Association. Dr. Altemeier is a world authority on wound healing and sepsis, and the wound infection rate in his hospital is one of the lowest in the nation.

Edward Berkich, M.D., received his medical degree from St. Louis University and then served six years' residency training with Dr. Altemeier. At present he is Instructor in Surgery at the University of Cincinnati and his field of special research interest is wound healing.

WOUND SEPSIS

The practice of surgery is singularly dependent upon the healing of wounds without serious complications. The development of wound sepsis, particularly in large wounds, is one of the most serious complications that can develop in critically ill patients. Indeed, it in itself may quickly lead to a critical state in a postoperative patient who has previously been in good condition. Sepsis occurring in postoperative wounds, accidental wounds, or wounds of violence may have a significant effect on the wounded patient's mortality and morbidity and on the final result of his operation. Its occurrence in wounded individuals who have been debilitated as the result of acute or chronic disease, severe or multiple injuries, or other similar factors may determine the issue of life or death. In addition, loss of limb and prolonged or permanent loss of function may be the results. Further destruction of tissues, beyond

that produced by injury, and suppression of the process of wound healing may be caused by the infection. Tissues thus destroyed must be replaced by scar tissue, and this may adversely affect function and cosmetic appearance.

History has shown that the prevention of sepsis in planned operative wounds represents one of the three greatest milestones in the development and practice of surgery. In the days before Lister, approximately 100 years ago, most, if not all, operative wounds became infected, and earlier surgeons felt helpless in dealing with septic processes which complicated most surgical procedures. The application of the principles of antisepsis, as developed through the work of Lister and Pasteur, paved the way for the prevention of postoperative infection in clean surgical wounds. Antiseptic technique was replaced by aseptic technique, and surgery, thus released of one of its three greatest scourges, rapidly extended its horizons. Thus it has become possible to explore the innermost cavities and recesses of the body with safety in the great majority of

*This work supported in part by USPHS Grant #5-PO1-GM-15428.

187

instances and without the development of serious postoperative infection.

Recent evidence suggests, however, that this heritage has probably been taken too much for granted. Wound sepsis has again become a problem of increasing importance in general hospital practice throughout the world. The continuing and apparently rising infection rate despite antibiotic prophylaxis has resulted in the appointment of committees by the American College of Surgeons, the U.S. Public Health Service, and the American Hospital Association to study this problem and make recommendations for its resolution.

Following the results of the introduction and general use of antibiotic therapy between 1942 and 1950, there was a widespread belief among physicians and surgeons that prophylactic antibiotic therapy had provided the answer for the prevention and control of wound sepsis. This misconception was probably inevitable, but it led to the general and indiscriminate use of the available antibiotic agents in clinical practice. The obvious limitations of antibiotic therapy soon became apparent, and the significance of factors in addition to bacteria as causes of wound sepsis came into sharper focus.

Recently there has been evidence to suggest that antibiotic therapy not only has failed to decrease the number of cases of wound sepsis but has also had a significant effect on the bacterial types of infections occurring in surgical patients.

It should also be remembered that the opportunities for sepsis in the modern general hospital are numerous and everthreatening. In addition to the reservoir of virulent and antibiotic-resistant bacteria and the hospital's personnel potential of patient cross-contamination and infection, there are other factors that contribute to this problem. There is a concentration of patients with a large variety of infections who have been admitted along with many other patients who are particularly prone to develop sepsis because of their unusual susceptibility. The latter include those hospitalized for treatment of recent trauma, debilitating chronic diseases, surgical conditions requiring operations, technical diagnostic procedures, steroid therapy or immunosuppressive therapy, and neoplastic diseases. The extension of complex surgical treatment to aged and debilitated patients and the widespread use of complicated diagnostic, therapeutic, and anesthetic procedures favor the development of hospital-acquired sepsis. In addition, the pressing demand of large numbers of patients in a short period of time and the inadequate supply of supportive nursing and paramedical personnel tend to produce compromises and administrative trends not in the best interest of infection control.

CAUSES OF WOUND SEPSIS

Bacteria, of course, are the basic cause of wound sepsis. Bacterial contamination of open wounds, whether produced by accidental injury or induced by surgical operation, usually can be demonstrated by careful bacteriological cultures of wound surfaces. Even clean surgical wounds that heal *per primam* are contaminated by airborne microorganisms. Some of the bacterial contaminants may be highly virulent, others less so and still others, saprophytic. Fortunately, only a small percentage of such wounds develop actual wound sepsis. Of great importance is the recognition of certain factors that influence the growth of bacteria in the wound and determine not only the development of a septic process but also its local and systemic characteristics. These factors have been under study at the University of Cincinnati Trauma Center and are listed in Table 8-1.

The number and types of contaminating bacteria can increase the probability and severity of wound infection. The premise that infection is the unfavorable result of the equation of dose multiplied by virulence and divided by resistance still is applicable. The mere presence of virulent bacteria in a wound *per se* does not make infection of that wound a certainty. The evidence indicates that the physiologic state of the tissue

TABLE 8-1. Etiologic Factors of Wound Sepsis

1. The virulence, types, and numbers of contaminating bacteria.
2. The presence and amount of devitalized tissue within the wound.
3. The presence and types of foreign bodies.
4. The nature, location, and duration of the wound.
5. The local and general immunity response of the individual.
6. The type, time, and thoroughness of treatment.
7. The general condition of the patient.

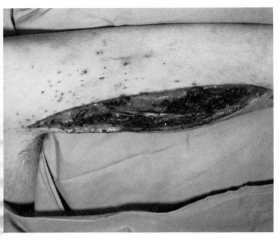

Figure 8-1. Infected shotgun wound of leg. Incision made for drainage reveals the extensive infection that had developed in the devitalized tissues in association with local foreign bodies.

within the wound before and after treatment is more important than the presence of bacteria. The presence of multiple bacterial strains with synergistic or symbiotic activity may also be an important determining factor of the nature and severity of the infection.

The presence of unhealthy, irritated, or dead tissue in wounds invites and supports the growth of virulent and nonvirulent bacteria since it has limited or little power of resistance to their growth and action. Conversely, healthy tissues possess a remarkable resistance and have the power to kill bacteria and to withstand their effects.

Foreign bodies, particularly those of organic composition, frequently carry large numbers of bacteria into wounds and increase the probability of infection by their heavy contamination and their local irritative action on tissues. This is the so-called foreign body effect. Suture and prosthetic materials buried within a wound may also act as foreign bodies and should be used intelligently, just enough being employed to approximate live tissues and obliterate dead pockets.

The nature of the wound is also an important factor. Wound sepsis is more prone to develop in extensive wounds containing large amounts of devitalized tissues, especially muscle, fascia, and bone (Fig. 8-1). As indicated previously, such wounds furnish excellent culture material for bacteria. Several pounds of damaged muscle tissue may be present in wounds of the thigh and buttocks, and these greatly devitalized masses may become septically involved. Wounds

produced by crushing or blast injuries and associated with heavy contamination are frequently multiple and are characterized by extensive tissue destruction, severe shock, and early wound sepsis.

The location of the wound is of significance because various tissues in different locations in the body are known to have different powers of local resistance to infection. Lacerations of the face and neck, for example, are prone to heal kindly unless they are in communication with the mouth and the pharynx. Wounds of the perineal area show a high tendency toward infection to some degree.

The multiplicity of severe wounds in one person may compromise his treatment and make adequate debridement of one or more of his wounds impossible. Because of severe shock, hemorrhage, or associated wounds of the chest and head, the local treatment of wounds may necessarily assume a relatively minor role in relation to the early over-all treatment of the patient. If the period of time required for the successful general treatment exceeds six to ten hours, infection may occur before local definitive treatment is possible.

The relative importance of the immunity response of the individual has become increasingly apparent in the past ten years as the limitations of prophylactic antibiotic therapy have become obvious. Resistance may be local, regional, or general. Local immunity depends partly on the type of tissue, especially on its vascularity. It is used to describe the resistance that the wounded area possesses naturally or that it acquires after overcoming an infection or reacting to a local antigen so that the same organisms can no longer invade at this point. Other important factors are the protective action of the regional lymph nodes and the development of phagocytosis and the intracellular digestion and killing of microbial organisms. The process of intracellular killing of bacteria after phagocytosis may be adversely influenced by severe injuries such as burns and by debilitating chronic diseases such as diabetes mellitus, uremia, and leukemia.

The type, time, and thoroughness of treatment influence the development of wound sepsis more than most surgeons realize. Of primary importance is the surgical excision and removal of all devitalized tissue and foreign bodies within the wound, preferably within four to six hours after injury in order

TABLE 8-2.   Factors Predisposing and Contributing to Wound Sepsis

1. Dehydration
2. Shock
3. Malnutrition
4. Anemia
5. Advanced age
6. Extreme obesity
7. Remote infection
8. Duration of operation
9. Duration of preoperative hospitalization
10. Associated diseases such as diabetes mellitus, uremia, and cirrhosis
11. Malignant neoplasms including leukemia
12. Debilitating injuries
13. Iatrogenic factors

to remove any potential pabulum before invasive bacterial growth can occur. Likewise, care must be exercised to prevent the development of devitalized tissue during the postoperative state. Impairment of the local blood supply by thrombosis or damage to large vessels, by the displacement of fractures, by the pressure of hematomas, by tourniquets or ill-applied casts, or by increased fascial tension due to swelling or tension by sutures favors the delayed development of devitalized tissues and decreases the local resistance of tissues. Thus bacterial colonization and the development of infection may be permitted.

The physical condition of the patient is an important predisposing factor to infection. Dehydration, shock, malnutrition, exhaustion, uncontrolled diabetes, anemia, and various associated diseases listed in Table 8-2 may lower his resistance sufficiently to increase the chances for bacterial growth and wound sepsis. Other contributing factors include advanced age of the patient, marked obesity, the presence of active remote areas of infection, the duration of the operation, the period of preoperative hospitalization, debilitating injuries, and various iatrogenic factors.

TABLE 8-3.   Clinical Types of Wound Sepsis

1. Cellulitis
2. Suppuration and abscess
3. Lymphangitis and lymphadenitis
4. Septic thrombophlebitis
5. Necrosis and gangrene
6. Toxemic
7. Bacteremia
8. Septicemia

CLASSIFICATION OF WOUND SEPSIS

Wound sepsis is the direct result of the entrance, growth, and metabolic activities of microorganisms in the tissues of a wound resulting from a planned operation or from injury. Surgical infections differ from medical infections in two principal ways. The surgical infection or primary focus is one which is unlikely to resolve spontaneously; instead, suppuration, necrosis, gangrene, prolonged morbidity, death, or other serious effects usually occur if not treated surgically. Secondly, the excision,

TABLE 8-4.   Etiologic Classification of Wound Sepsis

I. Aerobic bacterial infections
  A. Gram-positive cocci
    1. Staphylococcus
    2. Streptococcus
    3. Pneumococcus
  B. Gram-negative cocci
    1. Neisseria catarrhalis
    2. Neisseria gonorrhoeae
  C. Gram-negative bacilli
    1. Escherichia coli
    2. Aerobacter aerogenes
    3. Klebsiella
    4. Pseudomonas aeruginosa
    5. Proteus
    6. Alcaligenes faecalis
    7. Salmonella typhosis
    8. Haemophilis influenzae
  D. Gram-positive bacteria
    1. Bacillus anthracis
    2. Corynebacterium
    3. Diphtheroid
    4. Mycobacterium tuberculosis
II. Microaerophilic bacterial infections
  A. Gram-positive cocci
    1. Streptococcus
      a. Hemolyticus
      b. Non-hemolyticus
III. Mixed infections
  A. Gram-positive and gram-negative
    1. Aerobic and anaerobic
IV. Synergistic infections
V. Anaerobic bacterial infections
  A. Gram-positive cocci
    1. Streptococcus
  B. Gram-positive bacilli
    1. Clostridia
      a. Perfringens
      b. Novyi
      c. Histolyticum
      d. Septicum
      e. Sordellii
      f. Sporogenes
      g. Tetani
  C. Gram-negative bacteroides
    1. Melanogenicum
    2. Spherophorus necrophorus

incision, and drainage of the area of infection must be possible technically. Other characteristics of surgical infections are their frequent polymicrobic etiology and their invasiveness with rapid growth and spread of bacteria into the surrounding tissues or regional systems. In contrast, medical infections are characteristically monomicrobic, diffuse, and associated with little or no local tissue reaction but a marked systemic reaction.

When wound sepsis occurs it may be classified clinically according to its pathophysiologic types (Table 8-3) or bacteriologically according to its microbial etiology (Table 8-4).

The majority of wound infections start as a cellulitis, a diffuse inflammatory process without suppuration, which is characterized by hyperemia, edema, pain, and interference with function. Suppuration often follows and is the result of local liquefaction of tissue and the formation of pus with the production of an abscess (Fig. 8-2). The cellulitis usually continues and extends peripherally beyond and around the area of the abscess.

Wound sepsis may subside spontaneously, remain localized, extend to regional or distant areas, or become chronic. If the infections extend, they do so by direct extension, lymphatic spread, venous spread, or, rarely, arterial spread. Direct extension is most common by way of subcutaneous tissue, muscles, tissue planes, or tendon sheaths.

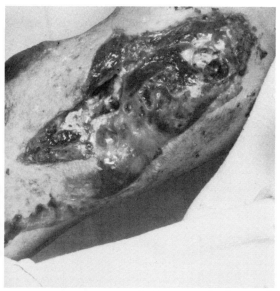

Figure 8-2. Compound fracture of ulna with staphylococcal wound sepsis.

They may also spread diffusely through cavities such as the peritoneal or thoracic cavities.

Rapid dissemination of the infection from the septic wound may occur along the regional lymphatics as a lymphangitis and lymphadenitis, particularly in septic lesions caused by the beta *Streptococcus hemolyticus.* The lymphadenitis may in turn become suppurative.

Septic thrombosis of adjacent and regional blood vessels may develop in association with some infections such as those caused by the hemolytic *Staphylococcus aureus,* the *Streptococcus hemolyticus,* the *Bacteroides,* or the anaerobic *Streptococcus.* Septic thrombophlebitis of neighboring veins may lead to thromboembolic disease, bacteremia, or septicemia.

Necrosis and gangrenous changes may be produced by bacterial action in a variety of ways, including inadequate blood supply resulting from the expanding pressure of marked edema (gas gangrene) (Fig. 8-3), liquefaction of tissues by necrotizing bacterial enzymes (staphylococcal and mixed synergistic infections), and ischemia secondary to vascular thrombosis (streptococcal and staphylococcal infections). (*See* Fig. 8-4.)

Severe toxemia without actual invasion of the bloodstream by bacteria may develop in patients with wound infections. This may be *nonspecific,* as in many mixed wound infections, or *specific,* as in tetanus.

When bacteria are distributed intermittently into the bloodstream from a septic wound, a *bacteremia* is generally considered to exist, with the blood cultures being only transiently positive. When the broadcast of bacteria from such a focus into the circulation is more or less constant, and the presence of bacteria is relatively constant in the cultures of the blood, a *septicemia* is considered to exist. In the latter instance metastatic abscesses and secondary areas of infection are prone to develop. These in turn may become foci, and the septicemia may become cyclic. In this regard it is important to recall that bacteria gaining entrance into the bloodstream make the circuit approximately every 25 seconds and usually are quickly removed from the circulation by the cells of the reticuloendothelial system.

Another useful classification of wound sepsis has been developed on an etiologic basis, as indicated in Table 8-4. Infections by the higher microorganisms such as

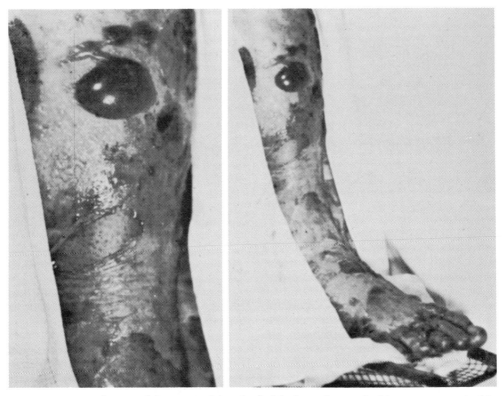

Figure 8-3. An open fracture of the proximal one-third of the lower leg resulted in gas gangrene in this patient. Note the brawny edema, the formation of bullae of the lower leg, and the ischemic wet gangrene developing in the toes. Above-the-knee amputation was the reoperative procedure necessary for the control of this infection, in addition to intensive antibiotic therapy with aureomycin and penicillin. (From Altemeier, W. A., and Wulsin, J. H.: Reoperative Surgery. New York, The Blakiston Division, McGraw-Hill Book Company, 1964.)

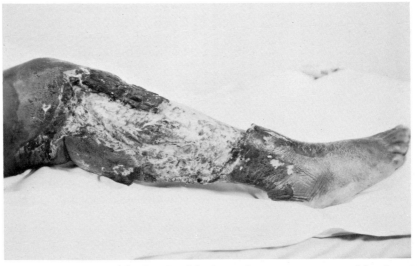

Figure 8-4. Hemolytic streptococcal infection of the leg with extensive necrosis of the skin and subcutaneou tissues associated with thrombosis of the superficial vessels.

Actinomyces, Blastomyces, Coccidioides, Candida, Aspergillus, and Entamoeba have not been included.

The three most frequently encountered bacteria responsible for postoperative wound sepsis in the series of 15,000 patients reported in the recent five-university collaborative study on the effects of ultraviolet irradiation were the *Staphylococcus aureus*, Proteus, and *Pseudomonas aeruginosa*. These three bacteria are also more or less ubiquitous in the hospital environment, are prevalent in the hospital personnel, and are inhabitants of the skin and the tracts of the hospitalized patients.

Throughout the years, however, the bacteria of most importance in wound sepsis have been the pyogenic bacteria: Staphylococcus, Streptococcus, Pneumococcus, Gonococcus, and Meningococcus. This term has also been applied to *E. coli, Pseudomonas aeruginosa*, and other gram-negative bacteria. The tubercule bacillus, although not considered a pyogenic bacterium, may produce typical thick, creamy pus in "cold" abscesses. Descriptions of representative types of some of the more important wound infections follow.

STAPHYLOCOCCAL WOUND SEPSIS

There is a tendency for staphylococcal infections to become localized with an initial area of cellulitis followed by central necrosis and abscess formation in the wound. The pus thus formed is thick, creamy, odorless, and usually yellow in color. Lymphadenitis or thrombophlebitis may complicate such lesions, making them systemically invasive. Thus they may act as distributing foci, invade the regional lymphatics and the bloodstream, and produce a bacteremia or septicemia.

The organism responsible in the majority of instances is the *Staphylococcus aureus*, which is hemolytic, coagulates human plasma, liquefies fibrin and gelatin, and produces yellow pigment in cultures. In closed wounds the symptoms and signs of staphylococcal infection consist of swelling, redness about the margins, and increasing local pain, which is throbbing in character and frequently synchronized with the pulse beat. Elevations of the temperature and leukocyte count are usually present. In the presence of bacteremia, the elevations of the temperature, pulse, and leukocyte count are greater as a rule.

In open wounds a purulent discharge is the principal sign of infection. Associated pain, redness, and swelling of the involved tissues vary with the severity of the process. There may be a disproportion between elevation of the temperature and pulse rates in infection of soft tissues as contrasted with those of the peritoneal or thoracic cavities. When the infection is regionally or systemically invasive, malaise, higher fever, lymphangitis, lymphadenitis, chills, and sweats usually develop.

The successful management of staphylococcal wound sepsis is dependent upon early diagnosis, antibiotic therapy, and surgical drainage of the infected wound. Other useful methods of treatment include application of the established principles of rest, heat, elevation, and general support. Each patient should be considered individually and treated according to his type of infection, his associated diseases, and his individual characteristics. In the presence of acute spreading infections with septicemia, surgical drainage of the area of infection should be temporarily delayed until appropriate antibiotic therapy has been established. Infected sutured wounds should first be reopened with the hemostat at the point of maximum pain, swelling, or fluctuation. The opening is then enlarged to the size of the cavity, irrigated gently with saline solution, and packed open, loosely, with fine mesh gauze. If pus and necrotic material are present, their removal by adequate drainage is important.

The antibiotics recommended for treatment of staphylococcal wound sepsis depend upon the antibiotic sensitivity of the infecting bacteria and any hypersensitivity of the patient to the antibiotics available. The following agents are generally useful and should be kept in mind: penicillin, methicillin, Prostaphlin, tetracycline, minocycline, Chloromycetin, and erythromycin. Penicillin is still the first choice unless the organism is resistant or the patient is hypersensitive. Resistance to methicillin by Staphylococci is being observed with increasing frequency in Great Britain and Sweden. It should be remembered that penicillin therapy alone in the presence of infected wounds with pus formation is inadequate. It must be supplemented by incision and drainage. It is recommended, however, that antibiotic therapy be started before surgical drainage in order that a bacteriostatic or bactericidal concentration can be produced in the blood and tissues to inhibit the growth of bacteria distributed by the operative manipulation. When the bloodstream has already been invaded, adequate penicillin therapy usually is followed by clearance of the organisms in blood cultures within 36 to 72 hours in association with a decrease in the signs of local invasiveness. The presence of devitalized tissue, prostheses, or foreign bodies usually limits the effect of the antibiotic therapy until they are removed.

STREPTOCOCCAL INFECTIONS

The majority of streptococcal infections in wounds are caused by the aerobic hemolytic Streptococcus. They tend to be invasive and to run a relatively short and rapid course. Characteristically, the local process is one of cellulitis with a large blood-filled local bleb and lymphangitis and lymphadenitis. There is little tendency to form abscesses. If local breakdown of tissue occurs, it is characterized by patchy gangrene of the overlying skin or the development of thin watery pus (See Fig. 8-4). Streptococcal invasion of the bloodstream is frequent and relatively early, particularly when operative intervention is made on a pyogenic process. Such trauma may result in the dissemination of septic thrombi into the general circulation. The systemic manifestations include chills, fever, tachycardia, sweats, prostration, and other signs of toxemia.

Variants of streptococcal wound sepsis are surgical scarlet fever and erysipelas.

The treatment of patients with streptococcal wound sepsis consists primarily of the control of bacterial invasiveness by rest, elevation, antibiotic therapy, and warm compresses and secondarily of adequate drainage for the removal of pus and necrotic tissue when they have formed. In invasive streptococcal infections, incisions or manipulations should not be made until the infection has been brought under control by antibiotic therapy, with the exception of cases of acute hemolytic streptococcal gangrene. This lesion is essentially an epifascial, spreading, subcutaneous gangrene with thrombosis of the nutrient vessels and patchy necrosis of the overlying skin. A longitudinal incision should be made as soon as possible through and beyond the gangrenous areas, contrary to the usual conservative treatment for streptococcal cellulitis.

Penicillin is still the treatment of choice for patients with streptococcal wound sepsis who are not sensitive. In addition, general supportive therapy consisting of adequate fluid and electrolytes and small daily transfusions may be of definite value. Frequent examinations are necessary to detect metastatic complications as early as possible and to treat any according to its individual location and characteristics.

PNEUMOCOCCAL WOUND SEPSIS

Pneumococcal infections of wounds are seen infrequently and usually are associated with infections of the lung and pleura, osteomyelitis, sinusitis, and meningitis. At first the pus in pneumococcal infections is usually thin. Later it rapidly becomes thick, creamy, and mucoid and exhibits clotted fibrin.

Treatment consists of antibiotic therapy, preferably with penicillin, and drainage of abscesses or infected cavities as indicated.

GRAM-NEGATIVE BACILLARY INFECTIONS

These have become more frequent and of greater importance during the past 15 years. Since the discovery and widespread use of penicillin, secondary or superimposed infections by gram-negative bacilli have tended to develop during treatment. In fact, gram-negative sepsis from a variety of sources has become a serious threat in modern surgical practice. During the past 12 years there has been a fourteenfold increase in the number of patients with gram-

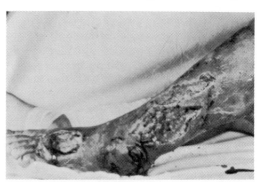

Figure 8-5. Extensive cellulitis of the foot and leg caused by a gram-negative bacillus, *Aerobacter aerogenes*, in a patient with severe diabetes. Reoperations for incision and drainage followed by skin grafting were necessary in addition to control of the diabetes and antibiotic therapy with chloramphenicol. (From Altemeier, W. A., and Wulsin, J. H.: Reoperative Surgery. New York, The Blakiston Division, McGraw-Hill Book Company, 1964.)

negative septicemia. Currently, approximately two-thirds of the cases of septicemia seen at the University of Cincinnati Medical Center are caused by gram-negative bacilli, whereas twelve years ago, two-thirds were caused by the gram-positive cocci, particularly the hemolytic *Staphylococcus aureus*. A similar shift in the incidence and importance of gram-negative infections has occurred in burn-wound sepsis.

The incidence of gram-negative sepsis has been strikingly progressive and particularly rapid. In a study of approximately 400 patients with this type of infection, the causes of this increase were not clear, but they seemed to have been related to rapid extension of new and complex surgical operations and diagnostic procedures to elderly and other poor-risk patients whose resistance was decreased by debilitating trauma, associated chronic diseases, and leukocyte suppression therapy (Fig. 8-5).

The bacterial most frequently identified in gram-negative sepsis were *E. coli*, *Aero-bacter aerogenes*, Proteus, *Pseudomonas aeruginosa*, and Serratia.

The sources of the infection leading to gram-negative sepsis included the urinary tract in over half the cases, the respiratory tract, the alimentary tract, and various iatrogenic factors.

Experience has indicated that prophylactic antibiotic therapy has not prevented gram-negative septicemia, particularly in poor-risk patients. Moreover, there has been a suggestion that intensive or prolonged antibiotic therapy may have contributed to the development and increasing incidence of this type of sepsis.

Between 1965 and 1970, a sharp increase in the number of cases of *Serratia marcescens* septicemia has been noted on the surgical services of the University of Cincinnati Medical Center. A series of 42 patients with this infection has been studied, and it is interesting to note that 80 per cent of the cases were related to antecedent or concurrent antibiotic therapy often in large

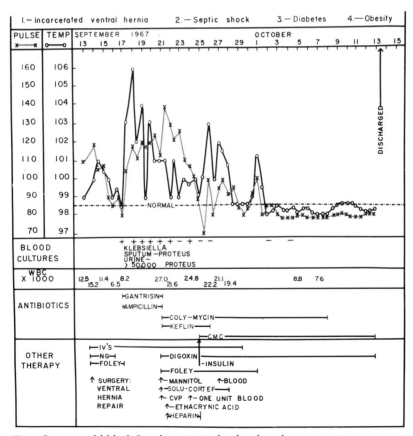

Figure 8-6. Forty-five-year-old black female patient who developed postoperative gram-negative sepsis caused by Klebsiella three days postoperatively after operative repair of a ventral hernia. Sepsis was associated with high fever, shock, and renal shutdown. Treatment with antibiotics, Solu-Cortef, mannitol, and insulin for the associated diabetes controlled the septic process and resulted in recovery.

dosage. This suggests that Serratia sepsis is an emergent secondary infection by an organism of otherwise low virulence or that the antibiotic therapy depresses the patient's resistance and permits invasive infections by such a microorganism.

The association of septic shock with gram-negative septicemia gives a poor prognosis. Treatment of such patients depends upon early diagnosis and early treatment, not only of the sepsis and its source but also of the associated shock. Prompt treatment with appropriate antibiotics administered intravenously, surgical drainage or excision of the source of infection, adequate supportive therapy, oxygen therapy, and the concurrent intelligent use of intravenously administered corticosteroids have been used by the authors (Fig. 8-6). Failure to drain obscure abscesses or similar foci contributing to the septicemia has usually resulted in death. The diagnosis of deep-seated or obscure abscesses can be made quite difficult by the masking effect of antibiotic or steroid therapy.

Microaerophilic bacterial infections

The principal microaerophilic bacteria associated with wound infections are the microaerophilic hemolytic streptococci and the non-hemolytic streptococci. The hemolytic microaerophilic streptococci characteristically produces burrowing sinus tract infections that are chronic active processes capable of penetrating any tissues in their pathway. The non-hemolytic variety may be associated with other bacteria to produce synergistic infections as the result of symbiotic metabolic activity. Peritoneal and retroperitoneal processes, putrid empyema, and chronic progressive cutaneous gangrene developing occasionally in abdominal and thoracic wounds are examples.

Surgical drainage of abscesses and excision of burrowing sinus tracts and areas of progressive cutaneous gangrene are essential methods of treatment. Antibiotic therapy, particularly with penicillin, is of adjunctive value to the surgical therapy.

Anaerobic streptococcal infections

Severe postoperative infections can be caused by the anaerobic Streptococcus with or without septicemia, particularly following operative procedures upon the genital, urinary, gastrointestinal, or respiratory tracts. The anaerobic Streptococcus is one of the important causes of septic abortions, puerperal sepsis, and tubo-ovarian abscesses. This microorganism is difficult to grow bacteriologically, and routine cultures are therefore inadequate in detecting its presence. Careful bacteriological studies, however, show that it is a frequent bacterial component of many infections seen in wounds and deep abscesses. The pus produced by the anaerobic Streptococcus characteristically has a fetid odor.

The treatment of infections produced by this organism consists of incision and drainage or excision of the area of sepsis, adjunctive antibiotic therapy usually with penicillin, and general supportive measures.

Mixed or synergistic infections

It is not generally appreciated that there is a large group of wound infections complicating surgical operations or trauma caused by a mixed bacterial flora. This group has a polymicrobic etiology consisting of a mixture of aerobic and anaerobic, gram-negative and gram-positive bacteria whose origin most often is a lesion or perforation of the gastrointestinal, respiratory, or genitourinary tracts. The aerobic and anaerobic bacteria often relate to each other in symbiosis, and their synergistic action determines the characteristic nature of these septic processes. They show the development of slough in the subcutaneous tissues, fascia, retroperitoneal tissues, and areolar tissues of the intermuscular planes (Fig. 8-7). The process spreads, producing thrombosis of the neighboring vessels, abscess formation, and extensive necrosis, particularly of the areolar tissue. Examples of such mixed infections are deep infections of the neck, postoperative peritonitis, retroperitoneal cellulitis, postoperative infection of abdominal operative wounds, and putrid empyema. Crepitation of the infected tissues may develop as a result of bacterial action of the clostridia, anaerobic streptococci, or aerobic aerogenic bacilli.

Successful treatment depends primarily upon early diagnosis and prompt and adequate surgical drainage. Roentgenograms for soft tissue detail may show the presence of progressive gaseous infiltration and aid

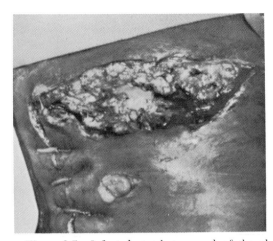

Figure 8-7. Infected gunshot wound of the abdominal and chest wall with extensive damage to soft tissues and intra-abdominal viscera previously repaired surgically. After control of the mixed infection, reoperation was successful in producing complete healing. (From Altemeier, W. A., and Wulsin, J. H.: Reoperative Surgery. New York, The Blakiston Division, McGraw-Hill Book Company, 1964.)

in the diagnosis of crepitant cellulitis or abscess. Antibiotic therapy with penicillin and an appropriate broad-spectrum antibiotic is helpful, particularly in overcoming the invasiveness of the infectious process. Septicemia by one or more bacteria may occur during the progress of this lesion. Bacterial destruction of tissue may be excessive, particularly in postoperative abdominal wounds.

The associated impairment of wound healing and intestinal ileus may lead to wound dehiscence.

GAS GANGRENE AND CLOSTRIDIAL INFECTIONS

Clostridial infections are serious complications that are most likely to occur in wounds with extensive damage to muscle masses, impairment of regional blood supply, gross contamination by dirt and other foreign bodies, and significant delay in adequate surgical treatment.

Fortunately they are relatively infrequent in modern clinical practice, but when they occur, they are usually spectacular in their development and course and serious in their threats to life and limb.

These microorganisms are anaerobic and the most important type is the *Clostridium perfringens.* It has been described as the

etiologic agent in from 56 to 100 per cent of various series of patients studied by MacLennan, Weinberg, and Seguin; Koukin; and Altemeier and Fullen. The *Clostridium perfringens* occurs either alone or in combination with other Clostridia such as *Clostridium novyi,* *Clostridium sporogenes,* *Clostridium septicum,* *Clostridium histolyticum,* and *Clostridium sordellii.* Less frequently, clostridial infections may be caused by only one of this latter group without the association of *Clostridium perfringens.*

Wounds of violence and war show a relatively high incidence of contamination by *Clostridium perfringens* and other clostridia. The incidence of gas gangrene and other severe clostridial infections in these wounds, however, is infrequent. The clostridial group of bacteria often shows a predilection for infecting muscle and areolar tissues, and the characteristics of the resulting lesion depend largely upon the type of tissue involved and the biological characteristics of the organism.

Gas gangrene is a spreading clostridial myositis which may occur as the crepitant, noncrepitant, mixed, or profoundly toxemic type. It is primarily an infection of the muscles that spreads rapidly and involves to a lesser degree the neighboring connective tissues. The accumulation of edema and gas in fascial compartments produces an expanding pressure, which aids in the lateral spread of the infection and contributes to further necrosis of the muscles. In this manner, groups of muscles, an entire limb, or the body may become successively involved.

During the early stages of the process, the muscles are hemorrhagic and friable. Later,

TABLE 8-5. Clinical Types of Clostridial Infections

I. Clostridial myositis
  A. Perfusing (true gas gangrene)
    1. Crepitant
    2. Edematous and noncrepitant
    3. Mixed
    4. Toxemic

II. Clostridial cellulitis

III. Synergistic infections
  A. Peritonitis
  B. Soft-tissue wounds

IV. Tetanus

they may become discolored and noncontractile, exuding a watery brown, foul discharge frequently containing bubbles of gas.

Occasionally, localized lesions of clostridial myositis are seen and these, too, may be crepitant or noncrepitant. This type of lesion is considerably less severe and does not show the tendency for rapid spread and the development of progressive toxemia.

The *Clostridium perfringens* is not infrequently found in cultures made of the exudate of peritonitis secondary to lesions of the gastrointestinal tract or from draining wounds of the peritoneal cavity. Under these circumstances the organism may be synergistically active as one of the group of symbiotic bacteria.

Bloodstream invasion by the Clostridia is relatively infrequent, and its occurrence is a particularly bad prognostic sign.

The most effective means of preventing gas gangrene and other clostridial infections is early and adequate surgery. Most experimental and clinical evidence indicates that antibiotic therapy alone cannot be relied upon to prevent the occurrence of clostridial infections. Prophylactic administration of gas-gangrene antitoxin has been of little or

no practical value in the prevention of gas gangrene. The evaluation of the prophylactic use of hyperbaric oxygen therapy has not been completed, and experimental studies in animals have shown equivocal results.

In the treatment of established gas gangrene, success depends upon early diagnosis and the institution of prompt emergency operative treatment with multiple incisions and fasciotomy for decompression and drainage of the fascial compartments, excision of the involved muscles, or open amputation when necessary (Fig. 8-8). Experience indicates that early and adequate surgery is the most reliable and effective primary treatment. Antibiotic therapy with penicillin in large doses intravenously and tetracycline in doses of 250 to 500 mg. intravenously every six hours or during and after operative treatment has been effective. There is evidence to indicate that the tetracyclines are the antibiotics of choice in the treatment of clostridial infections. Antibiotic therapy has been most effective as adjunctive treatment to operative procedures.

The administration of polyvalent gas-gangrene antitoxin pre- and postoperatively is also of equivocal value. Many surgeons doubt

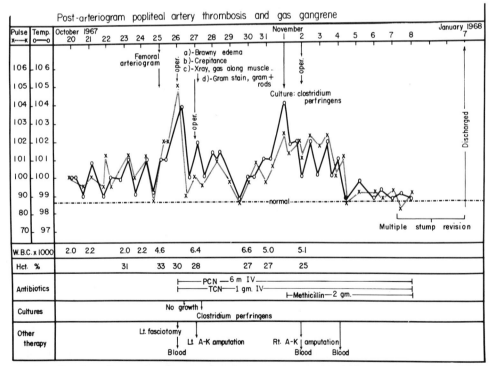

Figure 8-8. This chart depicts the course and methods of treatment of a 49-year-old white male who developed gas gangrene of the thigh following femoral arteriograms. Thrombosis of left popliteal artery and clostridial myositis developed within 24 hours, requiring open amputation above the knee. Five days later, a similar infection developed spontaneously in the right leg, requiring above-the-knee amputation. The patient was a diabetic.

the efficacy of gas-gangrene antitoxin; others use it in an effort to prevent death from toxemia allowing additional time for surgery and antibiotic therapy to bring the infection under control. Other supportive treatment consisting of the administration of blood plasma, electrolytes, and steroids in some cases with overwhelming toxemia and septic shock may become very important.

Since the introduction of hyperbaric oxygen in the treatment of gas gangrene and other clostridial infections by Brummelkamp and Boerema in 1961, numerous favorable reports have appeared indicating rapid, dramatic clinical improvement within the first day. Others have found hyperbaric therapy without surgical debridement or radical incision ineffective and have used the two modalities in conjunction. At this time, it appears that no type of chemotherapy, serotherapy, or hyperbaric oxygen therapy has replaced early and adequate surgery in the treatment of clostridial infections.

WOUND DEHISCENCE

Wound dehiscence (disruption) literally means the "splitting apart" or "bursting open" of a wound. In clinical practice, however, it may carry a number of other connotations, depending upon its completeness and location in the body. It is most frequently used in relation to abdominal wounds, but may include thoracic, various soft-tissue, and other incisions. Dehiscence is a serious and unfortunate complication and invariably leads to further morbidity and high mortality. Its occurrence is particularly significant in incisions involving the abdominal and thoracic walls. When it occurs in the postoperative period, the resulting loss of anatomic continuity, the escape of underlying tissues or organs into the wound, and the development of any pathophysiologic effects require urgent attention. Any wound, surgical or accidental, is susceptible to this potentially grave complication. Basically it represents failure of wound healing from some cause. It may thus include the disruption of any of its layers and become the circumstance that leads to the development of a postoperative incisional hernia, an incomplete or complete dehiscence, or only a superficial separation.

ABDOMINAL WOUND DEHISCENCE

Dehiscence of abdominal wounds may be *complete*, with separation of all layers of the abdominal wall, or *incomplete*, with separation of only some of the layers (Fig. 8-9). If complete, the dehiscence may be associated with extrusion of abdominal viscera and additional bacterial contamination, which may lead to further wound sepsis and secondary peritonitis. If incomplete, with separation of the fascial and muscular layers, a postoperative incisional hernia or obstruction of a herniated loop of intestine may occur. (See Fig. 8-9.)

The incidence of abdominal wound dehiscence is reported to vary from 0.5 to 3.0 per cent with an average of 2.5 per cent. Death may follow wound disruption in approximately 15 per cent of cases, particularly in patients debilitated by carcinoma and other chronic diseases. The incidence is related to age and is probably four to five times higher in the older age groups (over 50 years of age) than in the younger. Disruption may occur as late as a month postoperatively, but it is commonest between the fourth and twelfth days. The earliest sign is often the presence of serosanguineous drainage from the wound between sutures. The patient may volunteer the information that "something gave way inside" and may actually have heard or felt the tearing separation of the fascial layers.

Occasionally the skin closure will remain intact, and loops of bowel or omentum can be palpated herniating through the fascial defect. Intestinal obstruction may occur from incarceration of a bowel segment into the separation. This may be the only recognizable sign of wound disruption if the associated serosanguineous wound drainage has been absent or overlooked. Any mechanical postoperative bowel obstruction, with or without severe localized pain in the incision, should suggest the possibility of wound dehiscence and incarceration of the bowel.

The major cause of abdominal wound disruption is probably poor surgical technique in wound closure, but many other factors come into play and may be involved. These can be considered under two general categories—local factors and systemic factors.

A. *Local Wound Factors*

1. Poor surgical technique, with ex-

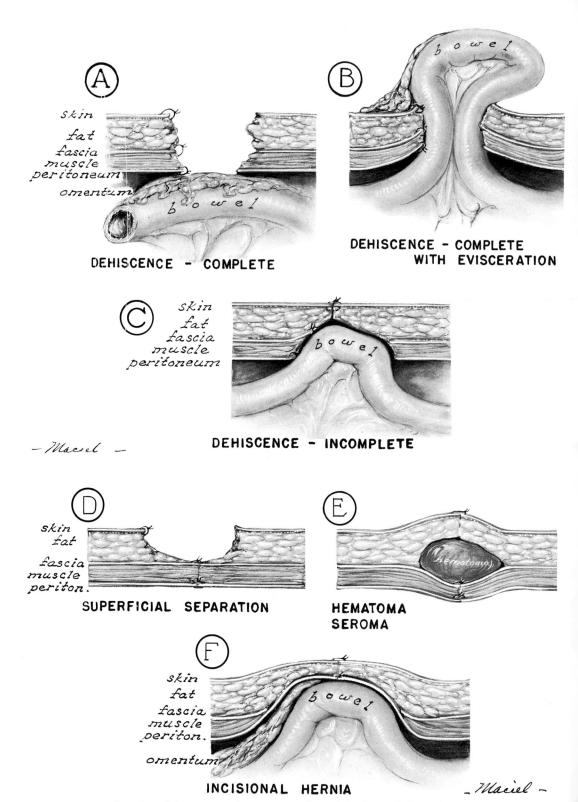

Figure 8-9. *A,* Complete dehiscence with tenuous sealing of the base of the abdominal wound by adherent omentum. *B,* The same wound with evisceration of the intra-abdominal contents predisposing to shock and infection. *C,* Incomplete dehiscence with displaced bowel in the subcutaneous tissues. Note the absence of a peritoneal sac. Removal of skin sutures would result in evisceration. *D,* Wound separation may be of varying depths without separation of fascia or peritoneum. It usually heals by secondary intention with fibrous union. *E,* Large hematoma or seroma predisposes to wound infection, superficial separation, or incisional hernia, unless removed by aspiration or evacuation. *F,* Incisional hernia with intact peritoneal layer protruding through separation of the muscular and fascial layers. This complication usually is not recognized in the immediate postoperative period. (From Altemeier, W. A., and Wulsin, J. H.: Reoperative Surgery. New York, The Blakiston Division, McGraw-Hill Book Company, 1964.)

cessive operative trauma to the tissues or improper closure.

2. Hemorrhage and hematoma formation.
3. Infection.
4. Sensitivity or idiosyncrasy to absorbable suture material.
5. Selection of the incision (vertical incisions are more likely to disrupt than are transverse incisions).
6. Weakening of the closure of the operative wound by bringing out drains, tubes, or intestinal stomas through it.
7. Failure to use available abdominal supporting dressings or abdominal binders postoperatively.

B. *Systemic or General Factors*
1. Preoperative and postoperative malnutrition.
2. Hypoproteinemia.
3. Chronic anemia.
4. Vitamin C deficiency.
5. Repeated coughing from pulmonary disease, hiccoughing, sneezing, or excessive movement.
6. Marked and unrelieved distention.
7. Abdominal ascites and other excessive accumulations of peritoneal fluid.
8. Debilitating diseases.
9. Prolonged adrenal steroid therapy.
10. Advanced age.

A knowledge of these factors is significant *only* if kept in mind by the surgeon and *used* for their recognition, prevention, or control during the preoperative, operative, or postoperative periods.

The failure to provide accurate closure of wound layers using good surgical technique, minimizing contamination, avoiding tension and other factors leading to tissue ischemia and necrosis is an important factor in wound separation. Sutures tied too tightly may cut through and thereby initiate the fascial defect or increase the defect around drains. Tubes, drains, or gastrointestinal stomas should be brought out through separate stab wounds when possible.

Careless hemostasis, the presence of dense scar tissue, or the persistence of residual dead spaces may lead to expanding hematomas, seromas, or infections. These, in turn, can produce separation of the tissue layers and seriously impair the process of wound healing, particularly large hematomas or

seromas. Usually, however, small hematomas are resorbed spontaneously.

In the case of wound sepsis, as has been discussed earlier, serious alterations in healing of the tissues and further necrosis of the tissues may occur and lead to wound disruption. The importance of minimizing wound contamination and avoiding infection is obvious.

The selection of the proper suture material for wound closure must include a consideration of the patient's hypersensitivities and idiosyncrasies. Any history of previous postoperative wound disruption following other operations should be obtained and kept in mind, for there is often a tendency for repetition.

Although dehiscence and evisceration may occur through any type of incision, they are less frequent in oblique or transverse incisions. Upper abdominal incisions are more likely to disrupt than lower abdominal ones, and long incisions are more prone to separation than are short ones.

Occlusive and supportive dressings are recommended not only for their supportive effect in minimizing disruption but also for protection against additional bacterial contamination and infection in the event of dehiscence and evisceration.

As indicated in the preceding listing, there are many more general or systemic factors than local factors that predispose to or excite the development of wound disruption. The presence of malnutrition preoperatively and postoperatively, with loss of weight, contracted blood volume, hypoproteinemia, vitamin-C deficiency, or chronic anemia, is a recognized complex factor of importance. Carcinoma of the stomach with pyloric obstruction is a lesion not infrequently associated with such states of malnutrition. In addition to carcinoma there are various other debilitating diseases that may be associated with impaired wound healing and lead to wound dehiscence such as adrenal insufficiency, collagen diseases, cirrhosis, malabsorption syndromes, advanced renal disease and uremia, and ulcerative colitis.

The presence of persistent postoperative ileus and abdominal distention is a threatening situation of considerable importance. Sudden, severe vomiting or retching may occur during recovery from anesthesia or later in the postoperative state, with resultant shearing or breaking of sutures in the fascia. Likewise, protracted hiccoughing, due to any one of many possible causes, may produce severe strain on the sutured wound. Sudden sneezing or repeated coughing from pulmonary disease are similarly important factors. Uncontrolled violent muscular activity can be seen in various psychiatric or neurologic patients in whom wound disruption occurs. Patients with convulsive seizures related to such diseases as tetanus are also very prone to wound disruptions. In fact, any uncooperative patient who voluntarily places undue stress on the incision by too early, sudden, or excessive physical activity should be watched carefully for this complication.

Large accumulations of fluid in the peritoneal cavity postoperatively may lead to unusual stress on the wound as well as a state of hypoproteinemia. In addition to ascites secondary to cirrhosis, other conditions, such as chylous ascites, may be contributory.

Treatment

The treatment of abdominal wound disruption depends upon whether the separation is minor or major. If only minimal disruption occurs, with separation of only the superficial layers and not the fascial layers, the treatment need consist of either the application of a dry sterile occlusive dressing with an abdominal binder or secondary suture. Caution is always indicated and, if there is doubt as to the extent of separation of the fascial layers, the wound should be examined under strict sterile procedures in the operating room. There the wound can be reopened and re-examined under anesthesia if indicated. As a general rule the extent of disruption of the deeper wound layers is usually greater than is grossly evident.

If major disruption occurs, the patient's condition will usually become critical as a result of this complication, if it was not previously. In the event of any sudden staining of the dressing with a profuse pink serous drainage, it is mandatory to remove all dressings under sterile conditions and examine the incision. A sterile dressing is applied until the patient can be moved into the operating room. In case of doubt, it may be necessary to remove skin sutures to inspect the deeper layers.

Even in poor-risk patients the authors prefer to correct any evisceration and close the wound with 22-gauge stainless steel malleable wire sutures through all layers. This can be accomplished under local anesthesia if the administration of a general anesthetic is contraindicated or too hazardous for the patient (Fig. 8-10). These wires should be placed approximately 3 to 4 cm. apart and back from the wound edges, as originally described by Reid, Merrel, and Zinninger. After careful placement of these sutures through all layers, including the perineum, the incision is closed by drawing together and twisting the wires at the proper tension. This method of closure is simple and rapid, providing security and a lower incidence of complicating wound infection. The fluids accumulating in the wound can easily escape into the dressings between the sutures with this type of closure. The use of drains in wounds closed by this method is discouraged. When drains are necessary, it is recommended that they be brought out through separate stab wounds.

If the tissue layers are not too friable, additional 00 chromic catgut interrupted sutures may be used to close the peritoneum and the fascia. Care must be taken to place the stay sutures properly and tight enough to prevent herniation of loops of intestine between them and not too tight, so as to avoid excessive tension and ischemia (Fig. 8-11).

This type of closure has been in routine use for such cases at the Cincinnati General Hospital for 35 years. Complications have been related to excessive tightening of the wires and placement of the stay sutures too close together or too far apart. Once properly applied, these through-and-through wire sutures give comforting assurance to the surgeon and the patient that the abdominal wound will not dehisce again.

If the patient does not have an indwelling nasogastric tube with suction, this should be instituted promptly to minimize the danger of vomiting with aspiration pneumonia and to decompress the gastroenteric tract and facilitate the secondary wound closure. These wire sutures are left in place for 21 to 23 days.

Antibiotic therapy is recommended before, during, and after the reoperative closure, using the appropriate antibiotic as indicated by Gram stain, culture, and sensitivity testing. Proper abdominal support with an

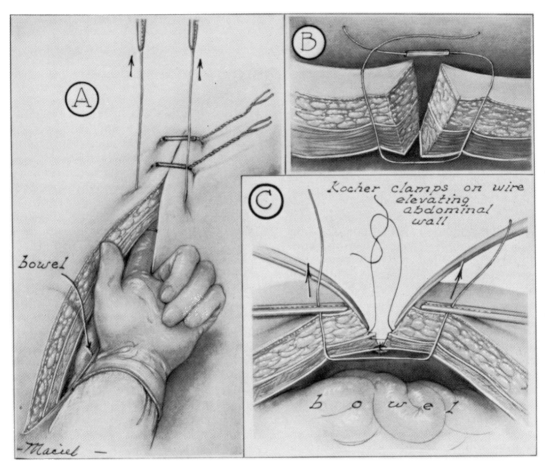

Figure 8-10. Through-and-through wire closure of the abdominal wall. *A*, *B*, Simple fast closure used for eviscerated or badly contaminated abdominal wounds. The wires are laid with a large hand needle and must be properly spaced. *C*, A layer closure can be added, if the condition of the patient and of the wound permits. Heavy clamps temporarily applied to the wires at the point of proper tension allow closure of the peritoneal and fascial layers before the wires are twisted. (From Altemeier, W. A., and Wulsin, J. H.: Reoperative Surgery. New York, The Blakiston Division, McGraw-Hill Book Company, 1964.)

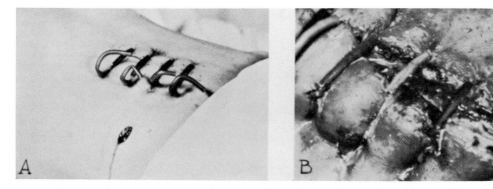

Figure 8-11. *A,* Correct and effective through-and-through wire closure of contaminated wound of the abdomen with stab-wound drainage of the retroperitoneal space. *B,* Incorrect wire closure, with ischemia, block necrosis, infection, and lack of healing. (From Altemeier, W. A., and Wulsin, J. H.: Reoperative Surgery. New York, The Blakiston Division, McGraw-Hill Book Company, 1964.)

occlusive protective dressing and an abdominal binder may be useful.

THORACIC WOUND DEHISCENCE

Disruption of the chest-wall closure during the post-thoracotomy period is an unusual, serious, and potentially lethal complication. It must be promptly recognized and treated, or it will be associated with a high mortality.

Fortunately this complication is of infrequent occurrence. Many of the factors that contribute to poor wound healing which were mentioned previously in the section on abdominal wound disruption may be contributory here also. In our experience, however, the single most important factor seems to be, again, poor surgical technique.

Thoracic-wound disruption usually occurs as a separation of the rib-cage closure, and the superficial soft-tissue layers may or may not remain intact. If separation of the rib-cage closure develops in the post-thoracotomy period, instability of the thoracic wall and herniation of the pleural space into the submuscular or subcutaneous areas within the chest wall occur. This results in a pathologic situation which may be similar to that associated with a flail chest, with paradoxic respirations and mediastinal flutter. This places an additional burden on the cardiopulmonary function of such patients, many of whom already have a limited reserve in the postoperative period. Effective ventilation is decreased, resulting in hypoxia and hypercarbia. The return venous flow to the heart may be impaired and the cough mechanism becomes inefficient. The sealing

of any raw lung surface to the parietal pleura is prevented by the to-and-fro movement of air and lung tissue with each respiration, and a prolonged air leak with tension pneumothorax may occur. In the same way, a progressive subcutaneous emphysema may be caused.

When chest-wall dehiscence includes the skin closure, there are additional dangers from the resulting sucking wound of the chest and infection.

For the successful treatment of postoperative chest-wall disruption, prompt recognition is particularly essential. The subtle nature of the early clinical signs of this complication may lead to a prolonged delay in diagnosis, and the accompanying altered physiological effects that may be present before its occurrence is recognized can be severe. The most important factors responsible for the delay in diagnosis are:

1. Failure on the part of the clinician to think of the possibility of this complication early in its development.

2. The tendency for the soft tissues to remain intact in the presence of disruption of the deeper layers of the thoracic wall.

3. The presence of a bulky dressing that obscures the wound and interferes with a close inspection of the wound and the recognition of the paradoxical motion of the chest wall early in its development.

The most important early clinical findings are instability of the chest wall, paradoxic motion and herniation of lung tissue into the thoracotomy wound space, dyspnea, cyanosis, ineffective coughing, subcutaneous emphysema, and pneumothorax. Radiographic findings may give an early clue to the presence of disruption of the chest wall. These include increasing subcutaneous emphysema, the presence of an air-fluid level in the soft tissues of the chest wall, and an expansion of the distance between the adjacent ribs of the thoracotomy wound.

The key to the *prevention* of a chest wall-dehiscence is the careful, secure, initial closure of a thoracotomy incision.

In this regard it is of interest to note that in the authors' experience, thoracotomy-wound dehiscence occurred only among the cases in which periosteal closure had been done with catgut rather than nonabsorbable sutures. Stabilization of the chest wall as part of the surgical procedure is an important aspect of the operation.

When disruption of the thoracotomy wound occurs, early diagnosis and immediate secondary closure are necessary. Restoration of the cardiorespiratory dynamics can thus be accomplished. The technique of secondary closure of this type of wound depends upon its nature and the condition of the tissues remaining. Our preferred method is the use of welded, 22-gauge stainless steel malleable wires passed through holes drilled in the adjacent ribs. This method is somewhat similar to that used in the closure of abdominal-wound dehiscence. In addition, absorbable sutures are recommended for closure of the intercostal muscles and the fascial layers. Appropriate antibiotic therapy is also recommended, depending upon the local and general circumstances.

Disruption of the median sternotomy wound presents similar problems and is treated similarly.

SOFT-TISSUE WOUND DISRUPTION

Disruption may also occur in various other types of wounds if the principles of wound care are violated and the normal process of wound healing is impaired.

The disruption or separation of a soft-tissue wound may occur as the result of a variety of factors. Frequently it will follow the removal of skin sutures too early and before adequate healing has occurred. This is particularly true for wounds in which healing is characteristically slower, such as those of the skin of the back or lower extremities. It may also occur in wounds over joints if motion is permitted too soon. Trauma, pressure, impaired blood supply, and sudden motions may precipitate the separation of the wound edges.

Treatment

When a disruption of a superficial soft-tissue wound occurs beneath an occlusive protective dressing early after primary closure, the incision can frequently be resutured successfully. Usually only skin sutures are required under these circumstances. If, however, infection is present or if gross contamination of the wound occurs, it is wisest to leave the wound open and allow it to either heal by secondary intention with granulation tissue or by delayed suture after three to ten days. Split thickness skin grafts or other plastic procedures may be necessary to correct any resultant cosmetic deformities or wounds with delayed healing.

At the time of disruption, contaminated and infected soft-tissue wounds may be converted gradually into clean wounds by the thoughtful debridement of necrotic tissue, incision and drainage of abscess cavities, correction of nutritional and metabolic problems, use of appropriate antibiotic therapy, and intelligent wound care.

REFERENCES

Alexander, H. C., and Prudden, J. F.: The causes of abdominal wound disruption. Surg. Gynec. Obstet., *122*:1223, 1966.

Altemeier, W. A.: Bacterial flora of acute perforated appendicitis with peritonitis; bacteriological study based upon 100 cases. Ann. Surg., *107*:517, 1938.

Altemeier, W. A.: Bodily responses to infectious agents. JAMA, *202*:1085, 1967.

Altemeier, W. A.: The pathogenicity of the bacteria of appendicitis peritonitis. Ann. Surg., *114*:158, 1941.

Altemeier, W. A., and Culbertson, W. R.: Wound Infections. Chapter 3, Reoperative Surgery. New York, McGraw-Hill Book Company, 1964, pp. 16–28.

Altemeier, W. A., and Fullen, W. D.: Prevention and treatment of gas gangrene. JAMA. (Accepted for publication.)

Altemeier, W. A., and MacMillan, B. G.: The Dynamics of Infection in Burns. Research in Burns, Publication No. 9, Amer. Instit. Biol. Sci., 1962, pp. 203–211.

Altemeier, W. A., and Stevenson, J. M.: Physiology of Wound Healing. Chapter 2. *In* Davis, L. (ed.): Christopher's Textbook of Surgery. 7th ed. Philadelphia, W. B. Saunders Company, 1960, pp. 22–41.

Altemeier, W. A., and Wulsin, J. H.: Wound Healing, Chapter 4, Reoperative Surgery. New York, McGraw-Hill Book Company, 1964, pp. 29–39.

Altemeier, W. A., Culbertson, W. R., Fullen, W. D., and McDonough, J. J.: Serratia marcescens septicemia. A new threat in surgery. Arch. Surg., *99*:232, 1969.

Boyd, A. D., Gonzalez, L. L., and Altemeier, W. A.: Disruption of chest wall closure following thoracotomy. J. Thorac. Cardiov. Surg., *52*:47, 1966.

Brummelkamp, W. H., Kogendijk, J., and Boerema, I.: Treatment of anaerobic infections (clostridial myositis) by drenching the tissues with oxygen under high atmospheric pressure. Surgery, *49*:299–502, 1961.

Findland, M., Jones, W. F., and Barnes, J. F.: Occurrence of serious bacterial infections since introduction of antibacterial agents. JAMA, *170*:2199, 1959.

Glenn, F., and Moore, S. W.: The disruption of abdominal wounds: A report of 22 cases. Surg. Gynec. Obstet., *65*:16, 1937.

Hartzell, J. B., and Winfield, J. M.: Disruption of abdominal wounds. Int. Abstr. Surg. (Supplementary to Surg. Gynec. Obstet., Abstracts), *68*:585, 1939.

Kukin, N. N.: The treatment of gunshot wounds complicated by anaerobic infection. Arch. Sci. Biol., Moscow, *62*:15, 1941.

MacLennan, J. D.: Anaerobic infections in Tripolitania and Tunisia. Lancet, *1*:203–207, 1944.

Mann, L. S., Spinazzola, A. J., Lindesmith, G. G., LeVine, M. J., and Kuczerepa, W.: Disruption of abdominal wounds. JAMA, *180*:1021, 1962.

Marsh, R. L., Coxe, J. W., III, Ross, W. L., and Stevens, G. A.: Factors involving wound dehiscence: Study of 1,000 cases. JAMA, *155*:1197, 1954.

Meleney, F. L.: The study of the prevention of infection in contaminated accidental wounds, compound fractures, and burns. Ann. Surg., *118*:171, 1943.

Reid, M. R.: Infections in surgery. Int. Abstr. Surg. (Supplementary to Surg. Gynec. Obstet., Abstracts), *69*:107, 1939.

Reid, M. R., Zinninger, M. M., and Merrell, P.: Closure of the abdomen with through-and-through silver wire sutures in cases of acute abdominal emergencies. Ann. Surg., *98*:890–896, 1933.

Thompson, W. D., Ravdin, I. S., and Frank, I. L.: Effect of hypoproteinemia on wound disruption. Arch. Surg., *36*:500, 1938.

Warren, R.: Hernia and the Abdominal Wall. Chapter 27, Surgery. Philadelphia, W. B. Saunders Company, 1963, pp. 879–900.

Weinberg, M., and Seguin, P.: La Gangrene Gazeuse. Monographes de l'Institut Pasteur, Paris, Masson et Cie., 1918.

CHAPTER 9

THE MASSIVE BURN WITH SEPSIS AND CURLING'S ULCER

by JOHN A. MONCRIEF, M.D., and
BASIL A. PRUITT, Jr., LIEUTENANT COLONEL, MC

John Arthur Moncrief, son of a distinguished Army family, received his college education at the Citadel and Cornell University and his medical degree at Emory where he was elected to Alpha Omega Alpha. Following residency training at Barnes Hospital in St. Louis under Carl Moyer, he served a conspicuously outstanding career with the U.S. Army, during which he developed an international reputation for the study and management of the burned patient. He was Commander and Director of the famed U.S. Army Surgical Research Unit from 1961 to 1968, at which time he became Professor of Surgery at the Medical College of South Carolina.

Basil A. Pruitt, Jr., received his formal education at Harvard College and Tufts University School of Medicine. Following his residency training at Boston City Hospital and Brooke Army General Hospital, he later served in Vietnam as Chief of the Trauma Study Section, U.S.A. Medical Research Team. His contributions to the improvement of burn management have been significant. He is currently Commander and Director of the U.S. Army Institute of Surgical Research, and Assistant Clinical Professor of Surgery at the University of Texas Medical School in San Antonio.

The extent and depth of burn determine the magnitude of thermal injury, and clinical experience clearly indicates that the greater the injury the more likely the occurrence of serious complications. Of these complications which so significantly affect the course of therapy and the ultimate outcome, acute ulceration of the gastrointestinal tract and sepsis are among the most significant and dramatic. This discussion is concerned with the large burn of over 40 per cent total body surface involvement with at least half of this full-thickness skin destruction (burn index 30 or greater); in patients so affected the incidence of Curling's ulcer and major sepsis is great. The complications of thermal injury and therapy for such trauma are myriad, but only these two will be considered; detailed discussion of resuscitation and rehabilitation are to be found elsewhere.

Although thermal injury may result from a variety of causes, such large burns are most frequently due to flame (ignition of clothing or bedclothes) or to an immersion scald. Though sometimes seen in the adult, extensive scalds are commonest among infants and young children as a result of careless parental action or lack of supervision of the activity of the child or his siblings. The most characteristic finding of such scald injuries is the sharp line of demarcation between burned and unburned skin and the uniform nature of the depth of tissue injury. This type of burn frequently proves to be much deeper than originally anticipated.

Extensive flame burns most commonly result from ignition of clothing, and the era of high speed vehicular transportation and serious accidents has generated great numbers of these patients. Irregular in outline, the distribution of this thermal injury may actually be spotty; full-thickness and partial-thickness destruction are characteristically mixed in the same general areas.

PRINCIPLES OF RESUSCITATION

Resuscitation of the patient with a very large burn differs from that of a patient with a smaller area of injury only in the volume of fluid replacement therapy required and the magnitude of the immediate associated problems which demand attention. The commonest of these latter is the necessity for maintenance of an adequate airway. Obviously an obstructing foreign body must be removed, but airway obstruction is more often due to accumulation of the patient's own secretions, which he is unable to clear from the tracheobronchial tree adequately by spontaneous coughing. The early effects of inhalational injury and its therapy and the requirements for tracheostomy, assisted or controlled ventilation, and upper airway toilet have been well described in other publications to which the reader is referred (Pruitt et al., 1970).

Fluid resuscitation therapy in patients with extensive burns must be initiated as soon as possible. Although much has been written favoring one type of fluid regimen or one rate of fluid administration, evidence shows that the important factors are not so much constituent quality, but rather the rate of fluid administration and the constant monitoring of the patient's response to this therapy. Data generated at the U.S. Army Institute of Surgical Research (Pruitt, Mason, and Moncrief, in press) would indicate that in the first 24 hours postburn a rapid administration of fluids (either Ringer's lactate, saline, plasma, or plasminate) exceeding 4.5 ml. per kg. per hour is necessary in order to effect any increase in plasma volume or rapid improvement in cardiac output. When there is an extensive burn and particularly when such injury occurs in the very young or the very old, rapid administration of large volumes of fluid must be accomplished with caution and with close monitoring of the response of the patient's cardiopulmonary circuit. Frequent auscultation of the chest, monitoring of the central venous pressure, close attention to rate of urinary output, and x-ray examination of the chest are of great value under these circumstances.

The administration of fluids at a rapid rate and in a large volume is predicated on clinical measurements which indicate that there is a marked increase in capillary permeability during the first 24 hours postinjury, as noted by Arturson in 1961. Subsequent to that period capillary integrity returns rapidly, and continued administration of large volumes of fluid is required beyond the first 24 hours only in unusual circumstances. Near the end of the first week, or sometimes sooner, rapid mobilization of the obligatory edema occurs and can result in a marked expansion of plasma volume, with precipitate pulmonary edema. This eventuality must be anticipated, diagnosed early, and treated expeditiously. The most effective therapy for such a situation is the restriction of any type of fluid intake and the immediate institution of diuresis by means of one of the potent, rapidly acting diuretic agents presently available (furosemide or ethacrynic acid).

It is worthwhile noting that during this period of fluid mobilization, there may be a precipitous drop in hematocrit. This is a reflection not only of hemodilution but also of the initial red blood cell hemolysis, which is proportional to the extent and depth of thermal injury. The presence of large amounts of pigment in the excreted urine in the earliest postburn period is a good clinical indication of a deep burn. Such protein and pigment loads can result in cast formation and obstruction of the renal tubule, with subsequent acute tubular necrosis. Preventive therapy should be directed toward clearing this pigment from the urine, and this can best be accomplished by fluid load so that the rate of urinary output can still be utilized as a means of measuring the response to fluid therapy. If, however, such a fluid load does not result in gross clearing of the urine, one should resort to some type of diuretic agent to produce a mechanical flushing of the renal tubules. Should the use of a diuretic be necessary, it is important to remember that urine will no longer be an accurate guide to adequacy of resuscitation since urine will be produced at the expense of blood volume.

CARE OF THE BURN WOUND

Initial care of the burn wound consists of thorough cleansing with soap and water and debridement of any loose devitalized tissue which can be easily removed. The entire burn wound and surrounding area should be shaved thoroughly to remove hair, as this is a significant source of contamination. The eyes should be inspected carefully for any evidence of thermal damage (which, however, is unusual except in chemical or contact burns), and care should be taken throughout the postburn period to maintain rigid cleanliness in the ocular area by means of irrigation and the use of a bland ointment. Antibiotic ointments may be preferred by some although, in the absence of frank conjunctival or corneal infection, the need for such medication is uncertain.

It should be remembered that, except in a few instances, the burn wound itself does not demand immediate attention in the early postburn period but becomes secondary to the efforts at resuscitation. The circumstances under which the burn wound per se demands early, if not immediate, attention are in the case of white phosphorus and other chemical burns or those in which the effects of a tight, constricting eschar jeopardize the unburned tissue deep or distal to the eschar. Embarrassment of the circulation to unburned tissue is particularly likely to occur in flame burns as a result of the dehydrating and shrinking effect of such injury on the eschar. Should this involve the area of the chest cage (particularly in children and infants), a marked restriction of the respiratory excursion of the thoracic cage occurs, with significant and sometimes fatal interference with respiratory exchange. Should the tight eschar be circumferential about an extremity, the edema forming beneath the unyielding eschar results in occlusion of first the venous and then the arterial supply to the distal tissues, with eventual ischemic necrosis. In both instances, the situation can be readily relieved by incision through the eschar down to the superficial fascia. Cutting this insensitive eschar requires no anesthetic, and relatively little bleeding is encountered. Relief is immediate and may be life- or limb-saving.

In recent years the advent of effective topical antibacterial therapy in the treatment of thermal injury has markedly improved the outlook for the patient with a burn involving from 30 to 60 per cent of the total body surface (Table 9-1) (Moncrief, 1969; Moncrief et al., 1966; Pruitt et al., 1968). In burns exceeding 60 per cent of the body surface in adults there appears to be little improvement in mortality rates, although even these patients no longer commonly die as a direct result of burn wound sepsis. In children, however, there does appear to be a definite improvement in mortality rates even in those with up to 70 per cent of total body surface involvement. The most commonly used agents are mafenide, silver nitrate, and gentamicin. Experience with the latter is limited,

TABLE 9-1. Burn Mortality

Years	% Burn				
	0-30	30-40	40-50	50-60	60-100
1962-1963	4.3	44.4	61.1	78.3	89.1
1964-1968	1.0	10.5	22.9	34.7	77.8

but that with mafenide and silver nitrate is extensive and both agents appear to be effective. The proper use of these agents has been thoroughly detailed elsewhere, and the reader is referred to those publications (Moncrief et al., 1966; Moyer et al., 1965; Order et al., 1965; Pruitt et al., 1968). Each of the agents has a wide spectrum of activity, is applied topically to the burn wound in either an aqueous or water-miscible vehicle, and each has its own peculiar advantages and disadvantages (Table 9-2). Mafenide (Sulfamylon) is cheap, clean, easy to apply, extremely effective in controlling burn wound sepsis because of its ability to actively penetrate the burn wound, and therapy can be instituted as late as the first week postburn with the expectation of control of the bacterial population. The main disadvantage is the strong carbonic anhydrase inhibition inherent in the drug which results in a blocking of the renal buffering mechanism with subsequent excretion of large amounts of bicarbonate, impaired ammonia production, and retention of chloride. The inhibition of carbonic anhydrase also impedes carbon dioxide transport, which can result in hyperventilation with a striking lowering of serum carbon dioxide, producing a picture of respiratory alkalosis. This hyperventilation may overshadow any tendency toward metabolic acidosis until the respiratory exchange is impaired by either pneumonia or some concomitant injury. This interference with respiratory exchange then results in a rapid shift of serum pH toward acidemia in these poorly defended patients with diminished serum bicarbonate levels.

Silver nitrate applied as a 0.5 per cent concentration in a distilled water vehicle is cumbersome and ultimately expensive to use; it stains fomites, hospital, and patient black or dark brown; but it is effective in the control of the bacterial population in the burn wound. Since contact with tissue fluids results in the immediate precipitation of silver chloride (the black discoloration), the

TABLE 9-2.   Therapy with Silver Nitrate and Sulfamylon* †

	Silver Nitrate	Sulfamylon
Availability	Readily available	Readily available
Chemistry	Inorganic silver salt	Methylated sulfonamide
Method of use	0.5% solution in distilled water, use to wet dressings q 2 h. Dressings changed b.i.d. Debridement with dressing changes	10% of drug in water miscible base applied once or twice daily without dressings Wash off drug daily and debride wound
Mode of action	Probably dependent upon free silver ions	Unknown
Spectrum of activity	Entire spectrum Bacteriostatic	Entire spectrum Primarily bacteriostatic
Local and systemic effects	Poor penetration Rapidly precipitated in local tissue as AgCl Very little absorption No argyria	Penetrates tissue well in active drug form Locally nontoxic Rapidly broken down in blood to inactive form of acid salt and excreted in urine No crystalluria
Biochemical changes	Hyponatremia due to absorption of distilled water and leaching of sodium Hypochloremia due to AgCl precipitation Methemoglobin elevation Correction by oral and i.v. NaCl	Acid salt breakdown product provides heavy acid load Carbonic anhydrase inhibition with HCO_3 excretion and chloride retention Compensation by hyperventilation and CO_2 depression
Advantages	Sensitivity not present Painless in application No antagonists No resistant organisms Wide spectrum	Active penetration allows delayed therapy to be effective Wound readily visible Easy to use and clean Nontoxic Wide spectrum Not inactivated by local substances Resistance does not develop Allows full joint motion
Disadvantages	Poor penetration prevents successful control of deep tissue and delay of therapy not tolerated Biochemical changes particularly in children Pain on changing dressings Messy and requires much work to use properly Dressings impede joint mobility Discoloration obscures the wound	Biochemical changes Pain of varying intensity on application 5% sensitivity manifest by rash

*Both substances if properly used can effectively control bacterial growth and eliminate burn wound sepsis as the major cause of death.

†From Moncrief, J. A.: The status of topical antibacterial therapy in the treatment of burns. Surgery 63:862-867, 1968.

substance does not actively penetrate tissues. Silver nitrate must, therefore, be used prior to bacterial invasion of subjacent unburned tissue and is perhaps best considered a prophylactic rather than a therapeutic agent. Although application is not painful, as is the mafenide, the changing of dressings twice a day results in intermittent painful stimuli to the patient. The biochemical derangements associated with the use of silver nitrate include hyponatremia and hypochloremic alkalosis, both of which are aggravated by a propensity to water intoxication as a result of the absorption of large quantities of the distilled water vehicle. The maintenance of biochemical homeostasis by means of oral or intravenous salt supplements is difficult to achieve, particularly in the very old or the very young.

Gentamicin has been used most extensively as an ointment in a petrolatum vehicle, but like most antibacterial agents is not released in effective concentration in such a form. Utilized with a water-miscible vehicle, penetration of the burn wound is much more effective (as reflected in high blood levels), and this would appear to be the most logical manner of application. Experience with the latter preparation in patients with extensive thermal injury has not been great, and interpretation of results must await further study. Significant is the fact that reports exist detailing the onset of burn wound sepsis while the patient was being actively treated with topical gentamicin (Stone et al., 1965). Both ototoxicity and nephrotoxicity have been reported following sytemic use of large doses of this drug in infants and children for the treatment of such diseases as meningitis and peritonitis; this should be kept in mind when treating patients with large burns.

In the therapy of any thermal injury the main objective is to secure an immediate favorable response to resuscitation and then to direct efforts to the control of the bacterial flora of the burn wound while various measures are directed toward converting the open, dirty burn wound to a closed, clean one. This latter is accomplished by means of frequent surgical debridement, topical antibacterial therapy, and initial coverage with skin from the same or a different species (Shuck et al., 1969), but eventually from the patient himself. It is during this period of burn wound closure subsequent to the resuscitation period that the complications of sepsis and Curling's ulcer most frequently appear.

SEPTIC COMPLICATIONS

The septic complications to which the thermally injured patient is heir are numerous and are the major identifiable causes of death among the burn population. An understanding of the etiology of these septic processes is essential for both their possible prevention and their effective treatment once they are established.

CELLULITIS

Though rarely life-threatening and quite readily controlled, a cellulitis of the unburned skin and subcutaneous tissue at the margins of the thermally injured tissue is frequently encountered. With rare exceptions this is due to either streptococci or staphylococci and may or may not be associated with a definite lymphangitis. A febrile response may also be noted. Since a zone of erythema (a chemical cellulitis due to the local absorption of altered tissue products) may be present at the periphery of any burn, unassociated with any indications of sepsis, therapy is not undertaken until the involvement becomes of significance, i.e., the area of cellulitis extends more than 2 cm. into unburned tissue and is associated with induration and edema. Lesser degrees of marginal cellulitis associated with lymphangitis or systemic toxemia may dictate much earlier therapy, however. Since the causative organism is rarely other than streptococci or staphylococci, surface or tissue cultures are not required with this entity, and a therapeutic trial with penicillin is instituted first. If a clinical response is not obvious within 48 hours, one may safely assume that the etiologic agent is a penicillin-resistant rather than a sensitive staphylococcus or a streptococcus, and appropriate antistaphylococcal therapy with a semisynthetic penicillin is the treatment of choice. It is the unusual patient in whom such therapy fails to bring about a prompt clinical resolution of the cellulitis.

THROMBOPHLEBITIS

Septic phlebitis involving veins which have been utilized as infusion sites is being recog-

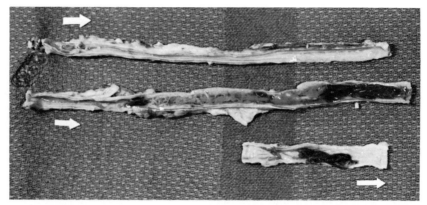

Figure 9-1. Note multiple foci of suppuration with intervening "skip areas" in this surgically excised vein with suppurative thrombophlebitis. From O'Neill, J. A., Jr., Pruitt, B. A., Jr., Foley, F. D., and Moncreif, J. A.: Suppurative thrombophlebitis — A lethal complication of intravenous therapy. J. Trauma 8:256-267, 1968.

nized with increasing frequency since the condition was first described as occurring in burn patients (O'Neill et al., 1968; Pruitt et al., in press). The presence of a constantly contaminated burn wound and the requirement for prolonged intravenous therapy predispose the burn patient to this complication. The incidence of this frequently fatal complication is directly related to the duration of therapy and the number of infusion sites. Discovery is often delayed until the second or third week postburn because of the frequent use of deep venous channels, the sometimes indolent initial septic focus (which later becomes rampantly virulent), and the failure to recognize this as a possible source of existing sepsis.

The presence of this disease is not always readily apparent and a high index of suspicion is mandatory. In any burn patient with otherwise unexplained sepsis, all previous cutdown sites should be opened, examined, and the site of cannulation inspected closely. The vein proximal to the cutdown site should be "milked" toward the site of cannulation; the extrusion of purulent material from the vein confirms a diagnosis of suppurative thrombophlebitis. Although both gram-negative and gram-positive organisms are cultured from burn patients, it is uncommon in the presence of effective topical therapy to isolate gram-positive organisms from the blood stream except in the presence of a septic phlebitis. The gram-negative organisms, on the other hand, may originate either in the burn wound or in a septic thrombus.

Systemic antibacterial therapy directed toward the control of suppurative thrombophlebitis is rarely of more than temporary benefit. The process may be controlled for a brief period of time, but eradication depends upon complete excision of the septic area. Such intravascular septic foci may be single or multiple, and skip areas of involvement of the vein are not uncommon (Fig. 9-1). Excision of any involved vein up to the point where it becomes a tributary of the next larger series of veins is the recommended treatment. If involvement is limited to superficial venous channels, surgical excision is readily accomplished and the wound is closed secondarily. If deep channels are involved, the origin is rarely discovered premortem. Should it be discovered prior to death, it would appear logical to resort to venous ligation and, if possible, thrombectomy.

PNEUMONIA

SEPTIC PNEUMONIA. With the successful control of burn wound sepsis a more frequent reality with effective topical antibacterial therapy, pulmonary sepsis manifested by pneumonia receives more attention in the clinical management of the burn patient (Pruitt et al., 1970 a and b). With diminution of burn wound sepsis as a cause of death, pneumonia has become a more common autopsy diagnosis (Foley et al., 1968), but has actually decreased in incidence in the entire burn population. With florid burn wound sepsis, hematogenous spread of the bacteria beyond the burn wound results in a miliary pneumonia (Fig. 9-2), which is characterized by subpleural septic lesions in the lung identical with the ecthyma gangrenosum seen in unburned skin. Such a hematogenous pneumonia is a portent of

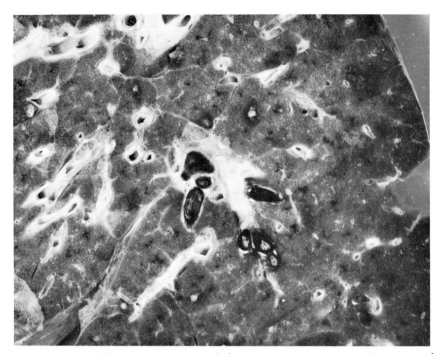

Figure 9-2. Cut section of lung from patient with hematogenous pneumonia. Note nonrandom "vascular" distribution of typical hemorrhagic lesions.

impending rapid demise, and recovery is extremely rare. Antibacterial therapy is directed at the burn wound and the control of miliary spread beyond the confines of the areas of thermal injury, but the presence of the bloodborne pneumonia indicates that such control has been unsuccessful.

BRONCHOPNEUMONIA. Another form of pneumonia encountered in the burn patient is that described as bronchopneumonia (airborne). This begins with patchy areas of infiltration noted on chest x-ray which gradually enlarge and coalesce (Fig. 9-3) and, in uncontrolled cases, is associated with a progressive impairment of pulmonary function and eventual death from a combination of sepsis and pulmonary insufficiency. A mixture of microorganisms (customarily the bacteria resident on burn wounds) may be cultured from the sputum, but ordinarily one or, occasionally, two strains predominate. To be successful, therapy must be directed at both eradication of the offending organisms and the prevention of the progressive pulmonary insufficiency. Systemic antibacterial therapy based on culture and sensitivity of the bacteria is coupled with efforts to improve ventilation. The tracheobronchial tree must be cleared of excess secretions by an effective and yet nontraumatic aspiration technique (bronchoscopy may be required). Administration of mucolytic agents and

ventilatory assistance may also be necessary. In advanced stages, use of volume cycled respirators may be necessary in order to

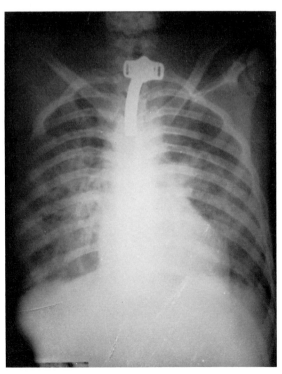

Figure 9-3. Chest x-ray of patient with airborne pneumonia showing the widespread patchy infiltration, with coalescence of pneumonic lesions noted in right lower lobe.

provide even minimal respiratory exchange. In the absence of inhalation injury such pulmonary complications rarely occur as an isolated happening in the course of the early postburn period; rather they are associated with deterioration of the burn wound and other body systems. Over-all therapy of the entire postburn syndrome must be accomplished in order to assure an optimum chance for recovery.

WOUND SEPSIS

PATHOPHYSIOLOGY. Teplitz's description of the pathophysiology of burn wound sepsis clearly identified the major cause of death in large burns and led to the more effective control of this fatal complication (Teplitz et al., 1964 a and b). Defined as the active proliferation of bacteria within the burn wound and active invasion of the subjacent unburned tissue in numbers exceeding 100,000 microorganisms per gram of tissue, this entity has satisfactorily accounted for the great majority of fatal septic complications subsequent to thermal injury. Of significance is the fact that, in many cases of fatal burn wound sepsis, the microorganisms are confined entirely to the burn wound or the immediately adjacent unburned tissue, and metastatic spread to other viscera has not occurred at the time of death. Thus, blood cultures may frequently be negative; autopsy examination to delineate the cause of death is incomplete unless the

burn wound itself is thoroughly examined both histologically and bacteriologically (Fig. 9-4).

A myriad of organisms may be cultured from the untreated burn wound, but those predominating during the different stages of development are readily identified. During the first three days staphylococci colonize the surface and the hair follicles of the burn wound; only later are they joined by the gram-negative bacteria. By five to seven days postburn the gram-negative organisms have become predominant and subsequent to this time may begin active invasion throughout the deeper layers of the burn tissue and into the subjacent unburned tissue, primarily by way of the lymphatics. Burn wound sepsis thus is a mixed infection in which the gram-negative organisms eventually predominate (Moncrief and Teplitz, 1964). Prior to the advent of effective topical therapy, *Pseudomonas aeruginosa* was the primary offending organism in burn wound sepsis, but with effective topical control other microorganisms, particularly the *Aerobacter-Klebsiella* group, are becoming more prominent and, indeed, in some centers the predominant organisms involved in burn wound sepsis.

SIGNS AND SYMPTOMS. Clinically such a patient may be noted to have a fever which is higher than usual or, in the severer and later stages of the complication, he may actually be hypothermic. Progressive changes in the sensorium beginning first with disorienta-

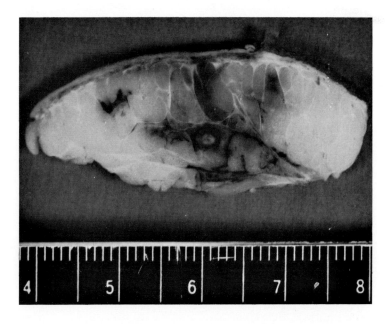

Figure 9-4. Section of burn wound above and underlying connective tissue showing bacterial invasion from the burn wound characterized by necrosis and hemorrhagic discoloration of the subcutaneous fat and connective tissue. Such extension of infection will only be apparent if this "third" dimension is examined.

tion and progressing to profound coma in the late stages are frequent. This is a less prominent symptom with gram-negative than with gram-positive infections. Varying degrees of intestinal ileus may be associated with the sepsis. One of the most reliable, but unfortunately most irreversible, signs is the appearance of deterioration of the burn wound itself with the onset of sepsis. If the onset is late in the postburn period when a clean, granulating wound has already formed, this previously healthy, firm, red tissue gradually becomes waxy, translucent, adopts a more orange-yellow color and begins to melt away. Soon the surface presents numerous small, black, punctate areas which gradually grow and coalesce until the entire surface is covered with what appears to be a new eschar (Fig. 9-5). Death occurs after a short interval of two to three days. Burn wound sepsis, however, frequently occurs prior to the separation of the eschar and long before a protective granulation tissue barrier has formed. Under such circumstances the intact eschar may very effectively hide the septic process advancing beneath it. An indication that such is occurring is the appearance of a dark red to purple margin on the burn wound which frequently is elevated above the surrounding tissue and, with the passage of time, may become frankly hemorrhagic. Tissue cultures of such border areas reveal overwhelming numbers of microorganisms and *Pseudomonas vasculitis* is frequently present.

THERAPY. The only really effective therapy for burn wound sepsis is its prevention, which has been detailed elsewhere and is covered briefly above. Therapy of established burn wound sepsis is usually a hopeless task. However, some effort must be made and, on rare occasions, will be met with success. The entire therapeutic effort is directed toward converting the open, dirty, septic burn into a closed, clean one by removal of the devitalized tissue and by grafting. This cannot be accomplished as a simple surgical exercise, however, and great risk is involved in any manipulation of the infected wound.

Although the immediate threat of spreading sepsis forces the issue, steps can be taken to bring about more effective local bacterial control. Use of the more actively penetrating topical agents (mafenide, gentamicin) should be instituted if not already begun, and installation of antibiotics directly beneath the eschar accomplished (Baxter et al., in press). The choice of drug depends upon the sensitivity of the organisms involved as determined by appropriate cultures and histologic examinations. A subeschar area of 7.5 cm. in diameter is infiltrated by 25 cc. of solution by means of clysis. The maximum tolerated daily dose of each antibiotic is administered beneath the entire area of invaded eschar in this fashion for those patients in whom the burn wound flora has escaped from topical control. These maneuvers are directed at securing local

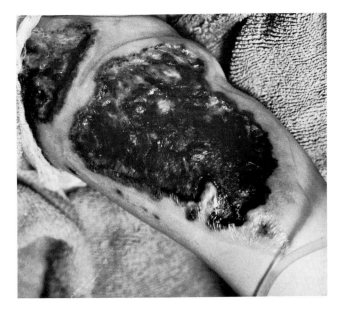

Figure 9-5. Burn wound sepsis of thigh with onset late in the postburn course. Note degeneration of the previously granulating wound bed and the raised hemorrhagic margin of unburned skin.

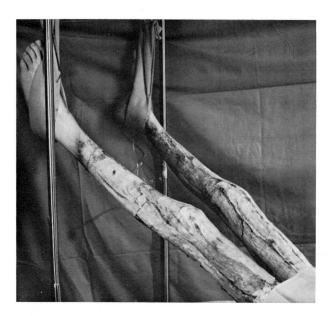

Figure 9-6. Coverage of burn wounds of both lower extremities following eschar removal with use of viable cutaneous homografts as temporary physiologic dressings.

control of the burn wound flora to a degree that will permit removal of the necrotic tissue with minimal risk of widespread dissemination of sepsis. Unless effective control is obtained, manipulation of the local wound results in a florid and rapid spread of the offending bacteria beyond the burn wound. Furthermore, surgical excision without prior bacterial control results only in rapid extensive invasion of the freshly exposed wound surface, with subsequent local tissue necrosis.

Systemic antibacterial therapy directed toward the predominant organism as identified by culture of appropriate wound biopsy tissue is worthwhile as a means of controlling distant spread of the septic process. This is effective at best for only a few days and, unless the septic feeding focus (i.e., the infected burn wound) can be eradicated, is doomed to ultimate failure.

Debridement of the burn wound must be accomplished with all haste; if intact eschar is present it should be removed as soon as possible. Many physicians are hesitant to attempt such a procedure because of the precarious condition of the patient but nonetheless, with full realization of the risk, it must be done if any type of favorable outcome is to be achieved. Blunt dissection is preferred, and extensive sharp scalpel excision should not be attempted under these circumstances since tissue planes are not readily identified at this postburn period and such procedures merely open up new chan-

nels for bacterial invasion. The more superficial layers of eschar and subcutaneous tissue are readily removed in the operating room and as much as possible of the underlying debris is cleared away. Topical antibacterial suppressive therapy should be continued throughout this period with daily progressive debridement of the burn wound. As soon as a viable tissue bed appears (granulation tissue per se is not necessary) some type of skin coverage should be attempted. Since the wounds are not usually ready for autografting, coverage of the wound at this stage is best accomplished by the use of a heterograft or a homograft (Fig. 9-6) (Shuck et al., 1969). Such physiologic dressings are initially changed with a frequency dictated by the rapidity of subgraft suppuration and lack of adherence to the wound. Serial applications of these biologic dressings should be made at least every five days until a firm, uniform take of the grafted tissue is realized. At that time autografting can be undertaken. Throughout the entire postburn period, but particularly during periods of systemic sepsis, intensive and broad general supportive care must be provided to the burn patient.

CURLING'S ULCER

As noted earlier, patients with large burns are particularly susceptible to the development of Curling's ulcer. This insidious, frequently life-threatening complication can occur suddenly and unexpectedly in any burn patient, even those with small burns who appear to be pursuing an uneventful course of recovery. The diagnosis of Curling's ulcer can be made at autopsy in up to 25 per cent of all burn patients who expire (Moncrief and Teplitz, 1964). In the past 15 years this diagnosis has been made in 281 of 2463 burned patients treated at the U.S. Army Institute of Surgical Research (formerly Surgical Research Unit), an incidence of 11.4 per cent.

INCIDENCE

Acute ulcerations of the stomach and duodenum have been encountered in burn patients from eight months to 82 years of age. In our series the males far outnumber females, a ratio that would be anticipated in our largely military patient population, but no sex predilection of this complication is evident. This form of stress ulcer may occur at any time from the first postburn day onward. Over half the patients with Curling's ulcer we previously reported had the onset of their disease within the first eight days postburn (O'Neill et al., 1967). In the past two years, however, the mean time of onset in 56 patients with Curling's ulcer has been delayed to the 14th postburn day.

ETIOLOGIC FACTORS

More than a score of causes of Curling's ulcer have been advanced, and each has been found lacking as being totally satisfactory for all cases. Only those which appear to be likely in light of present day surgical opinion will be considered here (Table 9-3). Absolute hyperacidity, the hallmark of chronic ulcerative disease, does not appear to be significant in Curling's ulcer disease.

TABLE 9-3.   Possible Etiologic Factors of Curling's Ulcer

1. Infection
2. Hyperacidity (? relative)
3. Elevated steroid levels
4. Decreased gastroduodenal blood flow
   A. Hemoconcentration
   B. Elevated catecholamines
   C. Hypovolemia
   D. Intravascular coagulation
5. Lytic effect of regurgitated chyme
6. Quantitative or qualitative change in mucus

O'Neill et al. (1967) studied the gastric secretion in 34 burn patients by means of overnight gastric analysis and could detect no absolute hyperacidity in the 20 patients who subsequently developed Curling's ulcerations. The frequent presence of microorganisms in the ulcer bed also mitigates against hyperacidity. It should be mentioned that comparison of the two study groups, that is, those with and those without later ulcer development, revealed a relative hyperacidity in the ulcer group. The only patients in the ulcer group with hyperacidity or even high normal levels, however, were those patients with pneumonia or other chest disease and hypercarbia. Although increased gastric acid secretion has been attributed to hypoxia and hypercarbia, a recent study by Passi and Vasko (1969) showed no such effect on basal acid secretion from innervated gastric pouches in dogs.

Decreased organ blood flow, an eventuality associated in the earliest postburn period with hypovolemia and increased peripheral resistance, may perhaps best be considered as a predisposing factor rather than a cause. This relative ischemia may damage the mucosal cells or at least render them susceptible to ulceration and may be followed by the rebound hyperemia and congestion noted previously. At any rate, mucosal cell integrity, rate of cell renewal, and mucus production may all be adversely influenced by ischemia early in the postburn course. Except for persistent or remote effects, this, of course, does not explain late ulceration. Late in the postburn period, a Curling's ulcer with hemorrhage may cause hypotension and decreased organ blood flow rather than result from it.

Hemoconcentration present in the immediate postburn period, as manifest by the usual hematocrit elevation, may similarly assist in "setting the stage" for later ulceration because of its effect on the rheologic properties of blood, further impairing organ blood flow. Excess catecholamine excretion present in the immediate postburn period would serve to intensify vasospasm and augment, both in severity and duration, the ischemia noted previously. The medullary secretions of the adrenal gland have no apparent direct effect on the gastrointestinal mucosa. The secretions of the adrenal cortex, on the other hand, do appear to influence gastric physiology directly through their effect on mucus and perhaps indirectly through their antiphlogistic action. Steroid hormones, according to McClelland (1966), have been reported by some to increase gastric acid secretion, and by others to have no effect on gastric acid secretion. An elevation of adrenal steroid hormones in the early postburn period has been documented by numerous investigators (Birke et al., 1957; Feller, 1962), and the known action of cortisone in decreasing antral mucus production (Menguy and Masters, 1963) may be the mechanism by which gastric mucus production was decreased in burned animals studied at this institute (O'Neill et al., 1966). If the protection of the gastroduodenal mucosa is impaired by either qualitative (Menguy and Desbaillets, 1968) or quantitative change in the mucus, normal or even low gastric acid content may be capable of producing mucosal injury. The interrelationship of gastric acid and gastric mucus has recently been emphasized by Wise and Ballinger (1969).

The influence of sepsis on the development of Curling's ulcer is still incompletely delineated. In an earlier publication, using recovery of a positive blood culture as an index of sepsis, we found no correlation between sepsis and Curling's ulcer (O'Neill et al., 1967). However, it appears that such a definition of sepsis may well be too restrictive. Careful review of the 56 cases of Curling's ulcer we have encountered in the past two years disclosed that 43 patients, or 77 per cent, had documented sepsis at the time of diagnosis of Curling's ulcer. This incidence varied from 52 per cent among patients in whom the diagnosis was made clinically (including eight operative cases) to 94 per cent among those with autopsy-confirmed diagnosis, reflecting in part the fact that the majority of the patients who die with Curling's ulcer die of sepsis (72 per cent), but also emphasizing the association of sepsis with this disease, either as a contributory factor or a permissive agent in an already susceptible, debilitated patient. The forms of sepsis encountered in these 56 patients, many of whom had more than one septic focus, are detailed in Table 9-4.

Another possible factor influencing the development of gastrointestinal ulceration in the burn patient, particularly in those in whom ileus is present, is the regurgitation of intestinal chyme into the first portion of the duodenum and the gastric lumen. A

TABLE 9-4. Sepsis Present at Time of Diagnosis of Curling's Ulcer in 56 Patients, 1967-1968

	No. of Patients	% of Patients
Pneumonia	32	57
Septicemia	30	54
Suppurative thrombophlebitis	21	38
Burn wound sepsis	12	21
Miscellaneous	6	11

recent study by Guilbert et al. (1969) has shown regurgitation of duodenal contents into the stomach, a constant finding in hemorrhagic shock, to cause reduction of gastric mucus and both gross and microscopic gastric ulcerations. Injection of a trypsin inhibitor or simple cross clamping of the pylorus during the period of shock reduced both the incidence and severity of the gastric lesions in the reported study, providing "a remarkable degree of protection against the development of gastric lesions." As noted previously, ileus is a common occurrence in the early postburn period of patients with extensive thermal burns and may, by this mechanism, predispose the mucosa to subsequent ulceration.

One possible etiologic factor which deserves special consideration is that of the local blood supply of the gastric and duodenal mucosa. The presence of arteriovenous shunts in the vessels supplying the gastroduodenal mucosa is well known. These shunts under the control of the autonomic nervous system can explain the occurrence of the focal ischemia in the earliest postburn period as well as the rebound hyperemia following closure of the shunt and engorgement of the previously ischemic mucosa (Fig. 9-7). Such local variation in blood supply might well explain impaired mucosal cell renewal rates as well as decreased mucus production and the absence of hyperacidity. One such shunt fortuitously encountered at postmortem examination in a burn patient is shown in Figure 9-8. Maintenance of the integrity of the gastroduodenal mucosa as opposed to ulceration can perhaps best be regarded as a balance between adequacy of blood supply, mucosal cell renewal, and mucus production on the one side, and gastric acid production, sepsis, and the influence of duodenal regurgitation on the other (Fig. 9-9).

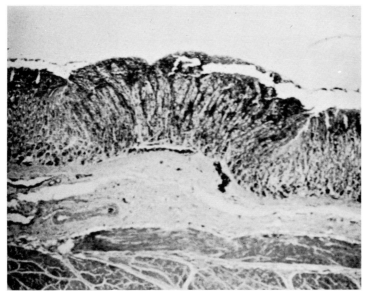

Figure 9-7. Extremely localized and sharply demarcated area of mucosal engorgement with beginning slough of surface. The necrosis and sloughing of such an area would result in a sharply punched-out lesion without inflammatory reaction characteristic of a Curling's ulcer. If such an area were to overlie an arterial channel, as in this section, significant hemorrhage would result. This human tissue was removed at autopsy two days postburn. The same lesion is readily produced in the experimental animal by burning and has been termed the "precursor lesion," since it is thought to be the forerunner of a Curling's ulcer.

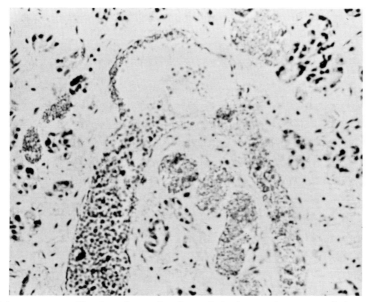

Figure 9-8. High power magnification of vascular channels in the gastric mucosa of a human stomach postburn. A mercury-barium mixture has been injected into the arterial tree and is seen here on the right side of this arteriovenous shunt, blending at the bulbous apex directly with the dark, heavy, granular blood of the venous side. Such bypassing of the capillary bed results in engorgement of the venous channels and, by back pressure, of the capillary bed also. Is this the basis for the vascular lesion seen in the gastric mucosa of the postburn period?

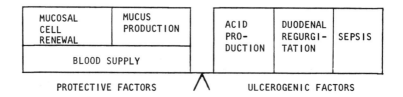

MUCOSAL CELL RENEWAL	MUCUS PRODUCTION	ACID PRO-DUCTION	DUODENAL REGURGI-TATION	SEPSIS
BLOOD SUPPLY				

PROTECTIVE FACTORS   /\   ULCEROGENIC FACTORS

ACCENTUATION OR DIMINUTION OF FACTORS SHIFTS "BALANCE" ACCORDINGLY

Figure 9-9. Diagram of protective ulcerogenic balance in burned patients.

PATHOPHYSIOLOGY

The typical lesion is small, shallow, rounded in configuration and sharply demarcated (Fig. 9-10). (Certain gastric ulcerations which may or may not be secondary to mechanical trauma appear linear in outline and may be hidden in the deeper mucosal folds.) Individual ulcers may be large, deep, and of irregular configuration. The largest in this group was 6 cm. in greatest dimension. These ulcers are characteristically acute, with little inflammatory reaction and essentially no fibrosis. The majority of these lesions extend only to the lamina propria, but those associated with bleeding have extended through the muscularis mucosa. An occasional ulcer may extend transmurally and perforate, or penetrate into the head of the pancreas. This may occur with or without hemorrhage. Recently, perforation appears to have increased in occurrence and has been noted at the time of diagnosis in 13 per cent of the last 56 cases. On histologic examination many of these ulcers contained, as noted by Sevitt in 1966, noninvasive bacteria or fungi. Erosions or ulcerations secondary to nasogastric intubation and drainage should be differentiated from Curling's ulcer. Such iatrogenic lesions are commonly linear and are located at the esophagogastric junction or along the lesser gastric curvature. They are rarely the source of clinically significant hemorrhage.

As noted by Artz and Moncrief (1969) and Ryan et al. (1965), gastric ulcers predominate anatomically and are commonly multiple whereas those which are duodenal in location are most often solitary. In children gastric and duodenal ulcers appear to occur with equal frequency. The fact that 22 per cent of patients encountered in the past two years had both gastric and duodenal ulcers is of great importance both diagnostically and surgically (Table 9-5).

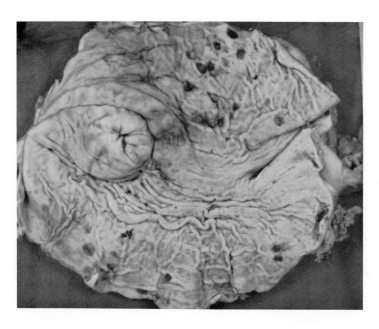

Figure 9-10. Autopsy specimen of stomach showing multiple, small, shallow, sharply demarcated lesions typical of Curling's ulcers.

TABLE 9-5. Location of Curling's Ulcer in 56 Patients, 1967-1968

Location	% of Patients with Ulcer	Single	Multiple	Total
Duodenum alone	46	13	6	19
Stomach alone	32	1	12	13
Duodenum and stomach	22	–	9	9

NOTE: Even though duodenal ulcers were more frequent in this smaller group, gastric ulcers have been more common in our total 15-year experience.

SIGNS AND SYMPTOMS

When ileus develops early in the postburn period in patients with burns covering 20 per cent or more of the body surface, clinical attention is frequently drawn to the gastrointestinal tract. This ileus is often associated with hemorrhagic gastritis with submucosal hemorrhage and even superficial mucosal ulcerations (Fig. 9-11). Erosive gastritis is a frequent observation in post-

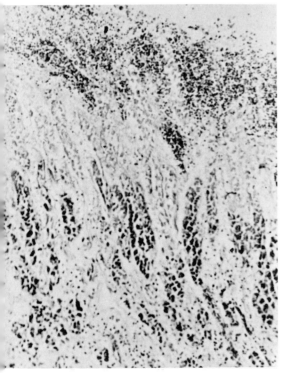

Figure 9-11. Section of the gastric mucosa of burned patient who died during the second postburn day. Note the marked engorgement of the mucosal capillaries, some of which have ruptured onto the surface. This accounts for "coffee-grounds" vomitus in the immediate postburn period.

mortem examination of patients with extensive thermal injury who expire in the early postburn period (Fig. 9-12). Such lesions are the frequent source of episodes of minor upper gastrointestinal hemorrhage manifested by coffee ground-like nasogastric returns or emesis in the immediate postburn period. Such bleeding is usually of short duration, relenting with restoration of intestinal motility (Kirksey et al., 1968). Treatment consists of withholding oral fluids, institution of effective nasogastric drainage, and adequate volume replacement. Gastrointestinal hemorrhage of any magnitude later in the postburn course is of greater importance and should suggest the diagnosis of Curling's ulcer.

Communication with and examination of the seriously ill and debilitated burn patient may be particularly difficult and may impede diagnosis of any complication. Confusion and a depressed state of awareness often occur in the severely burned patient with sepsis, making description of symptoms impossible. Tracheostomy required for the treatment of pulmonary complications or severe facial burns further limits effective communication. Lastly, burns of the abdominal wall make it virtually impossible to carry out an adequate abdominal examination.

It is subject to the above limitations that we state that up to 27 per cent of patients have no symptoms prior to the diagnosis of Curling's ulcer, and it is in this group that the diagnosis is first made at autopsy examination. The most frequent initial sign of Curling's ulcer in those in whom it is diagnosed during life is gastrointestinal hemorrhage, which is present in 66 per cent. It is massive and life-threatening in almost one-half of these patients, necessitating immediate therapeutic decisions and, in some, prompt surgical treatment (Table 9-6). Only 5 per cent of the patients in our series have complained of epigastric pain prior to the bleeding episode. Abdominal distention was noted in approximately 14 per cent of all patients with Curling's ulcer, but this finding is difficult to evaluate in the burn patient with sepsis who may have a coexisting ileus during a period of toxemia. It should be noted that nearly one-half of all patients requiring operation had ileus and distention shortly prior to their episode of hemorrhage. This paucity of prodromal symptoms and signs merely accentuates the sudden unexpected onset of this complication in the seriously

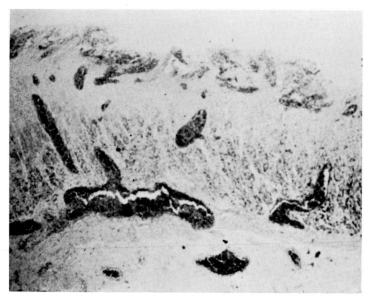

Figure 9-12.   Section of gastric tissue obtained postmortem two days postburn. There is extreme venous engorgement in both the mucosa and submucosa, mucosal capillary congestion, and surface bleeding.

ill burn patient. A few patients with massive hemorrhage have experienced unexplained restlessness and even a sense of impending doom immediately prior to hematemesis or melena, and certain of these patients have shortly thereafter exsanguinated before any effective treatment could be begun. The magnitude of the initial bleeding is illustrated by the fact that in approximately 29 per cent of all patients, hypotension, a 4 gm. per cent decrease in the hemoglobin, or a 10-point drop in hematocrit will occur with the upper gastrointestinal hemorrhage.

DIAGNOSIS

In the past two years 13 per cent of all patients with a diagnosis of Curling's ulcer have already experienced perforation of the ulcer at the time of diagnosis. This may be

manifest clinically as an abdominal catastrophe with the usual signs associated with a perforated viscus. Some perforations, however, remain occult, with an associated low grade peritonitis. Those which perforate into the lesser omental sac may be particularly difficult to diagnose, and the only clinical manifestations may be those of smouldering sepsis and impaired gastrointestinal motility. The appearance of clinical signs of gastrointestinal perforation, upper gastrointestinal bleeding, and otherwise unexplained ileus at any time in the postburn period demand that the diagnosis of Curling's ulcer be considered.

Conditions permitting, appropriate roentgenologic studies may be of assistance in confirming a questionable diagnosis of Curling's ulcer, in confirming the existence of a perforation, or in locating the ulceration prior to surgery. The diagnosis should not be dismissed in the absence of positive x-ray findings. The x-ray demonstration of a penetrating ulcer of the duodenum in a one-year-old child is shown in Figure 9-13. Penetration had occurred into the head of the pancreas, and continued upper gastrointestinal hemorrhage necessitated surgery. The cause of sudden shock or abdominal distention in the burn patient may be revealed to be a perforated Curling's ulcer if the alert physician will merely consider the diagnosis and obtain an upright abdominal or chest x-ray.

TABLE 9-6.   Signs and Symptoms of Curling's Ulcer in 56 Patients, 1967-1968

	No. of Patients	% of Patients
Hematemesis	17	30
Melena	20	36
Abdominal pain	3	5
Distention	1	2
No symptoms (perforation present at time of diagnosis)	15	27
	7	13

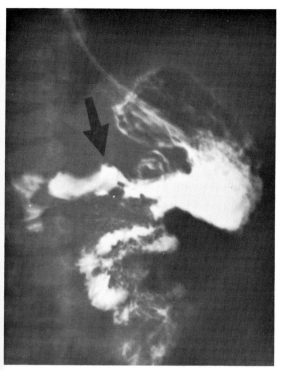

Figure 9-13. X-ray taken during upper gastrointestinal series in a small child with a penetrating ulcer of the duodenum (arrow) documented at subsequent operation.

THERAPY

The attending surgeon's reluctance to operate on the extensively burned patient with an infected burn of or near the abdomen and perhaps a superimposed pneumonia or other complication accounts for a natural preference for nonoperative management of such patients. A variety of such treatment has been employed by the authors and others in an attempt to staunch the bleeding and avoid surgery. It has been our experience, however, that one-third of the cases with massive hemorrhage treated by nonoperative means will rebleed, even if the initial hemorrhage stops with nonoperative therapy.

Hesitance to operate can lead to inappropriate delay in making the decision to intervene surgically. In general, one tends to treat these patients with nasogastric lavage, blood transfusion, and general supportive measures longer than the nonburned ulcer patient with hemorrhage. In an earlier paper from this institute, O'Neill et al. (1968) noted that an average of 5500 cc. of blood had been administered to those patients with hemorrhage from Curling's ulcer who ultimately went to surgery before operation was under-

taken. It was suggested then, and it is our opinion now, as it is of others (DeWeese, 1967; Dimick, 1967; Shaw et al., 1966) that such delay and prolonged anticipatory treatment is deleterious and adversely influences the outcome in these patients.

INDICATIONS FOR SURGERY. The indications for surgery in the burn patients with Curling's ulcer have been previously stated as: (1) uncontrollable hemorrhage, as defined later, (2) free perforation into the peritoneal cavity, or (3) perforation into the lesser omental sac with sepsis. Uncontrollable hemorrhage may present as sudden hypotension due to massive bleeding which is unresponsive to prompt blood replacement, or as failure of blood replacement to restore the hematocrit during several hours of therapy. In terms of chronicity of blood transfusion requirements, operative intervention is indicated when more than 2500 cc. of blood are required over a 12-hour period, or when bleeding of lesser magnitude continues for more than 48 hours. It must be emphasized that the paucity of symptoms can result in the existence of a significant blood volume deficit when bleeding is first noted clinically. As a result cardiovascular reserve is already compromised and little time can be devoted to nonoperative resuscitation. Early surgical intervention is, in actuality, conservative treatment in this situation.

The choice of operation, once the decision to intervene has been made, is predicated on the patient's condition, the existence of perforation, and the surgeon's experience and prejudice. Consideration of the pathogenesis of this disease, however, may allow one to select the best operation for each patient on a more physiologic basis.

PREOPERATIVE PREPARATION. Once the decision to operate has been made because of magnitude or persistence of hemorrhage, or because of perforation, the patient is prepared as any other patient, with particular care being taken to evacuate the stomach in order to minimize the possibility of aspiration as an additional complication in the already debilitated burn patient. The preferred incision is vertical and midline unless a paramedian or transverse incision would permit one to completely avoid incising the burned area of the abdominal wall. If the abdominal wall is unburned in the area of the incision, an impermeable adherent plastic drape should be used to minimize operative wound contamination. If the incision must be made through a burned abdominal wall, such a drape will not adhere to the burned skin and does not serve its intended purpose.

CHOICE OF PROCEDURES. Although one would prefer to perform an operation of lesser magnitude because of the frequently precarious status of these patients and because of the absence of chronicity of the disease process following recovery from the burn, our operation of choice is vagectomy with antrectomy and an antecolic gastro-jejunostomy. The vagectomy is advocated to decrease whatever acid secretion is present and for its beneficial effect on any gastric component. The resection is felt to be necessary to remove the ulcer if at all possible, to reduce gastric mass, and to minimize the chance of reulceration, and also because of our discouraging, albeit limited, experience with recurrence and rebleeding with lesser operations. It should be pointed out that our earlier experience with 60 to 80 per cent subtotal gastrectomy was equally successful. However, knowing that these patients are not more liable to chronic ulcer disease than the general population after recovery from their burns, we prefer the more limited resection to preserve as much stomach as is consistent with adequate control of this acute ulcer diathesis.

Because of the frequent presence of multiple ulcers, a generous gastrotomy is necessary, and thorough inspection of the entire gastric lumen is mandatory. In examination of the duodenum, palpation with the examining finger may rarely enable one to detect a sharply demarcated ulcer crater; in the case of extensive ulcers a slightly firmer, smooth, or finely granular ulcer bed may be detected in this manner. However, this is not a substitute for visual examination. The ulcer should be excised with the resected specimen if possible. Failure to remove the ulcer poses a great threat since the ulcer is a progressively enlarging necrotic lesion which can overnight double or triple in size. Fundal lesions are excised by wedge resection locally along with vagectomy and antrectomy. In the case of lesions too near the ampulla of Vater, careful, secure oversewing of the ulcer is a reasonable compromise; a compromise because it is precisely in these patients that significant rebleeding has occurred. The occurrence of both gastric and duodenal ulcers in 22 per cent of patients dictates that, even if the source of bleeding appears to be a duodenal ulcer, a search for associated gastric ulcers must be made.

In five patients with lesser operative procedures (vagectomy and pyloroplasty, three; drainage of lesser sac, one; and suture of ulcer with gastrostomy, one) there were two cases of massive rebleeding, one suture line disruption, and no survivors. Our unsatisfactory experience coincides with that of others, and we have reserved suture closure for those patients with perforation who are in extraordinarily precarious condition. Vagectomy and pyloroplasty might well be employed in those patients with fundal perforation and no evidence of hemorrhage. Posterior perforation with lesser-sac abscess formation requires drainage, but resection in the presence of established local infection is contraindicated.

The noninflammatory nature of these lesions is reflected by the fact that the duodenum can, in general, be closed primarily, but a rare case may require use of a tube duodenostomy. Meticulous closure is essential since a hastily and poorly constructed suture line will almost certainly leak, and the resulting peritonitis and disruption of the anastomosis will be poorly tolerated in an already seriously ill patient.

Any significant peritoneal contamination or coexistent sepsis apt to cause prolonged postoperative ileus suggests use of a gastrostomy in an attempt to minimize pulmonary complications which may occur with prolonged nasogastric intubation. The usual care in placement of the gastrostomy tube should be taken to avoid impairment of the blood supply of the anastomosis.

In an earlier report only one-fourth of operated patients developed postoperative wound infection. In the past two years, however, all the patients operated upon for Curling's ulcer, who survived longer than 48 hours following surgery, developed a postoperative wound infection. This fact, plus the hypoproteinemia and hypermetabolism

TABLE 9-7.   *Postoperative Complications*

Wound infection	10
Dehiscence	2
Rebleeding	5
Anastomotic leak	4
Gastrocolic fistula	1
Stomal obstruction	1
Obstruction 2° adhesions	1
Pneumonia	2

of the burn patient, recommends the use of retention sutures. Primary skin closure is avoided, and the wound can effectively and more safely be covered with homograft as described by Shuck et al. (1969).

POSTOPERATIVE COMPLICATIONS. Rebleeding has been infrequent in this series of patients undergoing resection and, aside from those patients in whom a duodenal ulcer has had to be left in place, has been associated with either suture line disruption and/or an intra-abdominal abscess or peritonitis.

Postoperative complications are common and are frequently related to conditions which existed preoperatively, as shown in Table 9-7. Operative mortality was closely related to complications which existed in these patients preoperatively, but in five patients appeared to be iatrogenic and directly related to a technical error (Table 9-8).

RESULTS. Sixty-eight per cent of all patients with Curling's ulcer in this series of 281 expired. Seventy-two per cent or 138 of the 192 deaths were due to sepsis and not to the ulcer per se. Approximately one-third of all cases of Curling's ulcer in this series were diagnosed at autopsy, having remained occult throughout the patient's entire hospital course. In these patients some other disease was felt to be the primary cause of death, usually a septic complication. In the group of 29 patients who underwent operation there were 17 who expired, a higher mortality than in the largely nonthermal stress ulcer series reported by Kirtley et al (1969). In seven of these patients the cause of death was felt to have been unrelated to the ulcer or the operation per se. There were 12 patients, or 41 per cent, who survived and were discharged from the hospital. The seven patients who survived operations but expired from other causes represent an additional 24 per cent of operated patients, for a total potential salvage rate of 65 per cent (Table 9-9).

TABLE 9-8. Causes of Death in
Operated Patients

Pneumonia	3
Septic phlebitis	2
Burn wound sepsis	1
Hepatitis	1
Cardiac disease	2
Renal failure	1
Massive bleeding	2
Intra-abdominal bleeding (technical error)	1
Anastomotic or stump leak	4

TABLE 9-9. Operative Results in 29 Patients

Operation	Total	Survived	Died
Subtotal gastrectomy	16	8	8
Vagectomy and antrectomy	8	4	4
Vagectomy and pyloroplasty	3	0	3
Drainage of lesser sac abscess	1	0	1
Suture of ulcer with gastrostomy	1	0	1
Total	29	12	17°

°Seven patients recovered from surgery but died of other causes.

SUMMARY

The extensively burned patient requires constant attention to a myriad of details of treatment to minimize the possibility of life-threatening complications. Topical mafenide chemotherapy is an effective means of controlling the bacterial population of the burn wound and significantly reducing the chance of invasive infection. A high percentage of these patients will nevertheless develop such complications, and the alert physician will anticipate and diagnose and treat in a timely fashion those septic complications which are most frequently encountered (suppurative thrombophlebitis, pneumonia, and burn wound sepsis). Although a direct relationship of sepsis to Curling's ulcer is uncertain, the association of the two suggests that sepsis is an additive stress contributing to acute gastrointestinal ulceration in the burn patient. Nonoperative treatment is initially employed in the burn patient with Curling's ulcer, but surgery should not be inordinately delayed in a deteriorating patient merely because a burn is present. Based on experience with 281 burn patients with Curling's ulcer, of whom 29 have been operated upon, our choice of operation is vagectomy with antrectomy.

REFERENCES

Arturson, G.: Pathophysiological aspects of the burn syndrome, with special reference to liver injury and alterations of capillary permeability. Acta Chir. Scand. (Suppl.), 274, 1961.

Artz, C. P., and Moncrief, J. A.: The Treatment of Burns. 2nd ed. Philadelphia, W. B. Saunders Company, 1969.

Baxter, C. R., Canizaro, P. C., and Heimbach, D. M.: Subeschar antibiotics: An adjunct in the prevention and treatment of burn wound sepsis. J. Trauma, In press.

Birke, G., Duner, H., Liljedahl, S. O., Pernow, B., Plantin, L. O., and Troell, L.: Histamine, catechol amines and adrenocortical steroids in burns. Acta Chir. Scand., 114:87, 1957-1958.

DeWeese, M. S.: Gastrointestinal ulceration. Symposium of Sixth National Burn Seminar. J. Trauma, 7:115, 1967.

Dimick, A.: Bleeding in children. Symposium of Sixth National Burn Seminar. J. Trauma, 7:119, 1967.

Feller, I.: A second look at adrenal cortical function in burn stress. In Artz, C. P. (ed.): Research in Burns. Washington, D.C., American Institute of Biological Sciences, 1962, p. 163.

Foley, F. D., Moncrief, J. A., and Mason, A. D., Jr.: Pathology of the lung in fatally burned patients. Ann. Surg., 167:251, 1968.

Guilbert, J., Bounous, G., and Gurd, F. N.: Role of intestinal chyme in the pathogenesis of gastric ulceration following experimental hemorrhagic shock. J. Trauma, 9:723, 1969.

Kirksey, T. D., Moncrief, J. A., Pruitt, B. A., Jr., and O'Neill, J. A., Jr.: Gastrointestinal complications in burns. Amer. J. Surg., 116:627, 1968.

Kirtley, J. A., Scott, H. W., Jr., Sawyers, J. L., Graves, H. A., Jr., and Lawler, M. R.: Surgical management of stress ulcers. Ann. Surg., 169:801, 1969.

McClelland, R. N.: Stress ulcers. In Shires, G. T.: Care of the Trauma Patient. New York, McGraw-Hill Book Co., 1966.

Menguy, R., and Desbaillets, L.: Gastric mucous barrier: Influence of protein-bound carbohydrate in mucus on the rate of proteolysis of gastric mucus. Ann. Surg., 168:475, 1968.

Menguy, R., and Masters, G. F.: Effect of cortisone on mucoprotein secretion by gastric antrum of dogs: Pathogenesis of steroid ulcer. Surgery, 54:19, 1963.

Moncrief, J. A.: Topical therapy of the burn wound: Present status. Clin. Pharmacol. Ther., 10:439, 1969.

Moncrief, J. A., Lindberg, R. B., Switzer, W. E., and Pruitt, B. A., Jr.: Use of topical antibacterial therapy in the treatment of the burn wound. Arch. Surg., 92:558, 1966.

Moncrief, J. A., Switzer, W. E., and Teplitz, C.: Experiences with Curling's ulcer. J. Trauma, 4:481, 1964.

Moncrief, J. A., and Teplitz, C.: Changing concepts in burn sepsis. J. Trauma, 4:233, 1964.

Moyer, C. A., Margraf, H. W., and Monafo, W. W., Jr.: Burn shock and extravascular sodium deficiency—Treatment with Ringer's solution with lactate. Arch. Surg., 90:799, 1965.

O'Neill, J. A., Jr., Pruitt, B. A., Jr., Foley, F. D., and Moncrief, J. A.: Suppurative thrombophlebitis: A lethal complication of intravenous therapy. J. Trauma, 8:256, 1968.

O'Neill, J. A., Jr., Pruitt, B. A., Jr., and Moncrief, J. A.: Surgical treatment of Curling's ulcer. Surg. Gynec. Obstet., 126:40, 1968.

O'Neill, J. A., Jr., Pruitt, B. A., Jr., Moncrief, J. A., and Switzer, W. E.: Studies related to pathogenesis of Curling's ulcer. J. Trauma, 7:275, 1967.

O'Neill, J. A., Jr., Ritchey, C. R., Mason, A. D., Jr., and Villarreal, Y.: Influence of thermal burns on gastric mucus production. Surg. Forum, 17:293, 1966.

Order, S. E., Mason, A. D., Jr., Walker, H. L., Lindberg, R. B., Switzer, W. E., and Moncrief, J. A.: Vascular destructive effects of thermal relationship to burn wound sepsis. J. Trauma, 5:62, 1965.

Passi, R. B., and Vasko, J. S.: Effect of hypoxia and hypercapnia on basal acid secretion from innervated gastric pouches in dogs. Surg. Gynec. Obstet., 128:322, 1969.

Pruitt, B. A. Jr., DiVincenti, F. C., Mason, A. D., Jr., Foley, F. D., and Flemma, R. J.: The occurrence and significance of pneumonia and other pulmonary complications in burned patients: Comparison of conventional and topical treatment. J. Trauma. In press.

Pruitt, B. A., Jr., Flemma, R. J., DiVincenti, F. C., Foley, F. D., and Mason, A. D., Jr.: Pulmonary complications in burned patients. A comparative study of 697 patients. J. Thorac. Cardiov. Surg., 59:7, 1970.

Pruitt, B. A., Jr., Mason, A. D., Jr., and Moncrief, J. A.: Hemodynamic changes in the early postburn patient—The influence of fluid administration and of a vasodilator (hydralazine). J. Trauma. In press.

Pruitt, B. A., Jr., and Moncrief, J. A.: Current trends in burn research. J. Surg. Res., 7:280; 332, 1967.

Pruitt, B. A., Jr., O'Neill, J. A., Jr., Moncrief, J. A., and Lindberg, R. B.: Successful control of burn wound sepsis. J.A.M.A., 203:1054, 1968.

Pruitt, B. A., Jr., Stein, J. M., Foley, F. D., Moncrief, J. A., and O'Neill, J. A., Jr.: Suppurative thrombophlebitis and life-threatening complications of intravenous therapy in burn patients. Arch. Surg. In press.

Ryan, R. F., Gay, J. S., Vincent, V., III, and Longnecker, C. G.: Stress ulcers of the upper gastrointestinal tract after burns: Curling's ulcer. Plast. Reconstruc. Surg., 35:385, 1965.

Sevitt, S.: Duodenal and gastric ulceration after burning. In Wallace, A. B., and Wilkinson, A. W. (eds.): Research in Burns, Edinburgh, E. & S. Livingstone Ltd., 1966.

Shaw, A., Symonds, F., Bush, J., and Wardlaw, L.: Surgical management of Curling's ulcer in children. J.A.M.A., 197:922, 1966.

Shuck, J. M., Pruitt, B. A., Jr., and Moncrief, J. A.: Homograft skin for wound coverage. Arch. Surg., 98:472, 1969.

Stone, H. H., Martin, J. D., Jr., Hugh, W. E., and Kolb, L.: Gentamicin sulfate in the treatment of Pseudomonas sepsis in burns. Surg. Gynec. Obstet., 120:351, 1965.

Teplitz, C., Davis, D., Mason, A. D., Jr., and Moncrief, J. A.: Pseudomonas burn wound sepsis. I. Pathogenesis of experimental Pseudomonas burn wound sepsis. J. Surg. Res. 4:200, 1964a.

Teplitz, C., Davis, D., Walker, H. L., Raulston, G. L., Mason, A. D., Jr., and Moncrief, J. A.: Pseudomonas burn wound sepsis. II. Hematogenous infection at the junction of the burn wound and the unburned hypodermis. J. Surg. Res., 4:217, 1964b.

Wise, L., and Ballinger, W. E., II: Effect of change in the hydrogen ion content of gastric juice on gastric mucus secretion. Surgery, 66:723, 1969.

CHAPTER 10

THROMBOPHLEBITIS AND PULMONARY EMBOLISM

by ROBERT H. JONES, M.D., and DAVID C. SABISTON, JR., M.D.

David Coston Sabiston, Jr., is a North Carolinian who was elected to Phi Beta Kappa at the University of North Carolina and Alpha Omega Alpha at Johns Hopkins University School of Medicine. After residency training at the Johns Hopkins Hospital he joined the staff, later spending a year in England in 1960–61, where he studied experimental thromboembolism at Oxford University. Returning to Johns Hopkins, he and his associates developed a body of information which greatly increased knowledge and understanding of clinical venous embolism, and he was made a full professor. In 1964 he was appointed Professor and Chairman of the Department of Surgery at Duke University where his imaginative leadership has been widely acknowledged.

Robert Howard Jones is a Kansan who gained his B.S. at Harding College and his M.D. at Johns Hopkins. During his medical school years he worked with Dr. Sabiston's pulmonary embolism research team. He served his internship at Duke University Medical Center, where he is currently a resident in surgery and a Scholar in Academic Surgery.

Delicate homeostasis maintains the fluidity of the blood essential for circulation, yet controls hemorrhage by rapid coagulation. Difficulty in achieving hemostasis in the occasional operative patient with deranged clotting mechanisms dramatically demonstrates the necessity of small vessel thrombosis in surgical wounds. However, tissue injury, increased clotting tendency, or blood stagnation, often associated with surgical disorders, may initiate potentially devastating venous thrombosis unrelated to wound hemostasis.

Thrombophlebitis and pulmonary embolism persist as common serious complications in surgical patients and they appear to be increasing in incidence. Often pulmonary embolic episodes add to gradual circulatory impairment, further complicating the postoperative course of critically ill patients. Without warning, massive and lethal embolism may suddenly conclude an otherwise uneventful postoperative recovery.

Appropriate management of the unique clinical setting of each patient with pulmonary embolism challenges the judgment of the most experienced clinicians but increases patient survival. The abrupt onset of cardiorespiratory symptoms may lead to therapy without diagnosis; proper treatment of pulmonary embolism, however, demands *accurate* diagnosis. This single most fatal pulmonary disorder is incorrectly diagnosed more frequently than any other common disease, and less than half of the fatal cases are recognized prior to autopsy. Clinical manifestations of pulmonary embolism are not specific and are easily confused with other pulmonary or cardiac disorders common to surgical patients. However, the systematic application of specific diagnostic methods has produced a marked increase in the number of cases recognized clinically. Objective documentation of pulmonary embolism through specific diagnostic procedures provides the basis for appropriate treatment. Aggressive exploitation of the preventive, diagnostic, and therapeutic methods presently available may produce the first decline in mortality of patients with pulmonary embolism since the recognition of the disorder, more than 100 years ago.

HISTORICAL ASPECTS

Two centuries after the classic observations of William Harvey confirming the direction of the circulation of the blood, the now obvious corollary of embolism was still foreign to medical thought. In 1819, Laennec distinguished hemorrhagic infarction, termed pulmonary apoplexy, from other causes of hemoptysis. He described hemorrhagic infarcts as swollen, dark red areas, discrete from the surrounding normal parenchyma, having granular cut surfaces and often showing central necrosis. In 1828, Cruveilhier treated a 44-year-old woman suffering from leg swelling; she developed sudden chest pain, dyspnea, and hemoptysis and died two days later with severe respiratory distress and venous distension. His surprisingly accurate autopsy observations and drawing clearly demonstrate pulmonary infarction (Fig. 10-1). Cruveilhier commented:

The lungs were studded with a large number of bloody areas. These areas disseminated here and there were

irregularly spheroid, but very clearly circumscribed, their color jet-black, their density, their friableness were in contrast to perfectly healthy adjacent pulmonary tissue. Their volume varied from that of a hazel nut to that of a large chicken egg. The largest number border upon the pleura which they raise and the smallest are situated immediately below this membrane. On sectioning, these hemorrhagic areas presented a granular surface. All arterial divisions ending at these areas were filled with thrombi with branching similar to the vessels. These thrombi were reddish in peripheral divisions and white in larger divisions, their side of origin furrowed, their side of termination occluding the vessels. These thrombi did not adhere to the arterial walls which scarcely presented traces of inflammation. Some of the larger pulmonary arteries contained thrombi equally furrowed.

Despite this detailed description, the true pathogenesis of pulmonary embolism was not appreciated, and the view prevailed that pulmonary apoplexy was a primary lung disorder producing secondary *in situ* thrombosis in pulmonary arteries.

Rudolf Virchow, observing thrombosis in veins of the legs and pelvis in patients with pulmonary embolism, postulated that the thrombi found in the lungs arose in the peripheral veins and subsequently dislodged

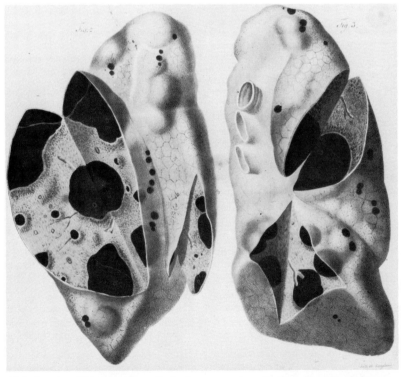

Figure 10-1. This drawing illustrates the pathologic appearance of lungs of a patient diagnosed and treated for pulmonary apoplexy by Cruveilhier in 1828. He described abnormal lung areas, discrete from healthy pulmonary tissue, with arterial branches leading to these areas filled with thrombi. However, Cruveilhier believed the thrombi to form in situ in pulmonary arteries and did not understand their embolic origin. (From Cruveilhier, J.: Anatomie Pathologique Du Corps Humain. Paris, J. B. Bailliere, 1829 to 1842. From the Trent Historic Collection, Duke University Medical Library.)

and passed into the pulmonary circulation as emboli. He confirmed the validity of his insight by inserting muscle, foreign matter, or human thrombi into the jugular veins of dogs and retrieving the material from the pulmonary circulation. In studies of human pathology he differentiated emboli of venous origin from *in situ* thrombi, which formed about the embolus in the pulmonary artery (Fig. 10-2). In an excellent review of embolism in 1899, William H. Welch commented on the significance of Virchow's observations:

> There is scarcely another pathological doctrine of equal magnitude the establishment of which is so largely the work of a single man. Between the years 1846 and 1856 Virchow constructed the whole doctrine of embolism upon the basis of anatomical, experimental and clinical investigations, which for completeness, accuracy, and just discernment of the truth must always remain a model of scientific research in medicine.

At the turn of the century, the diagnosis of pulmonary embolism depended upon the sudden appearance of respiratory distress, chest pain, and circulatory collapse. Little, if any, specific treatment was recognized. In 1908, Trendelenburg proposed direct surgical removal of emboli from the pulmonary arteries. He demonstrated experimentally the successful removal of an embolus from a calf and four months later, at the time of sacrifice, showed healing of the pulmonary artery. Three embolectomies attempted in man were reported by Trendelenburg to have

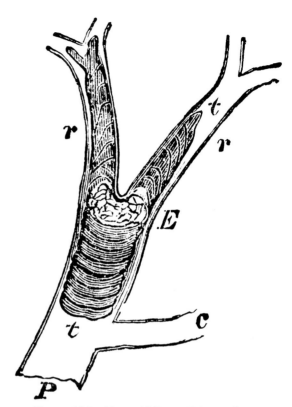

Figure 10-2. From 1846 to 1856 Virchow constructed the theory of embolism and differentiated emboli of venous origin from in situ thrombi forming about the embolus in the pulmonary artery (P) and a bifurcating vessel (C). An embolus (E) is lodged at a distal bifurcation and in situ thrombosis (T) has occurred proximal and distal to the occluding lesion. (From Virchow, Rudolph: Die Cellularpathologie. Berlin, A. Hirschwald, 1858.)

TABLE 10-1. Major Advances in Pulmonary Thromboembolic Disease

Date	Investigator	Contribution
1819	Laennec	Described hemorrhagic pulmonary infarct
1846 to 1856	Virchow	Defined pulmonary embolism with correct pathogenesis
1908	Trendelenburg	Experimental pulmonary embolectomy and first attempts in man
1918	Howell	Heparin purified
1922	Wharton	Chest film changes with pulmonary embolism reported
1924	Kirschner	First successful pulmonary embolectomy in man
1931	Moniz	Pulmonary angiography
1934	Homans	Prophylactic venous ligation
1938	Murray	Heparin therapy for thromboembolism
1942	Megibow	Circulatory alterations with pulmonary embolism measured
1964	Wagner	Radionuclide lung scanning

been unsuccessful, and it remained for Kirschner to report the first successful pulmonary embolectomy in 1924. The high mortality of early pulmonary embolectomies prompted a search for an effective way of preventing pulmonary embolism. Although venous ligation for suppurative thrombophlebitis was done as early as 1865, it was performed infrequently. In 1934 Homans reported early observations of venous ligation as prophylaxis for pulmonary embolism in patients with bland thrombophlebitis. Purification of heparin by Howell in 1918 permitted Murray, twenty years later, to report the effectiveness of anticoagulation in patients with thromboembolism. The introduction of methods to prevent and treat pulmonary embolism stimulated the refinement of procedures to increase diagnostic accuracy; such procedures included chest films, pulmonary arteriograms, electrocardiograms, and, more recently, radionuclide and serum enzyme studies. Measurement of hemodynamic alterations in experimental pulmonary embolism by Megibow in 1942 has been followed by extensive experimentation in mechanisms responsible for clinical and pathological manifestations of the disorder. Table 10-1 summarizes some of the major contributions to the clinical management and understanding of pulmonary embolism during the past century. Present active investigation into many aspects of pulmonary embolism will undoubtedly lengthen this list as continued progress is made to control this disorder.

MECHANISMS OF VENOUS THROMBOSIS

Virchow enunciated the three factors predisposing to thrombosis to be blood stasis, increased blood coagulability, and vessel injury. Subsequent investigation has validated this classic triad, and one or more of these factors are usually present in each patient with thrombosis. Patients with thrombosis show an increase in platelet adhesiveness and in the utilization of labeled fibrinogen that suggests an enhancement in clotting mechanisms (Hirsch et al., 1965; Izak et al., 1967). Although both platelet number and adhesiveness increase postoperatively, a clinically significant hypercoagulable state from the overactivity of normal blood-clotting mechanisms is uncommon in surgical patients (Bennett, 1967; Ardlie et al., 1967; Makin, 1968). Increased clotting tendency, encountered more frequently by the surgeon, results from altered blood elements with blood dyscrasias or polycythemia secondary to dehydration or cyanotic heart disease. Vessel injury from infection, trauma, or tumor invasion occasionally presents an obvious etiology for thrombophlebitis, but more often microscopic examination of the involved vessel reveals only mild intimal inflammation, which may represent a result rather than a cause of thrombosis. Stasis of blood is probably the most important clinical factor predisposing to thrombophlebitis. Shock, congestive heart failure, immobilization, anesthesia, and aging are some of the major reasons for a decrease in venous blood flow and are apparent in almost every patient with thrombophlebitis. Shock and congestive heart failure decrease arterial blood flow in the muscles, thereby depressing venous return from the extremities. Intermittent venous compression through muscle contraction accelerates venous blood flow in the extremities; inactivation of muscle pumping action, due to anesthesia, bed rest, or aging, may stagnate venous blood flow.

Clark and others (1968) used thermodilution probes during operation to measure flow in the deep leg veins of 14 patients. Immediately after the induction of general anesthesia, flow in external iliac and popliteal veins was reduced by half and remained depressed for the duration of anesthesia. McLachlin and associates (1960, 1962) assessed the effect of bed rest and age on venous flow by injecting the leg veins of patients for intravenous pyelography and determining the dye clearance time through radiographs. Patients injected while walking cleared dye from leg veins four times faster than those injected at bed rest. Dye clearance was prolonged in the elderly at bed rest more than in young patients. The risk of thrombosis is greatest in patients with multiple predisposing factors, such as a dehydrated elderly patient with chronic congestive heart failure who sustains shock from a severe injury to an extremity, necessitating general anesthesia and prolonged immobility. It is not surprising that more than 35 per cent of unselected patients with hip fractures show phlebographic evidence of venous thrombosis sometime during recovery (Freeark et al., 1967; Stevens et al., 1968)

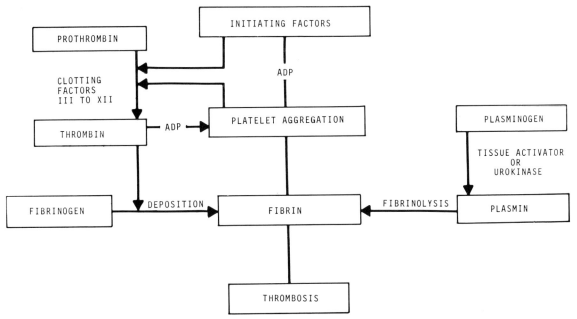

Figure 10-3. Factors that initiate venous thrombosis activate both platelet aggregation and fibrin deposition. Once activated these reactions are self-perpetuating. Tissue activator substance converts plasminogen to plasmin, which enzymatically degrades fibrin. If fibrin deposition exceeds the fibrinolytic action of plasmin, platelet aggregates are stabilized into a small intravascular thrombus. Blood, flowing about the site of aggregation, deposits successive layers of platelets and fibrin to form a white thrombus.

Patients with a high risk of thrombophlebitis deserve careful attention for the prevention and early diagnosis of pulmonary embolism.

Present knowledge of the process of venous thrombosis is summarized in Figure 10-3. Although predisposing factors are apparent in most patients with thrombosis, basic mechanisms initiating inappropriate intravascular clotting remain unclear. Experi-

mental studies suggest that some degree of vessel injury precipitates clotting in veins with stagnant blood flow. Collagen exposed to blood by intimal damage releases platelet ADP, initiating platelet aggregation at the site of injury. Platelet aggregates serve as foci stimulating coagulation, and the resulting thrombin generation further aggregates platelets by the release of ADP. This auto-

Figure 10-4. This illustration by Virchow depicts mechanisms of thrombus propagation in veins. Small venous channels (c, c') are occluded with thrombi (t, t'), which extend into a larger proximal vein. Extension of the thrombi into the current of blood flow (C) initiates further fibrin and platelet deposition in the proximal vein. (From Virchow, Rudolph: Die Cellularpathologie. Berlin, A. Hirschwald, 1858.)

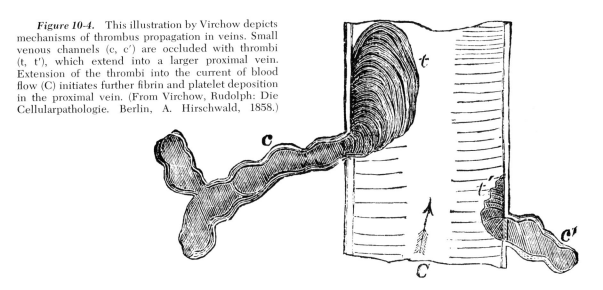

catalytic process deposits fibrin around platelet aggregates to form stable clots. However, an activator substance in endothelium converts plasminogen into plasmin, which enzymatically degrades fibrin. If fibrinolysis is sufficient to prevent fibrin deposition, platelet aggregates disperse and thrombosis is prevented. Injury partially depletes the vessels of the tissue activator substance and fibrinolysis may be insufficient to arrest thrombosis. Successive layers of platelets, fibrin, and leukocytes deposited by flowing form an ordered thrombus, which appears white because of selective platelet concentration and the paucity of erythrocytes.

In contrast to these white thrombi, red thrombi with no orderly arrangement form in association with the white thrombi in occluded vessels; these red thrombi resemble test-tube blood clots. The red thrombus extends proximally and distally to the occluding white thrombus in veins. Extension of the propagated thrombus into the lumen of the proximal vein again provides a site of partial obstruction for platelet and fibrin deposition (Fig. 10-4). Thrombus propagation may eventually occlude major veins, and the nonadherent red thrombus tail in these veins extends toward the heart and easily dislodges, becoming an embolus. If embolism does not

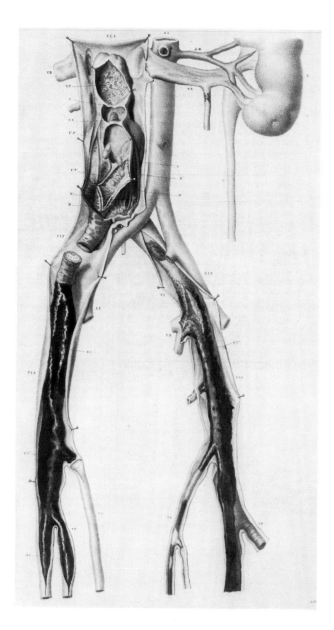

Figure 10-5. This illustration by Cruveilhier demonstrates postmortem findings in a patient dying with severe phlebitis. Suppuration is present in the center of an old organized thrombus in the vena cava. The femoral veins contain organizing thrombi, and fresh red and white thrombi are demonstrated in peripheral venous channels. (From Cruveilhier: J. Anatomie Pathologique Du Corps Humain. Paris, J. B. Bailliere, 1829 to 1842. From the Trent Historic Collection, Duke University Medical Library.)

rid the vein of the thrombus, an inflammatory response occurs within days after occlusion and, although usually mild, may occasionally progress to suppuration (Fig. 10-5). Eventually fibroblasts invade the thrombus, resulting in recanalization and restitution of venous flow. Thrombophlebitis scars the once delicate vein valves and the resulting increase in venous pressure may produce edema and skin ulceration typical of the postphlebitic leg.

PHYSIOLOGIC RESPONSE TO PULMONARY EMBOLISM

CIRCULATORY ALTERATIONS

Maturation or mechanical forces dislodge venous thrombi that may pass intact into a major pulmonary artery. However, right ventricular contraction may fragment the passing embolus and these fragments may become impacted in the pulmonary artery. Emboli may totally occlude pulmonary arteries, but those that do not completely conform to the geometry of the retaining vessel cause only partial occlusion and allow partial distal perfusion (Fig. 10-6). Embolic obstruction shifts blood flow to uninvolved areas of pulmonary circulation. Low vascular resistance characteristic of normal lungs permits severalfold increases in total pulmonary blood flow with small increases in pulmonary arterial pressure; therefore, severity of pulmonary arterial occlusion is not linearly related to the degree of resulting pulmonary arterial hypertension. Intraluminal balloon-tipped catheter occlusion of one main pulmonary artery in man may increase the arterial pressure proximal to the occlusion 20 to 30 per cent, but does not alter systemic arterial pressure or cardiac output. The active lives of most patients after pneumonectomy further illustrate the minor circulatory alterations resulting from removal of half of the pulmonary vascular bed. Occlusion beyond 50 per cent elevates pulmonary arterial pressure at an increasingly steep rate. Nevertheless, it has been shown experimentally that sequential ligation of major pulmonary arteries of dogs can continue until only 18 per cent of the pulmonary vasculature remains patent and capable of maintaining 75 per cent

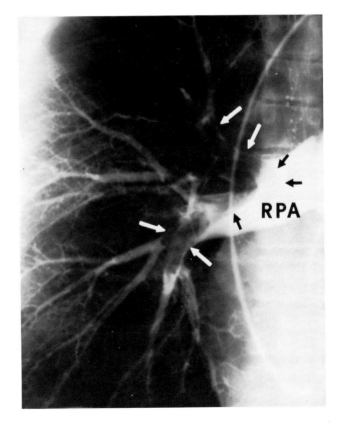

Figure 10-6. This pulmonary arteriogram in a patient with recent massive pulmonary embolism demonstrates an embolus in the right pulmonary artery (RPA) extending into all branches. Even this large embolus does not totally occlude the vessels, and dye seen in arteries distal to the embolus indicates blood flow to be diminished but present.

of control pulmonary blood flow, enough to sustain life several hours (Ebert et al., 1967).

In addition to the beneficial influence of low pulmonary vascular resistance, which rises slowly with arterial occlusion, normal right ventricular tolerance of outflow resistance also benefits patients with pulmonary embolism. In 1889, Cohnheim slowly tightened a ligature around the pulmonary artery of a dog and observed an immediate increase in right ventricular systolic pressure proportional to the degree of stenosis. However, systemic venous and arterial pressures remained stable until stenosis reached a marked degree. At the point of highest right ventricular pressure, arterial pressure suddenly fell and venous pressure suddenly increased. If stenosis was continued, heartbeat became irregular, and death rapidly ensued.

Since that time the observation has been made repeatedly that up to 60 per cent occlusion of the pulmonary vasculature does not cause failure of a normal heart (Haggart et al., 1923; Moore et al., 1927; Gibbon et al., 1932). Elevated right ventricular systolic pressure matches the increased pulmonary vascular resistance to maintain constant pulmonary blood flow. Increased perfusion of the right and left circumflex coronary arteries supports the added work of the right ventricle (Love et al., 1963; Guzman et al., 1964; Stein et al., 1968). Whereas a normal circulation tolerates significant pulmonary arterial occlusion, the capacity to withstand pulmonary embolism is limited by disorders that increase pulmonary vascular resistance or decrease right ventricular response to added work, and a small embolic insult may be fatal to patients with severe underlying cardiorespiratory disease. When pulmonary arterial occlusion exceeds the individual patient's capacity to compensate, heart failure rapidly ensues. Right ventricular diastolic pressure elevation, which marks the onset of heart failure, is manifested clinically by increased central venous pressure. Cardiac output diminishes and in both ventricles systolic pressure falls as diastolic pressure rises. Systemic arterial hypotension reduces coronary perfusion, and the heart dilates in ventricular fibrillation or arrest (Taquini et al., 1960).

In addition to mechanical arterial obstruction, pulmonary emboli have been suspected of initiating reflex circulatory alterations. In isolated dog lungs perfused at a constant rate, embolism with glass microspheres less than 250 microns in diameter causes an immediate rise in perfusion pressure followed by a further gradual increase, but embolism with larger particles causes an initial pressure rise without secondary increase (Niden et al., 1956; Caldini, 1965). These findings suggest that small pulmonary emboli cause initial pressure elevation through mechanical obstruction followed by more gradual pressure elevation due to pulmonary vasoconstriction.

Weidner and associates (1958) studied pulmonary embolism in dogs using plastic spheres of graded size to demonstrate vessels sensitive to occlusion. A 100 mg. embolic dose of 62- to 100-micron particles produced pulmonary hypertension, but a 750 mg. dose of 105- to 177-micron particles did not significantly change pulmonary arterial pressure. Dexter and associates (1964) injected sized particles into dog lungs and compared the number of particles required to reach a selected pulmonary artery pressure with the number of lung vessels of each corresponding caliber. The endpoint in pulmonary arterial pressure was attained by occlusion of a constant proportion of vessels *larger* than 170 microns, but the same pressure elevation was achieved by occlusion of a significantly lower proportion of vessels *smaller* than 170 microns.

Experimental pulmonary arteriolar embolism in dogs appears to evoke reflex vasoconstriction, which contributes a small amount to pulmonary hypertension caused primarily by mechanical vessel obstruction. Reflex pulmonary vasconstriction following pulmonary embolism has not been demonstrated in man, and, if it occurs at all, it appears to be of little clinical significance.

RESPIRATORY ALTERATIONS

Pulmonary embolism commonly causes dyspnea with rapid, shallow breathing. Mechanical stimulation of receptors in pulmonary arterioles initiates this ventilatory reflex, which is mediated through the vagus nerves. The quantity but not the distribution pattern of pulmonary arteriolar emboli determines the severity of reflex tachypnea (Horres et al., 1961). Bernthal and associates (1961) injected known quantities of 65- to 100-micron glass beads into dogs while continuously recording their breathing. He elicited significant respiratory changes with quantities of emboli insufficient to cause pulmonary arterial pressure elevation. The sensitivity of this reflex explains why dyspnea is the most frequent and often the sole clinical indication of pulmonary embolism. Dyspnea manifested by deep, labored breathing occurs in patients with massive embolism of large pulmonary arteries, but mechanisms responsible for this hyperpnea are unclear.

Boyer and associates (1944) observed a transient increase in intratracheal pressure and a simultaneous decrease in intrapleural pressure after experimental pulmonary embolism and suggested that these changes indicated transient bronchoconstriction. Subsequent investigation has elucidated two separate mechanisms which possibly effect bronchoconstriction after pulmonary embolism in man. Total balloon occlusion of one main pulmonary artery in both dogs and man increases pulmonary resistance and decreases compliance, functional residual capacity, and anatomic dead space in the involved lung (Severinghaus et al., 1961, 1962; Swenson et al., 1961). These changes indicating unilateral bronchoconstriction could be prevented by increased carbon dioxide content in the air ventilating the ischemic lung. Similar responses occur in autotransplanted dog lungs, indicating neural influence to be unimportant in bronchoconstriction after pulmonary artery occlusion (Allgood et al., 1968). In patients with embolic occlusion of major pulmonary arteries, ventilation of ischemic areas causes depressed alveolar carbon dioxide tension, which directly constricts corresponding bronchi. Bronchoconstriction partially corrects the ventilation-perfusion imbalance caused by embolism of major pulmonary arteries. Emboli scattered throughout smaller pulmonary arteries produce diffuse bronchoconstriction by means of a separate mechanism unrelated to alveolar carbon dioxide concentration.

Experiments by Thomas and associates (1964, 1965, 1966) have demonstrated in dogs that fresh platelets adhere to thrombi while passing into the pulmonary circulation and that release of serotonin by platelets into the lungs causes bronchoconstriction. Heparin, which inhibits platelet serotonin release, or drugs antagonistic to serotonin action prevent bronchoconstriction after autologous clot pulmonary embolism in dogs. Endo-

toxin, an agent releasing platelet serotonin, produces bronchoconstriction in dogs, a reaction which is prevented by the depression of blood platelets or heparin administration. Although serotonin release has not been demonstrated in patients, the fact that heparin partially reverses bronchoconstriction after pulmonary embolism suggests that serotonin release may occur in man (Gurewich et al., 1963). Inhibition of platelet serotonin release may contribute to the therapeutic effectiveness of heparin in acute pulmonary embolism, thereby relieving bronchoconstriction.

Mild hypoxemia commonly follows pulmonary embolism and, in 20 per cent of patients, is sufficiently severe to cause cyanosis. In a few patients pulmonary edema follows pulmonary embolism and accounts for the severe cyanosis. Experimental evidence suggests that this pulmonary edema results from pulmonary infarction and is unrelated to pulmonary arterial hypertension (Kabins et al., 1962). However, pulmonary edema is not consistently observed after lung infarction. Unless pulmonary edema occurs, the slight depression in diffusing capacity following pulmonary embolism is insufficient to cause hypoxemia. Mechanisms preventing complete oxygenation of blood after pulmonary embolism remain obscure in the majority of patients.

NATURAL HISTORY OF PULMONARY EMBOLISM

On pathologic examination the typical appearance of pulmonary emboli in patients dying soon after embolism is an irregular mixture of red and white thrombi loosely retained at a vessel bifurcation and extending into distal arterial branches (Fig. 10-7). In addition to this thrombus of venous origin, blood stasis in obstructed pulmonary arteries initiates *in situ* thrombosis distal and proximal to the site of occlusion (Sabiston et al., 1964). Usually, patients who survive the immediate effects of pulmonary embolism recover completely unless claimed by a repeated embolic insult or a second disease. Normal lungs can resolve quite large quantities of thrombus without permanent functional impairment.

Downing and associates (1967) ligated all the pulmonary arteries of dogs except the

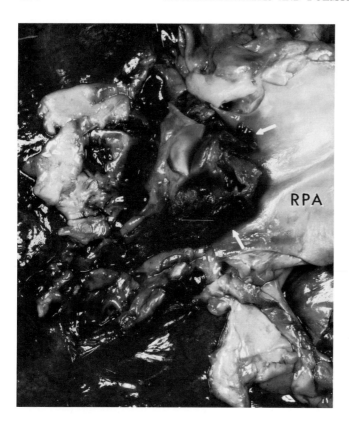

RPA

Figure 10-7. These postmortem findings are typical in patients with recent massive pulmonary embolism. The combined red and white thrombus appears irregular and is not adherent to pulmonary arteries into which it extends.

left lower lobe artery, and observed that autologous thromboembolism repeated at monthly intervals did not cause a sustained increase in pulmonary vascular resistance. Just-Viera and associates (1966) found that dogs tolerated ten times the usual amount of lethal autologous clot embolus administered intermittently over a four-month period.

Experimental and pathologic studies have defined the usual histologic response to pulmonary embolism, which effects thrombus resolution without impairing pulmonary function (Orell, 1962; Still, 1966; Sabiston et al., 1968). Inflammatory cells accumulate in the vessel at the site of embolus within two days. Within a week, fibroblasts and macrophages invade the retracted embolus and flat cells cover its surface (Fig. 10-8). After two to three weeks, capillaries are present within the thrombus, and a few firm cellular attachments to the vessel intima have formed. Further resolution reduces the thrombus to a fibrofatty subintimal plaque (Fig. 10-9). Thrombolysis is usually complete six weeks after embolism, and only endothelialized connective tissue webs or bands mark the vessel site originally occluded.

Partial blood flow through involved pulmonary arteries usually returns within one week after embolism, and within several weeks lung function may again be normal (Fig. 10-10) (Sabiston et al., 1965). However, individual patients vary greatly with respect to the average time course of resolution after pulmonary embolism. Restitution of blood flow in occluded pulmonary arteries has been documented within 30 hours of embolism, yet in some patients blood flow may not return for several months or longer after occlusion. Tow and associates (1967a) obtained serial lung scans on 33 patients with pulmonary embolism and observed, after four months, the significant return of perfusion in 64 per cent. Murphy and colleagues (1968), using serial lung scans in 25 patients, demonstrated some improvement in pulmonary perfusion in 63 per cent, one week after embolism, and only two patients showed incomplete resolution after 20 weeks.

Several factors influence the variable resolution of pulmonary emboli in patients. Emboli in large pulmonary arteries occasionally fragment and pass into smaller distal arteries, causing the early return of perfusion

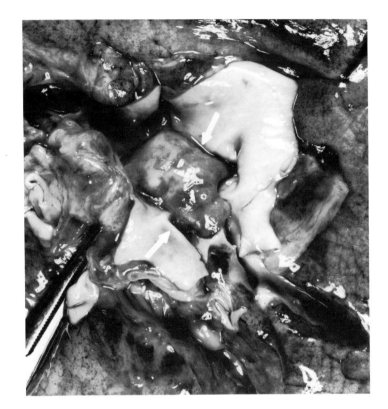

Figure 10-8. These postmortem findings in a patient sustaining pulmonary embolism one week prior to death illustrate partial resolution of the embolus. The embolus appears homogeneous and glistens with a smooth covering. Extensions of the embolus into pulmonary arteries have retracted to permit distal blood flow.

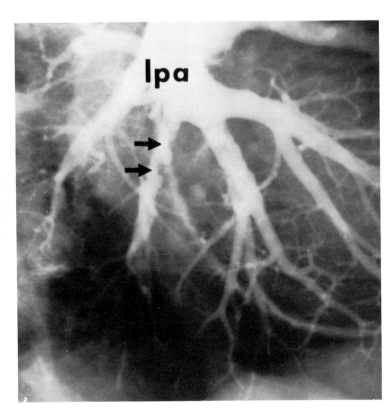

Figure 10-9. This pulmonary arteriogram in a patient several weeks after embolism demonstrates irregular pulmonary arteries with several discrete intimal plaques which represent residua of the previous pulmonary emboli.

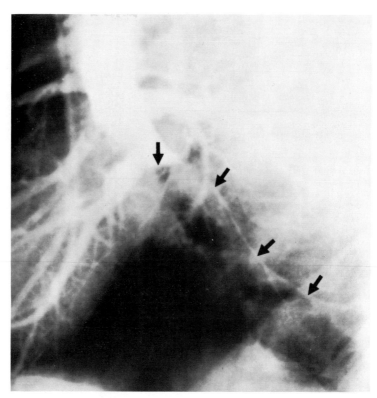

Figure 10-10. This pulmonary arteriogram demonstrates early recanalization in a pulmonary artery one week after embolism. A major vessel abruptly terminates and continues in only a thin line of contrast material contained in the small new channel (arrows).

to some lung areas. The lungs lyse fresh clot more rapidly than they lyse organized thrombi, and the age and composition of venous thrombi embolic to the lungs is variable (Marshall et al., 1964). Also, patients with underlying heart or lung disease resolve pulmonary emboli less effectively than other patients (Chait et al., 1967; Wechsler et al., 1969). Pulmonary emboli in occasional patients may fail to resolve, and pulmonary arterial occlusion may persist unchanged for several months and may remain permanently (Nash et al., 1968). Patients sustaining recurrent pulmonary embolism over a prolonged period may eventually develop pulmonary hypertension and cor pulmonale (Fleischner, 1967). However, the majority of patients completely resolve pulmonary emboli within several months with no significant lung impairment.

Normal lungs tolerate complete pulmonary arterial occlusion without infarction because of increased collateral circulation in the bronchial arteries. In the dog, bronchial flow greatly increases after pulmonary artery occlusion and, within 12 weeks, may equal

pre-occlusion pulmonary arterial flow (Gahagan et al., 1966).

Smith and associates (1964) used postmortem injection to study the bronchial circulation in six patients with recent pulmonary embolism. Within hours after embolism the bronchial arteries in areas of pulmonary arterial occlusion were dilated. Pulmonary embolism causes infarction in approximately 10 per cent of patients, and infarction, when present, is usually associated with congested heart failure or pulmonary suppuration. Although mechanisms leading to pulmonary infarction in patients remain obscure, recent experimentation suggests atelectasis may predispose to infarction after pulmonary embolism.

Edmunds and colleagues (1968) observed that bronchial artery occlusion causes severe alveolar hemorrhage in atelectatic lungs in dogs with ligated pulmonary arteries. When the lungs were ventilated with nitrogen to prevent atelectasis, alveolar hemorrhage was greatly reduced after ligation of the bronchial and pulmonary arteries. Sutnick and associates (1967) found no difference between the surface properties of normal lung extracts and lung extracts from patients dying after acute pulmonary embolism. However, lung extracts of patients dying with pulmonary infarction showed a great reduction in active surface properties. These studies suggest that altered cellular metabolism may diminish surfactant production in certain patients after pulmonary embolism causing atelectasis, which leads to pulmonary infarction. When infarction occurs, necrotic lung tissue is gradually replaced with contracted, nonfunctional scar tissue. Although pulmonary infarction, chronic pulmonary arterial obstruction, and pulmonary hypertension infrequently follow pulmonary embolism, most patients retain no evidence of embolism after recovery from the acute episode.

DIAGNOSTIC METHODS

INCIDENCE

Venous thrombosis that precedes pulmonary embolism usually occurs in veins of the legs or pelvis. Of 1920 unselected autopsies reviewed by Stein and associates (1967a), 809, or 42 per cent, demonstrated thrombosis in leg veins. Vein dissection was incomplete in many patients, and actual postmortem incidence of venous thrombosis probably exceeded 50 per cent. When both leg and thigh veins were examined, thrombi were present in 44 per cent of legs and 17 per cent of thighs. The lower incidence of thrombi in thigh veins alone suggests thrombophlebitis, which commonly begins in lower leg intramuscular veins and extends secondarily into thigh veins. The postmortem frequency of venous thrombosis suggests that pulmonary embolism occurs in a majority of severely ill patients, and thorough pathologic examination of lungs has shown emboli in over 60 per cent of adults dying from all causes (Freiman et al., 1965). Morrell and associates (1968) found pathologic evidence of embolism in 52 per cent of 263 *carefully* examined right lungs from unselected patients, while *routine* necropsy of the left lungs revealed embolism in only 12 per cent. Pulmonary embolism appeared to be the immediate cause of death in 21 per cent, and in 14 per cent of all patients, embolism caused death, which was otherwise not inevitable. Lethal pulmonary embolism followed 14 of

10,000 operations and caused death in 2.8 per cent of autopsies in reports of more than 3 million operations and 300,000 autopsies collected by DeBakey (1954). In most pathologic studies, pulmonary embolism is a leading cause of death and the most frequent fatal postoperative pulmonary complication (Andreasen et al., 1965). Some pathologic studies have indicated yearly increases in the incidence of pulmonary embolism. However, actual increases in incidence have not been clearly distinguished from apparent increases that may be due to more thorough pathologic lung examination.

Pulmonary embolism primarily afflicts the elderly, and more than 90 per cent of patients dying with the disorder are over 50 years old. However, no age group is totally free of the threat of lethal embolism. Pulmonary embolism is present in about one per cent of children who die between birth and age 15 (Jones et al., 1966). Pulmonary embolism has been reported in pregnancy and in otherwise healthy young adults (Evans et al., 1968; Fleming et al., 1966; Loehry, 1966). An interesting comparison of autopsy series with respect to age groups shows pulmonary embolism ten times more frequent in the United States than in Japan or India (Hirst et al., 1965). Incidence of myocardial infarction was equally unbalanced in the two populations, which suggests that some environmental variation, such as diet, may contribute to a common mechanism of increased thrombosis.

CLINICAL MANIFESTATIONS

Blood filtration is an important physiologic function of pulmonary circulation. The lungs rapidly resolve small thrombi that have been retained. The spectrum of thromboembolic disease extends from these asymptomatic episodes to massive embolism causing sudden death. Both the magnitude of embolic insult and the general condition of the individual patient determine the nature and severity of clinical indications of pulmonary embolism. It may be impossible to recognize minor embolic episodes in otherwise healthy patients or embolism of significant magnitude in seriously ill, obtunded patients, because of the absence or masking of suggestive signs. Occasionally sudden death from massive embolism precludes any diagnosis. Clinical manifestations of pulmonary embolism are vague and, even when quite typical, remain suggestive of other disorders. This variable, nonspecific clinical picture makes pulmonary embolism the most frequently misdiagnosed common disease — less than one third of the fatal cases are recognized prior to autopsy. It is common for circulatory or respiratory alterations in postoperative patients with pulmonary embolism to be incorrectly attributed to pneumonia, atelectasis, heart failure, or myocardial infarction. Institution of therapy specific for each of these serious complications demands an accurate diagnosis. Aggressive diagnosis of symptoms that suggest pulmonary embolism is often negative or identifies another disorder; only a high-index clinical suspicion will lead to early recognition of embolic episodes at the time when immediate treatment is most effective. Systematic application of a diagnostic protocol for all patients with symptoms suggestive of pulmonary embolism has been shown to increase from 30 to 70 per cent the fatal cases recognized clinically (Sasahara et al., 1967b).

Since most emboli arise in deep leg veins, accurate detection of thrombophlebitis could identify patients susceptible to pulmonary embolism and aid in prevention or early treatment. However, even thorough examination reveals clinical evidence of venous thrombosis in only a third of patients with pulmonary embolism. Thrombophlebitis is often asymptomatic and clinical indications are present in only 40 per cent of patients with venous thrombosis confirmed at autopsy (Sevitt, 1967). When present, the common signs of thrombophlebitis are leg pain and swelling, deep muscle tenderness, and fever. Kramer (1966) diagnosed deep vein thrombosis clinically in 454 patients and found pain in 440 (97 per cent), edema in 351 (77 per cent), induration in 146 (32 per cent), warmth in 122 (27 per cent), and redness in 98 (20 per cent). Of 365 patients examined, 237 (65 per cent) had calf tenderness and only 88 (24 per cent) had Homan's sign. Manifestations typical of thrombophlebitis have occasionally occurred in patients shown to have normal veins at phlebogram or operation. Phlebography is the definitive clinical method for accurately confirming presence or absence of venous thrombosis in the legs. Contrast material injected into superficial ankle veins is directed into deep veins with tourniquets while the patient maintains a semierect position. Sequential radiographs document the flow of dye through the veins and thrombi are visible as intraluminal defects or nonfilling vessel segments. Stein and associates (1967a) demonstrated a 90 per cent good correlation of phlebogram and postmortem findings in 47 limbs. Phlebography is safe and useful clinically when accurate documentation of the presence and extent of venous thrombosis might influence management. The absence of indications of thrombophlebitis provides no security from pulmonary embolism, but the presence of thrombophlebitis must be considered as a forewarning of subsequent pulmonary embolism.

The most constant symptom of pulmonary embolism is the abrupt onset of dyspnea, usually with rapid and shallow breathing. Dyspnea appears to be initiated by a sensitive reflex and is present in almost all patients with pulmonary embolism. Faintness or syncope commonly follows massive embolism and is particularly dramatic in otherwise healthy postoperative patients. Chest pain occurs in about one third of patients with pulmonary embolism and may be pleuritic, because of pleural reaction to the embolus, or of anginal origin, because of myocardial ischemia. It should be emphasized that hemoptysis, often regarded as a classic symptom of pulmonary embolism, occurs in less than 10 per cent of patients with the disorder (Sutton et al., 1969). Thus only one of three patients with pulmonary embolism displays either thrombophlebitis, chest pain, or hemoptysis, symptoms often considered specific for the disorder. Also, physical signs indicating pulmonary embolism in patients may be vague and inconsistent and so aid little in diagnosis. In a majority of patients with major embolism, acute pulmonary hypertension accentuates the pulmonary second sound, but concurrent sinus tachycardia often hinders the assessment of heart sounds. An elevated systemic venous pressure and gallop rhythm indicate right heart failure, and in massive pulmonary embolism systemic arterial hypotension may be severe. Tachypnea and respiratory distress are common. Lung examination occasionally reveals rales or wheezes but more commonly shows no abnormality. A pleural friction rub, although rarely present, is fairly indicative of pulmonary embolism. Cyanosis is present in approximately 20 per cent of patients after embolism and is usually mild.

Temperature is usually normal or mildly elevated and is only markedly elevated with septic pulmonary embolism.

Determination of serum levels of lactic dehydrogenase activity (LDH), glutamic oxaloacetic transaminase activity (SGOT), and bilirubin has been used in diagnosis of pulmonary embolism. About 75 per cent of patients with pulmonary embolism develop abnormally high serum values of one or more of these factors (Sasahara et al., 1967b; Polachek et al., 1968). The most frequent combination of alterations after pulmonary embolism is increased LDH with normal SGOT and bilirubin. Elevation of both LDH and bilirubin commonly follows embolism in patients with heart failure. The LDH elevation that occurs with pulmonary embolism is detectable in eight to 24 hours and may not peak for four days (Cugell et al., 1967). Inherent delay and inconsistent results make serum enzyme determinations of little practical value in diagnosing pulmonary embolism.

Chest films often appear normal but may be suggestive after experimental or clinical pulmonary embolism (Wolfe et al., 1968; Sutton et al., 1969). In 1928, Westermark described radiolucency and the decreased vascular markings in ischemic lung areas with prominent uninvolved vessels dilated by acute pulmonary hypertension; this finding remains the most helpful radiographic sign of pulmonary embolism. Other chest film abnormalities occasionally present with pulmonary embolism include atelectasis, pleural effusion, and dilatation of the right heart or major pulmonary arteries. Pulmonary infarction is visible on chest film as a half-spindle-shaped density based upon a pleural surface. In the absence of infarction, chest film findings may be suggestive but not diagnostic of pulmonary embolism, and often prove of greatest diagnostic usefulness in confirming absence of other pulmonary disease.

Massive embolism causes abnormalities on serial electrocardiograms in up to 80 per cent of patients, but less than a fourth of all patients with pulmonary embolism demonstrate abnormal initial electrocardiograms. When present, common abnormalities associated with pulmonary embolism include S–T segment depression, atrial arrhythmias, right axis deviation, prominent P waves, right bundle branch block, and inversion of T waves in right precordial beads (Weber et al., 1966; Winsor, 1968). It is frequently difficult to differentiate these electrocardiographic changes from alterations due to the coexisting cardiac disease common in patients with pulmonary embolism. The greatest value of electrocardiography in pulmonary embolism is the exclusion of the diagnosis of myocardial infarction, which itself may be difficult. Unless evidence of pulmonary *infarction* is present on the chest film, clinical manifestations and routine diagnostic procedures are inadequate to establish the definitive diagnosis of pulmonary embolism. However, careful clinical observation and judgment usually exclude atelectasis, pneumonia, and myocardial infarction as the causes of cardiorespiratory symptoms and provide a tentative diagnosis of pulmonary embolism. When feasible, specific diagnostic procedures should confirm the diagnosis of pulmonary embolism prior to institution of therapy.

Pulmonary Scanning

Wagner and associates reported pulmonary scanning in 1964 as a method of determining regional pulmonary blood flow. The lung scan is a rapid, simple procedure that inflicts minimal risk and discomfort and can be performed even in the severely ill patient. Aggregated radioactive human serum albumin is injected intravenously and particles disperse in pulmonary arterioles and capillaries in proportion to blood flow. The aggregates temporarily occlude a minute portion of small lung vessels and cause no pulmonary hemodynamic alteration. The external detection of radioactivity over the thorax outlines regional pulmonary perfusion.

Experimental pulmonary embolism demonstrated the reliability of lung scanning in defining alterations of pulmonary perfusion, and clinical experience confirmed its validity for determining pulmonary arterial perfusion in man (Sabiston et al., 1964). The lung scan *alone* is not diagnostic for any specific disease but defines abnormalities in pulmonary arterial flow caused by any disease process (Jones et al., 1967). However, the procedure is a valuable aid in diagnosing patients with pulmonary embolism when it is evaluated with proper consideration of all other clinical information. Figure 10-11 shows a typical lung scan in

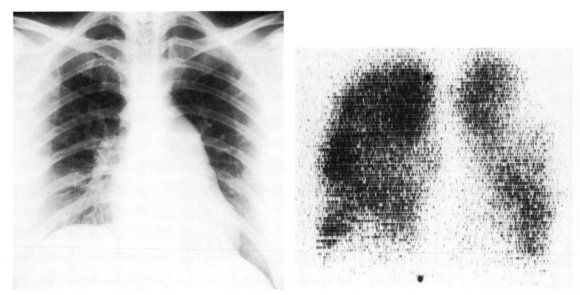

Figure 10-11. The chest film and lung scan illustrate the typical appearance of multiple pulmonary embolism. Crescent-shaped peripheral perfusion defects on scan are diagnostic of pulmonary embolism. The same areas on the chest x-rays are normal.

a patient with multiple bilateral pulmonary emboli. A concurrent chest film is essential for an accurate interpretation of the abnormal pulmonary blood flow depicted on the lung scan. Correlation between the position of scan defects and chest film densities suggests another pulmonary disease, and only decreased perfusion of lung areas appearing *normal* on the plain chest film indicates pulmonary embolism (Fig. 10-12). An infiltrate demonstrated on a chest film does not contraindicate the use of lung scanning for

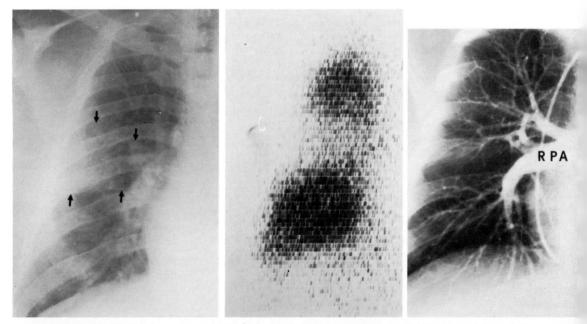

Figure 10-12. Various lung disorders that decrease pulmonary perfusion are demonstrated by lung scan defects This chest film (left) shows early pneumonia with minimal infiltrate in the right lung (arrows). A lung scan (middle indicates that capillary perfusion is decreased in the area of the infiltrate on the chest film, but the pulmonary arterio gram (right) shows the right pulmonary arteries to be patent and free of emboli. Lung scan perfusion defects in area corresponding to chest film infiltrates are not diagnostic of pulmonary embolism.

diagnosis of pulmonary embolism, since perfusion abnormalities indicating emboli may be present in the portions of the lungs not involved with infiltrate. Sensitive detection of abnormal pulmonary perfusion without significant patient risk or discomfort is made possible by lung scanning, making it an ideal diagnostic procedure for screening all patients with indications suggestive of pulmonary embolism. In addition to diagnosis, lung scans provide an estimate of the severity of pulmonary arterial occlusion, and serial scans record the return of blood flow to ischemic lung areas to aid in evaluating response to treatment.

Pulmonary Arteriography

Although less sensitive to small emboli than the lung scan, pulmonary angiography is another procedure quite helpful in the diagnosis of pulmonary embolism. The injection of intravenous dye occasionally produces satisfactory pulmonary arteriograms, but the injection of contrast material through a catheter in the pulmonary trunk is preferable for consistent, precise films. Moreover, the catheter technique allows measurement of the right heart and pulmonary arterial pressures. Rapid sequence films record the progression of dye through pulmonary circulation and accurately demonstrate anatomic abnormalities in pulmonary arteries. Pulmonary angiography, especially in severely ill patients, may inflict significant, although not prohibitive, risk from cardiac arrythmias, myocardial penetration by the catheter, and allergic reactions to the contrast media.

On a pulmonary angiogram morphologic findings specific for embolism can be identified in more than 80 per cent of patients with the disorder (Stein et al., 1967b). Intraluminal filling defects in pulmonary arteries containing nonocclusive emboli represent the most common angiographic abnormality (Fig. 10-13). Occlusive pulmonary emboli abruptly terminate the column of contrast material giving the vessel a cut-off appearance on the pulmonary arteriogram. If

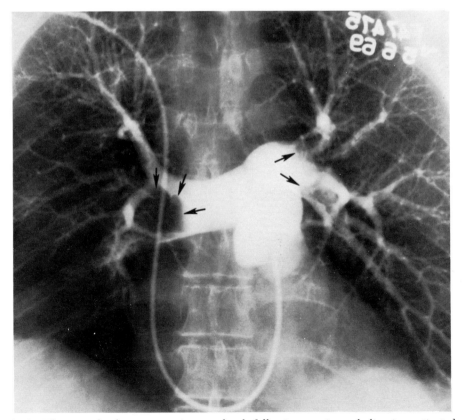

Figure 10-13. This typical pulmonary arteriogram, shortly following massive embolism in a patient, demonstrates multiple bilateral intraluminal filling defects and total occlusion of the right lower pulmonary artery (arrows).

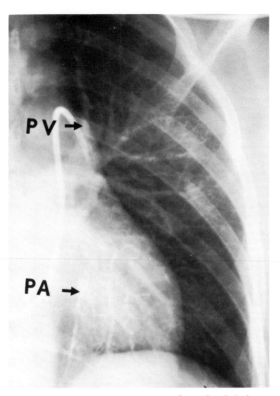

Figure 10-14. Dye is retained in the left lower pulmonary artery (PA) during the venous phase (PV) of this pulmonary angiogram. Slow transit of dye on pulmonary arteriograms indicates areas of decreased perfusion.

arterial occlusion begins at the point of bifurcation, the artery remaining patent may appear pruned of branching vessels on the arteriogram.

Less specific than morphologic demonstration of emboli by pulmonary angiography are indirect indications of circulatory alterations from pulmonary embolism. Dye retained in pulmonary arteries during the venous phase of the angiogram marks areas with decreased blood flow due to pulmonary embolism (Fig. 10-14). Pulmonary ischemia may be demonstrated on an angiogram by avascular areas or regions with small pulmonary arteries reduced in caliber. Pulmonary angiographic indications of altered pulmonary perfusion without anatomic demonstration of emboli may be suggestive, but not diagnostic, of pulmonary embolism.

Lung scanning and pulmonary angiography are complementary procedures for diagnosing pulmonary embolism, and each has certain advantages over the other. The procedures differ little in accuracy, and scan perfusion defects usually coincide with angiographic abnormalities (Fig. 10-15). Lung scanning determines regional pulmonary blood flow and sensitively detects small perfusion abnormalities but does not identify

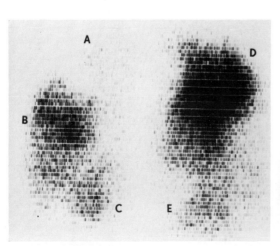

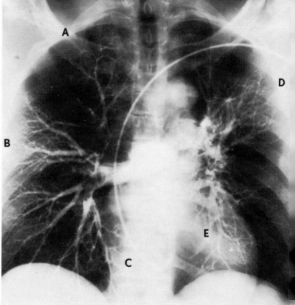

Figure 10-15. The lung scan and pulmonary arteriogram of a patient with bilateral pulmonary embolism demonstrate the usual correlation between the two studies in the determination of pulmonary perfusion. The letters on the two studies mark comparable lung areas.

their cause. Pulmonary angiography anatomically outlines embolic filling defects in major pulmonary arteries but only vaguely reflects pulmonary arterial blood flow, a limitation that prohibits accurate detection of peripheral emboli. Adequate pulmonary arteriograms require right heart catheterization, which entails significant risk in severely ill patients. Because a normal lung scan obviates pulmonary angiography, initial evaluation of pulmonary perfusion should usually be made by means of scanning. If scan diagnosis is equivocal because of a density on chest film or if an anticipated embolectomy demands anatomic localization of emboli and measurement of pulmonary arterial pressure, pulmonary angiography is indicated. Judicious use of both diagnostic procedures permits accurate diagnosis in almost all patients with clinically significant pulmonary embolism.

MANAGEMENT

Anticoagulation

The objectives of anticoagulation in pulmonary thromboembolic disorders are the limitation of venous thrombus extension and the inhibition of *in situ* thrombosis around emboli in the pulmonary arteries. Also, more than 30 per cent of patients with pulmonary embolism sustain a repeated episode, and anticoagulation seems to prevent recurrent venous thrombosis and pulmonary embolism. Heparin and coumarin compounds, the two most commonly used anticoagulants, differ in their route of administration and mechanism of action (Wright, 1969).

Heparin, a sulfate-containing mucopolysaccharide with a molecular weight of about 16,000, occurs naturally in man and is produced primarily by mast cells. It is obtained commercially from animal sources, especially beef lung. The complex actions of heparin affect most reactions in the clotting sequence. Heparin and an alpha-1 globulin cofactor form an inactive high molecular weight complex with thrombin, and the resulting thrombin inhibition inactivates much of the clotting mechanism (Shanberge, 1968). Basic polyelectrolytes, such as protamine and Polybrene, dissociate the heparin-cofactor-thrombin complex and provide a clinically important antidote to heparin anticoagulation (Porter et al., 1968).

A second action of heparin, which blocks platelet serotonin release, is possibly important in relieving bronchoconstriction in patients with pulmonary embolism. Although also degraded by liver heparinase, heparin is primarily eliminated by rapid renal excretion and must be administered with caution to patients with impaired glomerular filtration. Heparin is inactive by mouth and may be given intravenously or subcutaneously, but intramuscular injection must be avoided because of frequent hematoma formation at the puncture site. After a single intravenous injection, heparin activity peaks within minutes and clears from the circulation within a few hours at a rate inversely proportional to the dose. Subcutaneous heparin is absorbed more slowly and may not reach maximum effectiveness for up to 12 hours. Continuous intravenous heparin infusion provides immediate, predictable anticoagulation and is the preferred route of initial heparin administration (Gurewich et al., 1967).

Daily heparin doses as large as 120,000 units have been advocated for treatment of pulmonary thromboembolic disease, but experimental evidence suggests that heparinization, constantly maintaining a two- to three-fold increase in normal clotting time, is sufficient to prevent intravascular coagulation (Wessler et al., 1955). Therapeutic anticoagulation is best achieved by an initial high dose titrated down to therapeutic range rather than a gradual increase in heparin by small increments to slowly elevate the clotting time. A usual intravenous heparin dose for treatment of thrombophlebitis or pulmonary embolism is 40,000 units daily, but individual patients vary widely in response to the drug. O'Sullivan and associates (1968) observed in 100 patients a mean daily heparin dose of 26,500 units to maintain a 20- to 30-minute clotting time. However, individual patient requirements ranged from 10,000 to 60,000 units—22 per cent managed with less than 15,000 units daily and 20 per cent required more than 40,000 units daily. Also, the individual patient's response to heparin changes with time, and during nine days average treatment, the essential heparin dose increased in 33 and decreased in 25 of the 100 patients. The variable patient response to heparin and the changeable requirements of individual patients demand daily clotting time determinations throughout the therapy period in order to adjust the dose properly. After intravenous heparin maintains stable anticoagulation for several days, subcutaneous heparin administration every four or six hours may prove more convenient and equally effective. Clinical studies have not clearly defined an optimum anticoagulation period for the treatment of thrombophlebitis and pulmonary embolism, but they suggest that anticoagulation, prolonged a minimum of three months after an initial week of heparin therapy, provides effective protection.

Anticoagulants of the coumarin or indandione groups are effective by oral administration and, therefore, are the preferable agents for long-termed anticoagulation. These oral anticoagulants are synthetic compounds that have no direct action on the clotting mechanism but act by suppressing synthesis in the liver of prothrombin and other clotting factors. Because of this suppression, the blood concentration of the affected clotting factors gradually declines, and therapeutic anticoagulation levels are usually attained two days after institution of the drug. In treatment of thrombophlebitis and pulmonary embolism, heparin must be continued until adequate oral anticoagulation is achieved. Warfarin is the most commonly used oral anticoagulant, and an initial 30 mg. loading dose followed by a 5 mg. daily maintenance dose usually depresses prothrombin time to 25 per cent of normal, which is the optimum therapeutic range.

The variable patient response to coumarin compounds makes daily prothrombin time determinations essential during initial therapy and makes less frequent but regular determinations necessary throughout the duration of anticoagulation. Patients with liver disease are unusually sensitive to oral anticoagulation, and a variety of drugs alter coumarin action. Phenobarbital, chloral hydrate, glutethimide (Doriden), meprobamate, griseofulvin, and haloperidol (Haldol) potentiate liver degradation of coumarins, and withdrawal of these drugs with constant coumarin administration may depress the prothrombin time to dangerous levels. Anti-inflammatory steroids, salicylates, and diphenylhydantoin (Dilantin) displace coumarins from plasma proteins, enhancing anticoagulation. Oral antibiotics may also potentiate the lowering of prothrombin time by inhibiting gut bacteria vitamin-K synthesis. Oral vitamin K (5 mg.) is a rapid, effective coumarin antidote that may be used to increase the prothrombin time in anticoagulated patients prior to operation or that may be necessary in excessively anticoagulated or hemorrhaging patients.

In 1938, Murray and colleagues first reported the efficacy of *heparin* therapy in patients with thromboembolic disorders. Bauer (1964) reviewed 937 patients treated with heparin over an 18-year period. Bronchopneumonia caused the only two deaths in 59 patients heparinized for treatment of significant pulmonary embolism, and no recurrent embolic episodes were observed. Fatal pulmonary embolism occurred in five of the 878 patients treated with heparin for venous thrombosis, but heparin had been discontinued in three of these patients prior to embolism. Recurrence or extension of venous thrombosis was observed in only 24 of the 937 patients during or soon after heparin treatment.

Barritt and associates (1960) randomly assigned 35 patients, with the diagnosis of pulmonary embolism and without contraindication to anticoagulation, to control and treated groups. The treated patients received 10,000 units of heparin every six hours for 36 hours and oral anticoagulation for 14 days. Five of 19 untreated patients died and five others experienced nonfatal recurrent embolism. In 16 anticoagulated patients, the single death resulted from pneumonia and gastrointestinal bleeding, and no recurrent pulmonary embolism was observed. Because of these results, no further patients were left untreated. In 30 consecutive patients added to the anticoagulated group with pulmonary embolism, only one sustained a nonfatal recurrent embolic episode, and the single death resulted from acute tubular necrosis precipitated by oral anticoagulation.

O'Sullivan and associates (1968) treated 100 patients with venous thrombosis or pulmonary embolism with 26,500 units of heparin daily for nine days followed by oral anticoagulation, continued for three to six months. During heparin therapy only two minor and two fatal embolic episodes occurred, and two patients developed thrombophlebitis. While on oral anticoagulants, two patients sustained massive pulmonary embolism, which was fatal in one, and six patients demonstrated recurrent thrombophlebitis. These studies indicate anticoagulation to be highly, but not totally, effective in the treatment of thrombophlebitis and pulmonary embolism.

Anticoagulant efficacy in treatment of established thrombophlebitis and pulmonary embolism prompted investigation into its use to prevent venous thrombosis in high-risk patients. Prophylactic anticoagulation has been shown to reduce significantly thromboembolic complications in elderly patients with hip fractures, a group highly predisposed to venous thrombosis and pulmonary embolism. Sevitt et al., (1959), Salzman et al., (1966), and Eskeland et al., (1966) randomly assigned elderly patients with hip fractures and no contraindication to a control group or group treated with prophylactic oral anticoagulation. Table II summarizes data compiled from the 665 patients in these three studies. Prophylactic anticoagulation caused a three-fold reduction in venous thrombosis and a five-fold reduction in pulmonary embolism confirmed at autopsy, but doubled the occurrence of hemorrhage. Many patients in the treated group were inadequately anticoagulated when thromboembolism occurred, indicating that stable anticoagulation might prove even more effective in preventing thrombosis.

Use of prophylactic anticoagulation in high-risk operative patients has also been investigated. Harris and associates randomly separated 116 patients over the age of 40 into control and treated groups prior to elective hip arthroplasty. Patients with contraindications to anticoagulation remained untreated and patients with previous thrombophlebitis were added to the treated group, which began warfarin anticoagulation the day of operation. Of 70 treated patients, thrombophlebitis developed in five and none suffered pulmonary embolism. Seven incidents of pulmonary embolism and 23 episodes of thrombophlebitis complicated postoperative recovery in the 67 untreated patients.

Matis (1968) randomly separated all preoperative patients without history of thromboembolism and without contraindication to anticoagulation into a control untreated group of 5872 patients and a group of 5867 patients, who began taking oral anticoagulants after operation. The incidence of thrombophlebitis or pulmonary embolism diagnosed clinically was 0.003 per cent in treated patients and 0.017 per cent in the control group. Other studies without random controls also suggest that prophylactic anticoagulation causes a three- to five-fold decrease in thromboembolic complications in surgical patients (Shepard et al., 1966; Skinner et al., 1967). Anticoagulation reduces the incidence of thrombophlebitis and pulmonary embolism in surgical patients at the cost of an increase in hemorrhagic complications.

Anticoagulation approximately doubles the risk of hemorrhage in patients, and major hemorrhage occurs in about four per cent of patients anticoagulated (Table 10-2). Royston (1966), in 1250 treatment-years of 524 patients receiving heparin or oral anticoagulants, observed 66 episodes of hemorrhage, an average of one hemorrhage complication for every 19 treatment-years. Anticoagulation appeared relatively safe, and only ten deaths could be ascribed to bleeding. Gastrointestinal bleeding accounted for one third of the 66 episodes, and genitourinary and cerebral bleeding were also common. Blood pressure did not appear to be related to the frequency of hemorrhage from any site. Clinical judgment must determine whether the potential benefit of anticoagulation outweighs the increased risk of bleeding in individual patients. Recent or anticipated operations often confuse the relative merit of anticoagulation in surgical patients with pulmonary embolism. However, wound bleeding in anticoagulated patients is usually not severe, and if control of hemorrhage proves difficult, anticoagulation can be rapidly reversed with protamine. All patients should be carefully questioned for a history of bleeding before anticoagulation is initiated and repeatedly examined for evidence of hemorrhage throughout the treatment period. Controlled anticoagulation effectively and safely treats thrombophlebitis and pulmonary embolism in carefully selected patients.

Table 10-2. Prophylactic Anticoagulation in Elderly Patients with Hip Fractures

	Control Group Average	Treated Group Average
Total patients	333	332
Mortality	26%	19%
Patients given autopsy	69	42
Venous thrombosis at autopsy	72%	26%
Pulmonary embolism at autopsy	49%	10%
Minor Hemorrhage	9%	17%
Major Hemorrhage	2%	4%

Prophylactic anticoagulation significantly reduces the incidence of venous thrombosis and its routine use may eventually prove warranted in high-risk patient groups.

DEXTRAN AND FIBRINOLYTIC THERAPY

Recent clinical studies report experimental use of dextran and fibrinolytic therapy in patients with pulmonary embolic disease. Dextran 40 and 70 are antithrombogenic agents that decrease blood viscosity and physically interfere with normal clotting. Dextran does not prevent experimental venous thrombosis but does decrease thrombus propagation (Johnson et al., 1968). In a double-blind study, Bernard and colleagues (1969) treated 14 patients having thrombophlebitis confirmed by phlebogram with saline or dextran 70 solution. Seven days of treatment demonstrated no difference in clinical response or objective phlebogram improvement in the two patient groups. Atik and associates (1968) randomly separated 84 patients with hip fractures into 58 untreated controls and 26 who received daily dextran infusions during the acute phase of illness. None of the 26 treated controls demonstrated thrombosis or embolism, but of 58 untreated patients, two had thrombophlebitis and seven sustained pulmonary embolism. Until further evidence accumulates, the use of dextran for the prevention or treatment of thromboembolic disease must remain experimental.

Clot dissolution by activation of the normal fibrinolytic system theoretically appears to be a more direct treatment of pulmonary embolism than anticoagulation. Streptokinase, a potent fibrinolytic activator, has been shown to rapidly lyse pulmonary emboli in man (Hirsh et al., 1968). However, treatment with this protein foreign to man causes frequent febrile and antigenic reactions. Urokinase, a substance obtained from human urine, is identical or quite similar to intrinsic tissue activator that converts plasminogen to plasmin, a fibrinolytic enzyme (Fig. 10-3). Urokinase infusion in patients with pulmonary embolism has been associated with rapid lysis of the embolus. Reports of 36 patients with pulmonary embolism treated with urokinase are now available, and rapid resolution was observed in 25 of the 36 patients (Sautter et al., 1967b; Sasahara et al., 1967a; Tow et al., 1967b;

Genton et al., 1968). However, bleeding frequently complicates urokinase treatment and occasionally proves fatal. Several institutions are presently cooperating in a clinical study sponsored by the National Institutes of Health evaluating the relative merits of heparin and urokinase in treatment of pulmonary embolism. Data from this study should both define the incidence of bleeding with fibrinolytic therapy and differentiate drug-induced lysis from normal thrombus resolution by the lungs.

VENOUS THROMBECTOMY

In 1948, Leriche described iliofemoral thrombectomy as treatment for acute deep vein thrombosis and prevention of pulmonary embolism. Local anesthesia is usually adequate for femoral vein exposure, and iliac and femoral vein thrombi are extracted with forceps or Fogarty catheter and expressed by means of leg compression. Anticoagulation is begun postoperatively and patients are placed at bed rest with the leg elevated. Although venous thrombectomy appears uncomplicated, an average blood loss of one liter and a 20 per cent incidence of wound disruption indicate a significant morbidity, and mortality associated with the operation approaches five per cent. Fatal pulmonary embolism has occurred during, or soon after, the procedure in occasional patients, and iliofemoral venous thrombectomy has not been proved more effective than anticoagulation alone for the prevention of pulmonary embolism in patients with thrombophlebitis.

Prevention of the post-phlebitic leg is a second objective of venous thrombectomy, and several reports of the procedure in patients with acute thrombophlebitis claim absence of significant leg edema in 50 to 80 per cent of patients observed two or three years (Fogarty et al., 1966; Wilson et al., 1967; Palma, 1968). Haller and associates (1963) found normal legs in 84 per cent of 45 patients, who were observed at an average of 18 months after thrombectomy for acute thrombophlebitis. However, a five-year follow-up in 39 of these patients found edema requiring elastic stocking support in all but one patient, a six-year-old-boy (Lansing et al., 1968). Phlebograms performed on 15 patients demonstrated the absence of functioning valves in every patient. This interesting group of patients indicates that venous insufficiency may gradually develop several years after iliofemoral venous thrombectomy and suggests that the procedure may hold little, if any, advantage over anticoagulation for treatment of thrombophlebitis. The rare but serious occurrence of massive venous thrombosis unresponsive to aggressive anticoagulation, and causing *phlegmasia cerulea dolens,* does definitely indicate venous thrombectomy for the prevention of gangrene.

INFERIOR VENA CAVAL INTERRUPTION

Vessel ligation proximal to venous thrombi appears logical for the prevention of pulmonary embolism, and a variety of sites and methods for retaining thrombi in the venous system have been devised. Although venous ligation for suppurative thrombophlebitis was reported as early as 1865, Homans in 1934 advocated ligation of the superficial or common femoral veins in patients with bland thrombophlebitis for the prevention of pulmonary embolism. However, postmortem studies in patients with pulmonary embolism demonstrate about 50 per cent of venous thrombi to extend above the inguinal ligament, and femoral vein ligation would offer ineffective prophylaxis for these patients. Inferior vena caval interruption provides more effective protection from pulmonary embolism than femoral vein ligation and causes less morbidity and mortality (Dale, 1958). More than 90 per cent of venous thrombi in patients with pulmonary embolism arise in tributaries of the inferior vena cava and simple ligation of this vessel prevents recurrent embolism in most patients.

The inferior vena cava is usually approached using retroperitoneal dissection through a right transverse incision at the level of the umbilicus. The inferior vena cava is ligated immediately below the renal veins to prevent blood stasis in a *cul-de-sac* created proximal to the site of occlusion. A transperitoneal approach may be preferable in patients with pelvic thrombophlebitis in whom ovarian or testicular vein ligation should be added to vena caval interruption. Vena caval occlusion immediately decreases cardiac output, and marked peripheral venous pressure elevation dilates the vena cava distal to the ligation (Maraan et al., 1965; Benavides et al., 1967). Increased

venous pressure stimulates collateral formation, and large lumbar veins are apparent on inferior vena cavagrams within a week after ligation. Within several months, testicular, ovarian, omental, and periureteral veins dilate into large collateral channels, and peripheral venous pressure decreases. Some degree of leg edema frequently follows inferior vena caval ligation, and patients should be kept on bed rest with the leg elevated during the immediate postoperative period.

Amador and associates (1968) observed a 15 per cent mortality associated with inferior vena caval ligation in 119 patients with pulmonary embolism. Progressive heart failure was present in two-thirds of the deaths and was the most common cause of death associated with inferior vena caval ligation. Mortality was 55 per cent in patients with severe heart failure prior to inferior vena caval ligation, which suggests that the procedure is contraindicated in patients with uncontrolled heart failure. Thrombus was observed at the site of vena caval ligation in four of 37 patients studied at autopsy, and recurrent pulmonary emboli were reported in three patients at postmortem examination.

Parrish and associates (1968) reviewed reports of 703 patients undergoing inferior vena caval ligation for pulmonary embolism and totaled 22 nonfatal and six fatal postoperative embolic episodes, a failure rate of four per cent. Experimental embolism in dogs within two days after inferior vena caval ligation showed that emboli pass through large dilated collateral veins. Although pulmonary emboli may arise in the right heart or in veins that are not tributaries of the inferior vena cava, most recurrent emboli course through large collateral veins that develop after vena caval ligation.

Mozes and colleagues (1966) observed a 12 per cent mortality in 118 patients with inferior vena caval ligation for pulmonary embolism, and four of the 14 deaths appeared directly related to the operation. Pulmonary embolism recurred after the procedure in four patients and caused death in one. Postoperative leg pain and swelling were common, and four patients developed massive venous thrombosis requiring thrombectomy. Chronic leg edema continued in 58 per cent and was severe in 13 per cent of the patients. This high incidence of venous complications after vena caval ligation prompted the search for a less disabling but equally effective operation to prevent pulmonary embolism.

Of the large variety of methods devised for partial interruption of the inferior vena cava, plication and clip application are the two most useful procedures. Spencer and associates (1960) reported vena caval plication with a single row of mattress sutures spaced 4 to 5 mm. apart to divide the vessel into three or four small channels. Six of 39 patients (15 per cent) undergoing vena caval plication died within a month of operation, but none of the deaths appeared related to the procedure. Recurrent pulmonary embolism was not observed in the immediate postoperative period, but one patient sustained pulmonary embolism several months after inferior vena caval plication. Vena caval occlusion was demonstrated in only three of 23 patients in whom the vessel was studied radiographically or at autopsy. Extensive venous thrombosis, which developed in four of 39 patients soon after plication, represented the most significant postoperative complication. Chronic leg edema persisted in nine patients but in only three was it sufficient to require supportive stockings.

Burget and associates (1967) reported inferior vena caval plication in 24 patients with pulmonary embolism without an operative death or recurrent embolism. The vena cava remained patent radiographically in 14 out of 17 patients studied several months after operation, and only five of 24 patients required elastic stockings for venous stasis.

Teflon-clip application offers another method for partial interruption of the inferior vena cava. Miles devised a serrated Teflon clip that divides the inferior vena cava into 3- to 4-mm. channels. Clip application in 104 patients with pulmonary embolism was associated with ten deaths (9.6 per cent), and pulmonary embolism recurred postoperatively in four patients (Miles et al., 1969). The inferior vena cava remained

patent in 25 of 34 patients (76 per cent) studied radiographically or at autopsy. In the first postoperative month, acute thrombophlebitis developed in 18 patients, and leg edema occurred in a majority of patients but remained severe and persistent in only eight of 94 surviving patients. Moretz (1959) developed a nonserrated Teflon clip that narrows the inferior vena cava to a flat, three-mm. lumen. Application of this clip in 62 patients with pulmonary embolism was associated with 27 per cent mortality, but only four of the 17 deaths appeared related to operation. Recurrent pulmonary embolism was documented in four patients, and the inferior vena cava was occluded in eight of 31 patients studied postoperatively. Leg edema present in 24 of 25 surviving patients was severe in only four.

The effectiveness of partial interruption of the inferior vena cava in preventing pulmonary embolism prompted Carmichael (1967) to prophylactically plicate the inferior vena cava during abdominal operation in 36 patients with a high risk of pulmonary embolism. Nine of the 25 patients who survived developed thrombophlebitis, and postmortem examination in one patient demonstrated a fresh lethal pulmonary embolus believed to arise from the inferior vena cava, which was thrombosed at the plication site.

The results of the major methods of inferior vena caval interruption are summarized in Table 10-3. Mortality associated with each of the procedures ranges from 10 to 15 per cent, but patients were often critically ill prior to operation and the procedure itself appeared to cause a small proportion of deaths. Clinically obvious pulmonary embolism recurs in about four per cent of patients after any operation for inferior vena caval interruption, although some series demonstrate an appreciably higher incidence, up to 20 per cent (Gurewich et al., 1966). Because emboli smaller than 3 mm. in diameter are not retained by partial interruption of the

TABLE 10-3. Operations for Inferior Vena Cava Interruption

	Ligation (Mozes, 1966)	Plication (Spencer, 1965)	Serrated Clip (Miles, 1969)
Patients	118	39	104
Mortality	12% (1 week)	15% (1 month)	10% (1 month)
Recurrent emboli	3.5%	2.6%	3.8%
Vena cava patency	—	87%	76%
Persistent leg edema	58%	8%	9%

vena cava, ligation would appear to be the preferable surgical method in patients with septic embolism or recurrent embolism causing cor pulmonale (Collins et al., 1952). Except for these two uncommon situations, partial interruption of the inferior vena cava appears equally as effective as total ligation in the prevention of pulmonary embolism and causes fewer venous stasis complications. Vena caval patency after partial interruption is maintained in about 80 per cent of the patients, and various operative methods to achieve partial vena caval interruption do not differ significantly in effectiveness or risk. Increasing evidence supports the concept that vena caval interruption is associated with significant morbidity and mortality and should be reserved for quite firm indications.

PULMONARY EMBOLECTOMY

At the German Surgical Conference of 1908, Trendelenburg proposed direct removal of emboli from the pulmonary circulation. The pulmonary trunk was exposed through a T-shaped incision along the left sternal border and left second rib. A rubber tube elevated and occluded the pulmonary trunk, which was rapidly emptied of thrombus, and the pulmonary arteriotomy was clamped to permit pulmonary arterial flow during vessel closure. Trendelenburg demonstrated the healing pulmonary artery of a calf, sacrificed four months after the direct removal of a large experimental embolus. He reported three unsuccessful pulmonary embolectomies in man, and that one patient, in whom the operation initially appeared successful, died 37 hours after operation due to internal mammary artery bleeding. Kirschner performed the first successful pulmonary embolectomy in 1924. However, only seven of 300 pulmonary embolectomies attempted by 1930 proved successful, and the operation gradually fell into disuse.

Experimentation into methods of artificial blood oxygenation to safely divert blood from the pulmonary circulation during embolectomy stimulated the development by Gibbon of cardiopulmonary bypass in 1953. Sharp (1962) performed the first successful pulmonary embolectomy with support of cardiopulmonary bypass. Even with modern surgical technique, mortality of the original Trendelenburg method of pulmonary embolectomy remains 85 per cent, and use of

cardiopulmonary bypass offers a safer operative method (Vosschulte, 1965).

Pulmonary embolectomy is indicated for patients with massive embolism shown in pulmonary arteriograms who persist in uncontrollable shock and progressive right heart failure despite aggressive medical therapy. General anesthesia imposes significant operative risk in these patients with severe circulatory alterations, and cardiac arrest may occur prior to the establishment of a cardiopulmonary bypass. Partial circulatory bypass from the inferior vena cava to the femoral artery may be used to support the failing right heart before total bypass is instituted. It can be achieved rapidly, using only local anesthesia for the exposure of the femoral vessels. Portable oxygenation equipment has been devised to permit immediate bedside partial circulatory bypass in patients suspected of massive pulmonary embolism (Beall et al., 1965). In general, however, surgical procedures are best confined to an orderly, adequately-equipped operating suite.

Partial circulatory bypass is not mandatory prior to general anesthesia for pulmonary embolectomy, but it appears to be indicated in most patients with severe right heart failure from massive pulmonary embolism. Through a median sternotomy, the pericardium is incised to expose the heart, and the total cardiopulmonary bypass is instituted. Emboli are extracted through a longitudinal pulmonary arteriotomy using forceps and gentle suction. Both pleural spaces are entered, and lung compression extrudes additional peripheral emboli. Brisk back bleeding from the bronchial circulation indicates the patency of peripheral pulmonary arteries and is important in evaluating the prognosis.

After the completion of pulmonary embolectomy, the inferior vena cava is commonly interrupted to prevent further pulmonary emboli. Partial vena caval interruption causes minimal circulatory disturbance and is preferable to vena caval ligation, which immediately decreases cardiac output (Maraan et al., 1968). Postoperative anticoagulation adds to the prevention of recurrent embolism by partial vena caval interruption and is indicated after pulmonary embolectomy.

Cross and Mowlem (1967) tabulated the results of 137 pulmonary embolectomies gathered from 28 centers. Cardiopulmonary

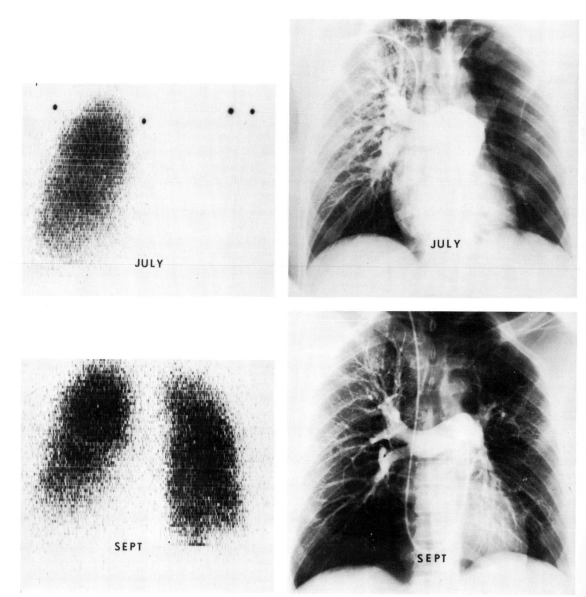

Figure 10-16. This figure illustrates the results of embolectomy in a patient with chronic pulmonary embolism (Moor and Sabiston, 1969). The patient had dyspnea on exertion and sustained recurrent pulmonary emboli. Total absence of pulmonary arterial perfusion to the left lung persisted unchanged on pulmonary arteriogram for several months. The lung scan and pulmonary arteriogram in July were completed just prior to pulmonary embolectomy for chronic arterial obstruction. The pulmonary arterial pressure preoperatively was 75/30 mm. Hg and fell to 40/20 following embolectomy. Studies repeated two months postoperatively indicate patency of the left pulmonary artery. Pulmonary emboli usually completely resolve spontaneously, but occasionally they fail to resolve and the patient demonstrates chronic pulmonary arterial occlusion. Embolectomy to restore pulmonary flow may be indicated for such patients.

bypass was used in 115 patients and the remaining 22 patients underwent some modification of the classic Trendelenburg pulmonary embolectomy. Initial operative mortality was 57 per cent, and late hospital deaths decreased the survival rate to 34 per cent. Pulmonary embolectomy proved fatal in all nine incorrectly diagnosed patients who demonstrated no emboli at operation. Subsequent reports of 67 patients undergoing pulmonary embolectomy with cardiopulmonary bypass averaged a 50 per cent operative mortality, and all seven of the patients in whom the diagnosis of embolism proved incorrect died following embolectomy (Beall et al., 1965; Khazer et al., 1967; Logan et al., 1967; Paneth et al., 1967; Sautter et al., 1967b; Stansel et al., 1967; Berger et al., 1968; Keon et al., 1969). High mortality in patients subjected to pulmonary embolectomy, with severe circulatory impairment resulting from a cause other than massive pulmonary embolism, makes mandatory an accurate diagnosis before operation. Although massive pulmonary embolism is often rapidly fatal, bypassing specific diagnostic procedures in order to perform immediate embolectomy is not justified, because of the high risk incurred by an inaccurate diagnosis.

Donaldson (1963) reviewed autopsy studies on 271 patients sustaining fatal pulmonary embolism and found that only 25 per cent of the patients survived longer than one hour after the onset of symptoms. A more recent autopsy study in 63 patients with fatal pulmonary embolism shows that 43 per cent of patients survived more than two hours after the first clinical manifestations of embolism (Berger et al., 1968). Many rapid deaths following massive pulmonary embolism reportedly occur in patients terminal because of another disease, and a majority of patients potentially able to be saved by pulmonary embolectomy can be sustained during the added short time required for pulmonary angiography.

The mortality in over 50 per cent of the operations indicates that pulmonary embolectomy should be reserved for patients who seem unlikely to recover without it. Lung scanning and pulmonary arteriography, with pulmonary artery pressure measurements, aid objective preoperative evaluation of the patient by documenting the severity of embolism. In most patients, pulmonary vascular occlusion exceeding 50 per cent and severe right heart failure, reflected in elevated end diastolic right ventricular pressure, are minimal indications for embolectomy. However, the final decision for pulmonary embolectomy rests upon the subjective clinical judgment that circulatory deterioriation progresses during a period of intense medical therapy. Most pulmonary emboli spontaneously resolve and embolectomy is usually not essential to restore normal pulmonary function. However, in some patients emboli remain occlusive in large pulmonary arteries and significantly impair pulmonary function. Elective pulmonary embolectomy using cardiopulmonary bypass has been shown to restore flow to *chronically* occluded pulmonary arteries with a corresponding correction of pulmonary hypertension (Fig. 10-16). This procedure may be useful in regaining adequate pulmonary function when spontaneous resolution of large pulmonary emboli fails to occur (Moor and Sabiston, 1969).

COMPOSITE MANAGEMENT

A systematic approach to the diagnosis and treatment of thrombophlebitis and pulmonary embolism is depicted in Figure 10-17. The variable clinical manifestations and broad spectrum of severity of thromboembolic disease require a flexible approach to treatment of the disorder, and clinical judgment must be used to adapt the general principles of proper management to the individual patient's situation. The risk and inconvenience of diagnostic procedures must be weighed against the potential benefit of accurately directed treatment. High-risk therapy, such as pulmonary embolectomy, demands an unequivocal diagnosis; but anticoagulation therapy, which is little associated with morbidity or mortality, is justified with only the clinical suspicion of thrombophlebitis or pulmonary embolism. Each of the accepted medical and operative methods of treatment has characteristic advantages and disadvantages and provides a complementary approach to managing this protean disorder. Prejudiced fixation on a single method of therapy for all patients with pulmonary embolism is not warranted, as is shown in available clinical studies, and should be avoided.

Prevention is the most satisfactory treatment of pulmonary embolism. It is important to have a gentle operative technique for all surgical patients, and to avoid vena caval compression through retraction during laparotomy. Also, constricting straps that impede venous flow should not be placed firmly over the legs of an anesthetized patient. Early postoperative ambulation stimulates venous flow and provides a simple but effective method for preventing venous thrombosis. For surgical patients with increased risk of venous thrombosis because of age, dehydration, heart failure, injury to extremities, prolonged immobility, or previous

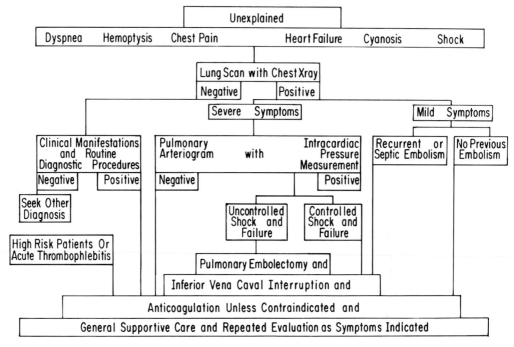

Figure 10-17. Management of pulmonary embolism from diagnosis to treatment.

thrombophlebitis, more intensive prophylactic measures should be taken. A 15-degree elevation of the foot of the bed accelerates venous flow almost as effectively as ambulation, and this simple expedient should be used whenever possible during and after operation in patients predisposed to thrombosis (McLachlin et al., 1960; Allison, 1967). The extremities of patients with increased risk of thrombosis should be examined regularly for signs of thrombophlebitis. In addition to these preventive measures, prophylactic anticoagulation is indicated in patient groups with an extremely high incidence of thromboembolism, such as the elderly with hip fractures. Treatment of patients with signs of thrombophlebitis should include aggressive heparin anticoagulation and bed rest with the legs elevated to prevent pulmonary embolism and the long-term sequelae common to postphlebitic legs. Lung scans of patients with the diagnosis of venous thrombosis are useful for detecting asymptomatic pulmonary emboli and for providing a base-line determination of pulmonary perfusion.

Most episodes of pulmonary embolism in surgical patients are minor and cause only mild, vague symptoms. However, these inconsequential minor episodes warn of the presence of venous thrombosis and permit early anticoagulation to prevent catastrophic recurrent pulmonary embolism. Clinical manifestations of pulmonary embolism are at best only suggestive, and all patients with unexplained dyspnea, chest pain, hemoptysis, or signs of right heart failure should receive a careful physical examination and a lung scan. A negative lung scan does not completely exclude the diagnosis of small peripheral emboli, and anticoagulation is still indicated if clinical diagnosis of this disorder appears relatively certain. Patients with positive lung scans require further evaluation only if symptoms appear sufficiently severe to warrant the consideration of pulmonary embolectomy. Thus, patients with mild symptoms and positive scans are spared the risk and discomfort of pulmonary angiography.

The majority of patients with mild symptoms of pulmonary embolism are best treated with anticoagulation, but occasionally patients with septic emboli or documented recurrence of embolism during adequate anticoagulation may require vena caval interruption. Anticoagulation is begun with 10,000 units of heparin in a liter of solution administered intravenously over a six-hour period. Determination of clotting time, obtained four hours after the institution of heparin and daily thereafter, aids in adjusting the dose in order to maintain clotting times in the 20- to 30-minute range. Heparin therapy is continued for a minimum of one week or until the patient is fully ambulant and adequately converted to oral anticoagulation. Follow-up lung scans are often useful to document the return of pulmonary perfusion after therapy and to assess patients for recurrent pulmonary embolism.

Patients with sudden, massive embolism develop acute respiratory distress with impending shock; therefore, pulmonary embolism must always be considered in surgical patients with unexplained cardiorespiratory arrest. After adequate ventilation and an effective heart action are established, a central venous catheter is inserted for monitoring venous pressure and administering essential drugs. Care is exercised to prevent excessive fluid administration to patients demonstrating right heart failure, and when necessary, systemic arterial hypotension is treated with isoproterenol (McDonald et al., 1968). Digitalis and oxygen are administered to patients with heart failure. Rapid, accurate evaluation of these critically ill patients is essential to confirm the diagnosis of pulmonary embolism, and an electrocardiogram and chest film are necessary to exclude the diagnosis of atelectasis, pneumonia, or myocardial infarction. When the clinical diagnosis of pulmonary embolism appears likely, heparin anticoagulation is begun prior to establishment of a definite diagnosis. *Inferior vena caval interruption or pulmonary embolectomy should not precede the objective documentation of embolism.*

Response of the patient to immediate therapy and practical considerations regarding the availability of either procedure determine whether lung scanning or pulmonary angiography should be used in diagnosing pulmonary embolism. Patients maintaining a stable clinical condition are best evaluated by means of lung scanning if the procedure is immediately available. A negative lung scan obviates pulmonary angiography and some other cause of the severe cardiorespiratory symptoms must be sought. However, patients with rapid circulatory deterioration, unchecked by medical therapy, require immediate pulmonary angiography to determine the need for pulmonary embolectomy. The objective documentation of the extent and course of pulmonary em-

bolism obtained by lung scanning and pulmonary angiography aids in the selection of appropriate therapy for the individual patient. Patients whose lung scans are diagnostic of pulmonary embolism but whose pulmonary angiograms are normal should receive anticoagulation therapy for small emboli that are detectable on a scan but not apparent on an arteriogram. When both lung scan and pulmonary arteriogram demonstrate pulmonary embolism, it is the severity of symptoms that determines the choice of treatment. Even patients with severe pulmonary embolism usually respond well to anticoagulation, the treatment of choice for the majority of patients with pulmonary embolism. However, inferior vena caval interruption may be necessary in occasional patients for whom an extremely high risk of hemorrhage accompanies anticoagulation therapy. Vena caval interruption may also be indicated for patients with septic embolism, cor pulmonale, or for those with severely altered circulation and judged to be unable to withstand even a minor recurrent pulmonary embolus. Pulmonary embolectomy is indicated in patients with massive embolism, shock, and progressive heart failure that fails to respond to intensive medical therapy. With this systematic approach, complete evaluation of patients with manifestations suggestive of pulmonary embolism requires a delay of only a relatively short time. The hazards of surgical therapy for pulmonary embolism justify this delay even in severely ill patients.

SUMMARY

Pulmonary embolism is a common and often fatal postoperative complication. Dyspnea is the most common clinical manifestation in pulmonary embolism, and other signs are frequently inconsistent and often vague. The chest film, electrocardiogram, and serum enzyme determinations are helpful in excluding other cardiorespiratory diseases, although they are frequently unreliable in establishing an objective diagnosis of pulmonary embolism.

Lung scanning is a safe, sensitive procedure for the initial evaluation of symptoms suggestive of pulmonary embolism, and pulmonary ateriography may be necessary in certain patients. Anticoagulation is effective in the prevention and treatment of pulmonary embolism and is successful in the vast majority of patients. Emboli that are not fatal gradually resolve in the pulmonary circulation. Vena caval interruption is occasionally beneficial in selected patients, especially those with septic emboli and cor pulmonale. Under certain circumstances pulmonary embolectomy is indicated: these are massive embolism, which abruptly increases pulmonary arterial pressure, and severe obstruction, which causes right heart failure and intractable shock. The hazards of these surgical procedures demand that a definite diagnosis of pulmonary embolism be made and a *systematic* approach to the diagnosis and treatment of pulmonary embolism should be followed.

REFERENCES

Allgood, R. J., Wolfe, W. G., Ebert, P. A., and Sabiston, D. C., Jr.: Effects of carbon dioxide on bronchoconstriction after pulmonary artery occlusion. Amer. J. Physiol., 214:772, 1968.

Allison, P. R.: Symposium on safe surgery. Circulatory and respiratory problems. Pulmonary embolism and thrombophlebitis. Brit. J. Surg. (Supple.), 54:466, 1967.

Amader, E., Li, T. K., and Crane, C.: Ligation of inferior vena cava for thromboembolism. JAMA, 206:1758, 1968.

Andreasen, C., and Lassen, H. K.: Fatal pulmonary embolism in a surgical department during a period of 15 years. Acta. Chir. Scand. (Supple.), 343:42, 1965.

Ardlie, N. G., Kinlough, R. L., and Schwartz, C. J.: In vitro thrombosis and platelet behavior after operation. Aust. Ann. Med., 16:269, 1967.

Atik, M., Hanson, B., Iola, F., and Harkness, J. W.: Pulmonary embolism: A preventable complication. Amer. Surg., 34:888, 1968.

Barritt, D. W., and Jordan, S. C.: Anticoagulant drugs in the treatment of pulmonary embolism. Lancet, 1:1309, 1960.

Bauer, G.: Clinical experience of a surgeon in the use of heparin. Amer. J. Cardiol., 14:29, 1964.

Beall, A. C., and Cooley, D. A.: Current status of embolectomy for acute massive pulmonary embolism. Amer. J. Cardiol., 16:828, 1965.

Benavides, J., and Noon, R.: Experimental evaluation of inferior vena cava procedures to prevent pulmonary embolism. Amer. Surg., 166:195, 1967.

Bennett, P. N.: Postoperative changes in platelet adhesiveness. J. Clin. Path., 20:708, 1967.

Berger, R. L., Gibson, H., and Ferris, E. J.: A reappraisal of the indications for pulmonary embolectomy. Amer. J. Surg., 116:403, 1968.

Bernard, H. R., Powers, S. R., Jr., Leather, R. P., and Clark, W. R., Jr.: A prospective double blind study of clinical dextran in thrombophlebitis. Surgery, 65:191, 1969.

Bernthal, T., Horres, A. D., and Taylor, J. T., III: Pulmonary vascular obstruction in graded tachypneagenic diffuse embolism. Amer. J. Physiol., 200:279, 1961.

Boyer, N. H., and Curry, J. J.: Bronchospasm associated with pulmonary embolism. Arch. Intern. Med., 73:403, 1944.

Brofman, B. L., Charms, B. L., Kohn, P. M., Edler, J., Newman, R., and Rizika, M.: Unilateral pulmonary artery occlusion in man. J. Thorac. Surg., 34:206, 1957.

Burget, D. E., Jr., Henzel, J. H., Smith, J. L., and Pories, W. J.: Inferior vena cava plication for prevention of pulmonary embolism: Results in 24 cases. Ann. Surg., 165:437, 1967.

Caldini, P.: Pulmonary hemodynamics and arterial oxygen saturation in pulmonary embolism. J. Appl. Physiol., 20:184, 1965.

Carmichael, J. D., and Edwards, W. S.: Prophylactic inferior vena caval plication. Surg. Gynec. Obstet., 124:785, 1967.

Chait, A., Summers, D., Krasnow, N., and Wechsler, B. M.: Observations on the fate of large pulmonary emboli. Amer. J. Roentgen., 100:364, 1967.

Clark, C., and Cotton, L. T.: Blood flow in deep veins of the leg. Recording technique and evaluation of methods to increase flow during operation. Brit. J. Surg., 55:211, 1968.

Cohnheim, J. F.: Lectures on general pathology. London. The New Sydenham Society, 1889, p. 50.

Collins, C. G., Norton, R. O., Nelson, E. W., and Weinstein, B. B.: Suppurative pelvic thrombophlebitis. IV. Results. Surgery, 31:528, 1952.

Cross, F. S., and Mowlem, A.: A survey of the current status of pulmonary embolectomy for massive pulmonary embolism. Circulation (Supple.): 86, 1967.

Cruveilhier, J.: Anatomie pathologique du corps humain. Paris, J. B. Bailliere, 1829.

Cugell, D. W., Buckingham, W. B., Webster, J. R., Jr., and Kettel, L. J.: The limitations of laboratory methods in the diagnosis of pulmonary embolism. Med. Clin. N. Amer., 51:175, 1967.

Dale, W. A.: Ligation of the inferior vena cava for thromboembolism. Surgery, 43:24, 1958.

DeBakey, M. E.: Critical evaluation of the problem of thromboembolism. Surg. Gynec. Obstet., 98:1, 1954.

Dexter, L., and Smith, G. T.: Quantitative studies of pulmonary embolism. Amer. J. Med. Sci., 247:641, 1964.

Donaldson, G. N., Williams, L., Scannell, G., and Shaw, R.: A reappraisal of the application of the Trendelenburg operation to massive fatal embolism. New Eng. J. Med., 268:171, 1963.

Downing, E., and Vidone, R. A.: Pulmonary vascular responses to embolization with autologous thrombi. Surg. Gynec. Obstet., 125:269, 1967.

Ebert, P. A., Allgood, R. J., Jones, H. W., III, and Sabiston, D. C., Jr.: Hemodynamics during pulmonary artery occlusion. Surgery, 62:18, 1967.

Edmunds, L. H., Jr., and Holm, J. C.: Effect of atelectasis on lung changes after pulmonary arterial ligation. J. Appl. Physiol., 25:115, 1968.

Eskeland, G., Solheim, K., and Skjoiten, F.: Anticoagulant prophylaxis thromboembolism and mortality in elderly patients with hip fractures. A controlled clinical trial. Acta. Chir. Scand., 131:16, 1966.

Evans, G. L., Dalen, J. E., and Dexter, L.: Pulmonary embolism during pregnancy. JAMA, 206:320, 1968.

Fleischner, F. G.: Recurrent pulmonary embolism and cor pulmonale. New Eng. J. Med., 276:1213, 1967.

Fleming, H. A., and Bailey, S. M.: Massive pulmonary

embolism in healthy people. Brit. Med. J., *5499:* 1322, 1966.

Fogarty, T. J., Dennis, D., and Kirppaehne, W. W.: Surgical management of iliofemoral venous thrombosis. Amer. J. Surg., *112:*211, 1966.

Freeark, R. J., Boswick, J., and Fardin, R.: Post-traumatic venous thrombosis. Arch. Surg., 95:567, 1967.

Freiman, D. G., Suyemoto, J., and Wessler, S.: Frequency of pulmonary thromboembolism in man. New Eng. J. Med., 272:1278, 1965.

Gahagan, T., Manzor, A., Isaac, B., and Mathur, A. N.: Reestablishment of pulmonary artery flow after prolonged complete occlusion. Studies in dogs. JAMA, *198:*639, 1966.

Genton, E., and Wolf, P. S.: Urokinase therapy in pulmonary thromboembolism. Amer. Heart J., 76:628, 1968.

Gibbon, J. H., Jr., Hopkinson, M., and Churchill, E. D.: Changes in the circulation produced by gradual occlusion of the pulmonary artery. J. Clin. Invest., *11:*543, 1932.

Gurewich, V., Thomas, D. P., and Rabinov, K. R.: Pulmonary embolism after ligation of the inferior vena cava. New Eng. J. Med., *274:*1350, 1966.

Gurewich, V., Thomas, D. P., Stein, M., and Wessler, S.: Bronchoconstriction in the presence of pulmonary embolism. Circulation, 27:339, 1963.

Gurewich, V., Thomas, D. P., and Stuart, R. K.: Some guidelines for heparin therapy of venous thromboembolic disease. JAMA, 199:116, 1967.

Guzman, S. V., Chavez, F. R., and Imperial, E. S.: Myocardial blood flow after experimental pulmonary embolism in the intact dog. Amer. Heart J., 68:66, 1964.

Haggart, G., and Walker, A. M.: The physiology of pulmonary embolism as disclosed by quantitative occlusion of the pulmonary artery. Arch. Surg., 6:764, 1923.

Haller, J. A., and Abrams, B. L.: Use of thrombectomy in the treatment of acute iliofemoral venous thrombosis in forty-five patients. Ann. Surg., 158:561, 1963.

Harris, W. H., Salzman, E. W., and Desanctis, R. W.: The prevention of thromboembolic disease by prophylactic anticoagulation. A controlled study in elective hip surgery. J. Bone Joint Surg., 49:81, 1967.

Hirsch, J., and McBride, J. A.: Increased platelet adhesiveness in recurrent venous thrombosis and pulmonary embolism. Brit. Med. J., 2:797, 1965.

Hirsch, J., Hale, G. S., McDonald, I. G., McCarthy, R. A., and Pitt, A.: Streptokinase therapy in acute major pulmonary embolism: Effectiveness and problems. Brit. Med. J., 4:729, 1968.

Hirst, A. E., Gore, I., Tanaka, K., Samuel, I., and Krishtmukti, I.: Myocardial infarction and pulmonary embolism. Arch Path., (Chicago) 80:365, 1965.

Homans, J.: Thrombosis of the deep veins of the leg, causing pulmonary embolism. New Eng. J. Med., 211:993, 1934.

Horres, A. D., and Bernthal, T.: Localized multiple minute pulmonary embolism and breathing. J. Appl. Physiol., 16:842, 1961.

Howell, W. H., and Holt, E.: Two new factors in blood coagulation—heparin and pro-antithrombin. Amer. J. Physiol., 47:328, 1918.

Hume, M.: Pulmonary embolism. Historical aspects. Arch. Surg., 87:709, 1963.

Izak, G., Galewski, K., and Eyal, Z.: Studies on the hypercoagulable state. II. The application of 131

I-labeled fibrinogen for the estimation of intravascular coagulation in human subjects. Thromb. Diath. Haemorrh., 18:544, 1967.

Johnson, D. C., and Reeve, T. S.: The effect and clinical significance of low molecular weight and clinical dextran on an experimental venous thrombus in sheep. Ann. Surg., 168:123, 1968.

Jones, R. H., and Sabiston, D. C., Jr.: Pulmonary embolism in childhood. Monog. Surg. Sci., 3:35, 1966.

Jones, R. H., and Sabiston, D. C., Jr.: The diagnosis and management of pulmonary embolism. Conn. Med., 32:814, 1968.

Jones, R. H., Goodrich, J. K., and Sabiston, D. C., Jr.: Radioactive lung scanning in the diagnosis and management of pulmonary disorders. J. Thorac. Cardiov. Surg., 54:520, 1967.

Just-Viera, J. O., Oster, W. F., and Yeager, G. H.: Recurrent pulmonary embolism. J. Thorac. Cardiov. Surg., 52:282, 1966.

Kabins, S. A., Fridman, J., Kandelman, M., and Weisberg, H.: Effect of sympathectomy on pulmonary embolism-induced lung edema. Amer. J. Physiol., 202:687, 1962.

Keon, W. J., and Heimbecker, R. O.: Massive pulmonary embolism: Modern surgical management. Canad. J. Surg., 12:15, 1969.

Khazei, A. H., Dembo, D. H., and Cowley, R. A.: Recognition and management of massive pulmonary embolism. A report of successful embolectomy. Arch. Surg., 94:884, 1967.

Kirschner, M.: Ein Durch die Trendelenburgische Operation Geheilter Fall von Emboli der Artialen Pulmonalis. Arch. Klin. Chir., 133:312, 1924.

Kramer, D. W.: Thrombophlebitis: Etiology and diagnosis. Vasc. Dis., 3:305, 1966.

Laennec, R. T. H.: De l'auscultation médiate ou traité du diagnostique des maladies des poumons et du coeur. Paris, Brosson et Chaude, 1819.

Lansing, A. M., and Davis, W. M.: Five-year follow-up study of iliofemoral venous thrombectomy. Ann. Surg., 168:620, 1968.

Leather, R. P., Clark, W. R., Jr., Powers, S. R., Jr., Parker, F. B., Bernard, H. R., and Eckert, C.: Five-year experience with the moretz vena caval clip in 62 patients. Arch. Surg., 97:357, 1968.

Leriche, R.: Y a-t-il des thrombosis primitives localisies à l'embouchure de la veine cava? A propos de la thrombectomie dans les phlebites, thrombose, et stase. Presse Med., 56:825, 1948.

Link, K. P.: The anticoagulant from spoiled sweet clover hay. The Harvey Lecture Series XXXIX. Lancaster, Pa., The Science Press Printing Co., 1944, pp. 162–216.

Loehry, C. A.: Pulmonary emboli in young adults. Brit. Med. J., 5499:1327, 1966.

Logan, W. D., Jr., Hatcher, C. R., Jr., Symbas, P. N., and Abbott, O. A.: Additional considerations in pulmonary embolectomy. Amer. Surg., 33:706, 1967.

Love, W. D., and O'Meallie, L. P.: Increase in coronary blood flow to the right atrium and ventricle in response to an acute increase in hemodynamic load. J. Lab. Clin. Med., 62:72, 1963.

Makin, G. S., Mayes, E. B., and Holyroyd, M. A.: Clinical and experimental studies on the effects of calf compression on deep venous flow rates and thrombosis. Brit. J. Surg., 55:859, 1968.

Maraan, B. M., and Taber, R. E.: The effects of inferior vena caval ligation on cardiac output: An experimental study. Surgery, 63:966, 1968.

Marshall, R., Sabiston, D. C., Jr., Allison, P. R., Bosman, A. R., and Dunnill, M. S.: Immediate and late effects of pulmonary embolism by large thrombi in dogs. Thorax., 18:1, 1963.

Matis, P.: Postoperative anticoagulant therapy. Clin. Obstet. Gynec., 11:281, 1968.

McDonald, I. G., Hirsh, J., Jr., Hale, G. S., Cade, J. F., and McCarthy, R. A.: Isoproterenol in massive pulmonary embolism: Hemodynamic and clinical effects. Med. J. Aust., 2:201, 1968.

McLachlin, A. D., McLachlin, J. A., Jory, T. A., and Rawling, E. G.: Venous stasis in the lower extremities. Ann. Surg., 152:678, 1960.

McLachlin, A. D., McLachlin, J. A., and Stavraky, W. K.: Venous stasis in the lower extremities — an evaluation of early ambulation. Canad. J. Surg., 5:385, 1962.

Megibow, R. S., Katz, L. N., and Feinstein, M.: Kinetics of respiration in experimental pulmonary embolism. Arch. Int. Med., 71:536, 1943.

Miles, R. M., Richardson, R. R., Wayne, L., and Elsea, P. W.: Long-term results with the serrated Teflon vena caval clip in the prevention of pulmonary embolism. Ann. Surg., 169:881, 1969.

Moniz, E., de Carvallio, L., and Limer, H.: Angiopneumographie. Presse Med., 39:996, 1931.

Moor, G. F., and Sabiston, D. C., Jr.: Embolectomy for chronic pulmonary embolism and hypertension. In press.

Moore, R. L., and Binger, C. A. R.: Observations on resistance to the flow of blood to and from the lungs. J. Exp. Med., 14:655, 1927.

Moretz, W. H., Rhode, C. M., and Shepherd, M. H.: Prevention of pulmonary emboli by partial occlusion of the inferior vena cava. Amer. Surg., 25:617, 1959.

Morrell, M. T., and Dunnill, M. S.: The postmortem incidence of pulmonary embolism in a hospital population. Brit. J. Surg., 55:347, 1968.

Mozes, M., Bogokowsky, H., Antebi, E., Tzur, N., and Penchas, S.: Inferior vena cava ligation for pulmonary embolism: Review of 118 cases. Surgery, 60:790, 1966.

Murphy, M. L., and Bullock, R. T.: Factors influencing the restoration of blood flow following pulmonary embolization as determined by angiography and scanning. Circulation, 38:1116, 1968.

Murray, G. D. W., and Best, C. H.: The use of heparin in thrombosis. Ann. Surg., 108:163, 1938.

Nash, E. S., Shapiro, S., Landau, A., and Barnard, C. N.: Successful thrombo-embolectomy in long-standing thrombo-embolic pulmonary hypertension. Thorax., 23:121, 1968.

Niden, A. H., and Aviado, D. M., Jr.: Effects of pulmonary embolism on the pulmonary circulation with special reference to arteriovenous shunts in the lung. Circ. Res., 4:67, 1956.

Orell, S. R.: The fate and late effects of non-fatal pulmonary emboli. Acta. Med. Scand., 172:473, 1962.

O'Sullivan, E. F., Hirsh, J., Jr., McCarthy, R. A., and DeGruchy, G. C.: Heparin in the treatment of venous thromboembolic disease: Administration, control and results. Med. J. Aust., 2:153, 1968.

Palma, E. C.: Early thrombectomy in phlebothrombosis: J. Cardiov. Surg., 9:161, 1968.

Paneth, M.: Pulmonary embolectomy. An analysis of 12 cases. J. Thorac. Cardiov. Surg., 53:77, 1967.

Parrish, E. H., Adams, J. T., Pories, W. J., Burget, D. E., and DeWeese, J. A.: Pulmonary emboli following vena caval ligation. Arch. Surg., 97:899, 1968.

Polachek, A. A., Zoneraich, S., Zoneraich, O., and Sass, M.: Pulmonary infarction and serum lactic dehydrogenase. JAMA, 204:811, 1968.

Porter, P., Porter, M. C., and Shanberge, J. N.: Protamine, polybrene and the antithrombin action of heparin. Clin. Chim. Acta., 19:411, 1968.

Royston, G. R.: The management of adequate anticoagulant therapy and its complications. Vasc. Dis., 3:295, 1966.

Sabiston, D. C., Jr.: Pathophysiology, diagnosis, and management of pulmonary embolism. Advances in surgery. Chicago, Year Book Medical Publishers, 1968.

Sabiston, D. C., Jr., and Wagner, H. N., Jr.: The diagnosis of pulmonary embolism by radioisotope scanning. Ann. Surg., 160:575, 1964.

Sabiston, D. C., Jr., and Wagner, H. N., Jr.: The pathophysiology of pulmonary embolism: Relationships to accurate diagnosis and choice of therapy. J. Thorac. Cardiov. Surg., 50:339, 1965.

Sabiston, D. C., Jr., and Wolfe, W. G.: Experimental and clinical observations on the natural history of pulmonary embolism. Ann. Surg., 168:1, 1968.

Sabiston, D. C., Jr., and Wolfe, W. G.: Pulmonary embolism. Ann. Rev. Med., 18:443, 1967.

Salzman, E. W., Harris, W. H., and DeSanctis, R. W.: Anticoagulation for prevention of thromboembolism following fractures of the hip. New Eng. J. Med., 275:122, 1966.

Sanders, R. J.: Venography in the diagnosis of thrombophlebitis. Amer. J. Surg., 116:696, 1968.

Sasahara, A. A., and Stein, M.: Pulmonary embolic disease. New York, Grune and Stratton, 1965.

Sasahara, A. A., Cannilla, J. E., Belko, J. S., Morse, R. L., and Criss, A. J.: Urokinase therapy in clinical pulmonary embolism. A new thrombolytic agent. New Eng. J. Med., 277:1168, 1967.

Sasahara, A. A., Cannilla, J. E., Morse, R. L., Sidd, J. J., and Tremblay, G. M.: Clinical and physiologic studies in pulmonary thromboembolism. Amer. J. Cardiol., 20:10, 1967.

Sautter, R. D.: The technique of pulmonary embolectomy with the use of cardiopulmonary bypass. J. Thorac. Cardiov. Surg., 53:268, 1967.

Sautter, R. D., Emanuel, D. A., and Wenzel, F. J.: Treatment of acute massive pulmonary embolism. Medical or surgical? Ann. Thorac. Surg., 4:95, 1967.

Sautter, R. D., Emanuel, D. A., Fletcher, F. W., Wenzel, F. J., and Matson, J. I.: Urokinase for the treatment of acute pulmonary thromboembolism. JAMA, 202:215, 1967.

Severinghaus, J. W., Swenson, E. W., Finley, T. N., and Lategola, M.: Shift of ventilation produced by unilateral pulmonary artery occlusion. Med. Thorac., 19:298, 1962.

Severinghaus, J. W., Swenson, E. W., Finley, T. N., Lategola, M. T., and Williams, J.: Unilateral hypoventilation produced in dogs by occluding one pulmonary artery. J. Appl. Physiol., 16:53, 1961.

Sevitt, S.: The acutely swollen leg and deep vein thrombosis. Brit. J. Surg., 54:886, 1967.

Sevitt, S., and Gallagher, N. G.: Prevention of venous thrombosis and pulmonary embolism in injured patients. Lancet, 2:981, 1959.

Shanberge, J. N.: The action of heparin as an anticoagulant. Acta. Haemat. Jap., 31:1, 1968.

Sharp, E. H.: Pulmonary embolectomy: Successful removal of massive pulmonary embolus with support of cardiopulmonary bypass: Case report. Ann. Surg., 156:1, 1962.

Shepard, R. M., Jr., White, H. A., and Shickly, A. L.: Anticoagulant prophylaxis of thromboembolism in postsurgical patients. Amer. J. Surg., 112:698, 1966.

Skinner, D. B., and Salzman, E. W.: Anticoagulant prophylaxis in surgical patients. Surg. Gynec. Obstet., 125:741, 1967.

Smith, G. T., Hyland, J. W., Peimme, T., and Wells, R. E., Jr.: Human systemic-pulmonary arterial collateral circulation after pulmonary thromboembolism. JAMA, 188:452, 1964.

Soloff, L. A., and Rodman, T.: Acute pulmonary embolism. I. Review. Amer. Heart J., 74:710, 1967.

Soloff, L. A., and Rodman, T.: Acute pulmonary embolism. II. Clinical. Amer. Heart J., 74:829, 1967.

Spencer, F. C., Jude, J., Reinoff, W. F., III, and Stonesifer, G.: Plication of the inferior vena cava for pulmonary embolism. Long-term results in 39 cases. Ann. Surg., 161:788, 1963.

Stansel, H. C., Jr., Hume, M., and Glenn, W. W. L.: Pulmonary embolectomy. New Eng. J. Med., 276:717, 1967.

Stein, P. D., and Evans, H.: An autopsy study of leg vein thrombosis. Circulation, 35:671, 1964.

Stein, P. D., Alshabkhoun, S., Hatem, C., Pur-Shahriari, A. A., Haynes, F. W., Harken, D. E., and Dexter, L.: Coronary artery blood flow in acute pulmonary embolism. Amer. J. Cardiol., 21:32, 1968.

Stein, P. D., O'Connor, J. F., Dalen, J. E., Pur-Shahriari, A. A., Hoppin, F. G., Hammond, D. T., Haynes, F. W., Fleischner, F. G., and Dexter, L.: The angiographic diagnosis of acute pulmonary embolism. Evaluation of criteria. Amer. Heart J., 73:730, 1967.

Stevens, J., Fardin, R., and Freeark, R. J.: Lower extremity thrombophlebitis in patients with femoral neck fractures. A venographic investigation and a review of the early and late significance of the findings. J. Trauma, 8:527, 1968.

Still, W. J. S.: An electron microscopic study of the organization of experimental thromboemboli in the rabbit. Lab. Invest., 15:1492, 1966.

Sutnick, A. I., and Soloff, L. A.: Pulmonary arterial occlusion and surfactant production in humans. Ann. Intern. Med., 67:549, 1967.

Sutton, G. C., Honey, M., and Gibson, R. V.: Clinical diagnosis of acute massive pulmonary embolism. Lancet, 1:271, 1969.

Swenson, E. W., Finley, T. N., and Guzman, S. V.: Unilateral hypoventilation in man during temporary occlusion of one pulmonary artery. J. Clin. Invest., 40:828, 1961.

Taquini, A. C., Fermoso, J. D., and Aramendia, P.: Behavior of the right ventricle following acute constriction of the pulmonary artery. Circ. Res., 8:315, 1960.

Thomas, D. P.: Treatment of pulmonary embolic disease. A critical review of some aspects of current therapy. New Eng. J. Med., 273:885, 1965.

Thomas, D. P., Gurewich, V., and Ashford, T. P.: Platelet adherence to thromboemboli in relation to the pathogenesis and treatment of pulmonary embolism. New Eng. J. Med., 274:953, 1966.

Thomas, D. P., Stein, M., Tanabe, G., Rege, V., and Wessler, S.: Mechanism of bronchoconstriction produced by thromboemboli in dogs. Amer. J. Physiol., 206:1202, 1964.

Thomas, D. P., Tanabe, G., Khan, M., and Stein, M.: Humoral factors mediated by platelets in experimental pulmonary embolism. In Sasahara, A. A., and Stein, M. (eds.): Pulmonary embolic disease. New York, Grune and Stratton, 1965, p. 59.

Tow, D. E., and Wagner, H. N., Jr.: Recovery of pulmonary arterial blood flow in patients with pulmonary embolism. New Eng. J. Med., 276:1053, 1967.

Tow, D. E., Wagner, H. N., Jr., and Holmes, R. A.: Urokinase in pulmonary embolism. New Eng. J. Med., 277:1161, 1967.

Trendelenburg, F.: Operative interference in embolism of the pulmonary artery. Ann. Surg., 48:772, 1908.

Virchow, R.: Die Cellularpathologie. Berlin, A. Hirschwald, 1859, p. 444.

Vosschulte, K.: The surgical treatment of pulmonary embolism. J. Cardiov. Surg., (Supple.): 197, 1965.

Wagner, H. N., Jr., Sabiston, D. C., Jr., Iio, M., McAfee, J. G., Meyer, J. K., and Langan, J. K.: Regional pulmonary blood flow in man by radioisotope scanning. JAMA, 187:601, 1964.

Weber, D. M., and Phillips, J. H., Jr.: A re-evaluation of electrocardiographic changes accompanying acute pulmonary embolism. Amer. J. Med. Sci., 251:381, 1966.

Wechsler, B. M., Karlson, K. E., Summers, D. N., Krasnow, N., Garzon, A. A., and Chait, A.: Pulmonary embolism: Influence of cardiac hemodynamics and natural history on selection of patients for embolectomy and inferior vena cava ligation. Surgery, 65:182, 1969.

Weidner, M. G., Jr., and Light, R. A.: Role of the autonomic nervous system in the control of the pulmonary vascular bed. III. Further studies in experimental pulmonary embolism. Ann. Surg., 147:895, 1958.

Welch, W. H.: Thrombosis and embolism. In Allbutt, R. C. (ed.): A system in medicine. New York, The Macmillan Company, 1901.

Wessler, S., and Morris, L. E.: Studies in intravascular coagulation. IV. The effect of heparin and dicumarol on serum-induced venous thrombosis. Circulation, 12:553, 1955.

Westermark, W.: On the roentgen diagnosis of lung embolism. Acta Radiol., 19:357, 1938.

Wharton, L. R., and Pierson, J. W.: Minor forms of pulmonary embolism after abdominal operations. JAMA, 79:1904, 1922.

Wilson, H., and Britt, L. G.: Surgical treatment of iliofemoral thrombosis. Ann. Surg., 165:855, 1967.

Winsor, T.: Electrocardiogram and pulmonary infarction. JAMA, 204:807, 1968.

Wolfe, W. G., and Sabiston, D. C., Jr.: A study of changes in the roentgenogram of the chest in experimental pulmonary embolism. Surg. Gynec. Obstet., 127:492, 1968.

Wright, I. S.: Anticoagulant therapy—practical management. Amer. Heart. J., 77:280, 1969.

CHAPTER 11

ESOPHAGEAL PERFORATIONS AND MEDIASTINAL SEPSIS

by THOMAS H. BURFORD, M.D., and THOMAS B. FERGUSON, M.D.

Thomas Hannahan Burford is one of the leading thoracic surgeons of his time. Born in Missouri and educated at the University of Missouri and at Yale University School of Medicine, where he took special work in endocrinology, he served his internship and residency training at Barnes Hospital under Dr. Evarts Graham and remained to become a foremost member of that staff. He later became Professor of Thoracic Surgery and Chief of Thoracic and Cardiovascular Surgery of the Barnes and Allied Hospitals. A Founder Member of the Board of Thoracic Surgery, he has been President of the American Association for Thoracic Surgery and the Society of Thoracic Surgery, and he was Acting Editor of the Journal of Thoracic Surgery. Diseases of the esophagus have constituted a special interest, and numerous publications have resulted from his large clinical experience and laboratory studies of esophageal lesions and their surgical management.

Thomas B. Ferguson was born in Oklahoma and was elected to both Phi Beta Kappa and Alpha Omega Alpha at Duke University. Following his thoracic residency training at Barnes Hospital, he joined the staff and is presently Associate Clinical Professor of Thoracic Surgery at Washington University School of Medicine. He is a member of the Board of Thoracic Surgery and has contributed significantly to knowledge of esophageal diseases.

Until the beginning of this century acute suppurative mediastinitis due to perforation of the esophagus was uniformly fatal; even today it is associated with high mortality or prolonged morbidity unless promptly diagnosed and properly treated. Table 11-1 classifies the major causes of esophageal perforation. Most inflammatory and neoplastic perforations are chronic rather than acute; however, this discussion will deal primarily with the traumatic category. Also, since penetrating esophageal wounds due to missiles or sharp instruments are covered in another chapter, they will be omitted from further consideration here.

HISTORICAL BACKGROUND

The following is a brief resumé of the publications which, in the opinion of the authors, are significant in the history of this disorder.

Virtually all the literature on esophageal perforation prior to 1900 relates to penetrating wounds from violent trauma, usually battle injuries. A notable exception was a paper published in 1724 by Hermann Boerhaave of Holland, which described in detail the first spontaneous rupture of the normal esophagus to be recognized. Boerhaave's

TABLE 11-1. Classification of Perforations of the Esophagus

TRAUMATIC
  Penetrating wounds (knife, bullet)
  Ingested caustics
  Ingested foreign bodies
  Iatrogenic injuries:
    Esophagoscopy and gastroscopy
    Bougienage, dilation or intubation
    Surgical
  Barogenic injuries:
    Normal esophagus (spontaneous or postemetic rupture)
    Diseased esophagus (diverticulum, etc.)
INFLAMMATORY
  Esophagitis
  Peptic ulceration
  Mediastinal granuloma
  Abscess
  Aneurysm
NEOPLASTIC
  Benign
  Malignant

patient, the Grand Admiral of the Navy of Holland, was given to excessive eating and drinking. He relieved the resulting discomfort by taking *Ipecacuanha* in a "copious infusion of blessed-thistle" to induce vomiting. An emetogenic rupture of the esophagus occurred and the patient died. At autopsy, Boerhaave was able to prove the barogenic etiology of the unfortunate incident. It was not until 222 years later, in 1946, that this condition was successfully treated surgically by N. R. Barrett of London. In the United States, attention was focused on postemetic rupture by Samson in 1951, and pertinent experimental studies were reported by Mackler in 1952.

Heidenhain (1899) is credited with the first cure for foreign body perforation (in this case a chicken bone) by means of surgical drainage of the neck. Von Hacker in 1901, however, was the first to advocate immediate surgical drainage of the mediastinum for all cases. Marschik of Vienna in 1916 described the technique of cervical mediastinotomy through an incision anterior to the sternomastoid muscle, and essentially his operation is the one used today. Gaudiani, also in 1916, showed that mediastinal abscesses above the body of the 4th thoracic vertebra can be drained satisfactorily through a cervical incision, whereas abscesses below this level require dorsal drainage. His observations were based on clinical cases as well as anatomic dissections of the cervicomediastinal fascial planes. The extrapleural posterior mediastinotomy described by Lilienthal in 1923 was a mainstay of surgical treatment throughout the years when antibiotic support was either nonexistent or

meager. The thoracic surgical techniques learned during World War II and the availability of antibiotics following the war made deliberate transpleural approach to the mediastinum the operation of choice, and relegated the extrapleural procedures to the history books.

Instrumental perforation of the esophagus has been a problem since the introduction of the first practical esophagoscope by Von Mickulicz of Vienna in 1881. Phillips in 1938 first outlined the symptom complex and the diagnostic studies necessary for early diagnosis. He emphasized that septic mediastinitis from instrumental perforation was a curable condition if recognized immediately and surgically treated. With the increasing application of esophagoscopy, plus the manipulative techniques of dilation and bougienage, instrumental perforations have increased in number year by year. Wychulis et al. (1969) reported a 0.4 per cent perforation rate among 8038 patients undergoing peroral gastrointestinal endoscopic procedures at the Mayo Clinic, and a literature survey indicates a range of 2 to 20 perforations per 1000 procedures. Mengoli and Klassen in 1965 advocated that instrumental perforations be managed by massive antibiotic therapy without initial surgical drainage. This view was supported in part by Hardin et al. (1967), but has met with spirited opposition from Groves (1966) and many others. Seybold et al. (1950) reported the first successful resection of the lower esophagus after perforation during a dilation for cardiospasm. The value of this approach was emphasized by Nealon et al. (1961), Webb and Burford (1962) and most recently by

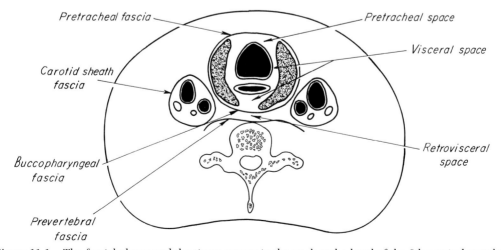

Figure 11-1. The fascial planes and the tissue spaces in the neck at the level of the 6th cervical vertebra.

Johnson et al. (1967), so that now, whenever possible, immediate surgery is recommended in instrumental perforations associated with diverticula, achalasia, carcinoma, stricture, and other kinds of esophageal pathology.

ANATOMIC CONSIDERATIONS

As an organ, the esophagus differs from other hollow viscera in a number of ways pertaining to infection. It lies in a bed of loose areolar tissue that extends from the neck to the diaphragm. There is no serosal covering to limit the extramural spread of disease. The lumen contains an abundance of oral pathogens, so that acute mediastinitis is most often caused by gram-positive organisms or a mixed flora, rather than by the gram-negative infections that occur when perforations are lower in the gut. These organisms produce a rapidly necrotizing process that may destroy portions of the esoph-

ageal wall and surrounding tissues. In perforations of the lower esophagus associated with vomiting, the highly irritating gastric contents produce caustic mediastinitis, and if a pleural tear has occurred, severe pleuritis. After perforation, rapid spread of infection is promoted by swallowed air and saliva being forced through the rent into the mediastinum. The negative intrathoracic pressure and the motions of respiration, plus the constant action of the heart and great vessels, all contribute to the dissemination of infectious material. Lateral extension of the process is limited only by the mediastinal pleural membrane; the frequency with which hydropneumothorax occurs indicates that this is only a moderately effective barrier.

Four layers of deep cervical fascia divide the structures in the neck into three compartments or potential spaces in which infection can occur: the pretracheal space, the visceral space between the trachea and esophagus, and the retrovisceral space between the esophagus and vertebral bodies

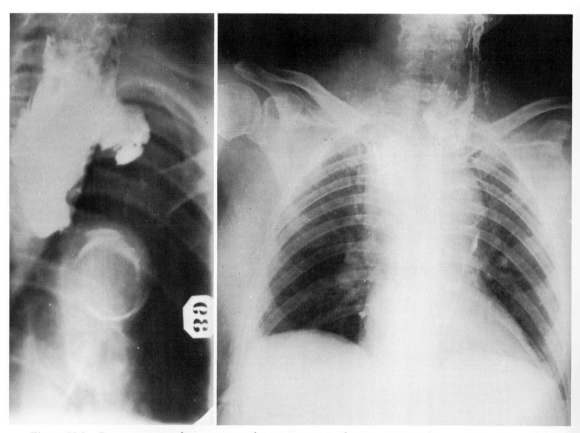

Figure 11-2. Roentgenogram demonstrating the extravasation of contrast material in a patient with perforation of the cervical esophagus. Note that the downward extension is limited by the aortic arch. The film on the right, taken later, shows widening of the mediastinum and further spread of the contrast material. Despite the delay in diagnosis, cervical drainage without closure of the perforation led to complete recovery.

(Furstenburg, 1929) (Fig. 11-1). The retrovisceral space is most frequently contaminated. Infections in the pretracheal space are rare, but may arise from perforations of the pyriform fossa (Seybold et al., 1950). These fascial layers lose definition as they extend down into the mediastinum. The transverse aortic arch forms a partial barrier to the caudad spread of infection, so that abscesses above the level of the 4th thoracic vertebra will for a time remain confined to the upper region, and can be satisfactorily drained through a cervical incision (Fig. 11-2).

PATHOPHYSIOLOGY

Suppurative mediastinitis due to esophageal perforation can occur in four ways: (1) immediate rupture of the entire wall; (2) laceration of the mucous membrane, accompanied by the development of an intramural abscess and subsequent rupture to the outside; (3) pressure necrosis of the wall, usually due to a retained or impacted foreign body; and (4) necrosis of an esophageal segment, deprived of its blood supply by intrathoracic surgery. The immediate perforations are most often associated with critical surgical illness. Intramural abscesses invoke a surrounding inflammatory response and often rupture back into the esophageal lumen. If treated by removal of the foreign body and antibiotic therapy, minute perforations from swallowed pins, fish bones, or dentures often do not lead to abscess formation. Esophageal necrosis due to compromised blood supply is dealt with in another chapter.

Perforations due to instrumentation in general fall into three groups, corresponding to the three levels of anatomic narrowing—at the cricopharyngeal sphincter in the cervical esophagus, at the thoracic constriction produced by the aortic nob, and at the cardioesophageal junction. Perforations of the cervical esophagus are not usually associated with pathologic conditions in this area. They are most often technical accidents, although such ruptures are seen with greater frequency in elderly individuals, in patients with adverse physical characteristics (such as hypertrophic spurs of the cervical spine, kyphoscoliosis, or cervical arthritis), or in the uncooperative patient under local anesthesia. The experience of the endoscopist, while a factor, is by no means the major one. Instrumental perforations of the midesophagus are most often seen in patients in whom a biopsy or attempted dilation for carcinoma has been performed. Also, stricture of the esophagus due to caustic ingestion occurs at the level of the aortic arch, and overzealous antegrade dilations frequently cause perforations at this level (Fig. 11-3). In the lower esophagus, endoscopic tears are seen following dilations for achalasia or esophageal stricture secondary to peptic esophagitis.

Barogenic rupture of the esophagus is associated with the highest morbidity and mortality of any type of perforation. In the literature these cases have been called spontaneous, postemetic, or emetogenic ruptures; however, vomiting is not an absolute requisite, since the condition has been reported to occur after defecation, lifting of a heavy weight, convulsive seizures, or the labor of childbirth. The physiologic process common to all these cases is a sudden pressure rise within the esophagus, and we therefore prefer the term barogenic rupture.

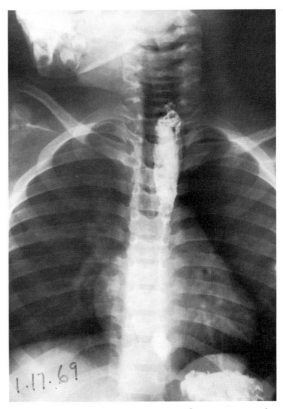

Figure 11-3. Roentgenogram demonstrating the onset of narrowing at the level of the aortic arch in a child with lye stricture of the esophagus.

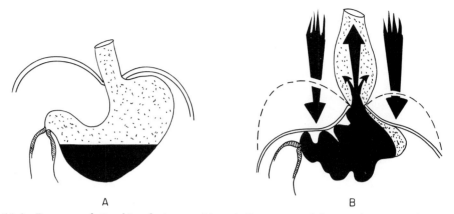

Figure 11-4. Pressure relationships during vomiting. *A,* Pre-emetic inhibition of gastric and cardiac sphincter tone. *B,* Forcible contraction of the diaphragm and abdominal muscles with resulting ejection of stomach contents into the esophagus. (After Mackler.)

Mackenzie in 1884 and Mackler in 1952 performed experimental studies on rupture of the esophagus and came to the following similar conclusions: (1) that the tear always takes place in a longitudinal direction, (2) that it always occurs in the lower half of the esophagus, (3) that the bursting pressure is about 5 pounds per square inch, and (4) that the mucosa is the most resistant layer. Mackler showed that the muscularis first splits in the long axis of the tube, and a diverticulum of mucosa balloons through the opening, and with further pressure bursts. He postulated that the lower esophagus is weaker because the upper portion is buttressed on all sides and contains an intermingling of striated and smooth muscle fibers, whereas the lower esophagus is unsupported and contains only smooth muscle. Duval (1921) showed that the rate of pressure rise is more important than the magnitude. This is probably the reason that the majority of barogenic rupture cases are associated with vomiting (Fig. 11-4). A history of alcohol ingestion is also frequently present, suggesting that muscular incoordination of the esophagus and acute esophagitis, both due to alcohol, are contributing factors. Zikria et al. (1965) postulated that the Mallory-Weiss syndrome (gastrointestinal bleeding from superficial mucosal lacerations in the lower esophagus), which also occurs after alcohol consumption and vomiting, and emetogenic rupture are but two stages of the same pathologic process.

Contamination of the pleural cavity occurs in perforations of the lower esophagus, most often on the left side. As the esophagus leaves the midsagittal plane and deviates to enter the esophageal hiatus, the left lateral esophageal wall is in direct contact with the mediastinal pleura. In their experience in treating 20 perforations of the lower esophagus, Seybold et al. (1950) noted pleural contamination in 16 (80 per cent). The left side was involved in 10 cases, the right in five, and one was bilateral. Bilateral empyema is usually associated with gross instrumental trauma or with the undiagnosed and neglected perforation. As might be anticipated, the occurrence of pleural contamination after perforation of the cervical esophagus is relatively rare.

SIGNS AND SYMPTOMS

The clinical features depend upon the site of perforation and the extent and character of the laceration of the esophageal wall. The cardinal signs and symptoms are chest pain, fever, pain on swallowing, and subcutaneous emphysema.

Pain is always the earliest symptom and in free perforations is continuous and severe. Any patient who complains of pain after a peroral endoscopic procedure must be considered as having an esophageal tear until proven otherwise, and immediate appropriate diagnostic steps should be taken. Initially the pain is fairly well localized to the third of the esophagus that is involved. A rent in the cervical esophagus causes pain in the neck, and swallowing or any motion of the larynx accentuates the pain. The patient will hold the head rigidly motionless, and refuse to raise up from the pillow. The pain is of maximal intensity along the anterior border of the sternomastoid muscle near the jugular notch. Palpation, medial and deep to the carotid sheath, causes intense discomfort. In neglected cervical perforations, after 24 to 48 hours the tissues become "woody," but redness and edema of the skin practically never appear, and the abscess does not "point" at the skin surface. Pain with a middle third perforation causes severe retrosternal discomfort. Any flexion, extension, or rotary motion of the thoracic spine aggravates the pain. Perforations in the lower esophagus, particularly barogenic ruptures, cause severe epigastric distress that is easily confused with a perforated peptic ulcer, acute pancreatitis, empyema of the gallbladder, or coronary disease. The intense reflex spasm of the upper abdominal musculature further focuses attention on the abdomen. A diagnosis of perforated peptic ulcer is likely to be made, particularly if rupture into the pleural space has not occurred, and a number of these patients have been subjected to exploratory celiotomy (Campbell and Cox, 1969). When a pneumothorax is present, irritation of the diaphragm will cause pain on respiration and referred shoulder pain.

Fever is the second abnormality to appear and is present in all cases. Although the temperature response is prompt, it does not suggest bacteremia. Chills are rarely present and elevations rarely exceed 102° F. Dysphagia is also invariably present, completing the diagnostic triad. Dysphagia here means painful swallowing rather than difficulty in swallowing, and is accompanied by excessive salivation.

Air in the mediastinum is pathognomic of perforation and does not occur in any other condition which may be considered in a differential diagnosis. Therefore a careful search for air must be made. Palpation of the neck should be repeated hourly in any patient suspected of having a cervical perforation. Any crepitation, however slight, immediately confirms the diagnosis. Air in the neck may not appear for 24 hours after the onset of pain, nor does it occur in all cases.

Wychulis et al. (1969) noted crepitation in 17 of 24 patients having instrumental perforation of the cervical esophagus. Samson (1951) called attention to the peculiar nasal twang that may be present in the voice, and noted that it often precedes by several hours the appearance of neck crepitation. Although occurring less frequently, this diagnostic sign is highly specific. Dysphonia and hoarseness are grave signs that herald the development of glottic edema. Mediastinal emphysema, which accompanies low esophageal perforations, is less common but nevertheless just as reliable when found. The earliest indication will be a mediastinal crunch, which must be listened for carefully with the stethoscope over the anterior and posterior chest. The air must dissect the tissue planes to reach the suprasternal notch before tissue crepitation can be palpated; therefore the time lapse is greater than with cervical perforations.

It should be emphasized that barogenic (emetogenic) perforations, in which gastric contents are spilled into the mediastinum or pleural cavity or both, result in a more striking clinical picture than that seen with endoscopic perforations of the lower esophagus. This condition is most common in males (85 per cent) between the ages of 35 and 55. A previous history of alcoholism, dietary indiscretion, malnutrition, or gastrointestinal symptoms is frequently present. The pain that follows a bout of vomiting is sudden and persists at an excruciating level. It is usually low retrosternal or epigastric in location. No position affords relief, and waves of accentuation occur with deep breathing, swallowing, and motions of the trunk. The patient appears severely ill with ashen color and cold moist skin. Cyanosis is frequently present. The pulse is thin and rapid, although the blood pressure may remain normal for several hours before hypotension and shock eventually occur. The signs of left hydropneumothorax are frequently elicited.

DIAGNOSTIC STUDIES

Roentgenographic studies will show positive findings very early in the course and should be obtained as soon as this diagnosis is suspected. In cervical perforations, posterior-anterior views of the neck and upper chest may show gas in the tissues and widening of the superior mediastinum (Fig. 11-5A). A lateral view of the neck will show fluid in the retrovisceral space with anterior displacement of the trachea (Fig. 11-5B). A swallow of radiopaque contrast material will confirm the diagnosis. It should be emphasized that there is not necessarily a correlation between the size of the rent and the

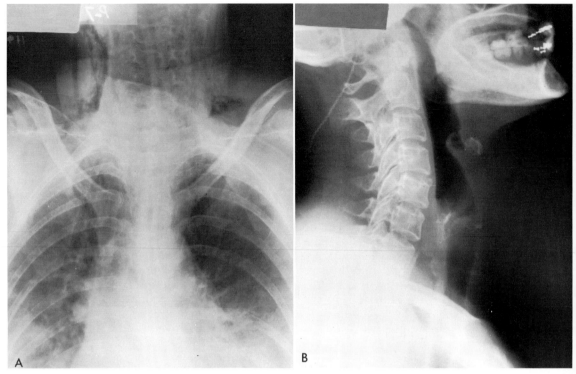

Figure 11-5. Instrumental perforation of the cervical esophagus following esophagoscopy in a patient with a hypopharyngeal (Zenker's) diverticulum. *A,* The air in the tissues is palpable as subcutaneous emphysema. *B,* Lateral view showing widening of the retrovisceral space, and anterior displacement of the trachea by air and fluid. Closure of the perforation, resection of the diverticulum, and drainage of the neck were followed by rapid recovery.

degree of extravasation. Because it is irritative to the tissues, liquid barium should never be used in suspected cases of perforations.

In perforations of the lower esophagus, the earliest roentgen sign is the presence of mediastinal air (Fig. 11-6). Naclerio (1957) described the linear air shadows, corresponding to air in the fascial planes of the mediastinal and diaphragmatic pleura near the region of the esophageal hiatus on the left, as the earliest indication of perforation. With extension of the process, air can be seen on both sides of the mediastinum extending up to the neck. Widening, due to edema of the tissues and retention of fluid, is usually also present. In the rare case in which the perforation extends below the diaphragm and penetrates the peritoneal-esophageal reflection, collections of air may be present and free in the peritoneal cavity, making differentiation from a ruptured abdominal viscus almost impossible.

In cases in which the mediastinal pleura remains intact, sympathetic pleural effusions are still common because of the intense inflammatory response. Approximately three-fourths of the perforations in the distal esophagus are associated with hydropneumothorax, and this complication provides additional clues to the diagnosis. Thoracentesis yields a dirty-brown fluid with a sour odor. These changes are due to the action of the gastric acid on the blood in the effusate. Particles of food and fibrin are usually present. The fluid should be tested for acid with litmus paper. The presence of a tear can be confirmed by having a patient swallow a dilute methylene-blue solution that is then recovered by needle aspiration of the thorax, or by Lipiodol or Hypaque swallow (Fig. 11-7). It must be emphasized that the lack of extravasation of the radiopaque medium does not rule out a perforation, since the contrast material may not pass through a small hole, or the perforation may seal prior to the diagnostic swallow.

The laboratory data are ordinarily of little value except that leukocytosis and a left shift in the hemogram are virtually always present. The white cell count is usually in the range of 15,000 to 18,000.

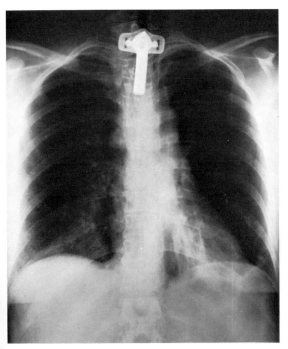

Figure 11-6. Roentgenogram taken immediately after instrumental perforation of the lower esophagus. Air is seen in the posterior mediastinum on the left behind the cardiac shadow. This patient had diffuse collagen disease with dysphagia. The tracheostomy had been done at an earlier time.

Esophagoscopy should not be performed in an attempt to establish a diagnosis. Visualization of a tear is very difficult. Many endoscopists are not aware that they have penetrated the esophagus, and this is one reason for the reluctance in accepting the diagnosis when the clinical picture suggests a perforation. Also there is the danger of enlarging the opening.

TREATMENT

Treatment of suppurative mediastinitis due to esophageal perforation is surgical. Ideally it consists of the prompt establishment of free dependent drainage, closure of the perforation, esophageal rest, and liberal antibiotic coverage. However, variations in the clinical situation, such as the size and location of the perforation, the presence or absence of associated pathologic conditions, and the delay in diagnosis, may make it advisable or necessary on occasion to deviate from these surgical goals.

As mentioned in the section on history, the principle of surgical drainage was first

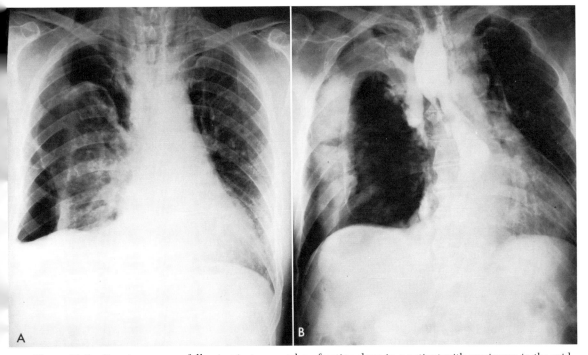

Figure 11-7. Roentgenograms following instrumental perforation done in a patient with carcinoma in the mid-third of the esophagus. *A,* Right pneumothorax. *B,* The extravasation of Hypaque from the esophagus into the pleural space. This patient succumbed.

advocated in 1901 by Von Hacker. All the papers of the pre-antibiotic era stressed drainage alone, with no mention of the desirability of closing the perforation surgically. In spite of this, drainage had a markedly beneficial effect—the mortality rate was reduced from approximately 60 to 70 per cent to about half that figure (Jemerin, 1948). The addition of antibiotic therapy has further decreased the mortality to around 20 per cent. Nealon et al. (1961) operated upon 18 patients with a mortality of 28 per cent. Mathewson et al. (1962) reported an overall mortality of 22 per cent in 76 patients. In 1968, Gerard reported 12 consecutive cases treated without a single death. As expected, the majority of deaths occurred with perforations of the lower esophagus. Wychulis et al. (1969), in a study of 33 patients with endoscopic perforation seen between 1961 and 1967, noted an overall mortality of 9 per cent. However, there were no deaths in 24 patients with cervical perforations, and 3 deaths among 9 patients with thoracic perforations. Closure of the perforation at the time of drainage further improved the results. Weisel (1952) described the surgical management of 7 cases without a death. He recommended closure of the perforation if at all possible, and indicated that the optimum period was within the first 6 hours, but showed that older perforations could be closed successfully in some cases. Paulson et al. (1960) treated 7 patients by means of drainage and antimicrobial therapy with no mortality but with a morbidity from 2 weeks to 2 years, the average being 9 months. Eight patients were treated by means of closure of the perforation, drainage, and antimicrobial therapy, also with no mortality and with an average morbidity of 2 months.

Hoover in 1944 was the first to suggest nonsurgical management of small perforations: "In a careful observation of medical treatment, many [minute perforations] will recover without mediastinitis, yet should symptoms develop, surgery must not be delayed." Mengoli and Klassen in 1965 presented 21 cases of endoscopic perforation, 18 of which were treated nonoperatively with massive antibiotic therapy (10 million units of penicillin and 1 gm. of streptomycin per day). There was one death in the series, making the mortality rate 6 per cent, which they felt compared favorably with immediate surgical intervention in every case. The site of perforation was the distal third in 14 cases,

the middle third in one, and the upper third in six. Hardin et al. in 1967 reported a similar experience in 20 patients with perforations due to various causes, with an overall mortality rate of 15 per cent.

Other surgeons have deplored this reliance upon antibiotic therapy and maintain that surgical drainage must be employed in every proven case. Groves (1966) believes that the "conservative" treatment of esophageal perforation is surgical drainage and repair, and that the "radical" treatment is the use of nonoperative methods. If the perforation is sizable, located within the thorax, and associated with a pneumothorax, the authors of this chapter agree.

One point of universal agreement is the necessity for immediate surgery in barogenic rupture of the esophagus. Derbes and Mitchell (1965) reviewed 71 patients with spontaneous rupture treated without operation. Of these, 35 per cent were dead within 24 hours and all were dead by the end of one week. Barrett in 1946 described the disease and recorded the case histories of three patients, all of whom died without surgical intervention, and he advocated surgery as the only possible hope for cure. In the way that chance favors the prepared mind, Barrett was presented with another case that very year, and in 1947 he reported the first successful surgical result. Even with modern techniques the mortality in this lesion is still appallingly high. Sealy (1963) states that the mortality rate varies between 34 and 50 per cent. Wychulis (1969) reported two deaths in four patients.

CURRENT CONCEPT OF MANAGEMENT

The preceding considerations have led to the formulation of the following concepts of management: There is a place for the immediate institution of massive antibiotic therapy, esophageal rest, and close observation in certain instances of esophageal perforation. This group will principally involve tears in the cervical esophagus due to foreign bodies or other agents which cause pinpoint openings (Fig. 11-8). In successful cases the signs and symptoms of mediastinitis never appear and the patient can safely be started on oral feedings by the fifth or sixth day. The decision regarding surgery

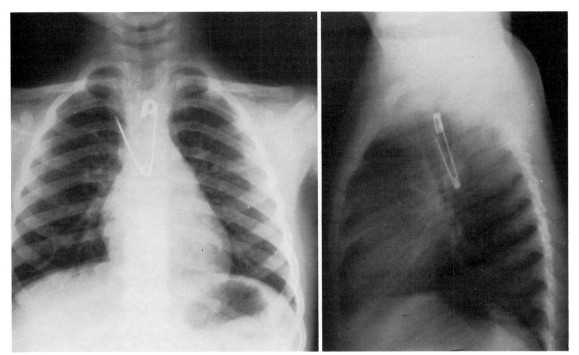

Figure 11-8. Roentgenogram showing a safety pin in the esophagus with obvious perforation of the wall. Treatment consisted of endoscopic removal of the foreign body, esophageal rest, and antibiotic therapy. The child made an uneventful recovery.

must never be made on the basis of the size of the opening as demonstrated by radiographic contrast material. Foster et al. (1965) reported an instance of a "pin-hole" perforation which at operation was found to be 8 cm. in length. Such cases will usually present other clear indications for operation. Perforations with mediastinitis require immediate surgical intervention (Fig. 11-9). This would include the majority of esophagoscopic perforations, and tears secondary to bougienage. Occasionally a penetration due to an esophageal biopsy can be managed conservatively. All barogenic ruptures require immediate surgery.

Iatrogenic (instrumental) perforations of the esophagus have occurred and will occur in the hands of the most qualified operators exercising the greatest precautions. Such cases, of course, frequently result in law suits to recover damages. On the whole the courts have been admirably enlightened in their decisions and have recognized the risk factor as inherent. What they have not condoned, and with this the authors agree, is the factor of negligence in failing to recognize very early the existence of a perforation. The patient who has undergone esophagoscopy, bougienage, or gastroscopy must be observed promptly and frequently. The presence of pain, excess salivation, or other un-

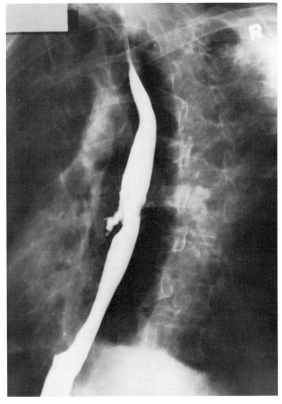

Figure 11-9. Barium swallow demonstrating perforation of the midesophagus by a chicken bone. This patient was successfully treated by thoracotomy, removal of the foreign body, and closure of the esophagus.

toward signs or symptoms demands a plain film of the neck, chest, and upper abdomen, and, if air is present, a Hypaque visualization of the esophagus from the cricopharyngeus to the stomach to exclude or confirm the presence of a perforation. There is no excuse for allowing more than three hours to elapse before discovering the existence of a perforation. The authors, in fact, routinely obtain chest films immediately after the instrumentation on all but the simplest esophagoscopies and frequently follow these with esophageal visualization with Hypaque.

When a perforation occurs in the presence of a distal obstruction of the esophagus, every attempt should be made to take care of the primary problem at the time the perforation is closed. Examples are a Heller esophagomyotomy for achalasia, and resection of a stricture secondary to the peptic esophagitis associated with hiatus hernia (Fig. 11-10). Malignant lesions should be resected and an esophagogastrectomy performed if at all

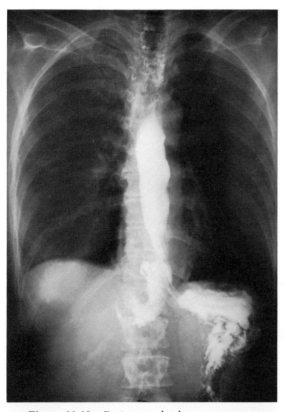

Figure 11-10. Barium study demonstrating extravasation of dye following dilatation for achalasia. Note extension of dye into the retroperitoneal tissues. The patient had immediate thoracotomy, closure of the perforation, and Heller esophagomyotomy with complete recovery.

possible, even if the resection is known to be noncurative. In this group of cases with additional surgical procedures time is of the essence, and every hour's delay in getting the patient to the operating room increases the probability of morbidity and mortality.

The problem of neglected perforations will require individualization, depending upon the condition of the patient and the degree of spread of infection. In general, however, these cases should be explored transthoracically whenever possible. This allows complete visualization and unroofing of the mediastinal abscess that is usually present. The edges of the tear should be carefully freshened and closed with a single layer of nonabsorbable sutures. The surgical principles followed are those which apply to secondary closure of any wound, i.e., the bites are taken fairly wide apart so as not to further compromise the blood supply, and the sutures are tied so as not to crush intervening tissue. Delayed closure of esophageal rents will not be successful in many cases. The results are unpredictable, however, and even if a fistula is re-established, the opening frequently will be smaller than the original tear. Foster et al. (1965) performed 13 suture closures within 2 to 24 hours after perforation and reported 11 successes and 2 breakdowns, whereas 3 suture closures performed 30 to 72 hours after perforation healed per primam. Paulson et al. (1960) reported a successful closure 27 days after perforation.

Other measures have been recommended for the subacute and chronic phases of esophageal perforation. Thal and Hatafuku (1964) used the fundus of the stomach as an onlay patch in successfully treating a case of emetogenic rupture (Fig. 11-11). They feel that parahiatal hernia, created by the operation, will not cause future difficulty. Dooling and Zick in 1967 described the use of a viable intercostal muscle pedicle graft for an esophageal disruption.

The treatment of persistent esophagopleurocutaneous fistulas is most difficult. Several authors have advocated total exclusion of the esophagus, as is done in other portions of the intestinal tract. Johnson et al. (1956) described three patients in whom the esophagus and the fistula were isolated by dividing and closing both the cervical esophagus and the esophagogastric junction, with exteriorization of the proximal opening as a mucous fistula. Continuity of the intestinal tract was later restored with a Roux-en-Y

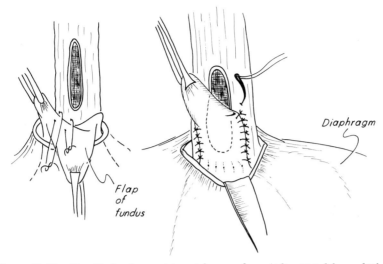

Figure 11-11. The Thal onlay gastric patch procedure. (After Hatafuku and Thal.)

jejunal limb, with success in two of the three patients. Keen (1968) deplored the "drain-and-hope" regime and urged an aggressive approach to this situation. He treated nine patients, seven of whom survived, by means of esophageal defunctioning as described above, with late closure of the fistula by omental wrapping or suture of the lung over the defect, and restoration of continuity by colon replacement if necessary.

SURGICAL TECHNIQUE

The technique for cervical mediastinotomy is shown in Figure 11-12. The incision and approach is the same as that used for repair of a hypophrenic (Zenker's) diverticulum. Local infiltration anesthesia is adequate in the cooperative patient. The incision is made parallel to the anterior border of the sternomastoid muscle and deepened between the thyroid gland and both the trachea medially and the carotid sheath laterally. Aside from skin and subcutaneous vessels, there are very few bleeders, and much of the exposure can be obtained by blunt dissection. The middle thyroid vein may require division. The retrovisceral space is entered, a culture is taken for both aerobic and anaerobic organisms to direct future antibiotic therapy, and the posterior pharynx and upper posterior pharynx and upper posterior esophagus are widely mobilized from the prevertebral fascia. This mobilization is necessary to make certain that all recesses are opened and to allow sufficient rotation of the

esophagus to visualize the point of rupture. Moist cottonoid sheets are used to protect the contents of the carotid sheath during lateral retractions of these structures.

The perforation is closed with a single layer of interrupted nonabsorbable sutures. Even in the freshest tears, it is probably unwise to perform a two-layer closure, since this further compromises an already marginal blood supply. Cervical perforations are virtually always in the transverse direction and should be closed this way. The entire wound is thoroughly lavaged with many changes of saline, and rubber tissue drains are placed into the depths of the wound and brought out through the lower margin of the incision. Care should be taken that the drains do not impinge directly upon the suture line. If the abscess pocket has dissected down into the upper mediastinum, a sump drain is placed to the bottom of the pocket (the newer plastic sump drains work very well) and attached to continuous low suction. The upper half of the wound is closed, leaving an opening of at least 3 finger breadths for drainage in the lower portion.

During the first 48 to 72 hours, the patient is kept supine and encouraged to position himself in bed so as to facilitate drainage from the wound. The patient must not be fed and the tissue drains must not be removed until it is certain that primary healing of the esophagus has been achieved. This requires from four to seven days. Prior to starting liquids by mouth, a swallow of radiopaque medium should be given to allow visualization of the area of closure.

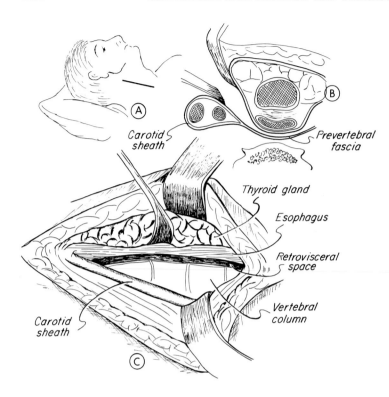

Figure 11-12. Operative approach for cervical mediastinotomy. See text for description. (After Seybold, et al.)

Many patients will develop a small fistula, as evidenced by drainage of saliva from the neck wound, but this need not portend protracted difficulty since many of these fistulas will close spontaneously within a few days. Usually the drains can be removed on the sixth to eighth day, after which the wound closes rapidly.

DORSAL MEDIASTINOTOMY

The principles of surgical exposure of the posterior-inferior mediastinum are shown in Figure 11-13. The vertical paravertebral incision is extended through the paraspinous muscles to the rib cage. Short posterior segments of the ribs and transverse processes overlying the abscess are resected and the pleura is reflected laterally until the pocket is fully exposed. The abscess is drained and packed with gauze, or tissue drains are inserted. Care must be taken not to injure the aorta, which usually forms one side of the cavity.

This procedure is of limited value because of the depth of the incision, the difficulty in avoiding the pleura, and the inaccessibility of the esophagus for definitive

repair. Though valuable in the past, it is now virtually an obsolete procedure.

DEFINITIVE TRANSPLEURAL REPAIR

The patient is prepared for the operating room as soon as the diagnosis is made. A nasogastric tube is inserted into the esophagus down to the region of the perforation and continuous suction is applied. Oxygen and fluids are administered and the patient is typed and crossmatched. A barogenic perforation is one emergency for which the surgeon cannot wait for complete resuscitation before proceeding with operation. Valuable time may be lost in attempting to get the systolic blood pressure above 100 mm. Hg, since many times this will not be possible until the chest is open.

An immediate and dramatic pressure response usually occurs as soon as the pleural cavity is opened and the fluid and air are removed. If hydropneumothorax is present, the operation is performed on that side; otherwise, a left thoracotomy is performed. The pleural cavity is opened through the bed of the resected sixth or seventh rib. The appearance of the pleural-mediastinal

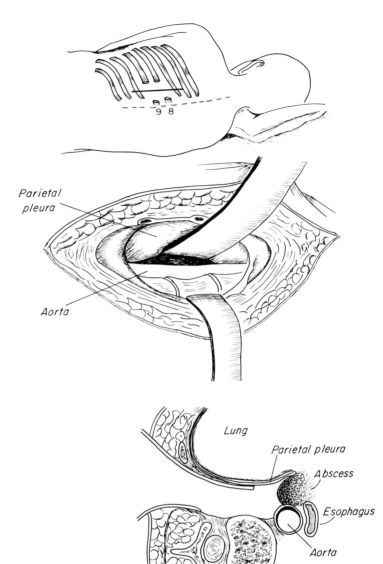

Figure 11-13. Operative approach for dorsal mediastinotomy. See text for description. (After Seybold, et al.)

surfaces is striking, since gastric contents evoke the most intensive inflammatory response to be seen anywhere in the body. The tissues vary from an angry red or purple to black, suggestive of early gangrene. The tear in the esophagus is readily apparent (Fig. 11-14). The mediastinal pleura is opened from the arch of the aorta to the diaphragm and the esophagus is mobilized with rubber tapes above and below the rent; care must be taken to avoid entering the right pleural cavity. The margins of the tear are defined and minimal debridement of the edematous mucosa is carried out.

The rent is always longitudinal and is closed in the same direction; attempts to increase the lumen size by transverse closure are unwise as the likelihood of breakdown is greater. If the perforation is fresh and all layers of the esophagus appear normal, closure can be accomplished by using two layers of interrupted, nonabsorbable suture material. If there is any degree of inflammatory response, closure should be accomplished by using one layer. Attempts at a more meticulous closure of the inflamed esophageal wall will only result in a higher incidence of postoperative leaks. It is strongly emphasized that the closure must be accomplished using nonabsorbable suture material, either fine silk or one of the newer synthetic materials.

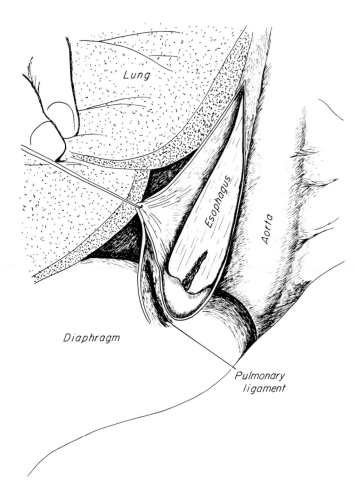

Figure 11-14. View obtained at left thoracotomy for barogenic rupture of the esophagus. See text for description of operation. (After Mackler.)

It is surprising how many papers in the older literature advocate full-thickness closure of the esophageal wall with catgut. Such closures are doomed to failure because the inflammatory fluids and particularly the gastric contents cause premature digestion of the catgut.

After the closure a nasogastric tube is passed under direct guidance into the stomach. The tissues of the mediastinum are debrided to remove all of the dirty-gray exudate, and mechanical cleansing of the pleural and diaphragmatic surfaces is performed with a dry gauze sponge to remove any residual particulate matter. If an inflammatory membrane has developed over any part of the lung, this is completely removed. The pleural cavity is then lavaged thoroughly with several quarts of warm saline. The lung is reinflated and three chest tubes are placed to assure complete expansion of the lung and removal of all post-operative fluid. The chest wound is closed primarily.

Postoperatively the patient is maintained on parenteral feedings until it is apparent that the esophagus will remain closed. Usually this will require seven days. The intactness of repair should be confirmed by a barium swallow before oral intake is started. It is also wise to leave the posterior intercostal drainage catheter in place during this period. Leakage is most likely on the fifth postoperative day; it is usually heralded by bubbling in the chest bottle or the development of pneumothorax. Lower esophageal leaks are less likely to close spontaneously than are cervical leaks, but continued esophageal rest and active expansion of the lung by vigorous suction through the intercostal catheters should be tried.

If the opening persists and it is apparent that an established fistula has developed, a jejunostomy is performed. Gastrostomy for the purpose of feeding should never be done in this situation, because the stomach contents pass back through the cardio-esophageal junction and into the pleural space. Large fistulas, in which quantities of saliva and gastric contents are lost, should be treated by performing a mucous fistula in the neck, a gastrostomy for continuous suction, and a jejunostomy for maintaining nutrition. Ultimately such patients will require an esophagogastrectomy or a colon bypass procedure.

REFERENCES

Barrett, N. R.: Report of a case of spontaneous perforation of the oesophagus successfully treated by operation. Brit. J. Surg., 35:216, 1947.

Barrett, N. R.: Spontaneous perforation of the oesophagus. Thorax, 1:48, 1946.

Boerhaave, H.: Atrocis, nec descripti pruis, morbi historia secundum medicae artis leges conscripta. Lugd. Bat. Boutesteniana, 1724, translated in Bull. Med. Libr. Assoc., 43:217, 1955.

Campbell, D., and Cox, W. A.: Spontaneous rupture of the esophagus presenting as an acute abdominal catastrophe. Surgery, 66:304, 1969.

Derbes, V. J., and Mitchell, R. E., Jr.: Rupture of the esophagus. Surgery, 39:688, 1956.

Dooling, J. A., and Zick, H. R.: Closure of an esophago-pleural fistula using onlay intercostal pedicle graft. Ann. Thorac. Surg., 3:553, 1967.

Duval: Bull. mém. Soc. Méd. Paris, 47:450, 1921.

Foster, J. H., Jolly, P. C., Sawyers, J. L., and Daniel, R. A.: Esophageal perforation: Diagnosis and treatment. Ann. Surg., 161:701, 1965.

Furstenburg, A. C.: Acute suppuration of the mediastinum. Tr. 35th Ann. Meet. Am. Laryng., Rhin., Otol. Assn., 35:210, 1929.

Gaudiani, V.: Surgical treatment of suppurative posterior mediastinitis. Ann. Surg., 63:523, 1916.

Gerard, F. P., Sabety, A. M., Trillo, R. A., and Fernando, M. B.: Esophageal perforation. Arch. Surg., 96:414, 1968.

Groves, L.: Instrumental perforation of the esophagus. What is conservative management? J. Thorac. Cardiov. Surg., 52:1, 1966.

Hacker von: Zur operativen Behandlung der Periodesphagealen und mediastinalen Phlegmone nebst Bemerkungen zur Technik der collaren und dorsalen Mediastinotomie. Arch. Klin. Chir., 64:478, 1901.

Hardin, W. J., Hardy, J. D., and Conn, J. H.: Esophageal perforations. Surg., Gynec. Obstet., 124:325, 1967.

Heidenhain, L.: Über einen Fall von Mediastinitis suppurativa plastica nebst Bemerkungen über die Wege, ins hintere Mediastinum einzudringen. Arch. Klin. Chir., 59:199, 1899.

Hoover, W. B.: Mediastinitis as a complication of esophagoscopy and instrumentation of the esophagus. Surg. Clin. N. Amer. 24:578, 1944.

Jemerin, E. E.: Results of treatment of perforation of the esophagus. Ann. Surg., 128:971, 1948.

Johnson, J., Schwegman, C. W., and Kirby, C. K.: Esophageal exclusion for persistent fistula following spontaneous rupture of the esophagus. J. Thorac. Cardiov. Surg., 32:827, 1956.

Johnson, J., Schwegman, C. W., and MacVaugh, H., III: Early esophagogastrostomy in the treatment of iatrogenic perforation of the distal esophagus. J. Thorac. Cardiov. Surg., 55:24, 1967.

Keen, G.: The surgical management of old esophageal perforations. J. Thorac. Cardiov. Surg., 56:603, 1968.

Lilienthal, H.: Posterior mediastinotomy. Arch. Surg., 6:274, 1923.

Mackenzie, M.: Diseases of the nose and throat. v. 2, 160, London, Churchill, Ltd., 1884.

Mackler, S. A.: Spontaneous rupture of the esophagus; experimental and clinical study. Surg. Gynec. Obstet., 95:345, 1952.

Marschik, H.: Mediastinotomia cervicalis superior. Wien. Klin. Wsch., 29:805, 1916.

Mathewson, C., Jr., Dozier, W. E., Hamill, J. P., and Smith, M.: Clinical experiences with perforation of the esophagus. Amer. J. Surg., 104:257, 1962.

Mengoli, L. R., and Klassen, K. P.: Conservative management of esophageal perforation. Arch. Surg., 91:238, 1965.

Von Mickulicz, quoted in Stevenson, R. S., and Guthrie, D.: History of oto-laryngology, Baltimore, Md., Williams & Wilkins, 1949, p. 131.

Naclerio, E. A.: The "V" sign in the diagnosis of spontaneous rupture of the esophagus (an early roentgen clue). Amer. J. Surg., 93:291, 1957.

Nealon, T. F., Jr., Templeton, J. Y., III, Cuddy, V. D., and Gibbon, J. H., Jr.: Instrumental perforation of the esophagus. J. Thorac. Cardiov. Surg., 41:75, 1961.

Paulson, D. L., Shaw, R. R., and Kee, J. L.: Recognition and treatment of esophageal perforations. Ann. Surg., 152:13, 1960.

Phillips, C. E.: Mediastinal infection from esophageal perforation. JAMA, 111:998, 1938.

Samson, P. C.: Postemetic rupture of the esophagus. Surg. Gynec. Obstet., 93:221, 1951.

Sealy, W. C.: Rupture of the esophagus. Amer. J. Surg., 105:505, 1963.

Seybold, W. D., Johnson, M. A., III, and Leary, W. V.: Perforation of esophagus; analysis of 50 cases and account of experimental studies. Surg. Clin. N. Amer., 30:1155, 1950.

Thal, A. P., and Hatafuku, T.: Improved operation for esophageal rupture. JAMA, 188:826, 1964.

Webb, W. R., and Burford, T. H.: Current concepts of the management of acute mediastinitis. Amer. Surgeon, 28:309, 1962.

Weisel, W., and Raine, F.: Surgical treatment of traumatic esophageal perforation. Surg. Gynec. Obstet., 94:337, 1952.

Wychulis, A. R., Fontana, R. S., and Payne, W. S.: Instrumental perforations of the esophagus. Dis. Chest, 55:184, 1969.

Wychulis, A. R., Fontana, R. S., and Payne, W. S.: Non-instrumental perforations of the esophagus. Dis. Chest, 55:190, 1969.

Zikria, B. A., Rosenthal, A. D., Potter, R. T., and Ferrer, J. M., Jr.: Mallory-Weiss syndrome and emetogenic (spontaneous) rupture of the esophagus. Ann. Surg., 162:151, 1965.

CHAPTER 12

MASSIVE GASTROINTESTINAL HEMORRHAGE

by JAMES H. FOSTER, M.D., ROBERT ALBO, M.D.,
and J. ENGLEBERT DUNPHY, M.D.

James H. Foster was born in New Haven, graduated from Haverford College and the Columbia College of Physicians and Surgeons, and served his internship at Barnes Hospital in St. Louis. Following his surgical residency under Dr. Dunphy at the University of Oregon he became Director of the Surgical Service at Hartford Hospital in 1966.

Robert J. Albo is a Californian. He received his baccalaureate and medical degrees and served his surgical residency at the University of California at Berkeley and San Francisco and is presently Assistant Clinical Professor of Surgery at that institution.

J. Englebert Dunphy was born in Northampton, Massachusetts, and received his medical degree from Harvard and his surgical training at the Peter Bent Brigham Hospital. Following outstanding military service in World War II he served on the Harvard faculty, rising to the rank of Professor of Surgery. He became Chairman of the Department of Surgery at the University of Oregon Medical School in 1959. In 1964 he became Professor of Surgery and Chairman of the Department of the University of California School of Medicine, San Francisco. Many signal honors have been awarded Dr. Dunphy in recognition of the intangible but nonetheless real force for excellence which he has imparted to American surgery. He has been president of most national surgical organizations in which he has participated, and his contributions to our knowledge of wound healing, gastrointestinal disease, and cancer are universally recognized.

UPPER GASTROINTESTINAL HEMORRHAGE

"Massive" is a relative word, but it is an excellent term to apply to the problem presented by a patient who is vomiting or defecating large amounts of blood. Not only is the hemorrhage massive; so are the reactions of the patient and his family; moreover a massive commitment is required of both physician and surgeon to meet the demands of modern management of this syndrome regardless of cause.

Surgical textbooks of 40 years ago ruled out emergency operation as a method of treatment for patients with massive gastroin-testinal hemorrhage. By 1940, improved techniques in anesthesia, blood replacement, and surgical skill allowed a selective operative approach which promised increased survival over medical therapy alone. This approach has been refined in the last two decades to the point that patients actively bleeding from peptic ulceration have a survival rate in excess of 95 per cent. However, the present treatment is not nearly as successful for patients hemorrhaging from esophageal varices, hemorrhagic gastritis, and "stress" ulceration. The patient with intermittent hemorrhage from an occult source remains an enigma, but diagnostic techniques are improving.

This chapter deals with the management of

patients with massive upper and lower gastrointestinal hemorrhage, with an emphasis on emergency and urgent measures. This discussion will be prejudiced strongly by our personal experience, some of which has been reported elsewhere (Dunphy, 1954; Dunphy and Hoer, 1948; Foster, unpublished data; Foster et al., 1963, 1966; Foster and Vetto, 1962, 1967; Hoerr et al., 1948). This personal prejudice is defended on the grounds that (1) there is no suitable experimental model with which to study this problem scientifically; (2) a review of the reported experience of others can be suitably arranged to defend almost any position on most of the controversial issues; and (3) the management of these patients depends to a large extent on the clinical experience of the attending physician. Current principles of treatment are more in the realm of "art" than "science." Most of the discussion is concerned with common problems, but reference is also made to recent reviews of the rarer causes of hemorrhage.

Clinical separation of patients bleeding from the upper gastrointestinal tract, i.e., above the mid-jejunum, can usually be made from those bleeding from lesions below this level. This chapter arbitrarily separates these two areas, although many of the features of management are common to both.

MASSIVE UPPER GASTROINTESTINAL HEMORRHAGE

ETIOLOGY

The reported causes of upper gastrointestinal hemorrhage vary according to different decades, authors, parts of the world, and age groups. Lesions that commonly cause mild bleeding may only rarely produce a massive hemorrhage. In Table 12-1 data from several recent surveys are tabulated to show the relative frequencies of the more common lesions that produce upper gastrointestinal hemorrhage.

These figures are subject to several criticisms. Palmer's (1965) report is based on endoscopic and roentgenographic evidence. Most of his patients never had a laparotomy to confirm the diagnosis. Many surgeons have reported that no bleeding lesion could be found in as many as 10 to 15 per cent of patients at operation; therefore they obviously missed the lesion and could not list it properly. In several of the reports listed in Table 12-1, no clear-cut definition of massive hemorrhage was given, so that a precise incidence of various causes of exsanguinating hemorrhage requiring operation is not recorded.

However, certain trends are apparent. Duodenal ulcer continues to remain the most common source of massive hemorrhage, although its percentage of the totals seems to be decreasing. Portal hypertension with bleeding from esophageal varices is on the increase, particularly in the large urban centers of the United States. Marginal or anastomotic ulcer is becoming less common because of better operative control of the ulcer diathesis.

Gastritis is a difficult diagnosis to evaluate. Most surgeons would place it low on their lists of causes of hemorrhage requiring emergency operation (and would like to place it even lower). On the other hand, endoscopists state that this diagnosis is responsible for as much as 26 per cent of the causes of massive upper gastrointestinal hemorrhage. If one includes in this general category all diffuse and superficial lesions, such as those caused by drugs, alcohol, and stress, then certainly the proportion of patients with bleeding gastritis seems to be increasing.

TABLE 12-1. Causes of Bleeding in Patients with Upper Gastrointestinal Hemorrhage

Authors	Duodenal Ulcer	Gastric Ulcer	Varices	Gastritis	Unknown	Other
	per cent		per cent	per cent	per cent	per cent
Zimmerman et al. (1956)	72.0		14.0	0.0	7.0	—
Gray et al. (1957)	65.0		9.0	11.0	10.0	5.0
Hirschowitz et al. (1963)	58.0		0.0	22.0	12.0	—
Katz et al. (1964)	25.0		19.0	26.0	19.0	—
Schiff (1964)	52.9		12.5	1.1	20.6	12.9
Balasegaram (1968)	34.0	25.0	13.0	1.0	12.0	15.0
Palmer (1969)	28.0	13.0	19.0	12.0	7.0	20.0

Other, rarer causes of massive upper gastrointestinal hemorrhage are listed in Table 12-2. Meticulous attention to details of the medical history often lead the alert clinician to consider these rarer lesions.

The cause of variceal rupture is debated in patients with portal hypertension. More often than not the hemorrhage occurs without preceding pain, but Simpson and Conn (1968) and Liebowitz (1961) have presented evidence suggesting that peptic esophagitis, perhaps on the basis of a gastroesophageal junction rendered incompetent by large submucosal varices, may cause the initial break in the variceal wall. The observation of Kern (personal communication) that cirrhotic patients with ascites, liver decompensation, or both often bleed *after* they have been hospitalized lends support to this theory. Orloff and Thomas (1963) present evidence that argues against reflux esophagitis as a cause of varix rupture.

The recent work of Menguy (1966) has led to a better understanding of the role of aspirin and adrenal steroids as causes of gastric hemorrhage. Rather than effecting an increase in the secretion of pepsin and hydrochloric acid, these and other agents apparently alter the gastric mucus and thus render the gastric mucosa more liable to peptic acid injury. The role of aspirin is thoroughly discussed by Salter (1968). Its importance as

TABLE 12-2. Unusual Causes of Massive Upper Gastrointestinal Hemorrhage

A. Lesions which may cause hemorrhage from any part of upper intestinal tract:	
Duplications	Hirsch et al. (1967)
Angiodysplasias	Halpern et al. (1968), Goldman (1964)
Rendu-Osler-Weber telangiectasia	Vetto (1962)
Angiomas	Bongiovi and Duffy (1967)
Leukemia	Hirsch et al. (1967), Cornes et al. (1961)
Suture lines	
Polyposis	Hittner (1966)
Aspirin	Parry and Wood (1967), Salter (1968)
Aneurysm	Foster and Vetto (1962)
Splenic	Matyus et al. (1966)
Hepatic	Gordon-Taylor (1943)
Cancer chemotherapy	Rousselot et al. (1965)
Anticoagulants	Klingensmith and Oles (1964)
Pseudoxanthoma elasticum	Robertson and Schroder (1959)
Amyloidosis	Dahlin (1949), Cooley (1953), Long et al. (1965)
Heterotopic pancreas	Abrahams (1966)
Polyarteritis nodosa	Lee and Kay (1958)
B. Bleeding from the esophagus:	
Hiatus hernia	Barrett and Reckling (1965)
Aortoesophageal fistula	Sloop and Thompson (1967)
Mallory-Weiss syndrome	Mallory and Weiss (1929)
Varices secondary to primary or metastatic	
hepatocarcinoma	Hirsch et al. (1967)
C. Bleeding from the stomach:	
Gastric ulcer in hiatus hernia	
Eroding myocardium	Arrants et al. (1968)
Eroding thoracic aorta	Couves et al. (1958)
Gastric arteriosclerosis	Frank (1946)
Retrograde jejunogastric intussusception	Foster (1956)
Gastritis	
Atrophic, with achlorhydria	Winower et al. (1967)
Hemorrhagic, alcohol and drugs	Nagel et al. (1967)
Curling and Cushing ulcers	Fletcher and Harkins (1954), Artz and Fitts (1966)
"Stress ulcer"	Grosz and Wu (1967)
D. Bleeding from the upper small bowel:	Netterville et al. (1968)
Duodenal varices	Richter and Pochaczevsky (1967)
	Rosen et al. (1967)
Pancreatitis	deKrester et al. (1966), Haller et al. (1966)
Duodenal diverticulum	Hirsch et al. (1967)
Hemobilia	Graff (1963), Sparkman (1953)
Tumors	Netterville et al. (1968), Schwartz (1966)
Jejunal diverticula	Wells (1967), Civetta and Daggett (1967)
Cholecystoduodenal fistula	Corry et al. (1968)

a factor in gastrointestinal hemorrhage is further demonstrated by Smith and Babb (1968).

Classification of the vascular anomalies of stomach and small bowel is variable. These seem to form a whole range of lesions from Rendu-Osler-Weber telangiectasis to serpentine arteriovenous malformations of mesentery and bowel wall. Angiomatous lesions may be single and quite large, but are more often small and multiple. Although such lesions are common, their association with massive upper gastrointestinal hemorrhage is rare.

A recent report (Evans et al., 1968) indicates that the tendency of patients with O type blood to bleed from peptic ulcer is related to a propensity toward hypersecretion which will lead to any or all of the complications of ulcer, only one of which is hemorrhage.

DIAGNOSIS

The clinical history is the most important factor in diagnosing the cause of massive upper gastrointestinal hemorrhage. The patient who has increasing fatigue and black stools for a week is not as urgently in need of help as the patient who suddenly vomits blood and faints. Hematemesis and liquid black stools usually indicate rapid bleeding. The word "melena" is derived from the Greek work meaning black, and is used properly to describe the black tarry stool typical of upper gastrointestinal hemorrhage. Hematochezia means a red, bloody stool. As little as 50 ml. of fresh human blood may produce a tarry stool. Hilsman (1950) showed that blood introduced into the cecum may result in a tarry stool in the presence of decreased colonic motility. The color of vomitus and stool relates more to the time the blood remains in the gastrointestinal tract than to the site of the bleeding lesion, but a copious "tarry stool" means upper gastrointestinal bleeding. Large amounts of bright red unclotted blood without evidence of shock indicate bleeding from the lower gastrointestinal tract.

We used to think that rapid hemorrhage probably meant penetrating peptic ulcer or ruptured varix, but it is now apparent that any and all of the lesions listed in Table 12-2, including aortoduodenal fistula, can produce any degree of hemorrhage from a slow ooze to rapid exsanguination.

Patients bleeding from peptic ulcer often have previously had characteristic symptoms of ulcer. This distress may not have been associated with the present bleeding episode, however. Schiff and Shapiro (1951) report that in 10 per cent of 399 patients bleeding from ulcer, no pain was present at or immediately before the onset of hemorrhage. In another 20 per cent of their patients distress was not typical of ulcer. They believe that if typical ulcer distress stops with the onset of bleeding, an inferential diagnosis of bleeding peptic ulcer can be made and substantiated in 90 per cent of all patients. Although personality factors may help the experienced clinician to detect the "ulcer type" of patient, the coexistence of major hemorrhage and shock will probably obscure these subtle differences. Melena without hematemesis or blood in the gastric aspirate strongly points to a diagnosis of duodenal ulcer, particularly in patients under 60 years old.

A past history of gastric operation will of course alert the clinician to the possibility of bleeding from marginal ulceration. The pathologist's description of the tissue previously resected should be checked to insure that duodenal mucosa was seen at the distal line of gastric transection.

If the bleeding comes from peptic esophagitis, there is usually a good history of "heartburn" and other symptoms characteristic of hiatus hernia. Vigorous nonbloody vomiting followed by the sudden appearance of hematemesis suggests the Mallory-Weiss syndrome. This lesion is more common in the alcoholic; therefore a history of retching without initial bleeding is a most important detail in differentiating the mucosal tears of the Mallory-Weiss syndrome from variceal hemorrhage.

A history of heavy alcohol consumption may not be obtained from the patient. Since this matter is so important in both diagnosis and treatment, it is wise to question another member of the family. Genteel old ladies, prominent business men, and civic leaders are not immune to the temptations of alcohol, and it is not unusual for a physician who specializes in the "carriage trade" to overlook this possibility when he is called upon to treat a professional colleague. If the alcohol was consumed recently, hemorrhagic alcoholic gastritis must be placed high on the list of possible causes of hemorrhage. If a history of chronic alcoholism is found, particularly in association with the characteristic physical stigmata of this condition, then portal hypertension with bleeding varices is the most likely cause of hemorrhage.

In our experience with portal hypertension in the nonalcoholic, there has often been no antecedent history of jaundice. Apparently an anicteric hepatitis has silently progressed to postnecrotic cirrhosis. Certainly a history of jaundice should be sought, but if the other signs of chronic liver disease are present, the absence of clinical jaundice in the past cannot be relied upon to rule out esophageal varices. The association of gastroduodenal ulceration with cirrhosis, either before or after portacaval shunting, is well documented, but as a general rule it is better to assume that hemorrhage is from varices in the known cirrhotic until other diagnostic tests document a second lesion.

The most important detail in the clinical history of the cirrhotic patient is whether bleeding has occurred at one end of a long course manifested by anorexia, lethargy, weakness, jaundice, and ascites. Such a history should stay the surgeon's hand, no matter what the liver function studies may show. Conversely, an acute episode of bleeding in a patient who has been working productively and has been feeling well, in spite of laboratory and clinical evidence of longstanding cirrhosis, suggests a favorable prognosis and justifies emergency intervention. The surgeon should also be encouraged if the patient gives historical evidence of previous hemorrhages without liver decompensation.

Hematobilia may occur weeks and even months after liver trauma. Aortoenteric fistulas are more common after aortic surgery, but spontaneous fistulas can occur anywhere in the gastrointestinal tract from midesophagus to rectum (Foster and Vetto, 1962). Aortoesophageal fistulas may arise from injury from a swallowed foreign body (Sloop and Thompson, 1967). Bleeding from an aortointestinal fistula, although usually massive, is commonly episodic. Spontaneous cessation of bleeding does not rule out an aortic fistula; indeed it is rather characteristic.

Bleeding telangiectases almost never cause hematemesis, but should be considered when there is no historical evidence of other gastrointestinal disease, particularly in the older patient. Textbooks mention the association of these gastrointestinal Rendu-Osler-Weber lesions with similar lesions in the mouth, but clinically this has not been of great help. Acute hemorrhagic pancreatitis and traumatic pancreatitis can cause massive gastrointestinal bleeding, usually by direct erosion of the digestive tract (deKretser et al., 1966; Haller et al., 1966). The more chronic form of pancreatitis is often associated with bleeding duodenal ulcer.

A careful history must also be taken to investigate evidence suggesting hemorrhagic diathesis. Nosebleeds, easy bruisability, and prolonged bleeding with minor lacerations should alert the physician and point to more intensive study of the coagulation mechanism.

Many drugs have been implicated as etiologic agents in upper gastrointestinal hemorrhage. Often this bleeding is not massive, but certainly aspirin can cause a diffuse hemorrhagic gastritis which can lead to exsanguinating hemorrhage. In a recent report Smith and Babb (1968) document the frequent association of aspirin ingestion with bleeding, often in association with other specific entities such as peptic ulcer or esophagitis. Butazolidin, ACTH, adrenal steroids, reserpine, indomethacin, and alcohol have all been implicated as precipitating causes of upper gastrointestinal hemorrhage in patients with and without peptic ulcer.

Massive hemorrhage from carcinoma of the upper gastrointestinal tract is rare. Although blood loss occurs, it is usually over a long period, and the patient presents with anemia. However, gastric tumors, particularly of smooth muscle, may present with massive hemorrhage. The syndrome of portal hypertension secondary to metastatic or primary liver carcinoma as a cause of hemorrhage is occasionally seen. An excellent review of gastrointestinal bleeding in infancy and childhood is given by Spencer (1964).

Physical Examination

The physical examination is only occasionally helpful in differential diagnosis of the bleeding lesion, although it may be of great importance in estimating operative risk and the degree of bleeding. Fever of 103° F. may be seen with blood in the gastrointestinal tract, and appears to be related to the rapidity of hemorrhage, rather than to the absorption of breakdown products of red blood cells (Schiff, 1964). Hyperperistalsis is often present with continuing massive hemorrhage. Green and Metheny (1957) have recommended the "tilt" test, in which elevation of the head of the bed will speed the pulse and perhaps lower the blood pressure in a patient with borderline blood volume compensation. This may be dangerous in geriatric patients. More helpful are the classic signs of restlessness, thirst, and apprehension that often accompany brisk bleeding. The nature of the pulse may tell as much as the rate. Warm, dry feet should encourage the clinician that the circulation is adequate, at least for the moment. The classic signs of hypovolemic shock indicate that treatment must assume a higher priority than diagnosis. Lowe and Palmer (1967) have reported seven cases of fatal upper gastrointestinal hemorrhage in patients who had not passed blood by mouth or anus.

Any evidence of petechiae or ecchymosis should alert the physician to the possibility of a coagulation defect. Early examination of the gastric and rectal contents for evidence of blood is important in helping to establish the level of the bleeding lesion.

The presence of spider hemangiomata, gynecomastia, and palmar erythema is not very useful in weighing the hepatic reserve of a patient with hepatic cirrhosis, but should draw the attention of the physician to the possibility of portal hypertension as a cause of hemorrhage. Muscle wasting is a most important physical sign and when present usually denotes serious chronic liver disease, probably associated with hypoproteinemia. The size of the liver and spleen should be carefully determined.

The classic intraoral lesions of the Peutz-Jeghers syndrome or the submucosal telangiectasia of Rendu-Osler-Weber disease suggests intestinal polyps or hemangiomata as the source of bleeding. The patient's sensorium must be evaluated by both the surgeon and the physician after admission to the hospital. A careful follow-up of the patient's mental status will be one of the most important factors in determining whether emergency operation can be safely performed. The patient's ability to construct a five-pointed star using ten matches or to write his name on a piece of paper are useful tests which may be used serially to evaluate the state of the sensorium. These signs often deteriorate before the patient loses his ability to remember the names of Presidents or subtract sevens.

Laboratory Tests

Every patient with signs or symptoms of upper gastrointestinal hemorrhage should have blood drawn for diagnostic tests as soon as possible after admission to the emergency room or hospital. Determination of the hemoglobin or hematocrit, white blood cell count, differential, platelet evaluation on smear, prothrombin time, activated clotting time, blood urea nitrogen, and typing and cross-matching of whole blood for transfusion should always be done. Elevation of the BUN to above 30 mg. per cent is seen in two-thirds of patients with massive hemorrhage and may reach above 50 mg. per 100 ml. After a single massive hemorrhage the BUN rises in a few hours, peaks at about 24 hours, and drops sharply to normal by the third day. Azotemia does not appear in hemorrhage from the colon (Schiff, 1964).

If the history and physical examination suggest any evidence of liver disease, the usual liver function tests should also be performed. Of particular use in the emergency evaluation of these patients is the determination of the serum albumin. The enzyme tests take longer to perform and are not quite as valuable initially, although they subsequently help evaluate the patient's liver function if elective operation is to be considered.

It has been our clinical impression that bedside determination of venous clotting time and careful observation of venipuncture sites for evidence of prolonged bleeding are useful measures in evaluating a hemorrhagic diathesis.

Initial hemoglobin or hematocrit levels will not be as helpful as physical examination in determining the need for replacement therapy. In one large series, the patients who had the highest hemoglobin values upon admission to the hospital manifested the most severe hemorrhage and had the highest mortality after operation (Foster et al., 1963). This is explained by the fact that the patient with very brisk hemorrhage and syncope has had no time to dilute his red cells before coming to the hospital. The patient with an admission hemoglobin of 5 gm. per 100 ml. has been bleeding longer and represents less of an immediate risk. Depression of platelets or white cells, particularly in association with a large spleen, is strong presumptive evidence toward the diagnosis of liver cirrhosis and portal hypertension.

Blood ammonia levels and Bromsulphalein retention have been recommended as useful tests in differentiating variceal bleeding from that of peptic ulcer. As more experience has accumulated, it has become apparent that these tests provide useful information only if they are normal. Patients bleeding from peptic ulcer and many other nonhepatic lesions may have increased retention of Bromsulphalein associated with an acute episode of hemorrhage. However, if the Bromsulphalein retention is less than 5 per cent, this does help exclude chronic severe liver disease or the presence of significant extrahepatic portal venous shunt. Belkin and Conn (1959) conclude that if both BSP and ammonia levels are elevated, a diagnosis of cirrhosis is confirmed; if both tests are within the normal range, cirrhosis is excluded, but if one test is abnormal and the other normal, no diagnostic value can be attached.

An electrocardiogram should be obtained for most patients over 30 years of age, and is particularly important in those who have had a syncopal episode. Myocardial infarction in relation to massive upper gastrointestinal hemorrhage is often painless and is a fairly common occurrence. Early detection of this lesion is of vital importance in weighing the risk of emergency operation. If posterior pituitary extract is to be used in the treatment of bleeding presumed due to portal hypertension, this drug is contraindicated in a patient with electrocardiographic evidence of coexistent coronary artery insufficiency.

When possible to obtain without excessive movement of the patient, it is useful to get a chest x-ray. This, together with the physical examination, helps the anesthesiologist give his opinion on operative risk. Aspiration of gastric contents is common in the patient with massive hematemesis, and preoperative appreciation of this condition may abort serious postoperative complications.

Other Diagnostic Maneuvers

NASOGASTRIC INTUBATION. Nasogastric intubation may have obvious therapeutic effects, but is also quite useful as a diagnostic tool. It helps establish the level of the bleeding lesion and also monitors the evidence of continuing hemorrhage. Gross blood in the stomach may be from lesions as far down as the upper third of the jejunum, but such distant reflux occurs only when hemorrhage is massive (Wells, 1967).

MEASUREMENT OF SPLENIC PULP PRESSURE. This has been recommended as an emergency diagnostic test for those patients in whom the suspicion of bleeding esophageal varices is strong. Panke et al. (1959)

state that a splenic pulp pressure of less than 250 mm. of saline rules out esophageal varices as a source of bleeding. A pressure over 290 mm. of saline was associated with hemorrhage from varices in every patient in their report.

TESTS TO EVALUATE THE LEVEL OF BLEEDING. The classic string test and its modification using fluorescein may have value in slow bleeding from an occult focus (Haynes and Pittman, 1960), but often is not useful in emergency situations (Brag, 1964). If the patient has had several previous episodes of bleeding from an occult source and is seen again without an obvious diagnosis, the passage of a long intestinal tube of the Kaslow or Miller-Abbott type has been recommended by Ross (1969). Simple aspiration as the tube proceeds down the gastrointestinal tract may locate the level of slow bleeding. Unfortunately, during rapid hemorrhage blood may reflux several feet in a retroperistaltic direction, negating the usefulness of this test. Lorimer (1968) has suggested using chromium-tagged erythrocytes to further define information gained from long-tube aspiration of gastrointestinal contents.

ANGIOGRAPHY. Several authors (Ashby et al., 1968; Baum et al., 1967; Boijsen and Reuter, 1967; Nusbaum et al., 1965; Reuter and Bookstein, 1968) have reported enthusiastically about the capability of selective visceral angiography in locating sites of blood loss into the gastrointestinal tract. Other reports (Halpern et al., 1968) credit arteriography with localizing vascular lesions such as aneurysms and angiomas, although no definite escape of contrast agent into the bowel lumen may be seen. This method may prove to have great merit, particularly in the patient who has bled previously and has undergone a thorough but unrewarding diagnostic work-up.

Our experience with this technique has not resulted in a single success to date, but improper case selection may be at fault. It would seem that the ideal patient for angiography would be one who is bleeding briskly but not rapidly enough to require continuous resuscitation or an immediate decision for operation. The most recent report of Nusbaum et al. (1969) indicates that it is deserving of much wider use.

ENDOSCOPY. Palmer (1961, 1969), Hedberg (1966), and many others have advised the routine use of esophagoscopy and gastroscopy in an aggressive approach to diagnosis. They would not delay use of these procedures during resuscitative efforts, and claim that more information will be gathered if the tests are done while the patient is actively bleeding.

The recommended technique involves irrigation of the stomach with an Ewald tube prior to endoscopy. This effects both a decrease in bleeding because of hypothermia and an irrigation of retained blood clots, whose continued coagulation is probably also inhibited by the cold temperature of the irrigant fluid. With little or no topical anesthesia the esophagoscope or gastroscope is passed quickly down into the suspected area. Complications from these procedures are closely but inversely related to the experience of the endoscopist (Hedberg, 1966). The diagnoses accumulated by endoscopy as causes of upper gastrointestinal hemorrhage differ somewhat from those gathered by other techniques. Obviously, barium contrast studies will result in few diagnoses of hemorrhagic gastritis and many of duodenal ulcer. With endoscopy the reverse proportion will apply.

The limitations of this diagnostic maneuver are several and are outlined clearly by one of its proponents (Hedberg, 1966). First, the endoscopist cannot visualize all those areas of the upper gastrointestinal tract that might be sources of hemorrhage. The most obvious lesion certain to be missed is the duodenal ulcer. If a definite lesion is seen with endoscopy, there is no real proof that this will be the only bleeding lesion. In spite of published reports to the contrary, there often are considerable technical difficulties in clearing the mucous membrane of either esophagus or stomach in the rapidly bleeding patient so that the endoscopist may see enough to be firm in his diagnosis. Conn et al. (1965) document disagreement among endoscopists about the presence of varices in the same patient.

It appears that an unselective routine use of endoscopy for the patient with massive upper gastrointestinal hemorrhage is not warranted at the present time. However, this technique has great application in selected cases. The following patients are most likely to benefit from an emergency endoscopy:

1. Patients with strong evidence of chronic liver disease and bleeding esophageal varices.

2. Patients with a history of recent alcohol ingestion.

3. Patients without historic or physical evidence leading toward a diagnosis of peptic ulceration.

4. Patients with a history of ingestion of aspirin, cortisone, reserpine, ACTH, butazolidin, or indomethacin.

Using these criteria we would advocate emergency endoscopy in approximately 50 to 60 per cent of our patients with massive upper gastrointestinal hemorrhage, assuming an experienced endoscopist is at hand.

BARIUM CONTRAST STUDIES OF THE UPPER GASTROINTESTINAL TRACT. Woodward (1967), Palmer (1969), and others continue to advise routine use of contrast radiography in the patient who is bleeding from the upper gastrointestinal tract. The fears of provoking hemorrhage by manipulation of the abdominal wall have largely been abandoned, and a vigorous, early, and complete study of the esophagus, stomach, and duodenum is recommended. The diagnostic reliability of emergency upper gastrointestinal x-rays in finding the bleeding lesion has been estimated at 42 to 90 per cent (Hedberg, 1966).

Again an unselective approach is inadvisable for several reasons: (1) subjecting an *unstable* patient with evidence of active and continued hemorrhage to a procedure that may inhibit resuscitative measures and isolates the patient, even for only a few minutes, from the responsible physician is unnecessarily hazardous, and its advantage to the patient remains undocumented; (2) it is often impossible to make an accurate radiographic diagnosis if the patient's stomach is full of clotted and unclotted blood; (3) unfortunately the lesions demonstrable by radiography are exactly those lesions that are evident to the surgeon at laparotomy; the diffuse and tiny bleeding lesions that surgeons find difficult to isolate at operation are also undiscovered by their colleagues in radiology; (4) another theoretical disadvantage which may become more important in the future is that barium in the upper gastrointestinal tract may obscure angiographic findings.

If hemorrhage has slowed or ceased and the patient's condition has become stable, early barium contrast studies should be obtained. Information gained will be helpful in determining the need for elective or emergency operation should bleeding recur.

A less than warm endorsement of radiologic assistance and a more enthusiastic selective endorsement of endoscopy need further explanation. Perhaps the bias can be best explained by looking at these procedures from the patient's viewpoint and asking three questions: Do these tests change the doctor's decision about operation? Do they help the surgeon at laparotomy? Will they make any measurable difference in the patient's survival?

The decision to operate is based mostly on clinical grounds, more specifically on evidence about the amount and rate of continued hemorrhage. Differential diagnosis takes a secondary place in this decision but is quite important if liver disease, drug ingestion (including alcohol), or the Mallory-Weiss syndrome is suspected. Endoscopy is helpful in establishing these diagnoses, whereas radiography usually is not. Clinical evidence suggesting duodenal ulcer, particularly in a patient without hematemesis, and certainly in a patient with no blood in his gastric aspirate, means that endoscopy will be of little help. If the patient's condition stabilizes, a contrast radiographic study of the upper gastrointestinal tract may be useful.

At laparotomy the experienced surgeon who knows the normal appearance of tissues and who knows which lesions are most likely to cause hemorrhage will quickly recognize pathologic findings that either radiology or endoscopy might "help" find. A preoperative diagnosis may help the surgeon find a bleeding lesion, but fixation on a predetermined lesion may also decrease the chances of finding other previously unrecognized disease.

There is no evidence that routine endoscopy has contributed to a lowering of the mortality in patients with massive hemorrhage. It is our feeling that there is no substitute for experience and clinical judgment in both the diagnosis and treatment of these patients. Pulmonary aspiration of gastric contents, unrecognized shock, esophageal and gastric perforation, and other complications of these diagnostic procedures do occur in a few patients and deter us from an aggressive unselective routine diagnostic regimen.

Could it be that these tests have brought out a fundamental kinship between physician and surgeon? Perhaps the diagnostician's aggressive support of endoscopy and radiology reflects an unexpressed and perhaps unrecognized need for the "surgical" approach to disease. Passing a large instrument down the alimentary tract in a hypotensive patient who is retching blood certainly might satisfy a need to "do something." On the other hand, when the surgeon insists on specific diagnosis prior to operation he may be sharing the physician's intellectual preoccupation with diagnosis, while postponing a difficult decision about the messy, uncertain business of treatment.

Perhaps physician and surgeon together should admit that neither approach alone suffices, and that the individual circumstances of any patient's hemorrhage must dictate the flexible priorities of diagnosis and treatment. Our bias toward clinical judgment is undoubtedly influenced by a selected exposure to massively bleeding patients who simply cannot wait for further testing.

The best management of the intestinal patient demands the team approach and selective use of appropriate diagnostic measures.

TREATMENT

Every patient with significant gastrointestinal hemorrhage should be hospitalized. The successful management of patients with massive upper gastrointestinal hemorrhage depends upon the ability of the physician to judge the patient's general condition and the degree of hemorrhage along with an aggressive approach to resuscitative therapy. Operative mortality correlates directly with the volume of blood transfusion required before operation, so that in most cases an early decision for or against operation should be made. This decision must be a joint one, shared by physician and surgeon; therefore the patient's best interests are served by a policy that requires combined medical-surgical consultation for every patient with significant upper gastrointestinal hemorrhage at the earliest possible moment.

The treatment of shock may take priority over diagnostic measures or specific therapy of the bleeding lesion. A large-caliber needle or intravenous catheter should be placed early for drawing of blood and for intravenous infusion of fluids. The advantages and dangers of replacing lost blood with crystalloid and colloid solutions (e.g. dextran) in patients with hemorrhagic shock has been well summarized by Eiseman and Carnes (1967). Type-specific but uncross-matched blood is safer to use in an emergency than transfusion with O-negative blood. Volume replacement should be performed aggressively when clinical signs indicate that a major hemorrhage has occurred. The blood pressure should not be allowed to remain at low levels in the hope that this may prevent recurrence of hemorrhage. Neither should blood transfusion be withheld pending hematocrit determinations. The patient with a very brisk hemorrhage and syncope has had no time to dilute his red cells, and therefore the first hematocrit determination is not a useful guide to the clinician in this situation. Serial hematocrit tests are often of some use, although clinical judgment and constant attention to the patient are the most important factors in determining volume replacement. A central venous pressure catheter can help greatly to evaluate the required speed of intravenous infusion. Urinary output should be monitored. When hypotension and other signs of shock do not respond quickly to resuscitative measures, an indwelling catheter should be used to measure hourly urinary outputs. Vasopressor drugs should not be used. If elevation of central venous pressure and other signs indicate cardiac failure, digitalis or an inotropic agent, such as Isuprel, should be used.

If the history is typical of peptic disease and the bleeding has obviously ceased, a regimen of frequent feedings and antacids may be prescribed. In all other instances a nasogastric tube should be passed into the stomach to remove blood and acid and to help in locating the lesion. Usually a Levin tube is used, although there are proponents of the Ewald tube, the Sengstaken-Blakemore or Linton tubes, and the gastric cooling balloons of Wangensteen and others. The use of these other tubes will be discussed later.

It is often difficult to clear the stomach of clotted blood. Attempts to do this with iced water or saline should be made, but only the aspiration of bright red blood correlated with other evidence of hypovolemia should lead the clinician to the firm diagnosis of continued hemorrhage. Palmer (1969) and others advocate continuous gastric irrigation with iced water. Irrigation with iced saline is satisfactory and results in an occasional slowing or cessation of hemorrhage. Objective scientific evidence that documents the value of this technique is still lacking.

Wangensteen et al. (1958) and many others Dollinger and Morgan, 1966; Schaller et al.,

1966; Wangensteen et al., 1963, 1966) have proposed a more controlled method of gastric mucosal cooling for the emergency treatment of massive upper gastrointestinal bleeding. A machine that continually irrigates the gastric balloon produces mucosal hypothermia in the range of 0 to 18° C. The procedure differs from gastric freezing, which has been advocated for the elective control of the peptic ulcer diathesis. Although initial reports were quite favorable, additional information has not established that this technique makes a significant difference in the patient's survival (Rodgers et al., 1966). The bleeding seems to be slowed or temporarily stopped by cooling but often recurs when the mucosa rewarms. Perhaps the greatest application of cooling is in the patient with diffuse superficial gastritis due to alcohol or other drugs.

Generalized hypothermia (Wheaton and Mark, 1967) and controlled hypotension (Hopkins et al., 1967) have been advocated for the emergency treatment of gastrointestinal hemorrhage. The results of the former are sufficiently encouraging to warrant continued use, especially when the general condition of the patient absolutely contraindicates operation.

Most patients will respond to initial vigorous resuscitative therapy. Many will have stopped bleeding before hospitalization. As soon as vital signs have stabilized, but not necessarily before cessation of bleeding, endoscopy and upper gastrointestinal x-rays should be made in selected cases.

The maximum amount of information that might contribute toward a decision to operate should be gathered as soon as possible, i.e., within a few hours of hospital admission rather than at the convenience of the hospital personnel the next day. More lives will be saved by the physician who anticipates the worst and prepares for it. Most patients will respond to the initial regimen of nonoperative therapy and may or may not become candidates for a subsequent elective operation. We offer the following guidelines for management of patients with continued bleeding.

Indications for Operation

If the patient does not have historic, endoscopic, or other evidence of portal hypertension, bleeding diathesis, or hemor-

TABLE 12-3.   Indications for Surgery in Gastroduodenal
Hemorrhage — Danger Signals

1. Repeated nausea and hematemesis
2. Persistent severe pain
3. Recurrence of bleeding after satisfactory medical therapy
4. Fainting, sweating, and weakness

rhagic gastritis, and the vital signs remain unstable after rapid transfusion of 1500 ml. of whole blood, a decision for emergency operation should be made. Even in the aged and debilitated patient, it has been established that the operative therapy of exsanguinating hemorrhage is superior to nonoperative support. Emergency operation is also advised if, after initial stabilization of vital signs and institution of adequate therapy, the patient shows evidence of recurrent hemorrhage or if prolonged slow bleeding occurs requiring daily transfusion of 1000 ml. or more of whole blood.

In the final analysis the primary indication for operation is the simple fact that the patient is presumed to be bleeding to death despite transfusions of approximately 500 ml. every eight hours after initial stabilization. Many other criteria have been recommended as definitive (Tables 12-3 and 12-4). In our experience the criteria in Table 12-3 should be regarded as danger signals. If any of these are present, the probability of an emergency operation being necessary is very great, and both physician and surgeon must be immediately available. In Table 12-4 are what can be termed contributing factors. These must be weighed in the balance in the assessment of each individual patient, but no one of them in itself is a primary criterion for operative intervention. Thus the aged patient is more likely to continue to bleed, but it is also in this instance that it is most desirable to avoid an emergency operation. The dangers of delay have been overemphasized. Delay in the face of continuing hemorrhage is

disastrous; but if the patient has stopped bleeding or bleeding is minimal, there is no biological significance to a chronological rule of 48 hours, as has been recommended by others. As will be pointed out later, the lower risk of pyloroplasty and vagotomy as compared to gastrectomy in the poor risk patient has contributed substantially to earlier decisions for operation.

Elective operation after bleeding stops should be performed (1) when the patient has a history of previous massive hemorrhage, perforation, intractable symptoms, or obstruction from ulceration, or (2) when roentgenograms of the upper intestinal tract show interval nonhealing or a gastric ulcer or an apparently malignant lesion.

If the patient has a history, endoscopic findings, or other evidence suggesting that portal hypertension, a bleeding diathesis, or hemorrhagic gastritis is the most likely cause of bleeding, then other rules apply concerning operative intervention. These will be discussed separately.

Emergency Operation for Nonvariceal Hemorrhage

PREPARATION. Once the decision for emergency operation has been made, all efforts should be aimed at getting the patient to the operating room at the earliest possible moment. Elective operating schedules may have to be cancelled or hospital personnel may have to be wakened in the middle of the night. To delay further for the convenience of hospital personnel is to court unacceptable risks for the patient. Hemor-

TABLE 12-4.   Indications for Surgery in Gastroduodenal
Hemorrhage — Contributing Factors

1. Age
2. Location of ulcer
3. Effect of delay
4. Number of previous hemorrhages
5. Accurate diagnosis
6. Complicating diseases

rhage requiring emergency operation also requires massive fluid replacement, and at least two large intravenous routes should be established before induction of anesthesia. Having a member of the surgical team in constant attendance adds several important benefits: first, immediate attention may be given to any sign of hypovolemic shock; second, technical preparations of the operating suite, including preparation and shaving of the patient's skin, may be expedited; and third, the anesthesiologist and the operating room personnel are kept closely informed about the nature and urgency of the problem.

If continuing blood loss requires transfusion under pressure, extraordinary precautions should be taken to avoid inadvertent air embolization.

If the patient has historic or other evidence suggesting that the bleeding lesion may be occult or may originate from the biliary tree, a cassette holder should be positioned beneath the patient on the operating table to allow x-rays to be taken during operation. Both angiograms and cholangiograms may be required.

Immediately prior to induction of anesthesia, careful, thorough aspiration and irrigation of the stomach should be performed. This will prevent pulmonary aspiration of gastric contents during intubation. Intubation often should be performed under local anesthesia with the patient awake. The early stages of anesthesia are liable to uncover continuing hypovolemia with cardiac arrhythmia, hypertension, or both. The electrocardiogram should be constantly monitored. Although certain anesthetic agents tend to produce venous hypertension and perhaps increased bleeding from surgical wounds, the anesthetic must be chosen by the anesthesiologist on the basis of multiple factors.

CHOICE OF INCISION. The fastest and driest way to enter the upper abdominal cavity is through an upper midline incision carried from the xiphoid process to beyond the umbilicus. This is true in most patients and is recommended as the usual emergency incision. In a few patients with a wide costal margin and a short distance between rib margin and iliac crest an upper abdominal transverse incision is preferred. A left thoracic approach to the upper gastrointestinal tract for massive bleeding is particularly helpful when there has been past evidence of multiple abdominal adhesions, when a marginal ulcer is suspected, after high subtotal gastrectomy, and when endoscopic or x-ray evidence of a fundal or gastroesophageal lesion has been found preoperatively.

As the incision is made and carried down through skin, subcutaneous tissues, and midline fascia, the surgeon should watch for excessive capillary oozing and non-clotting of shed blood. Evidence of collateral circulation as a result of portal hypertension may also be seen.

EXPLORATION. Osborne and Dunphy (1957) have emphasized the importance of an orderly and systematic exploration, including the absolute need for gastrotomy when a bleeding point is not evident.

Upon opening the peritoneal cavity, one should sense certain findings immediately. If there is no evidence of blood in the stomach, the highest level of blood in the small bowel should be immediately determined. Blood passes rather quickly through the small bowel, and within a few minutes this highest level may have moved down well beyond the bleeding lesion. The condition and size of the liver and spleen and the presence of an aortic aneurysm are quickly appreciated. Most patients with portal hypertension have obvious serpentine, tense visceral veins, but this is not always true. Palpation of the foramen of Winslow may reveal a common duct filled with blood clots. Rich vascular and lymphatic retroperitoneal collateralization in association with cirrhosis decreases the size of or obliterates this foramen.

If the patient's clinical condition suggests that hemorrhage is continuing and there is blood in the stomach, an immediate and direct approach to the gastroduodenal area should be made. However, the trip to the operating room and induction of anesthesia often seem to be followed by cessation of active bleeding. If there is no evidence of continued hemorrhage, a thorough abdominal exploration should be made prior to entering the gastrointestinal lumen. Visual and digital examination of the anterior surface of the stomach and duodenum reveals evidence of most peptic ulcers. Subserosal hemorrhage in the vicinity of the gastroesophageal junction suggests Mallory-Weiss lacerations. Manipulation of the serosal surface over a small peptic ulcer may result in the subsequent appearance of some petechial hemorrhage in an area of inflammation. Attention should be paid to those parts of the upper intestinal tract in closest contact with major arteries. Of particular concern are the posterior wall of duodenum over the pancreaticoduodenal artery, the lesser curvature of the stomach near the arcade formed by the right and left gastric arteries, and the area high on the posterior wall of the stomach where it overlies the splenic artery.

If there is no blood in the stomach and duodenum, the small bowel should be carefully inspected throughout its length. Telangiectases are fairly common in the older patient. We have found that these lesions disappear rather quickly with handling, so that the first look at the small bowel is most important in finding these lesions. Compression with a glass slide as described by Vetto (1962) is useful in defining this lesion. Palpation as well as visual inspection helps detect small tumors of jejunum and ileum. Transillumination of the small bowel has been helpful in locating several angiomatous lesions not evident by other techniques. In the occasional patient in whom isolation by segmentation has suggested one suspicious area of small bowel but when no discrete lesion can be found, the introduction of a sterile sigmoidoscope through an enterotomy has been useful in pinpointing the bleeding focus.

Jejunal diverticula are being documented with increasing frequency as a source of upper gastrointestinal hemorrhage (Civetta and Daggett, 1967; Shackleford and Marcus, 1960; Wells, 1967). These diverticula may be hard to find as they lie within folds of the mesentery, but if the bowel is distended by trapping and compressing intraluminal gas and fluid, the diverticula may become more evident. They usually occur in the upper third of the jejunum and may contain enteroliths.

If an aortic abdominal aneurysm is present, the third and fourth portions of the duodenum should be carefully dissected away from the anterior surface of such an aneurysm. If inflammation is found in this area, preparation for proximal and distal control of the aorta should be made prior to breaking into the ulcerative focus. Complete exposure of the anastomosis is essential to exclude a fistula. Moreover the degree of inflammation and induration is often so slight that the inexperienced surgeon is apt to rule out a fistula because "everything feels so normal."

Careful inspection of the rest of the abdominal contents may reveal other lesions, such as gallstones and tumors. However, correction of lesions other than those causing upper intestinal hemorrhage should not be attempted during emergency operation.

If at this point no obvious source of hemorrhage has been discovered, the lesser sac should be entered through the gastrocolic ligament. Careful palpation of the posterior gastric wall, the anterior surface of the pancreas, and the celiac axis will now be possible. By these maneuvers in the vast majority of patients, some lesion will have been found that is the probable cause of upper gastrointestinal hemorrhage. Further maneuvers depend on the location and nature of this lesion.

If the stomach is filled with blood clots and no definite gastric lesion is noted, the next step is to make an anterior longitudinal incision, 8 to 10 cm. long, which crosses the pylorus. Unless a lesion is immediately obvious, this incision should be longer than the usual elective pyloroplasty incision. It is particularly important to secure hemostasis along the gastroduodenotomy incision, because bleeding from this site may confuse subsequent exploration of the mucosal surface. Evacuation of clotted and unclotted blood from the lumen of the stomach and duodenum should be initially accomplished with a blunt metal suction tip of the sump type. After careful inspection of the duodenal and antral mucosa, this area should be palpated. The use of sharp instruments or dry gauze will provoke mucosal injury with hemorrhage and confuse the diagnosis. If a definite bleeding duodenal or antral ulceration is found, this should be controlled. It may be appropriate to biopsy the wall of a gastric ulcer prior to ligation of the bleeding point, but it is not necessary with duodenal ulcers. If an ulceration is found with a dry base, one should continue to search for another bleeding lesion. If the ulcer is not bleeding but has a blood clot in its base, this clot is disturbed and provoked until active bleeding follows.

If the stomach is filled with clots and no bleeding focus has been found at the antrum or duodenum, it is better to make a separate, higher gastrotomy than to extend the gastroduodenotomy incision (Fig. 12-1). A moist

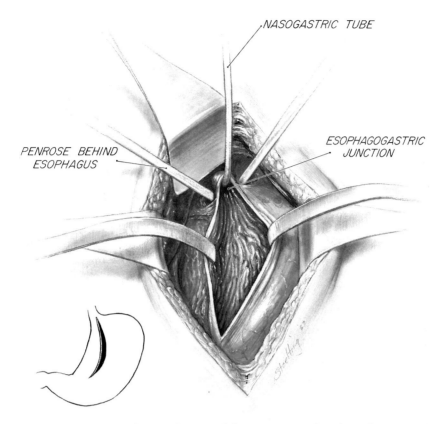

Figure 12-1. Gastrotomy incision for visualization of the upper stomach and esophagus. In a large stomach a high horizontal incision may be used, but we have found the one illustrated here to be more generally applicable. If a pyloroplasty incision has been made previously, the lower end of the gastrotomy incision should be well away from it. Mobilization of the lower esophagus and the passing of a Penrose drain behind it greatly facilitate inspection of the upper fundus and lower esophagus.

gauze plug is placed in the duodenum to prevent passage of blood up or down. Although a high transverse gastrotomy incision has been recommended, we have found more useful a curved gastrotomy that begins vertically at about the level of the incisura along the long axis of the anterior gastric wall and then curves up toward the gastro-esophageal junction. Suture control of bleeding vessels along this gastrotomy incision, placed as the incision is gradually extended cephalad, has helped with both visualization and retraction.

When the incision is large enough to allow entry of the surgeon's hand, manual evacuation of all clotted blood from the fundus and body of the stomach should be done. Gentle suction, irrigation, and eversion of the gastric fundal mucosa into the gastrotomy wound with a hand in the lesser sac permit inspection of most of the mucosal surface. Occasionally, it is necessary to divide the short gastric arteries along the greater curva-

ture of the stomach to allow complete inspection of the gastric wall. In several instances careful palpation of the mucosa has revealed a tiny bead-like nodule along the gastric wall which proved to be an ulceration of an arteriosclerotic artery. Palpation is also quite useful in picking up Mallory-Weiss lacerations at the gastro-esophageal junction. If mucosal tears without surrounding induration are found in this area after vigorous retraction, the lesion is most likely iatrogenic.

When the gastrotomy incision has been extended up to within 1 cm. of the gastro-esophageal junction, it is usually possible to see the very pale, smooth esophageal mucosa. The indwelling nasogastric tube is most useful in guiding the surgical incision to this point.

The passage of a second nasogastric tube has been advocated to allow separation of these two tubes to produce exposure of the distal esophagus. We have not found this maneuver as useful as direct inspection or the use of a sterile sigmoidoscope in visualizing the distal several centimeters of esophageal mucosa. Use of a sigmoidoscope to inspect the gastric mucosa is seldom helpful, because the many redundant folds of gastric mucosa prevent any thorough inspection or localization of lesions. Particularly in deep-chested patients, blunt dissection of the esophagus away from the diaphragmatic hiatus and passage of a Penrose drain through this channel for retraction allow better exposure of this poorly accessible area.

By these maneuvers nearly all gastroesophageal lesions will be found. Continued hemorrhage will lead the surgeon toward an undiscovered bleeding site, but when there is no further bleeding and no lesion has been found at this point, attention should be returned to the distal gastroduodenotomy. The sponge should be removed from the proximal duodenum. If blood wells up in this area, the bleeding lesion is probably distal to the papilla of Vater. Further dissection of the third and fourth portions of the duodenum and inspection of the proximal jejunum should be done. In one of our patients isolation of a bleeding duodenal varix was facilitated by placing a loose ligature around the jejunum just distal to the ligament of Treitz and watching reflux of blood through the proximal duodenum. In other patients a small jejunotomy incision has been made and the second and third portions of the duodenum irrigated to confirm bleeding in this area (Osborne and Dunphy, 1957).

Definitive Procedures After Diagnosis Is Made

Arbitrary recommendations will be made for the selection of appropriate operations for some of the lesions commonly causing massive upper gastrointestinal hemorrhage. These choices will be defended in a subsequent section that considers the results of operation.

BLEEDING DUODENAL ULCER. When an actively bleeding vessel is found at the base of a duodenal ulcer, either primarily or after provocation, definitive suture control is achieved by using heavy sutures of nonabsorbable material. Since the hemorrhage is often caused by a side hole in the artery,

sutures are necessary on both sides of the bleeding point (Fig. 12-2). The sutures should be placed deeply, even at some risk to the common bile duct, because rebleeding from a previously sutured ulcer has necessitated reoperation in several of our earlier patients.

The gastroduodenotomy is then closed transversely with one layer of silk as a Heineke-Mikulicz pyloroplasty. Soft tissue is interposed between this layer and the liver prior to wound closure. Bilateral truncal vagotomy is done with the usual care to insure transection of all vagal fibers.

BLEEDING GASTRIC ULCER. After biopsy of the wall of the ulcer and careful suture control of any bleeding points with nonabsorbable suture, vagotomy and pyloroplasty should be accomplished as previously described. Multiple ulcers are not uncommon and should be looked for. It has been our practice to close gastric ulcers from

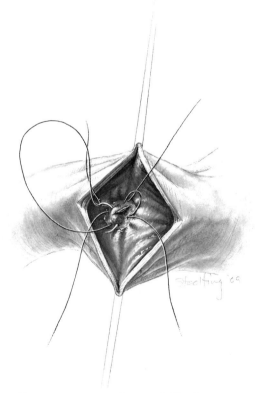

Figure 12-2. Transfixion of bleeding posterior duodenal ulcer through pyloroplasty incision. The needle should be a full half-circle in shape and sufficiently stout to permit deep penetration into the ulcer bed. Since the bleeding may be coming from a lateral hole in the artery, double ligation is recommended, as shown.

the mucosal surface rather than excising them, although the value of this procedure has not been established.

Occasionally technical factors, usually associated with giant gastroduodenal ulcers, will prevent simple vagotomy and an emptying procedure. In these cases posterior gastroenterostomy and vagotomy is recommended. On occasion, especially in the good risk patient, gastrectomy and vagotomy may be the procedure of choice. This is necessary in less than 10 per cent of patients bleeding from peptic ulcer.

In the past, recommendations have been made for the control of bleeding peptic ulcers by ligation of one or more gastric arteries. A consideration of the multiple interconnections between the various gastric arteries suggests that ligation of any individual vessel would probably not decrease arterial pressure at the mucosal level. Our own experience corroborates this impression (Foster et al., 1966). We now believe that there is no place for arterial ligation as an emergency operation to control massive upper gastrointestinal hemorrhage from peptic ulcer, diffuse gastritis, or multiple erosions.

PEPTIC ESOPHAGITIS. If a discrete ulcer or bleeding lesion is found in the distal esophagus of a patient with a sliding hiatus hernia, suture control of the bleeding focus with nonabsorbable material should be combined with hiatus herniorrhaphy, vagotomy, and Heineke-Mikulicz pyloroplasty. In the poor-risk patient a Nissen fixation of the stomach to the anterior abdominal wall is the method of choice. Early palpation of the distal esophagus after gastrotomy incision will alert the surgeon to this possibility. In the more common problem of diffuse esophagitis with oozing from multiple points, the bleeding usually stops after vagotomy and reduction of the hernia.

MARGINAL ULCER. If a subtotal gastric resection has been done previously, suture control of the bleeding vessel and bilateral vagotomy are recommended through either a thoracic or an abdominal incision. Careful inspection of the duodenal stump is indicated if there is some doubt about complete removal of antral mucosa. If no stomach has been previously resected, we would reperform the vagotomy and gain suture control of the bleeding vessel in older and poor-risk patients, but would probably also add a distal gastrectomy in the younger or good-risk patient bleeding from a marginal ulcer.

ALCOHOLIC OR DRUG-INDUCED GASTRITIS. The key to treatment in patients with drug-induced gastritis is a careful medical history with this diagnosis invariably in mind. Gastroscopy is essential in these patients. If a diffuse, edematous hemorrhagic gastric mucosa with petechial hemorrhage is seen, operation should be avoided if at all possible. Gastric cooling would seem to be an ideal solution to this problem, because the effects of these noxious drugs should be short-lived, and the gastric mucosa should subsequently heal. However, results have not been up to expectations (Wangensteen et al., 1963). Emergency operation in the acutely intoxicated alcoholic patient is fraught with danger. The use of balloon tamponade may help to separate this lesion from esophageal varices, but gastroscopy should precede passage of the balloon tube. A preoperative diagnosis of alcoholic or drug-induced hemorrhagic gastritis strongly favors nonoperative management with lavage, neutralization of acid, and massive transfusions. If exsanguinating hemorrhage forces the surgeon's hand, or if he stumbles upon this diagnosis at laparotomy, he should perform vagotomy and pyloroplasty plus ligation of obvious bleeding points. In our experience these patients often continue to bleed after operation. However, the rate of hemorrhage is decreased, is controllable by transfusion, and usually has not contributed to subsequent mortality (Foster et al., 1966).

MALLORY-WEISS LACERATIONS. Longitudinal suture of the mucosal tear with chromic catgut is recommended. The distal gastroduodenotomy is closed transversely, but vagotomy is not necessary unless there is a history or evidence of peptic ulcer.

BLEEDING GASTRIC NEOPLASMS. Bleeding gastric neoplasms, such as angiomas, leiomyomas, leiomyosarcomas, carcinomas, and carcinoids, should be excised in a definitive fashion, because anything less than total extirpation will probably result in continued bleeding. However, we have chosen not to get frozen sections on biopsies of small, clinically benign, bleeding gastric ulcers. Suture control with pyloroplasty and vagotomy is a much safer emergency operation. If a diagnosis of cancer is made from the permanent section, elective gastric resection should be done after an appropriate interval.

DIFFUSE "STRESS" ULCERATION. This will be discussed presently in more detail, but pyloroplasty and vagotomy are recommended.

DUODENAL OR JEJUNAL DIVERTICULUM. The solitary bleeding duodenal diverticulum should be excised. Multiple jejunal diverticula require segmental bowel resection, because resection or suture control of a single bleeding focus is made technically difficult by diffuse diverticular disease.

HEMATOBILIA. If the history, physical examination, and operative findings suggest a diagnosis of hematobilia, the common bile duct should be opened and blood clots evacuated. Often this clot forms a cast of the biliary tree. At this point the surgeon will appreciate having thought of the x-ray cassette-holder before operation. Operative cholangiography may demonstrate a definite defect in the duct system. Fogarty biliary balloon catheters may be helpful in the removal of clots and location of a lesion (Anderson et al., 1969).

Hematobilia is usually due to central hematoma, with infarction and necrosis of liver tissue after trauma, or to ruptured hepatic artery aneurysms. Control may require deep dissection and possibly hepatic lobectomy. Hepatic arteriography may assist in this difficult decision.

After control of bleeding, the common bile duct is drained with a T-tube. Antibiotics are given postoperatively, because infection probably plays an important role in recurrent hemorrhage, particularly when a foreign body is left in the common bile duct.

DUODENAL VARICES. This lesion requires direct suture control and a decision about emergency portosystemic decompression. This will be discussed later, but rebleeding is to be expected if the portal pressure cannot be reduced.

Special Problems

IN-HOSPITAL BLEEDING — "STRESS ULCER." The most desperate problems are presented by patients who bleed massively from the upper gastrointestinal tract while hospitalized for another illness. Patients who carry a high potential for this often lethal complication include those with renal failure, respiratory insufficiency, jaundice, head trauma, burns, severe cardiac problems, hepatocellular failure, overwhelming sepsis, and many other diseases resulting in maximum "stress." There is some confusion about the classification of these bleeding lesions. Many authors restrict the term "stress ulceration" to the diffuse, superficial ulcerations without induration, which are well defined by Fletcher and Harkins (1954). This lesion is described as a distinct pathologic entity, separate from Cushing's or Curling's ulceration, and perhaps requiring different management.

However, a clinical diagnosis of "stress ulceration" is often made in patients who are eventually found at laparotomy or autopsy to have single chronic indurated gastric or duodenal ulcers (1966). The "stress" of another illness has resulted in bleeding of these lesions. There is no conclusive evidence that hypersecretion of hydrochloric acid plays an etiologic role or that antacid therapy has a place either in prophylaxis or treatment of these ulcers. There is some evidence that in stress states the gastric mucosa has a decreased resistance to the corrosive action of pepsin and hydrochloric acid, or, perhaps more likely, a systemic decrease in the ability to react to injury and to heal injured tissue.

Clinically we may not be able to separate the patient with multiple acute bleeding ulcers from the patient with a more chronic lesion. Gastroscopy and barium x-rays may be helpful and should be done as early after the onset of hemorrhage as the patient's condition permits. Although there is no definite proof of merit, it does seem reasonable to keep the gastric pH as high as possible with continuous nasogastric suction or frequent antacid medication as a prophylactic measure in patients liable to develop stress ulceration.

When upper gastrointestinal bleeding does occur in the hospitalized patient or "in-hospital bleeder," several measures must be considered. Probably the most critical factor in the patient's eventual survival is the progress of his basic illness, be it sepsis, trauma, or organ failure. Treatment directed toward the underlying illness may do more to stop bleeding than measures aimed at the gastroduodenal mucosa.

Because the results of operation have been so poor in the in-hospital bleeder and even poorer in the small group of such patients with multiple superficial erosions, it has been our practice to delay operation until it becomes obvious that rapid blood transfusion is necessary to keep up with blood loss. If endoscopy or x-ray has demonstrated a discrete lesion, then early operation may be justified. If diffuse erosions are noted at gastroscopy, we would prefer to treat the patient with gastric cooling, continued nasogastric suction, and other supportive measures. We have seen many patients who stop bleeding after 1 to 8 liters of transfused blood.

Our enthusiasm for operation would be greater if we better understood the etiology of "stress ulcers" and therefore could plan treatment more rationally. A review of published reports suggests no clear solution to this problem (discussion appears later). Because our own results have been more satisfactory with pyloroplasty and vagotomy, and because we feel that emergency gastric resection carries a prohibitive postoperative mortality rate in the debilitated patient, our recommendation is for vagotomy and pyloroplasty for the treatment of diffuse superficial ulceration and for the treatment of bleeding silent chronic peptic ulcerations uncovered by an acute stressful situation (Foster et al., 1966). This would seem to be the reasonable course until evidence to the contrary becomes available.

CURLING AND CUSHING ULCERS. Curling, in 1842, reported acute duodenal ulcer in patients with severe burns, and Cushing described acute gastroduodenal ulcerations in patients with hypothalamic lesions in 1932. In the laboratory it seems possible to isolate at least two mechanisms for acute ulceration. Vagotomy will alleviate the hypothalamic or Cushing ulcer problem. It will not affect the "pituitary–adrenal axis" ulcer which can be relieved by adrenalectomy. Hemoconcentration, sludging of blood, and localized necrosis or infection may also play important roles in the causes of acute ulceration in burn patients. Davis and Brooks (1963) have reviewed the experimental background of Cushing ulcer. Artz and Fitts (1966) and Moncrief et al. (1964) have documented the Curling ulcer problem at burn centers.

The clinical separation into necrotic perforating ulcers or penetrating bleeding ulcers has also been attempted, but our experience and that of others would suggest that, in man, these "different" etiologic factors tend to merge together with "stress ulcers" unrelated to burns or intracranial lesions to form a spectrum of pathologic lesions, all of which may bleed. Our approach to Cushing and Curling ulcers, therefore, is similar to that outlined previously for stress ulceration. If operation is necessary, we advise definitive suture control of any bleeding points plus vagotomy and pyloroplasty. Reoperation and resection are necessary in a few patients, but more lives will be saved by beginning with a lesser operation.

WHEN NO LESION HAS BEEN FOUND. Continued bleeding will eventually lead the persistent surgeon to the responsible lesion. However, if hemorrhage has stopped and if no lesion is found after the extensive exploration outline described earlier, a difficult decision must be made. With historic evidence or old fibrotic changes in the stomach or duodenum suggesting peptic ulcer disease, pyloroplasty and vagotomy should be done. There is no longer a place for blind gastrectomy.

If no evidence of present or past ulceration is found, we recommend closure of gastroduodenal incision as in pyloroplasty. The missed lesion is probably a small ulceration in an arteriosclerotic vessel, or a small angiomatous malformation or tumor. The value of vagotomy is debatable. Operative angiography may be valuable. The experiences of Nusbaum, Baum, and Blakemore (1969) indicate that a wide use of both preoperative and operative angiography will reduce the number of unidentifiable causes of bleeding to a minimum.

Results of Operation

The results of emergency operation for bleeding peptic ulcer and other acute inflammatory conditions of the gastroduodenal area should be evaluated by considering *primarily* mortality rates related to the acute illness and *secondarily* the late sequelae, such as recurrence of ulcer disease, hemorrhage, or other postoperative complications, such as dumping and loss of weight.

A review of results reported after several types of emergency operation leaves us with the conviction that no author's series is strictly comparable with another's. There are few series that do not contain some bias toward a particular operation, some degree of patient selection, or some differences in the definition of massive hemorrhage or the criteria for emergency operation—in short, some uncontrolled factors that render the data less than "scientific."

It will always be thus, and should be. The emergency management of these patients must take into account so many different factors that no computer could be programmed to expect them all and to be of help. The patient's attending physician must weigh evidence and select therapy on the basis of incomplete information from the patient and inconclusive evidence from the reported experiences of others. Given this limitation we will attempt a defense of our recommendations listed in the previous section of this chapter.

DUODENAL ULCER. In the last 15 years the pendulum has swung away from subtotal gastric resection as an emergency operation to control hemorrhage from duodenal ulcer because of the high postoperative mortality rates after resectional surgery. Most authors would now agree that vagotomy should be part of any elective or emergency operation for duodenal ulcer. The controversy centers around whether a limited gastric resection should also be done or whether the results after the simpler vagotomy plus pyloroplasty, vagotomy, and emptying procedure or gastroenterostomy are sufficiently good to justify avoidance of resection.

In most reports the mortality rate after elective operation of any type for control of hemorrhage is acceptably low. It is no surprise that most of the postoperative deaths occur in the older and debilitated patients who have undergone emergency operation for the control of hemorrhage.

Our own experience and that of many others have demonstrated that pyloroplasty and vagotomy will result in a reduced number of postoperative deaths when compared with subtotal gastric resection as an emergency operation (Carruthers et al., 1967; Dorton and Hyden, 1961; Enquist et al., 1965; Fisher et al., 1966; Foster et al., 1966). The reporters of the largest experience with antrectomy-vagotomy agree that vagotomy and emptying procedure is indicated in the poor-risk patient, but they defend the addition of a limited gastric resection in the younger or healthier patient (Scott et al., 1966). This defense is based on their premise that antrectomy-vagotomy provides the best insurance against recurrent peptic disease in the future. Sedgwick et al. (1966)

and others continue to recommend subtotal gastric resection as an emergency operation on the grounds that "each surgeon must develop his own preference based on experience."

If elective vagotomy and emptying procedure was followed by recurrent peptic disease in a large percentage of patients, and if only the older and debilitated patients died after emergency operation for hemorrhage from duodenal ulcer, we would agree with some of the recommendations for emergency resection in selected patients. Since the long-term results of vagotomy and emptying procedure have been quite satisfactory (Farris and Smith, 1967; Weinberg, 1963), since "healthy patients" continue to die after any operation for massive hemorrhage, and since the evidence seems to indicate that any degree of resection significantly increases immediate mortality rates, we continue to recommend the "lesser" operation in the emergency situation. Read et al. (1965) conclude that early operation is necessary, whereas the study of Enquist et al. (1965) suggests that a selective approach to the timing of operation for massive hemorrhage is warranted.

It is difficult to compile impartially figures from the literature about the results of emergency operation for hemorrhage, but an attempt is made in Table 12-5 to outline some of the reports of treatment of gastric and duodenal ulcer.

Kelley et al. (1963) have reported a very high (36 per cent) incidence of postoperative bleeding in patients undergoing emergency vagotomy and emptying procedure. This has not been our own experience. In fact, postoperative bleeding has occurred as often after emergency subtotal gastric resection (9 per cent) as after vagotomy and emptying procedure (8 per cent) during the same hospitalization period (Foster et al., 1966). Carruthers et al. (1967) report postoperative bleeding in 11 per cent of patients after gastric resection and 14 per cent of patients after vagotomy and emptying procedure.

Long-term follow-up of patients who have been operated upon for bleeding peptic ulcers reveals a distressingly high incidence of recurrent bleeding after all types of operation. Farris and Smith (1967) have reviewed some of these reports. Palmer (1965), Moghadam and Haubrich (1967), Leape and Welch (1964) and Kozoll and Meyer (1964)

TABLE 12-5. Mortality Rates after Emergency Operation for Control of Hemorrhage from Peptic Ulcer

Author	Subtotal Gastric Resection per cent	Operation Antrectomy– Vagotomy per cent	Vagotomy and Emptying Procedure per cent	Comment
A. Duodenal ulcer				
Carruthers et al. (1967)	16.0		2.0	
Kozoll and Meyer (1964)	33.0			
Hampson et al. (1968)	6.9		11.1	Includes early elective operation
Dorton and Hyden (1961)			0.0	Twenty-seven patients — no deaths
Palumbo and Sharpe (1961), (1967)	13.0	4.7		
Foster et al. (1966)	31.0		11.0	
Farris and Smith (1967)			6.0	Massive hemorrhage but not necessarily an emergency
B. Gastric ulcer				
Carruthers et al. (1967)	20.0			
Kozoll and Meyer (1964)	37.0			
Stafford et al. (1967)	25.0			
Hampson et al. (1968)	2.2			Includes early elective operation
Foster et al. (1966)	26.0		11.0	
Dorton (1966)			7.0	
C. Gastric and duodenal ulcers together—"peptic ulcer"				
Enquist et al. (1965)	13.0			Immediate operation for all patients with hemorrhage
Paine (1962)	16.0			Elective and emergency blood loss over 1000 ml.
Brooks and Eraklis (1964)	21.0			
Harvey (1963)	9.0			
Kelley et al. (1963)		18.0		
Stewart et al. (1956)	11.0			18% over 70 years
Mead (1967)			12.0	34 patients
Darin (1961)	24.0			
Fisher et al. (1966)	20.0	11.0	6.0	
Foster et al. (1966)	30.0		9.0	66% over 60 years

have added new data. The combined reports indicate that from 6 to 50 per cent of patients will bleed again some time after any type of gastric surgery to control hemorrhage.

GASTRIC ULCER. Etiologic factors in gastric ulcer range from hypersecretory states to achlorhydria and ischemic conditions. It is no wonder that many different elective operations have "succeeded" in controlling gastric ulceration, or that every operation has been followed by some failures. We must look then to empiric results for guidance. Gastric ulcer occurs in older patients when the risks of any operation are greater. Our basic premise in poor-risk patients or in the emergency situation has been that we should do the easiest and fastest operation that will control hemorrhage. Immediate survival is again the most important criterion of success.

Ligation of gastric arteries or a simple suture of the ulcer has been followed by recurrent hemorrhage in a large percentage of patients. Table 12-5 documents some of the results of different emergency operations for bleeding gastric ulcer. Pyloroplasty, vagotomy, and suture of the bleeding bed seems to be at least as effective as gastric resection and perhaps more so. We believe that absolute suture control of the bleeding ulcer is even more important with gastric ulcer than with duodenal ulcer.

GASTRITIS, STRESS ULCER, AND ACUTE GASTRIC EROSIONS. Although these lesions may be separate, they are discussed together because the surgeon's ability to distinguish these pathologic processes, both preoperatively and at operation, has often been refuted by subsequent evidence gathered at autopsy. The results in terms of survival after any method of treatment for these several conditions are poor. The patient's underlying problem probably contributes more to mortality rates than does the gastric or duodenal lesion. In evaluating results we must concentrate on (1) whether the gastrointestinal bleeding recurs after operation, and (2) whether recurrent bleeding is a terminal incidental phenomenon or an important contributing cause of death.

Bartlett and Ottinger (1966) and Rosenkrantz and Bartlett (1961) have concluded that vagotomy should be added to gastric resection or other procedures for the emergency control of massive bleeding from gastritis. Sullivan et al. (1964) and others (Ferguson and Clarke, 1966; Menguy, 1969; Mixter and Hinton, 1957) report success with vagotomy and pyloroplasty for control of massive hemorrhaging from gastritis, but Hardaway and Castagno (1959) and Palmer (1959) believe that total gastrectomy may be necessary in this condition. Freeark et al. (1967) are unhappy with gastrectomy. Nagel et al. (1967) separate patients bleeding from gastritis into two distinct clinical groups: patients with mild bleeding not requiring operation, and patients with truly massive bleeding. Pyloroplasty with vagotomy has been the mainstay of operative treatment in the latter group, and there were no deaths in a series of 14 patients.

Goodman and Frey (1968) report 24 patients bleeding massively from stress ulcers treated by various operations. Only vagotomy with a drainage procedure was followed by significant survival. Grosz and Wu (1967) recommend 75 per cent gastrectomy for stress ulcers, but report survival of only one of four patients. Eight of 57 of their patients treated without operation survived. Fogelman and Garvey (1966) reviewed the results of treatment in 53 patients with hemorrhage from "stress" ulcer. Two thirds of their patients had single ulcers, half of which were in the duodenum and half in the stomach. Twenty-five of 41 patients (61 per cent) treated medically died, whereas four of nine patients with emergency operation died. Four patients had pyloroplasty and vagotomy; three died, two with recurrent gastrointestinal bleeding. Four patients had subtotal gastrectomy and one died. Bryant and Griffen (1966) and Silen (personal communication) on the basis of disappointment with small series treated with pyloroplasty and vagotomy believe that gastric resection is necessary for stress ulceration. Carruthers et al. (1967) treated four patients with diffuse erosions by gastrectomy; three had recurrence of hemorrhage, and two needed reoperation. One died of recurrent hemorrhage. They also treated nine patients with diffuse erosions with pyloroplasty and vagotomy. Three of these patients had recurrence of hemorrhage; two died from hemorrhage, and one died of other complications.

In summary, most reports include comparatively small numbers of cases of either gastritis or stress ulcer treated by operation. Most authors share our prejudice that when possible operation should be avoided, but all conclude that if any operation is to be done it should be done at the earliest possible moment. It is interesting that most of the reporting surgeons who began with gastrectomy for control of these lesions are unhappy with it and have shifted to pyloroplasty and vagotomy. A number of surgeons who have treated stress ulcer with pyloroplasty and vagotomy have had poor results and are now recommending gastrectomy. None of these reports are conclusive, but the balance, if anything, favors the lesser operation. Our own experience leads us to recommend pyloroplasty and vagotomy. If bleeding persists, a subsequent gastric resection may rarely be justified.

BLEEDING ESOPHAGEAL VARICES

When the clinical data, with or without the aid of roentgenographic and endoscopic techniques, have led to a probable diagnosis of hypertensive esophageal varices as the cause of bleeding, our principles of treatment and indications for operation differ from those recommended for the patient with ulcer. Many statistical studies have "shown" that such single factors as early operation, reliance on certain laboratory or clinical phenomena, one type of operation versus another, or the etiologic factors of liver disease make a critical difference in prognosis in the patient bleeding from esophageal varices. It is our firm conviction that no single factor can be depended upon to guide us. However, it is also our conviction that the experienced clinician can select appropriate therapy and, more specifically, can decide whether or not emergency operation is indicated in the vast majority of such patients by using a combination of criteria. Patients whose mortality rate after emergency operation will approach 100 per cent can be differentiated from patients whose emergency operation will be followed by a mortality rate of 15 to 30 per cent. The selection process depends on two factors: first, a thorough evaluation of the patient's condition on hospital admission, and second, a 36- to 48-hour period of observation.

Treatment should begin in the Emergency Room. In addition to the diagnostic and supportive measures already mentioned, careful attention should be paid to the coagulation mechanism. If the patient's condition permits, esophagoscopy should be done. Gastroscopy requires preliminary gastric irrigation and should be done if there is a history of recent alcohol intake and if no esophageal bleeding point was discovered at esophagoscopy.

Cathartics and antibiotics should be given by mouth or by nasogastric tube, and enemas are used to clear the gastrointestinal tract of blood to prevent ammonia formation and absorption. We have used magnesium sulfate and neomycin for this purpose. Vitamin K_1 oxide should also be administered, even in the presence of a normal prothrombin time. Adequate calories should be provided, usually in the form of large amounts of glucose given intravenously. These patients may be alkalotic and hypovolemic. Both conditions should be documented and reversed by appropriate fluid therapy. Sedatives should be used with great caution, because patients with chronic hepatic disease tolerate them poorly and because they may obscure evidence of changes in sensorium which might critically influence a future decision. Jackson et al. (1968a) have discussed the preoperative management thoroughly.

If the patient continues to show evidence of hemorrhage after admission and has tachycardia and perhaps hypotension after initial volume replacement, the first step in therapy is to insert a balloon tube to establish tamponade of the gastroesophageal junction. These balloon tubes have a very bad reputation, particularly among physicians. Many reviews have shown a high incidence of pulmonary complications associated with

their use (Conn and Simpson, 1968; Sherlock, 1965). However, most of the problems with balloon tubes are directly related to misuse and lack of information about this important diagnostic and therapeutic tool.

The Sengstaken-Blakemore tube has the advantage of an esophageal balloon, but esophageal tamponade is rarely necessary if proper gastric balloon placement and traction are achieved. The Sengstaken tube has the disadvantage of no lumen for esophageal aspiration. It can be modified by tying a Levin nasogastric tube to the tube just above the gastric balloon for esophageal aspiration. The Linton tube has an orifice for suction in the esophageal portion of the tube, a larger gastric balloon, but no esophageal balloon.

Every balloon tube should be carefully tested prior to insertion. Each balloon must be inflated fully in a pan of water to check for leakage. The gastric balloon should be tested with 500 to 600 cc. of air. The esophageal balloon should be tested with 50 mm. Hg pressure. The tip of the tube and the gastric balloon should be well lubricated with jelly and passed gently and quickly down through the esophagogastric junction so that the gastric balloon lies several inches beyond the gastroesophageal junction. Because cessation of hemorrhage is the first order of business, the physician should immediately inflate the gastric balloon with air to at least 400 to 500 cc. volume. The tube should be pulled back until the balloon lodges against the diaphragm, and then $1/2$ to $1^1/_2$ pounds of balanced traction are applied. Clinical estimates of correct traction and the practice of pulling the tube firmly and taping it to the nares are to be discouraged as hazardous and ineffective.

With the patient in a semi-Fowler position an overhead bar can be used with a central pulley so that the traction rope pulls in line with the nares and avoids erosion of the nasal cartilages. The second pulley at the foot of the bed allows passage of the rope to the foot of the bed where the appropriate traction weight can be hung. There is now commercially available a helmet type of apparatus which has a controlled tension traction device.

This maneuver will stop bleeding from gastroesophageal varices in a large majority of patients. Blood may have accumulated in the esophagus at this point and will be coughed up by the patient or can be aspirated if the capability for esophageal aspiration has been provided. No further accumulation of blood will ensue, but of course saliva cannot be swallowed and the patient must be provided with a basin for expectoration. In those rare instances when esophageal bleeding seems to continue, the esophageal balloon on the Sengstaken-Blakemore tube should be inflated to a pressure of 35 to 40 mm. Hg. This pressure should be monitored frequently. The position of the gastric balloon should be checked with a portable x-ray machine. The mechanical details of proper application of balloon tamponade are stressed because it is usually failure in technique that causes failure of control of hemorrhage from esophageal varices.

After tamponade has been accomplished, gastric irrigation and aspiration should be done. Large quantities of blood may be removed from the stomach, but it is usually impossible to irrigate sufficiently so that the returns are clear. Continued irrigation of bloody fluid should not discourage the physician. Only evidence of rapid aspiration of bright red blood or continued systemic evidence of blood loss, such as tachycardia and increasing hypotension, should lead to the conclusion that hemorrhage is continuing. If distal hemorrhage continues despite tamponade and the balloon has been shown to be properly positioned by x-ray, the bleeding must be from a source other than varices. In such cases it is usually obvious that tamponade has been ineffective from the beginning.

A prompt dramatic response to esophageal tamponade with a fall in pulse rate and rise in blood pressure is one of the best diagnostic criteria of bleeding esophageal varices.

INDICATIONS FOR OPERATION

Emergency operation in the sense of a procedure done within a few hours of the patient's admission to the hospital should rarely if ever be recommended for patients bleeding from esophageal varices. However, if the patient is well known to the physician, if he has survived other hemorrhages without evidence of liver decompensation, if esophageal varices are well documented, if, therefore, the patient is known to be a good but previously reluctant candidate for elective portosystemic shunt, and *if* massive hemorrhage continues after replacement of 1000 to 2000 ml. of whole blood, then emergency operation may be warranted without delay. Tamponade should be established even in this small group of patients to stabilize the patient's condition prior to and during operation.

In all other patients an arbitrary period, usually 36 to 48 hours, is selected for balloon tamponade. This will permit evaluation of the patient's liver function and sensorium which may deteriorate in a short period. Balloon tamponade with traction even if intermittent for more than 48 hours at a time leads to increasing morbidity and mortality. Blood volume should be replaced during this period, but overtransfusion is to be avoided, because hemorrhage often seems to recur when transfusion has been excessive. Deficiencies in coagulation factors and serum proteins should be corrected and other diagnostic and therapeutic maneuvers accomplished as if all patients were to undergo operation at the end of the period of observation.

Because all observers have noted that these patients deteriorate rather rapidly over a period of several days unless their bleeding stops and their nutrition is adequate, the decision about operation should be made by 48 hours after admission. Early or urgent operation should be offered to a small group of patients at this time.

We would exclude from the group of candidates for early operation patients who have had hemorrhage at the end of a long progressive history of hepatic failure, patients who have hemorrhage in immediate relation to an episode of acute alcoholism, patients who have exhibited signs of precoma or coma during the 36 to 48 hours of observation, and patients with very small livers or very large livers. Child (1964) quotes Mikkelsen who refuses emergency shunt operation to patients with nonpalpable livers because the salvage rate after operation in this group has been very low. Our experience prejudices us against offering operation to patients with huge livers that extend to the iliac crest. This is particularly true of the muscular young man who bleeds at the end of a massive alcoholic binge and who has an enormous liver. These patients tolerate surgery very poorly (Gall and Keirle, 1965). With proper medical therapy their livers may shrink rapidly, suggesting that much of the enlargement is due to acute fatty infiltration or "alcoholic hepatitis."

It is difficult to deny operation to a patient

with exsanguinating hemorrhage, but surgeons with the most experience with these problems have moved away from an unselective approach. Some of these desperately ill people will survive excellent medical management, but few will survive a major operation.

Also to be excluded from the group offered emergency operation are patients who stop bleeding with tamponade and have no recurrent bleeding after release of tamponade. These patients may be suitable candidates for an elective shunt operation at an appropriate interval. We used to wait at least six weeks, but now feel that seven to ten days of adequate nutrition may prepare a *good-risk* patient for elective shunt during the same hospitalization.

Recurrence of hemorrhage may follow release of tamponade but usually is not apparent for several hours or even days. It has been our practice to leave the deflated balloon tube in place for 24 hours after release of traction. Its presence will help monitor subsequent bleeding, and it can be used for giving cathartics, calories, and antibiotics. Measures are taken to prevent esophageal reflux of gastric contents, and adequate caloric intake is provided. Patients with no deterioration of liver function, whose hemorrhage seems to be associated with adequate liver function, and who bleed after release of balloon tamponade should be taken immediately to the operating room after reinstitution of balloon tamponade.

OTHER FORMS OF TREATMENT

Sheila Sherlock (1965) and others (Delaney et al., 1966; Nusbaum et al., 1967), partially because of their discouragement with balloon tamponade, have recommended the use of the posterior pituitary extract, vasopressin. This agent, when properly used, may lower portal pressure by decreasing the arterial inflow to the portal vein. The drug must be used in large doses, usually 20 units in 100 ml. of 5 per cent glucose and water, injected intravenously over a 10- to 15-minute period. If the material is pharmacologically active, the patient will turn white, defecate, and have intestinal colic. His portal pressure may fall, but so will his hepatic blood flow. By temporarily reducing portal pressure, one has also decreased the oxygen supply to the failing liver. This is a mixed blessing at best (Merigan et al., 1961). The decrease in portal

pressure is transient and will last up to one hour but no longer. Repeated doses of vasopressin are less effective. Recent studies by Kessler (1968) in man would seem to indicate that there is no predictable and consistent effect of vasopressin on the portal pressure of *human* subjects with chronic liver disease or with normal livers (Kelley et al., 1963). This drug may find a place in the initial emergency management of a patient prior to the institution of balloon tamponade. However, there is some evidence that its use does not affect patient prognosis at all, and eventually may prove to be of no value. Vasopressin cannot be used in patients with coronary artery disease.

Wangensteen and others have recommended gastric cooling for patients with massive hemorrhage from varices. This is done with a special balloon which has both gastric and esophageal portions. A recent review has summarized this experience (Wangensteen and Smith, 1965). Hemorrhage did stop in a majority of patients with cooling, but most of the patients died during the same hospitalization. More information will be needed before cooling can be recommended for general use.

Dumont and Witte (1965) and Bowers et al. (1964) have recently introduced a new concept into the emergency treatment of patients with portal hypertension and bleeding varices. They theorize that thoracic duct obstruction due to heavy lymph flow from an obstructed liver results in sinusoidal hypertension and obstruction to vascular flow through the liver. They postulate that external drainage of thoracic duct fluid will decrease pressure in the lymphatic system and liver sinusoid and thereby allow better blood flow through the liver, thus decreasing portal pressure. Only a small clinical experience with this technique has been reported to date, and the results have not been very good (Dumont and Witte, 1965).

Since the obstruction to venous outflow of the liver is the reason for the increased lymphatic flow, it is difficult to see how reducing lymphatic pressure can decrease vascular resistance. A recent article by Warren et al. (1968) considers this theory and should be read by all those interested in this new technique. We share Warren's conclusion that both the theoretical and practical usefulness of this method remain to be proved.

Extracorporeal shunting has been suggested as an emergency measure, but its clinical usefulness has not been demonstrated (White et al., 1968).

EARLY OPERATION

Many operations for the emergency management of patients with bleeding esophageal varices have been proposed and defended by statistical comparison with other reports. Each of the recommended operations carries a high mortality rate when used in the emergency situation. It is our opinion then that, when possible, an adequate portal systemic venous shunt operation should be constructed. All the procedures which involve ligation or interruption of venous collateral pathways are followed eventually by recurrent bleeding from esophageal varices. If the rationale for any operation is based on the surmise that these patients can tolerate no further hemorrhage, then we must also surmise that they are poor candidates for several operations. For this reason a single operation which may result in a permanent alleviation of their portal hypertension is to be preferred.

Should splenoportography be done routinely to document the patency of the portal vein prior to urgent operation? Since most portacaval shunts are done through a right subcostal incision and since splenorenal shunt cannot be readily done through this incision, we have felt in the past that x-ray evidence of the patent portal vein was essential for positioning the patient on the operating table. However, we have recently become discouraged with the long-term effectiveness of the smaller splenorenal shunt in preventing recurrent hemorrhage (Foster and Vetto, 1967). The splenorenal shunt is a more difficult and time-consuming emergency operation, and we now have several alternative venous shunting operations which can be performed through a right-sided abdominal incision. Therefore at present we seldom perform emergency splenoportography except when clinical and laboratory findings suggest extrahepatic portal venous obstruction, or when splenic pulp manometry is used for differential diagnosis.

Our practice has been to construct an end-to-side portacaval shunt when possible on the grounds that this decompressed the portal bed as well as any other operation, was easier technically than any other shunt, and resulted in no greater incidence of postoperative encephalopathy and other complications. Recently Turcotte et al. (1969) have reported lower operative mortality and better long-term results after side-to-side portacaval shunts when compared to end-to-side portacaval shunts in poor-risk patients and in emergencies. Reynolds et al. (1966) found end-to-side shunt preferable to side-to-side. Our clinical impression is that the patient's hepatocellular reserve affects the results of emergency operation much more critically than does the specific type of venous anastomosis.

TECHNIQUE OF OPERATION

The patient is placed on the operating table in a semilateral position with supports beneath the right back; the right arm is brought up and forward over the chest. The operating table is then turned so that the abdomen is flat for the initial abdominal incision. Although we have wished for angiographic capability on a few occasions, we have not routinely used a cassette-holder beneath the patient, because the ability to break the table to expose the portacaval area has been considered more important. The entire abdomen, anterior chest, and right posterior chest are prepared and draped into the operative field.

A right subcostal incision is preferred. This is carried down through peritoneum with careful control of hypertensive venous collateral vessels. An enlarged liver should not result in a lower incision, because the area of anastomosis will eventually be high on the posterior peritoneal surface. The incision should extend from the falciform ligament to the right posterior peritoneal reflection on the colon. The falciform ligament should not be divided unless gastroesophageal exposure is necessary. Interruption of large physiologic shunts will increase portal pressure and will not aid in exposure of the portal vein or inferior vena cava.

If exploration reveals the classic changes of cirrhosis and venous hypertension without any other obvious gastrointestinal disease, dissection of the great veins should begin after lateral rotation of the patient to the left and extension of the operating table to increase the distance between costal margin and iliac crest. If the usual peritoneal and retroperitoneal lymphatic and venous collateral vessels are not evident, early measurement of portal venous pressure is indicated. A hypertensive enlarged portal vein is usually ballotable on the posterior surface of the porta hepatis if the foramen of Winslow is open.

The technique for construction of portacaval venous shunts has been well described by Preston and Trippel (1966) and McDermott (1965). We would emphasize several additional points which we believe to be critical to the safe conduct of this operation. In many patients the pathologic anatomy does not obscure the normal anatomy, and venous shunting can be accomplished rather easily. In others the retroperitoneal inferior vena cava is buried in a firm but friable mass of lymphatic and vascular tissue which may measure up to 3 cm. in thickness and which bleeds vigorously at the slightest touch. Each patient presents a different technical problem, but the following principles are offered as guidelines:

1. No collateral vessels should be divided unless absolutely necessary for exposure. It is usually necessary to divide a few vessels which join the posterior edge of the right lobe of the liver to the prerenal fascia in order to retract the liver cephalad to expose the inferior vena cava as it enters the liver. It is not usually necessary to divide the falciform ligament or the retroperitoneal attachments of the hepatic flexure to the colon. Many descriptions of this operation begin with a recommendation for a Kocher maneuver. This requires a tedious bloody dissection and is entirely unnecessary in most cases. The portion of the inferior vena cava that needs to be exposed is above the duodenum forming the back wall of the entrance to the narrowed foramen of Winslow (Fig. 12-3).

2. Dissection of the anterior surface of the inferior vena cava often is more difficult and should precede dissection of the portal vein. Exposure of the low pressure outlet first will allow rapid decompression by shunt

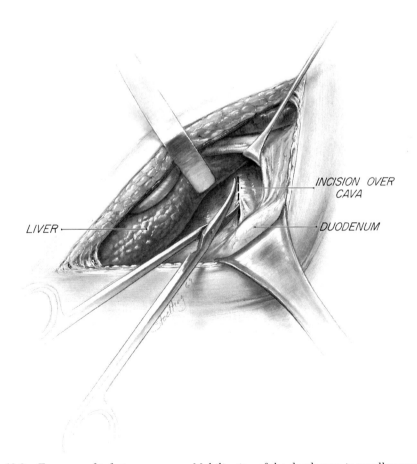

INCISION OVER CAVA

LIVER

DUODENUM

Figure 12-3.   Exposure of inferior vena cava. Mobilization of the duodenum is usually unnecessary.

construction should dissection of the portal vein result in a major venous laceration. Only the anterior two-thirds of the vena cava need be cleared. Circumferential dissection is not necessary for construction of most end-to-side shunts, but may be necessary to mobilize the veins enough for side-to-side anastomosis.

3. The dissection of adhesions and the exposure of the great veins require careful attention to operative technique. No other factor is more important in the safe conduct of this operation. It is our practice to tie every small or large vessel with fine silk ligatures *in continuity* during the great vessel dissection. Clamps may slip off, particularly in a deep hole. Hypertensive bleeding, even from small collateral vessels, can quickly obscure the operative field. The few extra moments required by this deliberate meticulous approach will eliminate hours of distress to patient and physician. Ligation of all tissue before transection will also result in occlusion of lymphatic channels. This certainly will keep the field drier during shunt construction and probably will decrease the postoperative formation of ascites.

4. The anastomosis should be made as high as possible on the inferior vena cava to prevent kinking of the portal vein. Liver enlargement may preclude adequate exposure of the anastomotic area. The surgeon should not hesitate to extend the incision into the thorax, usually through the right seventh or eighth intercostal space. An incision in the diaphragm will allow displacement of much of the liver into the chest and will result in better exposure. This thoracic extension will be necessary in less than 10 per cent of patients undergoing portacaval shunt. In many patients a selective enlargement of the caudate lobe will prevent high exposure of the inferior vena cava. This problem can be handled by resection of the tip of the caudate lobe distal to mattress sutures of catgut, or, preferably, by longitudinal incision between mattress sutures. The tissues on either side of such an incision will retract to allow placement of vascular clamps in the area of anastomosis.

5. An adequate portosystemic shunt will drop the measured portal pressure *at least* 10 cm. of saline. Often this results in a pressure still in the hypertensive range at the end of the operation. However, continuous monitoring has shown us that the portal pressure will continue to decrease into the normal range during the first few postoperative days. If unbreaking the operating table and restoring the viscera into their normal positions do not result in a post-shunt decrease in pressure of at least 10 cm. of saline in the presence of a normal central venous pressure, the shunt should be reconstructed.

If evidence of chronic peptic ulceration is found, we do not perform a definitive operation for ulcer in association with portacaval shunting. A few patients have urgently required portacaval shunting while still hospitalized after operation to control bleeding peptic ulcer, and a few patients with portacaval shunt have required emergency reoperation two or three weeks later for bleeding from gastric or duodenal ulcer, but we feel that patients will benefit most from a policy which attacks one disease at a time. We do give vigorous medical therapy for ulcer to postoperative patients whom we found had physical signs of ulcer disease during shunt operation. Since these ulcers are not usually related to hypersecretion, it is difficult to know whether this treatment is effective.

After construction of an adequate shunt, should the gastroesophageal varices be ligated? Although we have seen several transient episodes of postoperative hemorrhage from a presumed unhealed variceal rupture, these have been easily controlled with balloon tamponade. Transgastric exposure of the gastroesophageal junction through a right subcostal incision is difficult and suture control of submucosal varices may be uncertain. Therefore we do not recommend ligation of varices after urgent portacaval shunt as a routine. We usually deflate the balloon and release the traction after shunt construction, but leave the tube in place for two or three days to serve in place of a Levin nasogastric tube.

ALTERNATIVE OPERATIONS

If the portal vein is occluded by a thrombus or tumor, another shunting procedure is attempted. The mesocaval shunt is probably the easiest and largest of the alternative operations. If the retroperitoneal plane behind the right colon is not obliterated by venous collaterals, reflection of the right colon to the left will provide the best exposure for mesocaval shunting. If this is obliterated, a more narrow but direct exposure of the inferior vena cava can be made to the left of the small bowel mesentery. The technical details of this operation are well described by Zollinger and Zollinger (1967). Several other imaginative shunts have occasionally been effective in controlling hemorrhage from varices. Recommendations have been made for the following: central splenorenal shunt (Clatworthy and Boles, 1959); combined hepatic and portal decompression (McDermott, 1958); splenorenal shunt (Linton et al., 1961); portorenal shunt (Lasher, 1965); distal splenorenal anastomosis (Warren et al., 1967); and umbilical-saphenous shunt (Piccone and LeVeen, 1967).

If no suitable portosystemic shunt can be effected, what should be done to control the bleeding varices at urgent operation? Transthoracic displacement of the spleen into the left pleural cavity has proved effective in decompressing the portal system in children (Turunen et al., 1963). Splenectomy alone has not been an effective emergency operation in this country, although some English surgeons still advocate its use. Gastric transection, omentopexy, gastric resection, hepatic artery ligation, and many other operations have been suggested but cannot be recommended on the basis of results achieved.

We feel that direct attack on the gastroesophageal varices is the next step to take in the one adult patient in 50 or 60 in whom an adequate venous shunt cannot be constructed. If it is difficult to expose the gastroesophageal junction through a right subcostal incision, we would probably turn the patient on his right side and make a separate left thoracotomy incision after closing the abdominal incision.

POSTOPERATIVE CARE

After operative relief of portal hypertension has been accomplished, the most critical factor in survival of the patient is the reserve of his diseased liver. This reserve can be extended by careful metabolic support during the postoperative period. Many patients who show no sign of precoma or coma during the preoperative period of tamponade will lapse into coma after operation. If this is associated with other evidence of hepatocellular failure, it is a bad prognostic sign, but in some patients coma will be quickly reversible by treatment directed at hypokalemic alkalosis or drug intoxication.

Postoperative formation of ascites is common after shunt operations. This is probably not an avoidable complication in most patients, but careful balance of sodium and water metabolism may help to control the extent of ascites. A cirrhotic patient often clings to sodium very tightly. Intravenous albumin supplementation is useful in maintaining oncotic pressure and mobilizing ascitic fluid. We have tried to avoid the use of diuretics and paracentesis in the postoperative period.

Renal failure after portosystemic venous shunt operation is an almost universally fatal complication. Although some clinicians are reluctant to accept the concept of a hepatorenal syndrome, there certainly is a distinct entity characterized by progressive noninfectious renal failure associated with chronic liver disease which resists all attempts at correction. Its occurrence is unpredictable and prophylactic measures are uncertain.

Adequate nutrition should be provided. In addition to albumin supplementation, a minimum of 1500 to 1800 calories a day should be given to the adult patient. This always means hypertonic glucose solutions, and usually means a certain degree of osmotic diuresis. If this effect is not dehydrating, we have not restricted glucose intake because of losses in the urine.

Most patients carried successfully through operation do well for at least seven to ten days. Then some of them have a gradual decline over the second, third, and fourth weeks and die of progressive renal or hepatic failure. Patients who die of progressive liver failure in the first week almost certainly should not have been operated on.

RESULTS OF OPERATION FOR PORTAL HYPERTENSION

There is considerable disagreement in the literature about operation for portal hypertension. All will agree that portal hypertension due to extrahepatic portal vein obstruction should be corrected by venous shunt when possible, *if* the patient has had life-threatening hemorrhage and *if* the age of the patient and the anatomy of the great veins are suitable. When portal hypertension is due to cirrhosis of the liver, opinions differ. We shall consider evidence that contributes toward answers to three questions:

1. What is the natural history of a patient

with cirrhosis who bleeds from esophageal varices?

2. What is the place of elective portosystemic shunt in altering this natural history?

3. What is the place of emergency operation?

The studies of Conn and Simpson (1967), Grace et al. (1966), and Jackson et al. (1968a) are very helpful and should be consulted for a more thorough discussion of the place of portosystemic shunt operations.

NATURAL HISTORY

Since Ratnoff and Patek's classic paper in 1942 there have been few well-controlled studies among selected patients with known esophageal varices with which to compare operative results. Cohn and Blaisdell (1958) describe what happened to a selected group of San Francisco patients with cirrhosis who did not have portacaval shunts. Of 456 patients with hemorrhage from cirrhosis and varices, 290 died after their first hemorrhage. Of the remaining 118, only 40 met Linton's criteria (1951) for an elective shunt. Eight of these patients died of hemorrhage within one year, two more died from hemorrhage during the second year, 12 patients lived at least five years, and four who died before five years never had hemorrhage again. The early mortality rate after a first hemorrhage from varices has been reported as 54 per cent and 64 per cent (with and without operation) and 36 per cent (Satterfield et al., 1965) without operation. Conn and Lindenmuth (1968) collected ten reports and found a mean death rate of 63 per cent (range, 33 to 84 per cent) after the first

hemorrhage in patients treated in several ways.

Satterfield et al. (1965) and Garceau and Chalmers (1963) document the progressive decline in surviving patients over a period of five years after their first hemorrhage. It is certain that more than half of these patients will not survive for five years, and some of the evidence suggests that more than 90 per cent will die, although not necessarily from hemorrhage.

ELECTIVE SHUNT OPERATION

The reports of Satterfield et al. (1965) and Grace et al. (1966) suggest that portosystemic shunting operations do not significantly affect survival in cirrhotic patients. The prospective cooperative Veterans Administration report has helped greatly in clarifying this matter (Jackson et al., 1965, 1968b). Their last report suggests that prophylactic shunt is not of benefit, and that therapeutic shunt may be of only slight benefit in increasing survival.

There is no question that the survivors of a shunting operation are less likely to have hemorrhage. Grace et al. (1966) report that 2.8 per cent of patients had rebleeding after portacaval shunt and 19 per cent after splenorenal shunt. Any true comparison with nonoperative measures, however, must also consider operative mortality in the shunted group. Grace reported a series of 1,244 patients who had an elective therapeutic shunt with a mortality rate of 15.5 per cent. Edmunds and West (1964) noted that eight of 21 patients lived five years after shunting operation, whereas only two of 21 patients

TABLE 12-6.   Elective Portosystemic Shunt Operation — Operative Mortality Rates

Author	Number of Patients	Operative Mortality per cent	Comment
Grace et al. (1966)	1,244	15.5	Collected review of 20 groups
Gütgemann and Esser (1968)	234	14.5	
Myers (1967)	100	19.4	Includes 44 "early" operations
Sedgwick et al. (1966)	97	19.6	55 "good" risks, 42 "poor" risk
Turcotte et al. (1969)	77	19.0	
Foster (unpublished data)	70	9.0	
Jackson et al. (1968b)	37	13.5	Prophylactic shunts

lived five years without operation in an uncontrolled report. These and other results are listed in Table 12-6. The review articles of Grace et al. (1966) and Conn and Simpson (1968) are recommended for a more complete survey of the data that determine the place of portosystemic shunting operation.

We conclude from the preceding data that elective shunting operation may be offered to good-risk patients during a period of stable hepatic function. Only a controlled prospective study will prove the soundness of this policy. To offer elective shunt to poor-risk patients does not seem warranted on the basis of survival figures accumulated to date.

EMERGENCY SHUNT OPERATION

Conn and Simpson (1968) have collected operative survival data on the results of emergency shunting operations. These and other reports are listed in Table 12-7.

This table includes patients who have been selected by a number of criteria. It is dangerous to draw conclusions from the over-all figures. To compare operative survival rates with the results of medical therapy alone is to compare a group excluding the obviously unsalvageable with a group including patients with end-stage cirrhosis. We studied retrospectively a small group of 21 patients undergoing emergency portacaval shunt at Hartford Hospital (Foster, unpublished data). Using the usual historical, clinical, and laboratory criteria to evaluate preoperative liver function, we found the following correlation with the results of operation. Of 12 patients judged preopera-

tively to be "poor" risks, 11 died after emergency shunt. Of the nine patients judged preoperatively to be "good" risks, three died, all with recurrent hemorrhage. One had a thrombosed shunt, one had an overlooked bleeding gastric ulcer, and the third aspirated blood during vomiting.

Clinical classification of risk is valuable. Proper selection of operative candidates will render invalid any statistical comparison of operative versus nonoperative treatment, but until controlled evidence to the contrary is presented, clinical selection of candidates for operation is the best way to insure the greatest chance for survival in both the unoperated and operated groups. Even Orloff (1967) concludes in his paper about an "unselective approach" that the obviously decompensated cirrhotic patient with jaundice, ascites, and encephalopathy should not have portacaval shunt.

Conn and Simpson (1968) conclude from these figures that an aggressive application of emergency shunt operation to all possible candidates is warranted. We conclude from the same data that a carefully restrictive and selective approach to emergency operation should be used. Such is the state of the "science." An impartial observer would correctly conclude from the physician's enthusiasm about emergency operation and the surgeon's reluctance that neither specialist was very happy about what his own discipline had to offer these unfortunate patients.

Emergency transesophageal ligation has been recommended by Linton (1966) and Orloff (1962). However, the mortality is high after this operation, eventual rebleeding is

TABLE 12-7. Emergency Portosystemic Shunt Operation—Operative Mortality Rates

Author	Patients	Operative Mortality per cent	Comment
Conn and Simpson (1968)	302	39.0	20 to 17% in 14 series
Sedgwick et al. (1966)	5	60.0	
Gütgemann and Esser (1968)	50	48.0	
Turcotte et al. (1969)	25	56.0	
Foster (unpublished data)	25	60.0	
Grace et al. (1966)	173	31.8	Nine series (may include cases from Conn et al.)
Adson (1967)	30	27.0	

the rule, and the patient must then be subjected to a venous shunting procedure. It is our feeling (shared by others) (Mikkelson, 1962; Roussellot et al., 1960) that the mortality rate exceeds that of selective emergency shunt alone.

The problem of portal hypertension in children is a different subject and is well reviewed by Foster et al. (1963) and Shaldon and Sherlock (1962). Children with extrahepatic portal obstruction or congenital hepatic fibrosis do well after operation. Because they tolerate hemorrhage without liver decompensation, operation may be delayed until their veins enlarge enough to allow construction of a large shunt.

Children with varices secondary to cystic fibrosis or biliary atresia do poorly with or without operation.

LOWER GASTROINTESTINAL HEMORRHAGE

Massive lower gastrointestinal hemorrhage is presented separately to emphasize certain unique features of this entity in comparison with massive upper gastrointestinal hemorrhage. Hemorrhage from the lower gastrointestinal tract is defined as coming from below the ligament of Treitz. Only recently has a systematized approach to this surgical emergency been developed. The contributions of Smith and Berne (1964), Noer et al. (1962), Albo et al. (1963), and Judd (1969) indicate increasing recognition of the need for operative intervention in carefully selected cases.

ETIOLOGY

The many causes of lower gastrointestinal bleeding include inflammatory, traumatic, vascular, neoplastic, and numerous systemic disorders. *Massive* lower gastrointestinal bleeding occurs in a comparatively small number of conditions, particularly diverticulosis. Polyps and polypoid carcinomas of the colon are an important but comparatively rare cause. Meckel's diverticulum and tumors of the small bowel are occasionally associated with massive lower gastrointestinal hemorrhage. In a significant number of cases the exact etiologic factor is not identified. This often is the case in patients with hypertension, multiple systemic disorders,

and, particularly, renal insufficiency and uremia. As a general rule surgical intervention is not indicated in this group.

Advanced ulcerative colitis may be associated with massive exsanguinating hemorrhage, but other manifestations of this condition usually dominate the picture. Only rarely is acute massive exsanguinating hemorrhage the sole presenting sign of ulcerative colitis. Although pathologic documentation is difficult to obtain, small ulcerated arteriosclerotic lesions probably account for a significant number of severe colonic hemorrhages (Albo et al., 1966). It is of interest that in diverticulosis with massive hemorrhage, hypertension and arteriosclerosis are often present.

Tumors of the small bowel, ulcerations, and vascular anomalies commonly present as bleeding from the lower gastrointestinal tract. Erosions caused by ingestion of potassium may produce massive bleeding (Boley et al., 1965).

DIAGNOSIS

The commonest cause of profuse rectal hemorrhage is a bleeding duodenal or gastric ulcer. Bleeding from the upper gastrointestinal tract, which appears as bright red blood in the stool, implies massive blood loss and rapid transit. It is very unusual to have bright red blood by rectum from the upper gastrointestinal tract without accompanying signs of hypovolemia and shock. When a patient passes a copious amount of bright red blood by rectum without significant systemic signs of blood loss, the bleeding is almost certain to be coming from the colon. Burgundy-colored stools are typical of colonic bleeding, but very often come from the right colon or distal ileum. The term *pseudomelena* is used to characterize such stools. In true melena the stool is thick, black, and "tarry" because of the decomposition of blood during its passage through the upper small bowel. Repeated episodes of colonic hemorrhage result in shock, and often when the patient is first seen the site of the bleeding lesion may be uncertain. For this reason initial emergency treatment of patients with lower gastrointestinal hemorrhage should be identical to that described in the preceding section on massive upper gastrointestinal bleeding.

Initial management must be directed toward correction of shock and hypovolemia.

Nothing is more important, however, than for the physician to observe the stool himself. The distinction between bright red blood with clots, pseudomelena, and true melena provides one of the best clues toward localization of the bleeding.

Laboratory Studies

The same laboratory studies described in the emergency appraisal of the patient with massive upper gastrointestinal hemorrhage should be performed.

A nasogastric tube should be passed promptly. If blood is obtained, the bleeding site is obviously in the upper gastrointestinal tract. On the other hand, if bright red blood continues to be passed by rectum and no blood is aspirated from the stomach, it is unlikely that the bleeding is from the upper gastrointestinal tract.

Other Diagnostic Maneuvers

If the differential diagnosis between upper and lower gastrointestinal hemorrhage is not clear, as is often the case, the diagnostic maneuvers described in the preceding section are in order. If the evidence points toward a bleeding site in the lower gastrointestinal tract, the following studies should be undertaken as soon as the patient's circulation is stable.

SIGMOIDOSCOPY. Sigmoidoscopy with evacuation of blood from the rectum should be done first. In lower gastrointestinal bleeding one typically finds bright red blood coming down from above, but a specific site of bleeding will not be seen. On rare occasions an ulcer or a polyp or a suspicious-looking diverticulum may be identified.

X-RAY. A barium enema is a useful and important diagnostic procedure if the evidence points heavily toward lower gastrointestinal bleeding. As a rule the barium enema will not identify a specific bleeding point. Rarely it may show a polyp or carcinoma, but usually the examination is negative, or negative except for "the presence of diverticulosis." Diverticulosis, particularly if confined to the left colon, is an extremely important finding which will have great weight in the subsequent management of the patient.

Because bleeding from the lower colon so often quickly subsides, it has been postulated that a barium enema may actually be therapeutic and even contribute to control of hemorrhage. Although there is no substantial evidence to support this, bleeding often ceases following barium enema, at least temporarily.

ANGIOGRAPHY. Angiography has been discussed in detail in the preceding section. Several authors have reported that early selective angiography will localize massive upper or lower gastrointestinal bleeding (Margulis et al., 1960; Nusbaum et al., 1965, 1969). It is our practice, particularly in suspected lower gastrointestinal hemorrhage, to perform a barium enema examination as the first step. Frequently, bleeding is episodic and ceases without therapy, but the patient is subsequently readmitted because of recurrence. During the second admission angiography is used as the first diagnostic maneuver. Because of the very encouraging reports on selected visceral angiography, we believe that this should be undertaken promptly (Nusbaum et al., 1969). Patients who have had massive bleeding from the lower bowel are urged to return promptly to the hospital in the hope that angiography can be done before the bleeding stops.

Unfortunately no specific nonoperative management can be recommended for the treatment of the primary causes of massive lower gastrointestinal bleeding comparable to the surgical therapy appropriate in upper gastrointestinal bleeding. Several steps merit consideration, however. The potential therapeutic effect of the barium enema should not be overlooked. If the patient is severely hypertensive, appropriate control should be considered.

The primary direction of management, however, is toward replacement of blood volume and then maintenance of an adequate effective blood volume. As a general guide we have used the same estimate of the rate of bleeding as an operative indication as in upper gastrointestinal bleeding: namely, failure of the circulation to stabilize despite multiple transfusions. Because spontaneous cessation of hemorrhage is more common in lower gastrointestinal hemorrhage, we tend to be more conservative and to continue with transfusion longer than would be the case if the site of bleeding were thought to be in the stomach or duodenum. Knutsson and Risholm (1961) have urged conservative management on the grounds that often the bleeding point cannot be found at operation, and in approximately half of these cases no subsequent bleeding occurred.

As Hoar and Bernhard (1954) pointed out, in selected cases exsanguination occurs and operative intervention is mandatory. Many factors influence the final decision regarding operation, the most important being the presence of associated systemic disease. If the patient has significant renal or hepatic disease, laparotomy is almost certainly going to prove futile. Hypertension, advanced age, and associated pulmonary or cardiac insufficiency are not contraindications, although they may force continued conservative management. Continuation of conservative management is not hazardous providing that replacement is adequate and the patient does not go into shock. This type of delay is not critical, and there is always the hope of spontaneous cessation of bleeding.

OPERATIVE MANAGEMENT

Exploratory laparotomy for massive lower gastrointestinal hemorrhage is difficult, hazardous, and frustrating. Only rarely can the specific site of bleeding be identified by palpation or visualization. Characteristically, as soon as the abdomen is opened the colon will be massively distended with blood. There may or may not be blood in the distal small bowel. If there is blood in the distal small bowel, it may have come from higher in the gastrointestinal tract or may have refluxed from the colon. Nevertheless, a quick look at the distal small bowel is in order, because it is here that specific lesions,

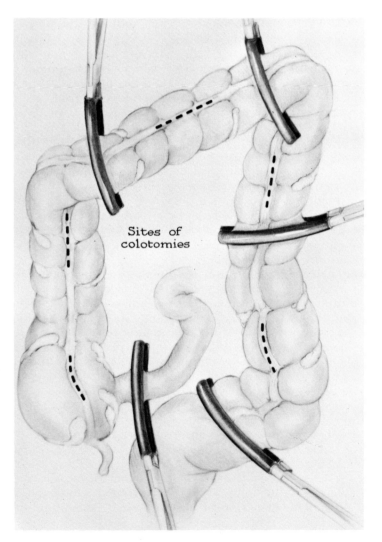

Sites of colotomies

Figure 12-4. Segments of large intestine isolated between noncrushing clamps; generous enterotomies allow visualization of the mucosal surfaces (From Albo et al.: Amer. J. Surg.)

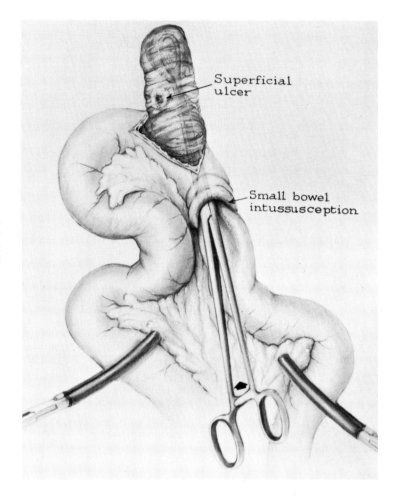

Superficial
ulcer

Small bowel
intussusception

Figure 12-5. Technique of intussusception may lead to the discovery of bleeding lesions by allowing direct visualization of the mucosa. (From Albo et al.: Amer. J. Surg.)

though rare, may be easily identified by the surgeon. Neoplasms, angiomas, or a bleeding Meckel diverticulum can usually be identified or excluded.

We prefer to segmentalize the colon with noncrushing clamps (Fig. 12-4). Hopefully, if bleeding continues it may be identified by progressive distention of a particular segment. Because bleeding so often ceases spontaneously we have practically never found this to be of value, and we now believe that prolonged delay to identify bleeding in this fashion is unwise.

If the evidence points strongly toward a small bowel lesion, both by preoperative findings and the presence of blood well up in the small bowel, several additional maneuvers may be helpful if the lesion cannot be identified. Transillumination of the bowel after gentle stripping and emptying it of blood clot may identify small tumors, ulcerations, or vascular anomalies. Suspicious vascular lesions may be identified more

clearly by pressing a clean sterile glass slide against the serosal surface of the bowel, as described by Vetto (1962). Occasionally we have carried out intussusception of long segments of small bowel to identify a lesion which could not be felt or seen by transillumination (Fig. 12-5).

Assuming that no lesion of the small bowel has been identified, the surgeon is faced with four choices: (1) right colectomy, (2) left colectomy, (3) subtotal colectomy, or (4) transverse colostomy. Which is to be used will be a highly individualized decision in each case, but there are some guidelines.

If the bleeding has always been bright red, it is very probable that the bleeding is in the left colon. Under these circumstances, therefore, we perform a blind resection of the sigmoid and descending colon. Hopefully, a bleeding site can be identified when the bowel is opened. Control of the hemorrhage may be evidenced by rapid stabilization of the circulation. This approach is used even if the diverticulosis involves the proximal colon.

If the bleeding has included clots, blood is often mixed with stool and is not consistently bright red, and if there are no diverticula, we prefer an initial resection of the cecum and ascending colon. Examination of the specimen may immediately show a small nonpalpable bleeding lesion such as a tiny polyp or a superficial ulcer. Nonspecific superficial ulceration of the right colon, possibly on a vascular basis, is being recognized more frequently as a specific cause of massive lower gastrointestinal hemorrhage (Albo et al., 1966; Corry et al., 1970).

If no lesion is found, the resection is continued across the transverse colon, usually resulting in a fairly radical subtotal colectomy. This approach is appropriate for the good-risk patient but may not be feasible in the obese, elderly, poor-risk patient with multiple system diseases.

If the condition of the patient is poor and if there are technical complications such as marked obesity and no clear-cut clue to localization has been obtained, a transverse colostomy may be the most conservative procedure. This will identify where in the colon the bleeding originates and will permit a more limited and more accurately selective resection. Because bleeding so often stops spontaneously, we have seen patients in whom no further bleeding occurred and in whom only at a subsequent admission did the bleeding site become evident. At times no lesion can be identified, no bleeding occurs, and closure of the colostomy is in order. Since this is a diagnostic rather than a therapeutic colostomy, it need not be completely diverting.

Finally, in some cases, after every maneuver including bowel resection, the bleeding point is still not identifiable. Hopefully, preoperative and operative angiography will reduce the number of such instances. The most frequent cause of massive bleeding appearing at the rectum continues to be duodenal or gastric ulcer, and the procedures and approaches outlined in the preceding section must be observed in every case of exsanguinating gastrointestinal hemorrhage.

REFERENCES

Abrahams, J. I.: Heterotopic pancreas simulating peptic ulceration. Arch. Surg., 93:589, 1966.

Adson, M. A.: Emergency portal-systemic shunts. Surg. Clin. N. Amer., 47:887, 1967.

Albo, R. J., Grimes, O. F., and Dunphy, J. E.: Management of massive lower gastrointestinal hemorrhage. Amer. J. Surg., 112:264, 1966.

Anderson, R. P., Leand, P. M., and Zuidema, G. D.: Uses of the balloon-tipped catheter in biliary tract surgery. Amer. J. Surg., 117:55, 1969.

Arrants, J. E., Green, J. R., and Hairston, P.: Peptic erosion of the myocardium. Ann. Thorac. Surg., 5:556, 1968.

Artz, C. P., and Fitts, C. T.: Gastrointestinal ulceration associated with central nervous system lesions and with burns. Surg. Clin. N. Amer., 46:309, 1966.

Ashby, E. C., Mott, T. J., and Starer, F.: Severe gastrointestinal haemorrhage: Haemangiomata demonstrated by selection visceral arteriography. Brit. Med. J., 4:737, 1968.

Balasegaram, M.: Haematemesis and melaena. A review of 326 cases. Med. J. Aust., 1:485, 1968.

Barrett, F. A., and Reckling, W. E.: Hiatus hernia and massive upper gastrointestinal bleeding. Rocky Mtn. Med. J., 62:32, 1965.

Bartlett, M. K., and Ottinger, L. W.: Vagotomy in bleeding gastritis. Surg. Clin. N. Amer., 46:613, 1966.

Baum, S., Nusbaum, M., Clearfield, H. R., Kuroda, K. and Tumen, H. J.: Angiography in the diagnosis of gastrointestinal bleeding. Arch. Intern. Med., 117: 16, 1967.

Belkin, G. A., and Conn, H. O.: Blood ammonia concentration and bromsulfalein retention in upper gastrointestinal hemorrhage. New Eng. J. Med., 260 530, 1959.

Boijsen, E., and Reuter, S. R.: Angiography in diagnosis of chronic unexplained melena. Radiology, 89:413 1967.

Boley, S. J., Schultz, L., Krieger, H., Schwartz, S. Elguezabal, A., and Allen, A. C.: Experimental evaluation of thiazides and potassium as a cause of small bowel ulcer. JAMA, 192:763, 1965.

Bongiovi, J. J., and Duffy, J. L.: Gastric hemangioma associated with upper gastrointestinal bleeding Arch. Surg., 95:93, 1967.

Bowers, W. F., McKinnon, W. M. P., Marino, J. M., and Culverwell, J. T.: Cannulation of the thoracic duct Its role in the pre-shunt management of hemorrhage due to esophageal varices. J. Intern. Coll Surgeons, 42:71, 1964.

Bray, R. S.: An improved gastrointestinal cord for the detection of upper gastrointestinal bleeding. Amer J. Proctol., 18:277, 1964.

Brooks, J. R., and Eraklis, A. J.: Factors affecting the mortality from peptic ulcer. New Eng. J. Med. 271:803, 1964.

Bryant, L. R., and Griffen, W. O., Jr.: Vagotomy and pyloroplasty: An inadequate operation for stress ulcer? Arch. Surg., 93:161, 1966.

Carruthers, R. K., Giles, G. R., Clark, C. G., and Goligher J. C.: Conservative surgery for bleeding peptic ulcer. Brit. Med. J., 1:80, 1967.

Child, C. G.: The Liver and Portal Hypertension. Philadelphia, W. B. Saunders Company, 1964, p. 47.

Civetta, J. M., and Daggett, W. M.: Gastrointestinal bleeding from jejunal diverticula. Ann. Surg., 166 976, 1967.

Clatworthy, H. W., and Boles, E. T.: Extrahepatic portal bed block in children: Pathogenesis and treatment Ann. Surg., 150:371, 1959.

Cohn, R., and Blaisdell, F. W.: The natural history of the patient with cirrhosis of the liver with esophageal varices following the first massive hemorrhage. Surg., Gynec. Obstet., 106:699, 1958.

Conn, H. O., and Lindenmuth, W. W.: Prophylactic portacaval anastomosis in cirrhotic patients with esophageal varices. New Eng. J. Med., 279:725, 1968.

Conn, H. O., and Simpson, J. A.: Excessive mortality with balloon tamponade. JAMA, 202:587, 1967.

Conn, H. O., and Simpson, J. A.: A rational program for the diagnosis and treatment of bleeding esophageal varices. Med. Clin. N. Amer., 52:1457, 1968.

Conn, H. O., Smith, H. W., and Brodoff, M.: Observer variation in the endoscopic diagnosis of esophageal varices. New Eng. J. Med., 272:830, 1965.

Cooley, R. N.: Primary amyloidosis with involvement of stomach. Amer. J. Roentgenol., 70:428, 1953.

Cornes, J. S., Jones, T. G., and Fisher, G. B.: Gastroduodenal ulceration and massive hemorrhage in patients with leukemia, multiple myeloma, and malignant tumors of lymphoid tissue. Gastroenterology, 41:337, 1961.

Corry, R. J., Barlett, M. K., and Cohen, R. B.: Erosions of the cecum. A cause of massive hemorrhage. Amer. J. Surg., 119:106, 1970.

Corry, R. J., Mundth, E. D., and Bartlett, M. K.: Massive upper gastrointestinal tract hemorrhage. A complication of cholecystoduodenal fistula. Arch. Surg., 97:531, 1968.

Couves, C. M., Howard, J. M., and Amerson, J. R.: Fatal perforation of the thoracic aorta by a gastric ulcer. Amer. J. Surg., 95:878, 1958.

Curling, T. B.: An acute ulceration of the duodenum in cases of burn. Med. Chir. Trans., 25:260, 1842.

Cushing, H.: Peptic ulcers and the interbrain. Surg. Gynec. Obstet., 55:1, 1932.

Dahlin, C. C.: Amyloidosis. Proc. Staff Meet. Mayo Clinic, 24:637, 1949.

Darin, J. C., Polacek, M. A., and Ellison, E. H.: Surgical mortality of massive hemorrhage from peptic ulcer. Arch. Surg., 83:55, 1961.

Davis, R. A., and Brooks, F. P.: Experimental peptic ulcer associated with lesion or stimulation of the central nervous system. Surg. Gynec. Obstet., 116:307, 1963.

deKretser, D. M. H., Bird, T., and McCollum, J. K.: Bleeding and pancreatitis. Brit. Med. J., 2:1306, 1966.

Delaney, J. P., Goodale, R. L., Jr., Cheng, J., and Wangensteen, O. H.: The influence of vasopressin on upper gastrointestinal blood flow. Surgery, 59:397, 1966.

Dollinger, M. R., and Morgan, L. R.: Local cooling in management of acute upper gastrointestinal bleeding. Amer. J. Surg., 111:651, 1966.

Dorton, H. E.: Vagotomy, pyloroplasty and suture for bleeding gastric ulcer. Surg. Gynec. Obstet., 122:1015, 1966.

Dorton, H. E., and Hyden, W. H.: Acute massive duodenal ulcer hemorrhage. Arch. Surg., 83:116, 1961.

Dumont, A. E., and Witte, M. H.: Thoracic duct cannulation: A new approach to the emergency treatment of bleeding esophageal varices. In Ellison, E., Friesen, S. F., and Mulholland, J. H. (eds.): Current Surgical Management. Philadelphia, W. B. Saunders Company, 1965, Vol. III, p. 264.

Dunphy, J. E.: The management of acute upper gastrointestinal hemorrhage. Amer. Surg., 20:1023, 1954.

Dunphy, J. E., and Hoer, S. O.: The indications for emergency operation in severe hemorrhage from gastric or duodenal ulcer. Surgery, 24:231, 1948.

Edmunds, R., and West, J. P.: Treatment of bleeding esophageal varices. Five year comparison of medical and surgical procedures. JAMA, 189:854, 1964.

Eiseman, B., and Carnes, M.: Hemorrhagic and traumatic shock. In American College of Surgeons: Manual of Preoperative and Postoperative Care. Philadelphia, W. B. Saunders Company, 1967, Chapter 6.

Enquist, I. F., Karlson, K. E., Dennis, C., Fierst, S. M., and Shafton, G. W.: Statistically valid ten-year comparative evaluation of three methods of management of massive gastroduodenal hemorrhage. Ann. Surg., 162:550, 1965.

Evans, D. A. P., Horwich, L., McConnell, R. B., and Bullen, M. F.: Influence of the ABO blood groups and secretor status on bleeding and on perforation of duodenal ulcer. Gut, 9:319, 1968.

Farris, J. M., and Smith, G. K.: Vagotomy and pyloroplasty. Ann. Surg., 152:416, 1960.

Farris, J. M., and Smith, G. K.: Appraisal of the long-term results of vagotomy and pyloroplasty in 100 patients with bleeding duodenal ulcer. Ann. Surg., 166:630, 1967.

Ferguson, H. L., and Clarke, J. S.: Treatment of hemorrhage from erosive gastritis by vagotomy and pyloroplasty. Amer. J. Surg., 112:739, 1966.

Fisher, R. D., Ebert, P. A., and Zuidema, G. D.: Peptic ulcer disease. Arch. Surg., 92:909, 1966.

Fletcher, D. G., and Harkins, H. N.: Acute peptic ulcer as a complication of major surgery, stress, or trauma. Surgery, 36:212, 1954.

Fogelman, M. J., and Garvey, J. M.: Acute gastroduodenal ulceration incident to surgery and disease. Amer. J. Surg., 112:651, 1966.

Foster, D. G.: Retrograde jejunogastric intussusception —a rare cause of hematemesis. Review of the literature and report of two cases. Arch. Surg., 73:1009, 1956.

Foster, J. H.: Unpublished data from Hartford Hospital.

Foster, J. H., Hall, A. D., and Dunphy, J. E.: Surgical management of bleeding ulcers. Surg. Clin. N. Amer., 46:387, 1966.

Foster, J. H., Hickok, D. F., and Dunphy, J. E.: Factors influencing mortality following emergency operation for massive upper gastrointestinal hemorrhage. Surg. Gynec. Obstet., 117:257, 1963.

Foster, J. H., Holcomb, G. W., and Kirtley, J. A.: Results of surgical treatment of portal hypertension in children. Ann. Surg., 157:868, 1963.

Foster, J. H., and Vetto, R. M.: Aortic intra-aneurysmal abscess caused by sigmoid-aortic fistula. Amer. J. Surg., 104:850, 1962.

Foster, J. H., and Vetto, R. M.: Fifteen years' experience with portasystemic venous shunting operations. Amer. Surg., 33:514, 1967.

Frank, W.: Hematemesis associated with gastric arteriosclerosis; review of literature with case report. Gastroenterology, 7:231, 1946.

Freeark, R. J., Norcross, W. J., and Baker, R. J.: Exploratory gastrotomy in management of massive upper gastrointestinal hemorrhage. Arch. Surg., 94:684, 1967.

Gall, E. A., and Keirle, A. M.: Portal system venous shunt. Pathological factors contributing to postoperative survival. Gastroenterology, 49:656, 1965.

Garceau, A. J., and Chalmers, T. C.: The natural history of cirrhosis. I. Survival with esophageal varices. New Eng. J. Med., 268:469, 1963.

Goldman, R. L.: Submucosal arterial malformation ("aneurysm") of the stomach with fatal hemorrhage. Gastroenterology, 46:589, 1964.

Goodman, A. A., and Frey, C. F.: Massive upper gastrointestinal hemorrhage following surgical operation. Ann. Surg., 167:180, 1968.

Gordon-Taylor, G.: Rare causes of severe gastrointestinal hemorrhage with note on aneurysm of hepatic artery. Brit. Med. J., 1:504, 1943.

Grace, N. D., Muench, H., and Chalmers, T. C.: The present status of shunts for portal hypertension in cirrhosis. Gastroenterology, 50:684, 1966.

Graff, R. J.: Considerations in the treatment of traumatic hemobilia. Amer. J. Surg., 105:662, 1963.

Gray, S. J., Olson, T. E., and Monrique, J.: Hematemesis and melena. Med. Clin. N. Amer., 41:1327, 1957.

Green, D. M., and Metheny, D.: The estimation of acute blood loss by the tilt test. Surg. Gynec. Obstet., 84:1045, 1957.

Grosz, C. R., and Wu, K. T.: Stress ulcers: A survey of the experience in a large general hospital. Surgery, 61:853, 1967.

Gütgemann, A., and Esser, G.: Portal hypertension, varicose vein bleeding and shunt operation. Minn. Med., 51:1517, 1968.

Haller, J. D., Pena, C., and Dargan, E. L.: Massive upper gastrointestinal hemorrhage due to pancreatitis. Arch. Surg., 93:567, 1966.

Halpern, M., Turner, A. F., and Citron, B. P.: Hereditary hemorrhagic telangiectasia. Radiology, 90:1143, 1968.

Hampson, L. G., Mulder, D. S., Elias, G. L., and Palmer, J. D.: The emergency surgical treatment of massively bleeding peptic ulcer. Arch. Surg., 97:450, 1968.

Hardaway, R. M., and Castagno, J. L.: Recurrent gastric hemorrhage due to idiopathic hemorrhagic gastritis which required total gastrectomy. Surgery, 45:780, 1959.

Harvey, H. D.: Emergency gastric resection for bleeding and perforation. Arch. Surg., 86:61, 1963.

Haynes, W. F., Jr., and Pittman, F. E.: Application of the fluorescein string test in 32 cases of upper gastrointestinal hemorrhage. Preliminary report. Gastroenterology, 38:690, 1960.

Hedberg, S. E.: Early endoscopic diagnosis in upper gastrointestinal hemorrhage. Surg. Clin. N. Amer., 46:499, 1966.

Hilsman, J. H.: The color of blood containing feces following instillation of citrated blood at various levels of the small intestine. Gastroenterology, 15:131, 1950.

Hirsch, E. F., Montero, G. G., and Gould, E. A.: Unusual causes of upper gastrointestinal hemorrhage. Amer. Surg., 33:453, 1967.

Hirschowitz, B. I., Luketic, G. C., Balint, J. A., and Fulton, W. F.: Early fiberscope endoscopy for upper gastrointestinal bleeding. Amer. J. Digest. Dis., 8:816, 1963.

Hittner, V. J.: Gastric polyposis with massive hemorrhage. Wisconsin Med. J., 65:204, 1966.

Hoar, C. S., and Bernhard, W. F.: Colonic bleeding and diverticular disease of the colon. Surg. Gynec. Obstet., 99:101, 1954.

Hoerr, S. O., Dunphy, J. E., and Gray, S. J.: Place of surgery in emergency treatment of acute massive upper gastrointestinal hemorrhage. Surg. Gynec. Obstet., 87:338, 1948.

Hopkins, R. W., Frationne, R. B., Abrams, J. S., and Simeone, F. A.: Controlled hypotension for uncontrolled hemorrhage. Arch. Surg., 95:517, 1967.

Jackson, F. C., Christopherson, E. B., Peternel, W. W., and Kirimli, B.: Preoperative management of patients with liver disease. Surg. Clin. N. Amer., 48:907, 1968a.

Jackson, F. C., Perrin, E. B., Dagradi, A. E., Smith, A. G., and Lee, L. E., Jr.: Clinical investigation of the portacaval shunt I. Study design and preliminary survival analysis. Arch. Surg., 91:43, 1965.

Jackson, F. C., Perrin, E. B., Smith, A. G., Dagradi, A. E., and Nadal, H. M.: A clinical investigation of the portacaval shunt II. Survival analysis of the prophylactic operation. Amer. J. Surg., 115:22, 1968b.

Judd, E. S.: Massive bleeding of colonic origin. Surg. Clin. N. Amer., 49:977, 1969.

Katz, D., Douvres, P., Weisberg, H., McKinnon, W., and Glass, G. B. J.: Early endoscopic diagnosis of acute upper gastrointestinal hemorrhage. Demonstration of a relatively high incidence of erosion as a source of bleeding. JAMA, 188:405, 1964.

Kelley, H. G., Grant, G. N., and Elliot, D. W.: Massive gastroduodenal hemorrhage. Arch. Surg., 87:22, 1963.

Kern, F., Jr.: Personal communication.

Kessler, R. E.: Effects of vasopressin on portal vein pressure in the unanesthetized man. Surg. Forum, 19:335, 1968.

Klingensmith, W., and Oles, P.: Surgical complications of dicumarol therapy. Amer. J. Surg., 108:640, 1964.

Knutsson, V., and Risholm, L.: Conservative treatment of melaena of unknown origin. Acta Med. Scand., 170:621, 1961.

Kozoll, D. D., and Meyer, K. A.: Massively bleeding gastroduodenal ulcers. Arch. Surg., 89:250, 1964.

Lasher, E. P.: Porto-renal shunt. Amer. J. Surg., 31:433, 1965.

Leape, L. L., and Welch, C. E.: Late prognosis of patients with upper gastrointestinal hemorrhage. Amer. J. Surg., 107:279, 1964.

Lee, H. C., and Kay, S.: Primary polyarteritis nodosa of of the stomach and small intestine as a cause of gastrointestinal hemorrhage. Ann. Surg., 147:714, 1958.

Liebowitz, H. R.: Pathogenesis of esophageal varix rupture. JAMA, 175:874, 1961.

Linton, R. R.: Selection of patients for portacaval shunts. Ann. Surg., 134:433, 1951.

Linton, R. R.: The treatment of esophageal varices. Surg. Clin. N. Amer., 46:485, 1966.

Linton, R. R., Ellis, D. S., and Geary, J. E.: Critical comparative analysis of early and late results of splenorenal and direct portocaval shunts performed in 169 patients with portal cirrhosis. Ann. Surg., 154:446, 1961.

Long, L., Mahony, T. D., and Jewell, W. R.: Selective amyloidosis of the jejunum: A case report of a rare cause for gastrointestinal bleeding. Amer. J. Surg., 109:217, 1965.

Lorimer, W. S.: Discussion of small bowel hemorrhage. Ann. Surg., 167:957, 1968.

Lowe, W. C., and Palmer, E. D.: Fatal gastrointestinal hemorrhage clinically unrecognized. Amer. J. Gastroent., 47:405, 1967.

Mallory, G. K., and Weiss, S.: Hemorrhages from laceration of the cardiac orifice of the stomach due to vomiting. Amer. J. Med. Sci., 178:506, 1929.

Margulis, A. R., Heinbecker, P., and Bernard, H. R.: Operative mesenteric arteriography in the search for the site of bleeding in unexplained gastrointestinal hemorrhage. Surgery, 48:534, 1960.

Matyus, L., Bodnar, E., and Littman, I.: Ruptured aneurysm of the splenic artery. J. Cardiov. Surg., 7:324, 1966.

Maynard, E. P., and Voorhees, A. B.: Arterial hemorrhage from a large bowel diverticulum. Gastroenterology, 31:210, 1956.

McDermott, W. V., Jr.: The techniques of portal-systemic shunt surgery. Surgery, 57:778, 1965.

McDermott, W. V., Jr.: The treatment of cirrhotic ascites by combined hepatic and portal decompression. New Eng. J. Med., 259:897, 1958.

McHardy, G., Bechtold, J. E., and McHardy, R. J.: Hemorrhage from primary disease of the mesenteric small intestine. Gastroenterology, 28:17, 1955.

Mead, P. H.: Experience with pyloroplasty and vagotomy. Amer. J. Surg., 114:910, 1967.

Menguy, R.: Surgical treatment of acute hemorrhagic gastritis. Summary of remarks given at Yale University, March, 1969.

Menguy, R.: Gastric mucosal injury by aspirin. Gastroenterology, 51:430, 1966.

Merigan, T. C., Jr., Plotkin, G. R., and Davidson, C. S.: Effect of intravenously administered posterior pituitary extract on hemorrhage from bleeding esophageal varices: A controlled evaluation. New Eng. J. Med., 266:134, 1961.

Mikkelson, W. P.: Emergency portacaval shunt. Rev. Surg., 19:141, 1962.

Mixter, G., Jr., and Hinton, J. W.: Gastroduodenal hemorrhagic diathesis: A report of ten cases treated by vagectomy. N. Y. State J. Med., 57:3803, 1957.

Moghadam, M., and Haubrich, W. S.: Long-term results of hemigastrectomy with vagotomy in the treatment of bleeding peptic ulcers. Amer. J. Digest. Dis., 12:1000, 1967.

Moncrief, J. A., Switzer, W. E., and Tepletz, C.: Curling's ulcer. J. Trauma, 4:481, 1964.

Myers, R. T.: Bleeding esophageal varices: A study involving 100 consecutive cases. Amer. Surg., 33: 919, 1967.

Nagel, C. B., Doering, R. B., Steedman, R. A., and Conolly, J. E.: Management of hemorrhagic gastritis: Analysis of 34 cases. Amer. Surg., 33:815, 1967.

Netterville, R. E., Hardy, J. D., and Martin, R. S., Jr.: Small bowel hemorrhage. Ann. Surg., 167:950, 1968.

Noer, R. J., Hamilton, J. E., Williams, D. J., and Broughton, D. S.: Rectal hemorrhage. Ann. Surg., 155: 794, 1962.

Nusbaum, M., Baum, S., and Blakemore, W. S.: Clinical experience with the diagnosis and management of gastrointestinal hemorrhage by selective mesenteric catheterization. Ann. Surg., 170:506, 1969.

Nusbaum, M., Baum, S., Blakemore, W. S., and Finkelstein, A. K.: Demonstration of intra-abdominal bleeding by selective arteriography. Visualization of celiac and superior mesenteric arteries. JAMA, 191:389, 1965.

Nusbaum, M., Baum, S., Sakiyalak, P., and Blakemore, W. S.: Pharmacologic control of portal hypertension. Surgery, 62:299, 1967.

Orloff, M. J.: A comparative study of emergency transesophageal ligation and nonsurgical treatment of bleeding esophageal varices in unselected patients with cirrhosis. Surgery, 52:103, 1962.

Orloff, M. J.: Emergency portacaval shunt: Comparative study of shunt, varix ligation and non-surgical treatment of bleeding esophageal varices in unselected patients with cirrhosis. Ann. Surg., 166:456, 1967.

Orloff, M. J., and Thomas, H. S.: Pathogenesis of esophageal varix rupture. Arch. Surg., 87:301, 1963.

Osborne, M., and Dunphy, J. E.: Identification of causes of obscure massive upper gastrointestinal hemorrhage during operation. Arch. Surg., 75:964, 1957.

Paine, J. R.: Immediate results of subtotal gastric resection for benign peptic ulcer. Surgery, 51:561, 1962.

Palmer, E. D.: Hemorrhage from erosive gastritis and its surgical implications. Gastroenterology, 36:856, 1959.

Palmer, E. D.: Diagnosis of Upper Gastrointestinal Hemorrhage. Springfield, Ill.: Charles C Thomas, 1961, p. 76.

Palmer, E. D.: Hemorrhage as sequel to gastric surgery. Amer. J. Med. Sci., 249:200, 1965.

Palmer, E. D.: The vigorous diagnostic approach to upper gastrointestinal tract hemorrhage. JAMA, 207:1477, 1969.

Palumbo, L. T., and Sharpe, W. S.: Partial gastrectomy for chronic duodenal ulcer with hemorrhage: Results in 450 cases. Surgery, 49:585, 1961.

Palumbo, L. T., and Sharpe, W. S.: Active bleeding duodenal ulcer (management during ten year period). Surg. Clin. N. Amer., 49:239, 1967.

Panke, W. F., Rousselot, L. M., and Moreno, A. N.: Splenic pulp manometry as emergency test in differential diagnosis of acute upper gastrointestinal bleeding. Surg. Gynec. Obstet., 109:270, 1959.

Parry, D. J., and Wood, P. H.: Relationship between aspirin taking and gastroduodenal haemorrhage. Gut, 8:301, 1967.

Piccone, V. A., and LeVeen, H. H.: Transumbilical portal decompression. Surg. Gynec. Obstet., 125:66, 1967.

Preston, F. W., and Trippel, O. H.: The technique of emergency portacaval shunt. Surg. Clin. N. Amer., 46:37, 1966.

Ratnoff, O. D., and Patek, A. J., Jr.: Natural history of Laennec's cirrhosis of the liver: Analysis of 386 cases. Medicine, 21:207, 1942.

Read, R. C., Huebl, H. C., and Thal, A. P.: Randomized study of massive bleeding from peptic ulceration. Ann. Surg., 162:561, 1965.

Reuter, S. R., and Bookstein, J. J.: Angiographic localization of gastrointestinal bleeding. Gastroenterology, 54:876, 1968.

Reynolds, T. B., Hudson, N. M., Mikkelsen, W. P., Turrill, F. L., and Redeker, A. G.: Clinical comparison of end-to-side and side-to-side portacaval shunts. New Eng. J. Med., 274:706, 1966.

Richter, R. M., and Pochaczevsky, R.: Duodenal varices. Arch. Surg., 95:269, 1967.

Robertson, M. G., and Schroder, J. S.: Pseudoxanthoma elasticum: A systemic disorder. Amer. J. Med., 27: 433, 1959.

Rodgers, J. B., Older, T. M., and Stabler, E. V.: Gastric hypothermia: A critical evaluation of its use in massive upper gastrointestinal bleeding. Ann. Surg., 163:367, 1966.

Rosen, H., Silen, W., and Simon, M.: Selective portal hypertension with isolated duodenojejunal varices. New Eng. J. Med., 277:1188, 1967.

Rosenkrantz, J. G., and Bartlett, M. K.: Hemorrhage from gastritis: An analysis of 44 proven cases. Ann. Surg., 153:617, 1961.

Ross, J. R.: Obscure gastrointestinal hemorrhage. Med. Clin. N. Amer., 53:417, 1969.

Rousselot, L. M., Cole, D. R., and Grossi, C. E.: Gastrointestinal bleeding as a sequel to cancer chemotherapy. Amer. J. Gastroent., 43:311, 1965.

Rousselot, L. M., Gilbertson, F. E., and Panke, W. F.: Severe hemorrhage from esophagogastric varices —

its emergency management with particular reference to porto-caval anastomosis. New Eng. J. Med., 262:269, 1960.

Salter, R. H.: Aspirin and gastrointestinal bleeding. Amer. J. Digest. Dis., 13:38, 1968.

Satterfield, J. V., Mulligan, L. V., and Butcher, H. R.: Bleeding esophageal varices. Arch. Surg., 90:667, 1965.

Schaller, R. T., Jr., Hessel, E. A., II, King, L. T., Jr., and Stevenson, J. K.: Gastric hypothermia for massive upper gastrointestinal hemorrhage. Experience with 24 patients and review of the literature. Arch. Surg., 92:707, 1966.

Schiff, L.: Hematemesis and melena. In MacBryde, C. M. (ed.): Signs and Symptoms. 4th ed. Philadelphia, J. B. Lippincott Company, 1964, chapter 20.

Schiff, L., and Shapiro, N.: In Sandweiss, D. J. (ed.): Peptic Ulcer. Philadelphia, W. B. Saunders Company, 1951, p. 623.

Scott, H. W., Sawyers, J. L., Gobbel, W. G., Herrington, J. L., Edwards, W. H., and Edwards, L. W.: Vagotomy and antrectomy in surgical treatment of duodenal ulcer disease. Surg. Clin. N. Amer., 46:349, 1966.

Schwartz, G. F.: Carcinoid tumor of the small intestine associated with acute gastrointestinal hemorrhage. Amer. J. Surg., 111:553, 1966.

Sedgwick, C. E., Poulantgas, J. K., and Miller, W. H.: Portasystemic shunts in 102 patients with portal hypertension. New Eng. J. Med., 274:1290, 1966.

Sedgwick, C. E., and Vernon, J. K.: Gastrointestinal bleeding. Diagnosis and management. Surg. Clin. N. Amer., 48:523, 1968.

Shackelford, R. T., and Marcus, W. Y.: Jejunal diverticula —a cause of gastrointestinal hemorrhage. A report of three cases and a review of the literature. Ann. Surg., 151:930, 1960.

Shaldon, S., and Sherlock, S.: Obstruction to the extrahepatic portal system in childhood. Lancet, 1:63, 1962.

Sherlock, S.: In Gamble, J., and Wilbur, D. (eds.): Current Concepts of Clinical Gastroenterology. Boston, Little, Brown & Company, 1965, p. 181.

Silen, W.: Personal communication.

Simpson, J. A., and Conn, H. O.: Role of ascites in gastroesophageal reflux with comments on the pathogenesis of bleeding esophageal varices. Gastroenterology, 55:17, 1968.

Sloop, R. D., and Thompson, J. C.: Aorto-esophageal fistula: Report of a case and review of the literature. Gastroenterology, 53:768, 1967.

Smith, V. M., and Babb, R. R.: Aspirin—Rosetta stone of gastrointestinal hemorrhage: A point of view. Military Med., 133:965, 1968.

Smith, W. R., and Berne, C. J.: Severe colonic bleeding. Calif. Med., 101:235, 1964.

Sparkman, R. S.: Massive hemobilia following traumatic rupture of the liver. Ann. Surg., 138:899, 1953.

Spencer, R.: Gastrointestinal hemorrhage in infancy and childhood. 476 cases. Surgery, 55:718, 1964.

Stafford, E. S., Ballinger, W. F., Zuidema, G. D., and Cameron, J. L.: Benign gastric ulcer with life-threatening hemorrhage. Ann. Surg., 165:967, 1967.

Stewart, J. D., Cosgriff, J. H., and Gray, J. G.: Experience with the treatment of acutely massively bleeding peptic ulcer by blood replacement and gastric resection. Surg. Gynec. Obstet., 103:409, 1956.

Sullivan, R. C., Rutherford, R. B., and Waddell, W. R.:

Surgical management of hemorrhagic gastritis by vagotomy and pyloroplasty. Ann. Surg., 159:554, 1964.

Turcotte, J. G., Wallin, V. W., and Child, C. G.: End-to-side versus side-to-side portacaval shunts in patients with hepatic cirrhosis. Amer. J. Surg., 117:108, 1969.

Turunen, M., Pasila, M., and Sulamaa, M.: Supradiaphragmatic transposition of the spleen for portal hypertension. Ann. Surg., 157:127, 1963.

Vetto, R. M.: The management of multiple diffuse telangiectasia of the small intestine. Surg. Gynec. Obstet., 115:56, 1962.

Wangensteen, O. H., Root, H. D., Jenson, C. B., Imamoglu, K., and Salmon, P. A.: Depression of gastric secretion and digestion by gastric hypothermia. Its clinical use in massive hematemesis. Surgery, 44:265, 1958.

Wangensteen, S. L., Orahood, R. C., Voorhees, A. B., Smith, R. B., and Healy, W. V.: Intragastric cooling in the management of hemorrhage from the upper gastrointestinal tract. Amer. J. Surg., 105:501, 1963.

Wangensteen, S. L., and Smith, R. B.: Esophagogastric cooling in the management of bleeding esophageal varices. In Ellison, E. H., Friesen, S. R., and Mulholland, J. H. (eds.) Current Surgical Management III. Philadelphia, W. B. Saunders Company, 1965, p. 259.

Wangensteen, S. L., Smith, R. B., and Barker, H. G.: Gastric cooling and gastric "freezing." Surg. Clin. N. Amer., 46:463, 1966.

Warren, W. D., Fomon, J. J., and Leite, C. A.: Critical assessment of the rationale of thoracic duct drainage in the treatment of portal hypertension. Surgery, 63:7, 1968.

Warren, W. D., Zeppa, R., and Fomon, J. J.: Selective trans-splenic decompression of gastroesophageal varices by distal splenorenal shunt. Ann. Surg., 166:437, 1967.

Weinberg, J. A.: Vagotomy and pyloroplasty in the treatment of duodenal ulcer. Amer. J. Surg., 195:347, 1963.

Weinberger, H. A.: Emergency portacaval shunt for esophagogastric hemorrhage. Arch. Surg., 91:333, 1965.

Wells, H. R.: Massive bleeding from jejunal diverticula. Amer. Surg., 33:663, 1967.

Wheaton, K. R., and Mark, J. B. D.: General hypothermia for massive gastrointestinal hemorrhage. Surg. Gynec. Obstet., 124:1018, 1967.

White, J. J., Slapak, M., and MacLean, L. D.: Extracorporeal portosystemic shunt for portal hypertension. Surgery, 63:17, 1968.

Winower, S. J., Bejar, J., and Zamcheck, N.: Recurrent massive hemorrhage in patients with achlorhydria and atrophic gastritis. Arch. Intern. Med., 120:327, 1967.

Woodward, E. R.: Stomach and duodenum. In American College of Surgeons: Manual of Preoperative and Postoperative Care. Philadelphia, W. B. Saunders Company, 1967, Chapter 22.

Zimmerman, S. L., Engel, E. F., Lapidas, B., Bradley, E. A., and Claytor, H.: Analysis of 200 admissions for massive upper gastrointestinal bleeding. Ann. Intern. Med., 45:653, 1956.

Zollinger, R. M., and Zollinger, R. M., Jr.: Mesenteric-caval shunt. Atlas of Surgical Operations, Vol. 2. New York, Macmillan Co., 1967.

CHAPTER 13

POSTRESECTIONAL GASTROJEJUNOCOLIC FISTULA AND ZOLLINGER-ELLISON TUMOR

by ROBERT M. ZOLLINGER, M.D., THOMAS T. VOGEL, M.D., *and* NEIL J. SHERMAN, M.D.

Robert Milton Zollinger is an Ohioan who received his premedical and medical education at Ohio State University, where he was elected to Alpha Omega Alpha. Following residency training at the Peter Bent Brigham Hospital he remained on the Harvard faculty. After distinguished World War II service, he returned to his alma mater as Professor and Chairman, Department of Surgery, and Director of the Surgical Services of the University Hospitals in 1946. He is a national and world leader in surgery and is also a former president of The American Rose Society. A great surgical teacher and clinician, he has made many original contributions to surgical science and literature. Perhaps his best known investigations deal with the discovery and metabolic effects of the Zollinger-Ellison tumor.

Thomas T. Vogel was born in Ohio and received his M.S. and Ph.D. degrees at Ohio State University. He received his M.D. degree from the Georgetown School of Medicine and served his surgical residency at Ohio State University.

Neil John Sherman received his baccalaureate and medical degrees at the University of Louisville and his surgical residency at Ohio State University. At present he is Chief of Hospital Services, Castle Air Force Base, California.

The diagnosis of gastrojejunocolic fistula implies a chronically ill patient, often metabolically depleted, and clearly points the suspicious finger of failure at a previous surgical procedure. Even the champions of posterior gastroenterostomy, when this was a popular operation in the treatment of duodenal ulcer, feared this complication. The chance of such a fistula developing in association with a marginal ulcer was considered to be lessened if the posterior gastrojejunal anastomosis was made in an opening in the mesocolon as far away as possible from the margin of the transverse colon. Others have since advocated an antecolic anastomosis to lessen the chance of fistula formation (Condon and Tanner, 1968). Gastrojejunocolic fistulas, however, do occur most commonly as a result of iatrogenic or extragastric factors which render control of the acid factor impossible.

The widespread appreciation of the importance of adequately controlling the acid factor to prevent marginal ulcer has no doubt dramatically reduced the current incidence of gastrojejunocolic fistula. The commonest cause is a gastrojejunal stoma placed too far to the left, allowing antral distention with continuous release of gastrin and subsequent gastric hypersecretion despite complete vagotomy (Fig. 13-1A). A second important cause of failure to control the acid factor is an overlooked vagus nerve, particularly the right or posterior trunk. An inadequate gas-

315

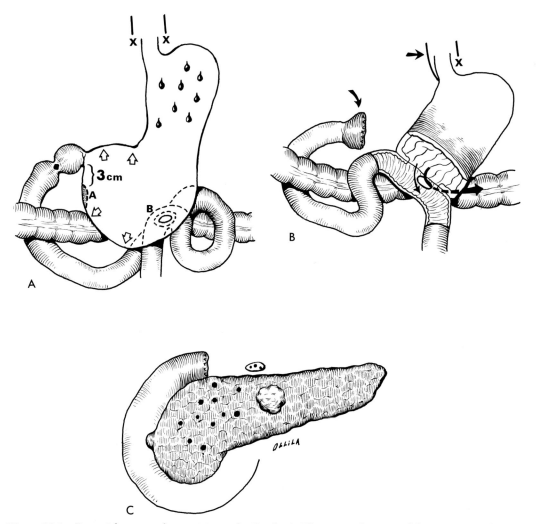

Figure 13-1. Potential causes of gastrojejunocolic fistula. *A,* The proper location of the gastrojejunal stoma after vagotomy should be within 3 to 4 cm of the pyloric outlet (A) instead of in location B. *B,* Failure to control the acid factor because of an overlooked posterior vagus nerve, inadequate gastric resection, or retained antrum are common factors leading to marginal ulceration and fistula formation. *C,* The gastrin-producing ulcerogenic tumor can occur anywhere in the pancreas or in the wall of the duodenum, with metastases to adjacent lymph nodes and the liver.

tric resection without vagotomy or a rim of retained antrum following a Billroth II anastomosis are additional causes of marginal ulceration and gastrojejunocolic fistula (Fig. 13-1*B*). Today the most likely causes of recurrent ulcer diathesis are inadequate control of the acid factor by the previous surgical procedure or extragastric causes such as chronic calcific pancreatitis or, more commonly, an ulcerogenic non-beta islet cell tumor of the pancreas or duodenum (Fig. 13-1*C*). In the presence of such a gastrin-

producing tumor, the acid factor will defy control by any means short of total gastrectomy.

HISTORY AND PREOPERATIVE EVALUATION

The diagnosis of gastrojejunocolic fistula associated with or without an ulcerogenic tumor of the pancreas should not be too difficult except that its rarity tends to assign it low priority in the differential diagnostic possibilities. The patients tend to be slight in build, or to have lost a considerable amount of weight, in addition to having a long and complicated ulcer history. They give a history of one-to-many surgical procedures, often carried out only a few days to a few months apart. They can demonstrate multiple surgical scars on the upper abdomen. Their discomfort is often persistent despite intensive antacid medication and, indeed, narcotics may have been required to control the ulcer pain. Their lack of confidence in additional operations to control the pain can be readily appreciated. Not uncommonly, after a bout of severe distress, they admit to a sudden relief of pain, followed by severe and persistent diarrhea. The pain pattern is altered and replaced in significance to the patient by the development of belching with a definite fecal odor, and the prompt passage of undigested food in the stool. The patient, as well as his close associates, is aware that something "serious" has developed. His appetite is impaired and, despite the best efforts, he tends to lose weight as the numerous stools filled with undigested food particles deplete caloric intake. The preoperative investigation and preparation of such patients must be energetic and carefully planned, particularly if an ulcerogenic tumor is suspected.

Since all these patients will have undergone one or many gastric operations, copies of the previous operative notes should be sought as the diagnostic evaluation is initiated. It is extremely important to know the details of all previous surgical procedures, including the gastric analyses performed before or after them, in searching for clues to both iatrogenic and extragastric causes of recurrent ulceration and subsequent gastrojejunocolic fistula formation.

Was the surgeon specific that both vagus nerves had been divided? Was there microscopic proof that both had been sectioned?

If vagotomy was not done, what about the extent of resection and the type of anastomosis?

Was there mention of considerable difficulty in freeing up the duodenum and closing the duodenal stump, suggesting a rim of retained antrum?

Did the surgeon pass his finger into the opened duodenum and palpate carefully for any irregularities which would suggest aberrant pancreas or one or more small islet cell tumors within the wall of the duodenum?

Was there evidence of an ulcer in the jejunum beyond the ligament of Treitz, or a past history of a free perforation of such an ulcer?

After mobilization of the head of the pancreas by a Kocher maneuver was there a thorough palpation of the pancreas from head to tail, including complete encirclement of the left half of the pancreas to permit palpation between the surgeon's thumb and index finger?

Was there a constant and copious output of gastric acid juice during the operation and/or the early postoperative period?

Did postoperative problems with gastric emptying lead to an enteroenterostomy as an emergency procedure?

Was there laboratory evidence of hyperparathyroidism and had the neck ever been explored because of hyperparathyroidism?

These are some of the many factors in the history which should be evaluated during the preoperative preparation of any patient suspected of having an ulcerogenic tumor of the pancreas and coexisting gastrojejunocolic fistula.

LABORATORY STUDIES

These malnourished patients require a thorough laboratory evaluation including, in particular, gastric analysis, blood volume determinations, prothrombin, and a complete profile of hepatic function. Repeated serum levels of calcium and phosphorus are important because of the high incidence of hyperparathyroidism in patients with ulcerogenic tumors. The possibility of hypo-kalemia associated with the diarrhea requires serial determinations of the serum potassium level.

The gastric analysis may provide significant evidence in favor of an ulcerogenic tumor if the ratio of basal to maximal acid concentration (BAC/MAC) equals or exceeds 0.6 after stimulation with histamine (0.04 mg./kg. histamine acid phosphate/body weight) (Ruppert et al., 1967). Often the analysis will not be valid, particularly if the colic fistula is large and allows significant alkaline neutralization of the stomach contents. The stomach should be washed out several times, the colon emptied by cathartics, and a clear liquid diet maintained for 24 hours, followed by placement of the nasogastric tube using fluoroscopic control. This is an ordeal for the patient, but all possible evidence for or against an ulcerogenic tumor should be sought since it may be necessary at operation to sacrifice the remaining stomach. The concentration of free hydrochloric acid in the one-hour fasting specimen may be almost as great as that following histamine stimulation, although the usual increased volume of gastric juice may be less than anticipated because of fluid losses through the fistula and associated diarrhea. A constant intravenous replacement with a balanced solution, such as lactated Ringer's, should be considered when 12-hour overnight gastric aspiration studies are performed. Cultures of the gastric juice and sensitivity studies should be made during the preoperative period of observation. Dye, such as brilliant blue (two 50 mg. tablets), can be given orally to provide an estimate of the rapid passage time of food from the stomach into the stool. Gross shading of the latter will be confirmation of the presence of undigested particles of food.

Adrenal hyperplasia or adenoma may often be associated with a non-beta islet cell tumor of the pancreas. Accordingly, serum cortisol and urinary 17-ketosteroid and 17-hydroxysteroid levels should be determined. If the clinical history and screening tests of parathyroid or adrenal function are suggestive, more subtle endocrine evaluation is warranted in addition to repetition of the usual screening tests.

ROENTGENOLOGIC STUDIES

Barium studies by mouth may or may not demonstrate the colic fistula, but they do pro-vide information as to the amount of stomach remaining and tend to identify the location and type of gastroenteric anastomosis. In the presence of an ulcerogenic tumor there should be evidence of marked thickening of the rugal folds and hypersecretion. It has been emphasized that the recurrent ulcerations are actually not marginal, but are more likely to be in the efferent loop along the mesenteric border (Christoforidis and Nelson, 1966). The barium enema will usually clearly define filling of the stomach and thereby confirm the presence of a gastrojejunocolic fistula. The colon may appear to be partially stenosed at the point of fistula formation.

Additional radiographic studies should include a chest film, cholecystogram, and intravenous pyelogram. Films should be made of those bones most likely to suggest evidence of hyperparathyroidism, such as the teeth, clavicles, and phalanges. A skull film may show the enlarged sella turcica of a pituitary tumor, which is occasionally associated with an ulcerogenic tumor of the pancreas. Technetium scans of the liver, selenomethionine scans of the pancreas and celiac arteriography may be helpful, when such facilities and experience are available, for determining the existence of a pancreatic mass or its metastases. However, micro-adenomatosis, small tumors in the wall of the duodenum, or metastases in the regional lymph nodes will require identification and definite histologic proof from surgical biopsies.

HORMONE ASSAYS

Hormonal assays, particularly immuno-assays, are valuable in the complete diagnostic workup of such patients because of the association of certain hormone-producing tumors with ulcer. Serum immunoassays may prove helpful in determining if there are increased levels of circulating parathormone (Egdahl et al., 1968). When an ulcerogenic tumor is suspected, but proof is lacking despite one or more previous operations, helpful supporting evidence may be sought with bioassays (Lai, 1964) to determine elevated levels of circulating gastrin (Moore et al., 1967). Precautions must be taken to avoid unauthorized eating by the patient in the middle of the night or the administration of drugs such as barbiturates, factors which can invalidate the assay. When the tracing is positive in two different laboratory animals, i.e., the patient's serum given intravenously results in a doubling of the baseline gastric secretion of the rat, the patient is definitely hypergastrinemic. A negative bioassay, however, does not exclude the existence of an ulcerogenic tumor since the size of the tumor as well as the probable cyclic release of gastrin makes the test quite variable (Wilson et al., 1968).

The radioiodine immunoassay developed by McGuigan is recognized as a more sensitive indicator for circulating levels of gastrin (McGuigan, 1968). In an earlier report serum gastrin levels in four patients with an ulcerogenic tumor of the pancreas exceeded by almost tenfold the mean serum gastrin level of 425 picograms/ml. in the control group (McGuigan and Trudeau, 1968). Determinations in a greater number of cases have reduced the lower limit of the ulcerogenic tumor range to 200 picograms/ml. Wider clinical application of the immunoassay should allow accurate diagnosis of the ulcerogenic tumor and more clearly define the necessity of total gastrectomy, particularly when all other evidence is in the gray or doubtful zone.

SURGICAL CONSIDERATIONS

GENERAL PRINCIPLES

The basic principles involved are to prepare adequately the patient for a safe operation, to close the fistula, and to control permanently the acid factor to prevent recurrence. It has been recognized since 1955 that when an incomplete, improper, or inadequate operation has failed to control the acid factor, removal of all acid-secreting surface by total gastrectomy is indicated if an ulcerogenic tumor is found (Zollinger and Ellison, 1955).

The management of gastrojejunocolic fistula has evolved from staged corrections to the present widely accepted subtotal gastrectomy and primary excision of the involved colon and jejunum as espoused by Marshall and Knud-Hansen (1957). The operative situation, however, may dictate selection of earlier techniques of staged repair. Wilkie (1934) recommended exclusion of the involved colonic loop as a first stage, to be followed by dismantling of the fistula. Lahey (1935) advocated primary

ileosigmoidostomy, then secondary en bloc resection of the fistula, the distal two-thirds of the stomach, and the right and transverse colon. Pfeiffer and Kent (1939) suggested proximal colostomy as the first stage, prior to dismantling the fistula three months later, during which time a good nutritional status has usually been re-established. The good response following colostomy was based on the concept that the severe gastritis and jejunitis caused by the constant irritation from the infected colonic contents was avoided. This procedure may be particularly appealing in a poor risk patient who is far below his ideal weight and lacks the operative findings of an ulcerogenic tumor of the pancreas.

The surgical management of a patient with an ulcerogenic tumor and associated gastrojejunocolic fistula is most complex. The patient has usually been sick for several years, has undergone one or numerous operations, and is thoroughly disenchanted with the prospect of facing yet another major operation. Although the procedure he now faces may be the first definitive one, it can also be the most radical and carries with it a calculated higher rate of morbidity and mortality.

The necessity of removing the entire remaining stomach in the presence of a gastrojejunocolic fistula is a procedure of such magnitude, because of the dense adhesions from previous, often multiple operations and potential contamination from the fistula, that the temptation to do a lesser, but ineffective, procedure is great. However, as long as any acid-secreting tissue remains, the tendency also remains for a fulminating ulcer diathesis with all the attendant complications. Recurrences tend to be prompt and are associated with high rates of morbidity and mortality, except in those few instances in which a solitary tumor has luckily been identified and removed. Although the ulcerogenic tumor always has the potential to produce ulceration and fistula formation as long as any acid-secreting surface remains, these tumors are too often unjustly accused, whereas the real cause is the failure of a previous incomplete or inadequate operation for duodenal ulcer.

Gastrojejunocolic fistula did occur in one patient in 25 of the more than 500 reported cases in the world literature tabulated by the Ulcerogenic Tumor Registry at The Ohio

State University. Sixteen of the patients with a gastrojejunocolic fistula were male and five were female. Pain was a significant factor in 14 patients, there was marked weight loss in nine, while hemorrhage and diarrhea were prominent in eight. The interval from the first operation to the development of the fistula was three weeks to 16 years; however, in seven cases it was one year or less. Twelve of these patients had two or more gastric resections. Five had recurrent fistulas after primary repair without the diagnosis of ulcerogenic tumor. Of the 14 patients who had an adequate operation for the ulcerogenic tumor, principally total gastrectomy, there were two postoperative deaths (hemorrhage and suture line leak) and two late deaths (insulin overdosage and esophageal stricture). All seven who did not have an adequate operation for ulcerogenic tumor died; four from the ravages of the syndrome, two from complications of surgery, and one from undescribed causes.

Ten days to two weeks should be considered minimal for preparation of the patient with a gastrojejunocolic fistula for operation. After gastric secretory and intestinal absorption studies are completed (viz., d(+) xylose and triolein uptake test), a nonabsorbable antibiotic, such as Sulfasuxidine (3 gm. four times a day) is started. A high calorie, low residue diet is begun, even though efforts to restore the patient's poor nutritional status before surgery are usually futile. However, if the patient tends to improve and the daily weight curve shows a persistent upward trend, surgery should be delayed, particularly in the severely malnourished patient. Fat-soluble vitamins should be given in high dosages because of incomplete absorption caused by the fistula. The blood volume should be measured and improved slowly with transfusions of whole blood. On the night before and the morning of surgery, the stomach should be irrigated with 1 per cent neomycin solution given through the nasogastric tube. The colon is emptied by saline enemas. Use of systemic, broad-spectrum antibiotics should be considered if there is a fistula.

Finally, a conference should be held with the patient and his family to ensure a thorough understanding and consent to the operative plan, which may include colostomy, with several surgical procedures, as well as total removal of the stomach, a portion of the pancreas, and possibly the spleen. The need to remove the entire stomach if an ulcerogenic tumor of the pancreas is found should be fully explained and the patient adequately reassured regarding his ability to eat and survive after the operation. The possibility of a colostomy, followed in several months by closure of the fistula and then closure of the colostomy, should be fully explained. This informed consent contributes significantly to better cooperation in the postoperative period and prepares all concerned for any complications which might ensue.

OPERATIVE TECHNIQUE

The exact operation can be determined only by the operative findings at the time of surgery, although the preoperative evaluation should provide strong guidelines for the surgeon. When a satisfactory cause for the persistent gastric hypersecretion is found, other than an ulcerogenic tumor, the colic fistula can be closed and the remaining stomach retained. However, the finding of an overlooked vagus nerve as well as a retained antrum does not rule out the possibility of an ulcerogenic tumor. Constant monitoring of the gastric juice output from the nasogastric tube is one means of determining the effects of the various procedures on acid control as they are carried out.

The severe nutritional and metabolic derangements, as well as the extent of the adhesions and inflammation which often accompany a gastrojejunocolic fistula, may dictate that a staged procedure be performed, unless an ulcerogenic tumor of the pancreas is found.

The surgeon must plan the operative approach in advance, basing it on what the primary diagnosis is thought to be. Having reviewed all the previous operative notes the surgeon will hopefully be able to decide when a staged procedure is necessary before committing the patient to a one-stage radical operation which includes total gastrectomy. In most instances the weight of evidence will suggest that the cause of the fistula is not an ulcerogenic tumor, but rather inadequate control of the acid factor by the previous operation. Exceptions are common, however, and patients who have undergone several gastric operations have an increased likelihood of an ulcerogenic tumor being present

The plan, therefore, depends on whether the patient has had vagotomy, gastric resection and/or gastrojejunostomy. Accordingly, the surgeon may suspect the failure to have resulted from inadequate gastric resection, retained vagus nerve following vagotomy, or gastroenterostomy placed too far to the left, allowing antral distention (Fig. 13-1). The fistula will often be surrounded by an intense inflammatory reaction, and dismantling it early during the procedure can result in substantial contamination. When iatrogenic causes of marginal ulceration are eliminated by thorough preoperative and operative investigation, staged procedures on the fistula can be considered, particularly in the patient with severe nutritional deficiencies or other systemic diseases.

Exploration of Duodenum and Head of Pancreas

If the previous operation was a vagotomy and resection with a Billroth II type of reconstruction, the first step should be to search for a retained antrum and, secondly, to inspect the esophageal hiatus for a retained vagal trunk. Finally, as much of the pancreas as possible should be laboriously explored for evidence of an ulcerogenic tumor. Usually the duodenal stump and head of the pancreas are first visualized and carefully explored. The presence of retained antrum should be suspected if the duodenal stump appears unduly elongated; it may include only a "nubbin" of antral mucosa. If the stump appears at all suspicious, it may be opened and a thorough search made for visual evidence of retained antral mucosa. Since intraluminal adenomata may occur in the wall of the duodenum, their suspected presence may be verified by exploring the duodenal lumen through the above-mentioned opening with the index finger. Ordinarily this is not done until the head of the pancreas has been mobilized as completely as possible by a Kocher maneuver. Further mobilization of the first portion of the duodenum can be affected if the peritoneum forming the lower border of the foramen of Winslow is divided. The middle colic vessels should be identified and gently mobilized medially in order to facilitate the mobilization of as much of the second and third portions of the duodenum as possible. The anterior surface of the head of the pancreas is cleared of omentum to permit visual inspection and more accurate palpation for a tumor mass in the head of the pancreas between the thumb and index finger of the surgeon.

Exposure of Lower Esophagus

Exploration of the esophagogastric junction to evaluate the completeness of vagotomy is especially important if it has not been possible to confirm positively the presence of an ulcerogenic tumor, retained antrum, or any obvious and likely cause for continuation of the gastric hypersecretion. Since many of these patients have had previous vagotomy, there tend to be very dense adhesions between the superior surface of the left lobe of the liver and the overlying diaphragm. Sharp dissection is required to avoid tearing the capsule of the liver and consequent troublesome bleeding. The undersurface of the left lobe of the liver is also very likely to be intimately attached to the underlying stomach in the region of the esophagogastric junction.

It is important that the left lobe of the liver be freed up and mobilized toward the midline to ensure adequate exposure of the esophagogastric junction. As the mobilized left lobe is brought toward the midline, it is covered with a moist gauze pad which is held in position with a large S-retractor. The gastrohepatic ligament is then divided, and the thickened uppermost portion, which contains a branch of the inferior phrenic artery, is clamped and ligated. This ensures a more direct approach to and exposure of the region posterior to the esophagus where the more commonly overlooked right vagus nerve is located. If the spleen is drawn into the general area of the fundus of the stomach by multiple adhesions, the short gastric vessels should be divided in the region of the fundus to facilitate mobilization of the esophagus without tearing of the splenic capsule. The sutures on the gastric side should be anchored to the wall of the stomach with transfixing sutures of 00 silk.

A secondary vagotomy is not so easy as the initial operation; for this reason, the peritoneum is carefully incised up over the esophagus after identification of its location by palpation of the underlying nasogastric tube. Since the usual cleavage planes tend to be obliterated by scar tissue attachments, less fraying of the muscular wall of the esophagus will result if blunt dissection is carried from above downward rather than using the usual blind, left-to-right finger dissection. It is important to maintain the usual integrity of the muscular wall of the esophagus for the subsequent anastomosis when total gastrectomy is necessary.

The tendency to displace the right or posterior vagus nerve posteriorly during the process of blind finger dissection to free up the esophagus no doubt accounts for the fact that this large nerve can be overlooked more than once, whereas the smaller filaments over the wall of the esophagus are very meticulously divided. The anterior vagus nerve is usually found superficially embedded in the anterior wall of the esophagus and is less commonly overlooked. After the nerve has been sectioned, the anesthesiologist may note a decrease in the volume of gastric acid output through the nasogastric tube.

After an unsuccessful search for or correction of iatrogenic causes of gastric hypersecretion, the ulcerogenic tumor is strongly implicated, especially if the patient has had two or more gastric operations. The presence of a gastrojejunocolic fistula limits the usual mobility of the stomach, jejunum, pancreas, and transverse colon; and the surgeon may have to rely heavily on palpation because the usual direct inspection of the body of the pancreas is likely to be obscured. Although division of the fistula would improve the exposure, the risk of contamination is high and the opportunity to perform a staged procedure is lost.

Search of Pancreas for Ulcerogenic Tumor

Exposure of the body and tail of the pancreas is particularly difficult in the presence of extensive inflammatory reaction about a retrocolic gastrojejunal anastomosis. Often only the head and left portion of the body and tail of the pancreas can be exposed for a thorough search for an ulcerogenic tumor. Usually the easiest approach into the lesser sac to visualize the left half of the pancreas is facilitated by freeing the omentum from the underlying left half of the transverse colon over to and including the splenic flexure. This is made easier by gentle downward traction on the left transverse colon as the omentum is retracted upward. The gastrocolic omentum is divided along the superior margin of the colon, permitting the omentum to be gently separated from the colon with entry into the lesser sac. The splenocolic ligament is divided to ensure clear visualization and examination of the region of the tail of the pancreas. As many adhesions as possible between the posterior wall of the stomach and capsule of the pancreas are divided to permit as wide and unobstructed view of the pancreas as possible without opening into the fistula. If room permits, the peritoneum along the inferior margin of the pancreas is incised, carefully avoiding the inferior mesenteric vein. The peritoneum along the superior surface of the pancreas is incised in a similar manner. It is not necessary to mobilize the spleen and, in fact, this may be hazardous in the presence of adhesions from previous operations. The surgeon may then completely lift the left half of the body and tail of the pancreas from the posterior parietes, using blunt dissection with his index finger, in order to carefully palpate for evidence of a small tumor mass. This site may be safely used later in the operation for biopsy of the inferior margin of the pancreas if no gross evidence of tumor is found elsewhere.

Biopsy of Lymph Nodes and Pancreas

When thorough exploration fails to uncover any evidence to support the diagnosis of ulcerogenic tumor, the surgeon must resort to biopsy of the peripancreatic lymph nodes, especially along the superior border of the pancreas. Occasionally the only evidence for ulcerogenic tumor is found in these normal-appearing lymph nodes. The pathologist should be alerted in advance of the operation that many frozen section examinations may be needed for determining the diagnosis of an ulcerogenic tumor or metastases in the lymph nodes. If these maneuvers fail, particularly in the presence of strong clinical and laboratory evidence favoring an ulcerogenic tumor of the pancreas, it is advisable to proceed with a generous biopsy of the inferior margin of the tail of the pancreas with frozen section examination in a search for microadenomatosis. However, frozen section studies of the pancreas are most challenging to interpret adequately, and gross inspection for evidence of small adenomata should not be overlooked.

In the presence of massive gastric hypersecretion, the continuous monitoring of gastric drainage during the operation can often determine the effect on acid production of various additional procedures, short of total gastrectomy. An abrupt decrease after one of these lesser procedures can confirm the adequacy of the approach. If an ulcerogenic tumor is present, however, the smallest amount of acid-secreting surface continues to produce acid, and recurrence of the ulcer diathesis tends to take place in a distressingly short period of time.

Principles of Surgical Treatment of Gastrojejunocolic Fistulas

There are two current concepts in the surgical treatment of gastrojejunocolic fistula. There is a growing tendency to perform a one-stage closure of the gastrojejunocolic fistula, providing the cause for the uncontrolled acid factor has been found and corrected. Secondly, when an ulcerogenic tumor is verified, a total gastrectomy should be done even in the presence of the gastrojejunocolic fistula. In the case of a very poor risk patient, particularly one with a history of repeated surgical procedures leading to dense adhesions in the upper abdomen which could be the source of considerable blood loss during exploration, it may be judicious to establish a diverting colostomy, using the right transverse or ascending colon.

The choice of operation, as emphasized by Maingot (1969), depends upon the patient's age and general condition, the extent of inflammatory reaction, and the nature of the primary operation. Finally, the type and extent of the operation will depend upon how well the surgeon believes he has identified the cause of the persistent acid factor and how effectively he has controlled it by completing the vagotomy, removing the antrum, etc. If an ulcerogenic tumor is found, he is committed to total gastrectomy.

When the fistula occurs in the presence of a previous gastrojejunostomy, with or without vagotomy, it may be adequate to complete the vagotomy, close the gastrojejunal anastomosis (which may have been placed too far to the left), perform pyloroplasty, and restore normal gastrointestinal continuity by closing the openings in the colon and jejunum. The scarred edges of the colonic fistula should be excised and the opening closed in two layers transversely to the long axis of the colon. This prevents stenosis of the colon at the point of closure.

It may be judicious to provide an additional safety valve in the form of a tube cecostomy. If the opening in the colon is quite large, it may be better judgment to to carry out a sleeve resection and perform direct end-to-end anastomosis. The same principle applies to repair of the remaining opening in the jejunum. A rather long jejunal opening may be closed by the Finney method or by two-layer closure at right angles to the long axis of the jejunum. A temporary gastrostomy should be added to this procedure, along with drainage of the left upper quadrant. Providing the acid factor has been adequately controlled, the malnourished patient should have a better chance for improved nutrition if normal gastrointestinal continuity has been restored. Care must be taken when the fistula is excised to minimize contamination through the liberal use of walling-off pads and noncrushing clamps on the stomach, jejunum, and colon.

Because of the seriousness of a gastrojejunocolic fistula, it is likely that the majority of surgeons would prefer to control both the cephalic and gastric phases of gastric secretion by ensuring the completeness of vagotomy and complete antrectomy. Under these circumstances a Billroth I reconstruction may be possible if the gastrosplenic vessels are ligated and the remaining gastric pouch is easily mobilized to the right. Some prefer to divide the splenorenal ligament and mobilize the spleen medially to remove tension from the suture line. Similar principles are involved when the patient has had a previous Billroth II type of anastomosis. The technical difficulties are greater when the original anastomosis was retrocolic rather than antecolic and a small gastric pouch remains. Once again, the colic fistula should not be disturbed until the completeness of vagotomy and the absence of either a retained antrum or an ulcerogenic tumor have been ascertained insofar as possible.

If an ulcerogenic tumor is found and its presence verified histologically, the decision to remove the tumor, the stomach, or both must be made. Local excision has been followed by dramatic recovery in a few isolated instances (Oberhelman, 1964; Rawson, 1960; Wolff, 1968), but this limited treatment should be considered only in special circumstances. The tumor must be benign, solitary, and located in a position which allows easy, complete removal. The highest frequency of successful local excisions has been in those patients with either solitary tumors in the duodenal wall or larger tumors of the pancreas with no evidence of adenomatosis or metastases. When less than total gastrectomy is performed, the incidence of recurrent ulceration is 55 per cent. When a gastrojejunocolic fistula *and* a tumor are present, total gastrectomy is the recommended procedure.

Surgical Technique

The operative maneuvers to be described are designed so that contamination of the operative field from the gastrojejunocolic fistula is held to a minimum. Accordingly, the fistula should not be opened until all dissection in the immediate subdiaphragmatic region is completed. The esophagogastric junction is exposed as described for vagotomy. Certain anatomic features differentiate surgical procedures on the esophagus from the remainder of the gastrointestinal tract. First, the esophagus has no serosa, and the muscular layers tend to tear when repaired and sutured. Secondly, the esophagus tends to retract into the mediastinum when divided from the stomach, even though it appears to extend well into the abdomen. The surgeon should not hesitate to extend the abdominal incision by removing the xiphoid process, splitting the sternum, or incising the appropriate costal cartilage. The wall of the esophagus can be anchored to the diaphragmatic crus to prevent rotation

and upward retraction (Fig. 13-2A). The esophageal wall can be given further substance by placing a series of interrupted, encircling, horizontal sutures of 0000 silk. Such fixation prevents fraying of the muscles and tends to give a firm cuff for the anastomosis. These sutures have not resulted in a compromised blood supply of the anastomosis (Fig. 13-2B). Medial and lateral angle sutures maintain proper orientation and prevent rotation of the esophagus as the anastomosis is carried out.

At this point the surgeon must isolate the gastrojejunocolic fistula in a manner to prevent major contamination, particularly in the subdiaphragmatic areas, and to allow for the simplest possible closure of the fistula into the colon. The gastric pouch should be completely freed of its blood supply before opening into the fistulous communication. The left gastric artery is doubly clamped and ligated, followed by division and ligation of the remaining gastrosplenic vessels. The decision must be made as to whether to remove the spleen. Splenectomy is indicated if there is troublesome bleeding from tears of its capsule. In the presence of tumor, or if there is a need for extensive biopsy of the tail of the pancreas, the splenic artery is doubly ligated at a readily accessible point along the superior margin of the pancreas. The splenorenal ligament is divided and the spleen mobilized into the wound to permit the double clamping and ligation of the splenic pedicle.

Since closure of the colonic opening is

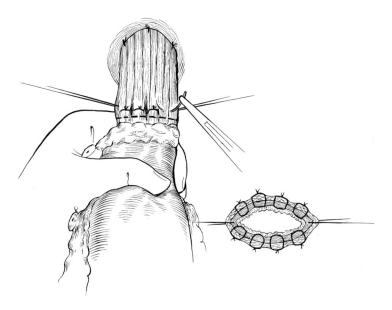

Figure 13-2. The esophagus is fixed to the crus of the diaphragm, and the esophageal wall is encircled by a series of interrupted silk sutures.

preferably delayed until completion of the esophagojejunal anastomosis, noncrushing intestinal clamps of the Scudder or a similar type are so placed as to seal off the communication between the stomach and the gastrojejunal anastomosis. The stomach is divided from the esophagus to permit removal of the remaining gastric pouch and freeing up of the jejunocolic openings without gross contamination from the colon. An attempt is made to free up as much of the jejunum as possible between the ligament of Treitz and the gastrojejunal anastomosis. When a sufficient length of jejunum is present, the noncrushing clamps are applied to the ascending as well as the descending jejunal limbs going to and from the fistulous area. The segment of jejunum involved in the fistula is divided, thereby further isolating and sealing off the colonic fistula from the adjacent remnants of gastric and jejunal walls.

Esophago-jejunal Anastomosis

After ligation of the mesenteric vessels going to the resected portion of the gastrojejunal anastomosis, the distal jejunum is prepared for the *Roux-en-Y* anastomosis to the esophagus, while the proximal end will be anastomosed to the ascending arm of the jejunum to restore gastrointestinal continuity. The distal jejunum is held outside the abdominal cavity and the arcades of blood vessels clearly identified by transillumination to facilitate preparation of the distal jejunum for anastomosis to the esophagus. To minimize the number of suture lines it is usually preferable to resect the involved, previous anastomosis unless the proximal segment is very close to the ligament of Treitz. If this is the situation, it may be necessary to trim away the gastric wall from the gastrojejunal anastomosis and the colonic fistula and close this sizable opening in the jejunum transversely to its long axis.

Every effort should be made to free up enough jejunum between the ligament of Treitz and the point of division of the jejunum so it can be safely anastomosed to the ascending jejunal arm brought up to the esophagus. Two or more arcades of vessels are divided, and the intervening devascularized segment that contains the gastrojejunal anastomosis is excised. An anchoring suture should be placed at the origin of the mesenteric incision to prevent retrograde tearing by traction of the peritoneum and trouble-

some bleeding. The limb is then passed through an opening made in the mesocolon to the left of the middle colic vessels. Care must be taken to avoid angulating or twisting the mesentery of the jejunum as it is pulled through. The jejunum is anchored to the defect in the mesocolon and the free margin of the jejunal mesentery is fixed with superficially placed sutures to the posterior parietes. The closed end of the jejunum usually faces the patient's left side before suturing is begun, and a final check is made to be certain that no tension is present and that active pulsations are present in the mesentery.

Care should be taken to avoid undue traction on the mobilized limb of the jejunum since this may result in tearing of the mesentery in its midportion, with devitalization of the proximal portion of the jejunum which is to be attached to the diaphragm. A row of 00 silk sutures fixes the end of the jejunum to the diaphragm on either side of the esophagus, as well as directly behind it. This suture line is designed to remove all tension from the subsequent esophagojejunal anastomosis (Fig. 13-3). The sutures must be placed more to the backside of the jejunum since there is a tendency to use the remaining jejunal

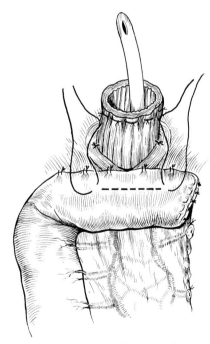

Figure 13-3. The esophagojejunal anastomosis consists of three layers anteriorly and three layers posteriorly to provide a firm anastomosis without tension on the suture line.

surface in the subsequent layers of closure. Horizontal mattress sutures are used in the posterior row, after which a small opening is made in the adjacent bowel wall. The opening in the jejunum is often made too large, rendering an accurate mucosal anastomosis difficult. When the posterior mucosal row is completed, the Levin tube is directed down into the jejunum. The presence of the tube in the lumen aids in the placement of the interrupted Connell sutures closing the anterior mucosal layer. The second layer is then placed and, when the jejunum is anchored to the diaphragm anteriorly, a three-layer closure has been effected. After completion of the anastomosis, the color of the jejunal limb should be re-evaluated. The peritoneal flap originally elevated from the lower end of the esophagus may now be used to cover the anastomosis.

Attention is now directed to the proximal jejunum from the region of the ligament of Treitz. It is anastomosed at an appropriate point to the jejunal limb with two layers of 0000 silk, and the several openings in the mesentery are closed to prevent subsequent internal herniation.

Closure of Colic Fistula

The final steps of the procedure are directed to closure of the colic fistula. The fibrotic margins of the fistula should be excised until flexible and normal-appearing colonic wall is available around the entire circumference. In the presence of severe stenosis it may be necessary to perform a sleeve resection of the involved segment with end-to-end anastomosis. Usually, however, it is possible to close the fistulous openings in the colon at right angles to its long axis. Traction sutures are placed in the seromuscular coat, both above and below the fistulous communications, to provide traction as the mucosal layer is closed with a row of interrupted Connell sutures of 0000 silk. A secondary reinforcing layer of interrupted mattress sutures of 00 silk is inserted. The patency of the anastomosis is tested between the surgeon's thumb and index finger. A tube cecostomy, using an 18 French Foley or mushroom catheter, can be carried out to provide a safety valve for the anastomosis. Because of the general condition of these patients it is advisable to provide liberal drainage, particularly of the left upper quadrant. Several large, rubber tissue drains

can be drawn out through a stab wound in the left upper quadrant, or Chaffin drainage can be instituted. However, the end of the drainage should not be in direct proximity to the esophagojejunal anastomosis. Before closure of the wound the adequacy of the blood supply to all portions of the mobilized jejunum should be verified and any abnormal openings about the mesentery double checked and closed with interrupted sutures. The closure of the wound should probably be supported with retention sutures.

POSTOPERATIVE MANAGEMENT

In the immediate postoperative period, constant drainage is maintained through the nasojejunal tube, which has been passed through and beyond the anastomosis. Alimentation is provided with intravenous fluids and vitamin supplements, although the patient is allowed sips of water by mouth for comfort. Because the pancreas may have been extensively mobilized, the development of postoperative pancreatitis, as indicated by increased pulse rate and backache, should be anticipated and, if present, treated appropriately with colloids, antibiotics, and blood transfusions.

Ambulation is begun on the first postoperative day, and a graded increase in physical activity is encouraged. The return of peristalsis may be hastened by the instillation of 30 ml. of mineral oil at regular intervals through the jejunal tube. Lactated Ringer's solution or water can be given through the nasojejunal tube on the first day. After the return of peristalsis, caloric intake can be maintained with frequent, small tube feedings.

The presence of fever, left upper quadrant pain, and leukocytosis should alert the clinician to the possibility of a subphrenic abscess. The location will usually be on the left side and can be confirmed by the usual roentgenologic studies.

The initial feedings should be small and low in carbohydrate and fat content to avoid dumping and diarrhea. These patients will have some difficulty adjusting to the diet and will require constant attention and many changes in regimen. The diet may be gradually increased to include soft, solid foods. The patient and his family, the surgeon, and the dietitian should meet as often as necessary prior to discharge to discuss and resolve any problems of diet. Supplemental vitamin B_{12} (500 micrograms/month) will be necessary, and oral iron may be required.

The patient should be admitted to the hospital at intervals of three, six, and 12 months postoperatively for evaluation. The esophagojejunal suture line may require dilatation, and the blood volume may need to be restored. More important, investigation of the patient's dietary habits, his nutritional status, and the presence of dumping or diarrhea can be ascertained. In most instances, within 12 months after total gastrectomy the majority of patients are able to eat almost all foods, including desserts; and, indeed, these patients enjoy a far better nutritional status than others who have undergone total gastrectomy for carcinoma. During these hospitalizations the patient as well as members of his family who come to visit him can be screened for polyglandular adenomatosis.

The following case report illustrates the management of co-existing tumor of the pancreas and postresectional gastrojejunocolic fistula by total gastrectomy and primary repair of the fistula as one operation.

CASE REPORT

F. D., a 33 year old white man, was admitted with the diagnosis of probable ulcerogenic tumor of the pancreas.

He was considered to be in good health until 1964, when he began to have intermittent nausea, vomiting, and vague epigastric pain. At that time he was drinking 10 cups of coffee and smoking two packs of cigarettes daily. Gastroduodenal examination showed an active duodenal ulcer (Fig. 13-4A). With the use of a bland diet and antacids, and the patient's abstinence from coffee and cigarettes, the ulcer healed promptly and his symptoms subsided. During the next two years the ulcer recurred several time, but strict dietary precautions and antacids always resulted in prompt healing.

In 1966 the recurrent pain and ulceration were accompanied by melena. The patient was hospitalized, and active ulceration was again found. Surgery was advised, but the patient refused and was discharged from the hospital. The pain became more frequent during the next year and required more frequent antacid therapy for control.

The melena recurred in the spring of 1967, and the patient was again hospitalized. The pain had been almost disabling for several months. Surgical exploration was undertaken, and a posterior duodenal ulcer penetrating into the pancreas was found. Vagotomy, gastric resection, and Billroth II antecolic gastrojejunostomy were performed (Fig. 13-4B). His postoperative course was uneventful and he was discharged from the hospital on the 12th postoperative day. Several days later, he began to vomit and to have early fullness with

meals and diarrhea. He passed some bright red blood per rectum and was readmitted to the hospital with a hemoglobin of 12.2 gm. per cent. The patient was treated symptomatically, but all attempts at oral feeding failed. Upper gastrointestinal examination showed gastric stasis and a stenotic gastrojejunal anastomosis. Nine days after admission, he vomited copious amounts of coffee-ground material and his hematocrit fell precipitously.

Emergency operation was performed, with the finding of a large hematoma in the posterior suture line of the gastrojejunostomy, but no definite marginal ulceration could be identified. A tremendous inflammatory reaction in the mesocolon made adequate exploration impossible. The anastomosis was taken down, an additional inch of stomach resected to include the old suture line, and a new gastrojejunostomy constructed (Fig. 13-4C). The tail of the pancreas was normal to palpation, although thorough exploration was not considered to be indicated at this time.

Postoperatively the patient rebled massively four times in the next eight days in spite of intensive antacid therapy; he received more than 50 units of blood replacement during this time. A repeat gastroduodenal examination demonstrated another ulcer, either gastric or marginal, but he progressed satisfactorily and experienced no further bleeding. An augmented histamine gastric analysis produced a basal to maximal acid *output* ratio of 0.65 (BAO/MAO). A 12-hour overnight gastric analysis contained 1000 ml. of gastric juice with a total of 9 mEq. HCl despite vagotomy and antrectomy. He had lost 30 pounds of weight in the two months preceding his discharge from the hospital.

For the next year he had daily epigastric pain and interscapular pain which was relieved for brief periods by milk and antacids. He gradually restricted his diet to Pablum, baby foods, one to two quarts of milk and a half gallon of ice cream per day. It became more difficult for him to work each month, and he obviously was worsening.

In July, 1968, the patient noted the rather sudden disappearance of the epigastric and high back pain and then he no longer required the large quantities of milk for comfort. However, he recognized a distinctly different set of symptoms which included intermittent crampy abdominal pain, increased flatulence with malodorous breath, diarrhea, and headaches. He began to resume a more normal diet and occasionally noted undigested food, such as beans and peas, in the stool. He obtained relief from the flatulence by self-induced vomiting, and the character of the vomitus was fecal. The diarrhea occurred several times a week, nine to ten times daily, and the stools were bulky, yellow, foul-smelling, and floating. His weight continued to fall, and although he now had relief from pain for the first time in three years, the flatulence and diarrhea forced him to stop working.

After two months of these symptoms, he was referred into our hospital with the diagnosis of ulcerogenic tumor of the pancreas (Fig. 13-4D). His past history included a concussion at age 10 years and four grand mal seizures during the past eight years. He was taking Dilantin 100 mg. three times a day for this disorder. He had passed a renal stone in 1959. Two siblings had a history of renal stones and perforated ulcer.

On physical examination he appeared thin and apprehensive. The blood pressure measured 170/70 mm. Hg, the pulse 84/minute; he was 63 inches tall and weighed 118 pounds. His breath had a fecal odor, and there was a large midline ventral hernia and slight epigastric tenderness.

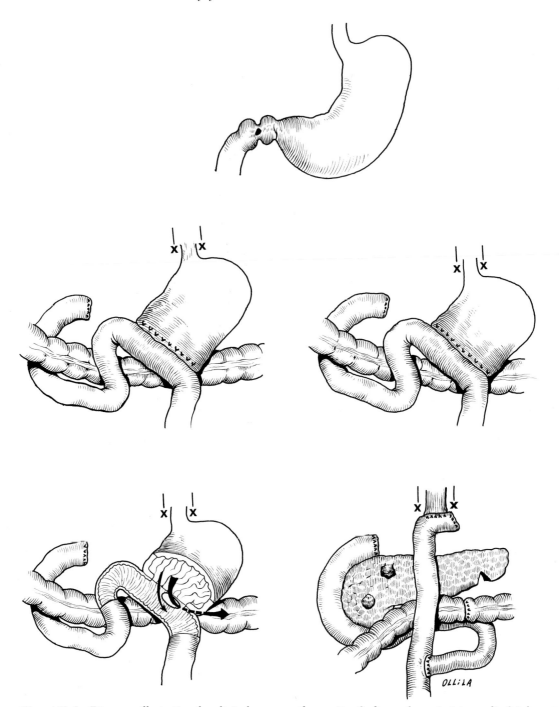

Figure 13-4. Diagrams illustrating the clinical course and operative findings of a gastrojejunocolic fistula associated with ulcerogenic tumors of the pancreas.

An extensive laboratory investigation was undertaken to determine the presence of any associated endocrinopathies. All studies of thyroid, parathyroid, adrenal, and pancreatic functions were normal. The stool guaiac was always positive for occult blood. The basal acid concentration (BAC) was 109 mEq./L., and after stimulation with histamine (histamine acid phosphate, 0.04 mg./kg. body weight), his maximal acid concentration (MAC)

was only 93.5 mEq./L. The BAC/MAC ratio of 1:2 was far into the range considered diagnostic of an ulcerogenic tumor despite some neutralization of all gastric analyses with stool content (Ruppert et al., 1967). A Hollander test was positive.

Gastroduodenal examination showed a normal afferent loop with a 4 cm. marginal ulceration in the proximal efferent limb. There was no evidence of gastrojejunocolic fistula, and the loops of small bowel were moderately dilated, suggesting gastric hypersecretion. On roentgenologic examination of the colon, the barium went from the midportion of the transverse colon into the stomach. The proximal colon could not be filled in retrograde fashion. There was an apparent stenosis of the transverse colon at the site of the fistula. Small bowel absorption studies could not be evaluated on a quantitative basis because of the gastrojejunocolic fistula. Radioisotope scans of the pancreas (selenomethionine-75) and liver (technetium-99m) were both normal.

In preparation for surgery the patient was started on Sulfasuxidine (3 gm. orally, four times a day, for five days), neomycin (1 gm./hr. for four hours, then 1 gm. with meals the day before operation), Gelusil, and multivitamins. His measured blood volume, depleted because of weight loss and poor nutrition, was replaced with 2000 ml. of whole blood over a six-day period. He consumed between 3000 and 4000 calories of a low residue diet and gained 6.6 pounds in the week prior to operation. Several conferences were held with him and his wife to explain the ulcerogenic tumor syndrome, the nature and possibility of a proximal colostomy, and the necessity of total gastrectomy and primary resection of the fistula if an ulcerogenic tumor were found. On the night before and the morning of surgery his stomach was irrigated with 1 per cent neomycin and his lower colon was emptied with a Fleet enema.

On the 12th hospital day surgical exploration was performed. The abdominal wall was reopened through the previous midline incision, which was extended well below the umbilicus. The gastrojejunocolic fistula was identified as a huge inflammatory mass between the gastric remnant and the transverse colon. The duodenal stump was first identified; no retained antrum could be demonstrated. With the utilization of a generous Kocher maneuver, the head of the pancreas was palpated anteriorly and posteriorly between the thumb and index finger. Two small pedunculated tumors 1 to 2 cm. in size were found—one attached to the head of the pancreas and the other near the closed end of the duodenal stump and near the inner border of the second portion of the duodenum. An adjacent lymph node was also removed for frozen section examination. Frozen section confirmed the diagnosis of ulcerogenic tumor of the pancreas with metastases to the lymph nodes. There were no tumor implants in the liver that could be seen or palpated. The duodenum was next opened; intraluminal exploration of the C-loop with the index finger was negative for aberrant pancreas or tumor nodules in the duodenal wall.

With the microscopic proof of ulcerogenic tumor, the decision to remove all the acid-secreting surface by total gastrectomy was mandatory. To minimize contamination of the lower mediastinum and subdiaphragmatic area, the esophageal hiatus was thoroughly dissected; no retained vagi could be found. Accordingly, the esophagus was divided and the gastric remnant mobilized inferiorly. The gastric remnant and gastrojejunostomy were removed and gastrointestinal continuity was re-established with a *Roux-en-Y* end-to-side esophagojejunostomy (Fig. 13-4E), with a gastric tube placed well beyond the site of the esophagojejunal anastomosis.

The gastrojejunocolic fistula had been isolated between noncrushing clamps to avoid contamination, and a jejunal ulcer was tailored away from the colon. The proximal colon, although appearing stenotic on x-ray, was adequate; after trimming the margin of the defect, a transverse closure was performed, avoiding resection but without narrowing the lumen.

The spleen was densely adherent in the left upper quadrant and therefore was not removed. The ventral hernia was repaired in a vest-over-pants fashion by wide relaxing incision in the rectus sheath. The subhepatic space was drained.

Nasogastric administration of water was begun on the first postoperative day, and by the fourth day the patient was receiving lactated Ringer's solution with potassium chloride and vitamins and a six-feeding, low glucose, and low roughage diet orally. The foods included were dilute fruit juice, poached eggs, and soft meats.

Within a week of operation the patient began to have a spiking daily fever, pain in the left upper quadrant and over the left shoulder. X-ray examinations confirmed the presence of an air-fluid level in the left upper quadrant, consistent with a subphrenic abscess. Because the position of the abscess seemed to be more anteriorly located, a subcostal approach was chosen for incision and drainage on the 13th postoperative day. Despite precautions for keeping the incision extraperitoneal, the colon was inadvertently entered at the time of draining the subphrenic abscess, which was actually located just superior to the transverse colon. The purulent and fecal drainage continued for several days, but within a week both had ceased. By this time the patient had resumed a regular diet and was improving rapidly.

At the time of discharge, 34 days after operation, he was eating 2500 to 3000 calories per day of a standard hospital diet in small feedings. He had no symptoms of dumping and no diarrhea, the headaches had disappeared, and he had gained 5½ pounds of weight.

Six months after operation, he has gained 40 pounds, has returned to full-time employment as a computer operator, and is having no intestinal problems.

SUMMARY

The serious complication of gastrojejunocolic fistula is relatively uncommon and it is difficult to establish its true incidence. This diagnosis usually implies failure of a previous surgical procedure to control the acid factor or the existence of an ulcerogenic tumor of the pancreas. If surgical causes (namely, retained vagus, retained antrum, improperly placed gastroenterostomy, or inadequate gastric resection) are excluded and many surgical procedures have already been performed, this is strong indication of the presence of an ulcerogenic tumor of the pancreas.

Confirmatory evidence is sought, principally with gastrin immunoassay or bioassay, histamine-stimulated or unstimulated gastric secretory collections, and barium study characteristics, as well as a historical review of all previous surgical procedures.

The patient should be prepared for a one-stage procedure which may well include total gastrectomy, or a multistaged procedure beginning with colostomy. There is a trend today to a one-stage approach for controlling the acid factor and closing the fistula. When an ulcerogenic tumor is found, a one-stage procedure including total gastrectomy to ensure complete control of the acid factor, is mandatory. The colonic fistula is isolated by noncrushing clamps until all other anastomoses have been completed in order to keep contamination at a minimum.

Careful preoperative planning, attention to operative detail, and enlightened postoperative dietary supervision should give a successful result in cases of postresectional gastrojejunocolic fistula with or without ulcerogenic tumor of the pancreas.

REFERENCES

Christoforidis, A. J., and Nelson, S. W.: Radiological manifestations of ulcerogenic tumors of the pancreas. The Zollinger-Ellison syndrome. JAMA, *198:* 511, 1966.

Condon, J. R., and Tanner, N. C.: Retrospective review of 208 proved cases of anastomotic ulcer. Gut, *9:*438, 1968.

Egdahl, R. H., Canterbury, J. M., and Reiss, E.: Measurement of circulating parathyroid hormone concentration before and after parathyroid surgery for adenoma or hyperplasia. Ann. Surg., *198:*714, 1968.

Lahey, F. H., and Swinton, N. W.: Gastrojejunal ulcer and gastrojejunocolic fistula. Surg. Gynec. Obstet., *61:*599, 1935.

Lai, K. S.: Studies on gastrin. Gut, *5:*327, 1964.

McGuigan, J. E.: Immunochemical studies with synthetic human gastrin. Gastroenterology, *54:*1005, 1968.

McGuigan, J. E., and Trudeau, W. L.: Immunochemical measurements of elevated levels of gastrin in serum of patients with pancreatic tumors of the Zollinger-Ellison variety. New Eng. J. Med., *278:*1308, 1968.

Maingot, R.: Anastomotic ulceration. *In* Maingot, R.: Abdominal Operations. 5th ed., pp. 522-538. New York, Appleton-Century Crofts, Inc., 1969.

Marshall, S. F., and Knud-Hansen, J.: Gastrojejunocolic and gastrocolic fistulas. Ann. Surg., *145:*770, 1957.

Moore, F. T., Murat, J. E., Endahl, G. L., Baker, J. L., and Zollinger, R. M.: Diagnosis of ulcerogenic tumor of the pancreas by bioassay. Amer. J. Surg., *113:*735, 1967.

Oberhelman, J. A., Jr., and Nelsen, T. S.: Surgical considerations in the management of ulcerogenic tumor of the pancreas and duodenum. Amer. J. Surg., *108:*132, 1964.

Pfeiffer, D. B., and Kent, E. W.: The value of preliminary colostomy in the correction of gastrojejunocolic fistula. Ann. Surg., *110:*659, 1939.

Rawson, A. B., England, M. T., Gillam, G. G., French, J. M., and Stammers, F. A. R.: Zollinger-Ellison syndrome with diarrhea and malabsorption. Observations on a patient before and after pancreatic islet cell tumor removal without resort to gastric surgery. Lancet, *2:*131 (July 16), 1960.

Ruppert, R. D., Greenberger, N. J., Beman, F. M., and McCullough, F. M.: Gastric secretion in ulcerogenic tumors of the pancreas. Ann. Intern. Med., *67:*808, 1967.

Wilkie, D. P. D.: Jejunal ulcer. Ann. Surg., *99:*401, 1934.

Wilson, S. D., Mathison, J. A., Schulte, W. J., and Ellison, E. H.: The role of bioassay in the diagnosis of ulcerogenic tumors. Arch. Surg., *97:*437, 1968.

Wolff, C. B.: Zollinger-Ellison syndrome. Proc. Roy. Soc. Med., *61:*960, 1968.

Zollinger, R. M., and Ellison, E. H.: Primary peptic ulceration of the jejunum associated with islet cell tumors of the pancreas. Ann. Surg., *142:*709, 1955.

CHAPTER 14

PROLONGED POSTGASTRECTOMY STOMAL DYSFUNCTION

by LARRY C. CAREY, M.D. and EDWIN H. ELLISON, M.D.†

Larry C. Carey is an Ohioan who received his college and medical school education at Ohio State University. Following surgical residency at Marquette University, he served with much distinction as Director of the Surgical Research Team, Navy Station Hospital, Da Nang, Viet Nam. In 1969 he joined the faculty of the University of Pittsburgh as Associate Professor of Surgery. A John and Mary R. Markle Scholar, he has published important reports in the surgical literature.

Edwin H. Ellison, Jr., was also born in Ohio and received his college and medical education at Ohio State University, where he was elected to Alpha Omega Alpha. Following residency training at that institution, he remained on the staff as one of its most respected members until he became Professor and Chairman of the Department of Surgery at Marquette University in 1958. He was an outstanding surgical teacher and investigator, and his contributions to surgical science and practice have been most significant and prolific. He had an abiding interest in nutritional problems following gastric surgery, and as co-discoverer of the Zollinger-Ellison tumor he had a profound knowledge of this field.†

---

†*(Dr. Ellison died in 1970.)*

GASTRIC EMPTYING

PHYSIOLOGY AND ANATOMY

Knowledge of the mechanism whereby the stomach empties under normal conditions is basic to appreciating the problems encountered in abnormal gastric emptying. The phenomenon of gastric emptying is difficult to study and a variety of techniques have been employed. Basically, the methods consist of the administration of a test meal followed by some method of assessment of its passage from the stomach. Direct sampling, radiography, and scintillation counting have all been employed.

Many variables influence gastric emptying, but most are inhibitory. The only natural stimulus known to speed gastric emptying is distention. Among the inhibitory influences are the type of food ingested, the state of distention of the duodenum and jejunum, and the solute load in the proximal gut.

Acid in the stomach has been demonstrated to inhibit gastric secretion. Contrary to what one might expect, the effect of acid on gastric emptying is not related to the strength of the acid but rather to the molecular weight. Acetic acid, a relatively weak acid, has nearly the inhibitory effect of hydrochloric acid. The higher the molecular weight, the less profound the effect on gastric emptying. This observation suggests that the anionic component of the acid is the factor that effects gastric emptying inhibition. The larger anions may diffuse to receptor sites more slowly, explaining this phenomenon. Receptors in the stomach, duodenum, and jejunum sensitive to acid have been postulated. Which of these sites is of most importance under normal conditions remains an unanswered question.

Fats are also known to inhibit gastric emptying. Fatty acids seem to be more potent than triglycerides in this regard, and unsaturated fatty acids are more potent than saturated ones. Carbon chain length has a decided effect on the ability of fatty acids to slow gastric emptying. Effectiveness increases up to a carbon chain length of 14 and then decreases again. Whether the effect of fat on gastric emptying is mediated neurally or hormonally remains unclear. The effect has been shown to be lessened by vagotomy.

Osmotic pressure has an effect on gastric

emptying. Shay and co-workers have shown that tap water leaves the stomach more slowly than isotonic salines. Hypertonic and hypotonic solutions of both electrolytes and crystalloids slow gastric emptying. It has been suggested that the osmoreceptors are located in the duodenum and proximal jejunum.

There seems to be a relationship between gastric anatomy and gastric emptying. Careful dissection of the distal gastric musculature discloses thickening of all three muscular coats in the prepyloric region. A basic question that remains unanswered is whether or not the pyloric area acts as a true sphincter. Various information compiled from radiologic observation, pressure measurements, and electrical activity suggests the following: The antrum and pyloric ring behave as one unit and the duodenal cap appears to function as another separate but perhaps partially related unit. A continuous peristaltic wave from stomach to duodenal cap is not a frequent occurrence. Once food reaches the duodenal cap, it is fed into the distal duodenum, which serves to convey it distally. Some feedback mechanism exists, so that if duodenal cap emptying is decreased, gastric emptying is also decreased. Most available evidence supports the view that the pyloric ring is not a sphincter in the sense of the esophagogastric sphincter. The pyloric-antrum region seems rather to serve as a pump, which produces episodic flow into the duodenal cap. Surgical interference with the pump, such as pyloroplasty, will prolong gastric emptying and this prolongation will be enhanced by vagotomy. Clearly, a great deal of work is needed to clarify these complex relationships. Their complexity serves to illustrate the difficulty in evaluating gastric emptying problems in patients whose physiology has been disturbed by both gastroduodenal disease and surgical alteration.

Failure of the stomach to empty following gastric surgery is an exceedingly distressing experience for both the patient and the physician. While more insidious than postoperative hemorrhage and anastomotic disruption, it is often no less devastating to the patient. The causes of gastric outlet obstruction are many. While a specific problem can usually be found, the etiology may be quite obscure. Sound surgical judgment is required in planning the management of the nonemptying stomach.

THE MAGNITUDE OF THE PROBLEM

Gastric outlet obstruction is a difficult problem to evaluate for several reasons. One major reason is the inability of surgeons to agree on its definition. The physician who routinely does not feed his patients for five to seven days identifies the problem differently than the one who starts alimentation on the second postoperative day. It would be agreeable to most to say that a patient whose hospitalization is prolonged by the failure of his stomach to empty has stomal dysfunction. A review of the literature has afforded data from a randomly selected group of 13,150 patients subjected to gastric surgery. Only a small percentage (less than 2) were operated upon for other than acid-peptic disease. A variety of surgical procedures were performed, including subtotal gastrectomy, hemigastrectomy or antrectomy, and vagotomy and vagotomy plus a drainage procedure. Approximately 60 per cent underwent subtotal gastric resection only, while 40 per cent had vagotomy combined with either limited resection or drainage procedure. The overall incidence of stomal dysfunction was 4.0 per cent, or 528 patients.

Of the 27 series reviewed, six did not describe the number requiring additional surgery and four described only those requiring additional surgery. There were 17 for which calculations could be made, and, of the 8562 patients, 429 (5.01 per cent) were reported as having some degree of gastric stomal dysfunction. There were 87 (1.01 per cent) who required additional surgery. Of the 429 with stomal dysfunction, the 87 reoperated upon represent 20.3 per cent. It must be emphasized again that the definition of gastric stomal dysfunction and the requirement for surgical intervention vary greatly among surgeons. Some authors have advocated re-exploration within 10 days. If no mechanical obstruction is found, then a feeding jejunostomy is performed. Others delay re-exploration for as long as one month. Fortunately, 80 per cent of the patients who have a postoperative emptying disorder will recover without operative treatment.

INCIDENCE RELATED TO TYPE OF PROCEDURE

Thirteen series from the available literature were analyzed in an attempt to evaluate the incidence of gastric stomal dysfunction after subtotal gastric resection. While not always the case, the vast majority (over 90 per cent) of this group of 6488 patients had subtotal gastrectomy and gastrojejunostomy; and 232 (3.6 per cent) had some degree of stomal dysfunction. Considering only those reports in which patients with reoperations were described separately, then 4189 patients had a 4.5 per cent (189) incidence of stomal dysfunction and 0.66 per cent (28) required a second operation.

There were 2349 patients who could be identified as having hemigastrectomy and vagotomy and 94 (4.07 per cent) had some degree of stomal dysfunction. Of those reports that listed patients with reoperations separately, the incidence was 4.32 per cent and 1.04 per cent required surgical correction. Wherever a comparison could be made, there was no difference between gastroduodenostomy and gastrojejunostomy.

Of the 1908 patients who had vagotomy plus drainage procedure, 65 (3.4 per cent) had emptying difficulties. Considering the experience of those who reported reoperative cases separately, the incidence was 6.8 per cent (61 out of 886) and 1.2 per cent (11) needed additional surgery. In defense of the pyloroplasty enthusiasts, it must be pointed out that eight of these 11 cases needing a second operation had vagotomy plus gastroenterostomy. The overall reoperative incidence for pyloroplasty and vagotomy was 0.46 per cent of 1515 patients. From these figures, it can be concluded that there is not a great difference in the incidence of stomal dysfunction between hemigastrectomy and vagotomy and subtotal gastric resection. Vagotomy and drainage procedure, and particularly pyloroplasty, results in a smaller number of clinically important gastric emptying problems.

CAUSES OF STOMAL DYSFUNCTION FOLLOWING GASTROENTEROSTOMY

Figure 14-1 diagrams the more common causes of emptying problems associated with gastrojejunostomy. It probably makes little difference whether or not the procedure is done in association with a partial resection or a vagotomy. The most common cause is obstruction of the efferent loop by an adhesive band or acute angulation just distal to the anastomosis. The distance between the point of obstruction and the anastomosis may be variable and, as a result, the patient's complaints may be quite different.

Efferent Loop Obstruction

Mrs. C. is a 43-year-old female who was admitted to Pittsburgh Presbyterian-University Hospital in May of 1969. Two years prior to admission, the patient had a vagotomy and antecolic gastroenterostomy in association with a hiatal hernia repair. Over the six-month period prior to admission, she had recurrent episodes of abdominal pain. The pain was crampy in nature, quite severe, located in the epigastrium and left hemiabdomen, and associated with nausea. The patient found that the pain was worsened by eating and so had decreased her food intake, seeking relief. Consequently, she lost 10 pounds. The pain episodes became more frequent and she was hospitalized.

She was a thin woman in moderate distress with pain as described. There was an area of tenderness in the left hemiabdomen just lateral to the umbilicus. The examination was otherwise unremarkable. There were no laboratory abnormalities. Upper gastrointestinal series disclosed delayed gastric emptying and a dilated loop of small intestine with an air-fluid level (Fig. 14-2).

Exploratory laparotomy was performed and the left transverse colon was bound to the right pelvic brim by an adhesive band. The band was divided and the gastroenterostomy was inspected. The efferent loop from the stoma distally for approximately 18 inches was dilated to a diameter of 7 cm., and was edematous and erythematous. Beyond the point of obstruction, the intestine was collapsed. The gastroenterostomy was divided, the stomach and intestine were closed, and a pyloroplasty was performed. Postoperatively, the patient had no further symptoms and was discharged from the hospital on the seventh postoperative day. She was now back on a general diet. Since that time, she has remained without symptoms and is gaining weight.

This patient exemplifies the variety of clinical manifestations of stomal obstruction. The variation occurs as a result of the different points of obstruction. If the efferent loop is obstructed near the gastric stoma and the stoma itself is patent, the equivalent of high small bowel obstruction occurs. Vomiting is a significant factor, and electrolyte and fluid disturbance may be profound. Bile in the vomitus is useful in indicating that both the afferent loop and gastric stoma are patent. If the obstruction is some distance below the stoma in the efferent loop, as in the case described, and particularly if the obstruction is a partial one, vomiting may be replaced by pain as the prominent feature of the problem.

It is extremely important that any patient having symptoms of abdominal disorder, following gastric surgery of any kind, be evaluated with maximum interest and sympathy. The easy course is to regard the

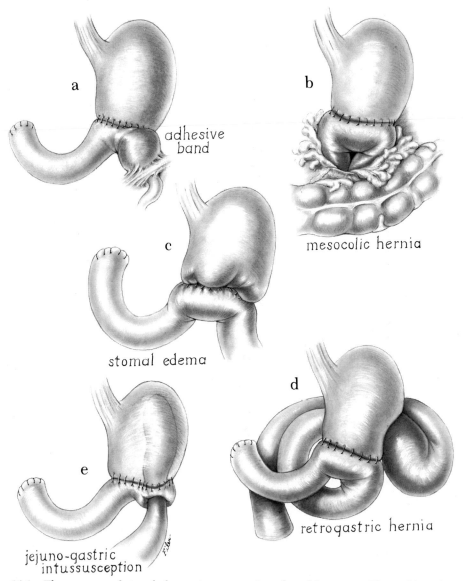

Figure 14-1. These causes of stomal obstruction are not in order of frequency. The problem described in the text for which no mechanical difficulty is found is not illustrated.

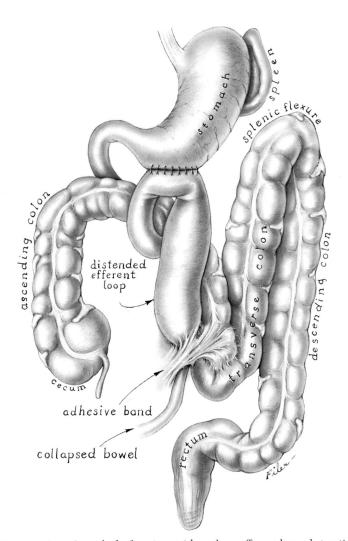

Figure 14-2. Stomal dysfunction with a long efferent loop obstruction.

symptoms as related to emotional instability, depriving the patient of a solution to a purely mechanical problem.

True gastric stomal obstruction occurs as the result of a variety of conditions. Some observers have suggested that a leak at the anastomosis precedes all or most anastomotic obstructions. An operative finding described by several authors supports this thesis. The finding is one of severe inflammatory reaction about the site of the stoma. This has been found following both Billroth I and Billroth II procedures. In retrocolic gastrojejunostomy, an encircling mass of necrotic mesentery has also been found. Whether this is related to devascularization of the mesentery or infection cannot be clearly determined.

Another cause for pure stomal obstruction is indelicate operative technique. If heavy sutures are used to invert large amounts of tissue, delayed stomal function may be expected. Occasionally an overzealous attempt to avoid dumping by creating a small gastrojejunostomy will result in a stoma that is compromised by a perfectly normal amount of postsurgical edema. This latter circumstance will usually subside in a few days and stomal dysfunction will not be prolonged.

The most alarming type of stomal dysfunction as yet has no explanation. It is the stomal problem most often described in surgical writing because it is the most puzzling, in regard to both understanding and treatment. After an uneventful course for six to 10 days, signs of stomal dysfunction occur. Early satiety, epigastric fullness, singultus, and vague pain precede frank vomiting. Gastrointestinal x-rays show a dilated gastric remnant with delayed emptying but no abnormality of the stoma. Gastroscopy will often reveal that the stoma is widely patent and appears normal. Typically, reinstitution of nasogastric suction will result in complete relief of symptoms only to have them recur when feeding is begun. The frustration of this problem can be well imagined. It is for this circumstance that a number of authors have recommended reexploration and direct examination of the external aspect of the anastomosis. If no abnormality is found to explain the symptoms, a feeding jejunostomy is performed and nothing more done. Nutrition is maintained with tube feeding and the surgeon and the patient wait. Cases of spontaneous stomal opening have been reported after 30 days with this regimen. Lillie has suggested an interesting theory (Fig. 14-3). A slight obliquity of the gastrojejunal suture line may cause mechanical dysfunction, which could

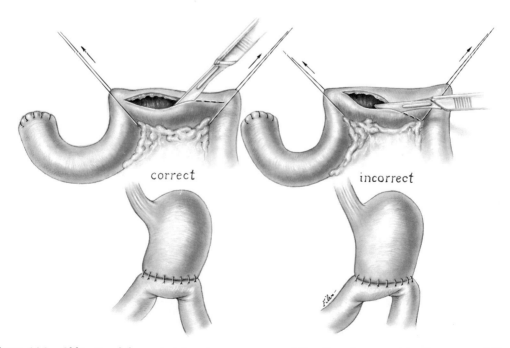

Figure 14-3. Obliquity of the gastrojejunostomy may account for otherwise unexplained emptying difficulty.

explain this phenomenon and could exist with no evidence of mechanical difficulty. Great care should be taken to construct the gastrojejunostomy exactly parallel to the long axis of the intestine to avoid this potential problem. Sachs, in describing two cases, suggested bougienage with a mercury-filled bag, while Narat performed an additional gastroenterostomy.

A secondary consideration in Billroth II construction is whether or not the addition of a so-called Braun modification is of benefit in stomal dysfunction. This modification is simply an entero-enterostomy distal to the gastroenterostomy. The theoretical advantages are to divert alkaline secretions, preventing bilious vomiting, and to improve the afferent loop emptying. There has been greater enthusiasm for this technique in the European clinics; and at the moment, it does not seem to be popular on the North American continent.

The procedure may offer little to prevent gastric stomal dysfunction, but it may have a significant role in protecting the duodenal stump closure by providing an emptying site below the point of efferent loop obstruction. The theoretical disadvantage is the shunting of protective alkaline juice away from the gastrojejunostomy.

RETROANASTOMOTIC HERNIA

Another and less common cause of stomal dysfunction following gastroenterostomy, with or without gastric resection, is retro-anastomotic herniation. Creation of a gastroenterostomy results in an opening behind the anastomosis through which small intestine and occasionally the omentum may herniate. The description by Petersen in 1900 of two cases has resulted in the condition being named "Petersen's hernia."

Both antecolic and retrocolic arrangements are susceptible, and there seems to be no greater incidence in one compared to the other. While herniation of both the afferent and efferent loops has been reported, the efferent loop is involved nearly twice as often. In at least one instance, herniation of both loops has occurred simultaneously. If gastric resection has been performed, the hernia is most likely to be from right to left, regardless of whether the afferent or efferent loop is involved. Antecolic anastomosis seems to predispose afferent loop herniation.

Strangulation with perforation is a disastrous complication and can be avoided by early operative intervention. There is some evidence that antecolic anastomoses are less likely to be associated with strangulation. If the herniation occurs early in the postoperative course, and they have been reported as early as the first day, the duodenal stump closure may be threatened.

The symptoms, as might be expected, tend to be those of small bowel obstruction; crampy abdominal pain, tenderness (not always in the upper abdomen), vomiting, and distention are classic. As opposed to stomal intussusception, a mass is not usually palpable.

Treatment consists of reduction of the hernia and decompression may be necessary before reduction can be accomplished. If perforation has occurred, simple closure may be possible. Any intestine of questionable viability must be resected. In some cases, fixation by entero-enterostomy between the afferent and efferent loops has been done. Closure of the hernial ring is indicated if possible. In several cases managed by reduction alone herniation has not recurred.

Jejunogastric Intussusception

Jejunogastric intussusception follows either gastric resection with gastrojejunostomy or, more rarely, gastroenterostomy. The condition is not common and between 150 and 200 cases have been described in the world literature. No improvement in the description of the clinical facets of the disorder has been accomplished since Aleman's classic description in 1948. His classification of the three types of jejunogastric intussusception is still valid. Type I, in which the afferent loop enters the stomach, would be expected to be most common, but is not. Type II (efferent loop) is the most frequent and accounts for nearly three out of four reported cases. Type III is the combined invagination of both the efferent and afferent limbs of jejunum into the stomach. In a variation of Type III, the anastomotic suture line enters the stomach (Fig. 14-4).

None of the various methods of gastrojejunal reconstruction are immune from intussusception, and cases following antecolic, retrocolic, Polya, Hofmeister, and gastroenterostomy procedures have been

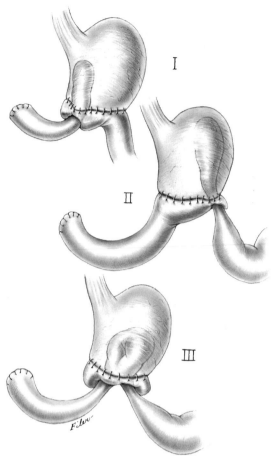

Figure 14–4. Jejunogastric intussusception of three types. Type II accounts for about 70 per cent of reported cases.

reported. The intussusception may occur from a few hours to 30 years postoperatively.

The classic findings of jejunogastric intussusception are those of abdominal pain, high-intestinal obstruction, a left upper quadrant or epigastric mass, and hematemesis. The radiographic findings are diagnostic if the films are taken when the intussusception is present. There is a mass visible in the gastric pouch on which striations, outlined with barium, suggest the mucosal pattern of the small intestine. Gastroscopy may also be very helpful in establishing the diagnosis.

When hematemesis or systemic toxicity occurs, surgical intervention is necessary to assure that strangulated intestine has not evolved. Some authors have suggested that those intussusceptions which occur in the early postoperative course are less likely to require surgical relief. Others have observed that a chronic recurrent type may be self-

limiting. Most agree that if symptoms persist or there is any evidence of impending strangulation, operation is indicated. Most surgical cases have been managed simply by reducing the intussusception. Other efforts have included resecting and performing another gastrojejunostomy. Gastroduodenostomy is the most certain method of cure, but with simple reduction recurrence is uncommon. A rational approach would seem to be simple reduction for those who have not had recurrent chronic symptoms and a more extensive procedure, such as gastroduodenostomy, for those who have.

CAUSES OF STOMAL OBSTRUCTION FOLLOWING GASTRODUODENOSTOMY

Since a number of possible causes of stomal obstruction possible in gastrojejunostomy are not possible in gastroduodenostomy, it might be expected that the incidence of stomal dysfunction in the latter would be less. This does not seem to be the case. Most authors who have reported extensive experience with both types of reconstruction have stated that no difference exists. The only place where a gastroduodenal stoma can become obstructed is at the suture line. Because the stomas tend to be small, great care must be taken to minimize edema. Herrington, who has had extensive experience, has reported several cases of adherence of the anastomosis to the underside of the liver. To prevent this problem, he has suggested interposing a portion of omentum between the liver and the suture line. As with gastrojejunostomy, suture line leak, albeit small, may result in perianastomotic inflammation and obstruction. Partial closure of the lesser curvature increases the likelihood of anastomotic leak. We prefer to reef down the cut end of the stomach to fit the duodenum end to end (Fig. 14-5).

As with gastrojejunostomy, a rare patient will manifest slow emptying and, at re-exploration, no apparent abnormality can be found. Under these circumstances, a feeding jejunostomy is performed after careful exploration. Tube feeding will allow maintenance of nutrition until stomal function begins. This approach is usually carried out after two weeks of nonoperative management. It must be remembered that gastric surgery provides no immunity from other common intra-abdominal disorders. Post-

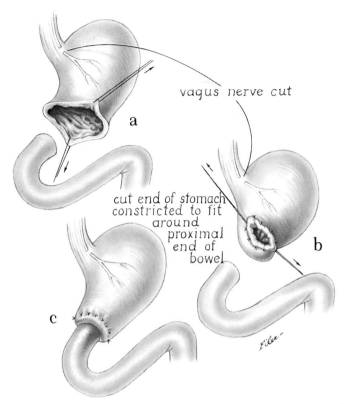

Figure 14-5. Von Haberer's gastroduodenostomy. The lesser curvature suture line is avoided and there are very few stomal dysfunction problems.

operative acute cholecystitis, appendicitis, or pancreatitis will occasionally result in poor gastric emptying. Accurate diagnosis, especially in the aged, may be very difficult and only established at laparotomy.

MANAGEMENT OF GASTRIC STOMAL DYSFUNCTION

VAGOTOMY

Transection of the vagus nerves results in a decrease in gastric tone as well as a decrease in both the strength and frequency of gastric peristalsis. At some variable time, both the tone and peristaltic activity of the stomach return; and while the recovery may not be complete, it is frequently adequate to allow near normal gastric emptying. The vagus nerve has both afferent and efferent fibers as well as fibers that both stimulate and inhibit gastric mobility. Stimulation of both afferent and efferent fibers has been shown to affect the stomach's muscular activity. Morrison has suggested that the inhibitory fibers require a stronger electrical stimulus than the stimulatory ones.

Effects of Vagotomy

There is no doubt that vagotomy has become a widely accepted procedure in the management of acid-peptic disease. While a great number of truncal vagotomies have been performed, still relatively little is known concerning the consequences of vagal section on gastric motility in man. Because of the disorders (mainly diarrhea) following truncal vagotomy, selective vagotomy was introduced several years ago. As might have been predicted, it has not become popular. There are three likely explanations for the relative unpopularity of selective vagotomy: 1. Most surgeons have had few unhappy patients following truncal vagotomy. 2. Many feel that they have trouble enough with the technical nuances of truncal vagotomy. 3. The benefits of selective vagotomy over those of truncal vagotomy have been somewhat obscure, but there seems to be no difference in their effects upon gastric motility.

Of interest in this treatise is the effect of vagotomy on gastric motor function. It has been postulated that vagal denervation of the stomach results in gastric stasis. It is clear that this reasonable assumption is not unequivocally true. Many patients have had vagotomy without drainage procedure and have had no apparent difficulty. These patients should be considered to be exceptions, since vagotomy without obviation of the pyloric sphincter will usually impair gastric emptying.

There has been considerable controversy over the effect of vagotomy on gastric emptying when either a gastric resection or an emptying procedure has been done. Animal investigation has indicated that vagotomy alone decreases gastric emptying and, when combined with pyloroplasty, even further decreases gastric emptying. This observation has been documented in man. While it has been possible to demonstrate decreased gastric emptying following vagotomy and pyloroplasty, the patients for whom this procedure has been carried out rarely have symptoms to suggest gastric retention. One must reflect on the efficacy of adding pyloroplasty to vagotomy for the treatment of peptic ulcer if gastric emptying is truly impaired by the procedure.

Nelson and co-workers found a decrease in both muscular and electrical activity in the stomach following vagotomy. In cases of both selective and truncal vagotomies, resting motor activity as well as response to feeding were impaired.

Barnes and Williams found no difference in postoperative emptying following vagotomy and drainage procedure, whether or not preoperative gastric obstruction was present. Other authors who routinely combine vagotomy with antrectomy or drainage procedure have had so little trouble with gastric emptying that they have recommended abandoning the routine use of postoperative gastric decompression. Other investigators have shown that while gastric tone is decreased by vagal section, positioning of the patient in a lateral position with the right side down greatly facilitates gastric emptying and gastric tone may return as early as six hours after vagal division.

Others have vigorously condemned vagotomy and drainage for patients who have had gastric outlet obstruction prior to surgery. It seems, however, that such sweeping conclusions drawn from only a few cases should not be readily embraced until either more clinical or experimental evidence is available. While there have been relatively few comparative studies done, the available information suggests, as previously stated, that vagotomy alone decreases gastric emptying and vagotomy plus pyloroplasty further decreases gastric emptying. Experimental evidence suggests that the type of pyloroplasty is of no consequence. Vagotomy plus gastroenterostomy or gastric resection results in a near normal gastric emptying time. Recalling the figures stated earlier, it seems that while there is evidence that pyloroplasty, when combined with vagotomy, decreases emptying, the incidence of clinically significant stomal problems is less than that following resection alone or resection plus vagotomy.

Weinberg has emphasized the importance of an adequate stoma with pyloroplasty and has strongly advocated one-layer closure.

The following case report demonstrates the problems occasionally encountered:

Mr. W. is a 50-year-old man who was admitted to Pittsburgh Presbyterian-University Hospital in June, 1969. He had been operated upon first in April, 1969 following a third episode of hemorrhage from a duodenal ulcer. A Heineke-Mikulicz pyloroplasty and vagotomy was performed. Following the operation, attempts to begin oral feeding resulted in fullness, singultus, nausea, and vomiting. After two weeks of repeated attempts at feeding and intermittent gastric suction, a gastroenterostomy was performed. Again following surgery, attempts at feeding resulted in distention and vomiting. Upon admission to Presbyterian Hospital, the patient had lost 20 per cent of his body weight (149 to 119 pounds). The findings were not remarkable, aside from the apparent weight loss. Upper gastrointestinal series showed little passage of the barium from the stomach after six hours. A Hollander test demonstrated incomplete vagotomy. At exploration the gastroenterostomy was found to be placed too high on the gastric wall for adequate function. The pyloroplasty was quite narrow (less than 0.5 cm. in diameter). Some edema of the stomach was present and the duodenum distal to the pyloroplasty was scarred by the ulcer. A 50 per cent gastric resection and end-to-end gastroduodenostomy were done along with division of a large posterior vagal trunk.

The patient made an uneventful recovery and was discharged on the eighth postoperative day. He was now back on a general diet. He had gained 10 pounds when seen one month following surgery and was without symptoms.

In general, a malfunctioning pyloroplasty is best treated by resection rather than gastroenterostomy. This case clearly points out the difficulty one can encounter in dealing with a "routine" duodenal ulcer.

Nutrition

The major problem to be solved in gastric outlet obstruction until food intake can be resumed is the problem of starvation. The average adult with limited physical activity requires between 30 and 40 calories per kilogram per day. Generally, for maintenance of body protein, 1 gm. per kilogram of protein is required and the remainder of the caloric needs are met with carbohydrates and fat. Approximately 25 per cent of the daily caloric intake should be fat. Caloric requirements are increased by the stress of surgery; and when this stress is increased by starvation, fever, infection, and healing wounds, the requirements may reach 60 to 70 calories per kilogram per day. Fever alone, for example, increases metabolic need as much as 13 per cent per degree centigrade above normal.

Normal adults excrete the same amount of protein nitrogen as they ingest under normal conditions. The stress of surgery, enhanced by any complication, results in protein utilization and nitrogen excretion exceeding intake, so that a state of negative nitrogen balance is said to exist. Protein is 16 per cent nitrogen; excreted and ingested nitrogen is multiplied by 6.25 to determine protein balance. Nitrogenous excretion is almost entirely via the kidney, so that, except in instances of unusual loss from the gastrointestinal tract, urinary nitrogen largely reflects total protein metabolism. The normal urinary nitrogen excretion is 10 to 15 gm. per day and may increase to as much as 50 gm. per day following major surgery or injury. In the usual patient after elective surgery, this protein loss ends quickly; but in the patient whose recovery is delayed, it may continue for weeks.

The protein lost following trauma or surgery is thought to be primarily from skeletal muscle. By maintaining high caloric intake, some of the protein loss can be abated. In the presence of gastric outlet obstruction, the maintenance of high caloric intake is a challenging problem.

Since fat emulsions have not proved to be clinically safe, parenteral caloric maintenance has been quite difficult. The ability to utilize intravenous glucose in humans is limited, and the administration of sugar at a rate greater than that which allows utilization results not only in loss of the sugar but in obligatory water loss as well by osmotic diuresis. The established glucose utilization rate for adult nondiabetics is about 0.5 gm. per kilogram per hour. Therefore, a 70-kg. man could be given 35 gm. of glucose per hour or 840 gm. in 24 hours resulting in 3360 calories. As glucose administration is gradually increased, tolerance develops and may be nearly tripled, 1.2 gm. per kilogram per hour. Various authors have suggested direct administration of concentrated glucose (50 per cent) solution into the vena cava by means of a catheter to supplement caloric intake.

Dudrick and associates have had extensive experience with parenteral feeding in adults and children with severe surgical problems. Their excellent studies have proved that positive nitrogen balance, weight gain, and growth can be accomplished entirely by parenteral means. These goals have been obtained by caval infusions via subclavian catheters. The solution used is one containing 200 gm. of glucose and 5 gm. of fibrin hydrolysate to which are added the necessary minerals, vitamins, and trace elements, according to the individual patient's need. Rush and co-workers have recently reported a series of patients treated in this way with excellent results. We have had some experience with this technique and have found it useful. However, in a discussion of Rush's paper, some patients were described in whom thrombosis of the superior vena cava had resulted.

Several surgeons have suggested re-exploration for gastric stomal dysfunction after 10 to 14 days. If no abnormality is found to explain the failure of the stomach to empty, a jejunostomy for feeding is performed. We prefer a simple Stamm jejunostomy over the Witzel type, since we feel that partial obstruction at the enterostomy site is less common with the former. It is important to tack the jejunum to the parietal peritoneum to avoid spillage into the abdomen or local infection.

Twenty-four hours after the jejunostomy is made, water is infused into it at a rate of 100 ml. per hour. For the second 24 hours, the infusate is changed to boiled skim milk. If this is tolerated then the tube feeding is advanced to a general hospital diet, homogenized and diluted with water to which is added enough fat in the form of corn oil to provide 1 calorie per milliliter. This is increased to 1.5 calories per milliliter after one or two days. Two or three thousand cubic centimeters of this diet is usually well tolerated and provides adequate caloric intake as well as a good balance of carbohydrate, protein, and fat. Vitamin and mineral content are easily adjusted to the individual's need.

The electrolyte disorder of gastric stomal dysfunction may be the same as that which occurs with obstructing peptic ulcer. If the gastric procedure has not eliminated acid production, the stomal obstruction will result in hypochloremic, hypokalemic alkalosis. Determination of the serum electrolytes will typically show an elevated carbon dioxide, depressed chloride, and normal or slightly depressed potassium. As treatment is begun and alkalosis corrected, the potassium may fall precipitously. Satisfactory correction of the problem can usually be accomplished with sodium chloride and potassium chloride. Ocassionally severe alkalosis will require a more acidifying salt, such as ammonium chloride, as described in a case reported by Gillespie. If the gastric surgery has resulted in near or total achlorhydria, then the electrolyte disorder may be no different from that associated with intestinal obstruction. A balanced salt solution will usually suffice for replacement, but additional sodium may be required. The most accurate way to replace electrolytes is simply to analyze the gastric aspirate and replace what is lost as it is lost.

Potassium replacement has tended to shorten postoperative hospital stay and stomal disorder. While there is not a great deal of experimental data to support the thesis, there seems to be decreased gastrointestinal motility with hypokalemia. Ravdin and others have felt that low serum protein levels led to stomal edema and prolonged ileus. The fact that these observations are primarily clinical, however, in no way lessens their validity. If serum protein levels are low, they may be corrected with plasma or commercially available solutions of serum protein in salt water.

SUMMARY

The problem of gastric stomal dysfunction is complex. It is indeed a systemic disease. The problems are those of maintaining nutrition and electrolyte balance until stomal dysfunction resolves. Five of every 100 patients undergoing gastric surgery will have some degree of emptying delay, and one in five of these will require reoperation. The procedure performed depends entirely upon the operative findings and may range from simple tube jejunostomy for feeding to gastric resection or reresection.

REFERENCES

Aleman, S.: Jejunogastric intussusception, a rare complication of the operated stomach. Acta. Radiol., 29:383, 1948.

Argyropoulos, G. D., and White, M. E. E.: Gastrointestinal function following vagotomy and pyloroplasty. Arch Surg., 93:578, 1966.

Baltartis, Yu. V.: Prophylaxis and treatment of evacuation disorders after gastric resection for ulcer. Arch. Klin. Chir., 4:65, 1965.

Barnes, A. D., and Williams, J. A.: Stomach drainage after vagotomy and pyloroplasty. Amer. J. Surg., 113:494-7, 1967.

Bastable, J. R. G., and Haddy, P. E.: Retro-anastomotic hernia. Brit. J. Surg., 48:183, 1960.

Belding, H. H.: Mechanical complications following sub-total gastrectomy. Surg. Gynec. Obstet., 117:578, 1963.

Borgstrom, S., and Arborelius, M.: Regulation of emptying of the stomach after gastric resection according to Billroth I or II. Acta Chir. Scand. (Supple.), 357:200, 1966.

Branch, C. D., and Adams, C. S.: Definitive surgery for duodenal ulcer in a community hospital. Amer. J. Surg., 105:317, 1963.

Buckler, K. G.: Effects of gastric surgery upon gastric emptying in cases of peptic ulceration. Gut, 8:137, 1967.

Coffey, R. J., and Lazaro, E. J.: Vagotomy, hemigastrectomy and gastroduodenostomy (Finney-Von Haberer) in the treatment of duodenal ulcer. Ann. Surg., 141:862, 1955.

Colp, R., and Weinstein, V.: Post-operative complications following sub-total gastrectomy for peptic ulcer. Surg. Clin. N. Amer., 35:383, 1955.

Devor, D., and Passaro, E., Jr.: Jejuno-gastric intussusception, a review of four cases, diagnosis and management. Ann. Surg., 163:93, 1966.

Dragstedt, L. R.: Supra-diaphragmatic section of the vagus nerves in the treatment of duodenal and gastric ulcers. Gastroenterology, 3:450, 1944.

Edwards, L. W., Edwards, W. H., Sawyers, J. L., Gobbel, W. G., Jr., Herrington, J. L., Jr., and Scott, H. W., Jr.: The surgical treatment of duodenal ulcer by vagotomy and antral resection. Amer. J. Surg., 105:352, 1963.

Eusterman, G. B., Kirklin, B. R., and Morlock, C. G.: The non-functioning gastro-enteric stoma: Diagnostic study of sixty-two surgically demonstrated cases. Amer. J. Dig. Dis., 9:313, 1942.

Gardner, B., Butler, E. D., and Goldman, L.: Early complications of gastrectomy with particular reference to delayed gastric emptying. Arch. Surg., 89:475, 1964.

Gillespie, J. A. L., and Sanders, R. I.: Sub-total gastrectomy complicated by mineral deficiency. Arch. Surg., 63:9, 1951.

Golden, R.: Functional obstruction of efferent loop of the jejunum following partial gastrectomy. JAMA, 148:721, 1952.

Hardy, J. D.: Problems associated with gastric surgery. Amer. J. Surg., 108:699, 1964.

Harper, F. B.: Gastric dysfunction after vagotomy. Amer. J. Surg., 112:94, 1966.

Harvey, H. D.: Complications in hospital following partial gastrectomy for peptic ulcer 1936 to 1959. Surg. Gynec. Obstet., 117:211, 1963.

Herrington, J. L., Jr.: Consideration of the factors responsible for stomal obstruction following Billroth I anastomosis. Ann. Surg., 157:83, 1962.

Herrington, J. L., Jr.: Elimination of routine nasogastric decompression following vagotomy-antrectomy and vagotomy with pyloroplasty or gastroenterostomy. Amer. J. Surg., 33:361, 1967.

Herington, J. L., Jr.: Methods of post-operative gastric decompression including an experience with the omission of its routine use. Amer. J. Surg., 110:424, 1965.

Herrington, J. L., Jr.: Vagotomy-pyloroplasty for duodenal ulcer: A critical appraisal of early results. Surgery, 61:698, 1967.

Hibner, R., and Richards, V.: Stomal or small bowel obstruction following partial gastrectomy. Amer. J. Surg., 96:309, 1958.

Hirai, T. et al.: Evaluation of early complications in gastrectomy. J. Therapy (Tokyo), 46:557, 1964.

Hopkins, A.: The pattern of gastric emptying: A new view of old results. J. Physiol. (London), 182:145, 1966.

Hunt, J. N.: Some properties of an alimentary osmoreceptor mechanism. J. Physiol. (London), 132:267, 1956.

Hunt, J. N.: Viscosity of a test meal, its influence on gastric emptying. Lancet, 1:17, 1954.

Hunt, J. N., and Knox, M. T.: A relation between the chain length of fatty acids and the slowing of gastric emptying, J. Physiol. (London), 194:327, 1968.

Hunt, J. N., and Knox, M. T.: Regulation of gastric emptying. Chapter 94 in: Handbook of Physiology. Alimentary Canal, Sec. 6, v. IV, Baltimore, Williams & Wilkins, 1968.

Irons, H. S., Jr., and Lipin, R. J.: Jejuno-gastric intussusception following gastroenterostomy and vagotomy. Ann. Surg., 141:541, 1955.

Johnson, L. P., and Magee, D. F.: Cholecystokinin-pancreozymin extracts and gastric motor inhibition. Surg. Gynec. Obstet., 121:557, 1965.

Jordan, G. L., Barston, H. L., and Williamson, W. A. A.: Study of gastric motility in the gastric remnant following sub-total gastrectomy. Surg. Gynec. Obstet., 104:257, 1957.

Kraft, R. O., Fry, W. J., and DeWeese, M. S.: Post-vagotomy gastric atony. Trans. West. Surg. Assoc., 71:287, 1964.

MacFee, W. F., and Sax, S. D.: Proximal duodenectomy with Von Haberer-Finney end to side gastroduodenal anastomosis for duodenal ulcer. Ann. Surg., 161:985, 1965.

Mathieson, A. J. M.: Prolonged delay in gastric emptying after partial gastrectomy. Brit. J. Surg., 59:657, 1965.

Mead, P. H.: Experience with pyloroplasty and vagotomy. A review of 184 cases. Amer. J. Surg., 114:910, 1967.

Narat, J. K., and Manilli, L. A.: Post-gastrectomy retention. Arch. Surg., 74:593, 1957.

Nelsen, T. S., Eigenbrodt, E. H., Keoshian, L. A., Bunker, C., and Johnson, L.: Alteration in muscular and electrical activity of the stomach following vagotomy. Arch. Surg., 94:821, 1967.

Nylander, G., and Wikstrom, S.: Gastric emptying and propulsive intestinal motility following partial gastric resection, gastro-entero anastomosis and abdominal truncal vagotomy in the rat. Acta Chir. Scand., 133:41, 1967.

Paine, J. R.: Immediate results of sub-total gastric resection for benign peptic ulcer. Surgery, 51:561, 1962.

Palumbo, L. T., Sharpe, W. S., Lulu, D. J., Bloom, M. H., and Porter, H. R.: Results in 300 cases of antrectomy with bilateral vagectomy for chronic duodenal ulcer. Surgery, 51:289, 1962.

Pearce, C. W., Jordan, G. L., and DeBakey, M. E.: Intra abdominal complications following distal sub-total gastrectomy for benign gastroduodenal ulceration. Surgery, 42:447, 1957.

Prohaska, J. V., Govostis, M. C., and Kisteen, A.: Mechanism of efferent stoma dysfunction following sub-total gastrectomy. Arch. Surg., 68:491, 1954.

Quigley, J. P., and Louckes, M. S.: The effect of complete vagotomy on the pyloric sphincter and gastric evacuation mechanism. Gastroenterology, 19:533, 1951.

Rachlin, L.: A rationale for post-gastrectic surgery care. Amer. J. Surg., 111:496, 1966.

Ramorino, M. L.: The motor activity and emptying mechanism of the stomach following sub-total resection with gastrojejunostomy. Radiol. Med., 50:972, 1964.

Ravdin, I. S.: Factors involved in retardation of gastric emptying after gastric operations. Penn. Med. J., 41:695, 1938.

Reyelt, W. P., and Anderson, A. A.: Retrograde jejunogastric intussusception. Surg. Gynec. Obstet., 119:1305, 1964.

Rhea, W. G., Killen, D. A., and Scott, H. W., Jr.: Long-term results in partial gastric resection without vagotomy in duodenal ulcer disease. Surg. Gynec. Obstet., 120:970, 1965.

Sachs, A. E.: Treatment of post-gastrectomy obstructed exit stoma. Arch. Surg., 70:449, 1955.

Savage, L. E., Stavney, L. S., Harkins, H. N., and Nyhus, L. M.: Comparison of the combined operation and Billroth I gastrectomy in the treatment of chronic duodenal ulcer. Amer. J. Surg., 107:283, 1964.

Sawyers, J. L., Scott, H. W., Edwards, W. H., Shall, H. J., and Law, D. H.: Comparative studies of the clinical effects of truncal and selective vagotomy. Amer. J. Surg., 115:165, 1968.

Schlicke, C. P.: Complications of vagotomy. Amer. J. Surg., 106:206, 1963.

Seifert, B., and Trefftz, F.: Mechanical obstruction due to post-operative pancreatitis following gastrectomy: Results in 2 cases. Chirurg., 36:401, 1965.

Sharp, W. V., Evans, D. M., and Burkhard, R. J.: Definitive gastric surgery for duodenal ulcer: A review of acute complications in an evaluation of 525 cases. Ohio State Med. J., 60:937, 1964.

Shoemaker, C. P., Jr., and Wright, H. K.: The rate of water and sodium absorption from the jejunum after abdominal surgery in man. Amer. J. Surg. In press.

Smith, E. T., Stephenson, W. H., and Damz, C. A.: Gastric resection for duodenal ulcer. Amer. J. Surg., 106:185, 1963.

Thoroughman, J. C., Walker, L. G., Jr., and Raft, G.: A review of 504 patients with peptic ulcer treated by hemigastrectomy and vagotomy. Surg. Gynec. Obstet., 119:257, 1964.

Wallace, R., DeChantal, J., and Mitty, W. F., Jr.: Morbidity and mortality of sub-total gastrectomy: A review of 500 cases. Amer. J. Dig. Dis., 9:745, 1964.

Weinberg, J. A., Stempien, S. J., Movius, H. J., and Dagadi, A. E.: Vagotomy and pyloroplasty in the treatment of duodenal ulcer. Amer. J. Surg., 92:202, 1956.

Welbourn, R. B.: Discussion on post-gastrectomy syndromes. Proc. Roy. Soc. Med., 44:173, 1951.

Welch, C. E., and Rodkey, G. V.: Partial gastrectomy for duodenal ulcer. Amer. J. Surg., 105:339, 1963.

Whittaker, L. D., Judd, E. S., and Stauffer, M. H.: Analysis of use of vagotomy with drainage procedure in surgical management of duodenal ulcer. Surg. Gynec. Obstet., 125:1018, 1967.

Wilder, T. C., Tobin, J. R., and Logan, A., Jr.: Functional efferent stomal obstruction following sub-total gastric resection. Arch. Surg., 72:719, 1956.

Williams, E. J., and Irvine, W. T.: Functional and metabolic effects of total and selective vagotomy. Lancet, 1:1053, 1066.

Williams, J. A.: Post gastrectomy problems. Brit. Med. J., 4:403, 1967.

Williams, J. A., Barnes, A. D., and Toye, D. K. M.: Tubeless vagotomy and pyloroplasty. Amer. J. Surg., 115:454, 1968.

CHAPTER 15

POSTOPERATIVE JAUNDICE AND HEPATIC FAILURE

by CHARLES G. CHILD, 3RD, M.D., JEREMIAH G. TURCOTTE, M.D., and S. MARTIN LINDENAUER, M.D.[*]

Charles Gardner Child, III, was born in New York City and received his degrees from Yale University and Cornell University Medical College. During college days he taught sailing, and he remains an avid practitioner of this ancient art. In the course of his residency and later staff membership at the New York Hospital-Cornell Medical Center, he established a sound basis for the signal contributions he has made to knowledge of liver disease and portal hypertension. In 1953 he accepted the Chair of Surgery at Tufts University School of Medicine and in 1959 he became Chairman of the Department of Surgery at the University of Michigan. Dr. Child is a broad scholar and a true leader in surgical science and in medical education.

Jeremiah George Turcotte was born in Detroit and graduated from the University of Michigan and the University of Michigan Medical School, where he was elected to both Phi Beta Kappa and Alpha Omega Alpha. Following his residency he remained on the staff of the University of Michigan Medical Center, where he is now Associate Professor of Surgery. The surgical management of liver disease represents a field of special interest for Dr. Turcotte.

S. Martin Lindenauer was born in New York City and graduated from Dartmouth College and Tufts Medical School. He served his residency at the University of Michigan, where he developed his active interest in hepatobiliary disease. At present he is Associate Professor of Surgery at the University of Michigan and Chief of the Surgical Service of the Veterans Administration Hospital at Ann Arbor.

Jaundice and hepatic failure, two manifestations of critical surgical illness, may occur after almost any surgical operation. They are most frequent after major operations performed upon one or more of the organs of the right upper quadrant of the abdomen, predominantly the gallbladder and common duct. They may be a fatal postoperative complication of operations performed upon patients with cirrhosis of the liver, the most common operation being portal decompression. Liver failure in patients with cirrhosis, however, may follow such lesser procedures as herniorrhaphy, cholecystectomy, or even operations performed outside the abdomen.

Occasionally postoperative icterus and hepatic failure reflect involvement of the liver in a general systemic disease, such as amyloidosis, lymphosarcoma or Hodgkin's granuloma, and, of course, in widespread metastatic cancer. These general hepatic ailments sometimes seem to be intensified by the stress of anesthesia and operation. In addition there are postsurgical problems related to operations of magnitude but not directly due to them. Here appear such entities as sensitivity to halothane, hepatotoxic drugs, such as chloroform, cholestatic drugs, of which there are a wide variety in common clinical use, hepatic infections and serum hepatitis.

Any intra-abdominal operation may, of course, be complicated by peritonitis and abscesses. When these are subdiaphragmatic, subhepatic, or intrahepatic, they too may be associated with jaundice and, if not successfully treated, even hepatic failure. For instance, suppurative appendicitis may be followed by jaundice and hepatic failure due to mesenteric pyelophlebitis, portal pyemia, and abscesses in the liver. These general complications of abdominal operations are omitted here, for they are considered in another chapter.

[*]Supported in part by N.I.H. Grant #HE-04260-10 and Brownell-Begole Surgery Research funds, University of Michigan Department of Surgery

345

PART I.

Jaundice Following Operations on the Biliary Tract and Contiguous Organs

by S. MARTIN LINDENAUER, M.D.

The largest group of patients who develop jaundice after operation are those whose primary disorder involves the gallbladder and the biliary drainage systems, both intrahepatic and extrahepatic. Here the commonest single surgical problem is calculus disease. The circumstances under which jaundice and, ultimately, hepatic failure develop are those of obstruction with and without infection. Sometimes these are transient, trivial, and self-correcting; on occasion, however, they are reflections of long, protracted illnesses, punctuated by acute exacerbations and many operations. In the early stages liver function is normal, but as the ravages of chronic obstruction and sepsis take their inevitable toll, biliary cirrhosis and hepatic failure appear and, for practical purposes, become new diseases grafted upon the old. In briefest terms, the problems that arise in connection with biliary tract surgery are mechanical and are usually relieved by a variety of surgical maneuvers. If these are successful, the patient is cured; if unsuccessful, critical surgical illnesses follow. These may terminate in hepatic failure early or late in the postoperative course.

CHOLECYSTECTOMY AND CHOLEDOCHOTOMY

The majority of patients undergoing cholecystectomy recover without incident. Postoperative jaundice, if it appears at all, may be due to a variety of technical circumstances associated with the operation itself. Bile may escape into the peritoneal cavity from the cystic duct remnant, from small biliary radicles extending directly from the liver to the gallbladder, or from tears in adjacent liver. Usually such bilious collections drain externally. However, when the gallbladder bed or the foramen of Winslow have been improperly drained or not drained at all, bile collects at the site of operation and is absorbed from the peritoneal surfaces.

Icterus, usually mild, appears postoperatively. Some of these collections drain spontaneously; others require reoperation, particularly if they are of sufficient magnitude to constitute a subhepatic or subdiaphragmatic abscess.

Another cause of temporary jaundice following cholecystectomy is cholangitis. This is believed to be a more or less universal accompaniment of cholecystitis and choledochitis. It may be exacerbated by the trauma of cholecystectomy and choledochotomy. In general, jaundice appearing for this cause will subside spontaneously as the patient recovers from his operation. If it persists, the need for appropriate antibiotic therapy becomes obvious.

When choledochotomy is added to cholecystectomy or performed alone, opportunities for extravasations of bile, common duct obstruction, and cholangitis increase. Once again these complications may be trivial and for the most part resolve spontaneously. On the other hand a whole gamut of complications of biliary tract operations may lead to jaundice and hepatic failure. These are always potentially serious and require careful thought, directed not only to their prevention but to their remedy as well.

COMMON DUCT STONE

In the course of cholecystectomy with or without choledochotomy, any surgeon may overlook a calculus in extrahepatic or intrahepatic bile ducts. Such a stone may, of course, produce postoperative jaundice by obstructing biliary drainage. The incidence of this misfortune is directly related to the age of the patient, surgical fortune, and the skill of the surgeon. It most often occurs in elderly patients, at the hands of surgeons who operate only occasionally upon the biliary tract, and in hospitals without modern roentgen facilities available in their operating rooms. The overall incidence of retained common duct stone lies somewhere between 8 and 10 per cent, and is about the same whether cholecystectomy is performed for acute or for chronic cholecystitis. The common duct is usually explored because of a history of jaundice, a dilated common duct, a palpable stone within the duct, chronic pancreatitis or the preoperative or intra-operative demonstration of calculi by cholangiography. In the majority of instances common duct stones are multiple and are recovered in from 28.5 to 63 per cent of patients undergoing choledochotomy.

The exact incidence of residual common duct calculi is difficult to determine. Glenn estimates this to be 25 per cent among patients with established choledocholithiasis, while Colcock and Perey report nine residual common duct stones among 1756 patients undergoing cholecystectomy for cholelithiasis. Literally volumes have been written on how to avoid leaving a common duct stone or two behind after what is often described as a routine cholecystectomy with or without choledochotomy.

Certainly a variety of methods are available today to avoid this serious postoperative complication. Intravenous cholangiography, transhepatic cholangiography, and intra-operative cholangiography are all extensions of a careful history and physical examination. The diligence with which these general and specific surgical rules are observed will contribute to decreasing the incidence with which common duct calculi are overlooked. No one surgical rule, however, will ever completely eliminate this hazard of cholecystitis, cholelithiasis, and choledocholithiasis.

Common duct stones manifesting themselves months or years after a biliary tract operation are not the concern of this chapter, for they really constitute a new surgical disease rather than a postoperative complication. The immediate problem, then, is the patient who becomes jaundiced after cholecystectomy with or without choledochotomy or after choledochotomy alone.

Most commonly residual common duct calculi occur in patients who have had a choledochotomy with retrieval of stones. Such patients usually undergo drainage of the common duct and jaundice may occur with clamping or elevation of the choledochotomy tube. Relief of the jaundice and the associated pain and fever can be readily accomplished by restoration of free drainage from the common duct T-tube or catheter. The diagnosis of a retained calculus can then be confirmed by performing a tube cholangiogram (Fig. 15-1).

Frequently, under these circumstances, the bile is infected. Forceful injection of contrast media into the common duct in the presence of infected bile should be avoided, for this can produce cholangitis and jaundice. Gravity alone should be utilized to fill the tube and the biliary drainage systems. The patient should be placed in the head-down position during injection in order to facilitate filling of the intrahepatic bile ducts. Prior to tube cholangiogram the bile should be

Figure 15-1. Tube cholangiogram demonstrating residual common duct calculus.

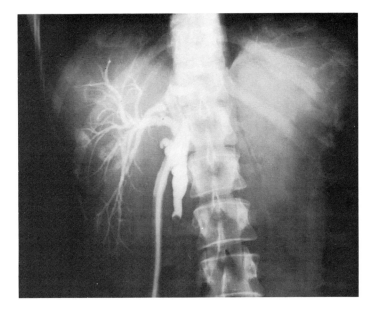

cultured and, if found to be infected, antibiotic sensitivity studies should be performed. Appropriate antibiotics are then administered the night before, the day of, and the day after the cholangiogram. Following uneventful cholangiography, the indwelling tube should be left in place and allowed to drain for 24 to 48 hours prior to its final removal. If, however, pain, fever, and jaundice follow roentgen visualization of the bile ducts, tube drainage should be continued until the patient tolerates periodic occlusion without complaint. When a patient progresses uneventfully with the tube occluded for two to three weeks and a free communication between the common duct and duodenum is demonstrated, his tube can probably be removed safely and without fear of subsequent difficulties.

In a patient with a residual common duct calculus, reoperation should be undertaken after a suitably short interval, preferably during the same hospital admission. If the patient tolerates clamping of the drainage tube and if the calculus is small, consideration may be given to deferring reoperation for four to six weeks. On occasion, small residual common duct calculi will be absent when cholangiography is repeated weeks or even months later. Presumably the offending stone has passed through the sphincter of Oddi. If, on the other hand, chills, fever, leukocytosis, and upper abdominal pain accompany every effort to clamp the drainage tube, reoperation should be prompt.

ROUTINE OPERATIVE CHOLANGIOGRAPHY

Surely it is far better to avoid leaving a common duct stone behind than to have to retrieve one at a later date. The routine use, therefore, of operative cholangiography is strongly advocated by many surgeons. When classic indications for common bile duct exploration are not present, intraoperative cholangiography has been demonstrated to reduce the incidence of residual stones. Letton and Wilson, and Jolly and his associates have recorded common duct calculi demonstrated by cholangiography in 5.7 to 6.3 per cent of patients undergoing cholecystectomy in whom no clinical suspicion of a common duct calculus existed. Overall, a greater degree of stone recovery is possible by the use of cholangiography than by the

use of the usual clinical criteria alone. Opponents of the routine use of operative cholangiography maintain that the procedure is time consuming, may produce pancreatitis, exposes the surgeon to excessive radiation, and adds unnecessary morbidity to cholecystectomy and choledochotomy. They also suggest that small unsuspected stones found on routine cholangiography would have passed through the sphincter of Oddi without difficulty. With care, experience, and good radiologic consultation, however, these objections have largely been overcome. There is no doubt that greater utilization of this procedure reduces the incidence of residual common duct calculi.

Consideration should also be given to selective operative cholangiography prior to planned common duct exploration. The number and location of biliary calculi may be determined and added assurance of their removal obtained. Similarly, operative T-tube cholangiography should be performed at the completion of every common duct exploration. This is a further aid in determining that all stones have been removed and that the ampulla of Vater is patent. Dilute Hypaque (20 to 25 per cent) should be utilized under these circumstances to avoid obscuring a residual small stone in a large duct. Particular attention should be paid to the distal duct in which a partially impacted stone may be overlooked. If there is question concerning the patency of the papilla of Vater, transduodenal exploration of the distal duct should be undertaken without hesitation.

INTRAHEPATIC CALCULI

A troublesome area in which stones may be overlooked is in the intrahepatic ducts. Fogarty and associates noted a 17 per cent incidence of intrahepatic calculi in patients with choledocholithiasis. The intrahepatic ducts should be adequately explored mechanically and completely visualized by cholangiography.

In jaundiced patients who have an extrahepatic biliary tract of normal size, a diligent search must be made for intrahepatic calculi before assuming that the etiology of the jaundice is not obstructive.

Most often intrahepatic calculi are located in the left hepatic duct. The right hepatic duct joins the common hepatic duct in an almost straight line, whereas the left duct

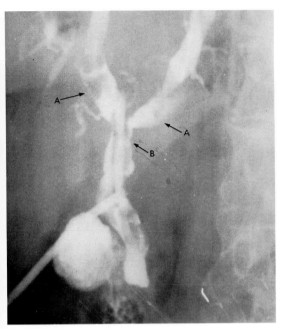

Figure 15-2. A, Tube cholangiogram demonstrating intrahepatic calculi, and B, stricture of left hepatic duct at junction with right hepatic duct.

enters at an angle of 30 to 45 degrees. Intrahepatic calculi will often be found in the left duct just proximal to this junction. There may also be an associated stricture (Fig. 15-2). On occasion, partial intrahepatic ductal obstruction may be due to localized cholangiocarcinoma. This can usually be identified by careful roentgen hepatography.

Intrahepatic stones are difficult to remove.

The balloon-tipped catheter described by Fogarty is helpful in retrieving a stone impacted deep within the liver. A large dilated duct proximal to an obstructing calculus and close to the surface of the liver is readily approached transhepatically and the stone extracted. If a stricture is tight and permanent, recurrent stone formation is likely. This can only be avoided by left hepatic lobectomy.

PANCREATICODUODENAL CANCER

Neoplasm of the head of the pancreas, papilla of Vater, distal common duct, or duodenum may be overlooked at the time of common bile duct exploration. These tumors may cause pain, fever, and persistent jaundice postoperatively as a result of common duct obstruction. Such symptoms and signs appear when the choledochotomy tube is temporarily occluded prior to its removal. Cancer is more readily overlooked if the neoplasm coexists with choledocholithiasis. If the stones are removed without proving patency of the distal duct, such a neoplasm may not be identified. Frequently the malignant nature of the distal obstruction is elucidated by a T-tube cholangiogram (Fig. 15-3). If the obstructing lesion cannot be distinguished from pancreatitis, tube drainage of the common duct should be maintained for three to four weeks. If the obstruc-

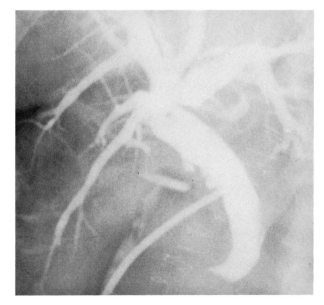

Figure 15-3. Tube cholangiogram demonstrating distal common duct obstruction due to carcinoma of the ampulla of Vater.

tion is due to neoplasm it will not relent. If due to pancreatitis, the obstruction will usually subside. If the obstruction persists and is thought to be due to pancreaticoduodenal cancer, the interval of temporary biliary decompression is valuable. Liver function improves and pancreaticoduodenectomy or permanent palliative biliary decompression can then be performed with less risk than is entertained in deeply jaundiced patients.

COMMON DUCT INJURY

Non-neoplastic stricture of the extrahepatic biliary tract is almost always due to operative injury (Fig. 15-4). This is likely to occur when there is inadequate surgical exposure, poor operative assistance, and suboptimal anesthesia. Acute inflammation, bleeding, and congenital anomalies sometimes obscure biliary tract anatomy. The stage is then set for inadvertent bile duct injury. The operative procedure during which a duct or vessel is injured is often described by the surgeon as routine and uneventful.

If a bile duct injury is recognized when it occurs, immediate repair is relatively easy. Too often, however, the injury is not appreciated. Jaundice is noted early in the postoperative period and is associated with fever and right upper quadrant discomfort. The injured duct is usually not completely occluded. Obstruction is partial and is associated with damage to the duct wall. This results in the escape of bile and excessive biliary drainage. The clinical course may suggest a retained common duct stone. Whether the gallbladder bed has been drained or not, bile peritonitis may ensue. This will be marked by severe abdominal pain and rigidity with fever, general toxicity, and dehydration. Bile peritonitis may be easily confused with postoperative pancreatitis. Normal amylase and serum calcium values tend, however, to exclude pancreatitis. Diagnostic paracentesis is helpful in this setting and the recovery of bile-stained peritoneal fluid is diagnostic of bile peritonitis. This differentiation should be made early, for bile peritonitis must be treated by prompt operation, external drainage of the bilious collection, and control of the

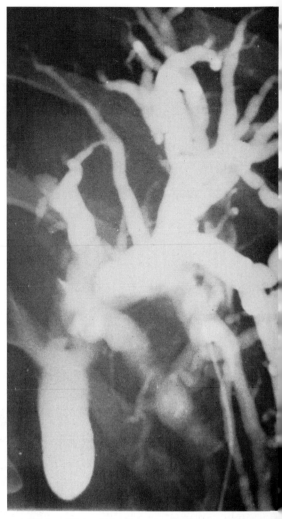

Figure 15-4. Transhepatic cholangiogram demonstrating complete obstruction of the common bile duct. This followed a so-called "uneventful" cholecystectomy.

extrahepatic biliary tract leak. The operation should not be extensive or prolonged, for most of these patients are too ill to tolerate anything more than the simplest of surgical procedures.

When the cholangitis and obstructive jaundice have subsided, the nutritional and metabolic status of the patient will usually have improved sufficiently to permit definitive repair of the stricture weeks or months later. In late reconstruction we favor end-to-side *Roux-en-Y* choledochojejunostomy. Many detailed articles are available on these subjects. They should be readily available in the working libraries of all abdominal surgeons.

INJURY TO HEPATIC VASCULATURE

One of the well-recognized but fortunately rare hazards of operations in the right upper quadrant is ligation of one or both of the hepatic arteries. When both are divided, one of the most critical of surgical illnesses may develop—ischemic necrosis of the liver.

Hepatic necrosis, however, does not invariably follow hepatic arterial interruption. In some individuals portal venous flow alone is sufficient to provide adequate oxygenation to the liver. Tygstrup and his associates have shown that the contribution of the hepatic artery to total hepatic blood flow is 35 per cent and that the arterial inflow supplies only 50 per cent of the oxygen utilized by the liver. Hepatic necrosis may follow arterial interruption in patients in whom nutrient portal flow is diminished (hypotension, shock, cirrhosis, portacaval shunt), in patients in whom oxygen demand is increased (pyrexia, sepsis), and in patients with prior or concomitant liver damage (trauma, cholangitis, and so on).

If injury to the right or left hepatic artery or to both is recognized at operation, repair should be undertaken without hesitation. If this is not technically possible, vigorous attempts should be made to avoid hypotension and fever and to insure maximum hepatic oxygenation in the postoperative period. Antibiotics should also be administered. Although infection probably does not play a significant role in the necrosis of a normal human liver following arterial interruption, this critical issue remains in doubt. Certainly with infection in the biliary tract, the potential role of sepsis in hepatic necrosis cannot be ignored when the blood supply to the liver has been compromised.

If hepatic arterial interruption is not recognized at operation, this catastrophe may be suspected postoperatively when a patient develops fever, jaundice, elevated transaminase levels, and low blood glucose in the presence of a low or normal blood urea nitrogen. Reoperation is imperative and reconstruction of the injured hepatic artery or arteries should be attempted. When this is not possible Karasewich and Bowden have suggested that death might be avoided by construction of an arteriovenous fistula between the portal vein and an adjacent small artery. The implantation technique of Shilling would probably be the surgical procedure of choice under these desperate circumstances.

An untold number of patients probably succumb to this tragedy and are never reported. When a single hepatic artery is occluded survival is more likely, for hepatic reserve is large. Such an accident is suspected of having occurred when, at some subsequent operation, disproportionate atrophy of one hepatic territory and hypertrophy of the other is observed.

ACUTE SUPPURATIVE CHOLANGITIS

Cholangitis may be due to reflux of intestinal contents into the biliary tract. Spontaneous or surgically created biliary-enteric fistulae, Vaterian papillary sphincterotomy, and choledochal cysts predispose to ascending cholangitis. Cholangitis is rare following a Roux-en-Y jejunostomy because of the defunctionalized jejunal limb. It is more common following choledochoduodenal anastomoses, particularly if the stoma is small. This may be troublesome in the early postoperative period but is more often a late problem.

Cholangitis is usually due to a combination of obstruction of the common duct and infection. If this misfortune is not promptly resolved, some patients progress to acute suppurative cholangitis. The clinical course of these individuals is marked by central nervous system symptoms, shock, and rapidly progressing sepsis. Patients who develop acute obstructive suppurative cholangitis are usually elderly and have a history of previous biliary tract disease. Pain is almost always severe and colicky, and often radiates to the back or scapular region. Chills, nausea, and vomiting are common and the temperature is usually elevated above 101° F. There is evidence of peritoneal irritation in the right upper quadrant and a tender, enlarged liver can sometimes be felt. Serum bilirubin levels are in the range of 5 to 15 mg. per 100 ml. The white blood count may be markedly elevated. In a few patients, body temperature may be subnormal, indicating lack of responsiveness to overwhelming sepsis. Hypotension is often a late manifestation and is frequently associated with the recovery of organisms from the blood. These are usually gram-negative and correspond to those found in the bile.

The central nervous system symptoms include lethargy, confusion, and disorientation. This manifestation of cholangitis as a distinct clinical entity was emphasized by Reynolds and Dargan in 1959. These authors believe that obstruction of the common duct with infected bile under pressure is responsible for the mental disturbances manifested by these patients. Such mental disturbances, with hypotension and septicemia, are ominous signs. In a series of 10 such patients reported by Dow and Lindenauer, a mortality of 60 per cent was encountered. In patients who did not manifest these symptoms, the mortality was 13 per cent. There appears to be an interval of a week or so between the onset of general symptoms and the development of septicemia. While preoperative supportive therapy is necessary, it should not be prolonged, since only prompt biliary decompression can reverse the disastrous course of acute suppurative cholangitis. These patients are usually refractory to all forms of nonoperative treatment. There are no reported survivals without operation.

At operation the biliary tract is uniformly dilated and inflamed. It contains purulent bile under pressure. This will often spurt dramatically from a choledochotomy incision, with immediate and striking improvement in an unstable patient who may be tolerating operative intervention poorly. The operation should be minimal and consist of the simplest and most direct method of obtaining decompression of the biliary tract, usually by T-tube drainage of the common bile duct. In patients operated upon late in the course of the disease, a brief search should be made for liver abscesses. These should be drained if this can be accomplished without extensive surgical manipulation. The mortality of acute suppurative cholangitis is in the neighborhood of 40 to 60 per cent. The only way this can be lowered is by early operation—hopefully before septicemia and hepatic abscesses materialize.

ACUTE POSTOPERATIVE PANCREATITIS

Acute pancreatitis occurring in the postoperative period is a dread surgical complication. Usually the preceding operation involves the biliary tract or other organs contiguous to the pancreas, particularly the stomach and duodenum. Less frequently, the operation precipitating this complication is remote from the pancreas, even extraabdominal. However, the majority of patients will have associated biliary tract disease. Among all patients undergoing biliary tract operations, the occurrence of pancreatitis postoperatively is fortunately uncommon. Colcock and McManus report five cases among 1356 patients undergoing biliary tract operations and Glenn, McSherry, and Dineen noted seven cases among 3217 patients undergoing biliary procedures.

The etiologic factors responsible for postoperative pancreatitis are sometimes not clearly definable. Operative trauma, biliary tract disease, manipulation of the pancreas, and pancreatic ductal obstruction appear to be the most important. Injudicious instrumentation and dilatation of the distal common duct and papilla of Vater cause spasm, edema, and inflammation in these structures, with subsequent obstruction of the major pancreatic duct. Large-caliber, long-arm T-tubes that extend through the ampulla may also cause acute pancreatitis. Vascular insufficiency, infection, anesthetic agents and narcotics have all been implicated for their role in certain patients manifesting acute postoperative pancreatitis. Inadvertent and forceful injection of bile into the pancreas is certainly one cause of acute pancreatitis. This may occur with operative cholangiography when a common channel exists between the common duct and pancreatic ducts. The direct injection of contrast media for operative pancreatography may rupture small ducts or acini and, in this way, cause pancreatitis. Nevertheless, underlying biliary tract disease appears to be the single most important factor predisposing to pancreatitis postoperatively.

The diagnosis of pancreatitis in the early postoperative period may be difficult. Jaundice, fever, leukocytosis, abdominal pain, tenderness, rigidity, intestinal ileus, dehydration, circulatory collapse, and oliguria may all be present. Increased serum amylase and calcium may, of course, be helpful in differential diagnosis. It should be remembered, however, that elevations of serum amylase occur with perforated peptic ulcer, intestinal obstruction, intestinal ischemia and with parotitis. Low or normal serum amylase values may occur if there is long standing chronic pancreatitis or if there has been extensive necrosis of the pancreas. Diagnostic paracentesis with the recovery of serous fluid with a high amylase content, is virtually diagnostic of acute pancreatitis.

The treatment of postoperative pancreatitis should be nonoperative. Therapy should include resting the gastrointestinal tract by nasogastric suction, analgesics, anticholinergics, adequate crystalloid and colloid replacement, whole blood when indicated, systemic antibiotics, and calcium replacement. Operative intervention should be considered if the diagnosis is in doubt or if massive pancreatic necrosis or abscess make their appearance.

Perforated peptic ulcer or intestinal infarction may be difficult to distinguish from pancreatitis and operative exploration should be rapidly undertaken if these two entities cannot be excluded. Occasionally pancreatitis may be complicated by hemorrhage, pancreatic abscess, or gastric outlet obstruction due to abscess or pseudocyst, and operation should be undertaken to deal with these problems.

If there is an associated acute cholecystitis or significant obstructive jaundice, operative intervention should also be undertaken. Operations on the biliary tract in the presence of acute pancreatitis should be minimal and as atraumatic as possible. Extensive ductal exploration is to be avoided and operative procedures should probably consist only of cholecystostomy or common duct tube drainage.

The mortality of postoperative pancreatitis remains high and has been reported to be from 35 to 48 per cent. Severe complications are common with postoperative pancreatitis. Oliguria or significant azotemia, hypocalcemia, low serum amylase values, and progressive jaundice are all ominous signs that are frequently present in patients succumbing to their disease. Death occurring in postoperative pancreatitis is most often due to renal failure and sepsis.

JAUNDICE FOLLOWING OPERATIONS ON THE STOMACH, DUODENUM, AND PANCREAS

Jaundice following gastrectomy, vagotomy, and pyloroplasty and distal pancreatectomy is almost always due to inadvertent injury to the common duct. When subtotal gastrectomy for duodenal ulcer was more common than it is today, one of the dread complications of duodenal dissection and closure was inadvertent ligature or laceration of the common duct. Protection of this structure during one of these operations is enhanced by threading a red rubber or woven-silk catheter throughout the length of the common duct and into the duodenum. In the course of a difficult dissection, one of these catheters not only helps prevent injury to the common duct but also assists in identifying such an injury the moment it occurs. As in common duct injury during cholecystectomy, repair is often readily performed if only the injury is recognized at the time of its occurrence.

REFERENCES

Part I

Brittain, R. S., Marchioro, G., Hermann, G., Waddell, W. R., and Starzl, T. E.: Accidental hepatic artery ligation in humans. Amer. J. Surg., *107*:822, 1964.

Cattell, R. B., and Braasch, J. W.: General considerations in the management of benign stricture of the bile duct. New Eng. J. Med., *261*:929, 1959.

Child, C. G., and Lindenauer, S. M.: Repair of bile duct strictures. Mich. Med., *65*:454, 1966.

Colcock, B. P., and McManus, J. E.: Experiences with 1,356 cases of cholecystitis and cholelithiasis. Surg. Gynec. Obstet., *101*:161, 1955.

Colcock, B. P., and Perey, B.: The treatment of cholelithiasis. Surg. Gynec. Obstet., *117*:529, 1963.

Cole, W. H.: Strictures of the common duct. Surgery, *43*:320, 1958.

Dow, R. W., and Lindenauer, S. M.: Acute obstructive suppurative cholangitis. Ann. Surg., *169*:272, 1969.

Fogarty, T. J., Krippaehne, W. W., Dennis, D. L., and Fletcher, W. S.: Evaluation of an improved operative technique in common duct surgery. Amer. J. Surg., *116*:177, 1968.

Glenn, F.: Choledochotomy in non-malignant disease of the biliary tract. Surg. Gynec. Obstet., *124*:974, 1967.

Glenn, F., and Beil, A. R., Jr.: Choledocholithiasis demonstrated at 586 operations. Surg. Gynec. Obstet., *118*:499, 1964.

Glenn, F., and Frey, C. F.: Re-evaluation of the treatment of pancreatitis associated with biliary tract disease. Ann. Surg., *160*:723, 1964.

Glenn, F., McSherry, C. K., and Dineen, P.: Morbidity of surgical treatment for non-malignant biliary tract disease. Surg. Gynec. Obstet., *126*:15, 1968.

Holm, J. C., Edmunds, L. H., Jr., and Baker, J. W.: Life threatening complications after operations upon the biliary tract, Surg. Gynec. Obstet., *127*:241, 1968.

Jolly, P. C., Baker, J. W., Schmidt, H. M., Walker, J. H., and Holm, J. C.: Operative cholangiography. Ann. Surg., *168*:551, 1968.

Karasewich, E. G., and Bowden, L.: Hepatic artery injury, Surg. Gynec. Obstet., *124*:1057, 1967.

Letton, A. H., and Wilson, J. P.: Routine cholangiography during biliary tract operations. Ann. Surg., 163:937, 1966.

Mays, E. T.: Observations and management after hepatic artery ligation. Surg. Gynec. Obstet., 124:801, 1967.

Monafo, W. W., Ternberg, J. L., and Kempson, R.: Accidental ligation of the hepatic artery. Arch. Surg., 92:643, 1965.

Peterson, L. M., Collings, J. J., and Wilson, R. E.: Acute pancreatitis occurring after operation. Surg. Gynec. Obstet., 127:23, 1968.

Popper, H., and Schaffner, F.: Drug induced hepatic injury. Ann. Intern. Med., 51:1230, 1959.

Reynolds, B. M., and Dargan, E. S.: Acute obstructive cholangitis. Ann. Surg., 150:299, 1959.

Subcommittee on the National Halothane Study of the Committee on Anaesthesia, National Academy of Sciences—National Research Council: Summary of the national halothane study. JAMA, 197:775, 1966.

Thorbjarnson, T., Mujahed, Z., and Glenn, F.: Percutaneous trans-hepatic cholangiography. Ann. Surg., 165:33, 1967.

Tygstrup, N., Winkler, K., Mellemgaard, K., and Andreassen, M.: Determination of the hepatic arterial blood flow and oxygen supply in man by clamping the hepatic artery during surgery. J. Clin. Invest., 41:447, 1962.

Walter, W., and Ramsdell, J. A.: Study of three hundred and eight operations for stricture of bile ducts. Follow-up of one to five and five to twenty-five years. JAMA, 171:872, 1959.

White, T. T., and Murat, J. E.: Treatment of the common bile duct in pancreatitis. Amer. Surg., 33:523, 1967.

Wise, R. E., and Twaddle, J. A.: Choledocholithiasis: Postcholecystectomy diagnosis by intravenous cholangiography. Surg. Clin. N. Amer., 38:673, 1958.

PART II.

Hepatic Cirrhosis in Surgical Patients

by JEREMIAH G. TURCOTTE, M.D.

Cirrhosis of the liver is now the tenth leading cause of death in the United States. In 1966, 26,692 deaths were attributed to hepatic cirrhosis in this country; since 1956 the mortality rate for this disease has increased from 10.7 to 13.6 per 100,000 population (National Health Education Committee, Inc., 1966). Surgeons can expect and should be prepared to manage patients with cirrhosis in both elective and emergent circumstances. An estimate of hepatic reserve before operation is helpful in the care of surgical patients with cirrhosis, but at times the first manifestation of hepatocellular disease is the insidious onset of jaundice in the postoperative period.

Deepening jaundice, although a most visible and dramatic sign of hepatic insufficiency, is only one of many derangements related to hepatic insufficiency. Proper management of the icteric patient requires a clear understanding of the pathophysiology induced by hepatocellular disease. In this section we review briefly some of the most important aspects of the disturbed metabolism and physiology observed in patients with cirrhosis. Special emphasis is given to the problems of those patients with cirrhosis and gastroesophageal varices who require portosystemic shunts.

JAUNDICE AND HEPATIC CIRRHOSIS

Each day about 250 to 300 mg. of bilirubin, derived mainly from the degradation of hemoglobin, is presented to the liver for excretion (Powell, 1967). The quantity of pigment which the normal liver is capable of excreting is uncertain. Bilirubin infusion studies indicate that at least a two- to threefold increase in the rate of red blood cell destruction must occur before plasma bilirubin rises above 3 mg. per 100 ml. With normal liver function the amount of pigment excreted increases in proportion to the square of its concentration in the serum. In most instances of hepatocellular disease, as well as with biliary obstruction of any etiology, plasma bilirubin is predominantly of the conjugated or direct reacting type.

With nutritional or postnecrotic cirrhosis, bilirubin concentration is usually not above 3 to 4 mg. per 100 ml., unless liver function is severely impaired. The hyperbilirubinemia accompanying cirrhosis is due to a combination of increased hemolysis of red blood cells and decreased ability of the liver to transport or conjugate bilirubin. We know that 50 per cent or more of the normal liver may be resected with only a transient rise in serum bilirubin (Bengmark, 1968).

The clinician can utilize this information in managing his patients. A serum bilirubin above 3 to 4 mg. per 100 ml. may indicate a severe disturbance in the intrahepatic metabolism of bilirubin. If massive hemolysis, extrahepatic biliary obstruction, and significant gastrointestinal or internal hemorrhage can be excluded, consideration should be given to instituting supportive therapy for the failing liver when bilirubin rises above the critical concentration of 3 to 4 mg. per 100 ml. Additional complications, such as ascites and congestive heart failure, can best be avoided by active early treatment of the patient with incipient hepatic failure.

WATER AND ELECTROLYTE ABNORMALITIES IN CIRRHOSIS

Total body water, plasma volume, and exchangeable sodium are often increased in patients with hepatic cirrhosis (Laragh and Ames, 1963). Conversely, total body stores of potassium may be depleted by as much as 500 milliequivalents (Casey et al., 1965). Serum electrolyte determinations do not routinely reflect these abnormalities, but often serum sodium concentration and sometimes serum potassium levels are low. In general, these abnormalities become more severe as hepatic reserve diminishes. The patient with a high-output cardiac systolic murmur, gross ascites, and pedal edema furnishes visible evidence of the severity of the disturbance in water and electrolyte balance that may accompany hepatic cirrhosis.

The pathogenesis of these derangements is not well understood. Secondary hyperaldosteronism, portal hypertension, and diminished intravascular oncotic pressure secondary to low serum albumin are important contributing factors, but do not fully explain the defect. We do know that the maximum renal excretion of sodium may be as low as 1 mEq. per day and frequently is below 30 mEq. per day with chronic hepatocellular disease (Orloff et al., 1967). So-

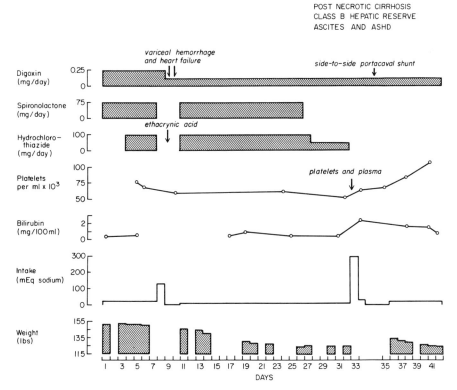

Figure 15-5. The combination of severe sodium restriction and therapy with hydrochlorothiazide, spironolactone, ethacrynic acid, and digoxin promoted the brisk diuresis of ascites in this patient with postnecrotic cirrhosis.

dium restriction may have to be severe and diuretic therapy intensive to diminish ascites and restore normal sodium and water balance. Potassium supplementation is indicated, but many patients with cirrhosis will not readily conserve added potassium. Renal excretion of sodium may be increased after the construction of a portosystemic shunt but does not return to normal.

Figure 15-5 illustrates a typical response to adequate therapy.

On February 7, 1969, a 69-year-old white woman with postnecrotic cirrhosis was admitted for an elective portacaval shunt. Gross ascites had been present for several years and massive variceal hemorrhage had occurred on two occasions. She was judged to be a moderate risk for portal decompression on the basis of estimated hepatic reserve (Class B, Table 15-3). In addition she was known to have arteriosclerotic heart disease, and pulmonary edema had complicated recovery from her last variceal hemorrhage. A serum creatinine of 2 mg. per 100 ml. indicated moderate impairment of renal function. Several days after admission, a third life-threatening variceal hemorrhage occurred. Again the patient lapsed into congestive heart failure and pulmonary edema. The hemorrhage was controlled by balloon tamponade. Replenishment of blood and fluid was carefully regulated by monitoring central venous pressure, urine output, and vital signs. Figure 15-5 illustrates that the combination of severe sodium restriction and therapy with hydrochlorothiazide, spironolactone, ethacrynic acid, and digoxin promoted a brisk diuresis of her ascites. A side-to-side portacaval shunt was constructed on March 12, 1969. Just prior to and at the close of operation, two units of platelet concentrates were rapidly infused to compensate for thrombocytopenia. During the procedure 1000 ml. of platelet-rich plasma was administered to supply additional platelets and prothrombin factors. The patient tolerated the surgical procedure well and only a transient rise in bilirubin occurred postoperatively. Following portal decompression the hypersplenic thrombocytopenia spontaneously improved.

Ascites did not recur despite the discontinuance of diuretic therapy.

CARDIORESPIRATORY DYNAMICS IN CIRRHOSIS

Arterial oxyhemoglobin saturation and oxygen tension are frequently low with advanced cirrhosis (Fritts, 1963). This seems primarily due to intrapulmonary shunts and communications between the portal and pulmonary venous systems, although disturbances in ventilation-perfusion relationships may be important in some patients. This venoarterial admixture has been reported to be equivalent to as much as 9 per cent of cardiac output (Mellemgaard et al., 1963). Cardiac output is usually increased with cirrhosis and has been measured as high as 15 liters per minute with severe hepatic insufficiency. Cardiac output or cardiac index are inversely related to reduced peripheral resistance. Table 15-1 summarizes some of the commonly observed cardiorespiratory disturbances accompanying cirrhosis together with frequently associated physical signs. The cause and effect interrelationship of these factors has not been well documented, but there can be no doubt that marked deviations from the norm often exist.

Even with our imperfect understanding of the pathogenesis of these abnormalities, some conclusions may be entertained. Increased "stroke work" is demanded of the myocardium in many patients with cirrhosis. When the stress of operation is added,

TABLE 15-1.   Abnormalities in Cardiorespiratory Physiology Common in Patients with Cirrhosis

Abnormalities Frequently Observed		Associated Pathophysiology	Common Physical Signs
Arterial oxygen tension and oxyhemoglobin saturation	↓	Portopulmonary and intrapulmonary shunts	Cyanosis, clubbing of fingers
Arteriovenous oxygen difference	↓	Arteriolar or capillary shunts	Palmar erythemia, spider telangiectasia
Total peripheral resistance	↓	Systemic and splanchnic arteriovenous shunts	Tendency to hypotension, hypertension unusual, widened pulse pressure
Cardiac output	↑	Low peripheral resistance Expanded plasma volume	Systolic ejection murmur, short circulation time, rapid pulse
Plasma volume	↑	Increased total body sodium and water, secondary aldosteronism, low peripheral resistance	Edema, ascites, high output cardiac failure if severe

cardiac failure may occur, especially if primary myocardial disease is also present (Greenspan and DelGuercio, 1968). The administration of ionotropic agents, such as digitalis or isoproterenol, and reduction in plasma volume by diuresis of sodium and water seem logical to support the failing heart. Postoperative hypoventilation or pneumonitis will likely further reduce oxygen saturation. The administration of nasal oxygen, or at times even a tracheostomy and respirator, may be necessary to maintain acceptable oxygen-saturation levels. Ideally, treatment should be monitored by serial blood gases. The true efficacy of these measures awaits confirmation.

BLOOD COAGULATION AND CIRRHOSIS

Surgeons caring for jaundiced patients should be cognizant of the common defects in blood coagulation associated with liver disease if hemorrhagic complications are to be anticipated and prevented (Deutsch, 1965; Penner, 1969).

The liver is essential for the synthesis of the "prothrombin group" of coagulation factors, that is, Factors II, VII, IX, and X. All of these factors require vitamin K to maintain normal levels, and they are frequently deficient in patients with liver disease. Vitamin K supplementation may reverse this deficiency if hepatic function is adequate. These factors are stable and the administration of large quantities of stored blood or plasma or a concentrate of prothrombin factors, which has recently become available, will temporarily replenish deficiencies. Factor V may also be reduced with severe liver disease. This factor is labile, and its activity will disappear from stored plasma in the period of a few days. Fresh plasma or blood is required for replacement. Factor XIII is reduced in 45 per cent of patients with cirrhosis. It is stable and can be replaced by stored blood or plasma. Table 15-2 lists the clotting factors important in liver disease, together with more complete current recommendations for specific replacement therapy.

Spontaneous hemorrhage will not occur in liver disease unless the prothrombin group of clotting factors are below 10 per cent of normal activity, or unless the defi-ciency is accompanied by another defect, such as severe deficiency in Factor V or significant thrombocytopenia. About 75 per cent of patients with hepatic cirrhosis have abnormal coagulation mechanisms, but clinical experience indicates that a spontaneous hemorrhagic diathesis develops infrequently.

Surgical dissection, however, inevitably produces many raw surfaces, which may continue to bleed with less severe coagulation abnormalities. A coagulation survey will indicate which abnormalities need correction. Fresh blood or plasma contains all the coagulation factors, including platelets, but combinations of blood products and platelet packs are more effective and avoid overexpanding blood volume or overtaxing the resources of a blood bank. Usually it is much easier to prevent a hemorrhagic diathesis than to reverse it. Consequently, blood products are often best utilized immediately prior to, during, and just after a surgical procedure. The objective of treatment is to raise rapidly the concentration of circulating clotting factors to a threshold that permits firm clot formation; effective concentrations cannot be reached if replacement is suboptimal or the rate of administration is too slow.

Occasionally a fibrinolytic and rarely an intravascular coagulation syndrome will be encountered in the surgical patient with liver disease. Patients with cirrhosis are prone to increased fibrinolysis because the diseased liver fails to clear fibrinolysin activators. A tendency toward intravascular coagulation may be related to the reduced levels of antithrombin and antithromboplastin accompanying cirrhosis. The differential diagnosis between these two disorders is not only difficult but also urgent, since divergent forms of therapy are required. Here the assistance of a hematologist is most helpful. A precipitous drop in blood platelets supports the diagnosis of intravascular coagulation. The administration of platelets and heparin is the treatment of choice. Circulating fibrinogen may be absent or reduced in either syndrome, so the differential diagnosis depends upon clinical judgment as well as evidence of increased fibrinolytic activity. When a fibrinolytic syndrome occurs, the administration of fibrinogen will raise fibrinogen levels and epsilon-aminocaproic acid will block fibrinolytic activity. Management of a patient

TABLE 15-2.   Clotting Factors Important in Cirrhosis*

Clotting factors	Synonym	With cirrhosis	Laboratory tests	Replacement therapy
Platelets		Moderate to severe decrease	Platelet count decreased, poor clot retraction	4 to 6 units of platelet concentrates
Prothrombin complex		Moderate to severe decrease	Prothrombin time and partial thromboplastin time prolonged	500 ml. of plasma or 10 units per pound of prothrombin complex (Konye-Cutter Laboratory)
II	Prothrombin			
VII	Serum prothrombin conversion acceler-ator (SPCA)			
IX	Christmas factor, plasma thrombo-plastin component (PTC)			
X	Stuart factor			
V	Accelerator globulin labile factor	Slight to moderate decrease, rarely significant	Prothrombin time and partial thromboplastin time prolonged	500 ml. of *fresh* plasma
XIII	Fibrin stabilizing factor	Moderate decrease, rarely significant	Clot soluble in dilute acid or urea	500 ml. of plasma
Fibrinogen		Slight decrease, in-significant unless very low	All clotting tests pro-longed if very low	6 to 8 gm. fibrinogen (Merck Company)
Fibrinolysin	Plasmin	Increased in some cases	Euglobulin lysin time shortened	10 mg. per pound of epsilon-aminocaproic acid every 2 to 4 hours

*The coagulation mechanism may be surveyed with a platelet count, prothrombin time, and partial thromboplastin time. If platelets are low then clot retraction is measured. Platelets should be supplied if the platelet count is below 50,000/mm.³, or below 100,000 mm.³ when clot retraction is poor. Deficiencies in prothrombin complex should always be corrected. The euglobulin lysis time is determined if fibrinolysins are suspected. (See text for discussion of fibrinolytic and intravascular coagulation syndromes.)

with liver disease and a coagulation defect is illustrated in Figure 15-5 and discussed in the accompanying case history.

PROTEIN AND CARBOHYDRATE METABOLISM IN CIRRHOSIS

The liver is the site of the synthesis of albumin, prothrombin component, and other essential proteins (Coon and Iob, 1964; Sherlock, 1968). The liver stores glucose by synthesizing glycogen and helps main-tain normal blood glucose concentrations by the slow release of glucose from its gly-cogen depot. With hepatic insufficiency defects in the metabolism of amino acids, the synthesis of urea from ammonia, and the production of energy-rich phosphates

by metabolism of glucose through the Krebs tricarboxylic cycle have been well docu-mented. Clinical manifestations of these derangements include a low-fasting blood sugar, an abnormal glucose tolerance curve, low serum albumin, muscle wasting, chronic hepatic encephalopathy, ammonium intoxi-cation, and a hemorrhagic diathesis. Occa-sionally hypoglycemia will be an early manifestation of impending hepatic coma.

No attempt will be made to describe in detail the biochemistry of these abnor-malities in these paragraphs. However, appreciation of the key role the liver plays in carbohydrate and protein metabolism provides the rationale for currently recom-mended therapy of patients with hepatic insufficiency. Glucose (or fructose or galac-tose) should be supplied in liberal amounts to prevent hypoglycemia, encourage glyconeogenesis, and provide substrate for adenosine triphosphate production through the Krebs cycle. Protein is needed for synthesis of albumin, hepatic enzymes, and other liver proteins, as well as for regeneration of hepatocytes if necrosis has occurred. Some authorities prefer to withhold protein from the jaundiced patient for fear of inducing encephalopathy and overtaxing the impaired pathways of protein metabolism. We prefer to provide 20 to 40 grams of dietary protein or intravenous albumin daily if there is no evidence of impending coma and to increase protein feeding to low normal levels, that is, 1.0 to 1.5 gm./kg. per day, as tolerated by the patient. In 1937 Patek demonstrated that feeding a nutritious diet, containing approximately 3600 calories, 139 gm. of protein, 175 gm. of fat, 365 gm. of carbohydrate, and vitamin supplements, was beneficial in the treatment of cirrhosis, but usually a well-balanced, normal diet will suffice (Patek, 1937). If coma appears, protein feeding is stopped and intestinal antibiotics and purgatives are administered to reduce bacterial production of ammonia in the gut.

RENAL FAILURE AND HEPATIC CIRRHOSIS

Oliguric renal failure may occur in the terminal phases of hepatic insufficiency. The term "hepatorenal syndrome" has been used to describe this association. However, no definite relationship between hepatic and renal function has been established and the concept implied by this expression may divert attention away from the identification of other specific etiologies for oliguria. Cardiac failure, hypovolemia secondary to variceal hemorrhage, septicemia with hypotension, and fluid and electrolyte imbalances are common causes for oliguria that may accompany cirrhosis. Appropriate specific therapy is required to permit recovery of renal function in these situations.

There remains a group of patients with advanced cirrhosis who become oliguric without any identifiable specific etiology (Baldus and Summerskill, 1968; Tristani and Cohen, 1967). Progressive ascites formation, hyponatremia approximating 120 mEq. per liter, and signs of hepatic precoma or coma characterize this condition. Injudicious removal of large quantities of

ascitic fluid by paracentesis may induce this clinical picture. Usually blood urea nitrogen is elevated and may even be disproportionately high compared to serum creatinine. In a few instances, presumably because of a severe impairment in the ornithine-citrulline-arginine metabolic cycle, blood urea nitrogen remains low. Renal histology is near normal in these patients and the pathogenesis of this form of renal failure has not been delineated. A low effective circulating blood volume or intrarenal shifts in blood flow away from the cortex and to the medulla of the kidney are currently the most plausible theories to explain the association of hepatic and renal failure. Ascites-induced increased renal vein pressure and partial obstruction of the inferior vena cava by a hypertrophied caudate lobe of the liver have also been implicated as causative factors. Cadaveric kidneys, obtained from donors who expired in hepatic and renal failure, have functioned promptly after being transplanted into uremic recipients. Cross-circulation between a patient with profound hepatic coma and oliguria and a normal baboon resulted in a temporary recovery of renal function in one reported experience. These latter two observations suggest that these kidneys are capable of normal function in the absence of hepatic failure.

The combination of hepatic and renal failure portends a high mortality. Management consists of correction of any underlying specific etiology and institution of a hepatic and renal failure regimen in the hope that renal function will return. Since most of these patients have elevated total body sodium and water, hyponatremia is best corrected by fluid restriction. Occasionally, with very low serum sodium, the cautious administration of hypertonic saline solutions may be indicated. Sometimes diuresis will be augmented by the use of intravenous mannitol. The usual indications for hemodialysis apply, but here the salvage rate is low despite correction of electrolyte imbalances and removal of waste products.

PORTAL DECOMPRESSION AND HEPATIC CIRRHOSIS

About one-third of patients with hepatic cirrhosis experience hemorrhage from gastroesophageal varices. Occasionally hepatic cirrhosis will be complicated by ascites that is intractable to vigorous medical therapy. These two complications of portal hypertension constitute the major indications for surgical construction of a portosystemic shunt. Commonly these complications do not occur unless cirrhosis is advanced. Survival statistics after development of a major complication of cirrhosis support this view. For instance, the probability of surviving five years after the discovery of esophageal varices is about 5 per cent (Fig. 15-6) (Garceau et al., 1963). Surgeons who manage these patients accept responsibility for performing a major operation in a patient with a diseased essential organ. Proper selection, preparation, and postoperative management are required if morbidity and mortality are to be kept to a minimum.

Operative mortality and longevity following construction of a portosystemic shunt are directly related to preoperative hepatic reserve. However, there is no single laboratory test of hepatic function that correlates well with prognosis. At the University of Michigan we have used a combination of laboratory tests and clinical features to classify patients according to hepatic reserve (Table 15-3). This classification system does separate patients into three distinct prognostic groups. For instance, in a recent analysis of our own experience with portocaval shunts in 102 cases of hepatic cirrhosis, the five-year probability of survival was 42 per cent for good risk (Class A), 33 per cent for moderate risk (Class B), and 18 per cent for poor risk (Class C) patients. These results include operative mortality (Fig. 15-6) (Turcotte et al., 1969).

Hyperbilirubinemia will almost invariably appear or increase in patients with cirrhosis who are recovering from a shunt. The depth of jaundice can be related to the preoperative hepatic reserve. Figure 15-7 shows a varying response of patients with cirrhosis undergoing portal decompression, dependent upon estimated hepatic reserve. Although a threshold level of hyperbilirubinemia cannot be selected from this data to predict the onset of hepatic coma, clearly the higher the bilirubin concentration the greater the chance of impending hepatic failure. A distressful and not uncommon sequence of events is for poor-risk patients to do well for 7 to 10 days and then slowly slip into hepatic coma and renal failure with deepening jaundice and progressive ascites accumulation, from which they do not usually recover.

The prevention and treatment of these complications requires the application of the principles discussed in the first part of this section. Preoperative evaluation should include not only liver function studies but clinical and laboratory estimates of cardiac, pulmonary, and renal status. Serum electrolytes and blood coagulation surveys are important. Diuresis by sodium restriction and the use of thiazides, aldosterone blocking agents, or furosemide singly or in combination, is indicated when ascites or edema is present. Proper diuresis of excess water and sodium greatly facilitates fluid and electrolyte management in the postoperative period. Reduction in blood volume reduces demands on cardiac work. Potassium supplementation may be helpful, especially when serum potassium is low. Digitalis is administered preoperatively if there is a history of congestive heart failure, residual edema or ascites, or evidence of myocardial or cardiac valvular disease.

Blood and blood products are used on the day of operation to prevent the development of a hemorrhagic diathesis when coagulation studies indicate the probability that this complication will develop. A central venous

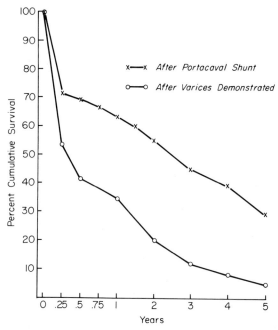

Figure 15-6. Cumulative survival in 102 patients at the University of Michigan with cirrhosis after the construction of a portacaval shunt, and 467 patients in Boston after the detection of esophageal varices (Garceau et al., 1963; Turcotte et al., 1969).

TABLE 15-3. Estimating Hepatic Reserve: Laboratory and Clinical Criteria[*]

Criteria	Good Risk A	Moderate Risk B	Poor Risk C
Serum bilirubin (mg/100 ml)	Below 2.0	2.0–3.0	Over 3.0
Serum albumin (gm/100 ml)	Over 3.5	3.0–3.5	Under 3.0
Ascites	None	Easily controlled	Not easily controlled
Encephalopathy	None	Minimal	Advanced
Nutrition	Excellent	Good	Poor

[*]Operative mortality and longevity can be predicted from these criteria for groups of patients with cirrhosis who require a portosystemic shunt (Turcotte et al., 1969).

pressure catheter together with urine output and vital signs are useful guides to fluid therapy. During operation and the first 48 hours postoperatively, sequestered fluid losses are replaced conservatively with balanced electrolyte solution. After this period usually no additional sodium is required, since sequestered sodium and water become available as

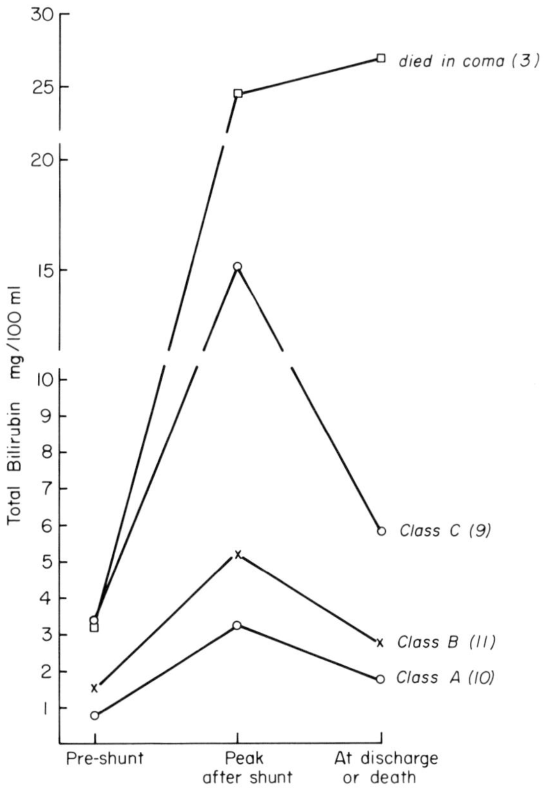

Figure 15-7. Serum bilirubin concentrations in patients with cirrhosis undergoing portacaval shunts dependent upon hepatic reserve (Table 15-3). The number of patients in each group is in parentheses. Cases were selected in which no factor other than hepatic decomposition was detected to account for the change in bilirubin concentration.

edema fluid is mobilized. Mannitol is a convenient intravenous diuretic which causes excretion of relatively greater proportions of water than sodium and thus tends to correct hyponatremia. During and after operation the liver is supported by the administration of liberal amounts of glucose. We also customarily administer 25 gm. of serum albumin daily when serum albumin is low. This improves intravascular oncotic pressure and supplies protein. Albumin administration is stopped if signs of encephalopathy appear. Obviously all of these supportive measures must be adjusted to the individual patient and circumstance. It is these judgments that require appreciation of the derangements in physiology which accompany hepatic insufficiency. Figure 15-5 illustrates the application of these principles.

SUMMARY

Jaundice has been considered in this section as only one of the more visible signs of hepatic insufficiency. The measures described to support the patient with a diseased liver are at best only partially effective. Newer experimental modes of therapy, such as exchange transfusion, hemodialysis or cross (parabiotic) dialysis, and cross-circulation, may prove to be more efficacious, but properly controlled clinical studies are needed to answer this question. Presently, correction of the physiologic and metabolic abnormalities known to accompany cirrhosis would seem to be the most rational approach to the management of the jaundiced patient with hepatocellular disease.

REFERENCES

Part II

Baldus, W. P., and Summerskill, W. H. J.: The kidney in hepatic disease. *In* Diseases of the Liver. New York, McGraw-Hill Book Company, 1968, pp.107-117.

Bengmark, S.: Liver Surgery. *In* Progress in Surgery. v. 6, New York, S. Karger, 1968, pp. 2–59.

Casey, T. H., Summerskill, W. H. J., Bickford, R. G., and Rosevear, J. W.: Body and serum potassium in liver disease. Gastroenterology, 48:208-215, 1965.

Coon, W. W., and Job, V. L.: The Liver and Protein Metabolism. *In* Child, C. G., 3rd (ed.): Liver and Portal Hypertension. Philadelphia, W. B. Saunders Company, 1964, pp. 127–151.

Deutsch, E.: Blood coagulation changes in liver diseases. Progr. Liver Dis., 2:69–83, 1965.

Facts on the Major Killing and Crippling Diseases in the U.S. Today. National Health Education Committee, Inc.: New York, New York, 1966.

Fritts, H. W., Jr.: Systemic circulatory adjustments in hepatic disease. Med. Clin. N. Amer., 47:563–578, 1963.

Garceau, A. J., Chalmers, T. C. et al.: The natural history of cirrhosis. New Eng. J. Med., 268:469–473, 1963.

Greenspan, M., and Del Guercio, L. R. M.: Cardiorespiratory determinants of survival in cirrhotic patients requiring surgery for portal hypertension. Amer. J. Surg., 115:43–56, 1968.

Laragh, J. H., and Ames, R. B.: Physiology of body water and electrolytes in hepatic disease. Med. Clin. N. Amer., 47:587–606, 1963.

Mellemgaard, K., Winkler, K., Tygstrup, N., and Georg, J.: Sources of venoarterial admixture in portal hypertension. J. Clin. Invest., 42:1399, 1963.

Orloff, M. J., Halasz, N. A., Lipman, C., Schwabe, A. D., Thompson, J. C., and Weidner, W. A.: The complications of cirrhosis of the liver. Ann. Intern. Med., 66:165–198, 1967.

Patek, A. J., Jr.: Treatment of alcoholic cirrhosis of the liver with high vitamin therapy. Proc. Soc. Exper. Biol. Med., 37:329, 1937.

Penner, J. A.: Blood Coagulation Laboratory Manual. Department of Postgraduate Medicine, University of Michigan Medical Center, 1969.

Powell, L. W.: Bilirubin metabolism and jaundice with special reference to unconjugated hyperbilirubinemia. Aust. Ann. Med., 16:343–357, 1967.

Sherlock, S.: Diseases of the Liver and Biliary System. Philadelphia, F. A. Davis Co., 1968.

Tristani, F. E., and Cohn, J. N.: Systemic and renal hemodynamics in oliguric hepatic failure: Effect of volume expansion. J. Clin. Invest., 46:1894–1906, 1967.

Turcotte, J. G., Wallin, V. W., Jr., and Child, C. G. 3rd: End-to-side versus side-to-side portacaval shunts in patients with hepatic cirrhosis. Amer. J. Surg., 117:108–116, 1969.

PART III.
Controversial Postoperative Jaundice

by CHARLES G. CHILD III, M.D.

Each year active surgical services that record the postoperative complications of their patients usually identify a number of patients who become jaundiced early or late after operation. In this section we will consider the records of 20 such patients. These have been culled from the files of our Department of Surgery not only to study the nature of their jaundice, but also in the hope that by reviewing them in detail something can be learned of this complication in cases in which its etiology was not readily apparent. Only one of these patients had cirrhosis of the liver, and none showed evidence of serious disease of the extrahepatic biliary tract. Eleven of these patients died in hepatic failure, while nine survived their bout of jaundice.

GENERAL OBSERVATIONS

Among these patients are a few whose signs and symptoms of hepatic failure were so classic that a diagnosis of fulminating hepatic necrosis was made before death. In a few jaundice was prolonged, and even critical study of necropsy and biopsy material and of their clinical courses did not fully disclose the etiology of their hepatic failure. In several the cause of the jaundice still remains wholly in doubt. Blood sugar levels below 44 mg. per 100 ml. were obtained in four patients (Deaths No. 1, 2, 5, and 8) and these results alerted us to the possibility of severe liver disease. A low or normal blood urea nitrogen in the face of high serum creatinine levels occurred in only one patient [Death No. 5]. We were perhaps disappointed that these two features of hepatic failure were not more prominent. Two explanations for this seem reasonable: One, glucose infusions are such an intimate part of postoperative care that hypoglycemia simply never became obvious; two, renal failure was such a consistent accompaniment of hepatic failure that nitrogen retention, in the blood urea form, always had an opportunity to appear. Apparently these classic concomitants, hypoglycemia and low or normal blood urea nitrogen, are rare clinically, for massive hepatic necrosis seldom appears rapidly enough to yield these signs with any regularity. High SGOT levels (1000 to 4000) were encountered in six patients who died and lesser increases (200 to 500) were seen in two similar patients. Among those who recovered, only two patients had high SGOT levels, while lesser increases were encountered in two other patients.

Serum bilirubin levels were consistently higher (3.3 mg. per 100 ml. to 52.0 mg. per 100 ml., with an average of 27.0 mg. per 100 ml.) in the patients who died. Among the survivors this serum value averaged 17 mg. per 100 ml. Those who died within a matter of a few days never developed high serum bilirubin levels (3.3 mg. per 100 ml. to 10.0 mg. per 100 ml.). Thus, these individuals never had time to develop the deep jaundice of those patients with more protracted illnesses. Renal failure (as judged from oliguria, elevated blood urea nitrogen, and serum creatinine) appeared terminally in all except four of the deaths. Slides of the microscopic sections of the kidneys of these patients failed to confirm the notion that their kidneys were badly damaged. The most consistent renal picture was one of glomeruli devoid of blood. This indicated a failure of renal perfusion rather than specific renal disease. In short, the degree of renal damage was less than that of hepatic damage in these patients. Transient renal failure was a problem in only one of seven survivors.

SPECIFIC OBSERVATIONS: DEATHS

Among the 11 patients who died, halothane anesthesia materialized as the most logical etiologic agent in six. The detailed protocols of these patients are summarized here with regard to diagnosis, number of operations, and types of anesthesias.

DEATH NO. 1

Here a tetralogy of Fallot was corrected on cardiopulmonary bypass under halothane. Later that same day the chest had to be re-explored for hemorrhage. This also was performed under halothane. This patient was well for ten days, then developed fever, delirium, coma, and jaundice. He died within 18 days of his first operation. His liver cells were diffusely necrotic. (See Figures 15-8 and 15-9.)

HALOTHANE (Death No. 1)

Date	Clinical Observations	Course of Illness (in days)	Serum Bilirubin (mg./100 ml.)	Blood Glucose (mg./100 ml.)	SGOT (Units/ml.)	BUN (mg./100 ml.)	Serum Creatinine (mg./100 ml.)
8/13/68	Admission		0.8		16	21	1.6
8/15/68	Tetralogy of Fallot corrected on cardiopulmonary bypass under halothane	1					
	Chest re-explored for hemorrhage under halothane						
8/25/68	Fever Temp. = 103° to 104° F.	10 12					
	Delirium	14	3.0	44		33	3.5
	Coma	16	6.5		1500	36	4.5
	Death	18	10.5			42	6.6

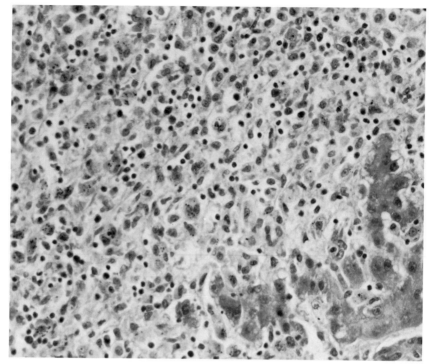

Figure 15-8. Liver (Death #1). In the necropsy specimen of this patient's liver the hepatic cells are diffusely necrotic, particularly in the peripheral zones. Interpretation of this specimen is difficult, for the pathologic picture can readily be interpreted as due either to halothane or to viral hepatitis. Since he died 18 days after two administrations of halothane anesthesias and cardiopulmonary bypass using whole blood, the proper etiologic interpretation favors halothane.

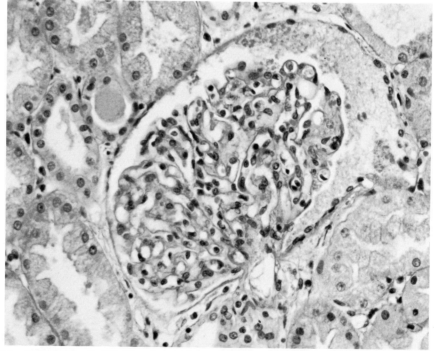

Figure 15-9. Kidney (Death #1). The glomeruli are diffusely ischemic and glomerular capillaries are swollen. Bowman's capsular spaces contain diffuse amorphous precipitate. There are rare bile casts. Renal failure, though evident terminally, did not seem to play a major role in this patient's death. His demise was much more hepatic than renal.

COMMENT

In this man, aged 20, cyanosis secondary to tetralogy of Fallot had been present since birth. His operation was uneventful but he had to be re-explored twelve hours later because of hemorrhage. Both operations were done under halothane. He was well for 10 days. He then developed fever, coma, jaundice, and renal failure, and he died.

FORMULATION

At necropsy the glomeruli were ischemic with marked glomerular precipitate within Bowman's capsular space. The liver was diffusely necrotic. This was interpreted as being due to halothane.

DEATH NO. 2

This patient's uneventful cholecystectomy was performed under halothane. At the time of operation her liver was grossly and microscopically normal. Two weeks later she became jaundiced, and died 24 days after operation. At postmortem examination her liver was diffusely necrotic. (See Figures 15-10, 15-11, and 15-12.)

HALOTHANE (Death No. 2)

Date	Clinical Observations	Course of Illness (in days)	Serum Bilirubin (mg./100 ml.)	Blood Glucose (mg./100 ml.)	SGOT (Units/ml.)	BUN (mg./100 ml.)	Serum Creatinine (mg./100 ml.)
11/20/60	Admission	1					
11/22/60	Cholecystectomy	2					
	Biopsy of liver	4					
	under halothane	6					
11/28/60	Recovered; discharged	8					
		16	11.8	43		62	
		18	19.0		150		
	Jaundice	20	13.0				
	Coma	22					
	Death	24					

COMMENT

This patient was admitted for a routine cholecystectomy. Her past history included many allergies. She recovered and was discharged on her eighth postoperative day only to be admitted one week later, jaundiced, in a coma, and in renal failure.

LIVER BIOPSY

No real liver disease, although mild centrilobular fatty infiltrates were present.

NECROPSY

Extensive necrosis of the liver. Glomerular ischemia with amorphous precipitate in glomerular and tubular spaces.

FORMULATION

This death was thought to result from halothane sensitivity.

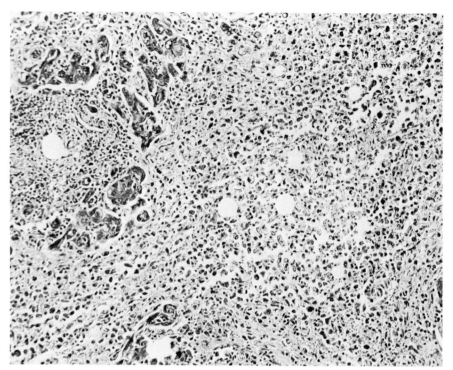

Figure 15-10.   Liver (Death #2). Twenty-two days after an uneventful cholecystectomy under halothane this patient's liver is diffusely necrotic.

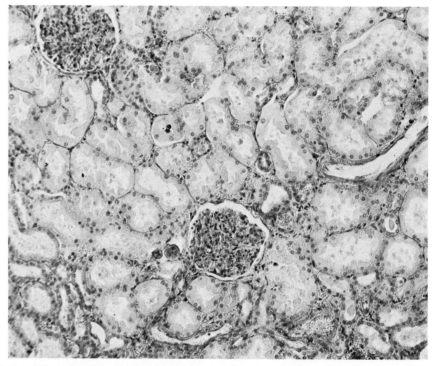

Figure 15-11.   Kidney (Death #2). The glomeruli are ischemic and there is some amorphous precipitate in both the glomerular spaces and in the tubules. Although this patient's renal function failed terminally, this is not the microscopic picture of severe renal disease. These are relatively normal kidneys. The changes reflect poor perfusion during this patient's terminal hours. The cause of death is hepatic, not renal, failure.

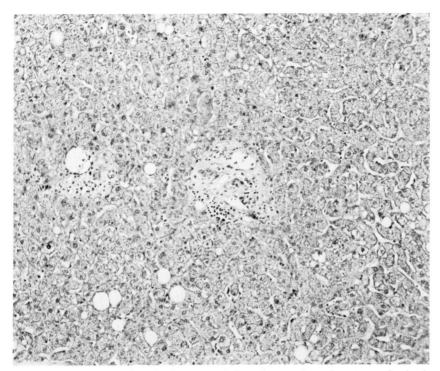

Figure 15-12.   Liver biopsy (Death #2). This patient's liver biopsy, 3 weeks prior to death, shows only slight fatty infiltrates and mild centrilobular fibrosis.

DEATH NO. 3

Again, this patient's uneventful cholecystectomy was performed under halothane. One month later she was in hepatic failure and she died 60 days after operation. Her liver at post-mortem was diffusely necrotic. (See Figures 15-13, 15-14, and 15-15.)

HALOTHANE (Death No. 3)

Date	Clinical Observations	Course of Illness (in days)	Serum Bilirubin (mg./100 ml.)	Blood Glucose (mg./100 ml.)	SGOT (Units/ml.)	BUN (mg./100 ml.)	Serum Creatinine (mg./100 ml.)
8/2/61	Admission	1					
		10	0.5	87			
8/22/61	Cholecystectomy and liver biopsy under halothane	15					
8/30/61	"T" tube cholangiogram	25					
	Chills, fever, acutely ill	30	1.6				
		35	14.0				
	Patient now chronically ill	40	32.4	90	330	5	
		45	30.6		130	21	
	Patient now comatose	50	42.4			25	1.5
	Death	60	52.0			45	

COMMENT

This elderly patient underwent an uneventful cholecystectomy under halothane. She did well for 10 days, but then began to develop progressive hepatic and renal failure. Her liver at the time of operation was normal except for mild cholangitis.

NECROPSY

Liver showed massive hepatic necrosis (halothane sensitivity).
Kidney evidenced ischemic glomeruli with some precipitate in the glomerular capsule. The renal failure appears to be more of a terminal event, since it occurred many days after hepatic failure.

CONCLUSION

An example, in our opinion, of slowly developing hepatic necrosis secondary to halothane sensitivity.

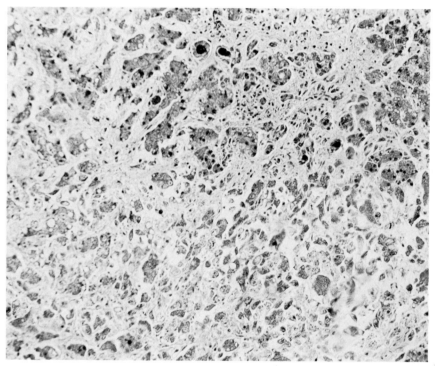

Figure 15-13. Liver (Death #3). Massive necrosis of liver cells. This is believed to be far more characteristic of halothane necrosis than of viral hepatitis.

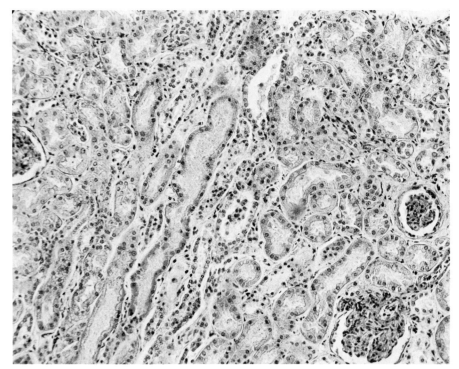

Figure 15-14. Kidney (Death #3). The glomeruli are ischemic, but otherwise this is a reasonably well-preserved kidney. Amorphous precipitate is present in both the glomerular spaces and in the tubules.

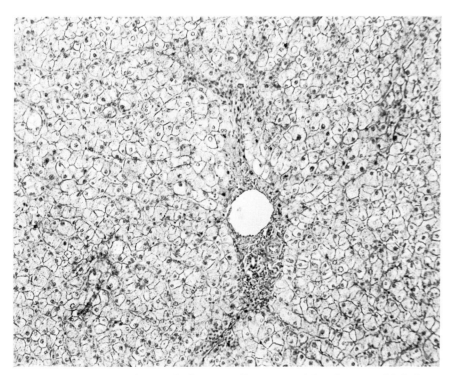

Figure 15-15. Liver biopsy (Death #3). The hepatic cells are normal, but there is mild cholangitis as reflected in round cell infiltrates in the portal triads.

DEATH NO. 4

This patient had two halothane anesthesias a week apart. Three weeks later she was in hepatic failure. She died 51 days after operation. Microscopic study of her liver suggested an early effort at recovery as reflected in regenerating hepatic cells. (See Figures 15-16 and 15-17.)

HALOTHANE (Death No. 4)

Date	Clinical Observations	Course of Illness (in days)	Serum Bilirubin (mg./100 ml.)	Blood Glucose (mg./100 ml.)	SGOT (Units/ml.)	BUN (mg./100 ml.)	Serum Creatinine (mg./100 ml.)
5/1/67	Cystoscopy under halothane	1					
5/6/67	Cholecystectomy under halothane	6					
	Fever 100° to 101° F.	7					
	" " "	8					
	" " "	9					
5/16/67	Recovered; discharged	16					
5/22/67	Jaundice, malaise	22	4.2				
5/31/67	Readmitted to hospital	31					
6/1/67	Patient acutely ill	32	28.0		280	5	
	" " "	37	26.5		240		
	" " "	42	15.5			19	3.7
6/16/67	Patient comatose	47	32.5		380		10.7
6/20/67	Death	51	40.0		200	46	8.8

COMMENT

This patient, aged 37, had two routine procedures under halothane. Some seven weeks later she was deeply jaundiced and in both hepatic and renal failure.

NECROPSY

The liver shows many proliferating bile ducts with obvious beginning cirrhosis. The liver cells appear much better preserved than one should judge from this patient's course. The kidneys are reasonably well preserved but show large numbers of bile casts. The thought is obvious: Had she lived only a few more days, she might have recovered.

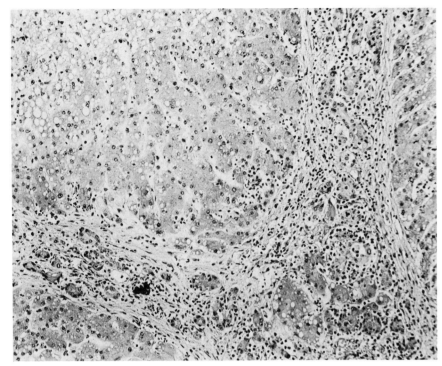

Figure 15-16. Liver (Death #4). The microscopic picture is primarily one of bile duct proliferation with regenerating liver nodules. The fibrosis of the hepatic triads suggests a form of biliary cirrhosis. There is some reason to believe that if this patient could only have been kept alive a week or two longer she might have recovered.

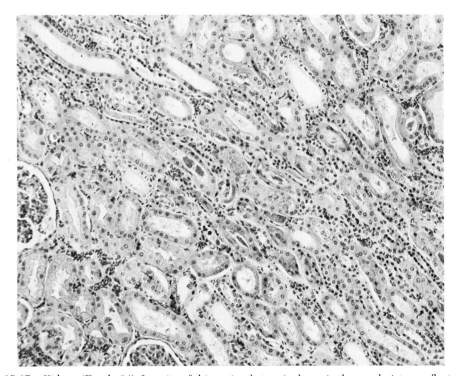

Figure 15-17. Kidney (Death #4). In spite of this patient's terminal anuria the renal picture reflects reasonable preservation. There are large numbers of bile casts consistent with this patient's longstanding jaundice.

DEATH NO. 5

This patient, a known alcoholic, died of massive hepatic necrosis five days after an uneventful gastrectomy under halothane anesthesia. (See Figures 15-18 and 15-19.)

HALOTHANE (Death No. 5)

Date	Clinical Observations	Course of Illness (in days)	Serum Bilirubin (mg./100 ml.)	Blood Glucose (mg./100 ml.)	SGOT (Units/ml.)	BUN (mg./100 ml.)	Serum Creatinine (mg./100 ml.)
3/19/68	Admission Patient in apparent good health						
3/20/68	Subtotal gastrectomy under halothane	1					
3/21/68	Patient well (Temp. = 100° F.)	2		109		12	
3/22/68	Patient acutely ill (Temp. = 102° F.)	3				25	3.5
3/23/68	Patient comatose (Temp. = 103° F.)	4	3.3	20, 20, 30 24, 27, 20	2000 1400	24, 30, 31	6.2
3/24/68	Death	5		100 to 200 by infusions		20	6.9

COMMENT

This patient, aged 56, underwent an uneventful gastrectomy under halothane. There was a long preoperative history of chronic alcoholism. Her fulminating illness was characterized by mild jaundice, low blood-glucose levels, near normal BUN levels and high serum creatinine values. An antemortem diagnosis of massive hepatic necrosis was made.

NECROPSY

Liver showed massive hepatic necrosis. Kidneys showed early destruction of the tubules but the glomeruli were well preserved.

CONCLUSION

A rapidly fatal halothane sensitivity of the liver with renal tubular failure. The clinical clues were low blood sugar and near normal blood urea nitrogen levels in the presence of increased high serum creatinine.

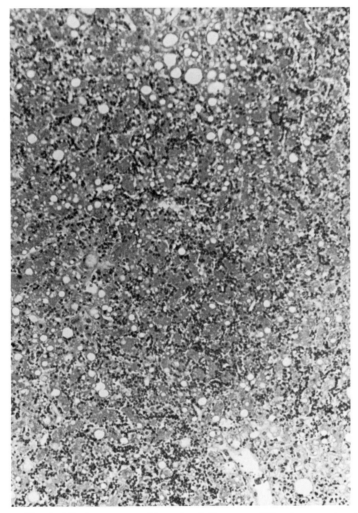

Figure 15-18. Liver (Death #5). At necropsy this patient's liver was diffusely necrotic without evidence of any viable liver cells. Following the administration of halothane, the rapid onset of low blood sugars, normal blood urea nitrogens, and high serum creatinine strongly suggests halothane sensitivity.

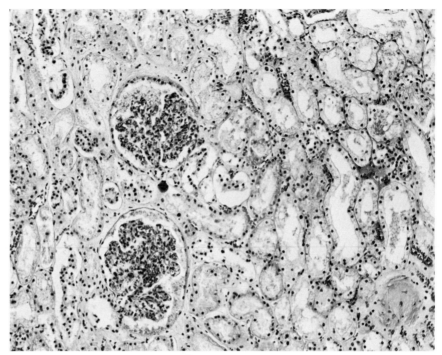

Figure 15-19. Kidney (Death #5). The glomeruli are reasonably well preserved, but the tubules are disrupted. There is amorphous precipitate in the glomerular spaces and in the tubules.

DEATH NO. 6

This patient had three exposures to halothane at approximately monthly intervals. He died in hepatic failure 98 days after his first exposure to halothane. (See Figures 15-20 and 15-21.)

COMMENTS

These six patients (Death Nos. 1, 2, 3, 4, 5, and 6) died five, 18, 24, 51, 60, and 98 days after both single and multiple exposure to halothane. Their operations were not excessively serious and, though blood transfusions were used in several of these patients, the deaths seem more closely related to halothane sensitivity than to any other possible cause.

HALOTHANE (Death No. 6)

Date	Clinical Observations	Course of Illness (in weeks)	Serum Bilirubin (mg./100 ml.)	Blood Glucose (mg./100 ml.)	SGOT (Units/ml.)	BUN (mg./100 ml.)	Serum Creatinine (mg./100 ml.)
10/10/61	Scleral imbrication under pentothal	1					
11/20/61	Scleral imbrication under halothane	5					
1/19/62	Scleral imbrication under halothane	10					
		13	42		1040	Jaundice— coma, urinary failure	
2/7/62	Death	14					

COMMENT

This patient was given three anesthetics—Pentothal, halothane, and halothane for scleral imbrication—and was febrile after none of these. After the third operation he was discharged without complaint. One week later he became jaundiced. Three weeks after his second halothane exposure he died, deeply jaundiced, in a coma, and in renal failure. At necropsy the kidneys were ischemic. The liver showed marked proliferation of bile ducts with early nodular regeneration of hepatic cells.

FORMULATION

It seems reasonable that this patient's first halothane exposure was associated with minimal damage and subsequent regeneration as reflected in regenerating bile ducts and hepatic nodules. Hepatic failure promptly followed the second halothane exposure.

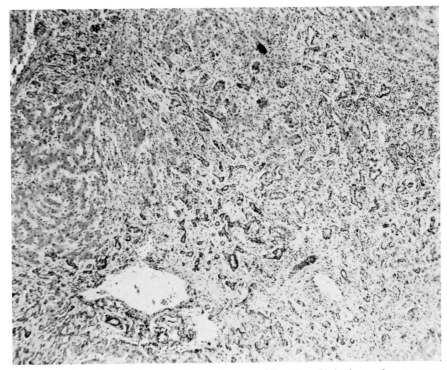

Figure 15-20. Liver (Death #6). This slide demonstrates proliferation of bile ducts, chronic passive congestion, and moderate central necrosis. There is early nodular regeneration with some fairly well preserved hepatic cells. Here again the impression is that if only the patient had survived a few weeks longer he might have recovered.

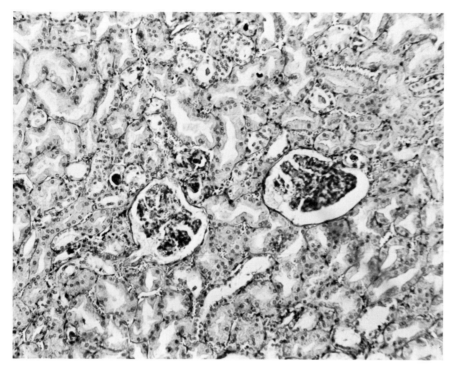

Figure 15-21. Kidney (Death #6). The glomeruli are ischemic but otherwise this kidney is reasonably well preserved.

DEATH NO. 7

This patient had four serious operations, the first of which was under halothane; the succeeding three were performed under cyclopropane. Here both halothane and blood transfusions might be implicated. The microscopic picture of the liver obtained at postmortem, however, suggested neither of these diagnoses. The liver was the site of severe chronic passive congestion with extensive central necrosis. (See Figure 15-22.)

CHRONIC PASSIVE CONGESTION WITH CENTRAL NECROSIS (Death No. 7)

Date	Clinical Observations	Course of Illness (in weeks)	Serum Bilirubin (mg./100 ml.)	Blood Glucose (mg./100 ml.)	SGOT (Units/ml.)	BUN (mg./100 ml.)	Serum Creatinine (mg./100 ml.)
2/15/67	Starr-Edwards valve inserted under fluothane	1		81		18	
2/20/67	Vein graft (superior mesenteric artery) under cyclopropane			100			
2/21/67	Second operation to examine abdomen under cyclopropane		2.5			58	
			3.1				
2/27/67	Small-bowel resection under cyclopropane	2	7.1				
		3	8.0		111	48	
		4	12.0		60	21	
		5	7.0				
3/24/67	Discharged	6	9.6	92	92	22	0.7
		7	7.5		73	45	
		8	26.0		1750	59	0.7
4/15/67	Death	9	45.0		550		

COMMENT

This man, aged 34, had a Starr-Edwards valve inserted under fluothane. His operation was complicated by partial aortic dissection secondary to femoral arterial cannulation. This may have temporarily compromised his hepatic arterial blood flow. He then survived three major abdominal operations all performed under cyclopropane. These were occasioned by superior mesenteric arterial occlusion, the etiology of which was never precisely determined. His entire postoperative course was associated with jaundice, which waxed and waned apparently with the degree of his cardiac compensation.

FORMULATION

At necropsy his liver showed widespread central necrosis, finally interpreted as secondary to chronic passive congestion.

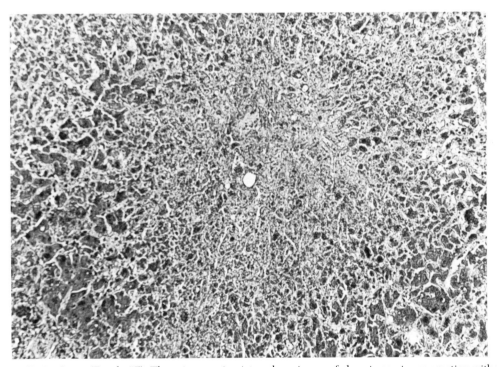

Figure 15-22. Liver (Death #7). The microscopic picture here is one of chronic passive congestion with severe central necrosis of hepatic cells.

DEATH NO. 8

This patient is included to give an example of the deleterious effect that longstanding colitis is thought to have on the liver. This was brought to light in the form of hepatic failure following two serious operations performed under cyclopropane anesthesia. At postmortem examination this patient's liver demonstrated extensive central necrosis. Had these operations been performed under halothane, we are sure that this anesthetic agent would have been assigned an etiologic role in this patient's death. (See Figure 15-23.)

CAUSE UNDETERMINED (Death No. 8)

Date	Clinical Observations	Course of Illness (in weeks)	Serum Bilirubin (mg./100 ml.)	Blood Glucose (mg./100 ml.)	SGOT (Units/ml.)	BUN (mg./100 ml.)	Serum Creatinine (mg./100 ml.)
10/28/68	Admission	1	0.3	114	23	5	1.0
			0.5	102		5	0.8
11/6/68	Colectomy and ileocolostomy						
	under cyclopropane	2					
	Fever (100° to 103° F.)	3					
	Stormy course						
		4	0.5		23	6	1.3
11/25/68	Ileostomy under						
	cyclopropane	5		143		10	1.0
	Fever		0.6	116		5	0.9
	Stormy course	6		10,25,25,10			
			4.4			6.5	0.6
12/7/68	Coma	7	5.2	180 (on glu-		25	1.6
	Death		5.7	cose infusion)			

COMMENT

This man had long-standing granulomatous colitis for which two serious operations were performed under cyclopropane. Hepatic failure was apparent when repeated blood sugars were 10 to 25 mg. per 100 ml. This was associated with low blood urea nitrogens. In spite of vigorous therapy the patient expired in a hepatic coma.

NECROPSY

The liver demonstrated chronic to acute central necrosis. The cause could not be identified.

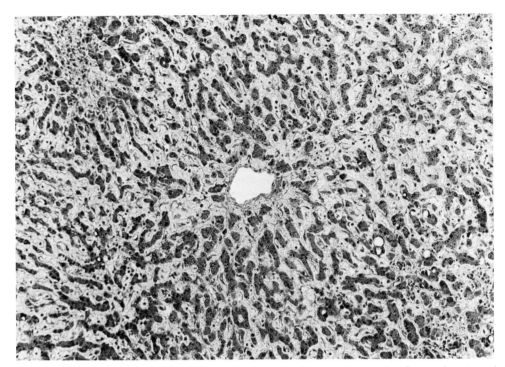

Figure 15-23. Liver (Death #8). The microscopic picture in this case is one of widespread acute and chronic central necrosis. This is not typical of halothane, chronic passive congestion, nor viral hepatitis.

DEATH NO. 9

Perhaps this patient should not be included in this study, for he was deeply jaundiced for many months prior to operation. He was thought to be suffering from viral hepatitis, but was explored to exclude extrahepatic biliary obstruction. A portal venogram (Figure 15-24) and intraoperative cholangiogram (Figure 15-25) were both normal. A liver biopsy demonstrated advanced amyloidosis of his liver with very few viable hepatic cells. His death, in hepatic failure following the stress of operation, was expected. (See Figures 15-24 and 15-25.)

AMYLOIDOSIS (Death No. 9)

Date	Clinical Observations	Course of Illness (in months)	Serum Bilirubin (mg./100 ml.)	Blood Glucose (mg./100 ml.)	SGOT (Units/ml.)	BUN (mg./100 ml.)	Serum Creatinine (mg./100 ml.)
October, 1958	Unexplained jaundice	1	5.0				
		5	7.1				
June, 1959	Admitted Univ. Hospital	9	11.6	100		17	
July, 1959	Exploratory celiotomy and liver biopsy under nitrous oxide and Surital	10 (Preop.	25.4	80		7	0.96
	Death in coma (3 days postop.)	(Postop.)	12.1	92		26	0.9

COMMENT

For nine months this man's jaundice went unexplained. Most clinicians thought that he was suffering from viral hepatitis.

LIVER BIOPSY AND NECROPSY

Demonstrated widespread amyloidosis.

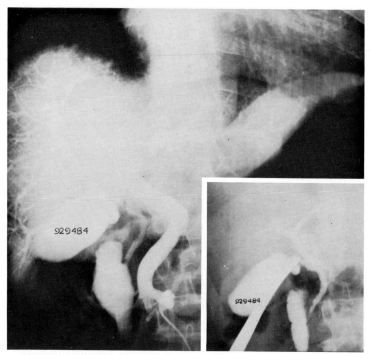

Figure 15-24.   Advanced amyloidosis of the liver. This patient (#9) was jaundiced before operation. Mere exploration of the abdomen, portal venogram, choledochography (*inset photograph*), and biopsy of the liver precipitated fulminant liver failure. He died three days after operation.

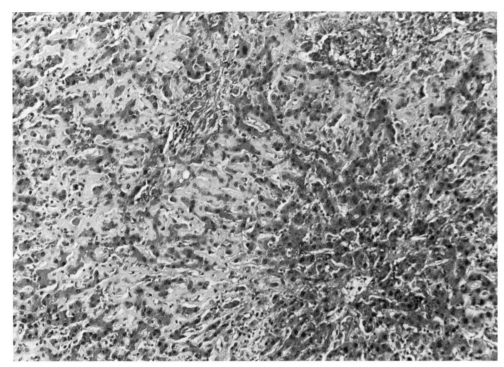

Figure 15-25. Liver (Death #9). Almost literally this patient's hepatic cells have been crowded to death by widespread amyloidosis.

DEATHS NO. 10 AND NO. 11

Of the last five deaths these two seem clearly due to viral hepatitis secondary to transfusion therapy; one died 14, and the other 16, weeks after transfusions of whole blood. Patient No. 10 was exposed to halothane twice for implantation of radium. Furthermore, she was mildly febrile after each procedure. Many might argue that this is a true halothane death. Dr. French, our pathologist, however, believes that the postmortem study of this patient's liver is more consistent with viral hepatitis than with halothane sensitivity. (See Figures 15-26, 15-27, 15-28, and 15-29.)

VIRAL HEPATITIS (Death No. 10)

Date	Clinical Observations	Course of Illness (in weeks)	Serum Bilirubin (mg./100 ml.)	Blood Glucose (mg./100 ml.)	SGOT (Units/ml.)	BUN (mg./100 ml.)	Serum Creatinine (mg./100 ml.)
12/2/66	Transfusions (4), Whole blood	1					
12/24/66	Cystoscopy under nitrous oxide	4					
1/16/67	Radium implant under Fluothane-F Fever (100° F.)	7					
1/30/67	Radium implant under fluothane	9	9.0				
	Fever (100° F.)	10	19.0		1590		
	Fever (103° F.)	11				15	0.9
	Delirium	12	38.0		300	14	1.4
	Coma	13	25.5		475	31	1.1
	Death	14					

COMMENT

This woman, aged 49, had four whole blood transfusions early in December, 1966. Eight and nine weeks later she had two fluothane anesthesias for radium application to the cervix. She then developed a rising serum bilirubin leading to hepatic coma and death. Terminal renal failure also occurred.

FORMULATION

The hepatic picture was one of postnecrotic cirrhosis. It was not considered possible to differentiate between viral hepatitis and fluothane sensitivity. Viral hepatitis, however, was favored. The glomeruli were without blood and there were many bile plugs.

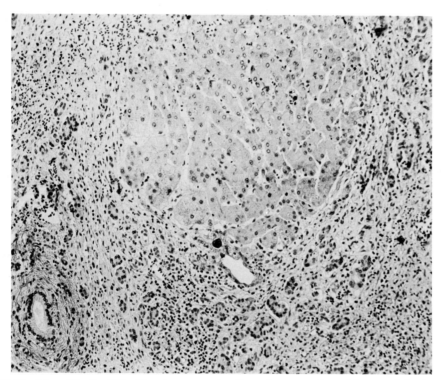

Figure 15-26. Liver (Death #10). Chronic progressive liver disease with proliferating bile ducts, round cell infiltrates, and early nodular regeneration. There are many bile plugs. This patient's prolonged course, following transfusions and two administrations of halothane, suggests either viral hepatitis or halothane sensitivity. Viral hepatitis appears more likely.

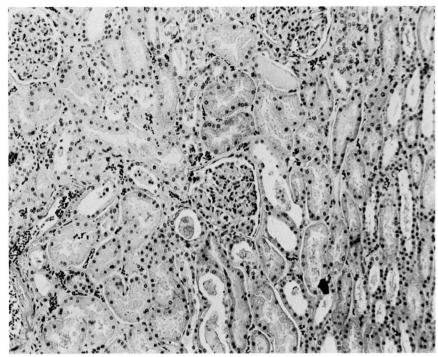

Figure 15-27. Kidney (Death #10). The glomeruli are ischemic and there are many bile plugs, but, otherwise, these kidneys are well preserved.

VIRAL HEPATITIS (Death No. 11)

Date	Clinical Observations	Course of Illness (in weeks)	Serum Bilirubin (mg./100 ml.)	Blood Glucose (mg./100 ml.)	SGOT (Units/ml.)	BUN (mg./100 ml.)	Serum Creatinine (mg./100 ml.)
2/15/68	Abruptio placentae under local anesthesia Transfusion (3), Whole blood	2					
March, 1968	Transient jaundice	4	6.8				
June, 1968		14	9.0		4000		
		15	13.0		3200	11	3.3
	Death—cardiac arrest	16	14.5		161	6	1.7

COMMENT

The liver at necropsy demonstrated marked hepatic necrosis typical of viral hepatitis. There were no viable liver cells. Kidneys were normal.

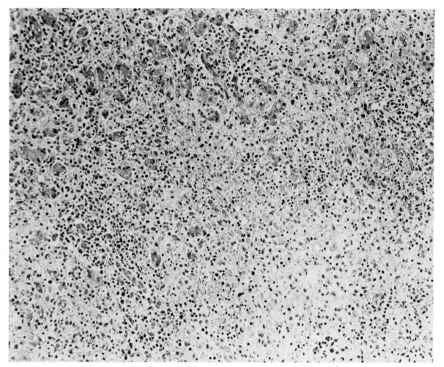

Figure 15-28. Liver (Death #11). The severe hepatic cellular necrosis in this patient leaves little doubt that her death was due to viral hepatitis.

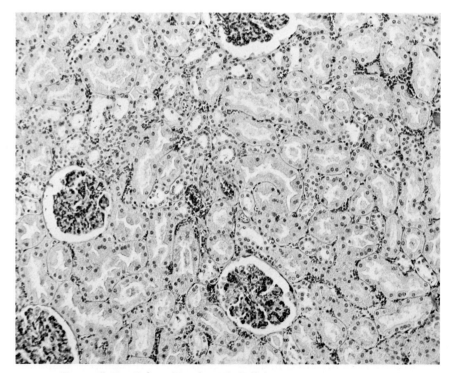

Figure 15-29. Kidney (Death #11). Cellular structure appears normal.

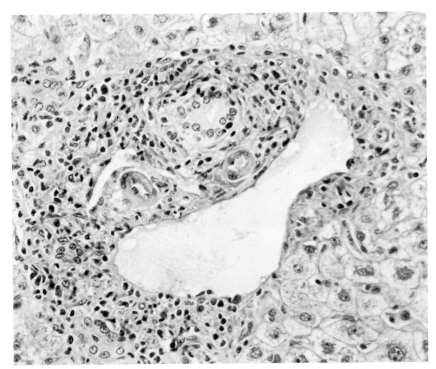

Figure 15-30. Liver (Survivor #3). Microscopic section of this patient's biopsy reflects mild chronic cholangitis. Hepatic cellular structure is normal.

SPECIFIC OBSERVATIONS: SURVIVORS

The charts of nine patients who survived a significant bout of postoperative jaundice have been abstracted. This phase of our study suffers from lack of hepatic tissue to be examined microscopically. The conclusions we have drawn have, therefore, necessarily been based on clinical conjecture. If these cases prove anything, they attest to the numerous choices that are often available as possible explanations for the patient's postoperative jaundice.

SURVIVOR NO. 1

This elderly man was admitted to the hospital for a large tumor in the left upper quadrant. At operation, under nitrous oxide anesthesia, this proved to be a large encapsulated neoplasm arising from the tail of the pancreas. It was resected easily. There was no evidence of metastasis. Postoperatively he became jaundiced, but without evidence of hepatic necrosis (SGOT was 50 to 60 units). There was no biliary tract disease. His jaundice subsided promptly and remains unexplained. Had this operation been performed under halothane this case would most certainly have been classified as one of halothane jaundice.

JAUNDICE OF UNKNOWN ORIGIN (Survivor No. 1)

Date	Clinical Observations	Course of Illness (in days)	Serum Bilirubin (mg./100 ml.)	Blood Glucose (mg./100 ml.)	SGOT (Units/ml.)	BUN (mg./100 ml.)	Serum Creatinine (mg./100 ml.)
9/20/68	Admission	1	0.3	92	42	11	1.1
9/24/68	Resection retroperitoneal tumor	5					
	Under innovar, nitrous oxide, Anectine, and curare	6					
	Jaundiced	9	15.0		60	12	1.2
		15	16.0				
		20	4.6		60	15	1.0
		25	2.1		60	14	0.9
10/19/68	Recovered; discharged	30	0.3		50	14	1.0

COMMENT

This 70-year-old man had a large retroperitoneal tumor of the tail of his pancreas resected without incident. On his fifth postoperative day he was noted to be jaundiced. Slowly this subsided without associated symptoms. His jaundice was never explained and he recovered and was discharged on his 25th postoperative day.

SURVIVOR NO. 2

This patient was explored twice for jaundice, once under halothane and once under nitrous oxide anesthesia. Each time her hepatic drainage system proved to be normal. Both liver biopsies demonstrated typical cholestasis, thought in retrospect to be due to Pyribenzamine. Arguments could readily be provided for excluding this patient from this study. She is included, however, to emphasize that jaundice of this kind may be a benign process as far as surgical intervention is concerned. Patients with it can survive operation quite uneventfully, even under halothane.

PYRIBENZAMINE JAUNDICE (?) (Survivor No. 2)

Date	Clinical Observations	Course of Illness (in months)	Serum Bilirubin (mg./100 ml.)	Blood Glucose (mg./100 ml.)	SGOT (Units/ml.)	BUN (mg./100 ml.)	Serum Creatinine (mg./100 ml.)
September, 1968	Jaundice believed associated with Pyribenzamine taken for allergies	1	15.0		120		
October, 1968	Exploratory celiotomy* under halothane Cholangiogram normal	2	12.2		125		
November, 1968	Exploratory celiotomy* under Demerol, nitrous oxide, and curare						
	Cholangiogram normal	3	10.1		25		
March, 1968		7	1.2		20		

COMMENT

This 71-year-old patient had taken Pyribenzamine for multiple allergies. She was operated upon twice, both times to show that the common duct was not obstructed. Neither halothane nor nitrous oxide intensified her jaundice.

*Both liver biopsies demonstrated typical cholestasis, believed, in retrospect, to be due to Pyribenzamine.

SURVIVOR NO. 3

This patient was jaundiced on admission. Preoperatively this was thought to be due to a common duct stone. At operation, however, the common duct was normal. The gallbladder was removed uneventfully but she became more jaundiced during the immediate postoperative period. A fortuitous liver biopsy demonstrated cholangitis. This probably accounted not only for the preoperative jaundice but the postoperative icteric exacerbation as well. Her elevated serum bilirubin subsided and she recovered and was discharged thirty-five days after operation.

We include this patient to emphasize once again that patients with chronic cholecystitis and cholelithiasis often have ascending cholangitis and jaundice, which do not resolve until the biliary tract disease is corrected, in this case by cholecystectomy. A favorite clinical diagnosis for this kind of patient is that a common duct stone has been recently passed. We believe, as do others, that chronic inflammation of the intrahepatic drainage system is a more logical explanation for jaundice in such patients. The question is often readily intensified by operation.

CHRONIC CHOLECYSTITIS AND CHOLELITHIASIS: CHOLANGITIS AND MULTIPLE ALLERGIES (Survivor No. 3)

Date	Clinical Observations	Course of Illness (in days)	Serum Bilirubin (mg./100 ml.)	Blood Glucose (mg./100 ml.)	SGOT (Units/ml.)	BUN (mg./100 ml.)	Serum Creatinine (mg./100 ml.)
9/29/68	Patient jaundiced on admission	1	8.7	100	800		1.5
			8.0	92			
10/3/68	Cholecystectomy under Penthrane anesthesia— common duct normal, no stones°	5		94			
		6	12.2		200		
	Uneventful post- operative course	8					
		10	10.2				
		15	2.1		800		
		20	1.0				1.6
		30	0.7		84		
11/11/68	Recovered; discharged	40	0.9		50		

COMMENT

This 43-year-old patient with known cholelithiasis was jaundiced on admission. The jaundice was attributed to common duct obstruction. At operation the common duct was normal and without stones. Though the serum bilirubin rose briefly it then subsided to normal and she recovered and was discharged.

°At the time of operation, the liver biopsy demonstrated a very real cholangitis together with bile stasis. Many eosinophiles reflected her long-standing allergies, primarily asthma.

SURVIVOR NO. 4

This patient became mildly jaundiced after insertion of a Starr-Edwards valve under halothane. The jaundice was unassociated with any increase in SGOT or SGPT and the alkaline phosphatase remained normal. He was febrile for the first two to three days after operation. Here there are two logical explanations for his postoperative jaundice—mild chronic passive congestion or equally mild halothane sensitivity. There does not appear to be any way of choosing accurately between these two alternatives.

HALOTHANE SENSITIVITY (Survivor No. 4)

Date	Clinical Observations	Course of Illness (in months)	Serum Bilirubin (mg./100 ml.)	Blood Glucose (mg./100 ml.)	SGOT (Units/ml.)	SGPT (Units/ml.)	Alkaline Phosphat. (King-Armstrong)
October, 1968	Admission		0.3		23	24	12
October, 1968	Starr-Edwards valve inserted under halothane	1					
	Fever (102° F.)	2	7.5		26	22	18
	Fever (101° F.)	3	8.0				
	Jaundiced	5	5.0		50	25	20
		7	3.1		30	25	25
		9	1.0		24	20	10
November, 1968	Recovered; discharged	15	0.8			15	10

COMMENT

Mild postoperative jaundice. This certainly could have been either mild passive congestion or halothane sensitivity.

SURVIVOR NO. 5

This patient had a Starr-Edwards valve inserted on cardiopulmonary bypass under nitrous oxide anesthesia. Two months later she became jaundiced, remaining so for the next two months. An elevation in enzymes and alkaline phosphatase is consistent with a diagnosis of viral hepatitis.

SERUM HEPATITIS (Survivor No. 5)

Date	Clinical Observations	Course of Illness (in months)	Serum Bilirubin (mg./100 ml.)	Blood Glucose (mg./100 ml.)	SGOT (Units/ml.)	SGPT (Units/ml.)	Alkaline Phosphat. (King-Armstrong)
September, 1967	Cardiac decompensation	1	1.4				
October, 1967	" "	2	0.3				
November, 1967	" "	3	1.4				
December, 1967	Starr-Edwards valve inserted under Surital, curare, and nitrous oxide	4	3.0				
January, 1968	Home, well	5					10
February, 1968	Home, well	6					
March, 1968	Jaundiced	7.0	5.0		400	150	8
	"	7.2	10.0		300	125	
	"	7.4	30.0		800	175	30
	"	7.6	30.0		200	200	
	"	7.8	38.0		1000	500	25
April, 1968	"	8.0	40.0		800	400	
May, 1968	Recovered; discharged	9.0	20.0		600	300	10
		9.2	10.0		50	100	10
		9.4	3.0		50	75	10

COMMENT

This patient became jaundiced but not severely ill about two months after her open-heart operation. All studies indicated serum hepatitis as the most logical diagnosis. She recovered slowly and was discharged two months later.

SURVIVOR NO. 6

One recognized cause of postoperative jaundice is shock. Not only was this patient in shock due to a ruptured aortic aneurysm, but, in addition, the aorta had to be clamped at the diaphragm for 25 minutes. Postoperatively he reflected both transient hepatic and renal failure but survived both, recovered, and was discharged from the hospital. Both of these failures can readily be explained upon a basis of poor perfusion in his liver and kidneys. It is perhaps remarkable that his SGOT didn't rise higher.

TRANSIENT HEPATIC AND RENAL FAILURE SECONDARY TO SHOCK (Survivor No. 6)

Date	Clinical Observations	Course of Illness (in days)	Serum Bilirubin (mg./100 ml.)	Blood Glucose (mg./100 ml.)	SGOT (Units/ml.)	BUN (mg./100 ml.)	Serum Creatinine (mg./100 ml.)
5/21/64	Admission Ruptured aortic aneurysm Blood pressure 40/0 Aneurysmectomy Aorta cross-clamped at diaphragm for 25 minutes under morphine, nitrous oxide,	1	1.2	100			
	Anectine, and Surital	2	3.6			33	1.8
		6	7.9				1.6
		8	10.0		126	58	2.3
		10	8.2		130		1.9
		12	6.8			46	1.65
		14	7.2			40	1.7
		16	7.6			40	1.5
		18	3.8			36	1.4
6/18/64	Recovered; discharged	22	1.4			19	0.5

COMMENT

This man was admitted in shock with a blood pressure of 40/0. In addition his aorta had to be cross-clamped at the diaphragm for 25 minutes before it was possible to cross-clamp just below the renal arteries. His transient hepatic and renal failure seems to be explained most logically on the basis of ischemia of these two organs.

Survivor No. 7

Here, two logical explanations for this patient's postoperative jaundice are available — halothane or chronic passive congestion of the liver. He suffered for many months preoperatively, off and on, from congestive heart failure. During this time he was consistently jaundiced. Insertion of a Starr-Edwards valve was followed by a period of increased serum bilirubin and SGOT levels, which both returned to normal within three months of the operation. There appears to be little basis for favoring one of these etiologies over the other. Most believe that his jaundice disappeared because his new valve enabled him to be rid of his heart failure.

CHRONIC PASSIVE CONGESTION OF THE LIVER: POSSIBLE HALOTHANE
(Survivor No. 7)

Date	Clinical Observations	Course of Illness (in months)	Serum Bilirubin (mg./100 ml.)	Blood Glucose (mg./100 ml.)	SGOT (Units/ml.)	BUN (mg./100 ml.)	Serum Creatinine (mg./100 ml.)
February, 1967	Congestive heart failure	1	3.0		70		
March, 1967	" " "	2	2.5				
April, 1967	" " "	3	2.8		83		
May, 1967	" " "	4	3.0				
June, 1967	" " "	5	3.4				
July, 1967	" " "	6	3.6				
August, 1967	Starr-Edwards valve inserted under halothane	7	11.6		100		
September, 1967		8	5.0		500		
October, 1967		9	2.5		100		
November, 1967		10	0.3		82		

Comment

This man, aged 39, had mitral insufficiency. He was repeatedly jaundiced during bouts of cardiac decompensation. Immediately following his operation he became jaundiced. This subsided to normal during his postoperative recovery period of several months. His period of increased jaundice could, of course, have been due to halothane sensitivity, but chronic passive congestion seems to be a more logical explanation.

SURVIVOR NO. 8

There are three logical explanations for jaundice in this patient: (1) cirrhosis of the liver secondary to chronic alcoholism, (2) transfusions, or (3) two halothane anesthesias. While on the medical service he was thought to be suffering from viral hepatitis until it was disclosed that the hemorrhoidectomy, performed at another hospital, was done under halothane. In any event he survived, and the explanation of his postoperative jaundice is still controversial.

CHRONIC ALCOHOLISM, THREE TRANSFUSIONS, AND TWO HALOTHANE ANESTHESIAS (Survivor No. 8)

Date	Clinical Observations	Course of Illness (in weeks)	Serum Bilirubin (mg./100 ml.)	Blood Glucose (mg./100 ml.)	SGOT (Units/ml.)	BUN (mg./100 ml.)	Serum Creatinine (mg./100 ml.)
2/27/67	Transfusions (3), whole blood	1					
3/23/67	Hemorrhoidectomy under halothane	4	0.3			6	1.0
4/6/67	Colectomy under halothane	8	6.5				
4/11/67	Jaundice	9	11.5		1205		
	Transferred to Med. Service	10	6.4		220		
			2.7		115		
	Slow recovery	11	1.9		82		
5/5/67	Recovered; discharged	12	1.6		70		
12/10/67	Follow-up	19	0.8		82		

COMMENT

This man, aged 44, was a known alcoholic. He received three transfusions and had two operations performed under halothane. A week after his second operation he became jaundiced but recovered. Three choices for the etiology of his transient hepatic failure are, therefore, available. Serum hepatitis seems most logical to us but halothane sensitivity cannot be excluded.

SURVIVOR NO. 9

This 19-year-old white female with end-stage chronic glomerulotubular nephritis received a renal transplant donated by her mother on October 24, 1966. She had been supported with peritoneal dialysis and hemodialysis, and had undergone bilateral recipient nephrectomy one month prior to transplantation. The Terasaki leukocyte-antigen match was "C" [incompatible]. Her recovery after transplantation was uncomplicated. However, serial intravenous pyelograms demonstrated progressive caliectasis in the allograft. On March 24, 1967 she underwent a third operation to correct this progressive hydronephrosis. The pelvis of the allograft was found to be dilated, but the ureter was of normal caliber and was patent to probing. No obvious cause for the obstruction could be demonstrated. A nephrostomy tube was inserted and this presently remains in place.

RENAL TRANSPLANT (Survivor No. 9)

Date	Clinical Observations	Serum Bilirubin (mg./100 ml.)	SGOT (Units/ml.)	SGPT (Units/ml.)	Alkaline Phosphat. (King-Armstrong)	Albumin (gm./100 ml.)	Serum Creatinine (mg./100 ml.)	Imuran (mg.)	Enovid (2.5 mg.)	Prednisone (mg.)
9/14/66	Pre-transplant	0.1/<.1	18		8.6		14.8			
10/24/66	Transplant	0.4/0.1	16		3.8		1.3	200	+	100
10/31/66		0.3/0.1			4.5	3.6	0.9	200	+	100
11/14/66							1.1	150	+	95
1/14/67							1.4	150	+	30
2/8/67	Imuran decreased 2/7	4.5/3.8	97		27.0				+	20
2/9/67		3.3/3.0							+	
2/10/67					61.0				+	
2/13/67		3.1/2.3			27.0				+	
2/20/67		8.0/7.5			24.0				+	
2/28/67		7.5/6.0			16.0				+	
3/7/67		1.7/1.4							+	
3/22/67	Imuran started 3/20	0.8/0.6			8.6	2.0		100	+	
3/29/67	Imuran decreased 3/23	0.9/0.4		20	7.9		1.6		+	
4/5/67		0.7/0.3						100	+	
4/11/67		9.5/8.5		1250	24.0			100	+	
6/10/67		3.1/1.6		686	16.0				+	20
6/20/67	Enovid decreased 6/24 to 8/8/67								+	
6/27/67		1.6/0.8		440	25.0					
7/11/67		1.4/0.5		480	16.0					
7/14/67		0.6/0.2		210	18.0					
7/15/67		0.7/0.2		114	16.0	2.4				
7/18/67		0.6/0.2		210						
8/8/67	Enovid started again 8/8 to 8/20/67	0.3/0.1		12.6					+	
8/22/67		1.8/0.3		290	12.2					
8/29/67		0.9/0.5		620	13.9					
9/5/67		0.5/0.3		350	10.4					
11/14/67				114	10.0		1.4			25
1/2/68		0.7/0.2	80							
2/13/68				121	7.5		1.4			20
3/19/68				121	7.5					
4/16/68			370		9.7	3.9	1.4			20
4/30/68				230						
6/11/68				128						
9/17/68				100	8.2		1.4			17.5
4/1/69										15

COMMENT

In February, 1967, three and one-half months after transplantation, jaundice first appeared. At this time the immunosuppressive regimen consisted of 150 mg. of azathioprine and 30 mg. of prednisone. The azathioprine was discontinued and liver function gradually improved after the bilirubin had reached a peak of 8 mg. per 100 ml. For one week in April another attempt was made to begin azathioprine dosage, but her serum bilirubin again promptly became elevated. Azathioprine has been withheld since that time. The dosage of prednisone has been gradually decreased from an initial dose of 100 mg. per day to her present dose of 15 mg. per day. Despite the discontinuance of azathioprine, renal function has continued to remain satisfactory with a serum creatinine of 1.4 mg. per 100 ml., two and one-half years after transplantation.

Currently, the patient's liver function is normal. This young girl had been started on Enovid birth-control pills prior to transplantation. These were discontinued in June, 1967, because there was some question that the sex steroids might be contributing to her hepatic dysfunction. However, prior to that time the patient's liver function had improved despite the continuing administration of Enovid; thus it appears that her drug-induced hepatitis was primarily due to azathioprine. This is the only example of azathioprine hepatotoxicity that we have encountered in 53 transplants performed at the University of Michigan Medical Center.

DISCUSSION

In reflecting upon these 20 patients, we confess that we have been unable to come to any very profound conclusions. It is obvious that hepatic failure, as manifest in jaundice, coma, and death, is a recognizable clinical entity. At necropsy, hepatic necrosis is evident and everyone is satisfied that the patient succumbed to a critical postsurgical illness. However, when it comes to defining the precise cause of the hepatic failure in a given patient, medical and surgical science today is simply not good enough. The reasons are obvious: death due to viral hepatitis will remain conjectural until the virus of this disease is isolated and Koch's postulates are satisfied. Most clinicians agree that a diagnosis of serum hepatitis is difficult to confirm accurately; most pathologists agree that the study of necropsy or biopsy specimens of the liver permits, under ideal circumstances, a reasonably accurate diagnosis of viral disease of the liver, but there are always cases in which doubts remain. Halothane jaundice is still a matter of wide controversy today despite many excellent studies on the subject (Fink (ed.), 1968; Medical News (JAMA), 1969; National Institutes of Health, 1969). The debate continues, since most investigations conclude that the evidence is insufficient to establish or refute a causal relationship between halothane and postoperative hepatic damage. Furthermore it is impossible to produce hepatic necrosis in animals by halothane. Klatskin (1968) is convinced that halothane is a sensitizing agent as far as the liver is concerned, and he may well be correct in this conviction. Certainly our study readily produced a number of cases, both deaths and survivors, for whom it is tempting to ascribe the hepatic necrosis encountered to both single and repeated exposures to this drug.

Catastrophic surgical illness certainly provides a likely setting in which hepatic failure may occur after operation. Often multiple transfusions, shock, halothane, alcoholism, and other less tangible events may all be identified as potential causes of a given individual's fatal hepatic disease. In its present state, medicine has great difficulty in defining precisely the etiologic agent or agents potentially involved in any given case. In the majority of instances there seems to be little hope that this perplexing postoperative complication will be resolved without new knowledge. When the virus of hepatitis is isolated, when the action of anesthetic agents is more fully understood, and when the precise effects of stress upon the liver are clarified, the problems presented by these representative 20 cases will be more clearly understood.

The subject of hepatic failure can hardly be left without some mention of concomitant renal failure (Dawson, 1967). Once again medicine and surgery are plagued with the clinical fact that renal failure often accompanies hepatic failure. This verifiable clinical relationship, conveniently designated many years ago by Heyd as the hepatorenal syndrome, has been the subject of innumerable studies and almost endless conjecture (Blakemore and Boyce, 1968). This obscure relationship is represented in most of our deaths and certainly in one of our survivors. Three general schools of thought prevail today; first, that the renal disorder is secondary to a vasoconstriction of vague etiology; second, that arteriovenous shunts within the kidney deprive it of adequate parenchymatous perfusion; and finally, that a fall in effective extracellular fluid volume due to splanchnic pooling is the cause of decreased renal blood flow. The demonstration that nonfunctioning kidneys, transplanted from a patient dying in hepatic failure to a recipient in renal failure, functioned immediately, sounded the death knell to a verifiable hepatorenal syndrome (Summerskill, 1966).

Perhaps the last general comment that is in order from this study relates to jaundice associated with cardiac decompensation. Logan, Mowry, and Judge (1962) have emphasized that cardiac failure may be associated with hepatic dysfunction. Furthermore these investigators emphasized that cardiac failure may be associated with a moderate elevation in serum bilirubin and serum glutamic-oxalacetic transaminase in excess of 1000 units. Often these patients are thought to have viral hepatitis, but in reality their hepatic failure is a reflection of chronic passive congestion of the liver with centrolobular necrosis. In three of our patients (Survivor No. 5, Survivor No. 7, and Death No. 7) this manifestation of heart disease is clearly evident.

What generalities are available with which to close this discussion? *First,* in all probability patients today should not be given sequential doses of halothane. Furthermore, when patients require more than one surgical procedure, it is now important to know not only the nature of the preceding operation but also the kind of anesthesia that was administered during its performance. In addition, it seems most important to ascertain whether a previous halothane administration was followed by fever or other manifestation of sensitivity to this drug. It seems unlikely that halothane would have been used for the colectomy in Survivor No. 8, had it been known that his hemorrhoidectomy had been performed under halothane.

Second, surgeons should probably be more aware of jaundice as a concomitant of cardiac decompensation, and thus avoid ascribing this kind of jaundice to halothane or to viral hepatitis.

Third, the whole subject of postoperative jaundice is going to have to await critical advances in virology, drug sensitivity, and toxicity, as well as other less predictable discoveries, before the causes of controversial jaundice are satisfactorily resolved.

THERAPY OF PATIENTS IN HEPATIC FAILURE

The therapy of patients in hepatic failure is unsatisfactory because so little is known of its etiology. Certainly the general rules of fluid, electrolyte, and protein therapy of patients with liver disease should be carefully observed. These have been outlined in detail in Part II of this chapter.

Once established, hepatic failure is most difficult to treat. Exchange transfusions, hemodialysis, and auxiliary porcine or human liver perfusions are all difficult technical procedures and of controversial benefit. Few would deny that a mode of therapy analogous to renal dialysis in kidney failure would be most valuable. To our knowledge, techniques for such treatment have not been devised.[*]

[*]Acknowledgment: The author wishes to express his appreciation of Dr. A. James French's great skill in interpreting the microscopic sections in this section.

REFERENCES

PART III   Controversial Postoperative Jaundice

Blakemore, W. S., and Boyce, W. H.: Is there a hepato-renal syndrome? Surgery, *64*:1138, 1968.

Bunker, J. P., Forrest, W. H., Mosteller, F., and Vandam, L. D. (eds.): The National Halothane Study. National Institutes of Health, National Institute of General Medical Sciences, Bethesda, Md., 1969. For sale by the Superintendent of Documents, U.S. Government Printing Office, Washington, D.C. 20402.

Dawson, J. L.: Acute postoperative renal failure in obstructive jaundice. Hunterian Lecture, March 21, 1967.

Fink, B. R. (ed.): Toxicity of Anesthetics. Baltimore, Md., Williams & Wilkins, 1968.

Klatskin, G.: Introduction: Mechanisms of Toxic and Drug Induced Hepatic Injury. *In* Fink, B. R.: Toxicity of Anesthetics. Baltimore, Md., Williams & Wilkins, 1968.

Logan, R. G., Mowry, F. M., and Judge, R. D.: Cardiac failure stimulating viral hepatitis. Ann. Intern. Med., *56*:784, 1962.

Medical News: Liver failure after repeated use rekindles halothane safety debate. JAMA, *207*:2197, 1969.

Summerskill, W. H. J.: Hepatic failure and the kidney. Progr. Gastroenterol., *51*:94, 1966.

CHAPTER 16
SUPPURATIVE CHOLANGITIS

by WILLIAM P. LONGMIRE, JR., M.D.

William P. Longmire, Jr., was born in Oklahoma and was elected Phi Beta Kappa at the University of Oklahoma and Alpha Omega Alpha at the Johns Hopkins Medical School. Under Alfred Blalock at Hopkins he began a brilliant career in surgery which was continued at U.C.L.A., when he became Chairman of the then new Department of Surgery in 1948. His impact on the total surgical scene in America has been impressive, and he has provided outstanding leadership in many capacities. Although his interests have been wide and varied, it is in the field of hepatobiliary disease that many of his most important contributions have been made.

Reduction in the normal rate of bile flow through the ductal system, usually due to stones, stricture, or neoplasm, combined with the presence in the bile of organisms such as *E. coli, Streptococcus faecalis*, and other bacteria commonly found in the intestine, leads to a wide range of acute and chronic disease states generally classified as cholangitis. If frank pus is identified in the biliary ducts, the diagnosis of suppurative cholangitis is justified.

The clinical picture of cholangitis may vary from a mild inflammatory process to the potentially lethal, acute, obstructive, suppurative form of the disease. The former, with intermittent, sometimes widely spaced, subacute episodes of jaundice, chills, and fever, is a rather bland disease; but if it continues unabated, it can eventually cause multiple intrahepatic abscesses or fibrosis and sclerosis of the intrahepatic ducts and secondary biliary cirrhosis. The latter, a relatively rare, potentially lethal form of suppurative cholangitis with a 30 per cent mortality rate, is characterized by the presence of complete biliary obstruction and distension of the intrahepatic and extrahepatic biliary system, with pus under pressure. The most consistent symptom is pain in the right upper quadrant. Chills, fever, mental confusion, and jaundice, although characteristically a part of the clinical picture, may or may not be present, and the absence of one or more of these typical symptoms may obscure the proper diagnosis. The sudden onset and rapid progression of septic shock, characteristic of the acute obstructive phase of suppurative cholangitis, is responsible for the unusually high mortality rate of this syndrome.

HISTORICAL DESCRIPTIONS

The first description of the clinical syndrome which we refer to as suppurative cholangitis is generally attributed to Charcot in 1877.

"I will end this discussion with a brief description of a form of intermittent symptomatic fever which accompanies the calculous obstruction of the choledochal canal or intrahepatic biliary lithiasis. This fever, called intermittent hepatic fever, does not necessarily occur exclusively with biliary lithiasis. It can appear with the typical features where there is a chronic or persistent obstruction of the choledochal canal whatever the cause, by fibrous stricture, by cancer of the head of the pancreas or other.

"The anatomical condition most favorable to the development of this fever appears to be the presence, in the dilated biliary ducts, of pus or purulent mucus mixed in stagnant bile.

"I propose the following hypothesis:

"The fever we are discussing has its origin in the presence of a septic substance in the dilated and inflamed biliary ducts, a marked fever-producing poison, resulting from an alteration of the bile. This substance is an unknown to the present, as are the conditions which govern its production. Actually, icterus may or may not be present. It is absent, for example, in cases of intrahepatic calculi accompanied by fever.

"One specific characteristic of hepatic fever would be . . . the diminution of the rate of urination during an attack in contrast to an attack of malarial fever."

Twenty-six years later, Rogers in 1903

emphasized the difficulties of diagnosis and reported the first common duct drainage for suppurative cholangitis. He observed at postmortem examination three cases of suppurative cholangitis with biliary abscesses that had not been diagnosed during life and reviewed 20 similar cases reported in the literature of that time, none of which had been diagnosed before death. The cause of the suppuration in 18 of these patients was gallstones in the hepatic or common duct; in one it was a hydatid cyst opening into an hepatic duct; in the remaining patient it was a primary cancer of the common duct. Rogers' removal of stones and drainage of the common duct with a glass tube in 1903 was the first reported antemortem diagnosis and operative decompression of the duct for this condition.

In 1904 Moynihan in his book, *Gallstones and their Surgical Treatment,* summarized the information presented by Rogers. He reported, in addition, that the offending organisms found in the pus were the *Bacillus coli* most frequently, *Staphylococcus pyogenes, aureus,* and *albus,* and various streptococci.

As suppurative cholangitis is, generally speaking, a relatively rare disease, it is little wonder that over the years isolated articles have appeared, repeating the pathologic findings of the syndrome, the difficulty of recognition, and the fact that the only treatment that might be regularly expected to terminate the disease favorably was surgical decompression of the common duct. Deaver, for example, discussed the subject in rather general terms in an article published in 1930 and recommended early surgical drainage of the common duct.

Grant in 1945 presented three well-documented cases of acute suppurative cholangitis relieved by removal of stones and common duct drainage. This constituted the first reported small series of such cases properly diagnosed and successfully treated.

Two years later Cole reviewed the clinical aspects of the process and reported five patients treated with biliary decompression, four of whom survived. None of the patients who survived were hypotensive, and only one had a positive blood culture. A liver abscess and bacteremia were responsible for the one death.

Reynolds and Dargan in 1959 identified a particularly lethal type of suppurative cholangitis which they labeled *acute obstructive cholangitis.* Mental confusion, lethargy, and profound shock were considered characteristic of the syndrome, in addition to the findings of suppurative cholangitis. They observed that these symptoms might occur in the course of recurrent cholangitis, in acute suppurative cholangitis, or, occasionally, as the first evidence of biliary tract disease. The bacterial flora was varied; coliform organisms, *A. aerogenes,* and *B. pyocyaneus* were the most common. Conservative treatment consisting of massive doses of antibiotics and the usual supportive therapy was characteristically unsuccessful in all cases. Dramatic improvement of even the most moribund patients was achieved by urgent surgical decompression of the common bile duct, and this was the only effective method of treating these patients.

Since the clear definition of the urgent importance of depression of the blood pressure and cerebral function by Reynolds and Dargan, subsequent reports have tended to emphasize the cases of suppurative cholangitis that would qualify for their definition of *acute obstructive cholangitis.*

REVIEW OF THE LITERATURE SINCE 1957

Hampson, Dickison, and Robertson (1960) reported two cases of acute suppurative cholangitis. One patient who was hypotensive and stuporous had a positive blood culture and died without operation. The second patient, who was operated upon and survived, did not become hypotensive or have septicemia. These two cases emphasize several major points: the difference between suppurative cholangitis and acute obstructive cholangitis, the lethal character of the latter condition unless the obstruction is relieved by operation, and the importance of operative decompression of suppurative cholangitis before the symptomatic effects of septicemia have become established.

Glenn and Moody in 1961 indicated that a wide variety of signs and symptoms may result from obstruction and infection of the biliary tract, depending upon the degree of obstruction and the virulence of the infecting organisms. When there is complete obstruction to bile flow in the common duct or one of the major hepatic radicles in the presence of pathogenic enteric bacteria, the stage is set for the sudden catastrophic onset of the syndrome of *acute obstructive suppurative cholangitis*. They recorded the course of eight patients, five of whom survived after operative decompression of the biliary tract, and three of whom succumbed to the disease without surgical intervention. Errors in diagnosis were related to an inability to distinguish obstructive cholangitis either from nonobstructive cholangitis when the patient was seen early in his illness or from far advanced infectious hepatitis when the patient was extremely ill.

The report of Ong presented in 1962 an analysis of 276 cases of recurrent pyogenic cholangitis, the largest published series. The particular diet of the Hong Kong population, possibly resulting in a high incidence of *B. coli* portal bacteremia, plus a high incidence of parasitic infestation, makes the clinical problems of this case material differ from those seen in this country, both in kind (such as strictures of the intrahepatic ducts) and in the advanced stage of the disease. The majority of the patients were treated conservatively until the acute stage was over and then were operated upon as elective cases.

Further information on this type of oriental cholangitis (sometimes referred to as cholangiohepatitis or Hong Kong disease) as encountered in the Chinese population of New York City has been reported by Mage and Morel in 1965.

The operative findings in 38 Chinese patients were compared with those in 378 occidental patients (Table 16-1).

T-tube drainage has been found to be inadequate in the treatment of this disease, and transduodenal sphincterotomy, choledochoduodenostomy, or choledochojejunostomy is the preferred method of treatment.

Altered biliary dynamics is the most frequent cause of cholangitis, according to Ostermiller, Thompson, Carter, and Hinshaw (1965), for infection rarely occurs unless major duct obstruction is present. Their eight patients all had right upper abdominal pain, jaundice, chills with fever, shock, and central nervous system depression. The blood culture was positive in all but one patient. *Klebsiella aerobacter* was cultured from the blood in four patients, *E. coli* in three, and *S. aureus* in one. The two patients who survived in the group of eight were treated by choledochostomy and cholecystectomy, but these authors advise using the simplest procedure that will adequately decompress the common bile duct.

Four of 51 patients with ascending cholangitis reviewed by Furey in 1966 had stenosis of a choledochoenteric surgical anastomosis. Regurgitation of intestinal contents through such an anastomosis is not considered injurious unless there is some element of stenosis at the ostium with biliary stasis. It is interesting how infrequently spontaneous biliary enteric fistulas result in suppurative cholangitis when there is biliary tract infection in all such fistulas. The answer probably lies in the fact that most fistulas form between the gallbladder and the intestinal tract, with the disease confined to the gallbladder and without stone or obstruction in the common duct.

Waddell, in presenting six cases of acute obstructive cholangitis in 1966, indicated that acute cholecystitis is not usually regarded as a surgical emergency in Scotland, and that obstructive jaundice due to stone is also treated conservatively initially while the diagnosis is established and the patient is prepared for the operation. He cautions, however, that close observation must be maintained and prompt drainage of the biliary system performed, should the clinical picture suggest acute obstructive cholangitis. The shock syndrome he observed in three fatal cases was strikingly similar to that occurring with gram-negative septicemia. *E. coli* was cultured from the blood in two of his three cases.

The 24 patients with acute obstructive suppurative cholangitis reported by Hinchey and Couper in 1969 were divided into five groups on the basis of their clinical patterns (Table 16-2). A reasonable period of time is allowed for resuscitation in preparation for emergency operation, but even if the patient

TABLE 16-1.   Operative Findings in Chinese and Occidental Patients

	Chinese	Occidental
Common duct exploration	30 (80%)	76 (20%)
Common duct stone	23 (60%)	46 (12%)
Stoneless cholecystitis	12 (30%)	3 (0.8%)

TABLE 16-2.   Clinical Patterns in 24 Patients with Acute Obstructive Suppurative Cholangitis*

Group	Clinical Patterns	Result
Group I, 2 patients	Admitted in shock; no improvement; no operation	2 died
Group II, 6 patients	Admitted in shock; no improvement before operation	2 died
Group III, 8 patients	Admitted in shock; improved but then deteriorated	4 died
Group IV, 3 patients	Admitted in shock; improved and operated upon when well	None died
Group V, 5 patients	Well on admission; deteriorated in hospital and emergency operation performed	None died

*Adapted from a report by Hinchey and Couper, 1969.

remains in shock, refractory to all attempts at stabilization, the operation is carried out. Resuscitative measures include replacement of blood volume with a colloid solution in the form of whole blood, plasma, or dextran, as well as Ringer's lactate solution. The amount is determined by the clinical response, urine output, and central venous pressure. Vitamin K_1 oxide, 20 mg., and fresh frozen plasma or fresh blood return the prothrombin content to a safe range for operation. Mannitol is given before and during operation to forestall acute renal failure. Kanamycin, 15 mg. per kilogram, is the antibiotic administered initially. Hypertonic glucose solutions are given because of the reports that glucose has brought about improvement of mental symptoms associated with lowered blood sugar levels in patients with suppurative cholangitis. Hydrocortisone is given intravenously, in doses of 2 to 4 gm., to moribund patients who remain refractory to other resuscitative measures before operation. These authors emphasize that the patient is still "at high risk" until decompression of the infected biliary tract is carried out.

Dow and Lindenauer in 1969 reported on their management of ten patients who exhibited (1) an acute illness characterized by abdominal pain, jaundice, and sepsis, (2) evidence of bile duct obstruction, (3) purulent bile proximal to the obstructing lesion confirmed by culture, and (4) the presence of hypotension or a positive blood culture or both during the acute phase of the illness. The bile duct was obstructed by stone in eight patients and by neoplasm in the other two. They consider the presence of hypotension or a positive blood culture necessary for the diagnosis of acute obstructive suppurative cholangitis, and they confirm the opinion of others that survival cannot be anticipated without operation.

Multiple hepatic abscesses were found at autopsy in a large percentage of their pa-tients, and it is emphasized that such abscesses cannot be effectively treated by biliary decompression. Even after biliary decompression these intrahepatic abscesses may continue as sources of sepsis and be responsible in part for the failures of duct decompression therapy.

The mean interval between the onset of symptoms and the development of septicemia was 11 days in their series. The use of this interval for the rapid institution of preoperative supportive therapy and early operation could be expected to improve the results by preventing the development of septicemia and possibly by lowering the incidence of intrahepatic abscesses. If the patient is operated upon late in the course of the disease and has developed septicemia, a search for liver abscess should be made.

GENERAL CLASSIFICATION OF CHOLANGITIS

Cholangitis may be classified into two main groups: first, that associated with a bacterial origin, and second, a nonbacterial or miscellaneous group, of minor clinical significance in this country today.

I. Cholangitis of bacterial origin
   A. Acute
      1. Acute cholangitis associated with acute inflammation of gallbladder without duct obstruction
      2. Acute nonsuppurative cholangitis
      3. Acute suppurative cholangitis
      4. Acute obstructive suppurative cholangitis
      5. Acute suppurative cholangitis with intrahepatic abscess
   B. Chronic
      1. Nonsuppurative
      2. Suppurative

II. Cholangitis of nonbacterial origin
   A. Parasitic invasion of the bile ducts
   B. Viral infections
   C. Chemical cholangitis
   D. Cholangitis due to allergic or hypersensitive state

To dismiss the nonbacterial types of cholangitis, which are of no further pertinence to this discussion, the following comments are made:

Parasitic invasion of the bile ducts rarely occurs in this country. In parts of the world where such infections are common, *Clonorchis sinensis, Trichuris trichiura,* and *Ascaris lumbricoides* are the most common contaminants of the biliary system. They may cause partial or complete obstruction of the secondary branches of the intrahepatic duct system and, with secondary infections of intestinal bacteria, may cause stenosis, abscesses, or sclerosis of the intrahepatic ducts.

It is doubtful if true viral cholangitis exists. Catarrhal jaundice, which at one time was thought to be a form of viral cholangitis, is a form of hepatitis and involves the hepatic cells rather than the cholangioles. Chemical cholangitis involving the finer intrahepatic ducts has been reported to occur from the ingestion of a wide variety of chemicals and chemical compounds, including phosphorus, arsenic, gold, manganese, sulfanilamide, and thiouracil. The cholangioles are affected rather than the major ducts.

The histologic picture of the bile duct wall in cases of sclerosing choledochitis presents evidence of submucosal inflammation and scar formation. Occasionally after operative exploration, bacterial infection may become established in the lumen of the duct. The process, however, is not primarily infectious in origin. Its exact cause is unknown, but there is some evidence to suggest that it may be related to an allergic or hypersensitive state.

PATHOPHYSIOLOGY OF BACTERIAL CHOLANGITIS

Cholangitis is defined in the twenty-fourth edition of *Dorland's Illustrated Medical Dictionary* as an inflammation of the bile ducts, but it would probably be more helpful in current usage if the disease process were defined in clinical rather than pathologic terms. The diagnosis should not be established simply on the evidence of inflammation in the wall of the ducts unassociated with the clinical manifestations of the disease. In clinical terms, cholangitis could be defined as a symptom complex characterized by fever and leukocytosis, usually associated with jaundice or other abnormal physical signs or laboratory tests suggesting obstructive disease of the biliary system. Such a definition would certainly fit more logically into everyday usage in clinical medicine and in most instances would correlate well with pathologic changes. It would additionally tend to identify those early, acute cases in which pathologic changes in the ducts may be slight or absent altogether and would also exclude those cases with mild cellular inflammatory reactions in the duct wall not associated with the clinical syndrome.

As previously indicated, nonbacterial types of cholangitis are rare and are not pertinent to our present discussion. In this chapter our interest centers on cholangitis of a bacterial origin.

BACTERIAL INVASION OF BILIARY SYSTEM

Edlund, Mollstedt, and Ouchterlony, in their extensive bacteriologic investigation of the biliary system in 1959, divided the organisms from the positive cultures they obtained into three main groups: aerobic intestinal flora, anaerobic flora, and contaminants (Table 16-3).

There are several potential pathways by which bacteria might enter the biliary ductal system. (1) A retrograde flow of duodenal bacteria through the sphincter of Oddi would be the most direct pathway, although there is little evidence to support the contention that such a mechanism is of clinical importance. Edlund and associates (1959) stated that it is not obvious how bacteria characteristic of intestinal flora reach the gallbladder and bile ducts, but they accept the theory of an ascending duct contamination by a process of excluding other pathways. They eliminate the possibility of spread by way of the portal venous system on the basis of a small number of negative portal blood cultures. (2) The passage of bacteria through the duct or liver lymphatics would require extensive retrograde flow through channels that normally maintain a forward movement of lymph by a system of

TABLE 16-3. Bacterial Strains Found in 305 Cases[*]

Strain	Number	Group
Escherichia coli	80	
Streptococcus faecalis	49	Intestinal aerobic flora
Nonhemolytic streptococci	19	
Atypical gram-negative rods	8	
Anaerobic gram-positive rods	34	
Anaerobic streptococci	25	Anaerobic flora
Lactobacilli	17	
Staphylococcus albus	67	
Diphtheroids	28	
Streptococcus viridans	12	
Staphylococcus aureus	12	Contaminants
Yeast	11	
Bacillus subtilis	4	
Streptococcus hemolyticus	1	

[*]From Edlund, Y. A., et al.: Arch. Chir. Scandinav., *116*:461, 1959.

competent valves. Primary bile duct contamination by this pathway seems unlikely, but it must be considered as one means of the extension of infection from an acutely inflamed gallbladder into the ductal system. (3) There is no evidence to support the theory of primary contamination via the hepatic arteries, except in cases of generalized bacteremia. (4) Finally, the spread of infection from the intestinal tract, via the portal venous blood, through the liver into the bile must be considered. The major objection to accepting this mechanism has been the negative results of repeated efforts to culture bacteria from the portal blood (Edlund et al., 1959). On the other hand, one of the most informative clinical investigations on this subject, is the report of Ong in 1961, previously referred to, concerning recurrent pyogenic cholangitis.

In this report 154 patients admitted in the acute stage of the disease had blood drawn for aerobic and anaerobic culture. Twenty-three of these cultures (14.9 per cent) were positive for intestinal organisms.

At the time of operation, aerobic and anaerobic cultures were taken of the portal blood. In 97 cases, 33 were cultured during the acute disease and 64 during a quiescent period; 39.5 per cent of the acute portal vein samples were positive, compared to 14.8 per cent of the acute peripheral blood samples. During a remission 6.25 per cent of the portal blood samples were positive, whereas the peripheral blood was negative in all cases.

Ong states, "The fact that all of the bacteria cultured so far are from the lower intestinal tract does suggest that the origin of infection is from the gut and the route by which it travels is probably the portal vein. . . . No matter what route it takes, the infection having reached the liver is excreted into the bile." If there is no obstruction, bactibilia of itself is of no serious consequence. If obstruction caused by tumor or especially by stones is present, however, all the factors required to initiate cholangitis are present. Ong goes on to point out that although most types of *E. coli* are well tolerated in the intestinal tract and in the unobstructed bile duct, there are certain serotypes of *E. coli* that cause enteritis in children and sometimes in older people, and it is proposed that repeated infections with these more virulent organisms could cause thickening, scarring, and stenosis, particularly of the smaller intrahepatic ducts, even in the absence of obstruction. The diet in certain sections of China, including a popular pickled vegetable from which pure cultures of *E. coli* can be grown, and the numerous attacks of gastroenteritis from which the people suffer may be precipitating factors in the production of portal bacteremia and the cause of the pyogenic cholangitis so common in the Chinese. Schatten and associates in 1955 obtained a 32 per cent positive portal blood culture in patients undergoing upper abdominal operation. As previously mentioned, Ong obtained a positive portal blood culture in 39.5

per cent of patients in the acute stage of cholangitis and positive lymph node cultures in 38.1 per cent. It has been suggested that the bacteria are actually in the lymphatics and that the positive cultures obtained from portal blood are contaminated by the surrounding infected lymph channels (Edlund et al., 1959).

Scott and Khan in 1967 indicated that ascending infection in the bile duct is rare except after reconstructive procedures. They suggested instead that the organisms in infected common duct bile are derived from the infected gallbladder and that the gallbladder wall itself is contaminated via a direct systemic hematogenous infection. In this manner they would explain the high incidence of infection in common duct bile associated with common duct stones and the invariably associated cholecystitis and lithiasis. If bile duct contamination comes only from an infected gallbladder, it would also explain the low incidence of common duct bile infection associated with obstruction due to tumor, in which condition infection in the gallbladder is rare. The theory does not explain infections in common duct bile, however, that sometimes occur years after the removal of the gallbladder.

Edlund and associates (1959) believe that infection of the gallbladder or bile by way of hematogenous spread from the general circulation is improbable on the basis of the types of bacteria found. They also point out that although it can be demonstrated at the time of operation that Evans blue dye injected about the duodenum will extend along lymphatics in the wall of the common duct to the gallbladder, this pathway of infection is rejected because of the higher incidence of intestinal flora bacteria in gallbladder bile than in the wall of the gallbladder.

In summary, although the evidence is by no means conclusive, it would appear that bacteria pass from the gastrointestinal tract by way of the portal vein to the liver, usually in such infinitely small numbers that positive portal blood cultures are rarely obtained. In man, a small number of bacteria remain in the substance of the liver, although most of those that survive pass innocently into the bile and back into the intestinal tract. Some bacteria may survive in the sluggish bile of the gallbladder or the gallbladder wall. Biliary obstruction, particularly when accompanied by a foreign body, such as a gallstone

in the duct, creates a favorable milieu for the growth and multiplication of any bacteria that survive this circuitous route.

DEVELOPMENT OF BACTEREMIA FROM CHOLANGITIS

The mere presence of bacteria in bile of the ductal system, bactibilia, may not provoke any specific systemic response or be associated with any detectable clinical symptoms. Edlund and associates (1959) cultured bacteria from the liver or biliary tract in 34 of 77 patients with chronic cholecystitis but without stones in the common duct. Flemma and associates in 1967 reported that cultures of intrahepatic bile at the time of percutaneous cholangiography revealed that 64 per cent of patients with partial common duct obstruction due to stricture, choledocholithiasis, and bile duct carcinoma had positive bile cultures. Only 10 per cent of patients with complete obstruction secondary to carcinoma of the pancreas or ampulla had positive cultures. Bacteria in concentrations of 10^5 per milliliter or more were found to exist in the presence of obstruction even though there were no symptoms such as chills and fever. Flemma and associates found that clinical manifestations of cholangitis could be precipitated by percutaneous, T-tube, or operative cholangiography. It was their opinion that the clinical signs of infection or cholangitis, i.e., chills, fever, and leukocytosis, occurred only when trauma disrupted the biliary tract mucosa and bacteria in the biliary system entered the bloodstream to produce septicemia. Although definite proof is lacking, it would seem that circumstances might frequently obtain whereby clinical symptoms of infection might result from a biliary tract infection with an absorption of "toxic products" without the passage of intact viable bacteria from the infected bile into the bloodstream. The transition from a bland bactibilia to cholangitis with systemic symptoms but without bacteremia and then to the full-blown picture of acute obstructive suppurative cholangitis with systemic effects not only of the cholangitis but also of the septicemia, is probably related to the pressure level of the contaminated bile within the ductal system and the virulence of the biliary organisms.

Mixer and associates, in their investigations conducted in 1947 of factors that might explain the occurrence of febrile reactions in patients undergoing direct or operative cholangiograms, observed that biliary pressures in the range of 200 mm. H_2O were necessary to initiate bacterial reflux from the biliary system to the bloodstream.

Hultborn, Jacobsson, and Rosengren in 1962 investigated the possibilities of regurgitation or reflux of choledochal contents into the circulation by recording the pressure pattern in the common duct during injection of contrast material for routine cholangiography, and during slow injection of radioactive substances into the blocked biliary tree while radioactivity in the blood was regularly checked. Their results were as follows:

1. Choledochal contents can be regurgitated to the circulation (blood and/or lymph channels) at pressures insignificantly higher than the so-called secretion pressure (cholangiovenous reflux).

2. Not only fluids and crystalloids pass over to the bloodstream at these pressures but also particles up to 200 or 300 Å., i.e., particles of virus size and probably somewhat larger.

3. The transition occurs under circumstances that cannot be explained by processes of diffusion or absorption but presuppose direct-artificial or preformed communications between the biliary ducts and the circulation (probably between bile capillaries and liver sinusoids).

The earlier observations of bacterial reflux by Mixer and associates (1947) were confirmed by the studies of Jacobsson and associates (1962), who injected a bacterial suspension into the blocked duct of three dogs while the intrabiliary pressure was continuously recorded. In two dogs nonlabeled bacteria were used, and in one the bacteria were labeled with radioactive cobalt (Co^{58}). In all cases the bacteria passed over to the blood at pressures which insignificantly exceeded the secretion pressure as recorded before injection. In the experiment with radioactive bacteria the findings suggested that most of the bacteria were filtered off in the liver, but that an estimated 10 per cent entered the bloodstream.

Leakage of bile and resorption were found by Barber-Riley (1963) to begin once the back pressure in the biliary tree exceeded 75 per cent of the maximum secretory pressure.

The exact pathway or pathways of regurgitation remain unsettled, for it cannot necessarily be assumed that the same process that results in an increased systemic level of liver enzyme (i.e., the serum alkaline phosphatase) in the face of biliary obstruction is also responsible for the regurgitation of bacteria from bile into the bloodstream. The observations of Edlund and Hanzon (1953) suggested a communication between the bile canaliculi and the sinusoids. Evidence of a direct communication between the bile capillaries and the space of Disse was proposed by the studies of Rouiller in 1956. The electron microscopic studies of the hepatic uptake and excretion of submicroscopic particles injected into the bloodstream and into the bile duct, reported in 1958 by Hampton, emphasized the action of the hepatic cells in the transport of foreign substances across their cell membranes and cytoplasm as a means of communication between the bile canaliculi and the bloodstream.

Huang, Bass, and Williams stated in 1969, "Under normal conditions, or even with a pressure gradient slightly above the secretory pressure, all particles are probably rapidly phagocytosed by the liver cells and transferred to the plasma or lymphatic compartments. The capacity of transfer may be enhanced by any increases in back pressure in the biliary tree."

In their experiments they readily isolated bacteria from the liver lymph at a pressure level that was approximately 70 per cent of maximum secretory pressure of the liver cells. Organisms began to appear in blood only at the pressure level above 250 mm. H_2O, and the number increased proportionally with subsequent increments in pressure. These authors suggested that it is also probable that any increase in the intrabiliary pressure could open potential or pre-existing communications between the terminal bile capillaries and the space of Disse.

Huang and associates (1969) pointed out further that an increased pressure within the biliary tract associated with obstruction is the primary factor in the pathogenesis of bacteremia and septicemia in cholangitis. They emphasized the importance of keeping biliary pressures below this level during diagnostic studies and the urgency of relieving acute, complete obstruction of the infected biliary tract.

ETIOLOGY

Cole (1947), in emphasizing, as had others, that suppurative cholangitis rarely occurs except when obstruction exists, listed the three conditions most frequently involved in producing the biliary blockage.

1. Stones in the common duct were the most common source of obstruction at the time of Cole's report. In a review of a total of 92 cases of suppurative cholangitis gleaned from the literature to date, 79 cases were associated with calculi (Tables 16-4 and 16-5; Fig. 16-1, part 1). The common bile duct was obstructed by calculi in 21 of the 24 patients reported by Hinchey and Couper in 1969. Seventeen patients gave a history of previous biliary disease. Such a history was apparently absent in four of their 21 patients. Six patients had had previous biliary tract surgery. Two of these had cholecystectomy without common duct exploration for chronic cholecystitis and cholelithiasis. Two others had had choledochoduodenostomies for recurring common duct stones. One patient had cholecystoduodenostomy for suspected carcinoma of the common bile duct, and one had a cholecystectomy and sphincterotomy.

Glenn and Moody (1961) found stones present in all their eight cases. In one patient the stones had formed in a congenitally dilated biliary tree, and in a second patient above a benign bile duct stricture. Three patients had undergone previous cholecystectomies, including one with a negative common duct exploration. Two other patients had had previous cholecystectomies plus repeated common duct explorations for removal of stones.

Howard, Martin, Stauffer, and Hallenbeck presented six patients in 1959 with common duct stones producing Charcot's hepatic fever without jaundice. Four patients had had a previous cholecystectomy, including one who had subsequently undergone a common duct exploration for stone without stone having been found. Two additional patients had not had a previous operation.

From these selected reports it can be seen that a previous history of biliary tract disease is common in these patients and retained or recurrent stones after cholecystectomy or even following repeated common duct exploration may be the cause of the obstruction. At the same time it must be repeated that suppurative cholangitis does occur without any antecedent history of abdominal disease, and under these conditions may provide a most difficult and confusing diagnostic complex. As Cole (1947) pointed out, obstruction by calculus may clear spontaneously, largely because of the ball-valve action of the obstructing stone or stones. This type of obstruction also may not be complete and persistent as it is in other types of obstruction, such as that caused by carcinoma of the head of the pancreas. As will be discussed later, however, despite the possibility of spontaneous improvement, emergency surgical treatment is usually indicated.

2. Carcinoma of the pancreas and other malignant tumors, such as carcinoma of the ampulla of Vater or primary carcinoma of the bile duct, frequently cause (in contrast to the type of obstruction usually produced by stones) complete biliary obstruction without the presence of infection in the obstructed biliary system above the tumor. This important characteristic has been discussed in the section on pathophysiology and is one of the strong arguments in favor of the theory of biliary infection arising from the duodenal contents and spreading up the common duct. Ascending cholangitis does occur, however, in the presence of malignant duct obstruction; a review of suppurative cholangitis in the current literature (Tables 16-4 and 16-5) revealed that malignant obstruction was present in six of the 92 reported patients (Fig. 16-1, part 2).

3. Strictures of the common duct will invariably give rise to suppurative cholangitis sooner or later. As the obstruction associated with strictures is usually not complete, the intensity of the infection and its systemic effects will vary from time to time with the degree of biliary blockage. Clear, thin, normal bile seems to find its way through the smallest of openings, occasionally no more than 1 or 2 mm. in diameter. Such small openings will periodically become obstructed, however, with plugs of mucus or pigmented debris which form in the sluggish bile above the narrowed lumen, and in the presence of bacteria this blockage will initiate an episode of cholangitis. The severity of the attack will depend upon (1) the completeness of the obstruction and thereby the pressure elevation in the ductal system, (2) the virulence of the contaminating organisms, and (3) the duration or persistence of the obstruction. Five of the 92 patients available for review developed

TABLE 16-4. Acute Suppurative Cholangitis with Shock Syndrome

Series	Age	Sex	Past History of Biliary Disease	Temperature, °F. or °C.	Jaundice	Chills and Fever	Right Upper Quadrant Pain	Shock	CNS Symptoms	Positive Culture: Blood	Positive Culture: Bile	Delay to Operation (Days)	Operation	Survival	WBC	Cause
Reynolds and Dargan (1959)	73	M	+	105	+	+	+	+	+	+	/	–	–	–	34,000	Stone
	54	F	+	102.6	+	+	+	–	+	/	+	–	+	+	16,100	Stone
	69	F	+	105	+	+	+	+	+	/	+	3	+	+	12,300	Stone
	62	M	+	104.6	+	+	+	+	+	/	+	7	+	–	/	Stone
	80	F	+	105	+	+	+	+	+	/	+	/	+	+	22,750	Stone
Hampson et al. (1960)	80	F	+	105	+	+	+	+	+	+	/	4	–	–	21,000	Stone
Glenn and Moody (1961)	55	F	+	38.5	+	–	+	+	–	/	/	1	+	+	/	Stone
	70	F	+	41	–	+	+	–	+	+	+	9	+	+	23,000	Stone
	64	F	+	40	+	+	+	+	+	+	/	36	–	–	37,600	Stone
	34	F	+	39	+	+	+	+	+	+	+	2	–	–	22,300	Stone
	20	M	–	40.2	+	+	+	+	+	+	+	3	–	–	20,100	Stricture of common bile duct and stone
Ostermiller et al. (1965)	39	F		106	+	+	+	+	+	+	/	–	+	–	33,800	Stone
	61	F		104.2	+	+	+	+	+	+	/		+	–	20,000	Stone
	72	F		104	+	+	+	+	+	+	+		+	–	13,700	Stone
	84	M		103.4	+	+	+	+	+	+	+		+	–	22,400	Stone
	76	F		103	+	+	+	+	+	/	+		+	–	47,900	Stone
	55	M	+	104	+	+	+	+	+	+	+		+	+	27,000	Stone
	82	F		101	+	+	+	+	+	+	+		+	–	24,500	Carcinoma
	77	F		105	+	+	+	+	+	+	+		+	–	36,800	Stone
Furey (1966)	5 cases	2/5		/	+	+	+	+	+	/	/	/	0	0	/	Stone, 5/5

Study	Age	Sex				Temp											WBC	Etiology
Waddell (1966)	68	M	+	−	−	103	+	+	+	+	+	+	+	+	−	−	−	60,500	Stone
	72	M	−	/	−	101	+	+	+	/	/	+	/	−	−	−	−	10,800	Stone
	63	M	−	+		102.6	+	+	+	+	+	+	+	−	−	−	−	12,900	Stone
Haupert et al. (1967)	3 cases		3/3	3/3		3/3	3/3	3/3	3/3	3/3	3/3	3/3	3/3	3/3	2/3	1/3	/	/	Stone, 3/3
Hinchey and Couper (1969)	24 pts.																		Stone, 21
	11	M				24/24	20/24	16/19	24/24	24/24	?	6/13	17/18	22/24	16/24	Elev. in 13			Carcinoma, 1
	13	F				>101													Stricture, 2
Dow and Lindenauer (1969)	65	M	+			102	+	+	+	+	+	+	+	−	−			5/10,	8/10 Stone
	70	F	+			101	+	+	+	/	/	+	+	+	−	−		<13,000	2/10 Tumor
	52	F	+			104	+	+	+	+	+	+	+	+	−	−		5/10, 20–	
	75	M	+			101	+	+	+	+	+	+	+	+	−	+		43,000	
	54	F	+			105	+	+	−	+	+	/	+	−	−	−			
	64	M	+			103	+	+	+	+	+	−	+	+	+	+			
	68	F	+			102	+	+	+	+	+	+	/	+	+	−			
	72	M	+			102	+	+	+	+	+	+	+	−	+	+			
	75	M	?			101	+	+	+	/	/	+	/	−	−	−			
	76	M	+			101	+	+	+	+	+	+	+	+	+	+			

Key to symbols:
(+) = condition present or test positive
(−) = condition recorded as absent or test negative
(/) = condition or test not recorded or evaluated

TABLE 16-5. Acute Suppurative Cholangitis without Shock Syndrome

Series	Age	Sex	Past History of Biliary Disease	Temperature, °F. or °C.	Jaundice	Chills and Fever	Right Upper Quadrant Pain	Shock	Positive Culture: Blood	Bile	Delay to Operation (Days)	Operation	Survival	WBC	Cause
Rogers (1903)	/	M	+	104	+	+	+	−	/	/	7	+	−	/	Stone
Grant (1945)	39	F	+	104	+	+	+	−	/	/	1	+	+	15,750	Stone
	31	F	+	102	+	+	+	−	/	+	2	+	+	25,000	Stone
	39	F	+	105	+	+	+	−	/	/	½	+	+	19,000	Stone
Cole (1947)	43	F	+	104	+	+	+	−	/	+	1	+	+	/	Stone
	45	M	+	105	+	+	+	−	+	+	3	+	+	26,500	Stricture of common bile duct
	45	M	+	102	+	+	+	−	+	+	/	+	+	14,500	Carcinoma of pancreas
Hampson et al. (1960)	41	F	+	101.6	+	+	+	−	/	+	1	+	+	9,400	Stone
Glenn and Moody (1961)	47	F	−	40	+	+	−	−	/	+	3	+	+	25,100	Stone
	65	M	−	37.9	−	−	+	−	/	/	1	+	+	30,200	Stone
	75	M	+	40.6	+	+	+	−	+	+	4-5	+	+	/	Stone
Furey (1966)	4 cases		2/4	/	/	4/4	4/4	/	/	/	/	0/4	0/4	/	1. Stone 2. Necrotizing pancreatitis 3. Cholecyst-duodenal fistula 4. Carcinoma of ampulla of Vater
Waddell (1966)	71	M	−	103	+	+	+	−	+	+	0	+	+	9,500	Incomplete stricture of distal common bile duct
	60	M	−	100	−	−	+	−	+	+	0	+	+	11,500	Stone
	70	F	+	99	+	+	+	−	+	+	0	+	+	11,000	Stone
Haupert et al. (1967)	10 cases		7/10	10/10	9/10	/	10/10	−	/	9/10	/	10/10	7/10	/	Stone, 10/10

Key to symbols:
(+) = condition present or test positive
(−) = condition recorded as absent or test negative
(/) = condition or test not reported or evaluated

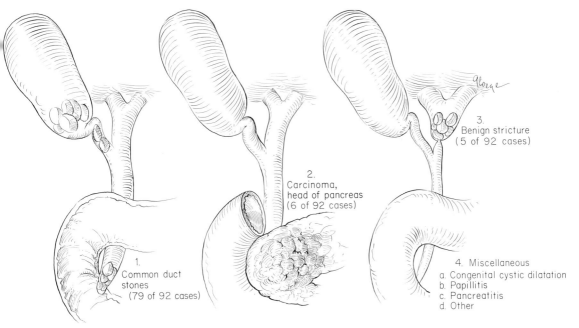

2.
Carcinoma,
head of pancreas
(6 of 92 cases)

3.
Benign stricture
(5 of 92 cases)

1.
Common duct
stones
(79 of 92 cases)

4. Miscellaneous
a. Congenital cystic dilatation
b. Papillitis
c. Pancreatitis
d. Other

Figure 16-1. Obstructive factors associated with purulent cholangitis.

suppurative cholangitis secondary to benign strictures of the extrahepatic ducts (Tables 16-4 and 16-5; Fig. 16-1, part 3).

As most strictures result from operative trauma, the interval between the onset of obstruction and the development of infection and cholangitis will depend upon the presence or absence of infection in the biliary tract, including the common bile duct at the time of injury. If the common duct is contaminated, the initial signs of obstruction will be accompanied by evidence of cholangitis. On the other hand, if the common duct contents are uncontaminated, there may be a prolonged interval between the signs of obstruction and the onset of cholangitis; this is supposedly sufficient time for bacteria to make the circuitous route up the portal venous flow, through the liver, and into the sluggish, obstructed bile where the presence of mucus and debris aids in the establishment of a persistent infection. Cole (1947) also mentioned regurgitation of intestinal contents into the common or intrahepatic duct as a cause of suppurative cholangitis. There can be no doubt that such reflux will carry bacteria into the ductal system. There is disagreement, however, as to the harmful effects of such contamination. The majority opinion holds that such a bactibilia *in the absence of obstruction* is innocuous. The chief point in question concerns the possi-

ble effect of this chronic infection on the duct wall and more specifically on the line of anastomosis between the duct and the intestine. Will the continued presence of bacteria in the lumen of the duct be prone to increase the development of scar at the anastomosis and thereby contribute to the development of obstruction with cholangitis? Although most surgeons would give a negative answer to this question, specific proof is difficult to obtain and it must remain an open question.

CLINICAL TYPES OF CHOLANGITIS

ACUTE CHOLECYSTITIS WITH CHOLANGITIS

CASE REPORT. M. V., a 38-year-old Mexican-American mother of three, was admitted to the hospital complaining of nausea, vomiting, and pain in the right side of six hours' duration.

With the exception of two brief periods of right upper quadrant pain about four and six months before and some fullness after fatty meals, she had been entirely well.

On physical examination, her temperature was 38.7° C., pulse 110 per minute, and respiration 26 per minute. She was a moderately obese patient who appeared acutely ill. There was questionable scleral icterus and the skin was warm and dry. There was marked muscle spasm in the right upper quadrant over a tender, smooth mass that moved with respiration.

Laboratory studies were performed with the following results: white cell count 18,250, urinalysis negative, serum bilirubin 3.8 mg. per 100 ml., alkaline phosphatase 18 KA units, serum transaminase 62 units. A chest roentgenogram was negative, and flat plate of the abdomen disclosed a 3 cm., rounded calcified shadow in the right upper quadrant suggesting a gallstone in the gallbladder.

Over the course of the next three days the patient was treated with appropriate sedation, intravenous fluid and electrolyte replacement, tetracycline, and nasogastric suction. There was no significant improvement of the tenderness in the right upper quadrant, however, or the size of the mass, the course of the temperature, the leukocytosis, or the serum bilirubin.

At operation on the third day after admission the gallbladder was acutely inflamed and distended and the wall was thickened and edematous. It contained a solitary stone, 3 cm. in diameter, impacted in the neck. There was some edema of the adjacent tissues of the hepatoduodenal ligament, but the common duct was of normal size. The head of the pancreas was not inflamed or edematous. A cholangiogram performed through the stump of the cystic duct was entirely normal. Because of the persistent elevation of the serum bilirubin the duct was opened and gently explored. It contained thin, yellow, normal-appearing bile. No debris or stones were present. A T-tube was inserted. A pure growth of *E. coli* was cultured from the gallbladder and common duct bile.

The postoperative course was uneventful. A cholangiogram one week after operation was also negative. The patient's subsequent three-year course has been without evidence of further biliary tract disease.

COMMENT. This case poses two questions in management. The first relates to the timing of operation in acute cholecystitis. In general, it has been our policy to institute initial nonoperative treatment. Early operation is performed if there is not definite improvement in the patient's condition within 72 hours or if there is worsening of the patient's condition before that time. In this particular patient there was evidence of failure to respond to the nonoperative therapy, and operation was performed about 72 hours after the onset of the attack.

The second question posed by this case, and one of particular pertinence to the subject of this chapter, concerns the presence of a persistent low-grade obstructive type of jaundice for which no adequate explanation was found.

It has been estimated that approximately 25 per cent of patients with acute cholecystitis have jaundice. The presence of common duct stones is an adequate explanation for the jaundice in some of these patients, but in others a variety of explanations for the occurrence of a type of mild, transitory jaundice have been advanced, such as small stones that obstruct temporarily and are passed spontaneously, external compression of the common duct by enlarged lymph nodes or inflammation in the head of the pancreas, edema and spasm of the sphincter of Oddi, edema of mucosa of the common duct, and hepatitis occurring either locally about the inflamed gallbladder or diffusely throughout the liver.

Glenn (1960) proposes that infection extends from the gallbladder by way of the lymphatic channels into the extensive intrahepatic lymphatic network to produce liver cell injury of sufficient degree to cause jaundice.

Except for those patients who are found to have small stones in the gallbladder and a papilla that is sufficiently patulous for a stone to have passed, or those cases with sufficient acute pancreatitis to have caused significant external pressure, it is not possible to define the exact cause of this type of jaundice at present.

Since the jaundice is of the obstructive, posthepatic variety, the interference with the pathway of bilirubin excretion must occur at or distal to the hepatic cell wall. The proposal of Glenn (1960) that the jaundice results from a diffuse intrahepatic process transported from the acutely inflamed gallbladder to the liver by way of either the lymphatic or the biliary system would seem to be the most plausible hypothesis at present (Fig. 16-2).

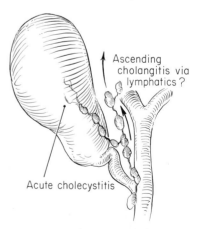

ACUTE CHOLECYSTITIS
WITH CHOLANGITIS

Ascending cholangitis via lymphatics?

Acute cholecystitis

Figure 16-2. Jaundice associated with acute cholangitis in absence of obstruction may be caused by ascending infection in extra- and intrahepatic lymphatics.

ACUTE NONSUPPURATIVE CHOLANGITIS

In nonsuppurative cholangitis, as the name implies, there is bacterial infection in the biliary system associated with the clinical signs of sepsis, but at the time of common duct exploration frank pus is not present (Fig. 16-3). The contents of the duct may vary from a normal-appearing thin yellow bile to a dark, thick bile that contains bits of debris. Intestinal-type bacteria are present. In "hematogenous cholangitis" infection is carried to the biliary tract by the hepatic artery. We have not recognized this type of infection in our cases and assume it is rare. The most common infecting organisms reported in hematogenous cholangitis have been pyogenic streptococci and Friedländer's and influenza bacilli (Wissmer, 1965).

From January, 1955 to December, 1968, there were 148 patients discharged from the UCLA hospital with a diagnosis of cholangitis. Thirty-five of these patients had a clinical course and operative findings that were compatible with the diagnosis of nonsuppurative cholangitis. These patients typically had a history of chills, fever, and mild jaundice. Pruritus was common, as was nausea and vomiting.

Pain in the right upper quadrant varied from a dull ache to severe biliary colic with radiation to the right subscapular region. The most prominent physical findings were evidence of sepsis, i.e., temperature elevation or chilling, jaundice, and tenderness in right upper quadrant and on some occasions an enlarged, tender liver. The confirmatory laboratory findings consisted of leukocytosis and elevation of serum bilirubin and alkaline phosphatase levels with minimal disturbances of the liver enzymes.

The moderate elevation of the serum bilirubin, usually 5 mg. per 100 ml. or below, and the presence of bile in the stools and urobilinogen in the urine, as frequently seen in this syndrome, are indicative of a partial biliary obstruction. In the majority of these patients the partial obstruction was due to stones in the common duct often associated with cholecystitis and cholelithiasis, but also included are patients with carcinomas of the pancreas or bile ducts and patients with obstruction due to benign stricture.

The following patient was found to have nonsuppurative cholangitis associated with a common duct stricture.

ACUTE NONSUPPURATIVE CHOLANGITIS

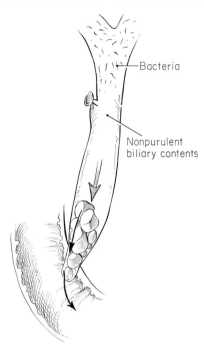

—Bacteria

Nonpurulent biliary contents

Figure 16-3. Common duct bile in acute nonsuppurative cholangitis contains bacteria but pus is absent.

CASE REPORT. M. S., a 69-year-old woman, was admitted to UCLA hospital on March 21, 1961, complaining of chills and fever and pain in the right upper quadrant.

She was first admitted to the hospital in August, 1960, with a 15-year history of right upper quadrant pain following the ingestion of fatty foods. There was also a two-year history of substernal "pressure on the heart" when she lay down after meals. General evaluation demonstrated cholelithiasis, possible choledocholithiasis, and a moderate-sized hiatus hernia. Cholecystectomy, exploration of a small, somewhat stenotic common bile duct, and repair of the hiatus hernia were performed.

Two months after operation, in October, 1960, the patient had several days of chills, fever, jaundice, dark urine, and light stools. An intravenous cholangiogram raised the question of common bile duct stone or distal bile duct stricture. She improved on conservative therapy. The same sequence of events recurred four months later in February, 1961.

Two days before the present admission the patient developed chills and fever, right upper quadrant pain, light stools, and dark urine. On physical examination, her temperature was 38.4° C., blood pressure 120/80 mm. Hg. She was a moderately obese, jaundiced female in mild distress. There was icterus of sclera and mucous membranes. There was severe right upper quadrant tenderness with rebound and guarding. The liver edge was 4 cm. below the right costal margin. Laboratory tests were performed with the following results: WBC 12,000, SGOT 127 units, serum bilirubin 2.3 mg. per 100 ml., alkaline phosphatase 53.2 KA units.

She was treated with intravenous fluids and Chloromycetin, 500 mg. every six hours, and she rapidly improved. An intravenous cholangiogram suggested the presence of a retained common bile duct stone.

Three days after admission a pronounced stricture of the distal third of the common bile duct was found at operation. Biopsies of the duct wall and surrounding tissues were negative for tumor. Cultures of the bile grew *Streptococcus faecalis*, although the bile itself was clear and light brown and contained a small amount of cloudy, muddy material. A *Roux-en-Y* choledochojejunostomy was performed. She has been asymptomatic for more than eight years.

Although the clinical differentiation may not be entirely distinct in each case, nonsuppurative is generally differentiated from suppurative cholangitis as indicated previously by the mild symptoms and signs of the nonsuppurative disease. The bacteria are from the intestinal flora, supposedly having been passed from the portal blood through the liver into the bile.

MEDICAL MANAGEMENT. Operation for relief of the biliary obstruction will eventually be necessary in most of these patients, but the initial treatment is designed to relieve the discomfort, usually with Demerol, to reduce the stimulation of bile production by instituting nasogastric suction and stopping oral intake, and to combat biliary tract infection with antibiotics: tetracycline, 250 mg. every 12 hours administered intramuscularly. If the symptoms promptly subside, operation is delayed for one to two weeks, and during this period the patient is maintained on a liquid or soft low-fat diet with restricted activities. On the other hand, if there is progression of the disease as evidenced by further elevation of the temperature and white cell count, deepening of the jaundice, or increase in pain or in the size of the liver, or if there is lack of improvement after 48 hours of treatment, operation is promptly performed.

OPERATION. The purposes of the operation in this condition are to (1) relieve the increased pressure in the biliary system, (2) remove the cause of obstruction, and (3) remove the gallbladder if it is inflamed or if it contains stones. These patients are rarely sufficiently ill from the effects of cholangitis that the operation must be limited to a simple maneuver to decompress the biliary system above the obstruction. The effects of cardiovascular or other concomitant diseases, however, may at times necessitate a simple biliary decompression if the patient's general condition is worsening during the course of medical management. T-tube drainage of the common duct above the site of obstruction is the most effective method of decompression. Although cholecystostomy performed under local anesthesia is a minimal, well-tolerated procedure, unfortunately it does not always provide adequate common duct decompression and should rarely be used.

An operation is most frequently indicated in the course of this disease to relieve a potential or partial biliary obstruction due to common duct stones after the acute febrile episode has subsided. If it has not previously been removed, the gallbladder will usually contain stones and will be inflamed. At operation after general visceral exploration, including a careful examination of the head of the pancreas for a possible neoplasm, the following steps are carried out:

1. The peritoneum of the hepatoduodenal ligament in the region of the junction of the cystic and common ducts is incised, and these structures are identified together with the cystic artery. If the inflammatory process has so distorted the tissues that identification of structures cannot be properly carried out, the dissection of the gallbladder is started at the fundus and continued downward. In most instances the cystic duct and artery are identified without undue difficulty. With the hepatic duct above and the common duct below visualized, the cystic duct and artery are divided.

2. The gallbladder is removed from below upward.

3. The clamp is removed from the stump of the cystic duct, and a small catheter is inserted through it into the common duct and tied in place.

4. Bile is drained from the catheter for culture and to release the pressure.

5. A cholangiogram is performed with the radiopaque dye injected with minimum pressure. Such a pre-exploratory cholangiogram provides a good "road map" of the biliary system with information concerning the location, size, and possible number of stones, as well as the presence of obstruction at the ampulla or at the hepatic end of the extrahepatic ductal system.

6. The duct is incised longitudinally between laterally placed stay sutures of fine silk, the incision being of sufficient size to permit passage of the largest stone in the duct.

7. The upper end of the duct is compressed with the fingers or with a bulldog-type, noncrushing, vascular clamp to prevent stones from entering the intrahepatic ducts; the lower end of the duct is then "milked" upward. The Fogarty bile-duct balloon catheter may be helpful in extracting stones from the lower end of the duct. Malleable

scoops and stone forceps are also useful implements. When it seems that all stones have been removed, the duct is thoroughly irrigated by injecting saline through a catheter. Dilators of increasing size are gently introduced via the duct through the sphincter of Oddi.

8. The occluding clamp is removed from the upper duct and the intrahepatic ducts are thoroughly explored with the Fogarty catheter, scoops, and stone forceps, and finally thoroughly irrigated with saline.

9. The choledochotomy is carefully sutured about a T-tube and a cholangiogram is repeated. If there is any question of retained stones, the duct is reopened and a further search instituted.

10. Stones impacted at the ampulla that cannot be removed from above require a duodenotomy and sphincteroplasty, so that the ampullary and intramural portion of the lumen of the common duct may be inspected and stones, if present, can be removed transduodenally or pushed retrograde and removed through the incision in the common duct. Duodenotomy adds significantly to the morbidity of common duct exploration and should not be undertaken lightly.

Antibiotic therapy is continued for three or more days after operation, depending upon the continued signs of sepsis. A septicemia may be produced by the manipulations of operation that cause an elevation of biliary pressure such as cholangiograms or duct irrigations. Blood pressure, pulse rate, and temperature must be closely observed during the first 12 hours after operation for signs of gram-negative septicemia and shock.

The treatment of cholangitis associated with tumors of the bile ducts, pancreas, ampulla, or duodenum depends primarily upon the extent of the neoplasm and the possibility of cure by resection.

If the tumor has metastasized beyond the limits of resection, the symptoms of biliary obstruction and cholangitis may be palliated by a bypass procedure, the simplest being a cholecystojejunostomy, unless there is a low intrapancreatic junction of the cystic and common ducts that is obstructed or about to be obstructed by tumor. If feasible, an anastomosis of the jejunum to the common hepatic duct will provide a maximum period of palliation.

On the other hand, if the extent of the tumor indicates that resection will be the best treatment, it may well be advisable in the face of an active cholangitis to perform a bypass cholecystojejunostomy to decompress the obstructed biliary system and bring the infection under control before embarking upon an extensive procedure such as a Whipple operation. In general we have not favored a two-stage operation for pancreatoduodenal resections (Longmire and Bruckner, 1969), but in the face of a progressive cholangitis superimposed on a resectable malignant duct obstruction, this would be recommended.

Mild attacks of nonsuppurative cholangitis associated with benign strictures of the bile duct may not be an indication for early operation. Treatment must be considered in light of the patient's previous history and progress. The condition of the remaining biliary ducts, the difficulties encountered at the time of previous repair if one has been performed, and the frequency and severity of these attacks of cholangitis are all factors which must be weighed. If one or two mild attacks of transitory jaundice and fever lasting less than 48 hours occur in the course of a year's time, and particularly if there has been a history of strenuous physical exertion just prior to an attack, operation would probably not be recommended. Such patients are cautioned against indulging in strenuous activities that may produce any degree of exhaustion. They are encouraged to drink six to eight glasses of water or fluids a day. If the attacks are mild but more frequent than indicated above, Zanchol, one tablet three times daily, may be prescribed continuously for three of every four weeks. An occasional patient may develop a mild stomatitis, indicating that the drug should be discontinued. This drug promotes the formation of thin bile in increased amounts and is said to be bacteriostatic as it is excreted in the bile.

In treating a more severe and progressive nonsuppurative cholangitis associated with biliary stricture, it is usually necessary to decompress the biliary system and to reconstruct a biliary passage at the same operation. This is particularly true for secondary repairs. So much time and effort are spent in exposing and identifying the stump of the proximal duct that it is usually preferable to complete the reconstruction once the duct has been identified. Our preference in reconstructive procedures has been for an end-to-side choledochojejunostomy utilizing a

Roux-en-Y jejunal limb. A rubber catheter or plastic tube is left in place through the anastomosis for one to six months, depending upon the security of the anastomosis. During the early postoperative period this tube provides a means of decompression of the intrahepatic biliary system if the lumen of the anastomosis should become compromised by edema of the mucosa and surrounding tissues.

ACUTE SUPPURATIVE CHOLANGITIS

Acute suppurative cholangitis, a severe, potentially lethal form of the disease, is fortunately rare (Fig. 16-4). Haupert and associates in 1967 found 52 cases reported in the American literature and added their 15 cases. There were 12 cases diagnosed in a four-year period at the Milwaukee General Hospital during which time there were 7429 admissions to the general surgical services, an incidence of 1.7 in 1000. In our current review of the literature the cases have been divided into those of acute suppurative cholangitis without the shock syndrome (characteristically these patients have biliary obstruction due to stones, tumor, or benign

ACUTE SUPPURATIVE CHOLANGITIS

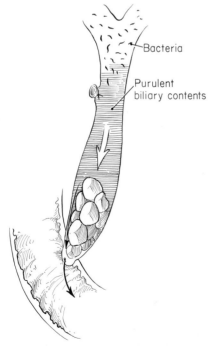

Figure 16-4. In acute suppurative cholangitis obstruction of common duct is not complete. Duct contents are purulent and contaminated with bacteria.

stricture, with jaundice, chills and fever, and right upper quadrant pain), and a second group of cases with similar etiologic factors and symptoms but with the additional symptoms of the shock syndrome, i.e., hypotension and mental depression. This syndrome was identified by Reynolds and Dargan in 1959 and called acute obstructive cholangitis. To fit this group of patients into the present classification we have used the term acute obstructive suppurative cholangitis, as have Dow and Lindenauer (1969). This syndrome will be discussed in the next section.

CASE REPORT. M. R., a 30-year-old woman, was admitted to UCLA hospital February 9, 1967, complaining of abdominal pain and vomiting.

Three years earlier she had had a brief episode of epigastric pain, nausea, vomiting, and transient jaundice. This cleared spontaneously and the cause of it was not pursued further. Three days before admission she had had moderate epigastric pain with nausea and vomiting that lasted a few hours and then subsided, only to return two days before admission and become progressively more severe, with radiation of the pain to the left back and shoulder and to the right subcostal area. For three hours the pain had been intense; she had vomited four times and had had chills and fever.

On physical examination her temperature was 37.8°C., pulse 130 per minute, and blood pressure 120/76 mm. Hg. The patient was a moderately obese, acutely ill woman who complained bitterly of epigastric pain. There was no scleral icterus. On examination the heart and lungs were normal. The abdomen was flat and soft with tenderness to direct palpation in the epigastrium. Murphy's sign was negative.

Laboratory studies were performed with the following results: hematocrit 43 per cent, WBC 21,000, total bilirubin 1.4 mg. per 100 ml., alkaline phosphatase 35 KA units. An x-ray of the abdomen in the supine position showed a few dilated loops of small bowel consistent with the diagnosis of ileus.

A diagnosis of acute cholecystitis with possible cholangitis was made and therapy was begun to bring the infection and the acute episode under control before operation. Intravenous fluids, antibiotics (Keflin and kanamycin), and nasogastric suction were instituted. Several hours later, however, her temperature increased to 39.2° C., and the pain became more intense in the right upper quadrant. Tenderness developed over the liver, along with a positive Murphy sign and scleral icterus. Eighteen hours after admission the patient became somewhat lethargic but the blood pressure was maintained. Results of repeat laboratory studies at this time were: WBC 52,000, bilirubin total 3.0 mg. per 100 ml., direct 1.8 mg. per 100 ml., alkaline phosphatase 28 KA units, SGOT 204 units. Blood cultures taken at this time were subsequently reported to be negative.

Thirty hours after admission an exploratory laparotomy was performed. Acute cholecystitis and cholelithiasis were found. A number of stones were present in the gallbladder and one was located in the distal end of the cystic duct. The common bile duct was dilated. Upon choledochotomy, gross pus, sludge, and small bits of stones gushed forth. A 10-mm. Bakes dilator passed through the sphincter of Oddi. No large obstructing stones were found in the common duct. The gallbladder was removed and the common duct drained with a T-tube. A cholangiogram at the conclusion of the operation showed dye to pass through the duct into the duodenum.

Postoperatively she did well and was discharged on the eleventh postoperative day with normal bilirubin and tests of liver function. After review of her postoperative cholangiogram, which demonstrated a slight residual dilatation of the intra- and extrahepatic ducts, the T-tube was removed six weeks after operation. She has had no further biliary symptoms since that time.

COMMENT. This case brings out some of the initial diagnostic difficulties that may be encountered in these seriously ill patients and the possible rapid progression of the disease. Upon admission this patient's temperature was normal and she had no icterus or elevation of the serum bilirubin. Her previous history and epigastric pain were the only indications of biliary tract disease. Yet, within eight hours, her temperature rose to 39.4° C., and the bilirubin to 3.0 mg. per 100 ml. The pain became worse and she became lethargic and more acutely ill despite vigorous treatment. The purulent contents of the common bile duct would indicate that infection had been present for some time, possibly going back to the previous attack three years earlier with a recent acute exacerbation of the infection of several days duration.

REVIEW OF COLLECTIVE PREOPERATIVE DATA. Twenty-eight cases of acute suppurative cholangitis without shock have been reviewed in the literature. The average age of patients whose ages were given was 60. Thirteen of the 23 patients were 70 years of age or above. The sexes were equally represented. Nineteen of the 28 patients had a previous history of biliary tract disease.

Right upper quadrant or epigastric *pain* was the most common symptom. It was present in all but one of the 28 patients and was a consistent initial complaint. Twenty-two had either clinical or chemical jaundice and chills and fever. Seventeen patients came for treatment with all three of these characteristic signs, but it should be emphasized that in 11 of the 28 patients, one or more of these characteristic features were missing. In the series of Haupert et al. in 1967, only two of 13 patients presented the complete triad. White blood cell counts ranged from 9400 to 30,200, and temperatures from 37.8 to 40.8° C.

Any patient suspected of having an acute cholecystitis should also be considered as a potential candidate for the development of acute suppurative cholangitis.

TREATMENT. The treatment of acute suppurative cholangitis is effective decompression of the common duct above the point of obstruction, with correction of the primary cause of the obstruction if the patient's condition permits. An effort should be made before operation to control the infection and to correct blood and fluid and electrolyte deficiencies. The patient's course is carefully monitored during the preoperative period, and if there is lack of improvement as indicated by lack of decrease in pain, tenderness, temperature, pulse rate, and white blood cell count, early operation (within a few hours) should be considered. If the patient's condition worsens, an emergency operation should be performed forthwith.

Ringer's lactate solution is initially given intravenously with additional colloid solutions in the form of whole blood, plasma, or dextran, as indicated. In these elderly, acutely ill patients, it is essential that the central venous pressure be carefully monitored and maintained in the range of 4 to 12 cm. H_2O. Replacement therapy is also evaluated on the basis of the clinical response, a urine output of 25 to 50 ml. per hour, and repeated hematocrit and serum electrolyte determinations. The serum sodium, chloride, potassium, and CO_2 are particularly pertinent. If urinary output does not rise when the patient seems to be hydrated, mannitol is given to provoke diuresis.

The most frequently encountered bacterial organisms in the reported cases have been *E. coli*, enterococci, *B. proteus*, *Staphylococcus aureus*, *Klebsiella aerobacter*, *Pseudomonas aeruginosa*, and *Streptococcus faecalis*. A combination of antibiotics has been recommended by a number of authors. Our preference would be for the intravenous administration of 500 mg. of ampicillin and 1 gm. of Chloromycetin intravenously three or four times daily, depending upon the patient's size and weight.

A nasogastric tube is passed and a Foley catheter is inserted into the bladder for continuous evaluation of urinary output. If jaundice has been persistent, 20 mg. of vitamin K_1 oxide are given intravenously.

OPERATION. In the case presented at the beginning of this section the patient was treated at operation by cholecystectomy, exploration of the common duct, and operative cholangiogram. The duct contained sludge and bits of stone. It is possible that a larger stone may have been passed just before operation. In any event, the obstructing process was relieved and there has been no further biliary tract disease. This represents the optimal surgical treatment for acute suppurative cholangitis caused by stones.

If the patient is desperately ill from the effects of the cholangitis or from secondary disease of the cardiorespiratory or other system, the operation may of necessity be limited to decompression of the common bile duct. Decompression should be performed in the most direct and simple manner, definitive operation being deferred until the patient fully recovers from his illness (Glenn and Moody, 1961).

The most effective emergency decompression is obtained by the insertion of a T-tube or a straight catheter into the duct above the obstruction, without any attempt to explore or to clean out the lumen of the duct or to perform a cholecystectomy. When the obstruction is caused by stones it is essential that the tube extend up the ducts above all the stones so that it will not become plugged.

The mechanism of the reported failure of cholecystostomy to provide adequate biliary decompression (Glenn and Moody, 1961; Hinchey and Couper, 1969) is also clearly demonstrated in the case report presented in this section. In addition to a number of stones contained in the inflamed gallbladder, there was also a stone lodged in the terminal end of the cystic duct just outside the common duct. Drainage of bile past this stone into the gallbladder for decompression of the common duct would have been impossible.

When suppurative cholangitis is encountered in a common duct obstructed by a neoplasm, it is advisable in most circumstances merely to provide T-tube decompression of the duct above the obstruction. If the gallbladder is distended and does not contain stones, drainage may also be provided by a cholecystostomy. The cystic duct will not be obstructed by stones or scarring in such cases, but the junction of the cystic and common ducts may be blocked by tumor invasion. The patency of this communication must be established at the time of operation. After the acute illness is resolved, a cholecystojejunostomy as a palliative procedure may be considered, or in rare instances a definitive resection of the neoplasm.

A benign stricture of the common bile duct was the obstructing mechanism in only two of the 28 reported cases of acute suppurative cholangitis. It may be difficult before operation to differentiate an obstruction resulting from a traumatic stricture from a retained stone. The previous history or operative report may or may not be helpful in this regard.

Every effort should be made to reduce infection in the patient with a benign stricture so that a reconstructive operation can be performed at the time of exploration, for, as previously indicated, the identification and isolation of the ductal system above such an obstruction constitutes a major dissection. It is desirable to proceed with a definitive operation if possible. If the patient is still running a septic course at the time of operation, however, decompression alone must be considered. After the proximal stump of the hepatic duct has been identified, a straight catheter is inserted for continuous drainage. Within one to two weeks the final procedure is performed if the patient's condition permits.

RESULTS.   An operation was performed in 24 of the 28 reported cases. Four of these patients did not survive. None of the four patients treated without operation survived.

ACUTE OBSTRUCTIVE SUPPURATIVE CHOLANGITIS

Reynolds and Dargan, in establishing this distinct clinical syndrome in 1959, stressed the urgency of decompression of the biliary tract. They pointed out that acute obstructive suppurative cholangitis is characterized by *complete* obstruction of the common bile duct with the accumulation of purulent material under pressure. The usual mechanisms of obstruction may be present. Stones are the most common (Fig. 16-5).

To the well-known clinical triad of chills and fever, jaundice, and right upper quadrant abdominal pain or tenderness characteristic of acute suppurative cholangitis, these authors added lethargy or mental confusion and shock to form a pentad of symptoms characteristic of acute obstructive suppurative cholangitis. The symptoms may occur in the course of recurrent cholangitis or in acute suppurative cholangitis or occasionally as the first evidence of biliary tract disease. They may also follow manipulations of an infected

ACUTE OBSTRUCTIVE SUPPURATIVE CHOLANGITIS

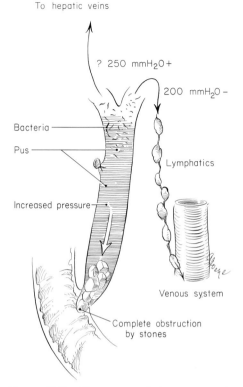

Figure 16-5. Obstruction of the common duct is complete in acute obstructive suppurative cholangitis and the duct contains bacteria and pus under pressure. When the pressure is at or above the secretion pressure of 200 mm. H_2O, bacteria pass into the lymphatic system. At the pressure of 250 mm. H_2O, bacteria may pass directly into the hepatic venous system. (Huang et al., 1969.)

biliary tree that cause an elevation of the intrabiliary pressure such as common duct exploration or percutaneous cholangiography.

CASE REPORT. R. T., a 63-year-old man, was admitted to the UCLA hospital on August 1, 1963, with a fever of undetermined origin and shock.

Eighteen months before admission a cholecystectomy had been performed for a "gangrenous gallbladder without stones." Six weeks before there was a sudden onset of shaking, chills, and weakness which he thought might be a recurrence of the malaria that he had had when he was ten years old. Despite quinine treatment, fever to 103° F., weakness, drenching sweats, and shaking chills persisted. He was hospitalized elsewhere for four days, and with antibiotic treatment his condition improved briefly. A recurrence of symptoms prompted a two-week rehospitalization and further treatment with antibiotics. Two days before admission his fever returned and reached 106° F., and he was hypotensive when he was again hospitalized. Cultures of blood and bone marrow grew *E. coli*. Despite intensive antibiotic therapy he failed to improve and was transferred to the UCLA hospital for further evaluation and treatment.

On physical examination, his blood pressure was 90/60 mm. Hg, pulse 82 per min., temperature 37° C. The patient was obtunded and lethargic. There was no scleral icterus. Examination of the heart and lungs was negative except for the presence of moist rales at the right posterior lung base. The bowel sounds were normal; there were no masses or palpable organs. There was no abdominal tenderness. The extremities were unremarkable.

Laboratory studies were performed with the following results: hematocrit 32 per cent, WBC 29,000, SGOT 20 units, bilirubin direct 0.3 mg. per 100 ml., total 1.2 mg. per 100 ml., alkaline phosphatase 14 KA units. Blood cultures grew *E. coli*, bacteroides, and *Streptococcus faecalis*. A barium enema demonstrated sigmoid diverticulosis and diverticulitis. Shortly after admission the patient's temperature rose to 39° C., and the blood pressure dropped below 80 mm. Hg. He was started on an Aramine drip, kanamycin, 300 mg., and Chloromycetin, 1.0 gm. intramuscularly every 8 hours. The blood glucose level at this time was 74.5 mg. per 100 ml.

A primary source of infection could not be determined. His course over the next nine days was variable, his temperature at times reaching 40° C. A number of antibiotics were added to the regimen, and an extensive laboratory and radiologic investigation was carried out without further specific definition of the problem.

An exploratory laparotomy in search of an intraperitoneal abscess was performed on the tenth day after admission. The liver appeared normal, without evidence of intrahepatic abscess. The porta hepatis was encased in dense scar tissue, and dissection in this area was bloody. No specific mass or abscess could be felt. The edge of the hepatoduodenal ligament felt free of abnormality, but the common duct was not specifically identified. A firm mass was present about an old sigmoid diverticulitis, but there was no sign of acute infection. The abdominal exploration was otherwise negative.

Postoperatively, the patient did well for two days. Then the septic fever returned and his condition steadily deteriorated with persistent hypotension and mental lethargy, until he died one week after operation.

At postmortem examination four pea-sized stones were found at the ampulla of Vater, appearing to completely obstruct the lumen of the common duct. Greenish-white pus under pressure filled the extra- and intrahepatic ducts. There was an intrahepatic abscess 3 cm. in diameter in the lower portion of the right lobe of the liver.

COMMENT. This patient's history demonstrates the extreme difficulty of arriving at a proper diagnosis in certain of these cases. The absence of pain or tenderness of the liver and of jaundice, despite the presence of a complete biliary obstruction and of a distended intrahepatic duct system with an intrahepatic abscess, indicates the unreliability of the characteristic diagnostic criteria. In retrospect, greater consideration might have been given to the history of a cholecystectomy 18 months before admission, a persistent slightly elevated alkaline phosphatase, and the dense vascular reaction about the porta hepatis and hepatoduodenal ligament at the time of operation.

The hypotension and mental obtundation which were prominent features throughout the final three weeks of the patient's illness were related to the constant septicemia.

Death has been the uniform result in all cases if the "pus under pressure" in the common duct has not been released. This patient may be considered somewhat unusual to have survived the repeated bouts of hypotension and multiple organism bacteremia for three weeks.

The small intrahepatic abscess probably did not play a significant role in the fatal course of this patient's disease, but such abscesses are a consistent finding in neglected cases and may contribute to the difficulty of eradicating the biliary tract infection if duct drainage is delayed until such septic sites have formed. This is discussed in further detail in the following section.

REVIEW OF COLLECTIVE PREOPERATIVE DATA. We have reviewed the data of 64 reported cases of acute suppurative cholangitis with the shock syndrome, or acute obstructive suppurative cholangitis. The average age was 65. There were 31 females and 25 males (in eight cases, sex was not specified). A previous history of biliary tract disease was obtained in 26 of the 32 patients whose records contained such information. Temperatures were elevated in all patients and ranged from 38.5 to 41.5° C. Jaundice was present in all but five of the 64 patients, chills and fever in all but four. Right upper quadrant pain was uniformly present in all cases reported. Shock was absent in three patients, and four did not have central nervous system symptoms. Bacteria were present in 27 of the 34 blood cultures and in 44 of 45 bile cultures (Table 16-6).

PREOPERATIVE TREATMENT. Once the diagnosis is established or reasonably suspected, operative decompression of the biliary tract is urgent. Vigorous supportive treatment is begun immediately; if there is improvement in the patient's condition, operation may be delayed for a few hours for the antibiotics to have their full effect and for adequate fluid and electrolyte replacement to be achieved. If there is no response to such treatment, one must proceed immediately with operation.

Treatment consists of *volume replacement* and efforts to *combat shock*. These patients are severely hypovolemic and, in most instances, anemic. Fluid replacement will be started with Ringer's solution, with the addition of blood, plasma or dextran as indicated by the hematocrit. If the hematocrit is under 30 per cent, blood is given; if it is over 30 per cent, plasma or dextran is used. The central venous pressure must be carefully monitored and maintained between 4 and 12 cm. H_2O. Digitalis is used if there is any concern of congestive failure. An effort is made to maintain the systolic blood pressure at 80 to 90 mm. Hg by volume replacement. If such a systolic pressure cannot be maintained after digitalization and despite a central venous pressure above 12 cm. H_2O, isoproterenol may be tried, 5 mg. Isuprel in 500 cc. of 5 per cent dextrose, infused at a rate of 0.25 to 2.5 ml. per minute or as required. If ineffective due to lack of blood pressure response, or if arrhythmias or tachycardia develop, the drug is stopped and a massive dose of corticosteroids is administered. A dose of hydrocortisone, 50 to 150 mg. per kilogram of body weight, is given in a single intravenous injection. This may again be followed by a lesser infusion of isoproterenol or levarterenol to maintain the systolic blood pressure in the 80 to 90 mm. Hg level.

If shock persists despite this therapy, it is essential that prompt biliary decompres-

TABLE 16-6.   Summary of Diagnostic Features — 64 Cases of Acute Obstructive Suppurative Cholangitis

Feature	No. Cases Reporting	Positive	Negative
Previous biliary disease	32	26	6
Fever	64	64	0
Jaundice	64	59	5
Chills and fever	64	60	4
Right upper quadrant pain	40	40	0
Shock	64	61	3
CNS symptoms	39	35	4
Blood culture	34	27	7
Bile culture	45	44	1

sion be performed by the simplest means possible.

Antibiotic treatment is begun immediately. According to the studies of Hinchey and Couper in 1969, Chloromycetin and kanamycin were the most effective antibiotics tested against the five most frequently encountered organisms in their series of 20 patients. They recommended the administration of kanamycin in a dose of 15 mg. per kilogram of body weight to all patients suspected of having this disease, with subsequent administration dependent upon the urine flow and the determination of kanamycin levels in the blood.

Haupert and associates in 1967 recommended a combination of antibiotics as preferable to tetracycline alone. They gave Chloromycetin to all patients and penicillin to most. Kanamycin and Chloromycetin were the initial drugs employed in the case reported in this section. The range of sensitive bacteria would be greater, however, if the combination of ampicillin and Chloromycetin were employed as indicated in the previous section. Until culture results are available, 500 mg. of ampicillin and 1 gm. of Chloromycetin are given intravenously three or four times daily, depending upon the patient's size and weight. Vitamin K_1 oxide, 20 mg., is given to all patients intravenously.

OPERATION. In these desperately ill patients the operation must be limited to the simplest procedure that will decompress the common duct above the obstruction. Cholecystostomy has been found repeatedly to give inadequate decompression and should not be used except when there is gross dilatation of the entire biliary system, including the gallbladder and cystic duct, in association with a neoplasm about the ampulla of Vater. Choledochotomy with the insertion of a straight catheter or T-tube well above the obstruction is the simplest effective procedure.

Only stones that present in the duct incision are removed unless the patient's general condition has been sufficiently improved by the preoperative treatment to permit a full-scale duct exploration. Under these conditions the gallbladder would also be removed if present.

The risk of an extended operation may be justified in some of the less acutely ill patients when the obstruction is due to a benign stricture, for, as previously indicated, the dissection and identification of the duct is such a major portion of the reconstructive operation that the procedure should be completed if possible. A drainage operation alone would add significantly to the difficulties of the final repair.

RESULTS. This disease is uniformly fatal if it is not recognized and biliary drainage performed. Even with operation the results have been very poor (Table 16-7). Of the 46 patients operated upon, 19 have died, a mortality rate of 41.3 per cent. Continued shock and sepsis, often associated with intrahepatic abscesses, have accounted in large part for the high mortality. As Hinchey and Couper pointed out in 1969, "The very best treatment is prophylaxis and the 33 per cent mortality associated with this benign disease might have been avoided had some of the patients had elective operations when the presence of gall stones was first diagnosed. It is also clear from the results of this study that the delayed or expectant method of treatment of acute cholecystitis exposes some patients to the risk of this more serious extension of the biliary tract disease."

ACUTE OBSTRUCTIVE SUPPURATIVE CHOLANGITIS PRECIPITATED BY MANIPULATIONS OF THE BILIARY TRACT. Septicemia and shock may follow any procedure that elevates the biliary pressure above the secretory pressure in the presence of infected bile within the ductal system. Elevation of the biliary pressure during percutaneous cholangiography or common bile duct exploration when suppurative cholangitis is present represents a real hazard of creating a gram-negative shock syndrome.

CASE REPORT. A. C., a 33-year-old man, was referred for treatment of an injury to the common bile duct. Five months before admission he had had a cholecystectomy and became jaundiced three days later. On re-exploration, an end-to-end repair was performed which functioned satisfactorily until the stent was removed three

TABLE 16-7. Review of Collected Results—Acute Obstructive Suppurative Cholangitis

	Number	Survived	Died
Not operated upon	18	0	18
Operated upon	46	27	19

months later. Jaundice and a spiking fever to 40° C. developed. Blood cultures grew gram-negative organisms. A second exploration was attempted, but the duct could not be identified. Despite his septic course, it was felt that a percutaneous cholangiogram might give pertinent information regarding the location and condition of the remaining ducts. *E. coli* was cultured from the blood and gentamicin was started. Six hours following the cholangiogram he developed a severe chill and his temperature rose to 40.7° C. Seven hours later he became hypotensive and lethargic, obviously in gram-negative septicemia with shock. Treatment consisted of massive doses of blood, plasma, fluids, digitalis, and Solu-Cortef. His condition improved somewhat, but the improvement was difficult to maintain. The temperature remained elevated, blood pressure was low, urine output was reduced, and the patient was obtunded. The cholangiogram had identified an obstructed stump of the hepatic duct. Despite his precarious state, plans were made for re-exploration. When the hepatic duct stump was opened there was a gush of purulent bile with sludge and debris from which *E. coli* was cultured. A choledochojejunostomy was performed.

Postoperatively cortisone therapy was gradually discontinued, his febrile course finally resolved over a period of four weeks, and the infected abdominal wall wounds began to granulate and eventually healed. One year later he is well and without complaints referable to his biliary system.

COMMENT. This case illustrates the violent reaction that may be precipitated by manipulation of the infected biliary system despite prophylactic antibiotic treatment. In certain situations the information to be gained from such an examination, as in this case, may be considered of sufficient value to justify the risk. It has been proposed that such cholangiograms should be followed by immediate operative decompression of the biliary system to prevent this type of gram-negative septicemia. Immediate operation will not prevent the bacteremia that occurs with increased pressure in the biliary system at the time of dye injection, and a severe septic shock reaction may be difficult to diagnose and treat during a prolonged difficult operation or in the immediate postoperative period. For this reason, operation immediately after cholangiography is not advocated.

In summary, acute obstructive suppurative cholangitis is a rare disease with a 40 to 50 per cent mortality. The typical case is characterized by a previous history of biliary tract disease and a pentad of symptoms consisting of right upper quadrant pain, chills and fever, jaundice, hypotension, and central nervous system depression. One or more of these characteristic symptoms may be absent, and lack of a clear clinical picture may delay the proper diagnosis. Urgent decompression of the biliary tract is essential. Preoperative

therapy includes the treatment of shock with volume replacement and possibly corticosteroid therapy and antibiotics. Operation consists of simple tube drainage by means of choledochostomy in most instances. Death may ensue following operation from shock or persistent sepsis, frequently associated with intrahepatic abscesses.

INTRAHEPATIC ABSCESSES ASSOCIATED WITH SUPPURATIVE CHOLANGITIS

Several reports have indicated that the number of intrahepatic abscesses secondary to cholangitis and distal duct obstruction has increased in recent years (Kinney and Ferrebee, 1948; Sherman and Robbins, 1960; Swartz, 1964; Joseph et al., 1968). Kinney and Ferrebee observed in 1948 that 22 per cent of pyogenic liver abscesses in their series occurred secondary to common duct obstruction, and that this type of intrahepatic infection continues to increase in older patients. Cholangitis was the disorder most frequently leading to hepatic abscess in the review of 130 cases in 1960 by Sherman and Robbins. More than 80 per cent had an intrahepatic infection secondary to distal bile duct obstruction. In the 70 cases reported by Swartz in 1964, 32 were due to cholangitis. Fifteen per cent of the 61 cases reported by Joseph and associates in 1968 were secondary to biliary obstructive disease. Eight of the 16 hepatic abscesses reported in 1969 by Dandurand, Saint-Martin, and Beaudoin were secondary to disease of the biliary system. Six of these patients died, and two survived (Fig. 16-6).

Thus it seems clear that today in most hospitals in North America intrahepatic abscesses due to intraperitoneal infections, i.e., appendicitis, perforated ulcer, diverticulitis, and tubovarian abscess, are undergoing a relative decrease as those intrahepatic abscesses resulting from cholangitis and septicemia increase.

Contrary to current views Cole (1947) believed that the wall of the common duct became infected first in cholangitis and that the infection then spread to the contents of the lumen of the duct and extended upward into the liver. His description of the pathologic changes in the duct wall seems accurate, however, regardless of the direction of the spreading infection. "The common duct wall becomes thickened, edematous and

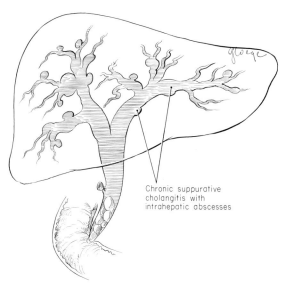

Chronic suppurative
cholangitis with
intrahepatic abscesses

Figure 16-6. The development of multiple intrahepatic abscesses associated with either a chronic or
acute suppurative cholangitis represents a serious and
frequently fatal complication of infection in the biliary
tract.

fibrosed. Microscopically invasion of polymorphonuclear and lymphocytic cells are
noted. Granulation tissue and fibrous tissue
are encountered in various stages of resolution. When the infection extends into the
liver there is a tendency for the development
of multiple liver abscesses. These start out
microscopically as small collections of polymorphonuclear cells at or near the termination of the bile capillaries and enlarge,
depending upon the degree of obstruction
and the treatment instituted. They may
coalesce into one large abscess but usually
there are numerous small abscesses scattered
throughout the rest of the liver, even though
coalescence does take place."

Ostermiller and associates commented in
1965 that in their eight cases (with stones as
the obstructing agent in seven cases and
carcinoma in one) the liver was diffusely
enlarged and congested with dilatation of
the intrahepatic bile ducts. Microscopically,
liver necrosis was found, varying from centrolobular degeneration to liver abscess.

Furey (1966) believes that the development of multiple liver abscesses is the most
serious complication of cholangitis; such
abscesses are most frequently seen in cases
with stones completely or nearly completely
obstructing the common duct. They are rare
in cases of obstruction due to neoplasm
unless accompanied by stones or unless

there has been a previous operation on the
biliary tract. In his 51 cases there were nine
patients who died without operation, and
multiple liver abscesses were found at
autopsy in all of them. Five of these patients
were admitted in a state of shock. All were
jaundiced and febrile and at autopsy were
found to have multiple liver abscesses with
associated common duct stones. From these
findings Furey concluded that jaundice,
fever, and cardiovascular collapse must be
regarded as indicative of suppurative cholangitis with multiple liver abscesses.

The seriousness of multiple hepatic abscesses cannot be doubted. This intrahepatic
complication is a frequent finding in the
acutely ill patient with an advanced stage
of cholangitis, particularly when the disease
has persisted for a matter of days or even
weeks. Cardiovascular collapse, however, is
usually indicative of a spread into the bloodstream of bacteria from suppurative cholangitis either with or without hepatic abscesses.
These signs do not necessarily connote a
syndrome peculiar to intrahepatic abscess
alone.

DIAGNOSIS AND TREATMENT OF INTRA-
HEPATIC ABSCESS. These acutely ill patients usually come to the hospital with a
history of chills, fever, and jaundice that
have been present for one to two weeks and
frequently give a history of previous biliary
tract disease. Shock, lethargy, and mental
depression may be present. A spiking temperature of 39 to 40° C. is common, and the
patient may complain of right upper quadrant pain. Physical examination reveals the
signs of acute illness, lethargy and jaundice.
The temperature is elevated and tachycardia is present. Blood pressure may be subnormal. The liver is enlarged beneath the
right costal margin, and there is tenderness
in the right upper quadrant. Laboratory
findings include a mild anemia, a leukocytosis of 20,000 to 40,000, and elevation of the
alkaline phosphatase and serum bilirubin.
These acute findings should arouse a suspicion of intrahepatic abscess but they are
by no means specific. The same acute picture
may be presented by acute obstructive suppurative cholangitis without hepatic abscess.
Prompt fluid and electrolyte replacement
and expeditious biliary decompression usually preclude the use of specific diagnostic
tests for hepatic abscesses. The usual radiographic aids are of limited assistance.
Posteroanterior and lateral roentgenograms

of the chest show evidence usually of hepatomegaly, but pleural effusions and air-fluid levels are rare in association with the multiple small abscesses of this disease process.

Hepatic photoscan is probably the most practical of the specific diagnostic studies unless the procedure is contraindicated by the general condition of the patient. Hepatic arteriography and splenoportography, although at times useful in the diagnosis and localization of the more chronic forms of hepatic abscess, have not been used in the diagnostic evaluation of the reported cases of suppurative cholangitis. Portal venography with dye injection through the obliterated umbilical vein has also been proposed (Piccone, 1968).

Operative cholangiography may be considered in the less acutely ill patient following complete decompression of the intra- and extrahepatic biliary tract. Abscess pockets will be demonstrated if cavitation has occurred. Care should be taken to insure a minimal intraductal pressure during the injection of the contrast medium. Postoperative tube cholangiography may also be helpful in establishing the diagnosis of intrahepatic abscesses. One postoperative death has been attributed to recurrent sepsis induced by a postoperative cholangiogram in a patient who was apparently progressing satisfactorily following common duct decompression (Haupert et al., 1967).

As in the treatment of suppurative cholangitis without liver abscess, there are several important factors that influence the result of treatment of the disease complicated by intrahepatic abscesses.

Failure to establish the diagnosis. Patients with intrahepatic sepsis are likely to have more of the characteristics of severe biliary disease than those without hepatic disease. They are more likely to have a history of previous biliary tract disease, jaundice, and a swollen, tender liver. The confusion here may be with a severe hepatitis.

Closely related to difficulty in establishing a diagnosis is the effect of *delay in decompression of the common duct.* An increased survival has been observed in all series of patients with suppurative cholangitis operated upon early as compared to those whose operation was performed after a significant delay. Delay in biliary decompression is of even greater hazard in the patient with hepatic sepsis because of the frequency of gram-negative septicemia. As Furey (1966) states, "This is a serious and frequently fatal condition, requiring immediate and vigorous therapy. Postponement of surgery may result in the patient's death."

Haupert and associates (1967) have correlated the mortality rate of suppurative cholangitis with the *nature of the antibiotic therapy.* As indicated in a previous section, our preference for initial antibiotic therapy is a combination of ampicillin and Chloromycetin. Administration of an effective antibiotic by way of the umbilical vein as reported by Piccone (1968) may have specific value for the patient with multiple intrahepatic abscesses.

Effective decompression of the biliary system is essential. A number of patients have died because the obstructed portion of the biliary tree was not adequately decompressed at operation. Ostermiller and associates in 1965 recommended using the simplest procedure possible that would adequately decompress the common duct in these critically ill patients. Choledochostomy is their preferred procedure. Dow and Lindenauer reported in 1969 that the multiple hepatic abscesses found at autopsy in a large percentage of their patients and in cases reported in the literature had not been effectively treated by adequate biliary decompression alone. Such abscesses contributed to continued postoperative sepsis and to the ultimate high mortality of the disease. Improvement of results could best be achieved, they advise, by interrupting the course of cholangitis with operative decompression of the biliary tree before septicemia and hepatic abscesses develop. The simplest and most reliable method of obtaining decompression of the extrahepatic biliary ducts is used. In most instances this is drainage of the common bile duct. If the patient is operated upon late in the course of the disease and has developed septicemia, a search for a liver abscess is made.

In summary it is clear that the group of patients with intrahepatic abscesses will include many of the most advanced and critically ill patients with suppurative cholangitis. Prompt diagnosis of the biliary problem, not necessarily including special studies to define intrahepatic disease, is essential, accompanied by expeditious supportive therapy and operation to provide effective decompression of the biliary tract above the site of obstruction. Coalescence of multiple abscesses into a single large collection is rare, but if this is detected at operation it should·be separately drained through the site nearest the surface of the liver. An operative cholangiogram performed with minimal pressure may establish the presence of intrahepatic suppuration and assist in postoperative treatment and prognosis.

Antibiotic therapy is instituted as a part of the preoperative supportive therapy. A combination of ampicillin and Chloromycetin should be used until drug sensitivity studies are completed in cultures obtained at operation. The administration of the appropriate antibiotic therapy by way of the umbilical vein (Piccone, 1968) may have merit in the treatment of the patient who does not respond to biliary decompression.

The outcome of the patient with multiple hepatic abscesses will rest on his response to general supportive measures, effective biliary decompression, and antibiotic therapy. The mortality of this complication has been high.

CHRONIC CHOLANGITIS

Most patients seen with the acute form of cholangitis and a history of previous biliary tract disease have an underlying chronic form of cholangitis with a persistent bactibilia and recurrent attacks of acute or subacute inflammation invariably associated with choledocholithiasis or stricture. Many of the minor attacks may be subclinical and not properly diagnosed or identified. Such persistent infection involves the finer radicles of the intrahepatic ductal system and, if undisturbed, will eventually provoke a sclerosis of the cholangioles and a secondary form of hepatic cirrhosis or the formation of multiple intrahepatic abscesses. The latter will eventually cause an acute generalized sepsis and the probable death of the patient. Colcock and Perey in 1964 noted a reduction in the incidence of common duct stones from 10.4 per cent to 7.9 per cent in a series of 1754 cholecystectomies reviewed approximately ten years after a similar earlier series. They felt that this decrease reflected the adoption of a policy of operating earlier for the removal of the gallbladder whenever a diagnosis of cholelithiasis was made.

Any steps that may be taken to reduce the incidence of choledocholithiasis will substantially lessen the opportunity for developing these potentially lethal forms of cholangitis.

Drainage of the common duct and removal of all stones and debris are indicated, of course, as soon as the diagnosis of choledocholithiasis is established. At the time of exploration care should be exercised not to cause an elevation of the intrahepatic ductal pressure or to needlessly traumatize the duct mucosa lest bacteria pass into the bloodstream and result in a gram-negative septicemia.

REFERENCES

Barber-Riley, G.: Rat biliary tree during short periods of obstruction of the common duct. Amer. J. Physiol., 205:1125, 1963.

Charcot, J. M.: Oeuvres Complètes de J. M. Charcot. VI, Leçons sur les maladies du foie et des reins. Bourneville, Sevestre et Brissau, p. 194. Paris, Vve. Babe et Cie., 1891.

Colcock, B. P., and Perey, B.: Exploration of the common bile duct. Surg. Gynec. Obstet., 118:20, 1964.

Cole, W. N.: Suppurative cholangitis. Surg. Clin. N. Amer., 27:23, 1947.

Danduraṅd, B., Saint-Martin, M., and Beaudoin, L.: Abcès microbiens du foie. Union Méd. du Canada, 98:63, 1969.

Deaver, J. B.: Cholangitis and hepatitis. New Eng. J. Med., 202:513, 1930.

Dorland's Illustrated Medical Dictionary. 24th ed. Philadelphia, W. B. Saunders Co., 1965, p. 295.

Dow, R. W., and Lindenauer, S. M.: Acute obstructive suppurative cholangitis. Ann. Surg., 169:272, 1969.

Edlund, Y., and Hanzon, V.: Demonstration of the close relationship between bile capillaries and sinusoid walls. Acta Anat., 17:105, 1953.

Edlund, Y. A., Mollstedt, B. O., and Ouchterlony, O.: Bacteriological investigation of the biliary system and liver in biliary tract disease correlated to clinical data and microstructure of the gallbladder and liver. Acta Chir. Scandinav., 116:461, 1959.

Flemma, B. J., Flint, L. M., Osterhout, S., and Shingleton, W. W.: Bacteriologic studies of biliary tract infections. Ann. Surg., 166:563, 1967.

Furey, A. T.: Ascending cholangitis. New York J. Med., 66:1299, 1966.

Glenn, F.: The liver and biliary system. In Davis, L. (ed.): Christopher's Textbook of Surgery. 7th ed. Philadelphia, W. B. Saunders Company, 1960, p. 759.

Glenn, F., and Moody, F. G.: Acute obstructive suppurative cholangitis. Surg. Gynec. Obstet., 113:265, 1961.

Grant, H. D.: Acute suppurative cholangitis. Permanente Found. Med. Bull., 3:175, 1945.

Hampson, L. G., Dickison, J. C., and Robertson, H. R.: Emergency surgery involving the biliary tract. Surg. Clin. N. Amer., 40:1171, 1960.

Hampton, J. C.: An electron microscope study of the hepatic uptake and excretion of submicroscopic particles injected into the blood stream and into the bile duct. Acta Anat., 32:262, 1958.

Haupert, A. P., Carey, L. C., Evans, W. E., and Ellison, E. H.: Acute suppurative cholangitis. Arch. Surg., *94:*460, 1967.

Hinchey, E. J., and Couper, C. E.: Acute obstructive suppurative cholangitis. Amer. J. Surg., *117:*62, 1969.

Howard, F. M., Jr., Martin, W. J., Stauffer, M. H., and Hallenbeck, G. A.: Common duct stone producing Charcot's hepatic fever without jaundice. Arch. Intern. Med., *103:*69, 1959.

Huang, T., Bass, J. A., and Williams, R. D.: The significance of biliary pressure in cholangitis. Arch. Surg., *98:*629, 1969.

Hultborn, A., Jacobsson, B., and Rosengren, B.: Cholangiovenous reflux during cholangiography. Acta Chir. Scandinav., *123:*111, 1962.

Jacobsson, B., Kjellander, J., and Rosengren, B.: Cholangiovenous reflux. Acta Chir. Scandinav., *123:*316, 1962.

Joseph, W. L., Kahn, A. M., and Longmire, W. P., Jr.: Pyogenic liver abscess. Amer. J. Surg., *115:*63, 1968.

Kinney, T. D., and Ferrebee, J. N.: Hepatic abscess: factors determining its localization. Arch. Path., *45:*41, 1948.

Longmire, W. P., Jr., and Bruckner, W. L.: Periampullary carcinoma. Proceedings, Sectional Meeting, American College of Surgeons, held in cooperation with the German Surgical Society, June 1968. Berlin, Springer-Verlag, 1969, p. 210.

Mage, S., and Morel, A. S.: Surgical experience with cholangiohepatitis (Hong Kong disease) in Canton Chinese. Ann. Surg., *162:*187, 1965.

Mixer, H. W., Rigler, L. G., and Gonzales-Oddone, M. V.: Experimental studies on biliary regurgitation during cholangiography. Gastroenterology, *9:*64, 1947.

Moynihan, B. G. A.: Gallstones and Their Surgical Treatment. Philadelphia, W. B. Saunders Company, 1904, p. 86.

Ong, G. B.: A study of recurrent pyogenic cholangitis. Arch. Surg., *84:*63, 1962.

Ostermiller, W., Jr., Thompson, R. J., Carter, R., and Hinshaw, D. B.: Acute obstructive cholangitis. Arch. Surg., *90:*392, 1965.

Piccone, V. A.: Discussion of paper by Joseph, W. L., Kahn, A. M., and Longmire, W. P., Jr.: Pyogenic liver abscess. Amer. J. Surg., *115:*63, 1968.

Reynolds, B. M., and Dargan, E. L.: Acute obstructive cholangitis, a distinct clinical syndrome. Ann. Surg., *150:*299, 1959.

Rogers, L.: Biliary abscesses of the liver with operation. Brit. Med. J., *2:*706, 1903.

Rouiller, C.: Les canalicules biliares: Etude au microscope électronique. Acta Anat., *26:*94, 1956.

Schatten, W. E., Desprez, J. D., and Holden, W. E.: A bacteriological study of portal vein in man. Arch. Surg., *71:*404, 1955.

Scott, A. J., and Khan, G. A.: Origin of bacteria in bile duct bile. Lancet, *2:*790, 1967.

Sherman, J. D., and Robbins, S.: Changing trends in the casuistics of hepatic abscess. Amer. J. Med., *28:*943, 1960.

Swartz, S. I.: Surgical Diseases of the Liver. New York, McGraw-Hill Book Company, Inc., 1964, Chapter 8.

Waddell, G. F.: Acute obstructive cholangitis. Scot. Med. J., *11:*137, 1966.

Wissmer, B.: Cholangitis. In Bockus, H. L. (ed.): Gastroenterology. Philadelphia, W. B. Saunders Company, 1965.

CHAPTER 17

ACUTE NECROTIZING PANCREATITIS

by ROGER D. WILLIAMS, M.D.

Roger D. Williams is a North Carolinian who attended both college and medical school at Duke University. His residency training in surgery at Ohio State University under Robert Zollinger was supplemented by a year in pathology. He subsequently progressed to full professor of Surgery at Ohio State and, in 1965, accepted the chair at the University of Texas Medical Branch in Galveston. At present he is in private practice and serves as Clinical Professor of Surgery at the University of Miami. Among his most significant works are those dealing with the biliary tract and pancreas.

Probably no other disorder is more often incorrectly diagnosed or inadequately treated than pancreatitis. This is in part due to its mimicking other diseases by its various forms. In order to simplify this discussion, no effort is made to define the several forms of pancreatitis, but rather to delineate acute hemorrhagic (necrotizing) pancreatitis and to present its complications and management. This surprisingly common catastrophic disorder, often associated with gallstones or alcoholism, occurs in all age groups and is easily confused with peptic ulcer, intestinal obstruction, dissecting aortic aneurysm, severe cholecystitis, acute coronary occlusion, or mesenteric vascular occlusion.

If considered, the diagnosis of acute necrotizing pancreatitis can be confirmed readily, and vigorous treatment can yield a low mortality. As Frey and others have reported, the mortality rate is from 12 to 25 per cent in retrospective reviews of clinical experience with this disease. A lower mortality can be achieved, as Elliott has shown, by adequate diagnostic studies in all patients with abdominal pain and by a diligent program of treatment in all cases of acute pancreatitis. Although still considered by many physicians to be a nonoperative disorder, the time has arrived to re-evaluate the complications due to necrotizing pancreatitis and to outline the indications for direct surgical as well as meticulous medical management.

ETIOLOGY

Let us first agree that we do not know the cause of necrotizing pancreatitis, except trauma, which cause, too, may not be self-evident. A relationship with biliary tract disease, particularly gallstones, and alcoholism is well established. What portion of necrotizing pancreatitis is actually related to these two disorders is difficult to discern from many reports which combine acute interstitial, hemorrhagic, acute recurrent, and chronic forms of pancreatitis for discussion.

Pancreatitis has been produced experimentally in numerous ways, as shown in Figure 17-1. Elliott and associates revised Opie's original theory of the relationship between pancreatitis and the simultaneous obstruction of the common bile duct and pancreatic duct by showing that bile and pancreatic juice, mixed together and incubated for 12 hours or longer, would readily enter the canine pancreas and produce hemorrhagic pancreatitis. Vascular disturbances have been implicated as a cause of pancreatitis. Block and associates relate this to combined ductal obstruction and vascular obstruction, while Thal and

425

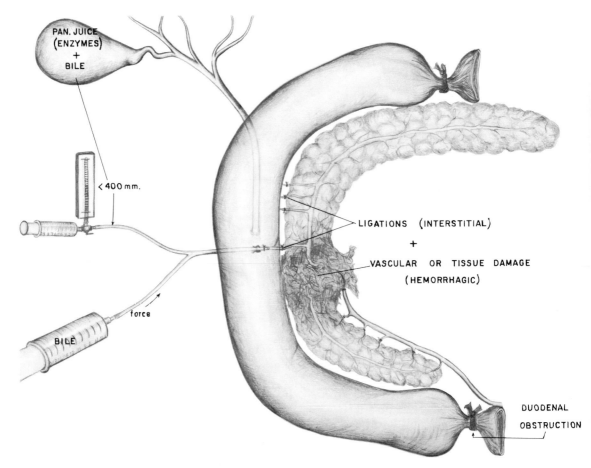

Figure 17-1. Methods of experimentally causing pancreatitis. See text for discussion.

Brockney produced pancreatitis by the Shwartzman reaction. Menguy and associates have produced pancreatitis by combined ductal ligation and splanchnic-nerve stimulation. Whether the pancreatitis resulting from duodenal obstruction as produced by Pfeffer, Stasior, and Hinton is due to bacteria, enzyme activation, or vascular factors is still debated by Byrne and associates. Epstein and Williams have shown experimentally that the effect of alcohol upon pancreatic secretion is through an increase in acid production, stimulating secretin release from the duodenum. It is assumed that alcohol may produce pancreatitis by causing edema of the ampulla of Vater and stimulating pancreatic secretion. Future attacks of both alcoholic pancreatitis and that associated with gallstones are preventable.

With the exception of a common channel obstruction by stone, it is difficult to relate pancreatic to biliary tract disease without assuming a relationship with the gallbladder. When stones exist, removal of the gallbladder alone usually prevents further episodes of pancreatitis; perhaps the gallbladder does serve as a container for incubation of bile and pancreatic enzymes, which then enter the pancreas at physiologic pressures to cause pancreatitis. Even so, most cases of acute hemorrhagic pancreatitis occur after long periods of alcoholism, in the presence of perhaps long-standing gallstones, as a catastrophic complication of surgery, or with no apparent associated disorder. This may leave us wondering in many cases what the specific causative factors really are.

A clinical relationship to other disorders is noted in approximately two-thirds of patients with acute necrotizing pancreatitis. As shown in Figure 17-2, the two most frequent associated diseases are gallstones and alcoholism. Mumps pancreatitis is uncom-

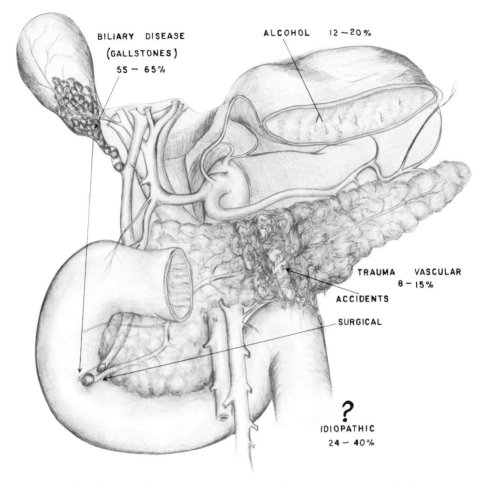

Figure 17-2. Related causative factors in acute pancreatitis. Percentage ranges are from literature reports.

mon, usually mild, and difficult to diagnose. The relationship between the rare, severe hyperlipemia and pancreatitis is well established, though the combined etiologic factors are not well defined. Trauma does not produce pancreatitis; but when the surgical management of pancreatic injury is inadequate, pancreatitis usually follows. This is not true for postoperative pancreatitis, which carries such a high mortality. Perhaps initially the largest number of cases of acute hemorrhagic pancreatitis will be considered idiopathic, since the associated disorder, excluding surgery or direct trauma, may not be obvious. The number which finally fall into the group of idiopathic pancreatitis will depend upon the adequacy of evaluation following recovery from the initial attack. While a second attack of hemorrhagic pancreatitis is rare when the cause is not found, future attacks of both alcoholic pancreatitis and that associated with

gallstones occur unless these disorders are corrected.

DIAGNOSIS

The diagnosis of hemorrhagic pancreatitis is made by careful history-taking and physical examination, combined with adequate, well-chosen laboratory study. It must be suspected when the differential diagnosis arises between all possible acute abdominal disorders. It must be considered in any patient not progressing satisfactorily after abdominal, particularly biliary and gastric, surgery.

Pain is the constant, and most often the first, symptom, although its location suggests other abdominal disorders. This is readily appreciated considering the location of the pancreas in relation to the celiac and mesenteric nerve plexuses (Fig. 17-3). Zol-

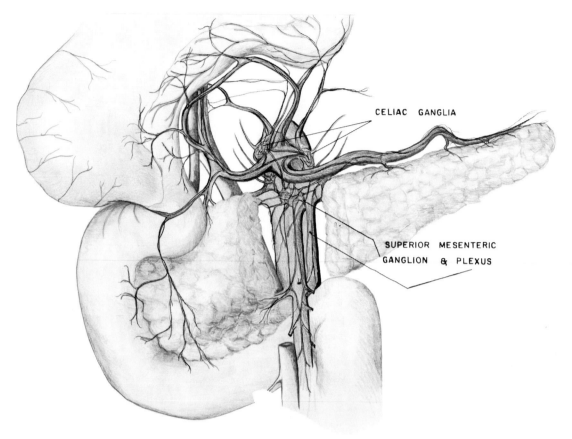

CELIAC GANGLIA

SUPERIOR MESENTERIC
GANGLION & PLEXUS

Figure 17-3.   The ganglia and rich nerve plexus in and around the pancreas account for the severe pain of necrotizing pancreatitis.

linger and associates stimulated the human pancreas electrically. When the head was stimulated, pain was felt in the right upper quadrant; body stimulation caused epigastric pain; the pain arising from the tail occurred in the left flank or left lower quadrant. Only maximal stimulation of all three sections of the pancreas produced band-like pain. This study helps to explain the lower abdominal and flank pain noted in the large series of Paxton and Payne. Clinically, pancreatic pain varies from a mild ache to a severe, constant, boring pain. It may be improved by sitting, leaning forward, or lying on the side or stomach. Unfortunately, its occurrence in the postoperative period is both uncommon and overshadowed by the pain from the surgical procedure.

Vomiting may be severe and unrelieved, even by a nasogastric tube, until pain is controlled. *Abdominal distention* is variable, but its persistence combined with prolonged ileus is perhaps the single most reliable indication that the inflammatory process in the pancreas is increasing its hemorrhagic necrosis, or that a complication is developing. *Gastrointestinal hemorrhage* occurs early or late in 5 to 10 per cent of these patients. *Diarrhea*, usually of unexplained cause, occurs almost as frequently. *Abdominal tenderness* is usually present but varies in location and severity from mild epigastric discomfort, when pressure is applied, to severe generalized tenderness and rebound tenderness.

Roentgenograms initially show nothing, but within hours to days they give evidence of paralytic ileus and, later, the complications of pancreatitis. Consequently, one evaluation is rarely sufficient. The so-called sentinel loops of small-intestinal gas and the colon cut-off sign due to paralytic ileus are helpful though not always found (Fig. 17-4). Recently, selective arteriographic studies have suggested that these changes may be due in part to arterial involvement in the inflammatory process. As the process continues, air bubbles from an abscess, a pseudocyst displacing the stomach, duodenum, or colon, elevation of the diaphragm, or fluid in the left chest may be noted.

Serum amylase determinations may be diagnostic early, but normal within hours or a few days after onset of symptoms. Although this enzyme may be elevated in nonpancreatic disorders, and some surgeons therefore consider it unreliable, the large number of determinations reviewed by Elliott and Williams defines its value: When above 500 Somogyi units, pancreatitis is almost definite; when between 250 and 500 units, there is rarely great difficulty in defining another cause for the elevation if it exists; when normal, other diagnostic methods should be sought.

Gambill and Mason, and Saxon and his associates suggest that *urine amylase determinations* may be more diagnostic than those of serum amylase. Urine is collected for two hours and reported in units cleared per hour which should normally be less

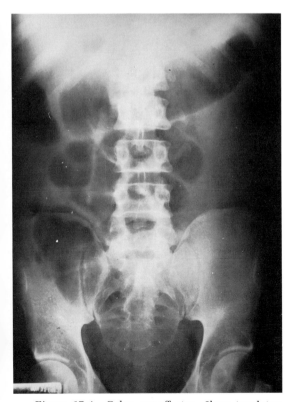

Figure 17-4. Colon cut-off sign. Ileus involving upper jejunal loops and transverse colon associated with distention ending with splenic flexure.

than 300 units. While amylase remains elevated longer in the urine than in the blood, there is general agreement that one urine determination when blood levels are normal is not diagnostic, and urine and blood determinations should be done simultaneously. Urine amylase may indicate severe hemorrhagic pancreatitis when seen late, after blood levels have returned to normal, but more often it is of value in diagnosing chronic pancreatitis. The urine amylase may be of value in following the course of pancreatitis when persistent elevation suggests continued inflammation, or the development of complications or both.

In severe pancreatitis, determination of the *serum calcium* may be as helpful as the serum amylase. Over half of these patients will have hypocalcemia. A low calcium level, particularly below 3.5 milliequivalents per liter, suggests severe pancreatitis and a poor prognosis. Calcium determinations are also important in pancreatitis because of the occasional association with hyperparathyroidism. *Glycosuria* and *hyperglycemia* are common findings early in the course of this disease, hyperglycemia occurring in over 70 per cent of cases. According to Akzhigitov and Strygina, diabetes is present in approximately 1.4 per cent and develops in another 2.3 per cent as a result of pancreatitis. *Hyperlipemia* is a less common associated disorder which should be evaluated if the serum is cloudy. Although old-fashioned, the *blood hematocrit* and the *urine specific gravity* tests are still useful in determining the state of hydration.

Trapnell considers the determination of *serum methemalbumin* levels to be helpful in differentiating interstitial from hemorrhagic pancreatitis. A recent study by Anderson and associates confirms this impression but shows that methemalbumin may be elevated in the serum in the presence of any intra-abdominal necrosis. Consequently, its elevation will not differentiate necrosis with intestinal infarction from that associated with hemorrhagic pancreatitis. This laboratory test, plus the repeated use of roentgenograms consisting of barium and air contrast studies and arteriographic procedures, may become important in following the course of patients with pancreatitis. Since it is impossible to determine the severity of pancreatitis at the onset, repeated observations are important to determine complications, such as increasing necrosis, abscess or pseudocyst formation, and intestinal obstruction.

Diagnostic paracentesis in pancreatitis has had insufficient use, probably because it was either incorrectly performed or mistakenly overrated. Keith and associates showed that peritoneal amylase remains elevated much longer than the serum amylase. Of more importance is the use of needle aspiration to exclude other diagnoses. The presence of bile, bacteria, or a low pH all point to a lesion which usually requires surgical intervention.

TREATMENT

The management of acute necrotizing pancreatitis must be vigorous, sustained, and frequently re-evaluated. As Trapnell has shown, the initial assessment of the patient's state gives no real guide to the prognosis. It is for this reason that the vigorous therapy advocated by Elliott seems preferable to selective management based upon an initial or early impression.

Nasogastric suction is used in all patients. A sump-type, double-lumen tube has been found to work better than the standard Levin tube. The volume of gastric aspirate is usually enough to require careful measurement and replacement. This tube is not removed until at least 48 hours after symptoms subside. While absence of bowel sounds and x-ray evidence of ileus are considered indications of continued or progressing pancreatitis, a well-functioning gastric sump will itself decrease bowel activity. The principle of gastric aspiration is to prevent acid from entering the duodenum and stimulating secretin release. Premature feeding is a major cause for flare-up of subsiding pancreatitis. Before the tube is removed, an overnight, 12-hour aspiration is measured for volume and free acid. Large volumes with high acid either suggest obstruction or may be of value in subsequent management. If tenderness, fever, or amylase elevation in the blood or urine persists, the patient should not be fed.

Fluid replacement is extremely important and the type of fluid is apparently specific. Some authors have simply advocated 3000 to 4000 cc. of glucose in water per day. Elliott's studies in animals and patients show that the protein-rich fluid in the pancreas and adjacent tissues is decreased when blood or serum albumin is administered and that the mortality is definitely lowered. More recently, Carey has shown that dextran is superior to albumin or saline in decreasing mortality due to experimental pancreatitis. There is also evidence that dextran decreases pancreatic secretions. It therefore seems preferable to give at least 500 cc. of dextran and 500 cc. of 5 per cent albumin solution plus 2 to 4 liters of Ringer's lactate during each of the first one to three days of therapy. As soon as symptoms definitely subside, dextran and albumin can be eliminated and subsequent fluid therapy can be based on daily basal requirements plus the replacement of estimated water and electrolyte losses. Should the hemoglobin and hematocrit drop to levels below 10 gm. and 30 per cent, respectively, blood transfusions are preferred. Urine output and serum electrolyte determinations are fairly good guides to the adequacy of fluid replacement, but repeated blood volume determinations are more helpful, particularly in elderly patients or those in whom the symptoms and signs of pancreatitis persist. Should the pancreatitis seem slow to resolve, chances are good that a complication is developing.

Antibiotics are given intravenously in sufficient dosage to decrease the incidence of secondary infection. Abscess formation is frequent enough to justify attempts to prevent it. Although staphylococcal abscesses are not rare, 1.5 to 2 gm. of either tetracycline or ampicillin per day in four to six divided doses until the course of pancreatitis has been determined is perhaps as efficacious as any antibiotic.

Pain relief is best accomplished with Demerol or morphine. Both produce spasm of the sphincter of Oddi; however, Butsch and associates have shown that this can be relieved by frequent sublingual glyceryl trinitrate. Stefanini and associates have found intravenous procaine to be quite effective. If these drugs do not suffice, blockage of the splanchnic nerves should be considered.

Calcium gluconate and occasionally parathormone may be required. In severe cases of pancreatitis it is important also to consider other metabolic derangements. In addition to serum electrolytes, base excess or deficit and blood-gas studies should be evaluated. Shock, hypovolemia, and marked tissue destruction cause major metabolic changes.

X-ray therapy has been found to be of

value in pancreatitis and the mortality is reported to be lower with this form of therapy than with others. While x-ray therapy may be helpful in the management of early pancreatitis, repeated observations should be made for complications not amenable to such therapy.

Anticholinergics, insulin, adrenocorticosteroids, and *Trasylol* are of no significant value and may even be dangerous. The dosage of *atropine, Pro-Banthine,* or *Pamine* recommended by most authors is ineffective in preventing pancreatic secretion or significantly reducing gastric secretion. To achieve this effect a "toxic" dose, producing tachycardia, marked dryness of the mouth, and even hyperpyrexia or mental confusion, is required; these signs cloud the clinical picture of pancreatitis and are uncomfortable for the patient. A well-functioning gastric tube decreases pancreatic stimulation and deserves more attention with less reliance on drugs. Despite frequent hyperglycemia, *insulin* is dangerous, since it may readily produce an excessive response with hypoglycemia. *Trasylol,* a trypsin and kallikrein inhibitor, has been found effective only when given before or concomitant with the production of experimental pancreatitis. There is no clear evidence to justify its clinical use, except perhaps in the prevention of anticipated postoperative pancreatitis after known surgical pancreatic trauma. *Adrenocorticosteroids* will decrease the inflammatory reaction in pancreatitis, but, as Stewart and associates have shown, the complications are increased. Since there is increasing evidence that steroids can also initiate pancreatitis, their use is not recommended.

POSTOPERATIVE PANCREATITIS

Pancreatitis after surgery deserves special attention since it is so difficult to diagnose and causes such a high mortality. It occurs more frequently after gastric and biliary procedures but has been an occasional cause of death after colon, aortic aneurysm, neurologic, cardiac, and pulmonary procedures, and many other types of surgery.

It is difficult to determine the true incidence of postoperative pancreatitis. Abasov in a recent review states that the severe form, producing a definite diagnosis through sufficient symptoms or death, is reported after 1.2 to 1.7 per cent of gastric operations. In less severe form, it is reported in 9 to 47 per cent of cases. He found an elevated urine amylase of over 500 Wohlgemuth units in one-fifth of his patients. It occurs even more often after biliary tract surgery. Bardenheier and associates found pancreatitis after 4 per cent of their biliary tract operations and an elevation of serum amylase above 200 Somogyi units in 9.5 per cent. They found a very high mortality, a finding confirmed by other authors. Peterson and associates also emphasize the higher incidence of pancreatitis when the common bile duct is explored and the high mortality, which was 36 per cent in their series. Although White and Murat suggest that careful avoidance of injury to the common bile duct, pancreas, and ampulla will decrease this serious complication of pancreaticobiliary surgery, there seems to be no better answer to pancreatitis following other surgery than earlier and more accurate diagnosis.

The diagnosis of postoperative pancreatitis can be improved, if it is looked for more often. Oliguria, jaundice, hyperglycemia, perhaps associated with obligatory dehydration from glycosuria, hypocalcemia, and shock should all suggest the need for considering pancreatitis. Unexplained hypotension is usually associated with the more severe form. Unfortunately all of these symptoms may be related to the surgical procedure.

Both blood and urine amylase determinations should be made. In view of the frequency of pancreatitis after biliary and gastric surgery, amylase determinations should always be performed when there are technical difficulties at surgery or when the patient is slow to recover. Although there are other causes for amylase elevations, blood levels above 300 units and urine levels above 500 units should be considered diagnostic of pancreatitis.

DIAGNOSIS AND TREATMENT OF COMPLICATIONS

Although the early management of necrotizing pancreatitis and the total management of interstitial pancreatitis are nonoperative, this disorder should not be considered medical. The complications of necrotizing pancreatitis are all surgical problems. These complications include jaundice, progressive pancreatic and surrounding tissue necrosis, hemorrhage, abscess and pseudocyst formation, and intestinal obstruction. There remains no method of regularly distinguishing either the initial severity of pancreatitis or whether it will progress to complications. Close observation with repeated studies and earlier direct surgical intervention may prevent some complications, notably abscess and hemorrhage. In the well-prepared patient there is no evidence that surgical intervention increases mortality.

Jaundice can occur as a result of initial combined obstruction of the common bile duct and pancreatic duct or as a secondary obstruction due to edema or necrosis of the head of the pancreas. Fish and associates have shown that pancreatitis is second only to a common-duct stone as the cause of unexplained jaundice associated with cholecystitis. If the jaundice and pancreatitis are both due to a common-duct stone, or if the jaundice is due to interstitial pancreatitis, the patient's condition should progressively improve with nonoperative therapy. Progression of jaundice may not only produce liver damage but may also imply that the inflammatory process is not adequately controlled. Surgical intervention seems imperative unless the process rapidly subsides and the jaundice clears.

The presence of an associated mass, whether it be considered gallbladder or pancreatic necrosis, is an indication for surgical intervention. In such cases necrotic pancreatic tissue should be removed by direct surgical excision combined with sump drainage. The gallbladder should be removed even in the absence of stones, since drainage of the common bile duct will be required. There is sufficient evidence that mixing of bile and pancreatic juice combined with obstruction of a main bile duct produces and accentuates pancreatitis, and this process can be controlled only by adequate biliary tract drainage.

Progressive pancreatic and surrounding tissue necrosis may be extremely difficult to determine. The continued presence of elevated pulse, temperature, white blood cell count, and serum amylase level all point to progression or continuation of the inflammatory process. A continued elevation of the amylase alone, occurring in 3.4 per cent of patients, is not a specific indication of pancreatic necrosis, progression of the process, or for surgical intervention. On the other hand, the development of a mass, temperature elevation, and continued tenderness suggest that pancreatic necrosis may lead to subsequent complications. Involvement of the duodenum and colon in progressive necrosis has been reported. This is preventable only by adequate surgical debridement. Although few authors have advocated primary excision of grossly necrotic pancreatic tissue, recent experience is in agreement with the report of Khedroo and Cosella, who have concluded that necrotic pancreatic tissue should be treated in the same way as necrotic tissue elsewhere—surgical debridement should be combined with adequate sump drainage.

Hemorrhage may occur directly from the pancreatic vessels involved in areas of necrosis or may occur from a duodenal ulcer. The incidence of hemorrhage from the gastrointestinal tract or into the pancreatic bed, as reported by Kirby and associates, is quite high. Bleeding was the most common cause of death in their more recent experience with pancreatitis. It may be prevented only by early surgical intervention, which is indicated in the presence of continued abdominal tenderness, development of a mass, or any evidence that the inflammatory process is not subsiding within a few days.

Abscess formation may be extremely difficult to determine but should be suspected in the presence of continued elevation of the white blood cell count, temperature, and pulse. An abdominal mass is present in approximately half of the patients. Occasionally air bubbles are seen on flat and upright films of the abdomen. This is often associated with moderate to marked accumulation of fluid in the left chest, which is usually sterile.

Although coliform organisms are more frequent, staphylococci have been reported in 13 to 50 per cent of abscesses. Evans states that antibiotics do not halt the progress of abscess formation, although there is no clear-cut evidence regarding their benefit from a prophylactic standpoint. The mortality is quite high, emphasizing the need for earlier diagnosis and surgical intervention in patients who continue to have temperature elevations and a mass. Survival is unlikely without adequate drainage.

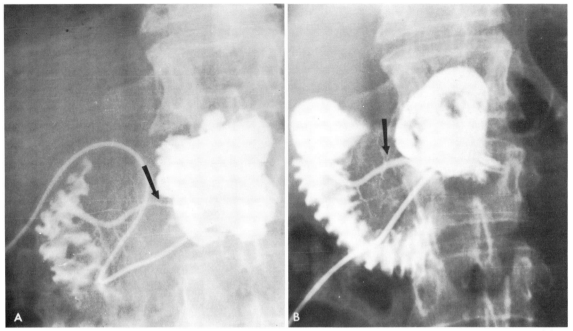

Figure 17-5. Note that, *A*, the pancreatic duct (arrow), which narrowed early, *B*, subsequently became normal, allowing the cyst to empty via the duodenum. See text for discussion.

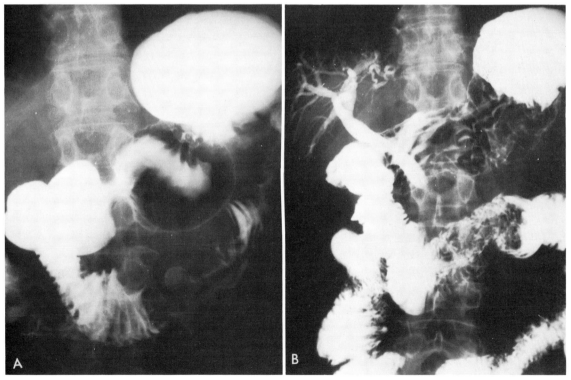

Figure 17-6. *A*, Almost complete obstruction of the fourth portion of the duodenum due to pancreatitis. *B*, Note that after choledochoduodenostomy and duodenojejunostomy to relieve both this and a lower partial common duct obstruction, the duodenal obstruction subsequently resolved.

Pseudocyst formation is a frequent complication of acute pancreatitis and usually indicates that the inflammatory process has initially subsided but that the main pancreatic duct or a branch remains obstructed. This can be differentiated from abscess by the presence of a high serum amylase associated with relatively few accompanying symptoms other than a mass. Many of these patients exhibit evidence of upper small-bowel obstruction. Oral administration of small amounts of barium, insufflation of air into the colon, and arteriography in a combined procedure will define precisely the location of the cyst and will permit an easier and more direct surgical approach.

Some reports advocate internal drainage as the choice treatment for pancreatic pseudocyst. This is not advised in all cases for two reasons: First, as Polk and associates have reported, these collections may be in reality abscesses and not uncomplicated pseudocysts. Even if the fluid is relatively clear, the cyst wall of an acute cyst is too thin and friable to be used efficiently for intestinal anastomosis; second, not only is external drainage easier and safer as a first procedure, in many acute pseudocysts it may be the only required surgery. Figure 17-5 illustrates why this is so. The pseudocyst, which was thin-walled and quite large, had decreased to less than half its original size in one week (Fig. 17-5A). The pancreatic duct, though narrowed initially, is open completely for drainage via the normal channel in two weeks (Fig. 17-5B). This cyst, with an open ductal communication, resolved without the need for another surgical procedure. If resolution fails in such cases because of continued occlusion of the route of internal drainage, it is much easier to perform a pancreaticojejunostomy for a smaller, thick-walled cyst.

Intestinal obstruction is not an infrequent complication of acute pancreatitis. Initially it results from edema and the inflammatory process, which produces severe paralytic ileus. Secondarily, it produces mechanical obstruction, as shown in Figure 17-6A, in which there is complete narrowing of the fourth portion of the duodenum due to marked constriction following an attack of acute pancreatitis. In this case, at the time of surgical intervention, the common bile duct was also found to be distended and surgical treatment consisted of choledochoduodenostomy in addition to gastrojejunostomy (Fig. 17-6B). Patients with intestinal obstruction will require surgical intervention if the obstruction persists more than a few days.

REFERENCES

Abasov, I. T.: Pancreatitis following operations on the stomach. Arch. Surg., 96:909, 1968.

Akzhigitov, G. N., and Strygina, T. A.: Interrelation between acute pancreatitis and diabetes mellitus. Klin. Med. (Mosk.), 46:70, 1968.

Anderson, M. C., Toronto, I. R., Needleman, S. B., and Gramatica, L.: Assessment of Methemalbumin as a diagnostic test for acute pancreatitis. Arch. Surg., 98:776, 1969.

Bardenheier, J. A., Kaminski, D. L., and Williams, V. L.: Pancreatitis after biliary tract surgery. Amer. J. Surg., 116:773, 1968.

Block, M. A., Wakim, K. A., and Baggenstross, A. H.: Experimental studies concerning factors in the pathogenesis of acute pancreatitis. Surg. Gynec. Obstet., 99:83, 1954.

Butsch, W. L., McGowan, J. M., and Walters, W.: Clinical studies in the influence of certain drugs in relation to biliary pain and to the variations in intrabiliary pressure. Surg. Gynec. Obstet., 63:451, 1936.

Byrne, J. J., Novogradac, W., Wilde, W. L., and Seifert, D. E.: The vascular factor in experimental hemorrhagic pancreatitis. Exp. Med. Surg., 22:332, 1965.

Carey, L. C.: Low molecular Dextran in experimental pancreatitis. Amer. J. Surg., 119:197, 1970.

Elliott, D. W.: Treatment of acute pancreatitis with albumin and whole blood. Arch. Surg., 75:573, 1957.

Elliott, D. W., and Williams, R. D.: A re-evaluation of serum amylase determinations. Arch. Surg., 83:130, 1961.

Elliott, D. W., Williams, R. D., and Stewart, W. R. C.: The role of trypsin and of bile salts in the pathogenesis of acute pancreatitis. Surg. Forum, 9:533, 1958.

Elliott, D. W., Williams, R. D., and Zollinger, R. M.: Alterations in the pancreatic resistance to bile in the pathogenesis of acute pancreatitis. Ann. Surg., 146:669, 1957.

Epstein, A. M., and Williams, R. D.: Pancreatic response to alcohol following antral-esophagostomy. Surg. Forum, 12:378, 1961.

Evans, F. C.: Pancreatic abscess. Amer. J. Surg., 117:537, 1969.

Fish, J. C., Williams, D. D., and Williams, R. D.: Jaundice with cholecystitis. Arch. Surg., 96:875, 1968.

Frey, C. F.: The operative treatment of pancreatitis. Arch. Surg., 98:406, 1969.

Gambill, E. E., and Mason, H. L.: One hour value of urinary amylase in 96 patients with pancreatitis. JAMA, 186:24, 1963.

Keith, L. M., Jr., Zollinger, R. M., and McCleery, R. S.: Peritoneal fluid amylase determinations as an aid in diagnosis of acute pancreatitis. Arch. Surg., 61:930, 1950.

Khedroo, L. G., and Cosella, P. A.: Acute hemorrhagic pancreatitis: beneficial effects of primary excision of grossly necrotic tissue. Ill. Med. J., *129*:61, 1966.

Kirby, C. K., Senior, J. R., Howard, J. M., and Rhoads, J. E.: Death due to delayed hemorrhage in acute pancreatitis. Surg. Gynec. Obstet., *100*:458, 1955.

Menguy, R. B., Hallenbeck, G. A., Bollman, J. L., and Grindlay, J. H.: Ductal and vascular factors in etiology of experimentally induced acute pancreatitis. Arch. Surg., *74*:88, 1957.

Morris, P. J.: Diagnostic paracentesis of the acute abdomen. Brit. J. Surg., *53*:707, 1966.

Opie, E. L.: Etiology of acute hemorrhagic pancreatitis. Bull. Hopkins Hosp., *12*:182, 1901.

Paxton, J. R., and Payne, J. H.: Acute pancreatitis: a statistical review of 307 established cases. Surg. Gynec. Obstet., *86*:69, 1948.

Peterson, L. M., Collins, J. J., and Wilson, R. E.: Acute pancreatitis occurring after operations. Surg. Gynec. Obstet., *127*:23, 1968.

Pfeffer, R. B., Stasior, O., and Hinton, J. W.: The clinical picture of sequential development of acute hemorrhagic pancreatitis in the dog. Surg. Forum, 8:248, 1957.

Polk, H. C., Zeppa, R., and Warren, W. D.: Surgical significance of differentiating between acute and chronic pancreatic collections. Ann. Surg., *169*:444, 1969.

Saxon, E. I., Hinkley, W. C., Vogel, W. C., and Zieve, L.: Comparative value of serum urinary amylase in the diagnosis of acute pancreatitis. Arch. Intern. Med., *99*:607, 1957.

Stefanini, P., Ermine, M., and Carboni, M.: Diagnosis and management of acute pancreatitis. Amer. J. Surg., *110*:866, 1965.

Stewart, W. R. C., Elliott, D. W., and Zollinger, R. M.: Cortisone in the treatment of experimental acute pancreatitis. Surg. Forum, 9:537, 1958.

Thal, A., and Brockney, E.: Acute hemorrhagic pancreatic necrosis produced by local Shwartzman reaction. JAMA, *155*:569, 1954.

Thomford, N. R., and Jesseph, J. E.: Pseudocyst of the pancreas. Amer. J. Surg., *118*:86, 1969.

Trapnell, J. E.: The natural history and prognosis of acute pancreatitis. Ann. Roy. Coll. Surg. Eng., 38:265, 1966.

White, T. T., and Murat, J. E.: Treatment of the common bile duct in pancreatitis. Amer. Surgeon, *33*:524, 1967.

Zollinger, R. M., Keith, L. M., and Ellison, E. H.: Pancreatitis. New Eng. J. Med., *251*:497, 1954.

CHAPTER 18

SUPPURATIVE PERITONITIS WITH MAJOR ABSCESSES

by **STEPHEN E. HEDBERG, M.D.,** and **CLAUDE E. WELCH, M.D.**

Stephen E. Hedberg was born in Boston and received his degrees from Harvard University and Harvard Medical School. He served his surgical residency at the Massachusetts General Hospital and then spent two service years at the Walter Reed Army Institute of Research. He is currently on the staff of the Massachusetts General Hospital, and diseases of the alimentary tract represent his field of special interest.

Claude Emerson Welch is a Nebraskan. He graduated from Harvard Medical School, was elected to Alpha Omega Alpha, and served his surgical residency at the Massachusetts General Hospital, where he remained to become a senior staff member and Clinical Professor of Surgery in the Harvard Medical School. A leader in multiple phases of American medicine, he also finds time for art and the piano. His scholarly contributions have been many, but he is above all a great surgical clinician. He has earned an international reputation in the physiology and management of surgical lesions of the alimentary tract.

Millennia have passed since ancient physicians described the signs and symptoms of the process that we now recognize as peritonitis. Surgical interventions not devised until early in this century finally reduced a near-total incidence of mortality to the range of 50 per cent. Unaided by parenteral therapy, sophisticated anesthesia, antimicrobial drugs, or physiologic understanding, surgical pioneers were forced to elucidate principles of management that permitted survival; violation of those principles meant almost certain disaster. Transperitoneal drainage of a mural iliac abscess was unthinkable. Failure to drain a subphrenic abscess properly meant death for nine out of ten patients. Expertly treated, appendicitis with peritonitis carried a mortality rate of 14.5 per cent at the Cincinnati General Hospital as recently as 1934 to 1938 (Altemeier and Culbertson, 1967).

Contrast these historical data with the postantibiotic experience. For example, the Cincinnati mortality rate was reduced by two-thirds in the next decade. Survival after drainage of subphrenic abscess had risen from the 52.6 per cent reported by Barnard in 1907 to only 63.2 per cent for 1,942 surgically treated cases collected by Ochsner and DeBakey in 1938. In the anti-biotic era, however, Boyd (1966) reported an extremely satisfactory clinical experience when he employed the traditionally "lethal" transserous approach; Moore, in 1963, treated ten consecutive cases without fatality following transpleural drainage.

Not all surgeons agree that antibiotics are important. Thus, Carter and Brewer in 1964 reported a mortality rate of 31.4 per cent in 70 operative cases, whereas the rate was 67.3 per cent in 55 patients treated vigorously with antibiotics. They concluded that the more circuitous extraserous route of drainage must be preferred and that antibiotics had not altered the mortality rate in subphrenic abscess. Boyd, in contrast, felt that antibiotic coverage rendered serous violation harmless and thus permitted the surgeon to use the most direct and effective (transpleural) route to the superior subphrenic space.

It is evident from this brief look at a little corner of critical surgical illness that important changes are occurring in the treatment of what might be considered a rather mundane problem, at least in comparison with spectacular surgical triumphs appearing regularly in other fields. In abdominal sepsis, the revolution still in progress is conceptual as well as technical.

Surgical practices that were once called "principles" are being challenged and revised. Patients are surviving previously fatal complications only to face new dangers that seem to reverberate through every organ and system. In the therapy of very ill patients, conflicts seldom before confronted are now seen daily: oxygen vital to the heart and brain is poisonous to the lungs; pressor amines essential for perfusion of kidneys blanch the intestines; water necessary for blood volume is lost to interstitial tissue spaces but floods the alveoli if replaced. With every step and advance of understanding or therapy, new problems are raised that seem to leave us only half a step ahead—or maybe even a little behind.

This then is justification for a new chapter on an old subject. Increased understanding of the pathophysiology of peritonitis, abscess formation, and other complications constantly needs to be reconciled with the great body of current and previous clinical experience. Furthermore, the overall approach to management of critically ill patients has been vastly altered by widespread employment of specialty units and teams. Thus, the surgeon in charge of a patient with peritonitis suddenly finds himself delegating responsibility to and cooperating with groups of experts in anesthesia, recovery room care, intensive care, respiratory physiotherapy, infectious disease, ventilatory assistance, renal failure and dialysis, and even emergency resuscitation.

Recognizing that this chapter can only be an interim report in a rapidly moving field, we nevertheless feel that it can serve as a practical guide for the surgeon in charge of patients who are critically ill with abdominal sepsis or its complications. We intend to consider the clinical problem in depth, including pathophysiology, clinical pictures, diagnostic methods, preoperative preparation, therapeutic options, and postoperative management. Special emphasis will be placed upon the detection and treatment of the frequent and potentially lethal sequelae of peritonitis. It has become quite apparent that peritonitis per se can rarely be implicated as a cause of death. It follows, therefore, that the complications of peritonitis are the real culprits; it is only by anticipating these difficulties and managing them effectively that the surgeon will be able to improve results significantly.

PATHOPHYSIOLOGY OF PERITONITIS

Like other serous cavities, the peritoneal cavity is lined with flattened cells of mesodermal origin. Parietal and visceral peritoneum is identical in form and function. Because every organ and crevice within the peritoneal cavity is covered or lined with peritoneum, the actual surface area is very large, equaling at least one-third that of the skin. This surface presents a tremendous absorptive potential; conversely, exudation and transudation can also occur at a rate that renders peritoneal dialysis a useful means of exchanging many of the constituents of blood.

Peritoneum has an almost total regenerative capacity. It is a common observation that, following Miles' resection or pelvic exenteration, the entire pelvis becomes covered by a new surface, indistinguishable from the original peritoneum. Though the peritoneum is responsible for troublesome adhesion formation, it is nevertheless surprising that on occasion small intestine that seems hopelessly involved with fibrinous adhesions of acute peritonitis may appear perfectly normal a few months later. Thus, under appropriate circumstances— which are not at all understood—the intestinal serosa is capable of dissolving fibrinous adhesions and healing itself without the formation of fibrous adhesions.

Like other mesothelial membranes, the regenerative power of the peritoneum is matched by the violence of its reaction to all varieties of physical and chemical trauma. The first response is that of congestion and edema of the vascular network immediately adjacent. Within two or three hours, the normally shiny and translucent surface becomes swollen, dull, granular, and sticky. There is an immediate outpouring of fluid that is at first a transudate with a low specific gravity. Later the fluid becomes turbid because of increasing amounts of leukocytes, protein molecules, fibrin shreds, and cellular debris. Antibodies may be released into the fluid. If the response is particularly vigorous, the fluid may become bloody very early even in the absence of bacterial invasion, as in hemorrhagic pancreatitis.

The type and quantity of fluid produced by offended peritoneum is quite variable, ranging from the thin, opalescent material seen in streptococcal peritonitis to the frankly purulent, thick, creamy fibrinous fluid of staphylococcal infection. When the fluid is thick, a fibrinous exudate glues the loops of intestine and omental parts together, thereby tending to wall off and exclude the focus of irritant from the remainder of the peritoneal cavity. In adults, this sealing function of inflammatory response may be perfectly effective in preventing widespread contamination, whereas in infants, early adhesion is rare and generalized peritonitis is the rule.

If the peritonitis progresses untreated, larger accumulations of seropurulent fluid collect in the walled-off spaces and abscess formation results as the peritoneal and fibrinous confines of the collection are organized into a pyogenic membrane. These collections tend to occur at the source of first contamination, of course, but also, very importantly, they form in the various folds and cul-de-sacs that comprise the peritoneal cavity. If walling-off is not immediate, the peritoneal fluid seems to have a surprising ability to flow to all parts of the belly.

Gravitation to the paracolic gutters and pelvis is easily understood; perhaps less apparent is the reason for migration to the potential space between the diaphragm and the liver. It is our opinion that the upward migration of fluid in apparent defiance of gravity is not a paradox at all, but is the indirect result of the elastic recoil of the lung. As we know, pulmonary elasticity creates a negative intrathoracic pressure great enough to pull the diaphragm upward on expiration. With a moment's reflection, we can quickly see that in a relaxed or sleeping patient, either standing or semisitting, the force of gravity will tend to pull the liver downward. Were it not for the negative pressure in the subphrenic space, the liver would fall away from the diaphragm. This "suction cup" effect seems an adequate explanation for the propensity of free peritoneal fluid to be drawn into the subphrenic spaces.

One of the more important effects of peritonitis is paralysis of the intestine, probably owing to the irritation of afferent sympathetic pathways and overstimulation of splanchnic inhibitory nerves. Later in the course of the disease, hypoproteinemia, hypokalemia, toxemia, and intestinal distention contribute further to an adynamic ileus. Profound homeostatic alterations in body economy involving all systems usually occur as a result of sepsis, electrolyte shifts, and hypovolemia; if uncorrected, these changes frequently lead to cardiac arrest. In more favorable situations in which the local and systemic response of the host is adequate to destroy the invader quickly, fibrin is absorbed and glistening serosal surfaces are restored in a few days. When the process is prolonged more than six to ten days, the exudate is usually organized with the resultant formation of dense vascular, then fibrous, adhesions. Pockets of pus may be absorbed or sterilized, or may go on to form a true abscess. In the following sections, it is proposed to discuss these physiologic events in terms of the therapeutic problems and opportunities that they pose for the surgeons.

ETIOLOGY OF PERITONITIS

Practically any foreign material introduced into the peritoneal cavity can induce peritonitis. Even chylous lymph—certainly the most "physiologic" and least irritating of fluids imaginable—can produce a clinical picture of generalized peritonitis. Obviously, most cases arise from diseases of the intraperitoneal organs; rarely do they arise from extraperitoneal structures. A very small proportion of cases are apparently primary without any provable intraperitoneal source. Acute cases that are obviously secondary to intraperitoneal disease are further subclassified according to whether the contaminating material is irritative or septic. These classifications are not artificial, but have considerable therapeutic import, as will be seen.

ACUTE PRIMARY PERITONITIS

Because acute primary bacterial peritonitis exhibits no identifiable source of infection or continuing contamination, surgical therapy theoretically has nothing to offer. If the diagnosis can be made without operation, most patients will respond favorably to vigorous antibiotic treatment. It is in these cases that peritoneal aspiration or lavage for diagnosis may be of great benefit. Most cases are actually diagnosed at laparotomy, for this procedure, which carries no great risk, is the only means by which more hazardous forms of secondary peritonitis may be positively excluded.

Pneumococcal peritonitis is unusual, except in prepubertal girls, but it may follow pneumococcal pneumonia in patients of any age. Recently, Epstein et al. (1968) proposed an association of pneumococcal peritonitis with cirrhosis and ascites, citing six cases. Entry is thought to be by way of the fallopian tubes (and is known to occur more commonly in children suffering from the nephrotic syndrome), but blood-borne infection must also occur. The onset is usually sudden, with only vague, initial localization in the lower abdomen. Penicillin is the treatment of choice, although the exudate tends to form abscesses that may later require drainage.

Streptococcal peritonitis is nearly as common as pneumococcal, and it almost always follows an upper respiratory infection. The onset is sudden, with chills, high fever, and much pain. It is unlikely that these patients will be treated without operation even if gram-positive cocci in chains are observed on a stained smear of the peritoneal aspirate. The exudate may be practically clear or bloody or purulent. Before antibiotics, thin fluid was regarded as a grave prognostic sign. Thick fluid was more apt to result in adhesion formation and localization, albeit with abscess formation. Occasionally, streptococcal peritonitis may be secondary to an unsuspected foreign-body perforation.

Coliform peritonitis may occur without obvious perforation. Various means can be proposed by which a tiny perforation may be sealed or overlooked by the surgeon, or perhaps some pathologic change in the bowel has permitted passage of organisms through the intact wall. In pure coliform infections, the pus is odorless. Following a diligent search for the source, as much pus as possible should be aspirated from the peritoneal cavity, which is then closed without drainage. A broad-spectrum antibiotic is given in high dosage, pending a report on the antibiotic sensitivity of the cultured organism.

Staphylococcal peritonitis is often found in association with other organisms. When a pure culture is identified, it is usually the result of metastatic infection from an abscess in some other location, for example, a perinephric abscess. There is severe toxemia as these patients tend to be in late stages of widespread systemic infection. At operation, thick creamy pus is found with a marked tendency toward adhesion formation and loculation in multiple areas. It is considered appropriate to close the abdomen with removal of as much pus as possible and drainage of the sites of greatest accumulation. Unless the organism is sensitive to an antibiotic, the prognosis is practically hopeless.

Tuberculous peritonitis that is truly primary must be very rare because usually the source of infection can be established as a hypertrophic bowel lesion, salpingitis, or a caseous, retroperitoneal lymph node. A protracted course is the rule, so that the diagnosis is commonly made on clinical grounds in a patient known to have tuberculosis. In this setting, laparotomy for definitive diagnosis is probably not justified, since adequate specimens are obtained on peritoneoscopy. If laparotomy is carried out, however, it is important that representative peritoneal nodules be biopsied, and especially important that the peritoneum be closed without drainage lest a persistent sinus result. Preferred treatment is an intensive course of antituberculous chemotherapy.

SECONDARY PERITONITIS

The usual cause of secondary peritonitis is the escape into the peritoneal cavity of intestinal contents or organisms. The causative lesion may be the result of infection, necrosis, trauma, or idiopathic perforation of any portion of the gastrointestinal tract or its appendages. The nature of the original lesion is of some importance both prognostically and therapeutically. For example, peritoneal soilage arising from infected or abscessed viscera should be considered to contain organisms that have already proved their virulence. These patients may be quite sick when first seen and frequently require considerable preparation before operation. They may test the surgeon's skill by presenting him with severe postoperative complications.

Quite a different picture is presented by the patient who is seen early in the course of chemical peritonitis. Though these patients may be prostrated with pain from a massive acid or alkaline insult, they are generally in the best condition when first seen. The peritoneal effusion, which may be practically sterile at first, rapidly becomes infected. Emergency surgery to close the leak is undertaken in these cases as part of the resuscitative effort. Another source of secondary peritonitis that may logically be considered separate from the rest is that which derives from gangrenous bowel. Here the organisms contained within the necrotic segment may not be particularly virulent, but necrosis of their habitat tends to favor the growth of microaerophilic and anaerobic organisms, while the bowel wall, physically intact though dead, may permit the passage of toxic fluids and organisms without exciting a vigorous peritoneal response.

Such a classification of secondary peritonitis into broad etiologic types is worthwhile only if we are considering the early case. Later cases are all septic, so that the clinical pictures and treatment become identical no matter what the original etiology may have been. The diagnoses listed in the following classification are not intended to be encyclopedic. They should suffice to support the validity of the classification and to convey features of therapeutic importance.

Suppurative Peritonitis

Though the material released from these sources usually contains virulent organisms, the quantity of material tends to be relatively small and its progress is slow, so that the peritoneum very often has a chance to react effectively in walling off the process.

Appendicitis is the commonest cause of suppurative peritonitis. Usually the patient is not seen until after the phase of appendiceal colic has been supplanted by the appearance of localized peritonitis. Perforation may occur in as short a time as six hours, and this event may bring relief of pain. Localized abscess formation may then occur, but if contamination becomes generalized, the patient may seek help at a time when he is toxic, dehydrated, febrile, hypovolemic, and oliguric or anuric. These patients require careful preoperative preparation and a well-timed operation, as will be discussed in a later section.

Salpingitis of gonococcal origin is an example of a condition leading to suppurative peritonitis of an entirely different significance. The typical patient experiences the rapid onset of severe lower abdominal pain associated with a foul vaginal discharge. Pelvic peritonitis of gonococcal origin does not result in severe toxemia, though much

pus may be produced and the local reaction may be very intense. As described by Carlos Stajano in 1919, this exudate not uncommonly finds its way to the right upper quadrant. Abscesses are rarely seen, but "violin-string" adhesions are the well-recognized sequelae described by Curtis in 1930. Diagnosis is made by the finding of gram-negative intracellular diplococci on a cervical smear. The treatment is penicillin in high dosage.Every effort should be made to control the infection promptly and completely, since this tendency to form adhesions may go on to produce a frozen pelvis with sterile, occluded fallopian tubes.

Diverticulitis may appear in many forms, ranging from mild, crampy left lower quadrant pain to sudden, free perforation with generalized peritonitis. Free perforations are not common, however, probably because the infection develops rather slowly at first around a diverticular stercolith. This sharply localized process may then extend in one of several ways. Abscess formation with perforation into the mesosigmoid is common. Rupture of the diverticular or mesosigmoidal abscess into the peritoneal cavity is a more frequent cause of suppurative peritonitis than free perforation of the bowel lumen. These abscess perforations also tend to become walled off in the pelvis or in the left gutter where they may subside, drain rectally, drain into the bladder with formation of a sigmoidovesical fistula, or finally lead to chronic narrowing of the bowel. Signs of spreading peritonitis or the appearance of a mass is an indication for early operation in diverticulitis. The question of exactly what operation should be performed is one that will probably excite debate among surgeons for some years more to come (Byrne, 1964; Watkins and Oliver, 1966; Rodkey and Welch, 1969).

Though many surgeons of experience are satisfied with their results in small series of primary resections and anastomosis, this procedure cannot be recommended for general use. The course of conservatism in a patient sick enough to be operated upon acutely would include, as a minimum, a transverse colostomy and drainage of the septic focus or abscess. Exteriorization often is impossible because of mesosigmoidal shortening. In the case of free perforation, a drain to the region of the perforation sometimes appears inadequate for proper drainage of semiliquid feces. In these cases it has been quite satisfactory to both plug and drain the perforation with a Foley catheter of appropriate size. A drain is placed next to the catheter and both are delivered through a stab wound in the left iliac region. Of course, a transverse colostomy is done.

Bacillary dysentery, amebic dysentery, and ulcerative colitis can progress to septic perforation of the bowel. In ulcerative colitis the only acceptable treatment for perforation is subtotal colectomy, with ileostomy and exteriorization or inversion of the distal rectal segment. Dysentery and amebiasis are treated with the appropriate antibiotics and emetine, respectively.

A very serious cause of septic peritonitis is secondary rupture of an intraperitoneal abscess. These abscesses are usually bacterial, arising as complications of previous peritonitis or surgery; if the abscess that ruptures is large, the resultant peritonitis may exhibit all the worst features of both chemical and septic insult. Immediate operation with evacuation of spilled material and drainage of the cavity are indicated. Intraperitoneal rupture of an amebic abscess is often heralded some days in advance by pain from stretching of the liver capsule or irritation of the diaphragm. If the diagnosis can be made, the preferred treatment is a carefully supervised course of emetine and percutaneous aspiration of the abscess. If rupture should occur, conservative treatment must be strongly considered, since the results of open drainage of hepatic amebic abscesses have been disappointing. Though the material released from the abscess is highly irritating, causing massive fluid shifts and profound ileus, it and the few amebae in it apparently do little real damage in the peritoneal cavity. Because there is some danger of secondary bacterial invasion, these patients should be given large doses of antibiotics in addition to all the general supportive measures that will be discussed later (Grigsby, 1969).

Chemical Peritonitis

In most of these cases, the material released into the peritoneal cavity is at first completely or nearly sterile. The peritoneal surfaces are overwhelmed with an irritating material that evokes a tremendous inflammatory response and outpouring of fluid. This is the case of the "peritoneal burn" in which there may be massive losses of plasma into the peritoneum. These cases are surgical emergencies and every effort should be made to control the source of contamination as soon as possible before infection supervenes. Several sources of chemical peritonitis are as follows.

ACID. This is the prime example of a chemical peritonitis. The perforation of a duodenal or a gastric ulcer floods the peritoneal cavity with caustic, though essentially sterile, gastric juice. Simple closure of the perforation, supplemented by an omental patch, yields such uniformly good results that serious consideration of conservative therapy need not be given, except in late cases or in patients who are gravely ill from some other cause, such as a recent myocardial infarct. Patients who have had a long history of ulcer and who are seen soon after perforation may be candidates for immediate gastrectomy. Very large ulcers in which there would be danger of obstruction following plication or in which gastrectomy would be hazardous can be handled satisfactorily with pyloroplasty and vagotomy; this is certainly a reasonable compromise procedure in this urgent situation.

MECONIUM. Neonatal peritonitis, manifested by distention and vomiting within the first day or two of life, must be considered to be due to meconium, and must be treated promptly because of the extremely irritant nature of the material and the borderline reserves of the newborn. As soon as blood volume is restored and the stomach emptied, operation should be undertaken using local anesthesia. At operation a perforation secondary to obstruction will be found in about 50 per cent of the cases. The obstruction may be caused by meconium ileus, atresia, stenosis, adhesions, volvulus, or intussusception. Trauma may be the cause in most of the remaining cases; in some, no cause is found. If perforation or diagnosis is delayed until after the third postnatal day, when bacteria reach the intestine, the mortality rate is exceedingly high (Fonkalsrud et al., 1966).

MUCUS. Ruptures of appendiceal mucoceles or pseudomucinous ovarian cysts usually produce a fairly vigorous peritonitis and serve as the origin of pseudomyxoma peritonei. Diagnosis will probably not be made preoperatively, but will be quite obvious upon entering the peritoneal cavity. Treatment consists of excision of the offending organ as well as meticulous removal of all mucinous material. It is sometimes difficult to predict the malignant potential of this lesion, since the clinical course often suggests malignancy even though the histologic appearance favors a benign lesion.

BLOOD. Though peritoneal hemorrhage may be accompanied by few if any irritative symptoms, it is more common for patients in this category to exhibit low-grade fever, leukocytosis, adynamic ileus, abdominal distention, and varying amounts of abdominal pain, tenderness, and rebound tenderness. Naturally, in the more severe cases, hypovolemic shock produces signs that lead rapidly to diagnosis or disaster. The archetype of this kind of peritoneal insult is the ruptured tubal pregnancy, though ruptures of graafian follicle and corpus luteum also are common. Mesenteric apoplexy, ruptured spleens, and ruptured abdominal aneurysms are also to be considered. The history is often essential in diagnosing the source of a hemoperitoneum; an exact diagnosis, however, is not necessary as an indication for surgery.

If peritoneal bleeding is suspected, a four-quadrant tap should be carried out with a #18- or #20-gauge needle. Nonclotting blood is diagnostic of hemoperitoneum, since blood in the peritoneum will have been defibrinated. Failure to obtain blood on aspiration obviously does not exclude the diagnosis, and in a deteriorating patient, exploration may have to be undertaken without the reassurance of a positive tap. If, by chance or design, peritoneal hemorrhage is treated conservatively, secondary infection of retained blood rarely results. Furthermore, breakdown and absorption of the blood are so rapid that prehepatic bilirubinemia may be produced by flooding of the processing capacity of the liver.

BILE. The peritoneal reaction to bile leakage is surprisingly unpredictable. Most cases, as expected, show an intense inflammatory and symptomatic response, but in a few there is an unaccountable tolerance of bile leakage that permits the eventual development of bile ascites. In general terms, a slow leak of sterile bile can be well tolerated, while a massive leak of bile that is infected or contaminated with intestinal contents is highly irritant. It was shown by McCarthy and Picazo in dogs that repeated introduction of bile into the peritoneal cavity was accompanied initially by a painful reaction, whereas after the first few injections there was little or no apparent discomfort. The usual causes of bile peritonitis are postoperative leakages, especially from choledochotomy and duodenal closure following gastrectomy. Nonpenetrating abdominal trauma may cause rupture of the gallbladder, common duct, or even hepatic duct. Spontaneous rupture of biliary tract components may occur secondary to cholangitis or cholecystitis, and often the basic defect is calculous obstruction of the cystic or common duct.

Idiopathic rupture is much less frequent; in these cases no cause for the appearance of a tiny perforation of duct or gallbladder can be found. Rarely, bile is found on exploration of the peritoneal cavity, but not even a biliary leak can be identified at surgery. In acute cases of whatever cause, the objective of surgery is to remove accumulated bile from the peritoneal cavity and to provide drainage of the biliary tree by means of cholecystostomy or choledochostomy. In late cases there may be so much inflammatory reaction that cigarette drains placed near the most probable sources of leakage are the only practical method of treatment. In most chronic cases, dissection of the ductal structures or even exposure of them may be very hazardous.

CHYLE. Chylous peritonitis or ascites is one of the rarest forms of chemical peritonitis. It may occur secondary to leakage from the cisterna chyli or from rupture of a mesenteric chylous cyst. Sometimes, as in chylothorax, no source can be found on exploration. Lymphoma is the most common tumor that obstructs lymphatics and leads to peritoneal chyle accumulation. Vasko and Tapper have reported 140 cases. Forty per cent occur in children. The major etiologic causes are congenital in children and inflammatory or neoplastic in adults. The degree of inflammatory response is variable, but may be acute and severe. Although the diagnosis sometimes is established by peritoneal aspiration and Sudan staining of the material, treatment by repeated aspiration is only rarely satisfactory, so that operation is usually necessary for diagnosis and treatment. Surgery for chylous peritonitis should be conservative. The desirability of external drainage is debatable. Dissection and ligation of the cisterna chyli is rarely feasible or indicated, and spontaneous closure is the usual course. Severe inanition may result if closure is unduly delayed (Krizek and Davis, 1965).

URINE. Urine peritonitis almost always follows rupture of the dome of the bladder by blunt abdominal trauma. Naturally, it is much more common in patients who have a full bladder at the time of wounding, so that relatively massive soilage is usual. Even if the urine is sterile initially, it soon becomes infected and early control of the leak is imperative. The diagnosis of bladder rupture can always be made by retrograde cystography in which dilute contrast medium is instilled into the bladder via the urethra. Laparotomy, closure of the perforation, and suprapubic cystostomy is the most effective method of treatment, though a few minor leaks can be handled by an inlying catheter.

These various forms of chemical peritonitis are by their nature frequently of traumatic origin. The nature of the trauma is often massive, as in highway accidents and serious falls. The prostration and shock that accompany a massive chemical insult to the peritoneum may become indistinguishable in these patients from hypovolemic and traumatic shock. In blunt or nonpenetrating trauma, the force of injury is commonly very energetic, so that these patients often have multiple injuries in addition to the crushing and bursting wounds that are hidden within the belly. With penetrating wounds caused by knives, shards of glass, and low-velocity bullets, the injuries are limited in area though they may be destructive in severity (Netterville and Hardy, 1967).

In abdominal trauma, then, the surgeon must constantly bear in mind the paradox that patients with intact integument must be suspected of having more extensive injury than those with an obvious penetrating wound. Furthermore, because of the multiple injury factor in blunt trauma, additional snares are set in the form of urgent problems involving brain, spinal cord, or airway, as well as the management and priority considerations of several surgeons and physicians of different specialties.

If patients with massive trauma are to be handled conservatively, they must be examined at frequent intervals by a general surgeon; we believe the general surgeon should assume leadership of the trauma team when such a team is necessary. These patients must be watched very closely for signs of peritonitis. The necessity for very frequent observations is enhanced in the hours immediately following the injury. This requirement leads to an obvious conflict of management if urgent surgery is required in another area, as, for example, with cord compression, epidural hematoma, or intrathoracic bleeding. In this situation, continued observation of the abdomen will be impossible, so that intraperitoneal hemorrhage and chemical peritonitis may go undetected for hours. The problems that can result in an anesthetized patient are so serious that the risk of an unnecessary laparotomy is obviously small by comparison. We have felt, therefore, that exploratory laparotomy is justified in such patients on the basis of indications that ordinarily would be considered inadequate.

Also to be considered among the traumatic causes of both chemical and septic peritonitis are undesirable after-effects of diagnostic and surgical procedures. Gastrointestinal endoscopy furnishes a small but steady supply of patients requiring emergency exploration. The gastroscope and peritoneoscope may cause massive lacerations or tiny leaks that are practically self-sealing, so that the onset of symptoms may be immediate or delayed 12 to 24 hours. When a sigmoidoscope perforates the colon, the event may not be readily apparent to either surgeon or patient (Befeler, 1967; Kiser et al., 1968). Urgent surgery is indicated because if these perforations are promptly treated before the inflammatory reaction becomes advanced, then usually a very simple procedure will suffice, such as simple closure of the viscus without drainage. After a few hours of leakage, hyperemia, exudation, and ileus, it will probably be necessary to perform some sort of decompression, drainage, or exteriorization, since a closure will not be trustworthy.

Another example of "iatrogenic" internal trauma that is typically seen in the later stages follows colonic perforation after irrigation of a colostomy. Here the clinical picture may vary all the way from a simple properitoneal abscess to the most virulent form of chemical and septic peritonitis that can follow evacuation of the fecal content or enema through a colonic laceration having free access to the peritoneum. One should not temporize longer than necessary to resuscitate these patients, since all will need advancement and resection of the colon or the construction of an entirely new colostomy (Spiro, 1966). One of the worst forms of chemical or septic peritonitis results when barium sulfate contrast material extravasates during radiographic examination. Even if operation is immediate, the mixture is found tightly adherent to many areas. Lavage and wiping with sponges are discouragingly ineffective in removing the material. The prognosis is poor because of the tendency toward recurrent abscess formation and intestinal obstruction (Westfall et al., 1966).

The literature is replete with traumatic exotica, such as air-hose injuries, blast injuries from an electric spark during electrocoagulation through a proctoscope, internal perforation from foreign bodies, and grisly impalements leading to peritoneal contamination. Many, but not all, require emergency surgery, and their management will be based on general principles derived from experience with more ordinary forms of chemical and septic peritonitis.

Apart from diagnostic and accidental perforations, the surgeon's own postoperative cases will in time furnish him with a great variety of experience in the handling of peritonitis. Here again the insult may be chemical or septic, depending upon the circumstances of contamination. Generalized peritonitis used to be a leading cause of death following laparotomy, even when the intestine was not violated. Its conquest awaited only the development of ordinary aseptic procedures. Asepsis in the strictest sense is impossible, however, when the bowel must be opened. There is always at least a little contamination; if the organism is virulent, a septic course follows, usually with the formation of a localized abscess, but occasionally with a more widespread process. The more common cause of postoperative generalized peritonitis is a massive intestinal leak rather than merely intraoperative deposit of a virulent organism. A free, upper intestinal perforation of this type sooner than 36 hours or later than seven days postoperatively is rare, whereas colonic anastomotic disruption typically occurs on the seventh or eighth postoperative day when walling-off is well established. The clinical characteristics of massive chemical peritonitis versus the septic type are suggested by our habit of referring to duodenal suture-line disruption as a "blowout," whereas perforation of a colon anastomosis is just a "leak."

The many factors responsible for postoperative peritonitis are obviously beyond the scope of this chapter; they are extensively discussed in other sources in which the role of prophylaxis is given deserved emphasis (Welch and Hedberg, 1967).

Intestinal necrosis due to interference with vascular supply constitutes another broad category in the etiology of peritonitis that perhaps deserves special mention because the pathophysiology of peritonitis in the presence of dead bowel may be different in several respects from the usual chemical or septic peritonitis (Cohn, 1964). Whether the cause is mesenteric thrombosis of an open-ended segment, or volvulus of a closed loop, or strangulation in a protective extraperitoneal sac, death of the bowel does introduce added complications. First of all, interruption of the circulation with lowering of oxygen tension enhances the emergence of microaerophilic and anaerobic organisms. The lack of circulation means that the organisms may multiply unimpeded by antibodies, leukocytes, antibiotics, or any of the other materials that are usually supplied in abundance to a nidus of infection. At the same time, death of the bowel wall furnishes a perfect culture medium for saprophytes. As the intestine dies, it becomes permeable to this army of microbes as well as to their abundant toxins. For some reason, inflammatory response around an intraperitoneal segment of dead bowel is commonly lacking, even 24 hours after onset. These various special features are reflected in a clinical picture dominated by profound toxemia. The shock-like state that results may be due as much to endotoxin absorption as to hypovolemia resulting from extracellular fluid shift. Though the systemic reaction may be massive, with high fever and leukocytosis, the local signs of peritoneal irritation may be so lacking as to be quite misleading. The surgeon's problems are not lessened by the fact that intestinal gangrene seems to be a disease of the very old and the very young; furthermore, even if they are not at these extremes in age, many patients are unable to give a coherent history simply because they are too sick. The overall mortality rate is high because included in this group are not only patients with volvulus of Meckel's diverticulum and strangulated hernia, but also those with such lethal conditions as massive small bowel infarction, segmental infarctions due to arteritis and collagen diseases, and that large group of infarctions due to low blood flow states of all types.

DIAGNOSIS OF PERITONITIS

It is interesting that the diagnosis of peritonitis must often await the actual clinical examination, whereas the etiology of the disease is usually determined on the basis of history, especially if a perforated viscus is the source. When peritonitis is found unexpectedly at operation, it is usually the result of walled-off perforations of ulcer, gallbladder, or appendix. It is important to go beyond merely diagnosing the existence of peritonitis because a preoperative understanding of the etiology, extent, duration, and bacteriology are major determinants in deciding the timing of operation or, indeed, the necessity for operation.

HISTORY

History taking will not be dwelt upon at length in a treatise aimed at the practicing surgeon. A few general points, however, do deserve emphasis. As peritonitis is usually a consequence of visceral disease, the history usually consists of a merging of the symptoms of the original process with those of peritonitis, and the different sequences that evolve may be very helpful in diagnosis and localization of the source. Pain is the most important symptom in peritonitis. The exact chronology of the onset of pain, its location, radiation, spread, and progression with time are usually diagnostic. The history of previous similar episodes of pain may be difficult to elicit because the patient, concentrating on his present problem, will tend to minimize all previous events in his eagerness to convey the unique character of the presenting complaint. On the other hand, the patient who denies any pain may do so because of reluctance to use the word "pain" at all. This patient is not anxious to get on with treatment; he would rather forget the whole thing. Sometimes patients who refuse to acknowledge pain will freely discuss "gas," a synonym that seems to produce less anxiety.

If blunt or penetrating abdominal trauma has been involved, an exact history of the nature of the contact is essential. Road accidents have produced classic patterns of injury in driver, passenger, and pedestrian.

Wounds that penetrate the trunk in any location can also extend into the peritoneal cavity. In woundings, one must discover the instrument used, the velocity of the missile (if a bullet), and the spatial relations of assailant and victim in order to predict accurately the likelihood of injury to specific viscera.

In postsurgical cases, history is no less important, for here it refers to the exact findings and happenings of the original operation as well as to the timetable of postoperative events that led to a consideration of peritonitis. Unfortunately, in many cases the surgeon is unable to recall anything untoward that was observed; this fact may serve to emphasize the value of the precautionary measures such as drainage, intubation, and diversion that are taken when complicating features can indeed be recognized and dealt with appropriately.

PHYSICAL EXAMINATION

Depending on the extent and duration of the process, the patient with peritonitis may vary in appearance from robust to moribund, from unconcerned to immobilized by pain. Differences in the general state depend not only upon the basic age and vigor of the patient, but also upon the degree of toxemia, presence or absence of fever, possible contraction of blood volume, and the location and duration of the process. A small abscess or acute inflammatory process in contact with the abdominal wall will produce more marked local signs than a very large retroperitoneal or subdiaphragmatic abscess, whereas patients with the latter may appear more anemic, dehydrated, wasted, and toxic.

In patients with abdominal pain, it is important to observe the character of the breathing and of the patient's voluntary motor reaction to the pain. Peritoneal irritation typically produces splinting of the diaphragm and costal margin, so that respirations tend to be shallow and rapid and employ the intercostal muscles of the upper chest and the accessory muscles of breathing in the shoulder girdle. Patients with painful peritonitis lie very still—supine or prone, or often in the fetal position. In contrast, patients who may be experiencing even more severe pain from blocked intestine or passage of a stone will often thrash about as their colic waxes.

Physical examination of the abdomen should be done first in patients suspected of having peritonitis. This violation of the usual order is recommended for a number of reasons. First of all, it is the most important part of the examination and it should be carried out before the patient has been agitated physically and emotionally by other procedures. This is particularly important in pediatric patients, but adults also respond to irritation with increased abdominal guarding and lowering of the pain threshold. Prior examination of the abdomen may make it obvious that any motion is extremely uncomfortable for the patient, so that the remainder of the physical examination can be modified to minimize sitting, turning, and the like. Finally, immediate examination of the abdomen permits a second look if it is examined again; sometimes the patient whose guarding is largely psychologic can be reassured to the point where a second abdominal examination at the end of the interview is much more revealing than the first. On the other hand, patients who actually do have chemical peritonitis may have such rapidly progressive symptoms that the second inspection may confirm what was only a strong suspicion before.

In appearance, the abdominal skin reflects the internal milieu in many respects. Blood volume contraction and poor circulatory status cause the ominous looking livedo reticularis so often seen in very ill patients. The broad expanse of skin manifests jaundice and the ecchymoses of trauma, retroperitoneal hemorrhage, and pancreatitis. Shape of the abdomen may vary from rigidly flat in early chemical peritonitis to frog-like, with bulging flanks in cirrhotic patients with infected ascites or mesenteric venous occlusion. The more typical patient with moderately advanced peritonitis exhibits a uniformly rounded belly, possibly somewhat shiny owing to recent stretching of the skin.

Percussion of the abdomen is sometimes startling to patients in great pain, so that it may be delayed until after auscultation and palpation. A tympanitic area overlying the liver is practically diagnostic of intraperitoneal air. In ausculting the belly, the listener must not draw profound conclusions from what he hears. Obviously, a perfectly silent abdomen is practically diagnostic of peritonitis. The reverse, however, does not hold and bowel sounds may persist for sev-

eral hours after the onset of severe generalized peritonitis.

Tenderness is the most important sign of all. Without tenderness it is virtually impossible to make a diagnosis of peritonitis or inflammation of any intraperitoneal viscus by physical examination. Exceptionally troublesome, therefore, are unconscious patients and patients who are too sick or too old to respond appropriately to pain. Another group of patients in whom the absence of tenderness may be misleading are those taking steroids, in whom even free perforation of an ulcer may exhibit few of the expected signs. When definite abdominal tenderness is present, peritonitis is the first diagnosis to be excluded. In the case of a child or a male of any age, for example, well-localized tenderness in the right lower quadrant ordinarily must be presumed to be due to appendicitis, no matter what the history, temperature chart, or white blood count may reveal. Rebound tenderness as a sign of peritonitis has been somewhat overemphasized, since a very significant rebound tenderness is present in many diseases of the intestine, such as intestinal obstruction and various forms of enteritis. When direct tenderness is minimal, however, as in very early cases, then rebound tenderness may become an extremely valuable sign, especially if it can be elicited from a distant point not tender to direct palpation. If peritonitis is not generalized, then the location of the tenderness becomes of the utmost importance in establishing an exact etiological diagnosis. Given a reasonably typical history, very often the touch of one hand is enough to confirm the presence of appendicitis, cholecystitis, or diverticulitis. Tenderness need not necessarily overlie the source of the inflammation, but may lie chiefly at the point to which fluid gravitates after perforation of a viscus; for example, tenderness in the early perforation of a duodenal ulcer may be most prominent in the right-lower quadrant, owing to the watershed of leaking contents descending into the right paracolic gutter.

Sometimes it is difficult to determine whether abdominal tenderness arises from an intraperitoneal or retroperitoneal structure, or from the abdominal wall itself, as in rupture of the rectus muscle or a rectus sheath hematoma without rupture. In these cases we have found it useful to palpate the area of tenderness (or mass if one is present) and then, while still palpating, require the patient to contract his abdominal muscles by slowly raising his head or head and feet. If the mass or the tender area lies deep to the muscle, it will either disappear or become protected as the muscle tightens.

Spasm of the abdominal musculature is certainly not the most valuable of signs, nor always the easiest to elicit. In older patients or obese patients especially, spasm may be practically nonexistent. On the other hand, voluntary or involuntary guarding in young and muscular patients may be so marked as to be almost indistinguishable from true spasm.

Rectal examinations and vaginal examinations, whenever anatomy permits, are mandatory because these apertures provide the only possible contact with the peritoneum in an area unprotected by overlying musculature.

A very thorough general physical examination must be done to exclude "medical" and extraperitoneal causes of peritoneal signs. In postoperative patients, the sudden appearance of peritoneal signs three to eight days after operation must lead first to suspicion of an anastomotic leakage, but one should not proceed to laparotomy without first excluding embolism, pneumonia, myocardial infarction, or pancreatitis. By the same token, in patients who have not been operated upon, chest disease frequently leads to reflex inhibition of peristalsis, abdominal spasm, and even rebound tenderness.

The differential diagnosis of peritonitis is raised in many patients with gastroenteritis and renal colic because of so-called peritoneal signs. Many acute fevers of bacterial or viral origin can present with nausea or vomiting and abdominal pain. One of the most dangerous forms of peritonitis is that which occurs in patients who are already hospitalized for some unrelated disease. Although hospitalization for any cause is known to increase the risk of developing an acute abdomen, nevertheless, it is a fact that the medical ward remains one of the most hazardous places for the patient who develops peritonitis. This, of course, in defense of our internist colleagues, is because the symptoms tend to be masked by medications, diets already restricted or nonexistent, and the administration of antibiotics. Sometimes even more important is the "labeling" phenomenon, in which the appearance of

new symptoms or signs is naturally ascribed to a new manifestation of a previously known condition.

Miscellaneous diseases in which abdominal pain may be a prominent and confusing feature include herpes zoster, tabes dorsalis, porphyria, periodic familial peritonitis, diabetes, epilepsy, migraine, hemolytic crises, lead colic, and mesenteric adenitis of viral origin. The diagnosis of most of these conditions is not really too obscure if they are considered even briefly, as most of them exhibit some pathognomonic feature in history, physical examination, or laboratory result.

Basic laboratory work in suspected peritonitis always includes a leukocyte count and differential, a hematocrit or hemoglobin determination, a urinalysis, and a serum amylase. Depending upon the patient's age, an electrocardiogram may be considered a portion of the minimum laboratory work. It is for this reason as much as any other that the practice of home visits to patients complaining of abdominal pain is to be discouraged; most patients readily accept the explanation that these tests are now considered essential in proper evaluation of abdominal pain, and they can well see that it would be impractical to bring to the home all the equipment necessary to make these tests. If the patient or his parents are still unconvinced that the hospital is now the setting in which to establish or exclude a diagnosis of peritonitis, then one may point out that house calls for this purpose have become an anachronism for many of the same reasons that kitchen table appendectomies have fallen out of fashion.

Once hospitalized, a patient with any but the most straightforward diagnostic problem will undoubtedly be subjected to somewhat more than the minimum diagnostic work alluded to above. Depending on circumstances and apparent diagnostic possibilities, blood for many other chemical tests will be drawn at the same time as aliquots for the basic work. A blood culture should be started on the markedly febrile patient or the patient experiencing shock; blood gases, electrolytes, liver function tests, or coagulation parameters will be necessary for other patients.

Certain radiographs have become practically routine in patients suspected of peritonitis. Calculi, subdiaphragmatic air, and gross pulmonary or cardiac changes may be excluded by plain and upright films of the abdomen and chest. Again, depending upon particular diagnostic considerations, various types of contrast studies may be indicated. When one is attempting to exclude perforations of the upper or lower gastrointestinal tract, barium studies are very definitely contraindicated because of the lethal effects of intraperitoneal spillage of barium sulfate suspensions. Aqueous solutions of iodinated compounds will do the job equally well and much more safely. In patients with abdominal or diffuse trauma, cystography may be carried out to exclude rupture of the urinary bladder, and an intravenous pyelogram is often very helpful and even mandatory when gross or microscopic hematuria is present. In stab wounds of the abdomen, demonstration of peritoneal penetration may be possible in the majority of cases by filling the wound sinus with sterile contrast medium injected through an occluding balloon catheter, according to Cornell et al. (1967). Our experience, however, has not been so satisfactory.

Peritoneal paracentesis for diagnosis of peritonitis has many enthusiastic adherents, who point out the elegance of diagnosis by means of a simple tap that may yield bile, chyle, blood, pus, or gastric juice. If fluid is obtained, it may be subjected to many simple but incisive tests, such as Gram stain, culture, and determination of amylase content. Those who oppose the use of peritoneal aspiration point out that aspiration of bilious material or intestinal contents may mean only that the needle has penetrated a viscus, and it is perfectly possible to obtain a falsely dry tap. They suggest rightly that the diagnosis of peritonitis should not depend upon a positive result from paracentesis, nor should a decision against operation be based upon a negative result. In rejoinder, the proponents of tapping might state that a properly performed needling hardly ever penetrates the bowel and that the admitted uselessness of a negative result is no contraindication to the performance of a test that yields very valuable results if positive. For a more complete discussion of this maneuver and the technique of its performance, the reader is referred to several recent publications (Morris, 1966; Veith et al., 1967).

We might mention here a "sniff" test that recently proved diagnostically valuable in one of our patients, a 340-pound, 68-year-old man with generalized peritonitis, subdia-phragmatic air, and a history of one week of infra-umbilical pain preceding the sudden onset of excruciating generalized pain. With the patient in the supine position, the bubble of free air was readily percussed and entered with a long spinal needle. As air gradually hissed from the needle, the bystanders sniffed it, and all agreed that it was odorless. The preoperative diagnosis of perforated ulcer was confirmed at operation.

The final diagnostic maneuver to be considered is, of course, laparotomy. Years ago the inclusion of this procedure as a diagnostic test would have been considered unjustifiable because of the attendant morbidity and mortality rates. Now the risk of exploratory laparotomy or appendectomy has been reduced to a fraction of 1 per cent by preoperative nasogastric drainage, and by improved anesthetic, operating room, and recovery room procedures. Thus, laparotomy is quite comparable in safety to many other widely accepted endoscopic and radiologic diagnostic procedures. In terms of diagnostic yield, the results of laparotomy are variable depending upon the clinical indication; but when the reason for laparotomy is suspected peritonitis, the yield of positive diagnoses exceeds that of any other diagnostic maneuver, and the incidence of false-positive and false-negative results is, for all practical purposes, zero. One may conclude that, as a purely diagnostic maneuver, exploratory laparotomy ranks very high in both validity and safety when compared with many other widely used techniques.

TREATMENT OF PERITONITIS

The treatment of peritonitis must be considered from the point of view of both operative and nonoperative methods. Some form of nonoperative or supportive therapy usually precedes, or may even supplant, operation, but the vigor and extent of nonoperative therapy obviously varies considerably, depending upon the exact nature of the clinical problem. A patient with an obvious diagnosis of early appendicitis or perforated ulcer will fare better if brought to the operating room with a minimum of time-consuming diagnosis and preparation. In the moribund neglected patient, however, the operating room experience may be just a punctuation mark in a resuscitative saga. Nevertheless, the importance of operative technique must not be minimized; for the critically ill patient the speed, accuracy, judgment, and skill of the operator are the crucial (but soon hidden) factors on which depends the success or failure of a massive multidisciplinary effort. In other patients, for example, those with primary pneumococcal or tuberculous peritonitis or peritonitis following rupture of an amebic abscess of the liver, totally nonoperative treatment may be an ideal seldom attained.

The discussion of modes of therapy necessarily includes general support measures used in many other forms of critical surgical disease so that some overlap with the material covered in other chapters is inevitable. Also, there will be some repetition within this chapter of general remarks concerning treatment that have already been made about certain types of peritonitis. In general, the treatment of late peritonitis of either chemical or septic etiology consists of applying the entire armamentarium of preparatory, operative, and postoperative techniques, whereas in early cases the preoperative and postoperative care may be greatly simplified.

NONOPERATIVE OR PREPARATORY THERAPY

This mode of therapy begins with preparations for monitoring the status and progress of a patient. In addition to a large-bore intravenous cannula for rapid administration of fluids, the very ill patients will require a bladder catheter and a central venous pressure catheter. If cyanosis or respiratory insufficiency is present when the patient is first seen, then an arterial catheter may greatly simplify the monitoring of blood pressure and the procurement of blood samples for gas determinations. As the various cannulas are inserted, samples are drawn for initial laboratory work, which should include, as a minimum, a hemoglobin and hematocrit, leukocyte count and differential, urinalysis, measure of blood electrolytes, serum amylase determination, and measure of blood urea nitrogen (BUN). Other chemical tests, of course, will be done on specific indication, such as liver function tests in patients suspected of having bile peritonitis or incidental liver disease. Urinary electrolytes should be measured in the specimen of urine obtained on initial catheterization if anuria is suspected.

All of these measures, of course, are extensions of the diagnostic maneuvers discussed in the previous section, but they are mentioned here because they relate so directly to the initial resuscitative efforts. Resuscitation per se, however, logically begins with attention to the respiratory system; if the patient is very sick, oxygen should be administered immediately by face mask. Moribund patients may require intubation of the trachea and artificial ventilation. In all patients, Levin tube decompression of the stomach should be started early, and in those with respiratory problems, aspiration of the stomach may produce significant lowering of the diaphragm and improvement of the respiratory status. Monitoring of the gastric tube output is, of course, essential for appropriate replacement of fluid.

Intravenous replacement therapy constitutes a major portion of the early resuscitative regimen. The large quantities of water, colloid, and salt that are lost into the peritoneal cavity with the initial insult of chemical peritonitis should be replaced as quantitatively as possible. Patients with even moderate degrees of septic peritonitis likewise lose several liters of fluid, with resultant oliguria.

If losses are minor, replacement can consist mainly of water and salt, and the colloid portion can be ignored since the total loss is not great. In late peritonitis of both types, the loss of colloid that results from the peritoneal burn stabilizes, but electrolyte and water losses continue into the lumen of the paralyzed gastrointestinal tract. Patients who are moribund when first seen must be treated with great vigor if kidney function is to be rescued. These dehydrated patients can and should immediately be given massive quantities of lactated Ringer's solution, to which may be added plasma or type-specific blood when these become available. The first object of therapy, however, is to restore urine output with a water load. When the first several hundred milliliters of water have failed to bring about a response, osmotic diuresis should be attempted by the addition of 50 gm. of mannitol to the intravenous fluid.

Many other drugs also have to be considered. Of primary importance are the antibiotics; though one hesitates to use the word "always," it is difficult to imagine a case of peritonitis being managed today without antibiotics. The value of antibiotics in the treatment of peritonitis has been accepted by the profession for many years. However, the clinical studies that have been reported are far from satisfactory from a scientific point of view with respect to adequate control, and they actually do little to solve the problem as to whether or not antibiotics are truly effective.

A far better approach has been provided in the laboratory. For example, Barnett has developed a standard method of inducing peritonitis by the injection of a fecal suspension into the peritoneal cavity in dogs. With such a preparation, control animals can be compared with those animals receiving various antibiotics. As Artz, Barnett, and Grogan have reported, survival in control dogs with such a preparation was only 10 per cent. In those treated immediately after the fecal injection with either penicillin or kanamycin survival was just over 50 per cent, whereas in those who had a combination of the two survival was 100 per cent. Similar studies in the laboratory by other investigators, such as Zintel et al., Yaeger et al., and Wright et al., have shown the beneficial effects of many other antibiotics compared with control groups. The main problem has been to determine which agents have the greatest effect with the least toxicity. For example, kanamycin or neomycin administered intraperitoneally may lead to very marked respiratory depression.

In a similar way, experimental evidence has been found concerning the best mode of administering antibiotics. Artz et al., in a summary of this material, have concluded that the intravenous route is decidedly better than the intramuscular, though there was not a great deal of difference between the intravenous route and the intraperitoneal.

Similarly, the value of irrigation of the peritoneal cavity with saline in early cases of experimental peritonitis has been established by Burnett et al. and by Barnett and Hardy. It would seem reasonable that in clinical practice late cases of peritonitis would respond less well because shaggy coats of fibrin would prevent removal of infected material. In clinical practice the effects of irrigation of the peritoneal cavity with antibiotics, insofar as death was concerned, have not been shown to be significantly different from those in a control group, according to Noon et al.; the incidence of infection, however, was seen to be reduced significantly, particularly in the wound, since the incidence of infection after the use of saline irrigation was 24 per cent and after irrigation with antibiotic solutions was only 12 per cent.

Antibiotic treatment should be started intravenously as soon as the diagnosis can be established beyond reasonable doubt. Selection of the proper antibiotic is more difficult. With the exception of primary peritonitis, pure cultures are rare, so that it is quite common for the various organisms involved to exhibit differing antibiotic sensitivity spectra. For this reason, unless a pure growth has been demonstrated by Gram stain or culture, it is preferable to treat with a broad-spectrum antibiotic or combination. The selection of the proper antibiotic has been discussed at length in the chapter on postoperative fever. Our usual selection in the case of a culture as yet unreported is a combination of penicillin and chloramphenicol, with Keflin as a second choice.

Barnett's studies in experimental animals would indicate that many antibiotics have a therapeutic effect; at present, however, he prefers Keflin. We prefer to administer the antibiotics intravenously and intermittently in doses of high concentration rather than continuously in lower concentration. The "pulsed" therapy method allows much more flexibility in the administration of other drugs and blood products intravenously, and seems to be more effective therapeutically (Moore, 1969). Although the initial choice of antibiotic is guided by the suspected diagnosis, there should be no hesitation in changing to a different combination on the basis of smear or culture report unless the patient is getting along particularly well.

Other drugs important in resuscitation are cardiac, autonomic, and steroid. Digitalis preparations are used whenever signs of congestive failure are present, but they may also be indicated when massive fluid therapy is anticipated in the elderly patient. Again, the intravenous route is preferred when peripheral circulation may be unreliable. Vasoactive drugs, such as isoproterenol, are used in counteracting the hypotensive effects of septicemia (Hermreck and Thol, 1969), but they are not generally indicated until the response to intravenous replacement of volume can be assessed (MacLean et al., 1965). Although we are reassured by the statements of our internist and cardiac consultants that the dangerous effects of vasoconstrictive drugs on the intestine may have been overemphasized, we are still very cautious in their use until we are satisfied that blood volume is adequate. It is important to realize that the vasodilatory, cardiogenic, alkalotic, and acidotic aspects of shock may be crucial in an individual case even though the etiology of shock may have been primarily hypovolemic or septic. Thus, in advanced shock, the treatment must be directed at some of the potentially lethal results of shock, as well as at the basic cause.

Steroid therapy in peritonitis is still of undetermined value (Lillehei et al., 1967; Thomas and Brockman, 1968). It is recognized that adrenal failure is an extremely rare condition and yet adrenal hemorrhage is not uncommon in patients dying of sepsis from any source. Steroids, then, may have a place in the treatment of shock though the exact position is not yet clear. Similarly, the anti-inflammatory effects have yet to be evaluated; in overwhelming sepsis, steroid therapy has seemed on occasion to furnish a little additional time to allow for antibiotic control. Steroids may also be useful in inhibiting the formation of postoperative or postperitonitic adhesions. However, sepsis appears to progress more rapidly under the influence of steroids, while colonic anastomoses are more likely to perforate (Hawley, 1969). At present, most authorities oppose the use of steroids in peritonitis.

Intestinal intubation and decompression are important not only from the point of view of ventilatory efficiency, as mentioned above, but also for the local effect upon the stomach and intestine. Relief of painful distention and avoidance of vomiting are symptomatic dividends. When gastric suction relieves or prevents distention of the small bowel and colon, the blood supply to the bowel is improved and the risk of necrosis and perforation is thereby lessened (Boley et al., 1969). When the bowel is distended, it not only increases in transverse diameter, but it also elongates, so that kinking of the bowel is apt to occur between the sausage-shaped areas of stretching and lengthening. When this distention and kinking occur in peritonitis, the inevitable adhesion formation is apt to fix the bowel in this angulated disposition; by this means the unrelieved distention of adynamic ileus may lead to mechanical bowel obstruction (Smith, 1964).

The use of rectal tubes has little theoretical advantage in the ileus of peritonitis. It is observed, however, that patients are often made more comfortable when they are relieved of that portion of gas that distends the rectum and which they are unable to expel voluntarily, so that a rectal tube should be given a trial if the patient complains of tenesmus or gas pains.

Long intestinal decompression tubes, such as the Miller-Abbott, Cantor, or Kaslow varieties, have their place in the treatment of mechanical small-bowel obstruction, especially in those patients subject to repeated bouts of obstruction and in whom the obstruction seems to be partial. By decompressing the distended loops proximal to an obstruction, the long tube may relieve just enough kinking to permit the narrowed segment to function adequately. The use of long intestinal tubes in peritonitis, however, is restricted because of the adynamic nature of the ileus. In general, the place for long intestinal intubation is in the postoperative patient who may be exhibiting signs of early mechanical bowel obstruction. Similarly, there would seem to be no place for any form of chemical or electrical bowel stimulation in the early stages of peritonitis. Even if such therapy should be successful in producing peristalsis, it is doubtful that active peristalsis in the presence of acute peritonitis would serve any useful purpose.

Symptomatic relief of pain in patients with peritonitis may be considerable following the use of only those measures discussed above. However, if pain persists, then it is justifiable to use narcotics even though the need for a laparotomy may not have been definitely settled upon. As long as one is aware that analgesic medication has been given, evaluation of the abdomen is not unduly difficult provided the patient is not completely unresponsive or unreliable, though one must make allowance for the increased pain threshold. Sometimes the simple application of a heating pad or packs to the abdominal wall is sufficient to relieve pain.

Much has been written about the position of the patient being treated conservatively for suppurative peritonitis. The semisitting position of Fowler is usually recommended in the hope that pus might thereby be encouraged to gravitate to the pelvis. It has been shown, however, that the pressure in the lower part of the abdomen is three times that in the upper part when the patient is in the sitting position (Drye, 1948). Hydrostatic pressure alone would account for this difference, perhaps, but would not in itself explain the upward migration of fluid that is observed. For this we must invoke the principle that the liver is not simply resting upon the viscera beneath it but that it is actually being held in its subdiaphragmatic position by a negative pressure from above. Despite these physiologic considerations, tradition dictates that Fowler's position is to be preferred in suppurative peritonitis when abscess formation is a possibility. While it is undoubtedly correct that a pelvic abscess is much easier to handle and much less dangerous than a subphrenic abscess, the irrationality of Fowler's position might suggest that the supine or very slightly elevated position could encourage the formation of a paravertebral gutter abscess, which would also be relatively simple to manage.

One should not leave a discussion of nonoperative treatment of peritonitis without mentioning the nutritional care of the patient, since the only organ that is rendered consistently nonfunctional by peritonitis is the alimentary tract. Fortunately, the nutritional reserve of most patients is sufficient to carry them for several weeks without additional supplementation, so that nutrition is never a problem in the acute case. In a referral practice, however, in which the surgeon sees numbers of chronically and acutely ill patients suffering from the complications of peritonitis, malnutrition may be an extremely urgent problem. In the past, refunctionalization of the intestine offered the only means of salvation for these patients, but now, as will be discussed later, the intravenous hyperalimentation techniques of Dudrick offer the possibility of a more leisurely and controlled approach to the problem.

OPERATIVE TREATMENT OF PERITONITIS

The operative treatment of peritonitis may be of little help or may even cause harm in late cases in which the walling-off of a perforation or the construction of an abscess has already begun. If the diagnosis of such localization can be somehow established, it may very well be better to give general nonoperative support and not disrupt the barriers that are forming just as a balance between bacterial invasion and host resistance is begin-

ning to swing in favor of the patient. Continual soilage, however, is incompatible with life, and the control of a septic focus by some means – natural or operative – is mandatory.

Basically, the decision to operate is founded upon an assumption that the focus of soilage will probably not be otherwise controlled. The decision, then, is not based solely on the result of nonoperative efforts, but must be arrived at very early in the course of evaluation of the patient. An estimation of the potential for localization is reliable only if it is based upon actual evidence of beginning localization rather than upon a vague hope or wish that localization may occur. Modern methods furnish the surgeon with much more leeway in this regard than in former times, when the presence of generalized peritonitis was often considered a relatively strong contraindication to surgical intervention. Until recently, the conservative surgeon might prefer to attempt "ochsnerization" rather than run the risk of operating in the face of generalized peritonitis. Actually, some of the essentials of the Ochsner treatment – i.e., nothing by mouth and intravenous fluids – are most valuable; other essentials such as immobilization in Fowler's position and morphine by the clock have been shown to have dangerous consequences.

Today we may utilize the valuable techniques found useful in ochsnerization and anticipate the patient's dramatic response to nasogastric suction, restoration of blood volume, blood pressure, urine output, and the control of septicemia with antibiotics. Thus, in an advanced case, one may rely heavily upon resuscitative and nonoperative methods in the early hours of therapy even though the decision to operate may and should already have been made. By making the decision to operate very early and rather liberally, the surgeon will not let pass the golden moment when relative homeostasis is restored and the patient is in as fit a condition for surgery as he will ever be. The experienced surgeon will not be cozened into believing that an excellent response to nonoperative therapy has obviated the need for operation, but will recognize that this moment is apt to be ephemeral, and that if the patient is allowed to slip back into toxemia and shock he may well not be responsive to a second round of vigorous preparation. How much preparation is required, of course, depends upon the stage at which the patient is seen. In acute chemical peritonitis or in a postoperative patient in whom a leak from the upper gastrointestinal tract or biliary tract is suspected, one should proceed promptly with the operation. In late cases, whether original or postoperative, immediate operation is never indicated without adequate preparation. Errors in timing are possible in both directions, in both early and late cases. Generally speaking, the worst errors will be the result of operating too late in early cases and too soon in established cases.

It is unnecessary to discuss preoperative preparation extensively, since it may well include all of the measures described under the nonoperative treatment of peritonitis. There is always a tendency to do more than is necessary in the early or relatively straightforward case. For example, in early appendicitis or in a patient seen immediately after perforation of a peptic ulcer, application of the full armamentarium of nonoperative treatment will probably do more harm than good. Delay will be inevitable on the one hand, while, on the other, one cannot overlook the small but troublesome incidence of complications resulting from central venous pressure catheterization, Foley catheterization, abdominal paracentesis, antibiotic therapy, and so forth.

Apart from all the measures previously discussed, patients scheduled for operation generally are prepared with intramuscular or intravenous atropine and meperidine or morphine. Because they are in pain, a narcotic is preferred to the usual preoperative barbiturate or phenothiazine. Of great importance, also, is the reduction of fever before submitting the patient to anesthesia. Every effort, including alcohol sponging, should be made to reduce the temperature below 101° F. because the incidence of cardiac and convulsive complications is dangerously increased in the febrile patient.

Likewise, anesthesia is variable according to the needs of the patient. Spinal anesthetics are excellent for appendectomy and other emergency lower abdominal procedures in which the patient has not been prepared by fasting, so that preservation of gag, cough, and vomiting reflexes is desirable. The sympatholytic effects of spinal anesthesia, however, may be so profound that some other anesthetic is preferable in patients whose blood pressure may be unstable for one reason or another.

Better control of all parameters is perhaps offered by a general anesthetic in which the anesthetist can apply the full range of the various techniques of monitoring and life-support that characterize his specialty. While it is true that many patients are maintained in a much more physiologic state under anesthesia than they were able to generate on their own preoperatively, nevertheless one cannot lose sight of the fact that general anesthetics are poisonous rather than therapeutic drugs, and a patient who is desperately ill will be better off in many cases without them. It is sometimes difficult to persuade an experienced anesthetist of this fact, especially when the anesthetist is able to blandish the surgeon with the promise of perfect relaxation, ideal operating conditions, perfect control of airway and ventilation, and perfect comfort for the patient. However, the ultimate interest of the very sick patient, particularly the very old and very young, is not served by the imposition of a general anesthetic upon his already precarious homeostatic balance. In these desperate situations, it is better to persuade the anesthetist to forego the convenience of a general anesthetic and to stand by, paying close attention to monitoring and life-support, while the surgeon foregoes the convenience of relaxation to proceed with laparotomy under local infiltration anesthesia. There is no question that this technique has proved lifesaving on many occasions. Nor can one question the fact that desperately sick patients sometimes fail to awaken from a general anesthetic for no presently measurable reason.

The choice of incision in operations for peritonitis inevitably generates discussion among surgeons, so that a few general comments on this subject are irrepressible. In infants the entire peritoneal cavity may be easily explored through a transverse mid-abdominal incision, whereas a long vertical incision is subject to great risk of dehiscence. In patients up to approximately the age of two, then, it is clear that transverse incisions should be employed even when the diagnosis is in doubt. Patients over two who are of average build should be explored through a right paramedian incision with retraction of the rectus muscle laterally. This incision is capable of extension to the xyphoid or pubis if need be, so that any procedure may be performed through it with ease, whether the surgeon has been correct in his preoperative diagnosis or not. Wound dehiscence should be no problem, provided that anterior fascial stays or all-layer retention sutures are used properly and appropriately.

Exploration of the abdomen in patients with peritonitis may be a rather variable procedure depending upon whether the process is local or generalized. A great deal has been written about the inadvisability of breaking down established fibrinous and early fibrous adhesive barriers. Actually, however, the decision should be based upon the surgeon's estimation of the extent of peritonitis. If the process is localized, then it may very well be inadvisable to risk contamination of the general peritoneal cavity by breaking down established adhesions. If, on the other hand, general peritonitis exists already, with adhesion and loculation in many areas of the peritoneum, it is probably better to break down all barriers, so that complete evacuation of toxic and purulent material may be assured. Complete removal of all available material seems sensible, although we are by no means convinced that washing or irrigation for the purpose of such removal is advisable. At any rate, irrigation should not be performed initially and will be discussed more extensively later.

The primary purpose of the operation for peritonitis is to control the focus of infection. Control may be achieved by removal, exteriorization, plication, drainage, debridement, defunctioning, or decompression. Specific methods have already been mentioned in connection with discussions on the various causes of peritonitis.

The most direct means of controlling a focus is to remove it. This, for example, is accomplished in appendectomy or Meckel's diverticulectomy. When removal of the focus involves more extensive operation, such as gastrectomy or colectomy, the surgeon must accept a far higher operative risk, and he must then decide whether some compromise procedure would be safer. For example, subtotal gastrectomy is by no means to be universally recommended in perforated ulcer, although it may reasonably be carried out in good-risk patients who are seen early in the course of their disease and who have a prior indication for gastrectomy. Though many perforated peptic ulcers may be perfectly controlled by plication or patching, this technique is not effective for leakage from other causes or in other areas. Exteriorization is most often proposed in patients with colonic perforation. Very frequently, however, the area involved through perforation is so fixed by inflammatory changes that elevation to the abdominal wall is impossible. In these cases one may decide upon resection with or without anastomosis and with or without proximal decompression, or even upon simple drainage and decompression.

With so many options available, it is obvious that an exercise of judgment is required in the selection of the optimum procedure. Such discrimination is acquired only through experience, but certain guidelines are possible. The surgeon must always have several factors clearly in mind, the first of which is the condition of his patient. If the patient is in critical condition, then the procedure must be one that can be performed quickly, with a minimum of disruptive dissection and a minimum of reparative work, while at the same time it must assure absolute control of the focus. By and large, rapid resection with exteriorization of the cut ends of the bowel is the most expeditious, safest, and most effective. When bowel cannot be resected, then simple intubated drainage of the viscus, be it colon, stomach, duodenum, or gallbladder, may be the wisest choice. Colonic perforations should be not only drained but also decompressed proximally. Small-bowel perforations should, as a rule, be closed or resected, though exteriorization of the terminal ileum may be done if anastomosis is considered hazardous. Duodenal or biliary tract perforations are never subject to exteriorization but they respond well to closure with intubated drainage. Debridement of devitalized or badly infected tissue is mandatory despite the increased risk of extensive resection. Drainage of necrotic bowel is seldom effective; these foci must be excised even though the procedure may appear formidable.

After the focus of infection has been controlled by some means or other, preparations must be made for leaving the intestinal tract in as functional a condition as possible. The first order of business is decompression of the bowel. While many surgeons enthusiastically advocate doing away with routine Levin-tube decompression of the bowel after abdominal surgery, and while such enthusiasm for discriminatory treatment is commendable, it would be unfortunate to allow this experimentation to extend to patients with peritonitis. We feel that the intestine of these patients should always be decompressed, at least with Levin-tube or gastrostomy-tube drainage, and that many of them with established distention will benefit from operative decompression of the bowel.

For many years we have employed the Hodge sump-suction apparatus for operative decompression of the small intestine. More recently, we have come to recognize the advantage in many situations of intubation, decompression, and splinting of the small intestine, using the tube described by Joel Baker (Baker and Ritter, 1963). Like Baker, we have enjoyed excellent results following the use of this tube in the worst possible situations in which the entire small bowel was not only obstructed but infected, as, for example, when it forms part of the wall of an intraperitoneal abscess. In these situations the Baker tube not only affords decompression of the bowel but also, when left in place, provides a kind of "internal Noble plication" or intraluminal splinting that is effective in preventing postoperative obstruction. The Baker tubes are so constructed that they are neither so stiff that they inflict undue pressure upon the wall of the bowel nor so flexible that they kink; instead, the tubes form gentle curves so that the intubated bowel, although it may become thoroughly encased by adhesions, nevertheless may function normally because it is not kinked.

Another method of decompression that has proved quite satisfactory is a closed method of "milking" the bowel contents proximally to the point at which they may be removed by a previously placed Levin tube or long intestinal tube. Or, in a few cases, the contents may be milked distally to the colon and then around the colon to be forced manually through the rectum by compression of the rectosigmoid. By whatever means decompression is accomplished, we are convinced that it not only affords easier, safer, and more secure closure of the wound but also provides a situation in which the most rapid return of effective bowel function may be expected.

Even before decompression is attempted or as it is being carried out, the entire small intestine should be thoroughly examined and inspected to make certain that no points of obstruction exist. In late cases of peritonitis, abscesses will frequently be encountered in the course of small-bowel dissection;

these are drained as they are encountered and appropriate specimens are taken for culture. Naturally these remarks do not apply to the early cases in which exploration takes place before such extensive adhesion formation has had time to occur, but in the late case, very extensive dissection may be justified, so as to assure evacuation of all abscesses and discovery of all foci of infection and obstruction. If certain areas of the bowel have been badly damaged by the dissection, it may be necessary to resect them. Serosal and seromuscular tears are probably better left alone, so long as the mucosa is intact, for it is well shown that these traumas are quite capable of repairing themselves, whereas if they are repaired with sutures, adhesion is almost certain to result.

After control of the focus, decompression of the distended gut, if appropriate, and restoration of bowel continuity, if necessary, are achieved, the question of peritoneal lavage with or without antibiotics will arise. Much has been written on the subject, both for and against. Our own position on this matter is a compromise. We feel that there is a definite contraindication to irrigation when the infectious process seems to be localized, because there can be no doubt that the infectious material is widely distributed by lavage (Thoroughman et al., 1968). On the other hand, in generalized peritonitis or in patients in whom the dissection has necessarily involved all quadrants of the abdomen, then dissemination of infection by lavage is no longer a matter of concern, since the surgeon has already accomplished this with his fingers (Noon et al., 1967). In these cases there is no contraindication to lavage with saline, and a good deal of material may be removed in this manner.

It should be noted that Noon's controlled clinical trials showed no advantage in mortality if peritoneal irrigation was employed; however, previous experimental work had shown an advantage (Barnett and Hardy, 1958). We do not irrigate the peritoneal cavity with antibiotics, since it has been shown that the intraperitoneal route of administration is less effective than the intravenous route (Shear et al., 1965; Burke, 1967; Sandusky, 1964). As has been mentioned, all of our patients who are seriously ill with peritonitis are already being treated vigorously with intravenous antibiotics before they arrive at the operating room.

Another topic to be considered as preparations are being made to close the abdomen is the question of drainage. It is generally accepted that the peritoneal cavity cannot be drained effectively; there is no advantage in drainage of the peritoneal cavity at an early stage of generalized peritonitis. The reason for this is that within 12 to 24 hours the foreign body represented by the drain will have been perfectly walled off from the general peritoneal cavity, so that it will furnish drainage only for its own tract. This fact has at least two implications: First of all, in peritonitis of septic etiology, even though there has been no actual abscess formation, drainage of the region of the focus of peritonitis via the incision will not only provide egress for material that may accumulate in the heavily contaminated focus but may also prevent the formation of a wound abscess. The second implication is that drainage of an established abscess by exteriorization with a wick is a very effective and worthwhile procedure. Whenever the tip of a drain can be placed in contact with an evacuated abscess, any remaining infected or necrotic tissue will tend to become localized to the drain tract and will find egress through the tract. A final implication might be that in chemical peritonitis there is no real advantage to drainage if the point of leakage has been controlled. Of course, if there is some doubt as to the efficacy of control, then a drain should be placed in the region of leakage, though certainly not in contact with the point of closure (Goldstein et al., 1966). There is some evidence that drains placed next to suture lines or closures do cause or encourage the formation of fistulas (Berliner et al., 1964). The presence of peritonitis must enhance this liability. Nevertheless, if there is considerable doubt concerning the adequacy of any closure or suture line, there is certainly less difficulty to be expected from a controlled fistula via a drainage tract than from a spontaneous fistula or even generalized peritonitis that might occur if no egress had been provided.

Before the abdomen is closed, the advantages and disadvantages of intubated drainage of various organs and conduits should be considered; examples are drainage of the common bile duct, gastrostomy, and cholecystectomy. The disadvantages of properly placed tubes are very few, whereas failure to decompress by means of a tube may permit the development of a leak that need not have occurred.

There are certain areas in which we use tubes almost routinely, such as following exploration of the common bile duct for any reason. In postgastrectomy or gastrojejunostomy patients who have severe nutritional problems or in whom bleeding has been the indication for operation, we feel that the insertion of feeding and draining jejunostomy tubes is indicated. The proximal drainage tube is positioned so as to traverse the gastrojejunal anastomosis, thereby draining the stomach. Intubated colostomy has been proposed as a temporary alternative to transverse colostomy; however, catheter intubation of the colon may prove unreliable because of the thickness of some of the contents. We prefer, therefore, to perform the colostomy by one of the standard methods, bringing the bowel out over a plastic rod through a small and appropriately placed counter-incision.

Another kind of tube that sometimes proves useful in these patients is the dialysis catheter; these are most expeditiously positioned while the peritoneum is still open in patients who, because of toxemia or a shock-like state, have entered into an oliguric or anuric phase. Peritonitis seems to be no contraindication to peritoneal dialysis; in fact, the membrane is considered to be more permeable and more efficient in the presence of inflammation.

As the wound is closed, every effort should be made to achieve as strong and secure a closure as possible. We believe that anterior fascial or all-layer retention sutures should, with one exception, always be employed in open-bowel cases or in patients found to have peritonitis. The single exception is in the case of McBurney's muscle-splitting incision, in which dehiscence is practically unknown. Delayed primary closure is still employed to a small extent, but in most cases primary closure is preferred, often with irrigation of the wound with 0.5 per cent neomycin solution.

In contaminated wounds, it is important to use absorbable suture material in the anterior fascia as well as in the peritoneum; even in the heavily contaminated procedures we have observed no increase in the incidence of wound dehiscence. The results have been very satisfactory with the catgut and wire-retention suture method. For example, in a recent study of 111 consecutive operations in patients 80 years of age or over, only a single instance of evisceration was encountered. When wound infection does occur in these patients, skin sutures, if they have been used, are removed and the pus is allowed to drain between one or more pairs of retention sutures. It is unnecessary and unwise to remove the retention sutures or to lay the wound open completely. We refer the reader to W. A. Altemeier's chapter on wound separation and infection, though we feel obliged to share with the reader our very satisfactory experience with both the catgut-subfascial stay method as well as with the practically foolproof single-layer wire closure. It should be mentioned perhaps that in the single-layer wire closure the wires should be twisted together rather than tied, so that they may be loosened on the second and third postoperative days of maximum wound-swelling, and then perhaps tightened again as wound edema subsides.

POSTOPERATIVE CARE

The postoperative care of patients with peritonitis has become a team affair, involving cooperation between many specialty groups within the hospital—the nursing service, recovery room team, intensive care unit, anesthesia service, cardiac, renal, and infectious disease consultants, and, it is hoped, the dietary department. All biochemical and physiologic parameters are monitored and appropriate adjustments are made in replacement therapy, support, or medications. Intestinal-tube or gastric-tube aspirate is replaced quantitatively with saline solution, with the addition of 20 milliequivalents of potassium chloride per liter. Unless the patient is on a humidified respirator—in which case insensible water loss may approach zero—the usual insensible loss is replaced with a liter of water per day. Following a massive peritoneal insult, or an operation in which gross contamination of the peritoneal cavity has been discovered or has been necessary, large quantities of plasma may be required to replace that which is lost into the peritoneal cavity. Arterial pressure, central venous pressure, hematocrit, and urine output are monitored constantly in order to estimate this plasma requirement, which may reach several liters during the first two or three days postoperatively. Salt-poor albumin may be substituted for plasma, but dextran is not a satisfactory substitute except in an emergency.

If blood pressure and urine output fall, in the face of a rising hematocrit, a normal or elevated central venous pressure must be viewed with suspicion (Stahl, 1965). This combination suggests either that the central venous pressure line is malfunctioning, that right heart failure is present, or that pulmonary congestion has occurred. Heart failure may be treated temporarily with infusions of isoproterenol, carefully titrated so as not to raise the arterial pressure above 110 mm. Hg or to induce ventricular irritability. Simultaneously, digitalization should be undertaken with intravenous digoxin or Cedilanid. These measures should not be undertaken before the central venous pressure line has been carefully checked, both as to position in the superior vena cava (by x-ray) and as to function (the observation of free fluctuations with heartbeat and respiration).

One of the most important measurements of the patient's overall status is arterial oxygen saturation. A fall in the partial pressure of arterial oxygen is viewed as a grave sign because it usually indicates either that the patient is becoming worn out, with loss of ventilatory efficiency, or that serious alveolar-capillary dissociation is occurring from one cause or another.

Corrective measures applicable to treatment of these various combinations will be discussed in another section. Before leaving the question of routine postoperative care, however, two other points should be made. First, the postoperative phase is simply an extension of the intensive care initiated in the preoperative preparation of the patient. Preoperative and postoperative care should be regarded as a continuum whose success is practically assured if the surgery has fulfilled its single real purpose—namely, control of the focus of infection. However, this is true only if new or persistent or metastatic foci are not overlooked in the postoperative period.

This brings us to the second point: The role of the physician is more important than that of all the monitoring devices and paraphernalia surrounding the patient. Frequent physical examination is still the best method for determining the overall progress of therapy. The patient's personal physician—the surgeon in this case—must not allow himself to become displaced in any way by the impressive array of gleaming instruments, fancy tests, and monomaniacal teams of specialists that have suddenly come to bear on his patient. As the surgeon surveys the multidisciplinary melee from a distance, he may feel that his consultations have created a many-headed monster, or, alternatively, he may resign himself to obsolescence in the presence of such mass intelligence. Neither conclusion does justice to the surgeon or to the patient; the advantages of the team approach are great, but two glaring disadvantages stand out—namely, lack of responsibility and lack of leadership. The surgeon must realize that by calling in several teams of experts he has in effect created a new team, a super team, and he has, furthermore, automatically become captain of that team. If he does not assume that responsibility it is quite likely that no one will assume it. The kidney man will attend to the kidneys and the chest therapist will attend to the lungs, but the surgeon must still attend to the patient. His close attention in the postoperative phase may prevent or minimize many complications of peritonitis.

Despite his best efforts, however, complications following exploration for suppurative peritonitis tend to be multiple, so that these patients may run the entire gamut of cardiac, respiratory, neurologic, renal, and circulatory problems. It could almost be said that the treatment of peritonitis itself is relatively simple and that most patients who fail to survive succumb to one of the many complications of peritonitis rather than to peritoneal suppuration itself. Thus, the overall success of therapy depends to a great extent on the detection and management of postoperative complications. Since complications are so frequent, perhaps the single most important factor in recovery is frequent examination of the patient, for many complications can be treated successfully only in the early stages of their development.

COMPLICATIONS OF PERITONITIS

In this section the complications of peritonitis will be discussed more or less in order of their usual appearance. Wide variations in onset, severity, symptoms, and signs demand alert, careful, and continued observation. The early sequelae of peritonitis are essentially inevitable; they are not actually complications. These early sequelae tend to be self-limited but they may merge subtly or progress dramatically into later complications. Following control of a septic focus, the patient's course of improvement should be progressive and obvious. If not, a dangerous complication is all too likely at fault, and vigorous diagnostic measures, or even another operation, may be justified.

EARLY SEQUELAE

Among the earliest complications of peritonitis are those having to do with the respiratory system. The onset of pain leads to tachypnea, with decreased tidal volume and inhibition of cough reflex. Tachypnea causes an immediate decrease in the partial pressure of carbon dioxide in the blood, so that respiratory alkalosis rather than acidosis is the first sign of derangement. The shallowness of respiration and inhibition of respiratory reflexes cause an accumulation of secretions within the larger air passages. This effect is much more prominent, of course, in smokers, who may experience considerable distress within a short space of time. As the terminal bronchioles become blocked with secretions, alveoli distal to them collapse and atelectasis is produced. Pulmonary circulation continues through the areas of collapsed alveoli, so that the oxygen saturation of the blood is decreased. Thus, in this phase of respiratory difficulty, it is not uncommon to observe respiratory alkalosis and hypocarbia in the presence of hypoxemia (Pontoppidan et al., 1969).

Proper respiratory care of the preoperative patient with peritonitis may be quite impossible because of his pain and inability to cooperate. If possible, however, the patient should be encouraged to take deep breaths at intervals, to cough if secretions are present within the upper airway, and to submit to intermittent positive pressure breathing or tracheal aspiration if necessary. If considerable secretion is present, it should be cultured preoperatively. In the early postoperative phase, atelectasis is quite likely, especially if general anesthesia has been used. All the various techniques of respiratory physiotherapy should be employed, and the patient's work in breathing should be lessened by the administration of oxygen via nasal catheters or face tents. Though sputum cultures are taken early, antibiotic therapy is directed toward the peritoneal cavity rather than the chest, at least in the initial stages. Later pulmonary complications may become superimposed upon atelectasis and these may require vigorous therapy.

Sequestration of fluid always occurs to some extent in peritonitis. The sequestration may be the result of several conditions operating simultaneously. Foremost is the chemical irritative effect on the very large peritoneal surface.

There are very many points of similarity between peritonitis and cutaneous burns. Peritonitis is similar not only in its fluid losses into the injured area, but also in the less specific stress effects. Water retention results in dilutional hyponatremia and an increase in extracellular fluid, in addition to that actually lost into the peritoneum. The hyponatremia resulting from increased total body water is physiologic and does not represent a real clinical problem unless the lungs become affected. Any contraction of intravascular volume that results, however, must be corrected, because it may lead to profound hemodynamic abnormality with hypotension, anuria, and finally irreversible shock. There may be a limit to the amount of protein and fluid that is destined to be lost into the peritoneal cavity or extracellular tissue spaces, but this limit is not a function of blood volume or blood pressure. In other words, extracellular loss respects no homeostatic equilibrium with regard to blood pressure or blood volume. If the injury is a small one, the extracellular fluid expansion may be easily accommodated without compromising the total body economy; in massive injury in which the capillary permeability increases markedly in many areas, loss of blood volume to the tissue spaces will continue even as blood pressure and blood flow approach zero.

With the response to injury so variable, the danger of overtreatment or undertreatment is great. As alluded to in the previous section on postoperative care, flexibility in therapeutic response must be guided by continuous monitoring of the body functions. Frequent measurements of urine output, hematocrit, and blood pressure, however, will not reveal the fact that the fluid that is being lost and must be replaced is essentially plasma. If plasma is replaced with large quantities of lactated Ringer's solution, as has been the fashion recently, urine output and blood pressure may be maintained, but a huge water overload results from the omission of colloid replacement. Consequently, one may observe pulmonary edema in the presence of a normal central venous pressure. This is another situation in which the central venous pressure measurement, valuable as it is, may lead one astray unless it is interpreted in light of all the other clinical findings. A gain in weight at this time, as Pontoppidan has pointed out, is a very important sign, and may be the first and only indication of incipient pulmonary edema.

The fluid sequestration of the early postoperative, posttraumatic, or postburn period runs its course in three or four days. Quite often, there is a dramatic point at which the direction of fluid shift across the capillary membranes reverses itself, and the diuretic phase is then under way. The cardiovascular-renal system of the elderly patient may be unable to compensate for the increasingly rapid return of extracellular fluid into the bloodstream, so that massive overload and pulmonary edema may occur just as the patient ought to be starting to improve. Usually this situation is alleviated promptly by the brisk induction of diuresis with ethacrynic acid or furosemide although sometimes more vigorous measures may be required. The essential point is that the surgeon be aware that the patient who has been requiring massive fluid replacement may at some point require strict limitation of fluid and perhaps even diuresis. There is real danger if the change in requirement occurs in the middle of the night, while the previous day's estimated fluid and colloid needs are still being rapidly administered. The sudden appearance of slight dyspnea, a few fine rales at the bases, and a fall in the PaO_2 will signify the start of interstitial edema to the alert observer, who may then reduce intravenous intake and induce diuresis appropriately.

Adynamic ileus is to be expected for two to four days, even after very minor and completely controlled episodes of peritonitis. Adynamic ileus has traditionally been regarded as a protective mechanism, though it is difficult to actually conjure any particularly beneficial results of ileus. Teleology aside, adynamic ileus presents certain therapeutic problems that have to be dealt with even in the most routine cases. First of all, there is the danger of intestinal distention, which can lead to such stretching of the bowel that profound incompetence and very prolonged ileus may ensue. Distention may be absolutely avoided by a properly functioning tube; unfortunately, there is no tube devised that functions properly all the time. The Levin tube, gastrostomy, and long intestinal tube must be repeatedly irrigated to make sure that they are working, and the nursing staff must understand that a malfunctioning tube is a relatively urgent situation. Many patients, accustomed to the sense of release that accompanies vigorous eructation, seem inclined to swallow air unconsciously at the slightest epigastric provocation. Thus, it is quite possible on morning rounds to discover that the first indication of a kinked or plugged Levin tube is a massively distended abdomen.

Whether the belly is distended or not, the adynamic ileus of the first few postoperative days is resistant to all treatment, so that vigorous measures are irrelevant. Vitamins, hormones, cholines, laxatives, and electrical stimulation have all proved to no avail. The best thing to do, and indeed the only thing to do, in the presence of adynamic ileus is to wait. This is not to say that one should not recognize the inhibitory effect of certain deficiencies, or the permissive effect on peristalsis of certain substances, such as thiamine, piridoxine, pantothenic acid and ionic potassium. Their replacement will not stimulate the bowel but will only permit it to function when the time is right. Return of bowel function after a period of profound ileus is probably always segmental, so that certain areas and sections of the bowel resume function before others. This circumstance quite possibly accounts for many of the cramps of which patients complain as function resumes, and certainly must explain the persistence of dilated loops of bowel for several days or even a few weeks after the gastrointestinal tract as a whole is functioning fairly well.

By the same token, a return of peristaltic sounds is not a sign that the gastrointestinal tract is functional again and certainly should not of itself suggest a removal of or clamping of a decompression tube. The best prognostic signs are a decrease in the quantity of gastric drainage and the spontaneous passage of gas by rectum. Even these are not infallible signs; perhaps it does not have to be pointed out that a Levin tube that slips beyond the pylorus may return a liter or two of fluid a day, even on gravity drainage rather than suction, while the rectal passage of gas can occur when a dynamic ileus subsides despite possible organic obstruction at a higher level.

If paralytic ileus has not become resolved in five to seven days, the surgeon's increasing concern is justified, for the indolence of the intestinal tract may indicate the development of one of the more unpleasant later sequelae of peritonitis.

Sepsis

Whether the peritonitis is obviously septic or technically "chemical," a certain amount of infection is to be expected whenever there is intraperitoneal leakage from the gastrointestinal tract or its tributaries. Chyle, blood, and mucus, however, are examples of chemical peritonitis in which infection is not inevitable but may readily be introduced at the time of exploratory or corrective surgery. If one considers the usual case of ruptured appendix or perforated viscus, then a certain septic course is to be expected postoperatively. If inflammatory barriers have been broken down at operation and if the previously uncontaminated peritoneal cavity has been soiled, then there may be a very brisk response in terms of pyrexia and fluid sequestration. The postoperative increase in temperature may not always signify bacteremia, though such is frequently the case. Even a short period of septic shock immediately after operation for peritonitis falls within the range of expected events.

The response of a patient to postoperative septicemia depends, first of all, upon the adequacy of operation in controlling the focus of infection, but also very definitely upon such factors as the virulence of the organism, the propriety or luck in choice of an effective antibiotic, the immeasurable quantities determining host resistance, and how well the patient's homeostatic balance is maintained in other respects. Normally, one should see improvement in six to twelve hours after operation, though indeed it frequently takes longer. However, if fever, leukocytosis, and hypotension, or abdominal pain and spasm persist, then a search must be made in order to discover and treat one of the later sequelae of peritonitis.

LATER COMPLICATIONS OF PERITONITIS

The later sequelae or true complications of peritonitis include persistent general or localized peritonitis, spreading sepsis, respiratory failure, intestinal obstruction, and major abscess formation. Each of these complications is really an outgrowth or extension of one of the early sequelae discussed in the previous section. It is difficult to define the point at which an inevitable sequela becomes an actual complication; no less difficult is detection. This is why it has been stressed repeatedly that frequent postoperative examination is essential to good care. Complications discovered early can usually be treated successfully; complications that are overlooked until they become obvious are more difficult or impossible to treat.

Persistent, Generalized, or Local Peritonitis

Intransigence, worsening, or spread of peritoneal signs is of grave significance. The local signs may be very difficult to detect before 24 to 36 hours postoperatively because of the usual incisional pain and because patients who are sick with persistent peritonitis are often unable to cooperate. Persistent elevation of temperature beyond 12 hours postoperatively is also cause for great concern and for even more frequent examinations of the abdomen.

The possible causes of persistent peritonitis are, first of all, an uncontrolled focus of infection. This may result from an inadequate operation, and all the various possibilities certainly could not be listed. A few of the more common inadequacies, however, are the failure to control sigmoid diverticulitis by means of transverse colostomy alone and the very common failure of resuturing to control postoperative anastomotic leakage from any source. Other causes are inadequate debridement of dead or infected tissue, and the failure to function of an intraperitoneal drain placed near the infected focus. Another form of uncontrolled focus is seen when there is development of a new source of contamination or when one source is controlled but another is missed, as may occur in violent abdominal trauma. In this category may also be included such conditions as postoperative pancreatitis or postoperative intestinal gangrene, representing causes of peritonitis that were not actually present at the original operation but may commonly follow operation. In some respects uncontrolled sepsis in the postoperative patient is not the same disease as it is in the patient not yet operated on, because there exists the possibility of fistula formation and

decompression through the surgical incision. Though fistula formation itself may present very serious problems (as discussed in Chapter 20), fistulous drainage is nevertheless preferable to the release of the same material into the peritoneal cavity.

If an organism of unusual virulence is deposited in the peritoneum, then peritoneal sepsis may persist despite control of the original focus. In these situations the surgeon must rely heavily on the bacteriology laboratory to quickly furnish him with the antibiotic sensitivity spectrum of the organisms found on culture. As Altemeier pointed out in 1938, however, it is rather unusual to obtain a pure culture in secondary peritonitis; it is entirely possible, therefore, that an organism predominating on a culture plate may not be the virulent and predominant organism in vivo. Repeated cultures may be necessary after persistent infection becomes manifest. Even in these cases, synergism between different types of bacteria may finally appear to be the true reason for the persistence of the infection.

Patients who have cancer, hepatic cirrhosis, hypogammaglobulinemia, or who are taking steroid medication for any reason, may be unusually susceptible to infection, even with organisms of low virulence. The resistance of the host is a difficult thing to measure and one is certainly reluctant in any case to blame failure of therapy on such questionable grounds. If some specific cause of low resistance can be discovered, of course it can be treated. If none is found, conventional treatment must be pursued with increased vigor.

Involved with all of the above, but not really relating directly, is the appropriateness of the particular antibiotics selected for coverage. In most cases the sensitivity spectrum of the infecting organism is not known at the time antibiotics are started. It is always difficult to switch to a new drug or combination, especially if the laboratory reports have not yet been returned. It is impossible to lay down any rules governing the decision to change drugs, though an extensive discussion of the subject may be found in Chapter 4, "Postoperative Fever," by Allison.

Spreading Sepsis

When infection spreads beyond the confines of the peritoneal cavity, one may assume a further degree of invasiveness and virulence of the organism. This extension used to be common with the streptococcus before antibiotics; now it is more commonly seen with resistant gram-negative infections and synergistic infections. The possibilities for spreading sepsis are cellulitic, metastatic focal, neighborhood, and generalized. Wound infection, being of an obvious cause and of usually small significance as a diagnostic or therapeutic problem, is only mentioned here, but is discussed fully in Chapter 8 by Altemeier.

Cellulitic infection of the retroperitoneum or abdominal wall demands specific antibiotic therapy. Drainage is usually of little value, since the infection spreads along tissue planes into inaccessible areas. Clostridial infections that begin in devitalized tissue and then extend into normal tissue by way of their necrotizing toxins may be very difficult to reach with antibiotics because of the vascular injury that accompanies the infection. Extensive incision and debridement may be the only method offering control in these cases. Fortunately they are now very rare. Another group of anaerobes being encountered more frequently in surgical infections are the Bacteroidaceae, which are normal inhabitants of the lower gastrointestinal tract. They are often involved in mixed infections but remain undiscovered unless cultured anaerobically. They are sensitive to chloramphenicol and tetracycline (Saksena et al., 1968).

Infective organisms may metastasize by way of the lymphatic system or bloodstream, and septic emboli may be found in the lung, brain, kidneys, surgical incision, or other areas. It is interesting that when mixed infections are present within the peritoneal cavity, the organisms grown from metastatic abscesses are usually also found to be mixed, suggesting either embolization of fairly large particles or perhaps simultaneous bacteremia involving several types of organisms (Altemeier, 1938).

A special form of metastatic infection peculiar to peritonitis is pylephlebitis. Despite the persistent frequency of peritonitis in all its forms, pylephlebitis has become extremely rare. The decrease in frequency must be due in part to better surgical methods, but primary credit must go to antibiotic therapy for covering those cases in which surgery was inadequate. Many patients still die of complications following peritonitis, but very few succumb to this particular one. No doubt prompt intervention in cases of suspected appendicitis is responsible for the marked reduction in incidence of this classic complication. The clinical picture of pylephlebitis is that of septicemia with recurrent chills and fever spikes. The appearance of jaundice introduces the possibility of secondary liver abscess and is of very grave prognostic significance. Multiple small abscesses developing from pyelephlebitis are almost always resistant to antibiotic treatment and are usually fatal. Large single abscesses that develop later, following successful treatment of the septicemia, may be surgically correctible. An intrahepatic abscess may be impossible to differentiate clinically from a subphrenic abscess. As a matter of practicality, and also of organizational convenience, the diagnosis and treatment of subphrenic, hepatic, and subhepatic abscesses will be discussed together in a later section.

Spread of infection to a neighboring area is best exemplified by the development of thoracic empyema secondary to subdiaphragmatic abscess. Though the diaphragmatic pleura and peritoneum may be intact, lymphatic drainage from below upward is known to occur, and the appearance of fluid in response to subdiaphragmatic sepsis is commonly seen. The exact mode of passage of organisms into the pleural fluid is not definitely known, though it is assumed that lymphatic drainage is responsible. The appearance of infection in pleural effusion may be quite undramatic, perhaps because the patient is already running a course that is septic owing to primary infection beneath the diaphragm. Aspiration of the pleural fluid is diagnostic and should always be done if fluid is known to be present in a patient with undiagnosed fever. The method of treatment of secondary empyema depends upon the stage in which it is discovered and upon the physical characteristics of the fluid. Thin fluid is removed by needle aspiration; thicker fluid may require placement of a drainage tube with constant suction. In advanced cases the empyema content may be so thick that resection of a segment of rib and insertion of a large rubber tube will be necessary for satisfactory drainage. In these cases pleural thickening and adhesion effectively isolate the abscess cavity from the remainder of the pleural space. If such adhesion and loculation have not occurred, pneumothorax will result when open drainage is attempted. There is little danger of this complication, however, if empyema is treated initially by aspiration and intubated drainage.

Generalized bacteremia and septicemia following peritonitis are usually the result of a breakdown of host resistance or the development of bacterial insensitivity to antibiotics. As with other manifestations of extraperitoneal spread of sepsis, generalized septicemia, disseminated abscess formation, and bacterial endocarditis usually result from failure to recognize and drain some primary or secondary intraperitoneal focus. In other instances, however, this generalization does not hold; at postmortem examination the lack of findings in the peritoneal cavity is presumptive evidence that dissemination of infection must have occurred prior to or at the time of corrective surgery. As with multiple liver abscesses following pylephlebitis, generalized septicemia responds poorly or not at all to vigorous antibiotic therapy, and the mortality rate is consequently very high.

Respiratory Failure

This fascinating subject has received extensive treatment in the literature over the past several years, largely as a result of the interest and accomplishments of specialized units and teams devoted to the care of respiratory problems of all kinds (Skillman et al., 1969).

From a pathophysiologic point of view, the respiratory failure associated with peritonitis represents an extension of the processes operative in the early phase of peritonitis both preoperatively and postoperatively. The segmental atelectasis that regularly accompanies suppression of normal respiratory reflexes may be abetted by chronic bronchitis, prior structural emphysema, and prior lung disease due to smoking or other causes, or to aspiration of regurgitated gastric juices. Other influencing factors are the deranged respiratory physiology that accompanies general anesthesia, the presence and degree of postoperative pain, the age and general strength of the patient, the depressant effect of analgesic medication, and the extent of body temperature elevation. Pain, medication, frailty, toxemia, and anesthesia reduce the efficacy of the sum total of the ventilatory mechanisms, while atelectasis and the increasing accumulation

of secretions tend to prevent inspired oxygen from reaching the blood that is circulating through the lung. The net effect is desaturation of the blood with respect to oxygen at a time when pyrexia and tachypnea have increased the oxygen requirement. As long as the patient is able to satisfy his oxygen demands by an increase in ventilatory effort to compensate for the decrease in efficiency, a state of equilibrium is possible. However, when the point is reached that increases in ventilatory work and cardiac output require more oxygen than they produce, an unstable situation results that Burke, Pontoppidan, and Welch in 1963 termed "high output respiratory failure." In simple terms it means that total oxygen requirements, including the requirements of the work of breathing, have outstripped the ability of the total breathing mechanism to supply oxygen; the resultant hypoxemia reflexively induces an even greater breathing effort so that a vicious cycle is begun that, unattended, can result only in exhaustion and death. The diagnosis of high-output failure depends upon the observation of increased ventilatory effort despite decreasing arterial oxygen saturation. Hypocarbia and respiratory alkalosis may be present in the early stages; the alkalosis, of course, makes matters worse by interfering with the acquisition of oxygen from oxyhemoglobin by the tissue.

When oxygen desaturation is diagnosed at an early stage, it may be possible to reverse the vicious cycle by vigorous intervention with measures aimed at the various operative factors. Basically, this means an increase in respiratory efficiency and a decrease in oxygen requirement. Specifically, attempts are made to improve efficiency by the following: (1) The administration of morphine for the relief of pain may relax the abdomen sufficiently to permit diaphragmatic rather than chest-wall ventilation with a marked increase in tidal volume and reduction of dead space. At the same time a moderate inhibition of the respiratory center will actually improve the efficiency by reducing the rate of breathing. (2) Maximum oxygenation of the inspired air is achieved by use of a flutter-valve face mask and a high flow of humidified oxygen. (3) Deep breathing, coughing, sighing, and changes in position are used to induce clearing of secretions from the bronchi and bronchioles as well as inflation of collapsed, but still vascularized, alveoli. (4) Tracheal suction, though regarded as a stigma of unsuccessful treatment by the chest physiotherapist, may nevertheless prove very helpful to induce coughing, deep breathing, and the clearing of secretions in an overly medicated or otherwise uncooperative patient. (5) Intermittent positive pressure ventilatory assistance is applied by means of a hand-held face mask and hand respirator in most cases; but in a particularly cooperative patient the nostrils may be pinched while a mouthpiece is held tightly between the teeth and lips. The pressure thus applied at the end of inspiration serves to increase the tidal volume while resting the ventilatory muscles. Atelectatic areas are forced open and if this ventilatory assistance is applied for a minute or more the arterial oxygen saturation may be increased to the point at which the muscles of breathing may work more efficiently.

Intermittent positive pressure assistance should not be mentioned without calling attention to the importance of a functioning nasogastric tube or gastrostomy, if any type of face-mask or mouthpiece ventilation is applied. Though we have referred repeatedly to the many adverse effects of intestinal distention, they are at no time more dramatic than the acute gastric dilatation caused by assisted ventilation in a patient already precarious from a respiratory point of view.

In addition to these measures aimed at increasing arterial oxygen content, the therapy of incipient high-output respiratory failure is also directed at reduction of oxygen need. Reference has already been made to the relief of breathing effort and, hence, the oxygen requirement provided by ventilatory assistance. It is not practical, however, to carry out face-mask assistance more often than every 30 minutes.

Another method of reducing oxygen consumption that comes to mind immediately, of course, is lowering the patient's temperature. In addition to treatment of the causative infection, an attempt should be made to treat fever by means of aspirin or acetaminophen. The traditional alcohol sponging or the newer refrigerated blankets must be used with care, both because they can be uncomfortable and because they actually may increase the oxygen need if shivering is produced.

The considered application of these measures usually will reverse early respiratory decompensation. However, they may be inadequate for patients with extreme obesity, prior lung disease, severe debility, or a history of heavy smoking. If the arterial oxygen saturation fails to improve or at least stabilize at a level that is reasonable for the particular patient, then much more vigorous measures are required, in the form of continuous inspiratory assistance. Formerly this meant tracheostomy and artificial ventilation. In recent years, however, tracheostomy is almost never justified as an initial procedure; instead an endotracheal tube is inserted under local anesthesia. With moderate to large doses of morphine or curare, patients can tolerate not only the irritating presence of the tube but also artificial ventilation almost indefinitely. The destructive effects of the tube upon the larynx and trachea, however, are another matter; the very serious and potentially lethal complications must be obviated by substitution of a tracheostomy tube after a few days. The hazards of emergency tracheostomy are thus completely avoided, since the procedure is carried out in a perfectly controlled manner while the patient is perfectly ventilated through the endotracheal tube.

Current practice in our postoperative recovery rooms has resulted in the infrequent appearance of high-output respiratory failure, which, it is now recognized, must have been a very frequent cause of death prior to its elucidation. For patients who are seriously ill or who have fallen into one of the high-risk categories, it is now quite common to anticipate ventilatory failure and prevent its occurrence by maintaining assisted ventilation through the endotracheal tube during the early recovery period. As the faculties are gradually regained following anesthesia, a very precise estimation of ventilatory capability is made by measuring tidal volume, vital capacity, maximum inspiratory pressure, and, of course, arterial gas saturations or partial pressures. Thus the surgeon and the anesthetist are practically relieved of the necessity for guesswork in determining the optimum time for extubation or, if necessary, elective tracheostomy.

Although the causes, prophylaxis, and treatment of high-output respiratory failure have been reasonably well worked out, there is another much more difficult respiratory complication that is only recently coming under close scrutiny. Because the condition is so poorly understood, it does not even have a name, or perhaps one might say that is has a number of names, such as "respirator lung," "pump lung," "congestive atelectasis," and "interstitial pneumonitis" (Berry and Sanislow, 1963). The pathologic lesion has been well described as including congestion, edema, and early fibrosis of the pulmonary interstitium combined with hyaline membrane formation and alveolar cell hypertrophy. Pontoppidan points out rightly that these changes may occur in a great variety of conditions including septic shock, hemorrhagic shock, oxygen poisoning, uremia, and the hyaline membrane disease of infancy.

Moore (1969) also emphasizes that the pulmonary lesions are not pathognomonic but that they are also seen in uremic pneumonitis, rheumatic pneumonitis, cholera, and viral infections. In his excellent book, Moore reviews the case histories of patients succumbing to several types of clinical emergencies; nonsurvivors all demonstrated the pulmonary changes at postmortem examination. In attempting to delineate the pathogenesis of pulmonary lesion, Moore discusses a number of possible etiologic factors, including massive transfusion, water overload, fat embolism, thromboembolism, aspiration of gastrointestinal contents, abdominal distention, failure of ventilatory mechanics, endotracheal intubation and tracheostomy, oxygen toxicity, bacterial colonization, and the use of antibiotics. Though Moore does not mention suppurative peritonitis or peritoneal abscess as possible etiologic factors in the development of this lesion, it is of interest that though his nonsurvivors were selected to illustrate a variety of clinical situations terminating with a single pulmonary lesion, they all also shared one other common characteristic that in the analysis was ignored or perhaps dismissed as insignificant—the patients all had focal or generalized peritonitis.

Experience with a number of our own nonsurvivors had already suggested that progressive pulmonary insufficiency may, indeed, be of diagnostic import in patients whose peritoneal infection is not otherwise manifest. Thus, the clinical characteristics of hypoxemia resistant to ventilatory assistance sufficient to correct hypercarbia, decreased lung compliance, and normal or increased cardiac output may well be more significant in pathologic terms below the diaphragm than above. This brings us back again to the critical and continuing responsibility of the operating surgeon, even though a major portion of daily care is delegated to the respiratory physicians, nurses, and therapists. If the surgeon overlooks the peritoneal abscess in his unconscious or paralyzed respiratory patient, it is virtually certain to remain hidden until revealed by the pathologist.

Intestinal Obstruction

The treatment of intestinal obstruction or peritonitis, when either exists alone, is fairly well standardized; when they are present in combination, the problem is much more difficult and the mortality rate rises sharply. Measures usually effective for intestinal obstruction, for example, lysis of adhesions, may be relatively contraindicated by the coexistence of peritonitis. The contraindication is only relative, however, because persistent intestinal obstruction is absolutely incompatible with survival, and restoration of continuity, therefore, is mandatory, whatever the risk. Such a bold philosophy implies an ability to diagnose persistent intestinal obstruction and to distinguish it from prolonged adynamic ileus in slowly subsiding peritonitis (Welch, 1958).

Returning for a moment to the pathophysiology of peritonitis, one may readily understand how the processes of fibrin deposition and fibrosis can lead to kinking of the bowel. It is not so easy to understand how the whole process may be spontaneously resolved, although this is well known to occur. Better understood are the adjuvant factors which, when added to the fibrin deposition of peritonitis, will quite regularly produce potentially obstructing adhesions. Intestinal distention, suture material of all kinds, serosal tears, foreign bodies, and abscess formation may all be implicated. Abscesses may produce obstruction by direct compression of the bowel lumen or by angulation due to plastic adhesions that form when a loop of intestine actually constitutes one wall of an abscess. The other possibility is, of course, that proximity to an abscess would be expected to produce at least a segmental adynamic ileus. Inflammatory edema of adjacent loops must also narrow the lumen of the bowel and reduce the leeway.

The diagnosis of intestinal obstruction

following suppurative peritonitis reduces itself to a differentiation between persistent adynamic ileus and significant mechanical interference with function. The differentiation obviously is not always possible because in a significant proportion of cases the classic signs may be absent. Absence of bowel sounds postoperatively is to be expected for at least three or four days. An abdomen that remains silent for longer than five to seven days becomes a cause for concern and for grave concern if the patient is not doing well in other respects. Conversely, the reappearance of intestinal sounds can occur in the presence of persistent adynamic ileus of a segmental nature as well as in frank mechanical obstruction. The usual and expected appearance of hyperperistalsis and cramps may be inhibited by residual inflammation, and abdominal distention will be prevented by an effective suction tube.

Fortunately, other parameters are available to support a diagnosis of obstructive peritonitis. Foremost are persistent signs of sepsis, such as fever, leukocytosis, and tachycardia. Continuing abdominal tenderness is a very important sign indicating that infection is not subsiding properly. The most important sign of all, of course, is the failure of gastrointestinal absorptive and peristaltic function. Continued large losses of intestinal fluid through the drainage tube suggest a mechanical problem; the losses in adynamic ileus are often in the neighborhood of a liter a day, whereas with obstruction gastric drainages of 2 or 3 liters in 24 hours are often seen. The passage of gas is an infallible sign of the return of bowel function but it does not exclude the possibility of obstruction.

Radiologic examination of the postoperative (or nonoperative) patient may yield valuable information. Plain and upright or lateral decubitus films may show disseminated collections of gas in many intestinal loops, including the colon, or perhaps marked distention of a few loops with air-fluid levels of differing heights, as seen in obstruction. Sometimes the instillation of thin barium or Gastrografin via the intestinal tube will delineate a point of obstruction; more often, however, the opaque medium simply parks in a few distended loops in both adynamic and mechanical ileus.

With all diagnostic parameters equivocal, the diagnosis and decision to operate become matters of exclusion. All possible factors that may contribute to intestinal paralysis are systematically excluded. Dehydration and electrolyte imbalance are corrected. Blood volume and hematocrit are restored. Serum albumin is restored to normal and intravenous hyperalimentation is begun. A long intestinal tube is passed and closely supervised until it reaches the ligament of Treitz. Successful passage of the tube may relieve any intestinal distention without relieving the obstruction. If improvement is to occur, it should do so in a few days.

As clinical progress is observed, the patient is constantly appraised and reappraised as a possible candidate for secondary surgery. If definite signs of mechanical obstruction or recurrent peritonitis appear, operation should be undertaken as soon as the patient can be restored to reasonable balance. If, however, as is more common, the course is an indolent one, the timing of operation becomes a most important factor and the decision to operate is often a matter of the nicest judgment.

Several considerations must be borne in mind. One is the condition of the patient's veins. Patients who die early in the course of peritonitis do not live to develop intestinal obstruction. Conversely, most obstructed patients are already in their second postoperative week when the question is raised. If veins are few or if they have been poorly nurtured, the surgeon must anticipate the fact that the patient faces at least another five to seven days of starvation as a result of adynamic ileus after the second operation. Newer techniques in intravenous therapy, including meticulous local treatment of intravenous cannulas, new methods of percutaneous central venous cannulation, and the long-awaited practicality of intravenous alimentation, have, to a great extent, relieved us of the burdensome problem of nutrition as a factor in the timing of reoperation (Wilmore and Dudrick, 1967; Mogil et al., 1967; Dudrick et al., 1968).

The method in current use at the Massachusetts General Hospital involves caval or atrial placement of a venous catheter through which hypertonic nutriment solution is given continuously. With meticulous daily dressings, the catheter sites may be maintained free of infection for weeks. The feeding solution we employ is composed of 1000 ml. water with protein hydrolysate (29 gm.), glucose (280 gm.), ethanol (14 gm.), potassium chloride (20 milliequivalents), and vitamin B complex. A saline solution is made by adding 70 milliequivalents of sodium chloride to the above. The caloric content is 1300 per liter and we try to give 2 or 3 liters per day. We recognize that intestinal continuity is essential to ultimate survival, but the great urgency for the earliest possible restoration no longer need take precedence. In other words, the timing of therapy may be adjusted to respect more fully the surgeon's assessment of the peritoneal sepsis instead of subordinating his best judgment on that matter to alimentary requirements. As the various measures of treatment are carried forth and the surgeon contemplates the status of homeostasis, ileus, sepsis, and veins, the passage of another two to four days should make apparent whether or not the patient is improving.

It is to be recognized that there is no ideal time for reoperation. From a technical point of view, however, there can be little question that earlier operations are far easier than later ones. The turning point seems to occur sometime around the seventh to tenth day, when adhesions become vascularized and fibrotic. When signs of peritonitis and mechanical obstruction remain vague but the patient is simply not doing well, the decision to reoperate may be one of the most difficult in surgery.

Once the decision is made, however, there is a sense of relief. The patient is prepared for a general anesthesia. Adequate blood and plasma are ordered. In addition to all the other tubes and cannulas that should already be functioning, any intestinal fistulas are intubated with catheters in order to provide easy identification. A generous incision is made, usually reopening the previous wound. The objectives of operation are to relieve obstruction, to preserve small intestine, to close or excise sources of peritoneal contamination, to locate, open, and drain all loculations of pus, to excise necrotic tissue, to relieve distention, and finally, but often most important, to prevent angulation during the phase of healing.

The procedure begins with evisceration of all dilated loops of small bowel. A point of major obstruction, marked by transition to collapsed bowel, is thus easily identified and dealt with. Often a very difficult dissection of the entire small bowel is necessary, since multiple points of adhesion and obstruction are frequently present. Distended small bowel is then emptied either by milking the contents upward or distally,

by enterotomy and sump suction, or, very satisfactorily, by means of the Baker tube. Passage of the Baker tube or a long intestinal tube, previously placed in the stomach or proximal small bowel, will demonstrate the adequacy of the small-bowel lumen. If the partially inflated catheter balloon cannot be passed through a kink or crimp, the situation must be corrected by either lysis of adhesions or resection, if necessary.

Primary anastomosis, inverting, in two layers, can be undertaken with nearly perfect safety in the small bowel, provided there is no distal obstruction. The same cannot be said for the colon, where fistula formation in the presence of peritonitis is common enough to mandate proximal decompression. Bypass enteroenterostomy or enterocolostomy may be preferable to resection if the entire small intestine cannot be mobilized. Even a jejunocolostomy would be preferable as a first stage to any lesser procedure that left the intestine in a state of obstruction. In desperate situations the construction of an ileostomy or colostomy may be preferable to an anastomosis. Since many of these patients may expect even more prolonged ileus following the second operation, the insertion of a gastrostomy drainage tube may be most beneficial.

These drastic operative measures will often succeed in cases in which any conservative method would probably be doomed to failure. In an early study, we employed as indications for surgery the presence of peritonitis, intestinal obstruction, failure of conservative measures, and the prospect of almost certain death unless the situation could be improved, and we carried out these extensive operations on 17 patients. Fourteen of them recovered after this refunctionalization of the intestine (Welch, 1955).

Major Abscess Formation

The pathophysiology of intraperitoneal abscess formation has already been discussed and the etiologic factors are now well known. Less obvious are the reasons why many patients have localized intraperitoneal sepsis, but relatively few form abscesses. The factors are not well understood, especially in the relationship of abscess to phlegmon, cellulitis, and suppurative peritonitis. In this section we will discuss the locations and nomenclature of major abscesses, their diagnosis, the timing of operation, and various operative approaches to these several major abscesses.

Retroperitoneal abscesses cannot logically be omitted from a consideration of intraperitoneal abscesses because they may arise from the same organs, diseases, and operations. Furthermore, a thoroughly walled-off abscess may from a physiologic point of view behave as if it were extraperitoneal, whereas an abscess that is anatomically retroperitoneal may produce extensive intraperitoneal effects. It is thus probably better to consider all major intra-abdominal abscesses together, dividing them into retroperitoneal and intraperitoneal for purposes of convenience in discussion and in deference to tradition.

Retroperitoneal Abscesses. Included among retroperitoneal abscesses are the retrocecal, psoas, perinephric, retrohepatic, and pelvic. Numerous subdivisions of these spaces are possible, but the major functional distinction is in terms of anterior retroperitoneal versus posterior retroperitoneal. Essentially, the posterior space lies behind the renal and transversalis fascia, and the anterior space lies behind the peritoneum and anterior to the transversalis fascia. Retrofascial abscesses, such as the psoas abscess, lie in a space that extends from the mediastinum to the upper leg. The renal fascia is formed by a special envelopment of the transversalis fascia. The perinephric space is closed superiorly, but communicates with the pelvic retroperitoneal spaces below. In terms of etiology, pyelonephritis is by far the most common single cause of perinephric abscess, although retroperitoneal perforation of a viscus is occasionally responsible.

The majority of anterior retroperitoneal space abscesses develop from perforations of the abdominal viscera. Perforative diverticulitis is the usual antecedent of left-sided anterior retroperitoneal abscesses; the retrorectal space may accumulate as much as 500 cc. of pus migrating downward from perforative sigmoid diverticulitis (Levy, 1965). In 1969, Stevenson and Ozeran reported a series of 48 patients with retroperitoneal space abscesses, and found that the condition was misdiagnosed in 44 per cent of the patients. The commonest symptom was lower abdominal or flank pain, although in some cases it was located in the back, hip, or thigh. Other common symptoms are chills, anorexia, weight loss, and limp. Systemic signs of infection, such as pyrexia and leukocytosis, are present, but the absence of peritoneal involvement may possibly lead to the high incidence of misdiagnosis and the equally high mortality rate.

Intraperitoneal abscesses also suffer from an extensive nomenclature, although in recent years there seems to be a trend toward simplification of the terminology (Davis et al., 1968; Boyd, 1966). Major intraperitoneal abscesses may occur in any of the numerous pockets, infoldings, and crevices that characterize the peritoneal cavity. Many of these nooks have special names, and the abscesses, naturally, are named after the spaces.

Before discussing the different abscesses, however, we should first mention the term "mural." A mural abscess is defined as one that is in contact at some point with the abdominal wall. Any abscess may become mural, even if it originates deep within the pelvis or high under the diaphragm. The only requirement is that it grow large enough to present above the pubis or beneath the costal margin. Iliac and paracolic abscesses, on the other hand, are mural from their inception and may present as palpable masses while still very small. The mural nature of an abscess has great significance with respect to surgical drainage, since it is always possible to evacuate such an abscess without entering the uninvolved peritoneal cavity.

In a strict semantic sense, all intraperitoneal abscesses are subphrenic. This facetious comment is made to point out the fallacy of expecting intraperitoneal abscesses to conform in extent to any anatomic description of their space of origin. The peritoneal cavity is one space, and all areas communicate freely with all others. The first definitive study of the subject of subphrenic abscess was made by Barnard in 1908. His original descriptions of the subphrenic spaces have colored surgical thinking and teaching ever since, though, as Boyd points out, Barnard's descriptions are based on an erroneous impression that the coronary ligaments suspend the liver from the dome of the diaphragm rather than attach it to the posterior abdominal wall, as is actually the case. Thus the anterior and posterior superior spaces described by Barnard are actually only one space—the right suprahepatic or subdiaphragmatic space. Likewise, the posterior inferior space has classically been divided into anterior and posterior divisions, although in reality it is all just one space and is probably more appropriately termed subhepatic than subphrenic. The posterior portion of this space corresponds to the hepatorenal pouch of Morison, whereas the anterior portion is represented by the surface of contact between colon and liver. If we accept the usual definition of a subphrenic abscess to be any localized collection of pus below and in contact with the diaphragm, we can readily see that the right subhepatic space does not fit the definition, classical descriptions notwithstanding. There is one other legitimate subphrenic space on the right, and that is the retroperitoneal space comprised by the bare area between the superior and inferior leaves of the coronary ligament. Abscesses may develop in this area either as a result of extension of an intrahepatic abscess or as a result of upward tracking of a retrocecal appendiceal abscess. Thus, from an anatomic viewpoint, on the right side there is one suprahepatic or subphrenic intraperitoneal space, one right extraperitoneal space, and one right subhepatic intraperitoneal space. From the clinician's standpoint, however, there is merit in considering anterior and posterior suprahepatic abscesses as distinct clinical problems. This is true also for abscesses located anteriorly or posteriorly in the subhepatic space; not only do the signs and symptoms differ, but the approaches to drainage are also quite different.

The falciform ligament divides right from left subphrenic spaces. The left lobe of the liver is so much smaller than the right and has such a short coronary ligament that it is impractical to establish any formal subdivision of the left subphrenic space, although this has been done in the past because of an inaccurate understanding of the placement of the coronary ligament. It is better to think of the left subphrenic space as being one big space in any portion of which an abscess may develop. The most definable space of all is the lesser omental bursa, which communicates with the right subhepatic space only by means of the foramen of Winslow. Abscesses in this sac are uncommon and usually follow direct contamination by a perforative gastric ulcer or by pancreatitis. The other abscesses are generally the result of upward migration of fluid from any source of intraperitoneal suppuration.

Right subphrenic and subhepatic abscesses following appendiceal rupture used to be fairly common and comprised 30 per cent of the series reported by Ochsner and Graves in 1933. More recent series demonstrate an increasing frequency of left subphrenic abscesses reflecting the increasing frequency of gastric, splenic, and pancreatic surgery. Five to ten per cent of subphrenic abscesses are primary or metastatic without any known antecedent trauma, perforation, or operation. This group of idiopathic abscesses is often very difficult to diagnose and, in consequence, carries a very high mortality rate. Even as recognizable sequelae of generalized or localized peritonitis subphrenic accumulations are sufficiently distinct from other intraperitoneal abscesses in terms of symptomatology, diagnosis, and treatment to merit separate consideration along those lines at this point.

Though the patient with a subphrenic or subhepatic abscess will usually demonstrate the general signs and symptoms of a closed-space infection, the local signs may be very obscure because of their deep-seated location. They are inaccessible not only to physical examination, but often have no contact with hollow viscera, so that irritative gastrointestinal symptoms are absent.

The interval before the appearance of signs and symptoms of subphrenic abscess after operation for peritonitis is unpredictable. In some patients, the expected subsidence of pyrexia does not occur, although the peritoneal signs may improve as expected. In other patients, especially those for whom antibiotic treatment has been more effective, there may be a period of improvement varying from days to weeks before a relapse, indicated by recurrence of fever. The sign of fever following a bout of peritonitis from whatever cause, should always arouse the suspicion of subphrenic abscess. Wound infection, urinary tract infection, atelectasis, phlebitis, and local operative complication are far more common, but when these have been excluded and the fever persists, then subphrenic infection becomes a distinct possibility. Chills, sweats, and spiking fevers indicate the necessity for a vigorous diagnostic approach.

Patients should be quizzed closely on the presence of costal margin or shoulder pain upon breathing or coughing. Hiccup may also indicate diaphragmatic irritation. Upper abdominal pain, chest pain, and flank pain are common, but by no means universal, abdominal symptoms (Carter and Brewer, 1964). Despite the deep position of many of these abscesses, it is unusual not to elicit tenderness either in the epigastrium or subcostal areas or by percussion over the costovertebral angles. Enlargement and tenderness of the liver may be discovered, or there may be only a vague impression of upper abdominal fullness, even with very large abscesses.

A variety of indirect diagnostic methods are now available by which the diagnosis should be established in the vast majority of cases in which it is suspected and sought. Plain films and fluoroscopic examination of the chest and abdomen in various positions will reveal evidence of subdiaphragmatic infection in nearly 100 per cent of cases (Carter and Brewer, 1964). Basilar atelectasis and congestion are common. Elevation of the affected diaphragm with diminished or paradoxical motion on breathing is one of the most reliable x-ray findings. A pleural effusion is universal in the true subphrenic accumulation, though subhepatic and lesser sac abscesses may produce no identifiable thoracic symptoms or signs. Plain films taken in various positions may reveal a subphrenic or subhepatic collection of air that is most suggestive, or even an air-fluid level that would be acceptable as diagnostic. It must be remembered, of course, that the persistence of air without a fluid level can be seen for ten days to two weeks following laparotomy.

At this point the diagnostic technique of pneumoperitoneum should also be mentioned, in which failure of air to enter the subphrenic space is considered to indicate abnormal adhesion and probably infection. This negative evidence is of such limited value that the method hardly seems worthwhile in relation to the more informative tests which can be done. One such test that has become rather simple in performance is radioactive scintiscan of the liver, or of the lung and liver simultaneously (Brown, 1966). An abnormal separation between the two, or an indentation of the dome of the liver beneath the high but normally rounded diaphragm, will indicate very nicely the extent of a suprahepatic or intrahepatic abscess.

Intrahepatic abscesses may be delineated by barium enema or upper-gastrointestinal barium studies and left-sided ab-scesses can almost always be suspected on the basis of their impingement upon the stomach from one direction or another. In one of our cases, a lesser sac abscess presented, several weeks following left colectomy, as a mildly tender epigastric mass very few systemic signs. An upper-gastrointestinal series revealed huge, gastric mucosal folds that were assumed to further indicate gastric lymphoma; their complete subsidence after drainage of the abscess, however, indicated their true edematous nature.

Because it is often impossible to distinguish subphrenic from intrahepatic abscesses, and because their clinical significance following peritonitis is not dissimilar, the method of differentiation by means of hepatic arteriogram should be considered (Pollard and Nebesar, 1966). If positive, the results are practically unequivocal and delineate very precisely the size and position of abscesses.

With the mortality rate for undrained subphrenic or subhepatic infection still in the range of 85 per cent (Sherman et al., 1969), it seems prudent to exhaust every diagnostic method for the patient with appropriate clinical findings in an effort to exclude a possible second abscess. This is particularly important if an extraperitoneal or transpleural approach seems indicated because of the suspected position of the abscess. In some cases, the situation will remain dubious, owing to the equivocal nature of all the diagnostic efforts. In these cases a diagnostic surgical exploration may be indicated if the systemic signs are sufficiently worrisome. Though extraperitoneal drainage of known abscesses is preferred, when the location or presence of the abscess is only suspected, a formal laparotomy is more likely to disclose the source of infection. The danger of transserous drainage has probably been overrated and even without antibiotic coverage is much to be preferred over inadequate drainage or no drainage at all.

The treatment of established subphrenic abscesses is entirely surgical, although on rare occasions even such deep-seated abscesses may drain spontaneously to the surface or into an adjacent loop of bowel, or they may even achieve drainage through a bronchus by penetration of the diaphragm. The chief point of interest regarding conservative treatment, however, is that it is so seldom effective. The only consistent exception to this dogma is the amebic abscess, either intrahepatic or subdiaphragmatic, in which perfectly satisfactory cures are achieved in almost all cases through adequate emetine and chloroquine therapy combined when necessary with needle aspiration of the abscesses. Secondary bacterial invasion and troublesome or fatal wound and peritoneal infections involving amebic-bacterial synergism are so common after open exploration that it is probably preferable to wait out even intraperitoneal rupture of an amebic abscess without surgery, *provided* it can be established that the ruptured abscess is amebic rather than bacterial.

Surgical drainage may be accomplished through the chest or through the abdomen, and in either case the approach may be "extraserous" or "transserous." More specifically, the posterior abscesses are drained extrapleurally or transpleurally, whereas the anteriorly placed abscesses may be drained extraperitoneally or transperitoneally. There continues to be a good deal of controversy in the literature regarding the advantages and disadvantages of the various operations. It seems clear from our own experience and from the experiences reported by Moore in 1963, Boyd in 1958 and 1966, and others that the method offering the best drainage in a given case is the best method. Thus the posterior (superior) subphrenic abscesses may be drained most directly by a transpleural approach through the bed of the resected tenth rib (Boyd). The posteriorly placed subhepatic abscess is simply and easily reached through the bed of the twelfth rib according to the safe extrapleural and extraperitoneal approach described by Nathan and Achsner in 1923. Anterior subphrenic abscesses are drained by the Clairmont technique, in which a subcostal incision is carried down to but not through the parietal peritoneum (Clairmont and Ranzi, 1905). The peritoneum is then stripped upward and away from the fascia until the abscess is encountered and entered, thus preserving the integrity of the general peritoneal cavity. Anterior subhepatic abscesses are usually mural, so that their drainage through a subcostal incision is effortlessly extraperitoneal.

Abscesses in the left subphrenic space can almost always be drained extraperitoneally through a left-sided Clairmont incision. Only the lesser-sac abscess does not lend itself readily to an extraperitoneal drainage. In a rare case, the abscess may be drained extrapleurally and extraperitoneally through an Ochsner incision on the left. Before leaving the subject of drainage, it should be mentioned that the extraperitoneal (bare area) subphrenic abscesses usually are drained through a posterior approach. However, when these abscesses become large, they may present anteriorly through the falciform ligament. When this occurs, a very direct and excellent drainage tract may be achieved through a simple midline extraperitoneal incision into the space between the leaves of the falciform ligament. This procedure should be used, however, only if tenderness and fluctuation are present anteriorly.

Special precautions to be taken in the drainage of subphrenic abscesses include measures against the possibility of pneumothorax if the chest is inadvertently entered or of flooding of the tracheobronchial tree with pus if an unsuspected bronchopleural communication with the abscess is encountered. Needless to say, general anesthesia with endotracheal tube intubation is preferable for the posterior approaches. In very ill patients, the anterior extraperitoneal incisions may be made under local anesthesia.

The abscess cavities should be drained with ¾-inch cigarette wicks or by the insertion of a soft rubber tube. These abscesses usually close very slowly. Recurrent infection is the rule if the drainage apparatus is removed too soon. The proper time for removal of drains can be determined by fluoroscopic injection of the cavity with radiopaque fluid.

Systemic response to drainage is usually rapid. If the patient does not improve immediately or if after initial improvement a second relapse occurs, then some other local collection must be suspected, such as another subphrenic abscess or, rather frequently, the development of thoracic empyema in a previously sterile pleural effusion.

Recent articles on subphrenic abscess indicate that this is still a very important and lethal clinical problem despite the widespread use of antibiotics (Carter and Brewer, 1964; Sherman, 1969; Magilligan, 1968). Antibiotics undoubtedly are beneficial in these serious infections, but the persistent high mortality rates broadly attest to the fact that the most massive antibiotic therapy can in no way substitute for prompt diagnosis and effective surgical drainage.

The various other types of major intraperitoneal abscess fortunately are much less troublesome in terms of diagnosis, treatment, and prognosis than are abscesses in the subphrenic spaces. Again it is emphasized that the boundaries of these spaces are not fixed or well defined, so that any given abscess may be somewhat difficult to name if, as is often the case, it either lies between two spaces or actually extends to occupy more than one space.

SUPRACOLIC ABSCESSES. The supracolic space is a poorly defined compartment that is divided roughly into right and left halves by the falciform ligament. On the right these abscesses are anterior to the gallbladder and the duodenum, and on the left, anterior to the stomach. They may extend downward, anterior to the greater omentum, or upward, in which case they occupy the anterior subphrenic position. They generally follow upper abdominal surgery or may result from perforation of any of the upper abdominal viscera. Because of their position immediately beneath the anterior abdominal wall, they are relatively easy to diagnose on the basis of local signs in the patient with the general signs and symptoms of infection. Their location is virtually always mural, so that an anteriorly placed incision must enter them directly without violation or contamination of the free peritoneal cavity.

CENTRAL PERITONEAL OR INTERLOOP ABSCESSES. These abscesses are more difficult to diagnose because they are located behind the greater omentum and may be enclosed between folds of mesentery and loops of small intestine. Because segments of small bowel may be intimately involved or actually form a portion of the wall of an interloop abscess, there may be marked gastrointestinal signs and symptoms such as diarrhea, intestinal bleeding, or intestinal obstruction. The abscess may occasionally drain itself into an eroded loop of small bowel. Most patients, however, eventually require surgical drainage because of persistent severe toxemia and signs of gastrointestinal tract irritation, even though they may never develop a palpable mass. Drainage is necessarily transperitoneal. If signs of intestinal obstruction have been present preoperatively, then the dissection of the intestinal segments caught up in the abscess wall may

have to be very extensive. Badly damaged loops may have to be resected or bypassed if resection appears too dangerous. Resection is preferable to bypass unless the involved segment is very long, but in any case the first consideration is that all infection be drained and all obstruction relieved.

PARACOLIC ABSCESSES. With the patient in the usual supine position, the right paracolic gutter is a locus of gravitation of pus from perforations of the appendix, right colon, and duodenum, whereas the left paracolic abscess usually follows diverticulitis. In stout patients a paracolic abscess may be difficult to detect by physical examination but ordinarily there should be little difficulty. One sign that may be of value even in the obese patient is the gravitation of edema fluid to the posterior flank, where it may be readily felt in the subcutaneous tissue on the affected side. These collections are easily drained through a flank incision.

ILIAC ABSCESSES. The paracolic gutters communicate freely with the iliac regions on each side as well as with the supracolic spaces above. In localized appendicitis and diverticulitis, however, an abscess may remain confined to the iliac area. As it enlarges, it may present immediately above the inguinal ligaments, where it may be readily evacuated through a relatively small incision under local infiltration anesthesia. Appendectomy need not and should not be attempted at this stage. In diverticular disease of the left colon, the need for concomitant exploratory laparotomy and transverse colostomy is determined by the degree of systemic and general peritoneal involvement.

PELVIC ABSCESSES. Pelvic abscesses are probably the most common site of localization following generalized or local peritonitis or open-bowel operations of any sort. The purulent collection accumulates in the most dependent portion of the peritoneal cul-de-sac, where they may be detected at a very early stage by rectal examination in male or female. Larger abscesses may present anteriorly in the suprapubic region, or they may extend upward and laterally in either direction to the iliac or even to the paracolic gutters. Actually there is no upward limit of extension; one patient recovered after extensive drainage of an abscess that extended from the pelvis via the left paracolic gutter to the left subphrenic space.

Of all intraperitoneal abscesses, the pelvic

abscess is perhaps the only one that can usually be regarded as a beneficial development. Although local irritation of the rectum may cause diarrhea, the systemic signs and symptoms seem less marked than with other abscesses in higher parts of the abdomen, and there is also perhaps less tendency to intestinal obstruction, since the small-bowel loops tend to float over the purulent accumulation.

Often it is difficult to distinguish pelvic phlegmon or cellulitis from actual abscess formation, since both may present as tender pelvic masses with systemic signs of toxemia. These cellulitides may subside gradually without treatment, though antibiotics would doubtless be recommended in every case today. Similarly, true collections of pus may resolve spontaneously either by absorption or by rupture into the rectum or posterior vaginal fornix. Abdominal pain, rectal tenesmus, bladder irritation, or small-bowel involvement constitutes a relative indication for surgical intervention. A patient who is moderately or markedly toxic has an even more pressing indication for drainage after a period of observation.

It should be emphasized strongly that even though surgical drainage of a pelvic mass may be indicated on the basis of systemic effects, nevertheless this mass should not be approached through the rectum or vagina unless there is very definite evidence of fluctuation. If the mass has neither softened in the rectum nor enlarged to an extent that it may be palpated suprapubically, then it may be better to await further developments while maintaining the patient on antibiotic coverage. It is interesting that many of these masses that at first seem certain to drain into the bowel may either disappear spontaneously or later present suprapubically or in an iliac position. Any attempt to hurry the process by a rectal or vaginal incision runs the risk of unnecessary disruption and contamination of a slowly resolving phlegmon or, even worse, a useless injury to a loop of small intestine. When fluctuation does become apparent, then the surgeon may safely proceed with rectal or vaginal drainage under general anesthesia.

The patient is placed in the lithotomy position, and the area of fluctuation is again palpated very carefully, including bimanual abdominopelvic palpation. The tip of a long spinal needle is then guided with the finger into the center of the fluctuant area. When pus is obtained, a slightly opened hemostat or scissor may be slid along the needle and so forced accurately into the collection. We believe that the precaution of prior aspiration with a needle is worthwhile because it assures accuracy in the placement of the larger instrument and because we have seen no instance of fistula formation even when small-bowel content rather than pus is obtained by aspiration. Naturally the procedure is abandoned if needle aspiration yields chyme rather than pus. When an abscess is opened, however, and the opening is enlarged by spreading the clamp or scissor, it may then be explored very gently with the finger. It is unnecessary and may possibly be damaging to break up adhesions or loculations. A large-bore rubber tube is inserted and sutured to the anal verge, or a Foley catheter makes an excellent self-retaining drainage and irrigation tube as recommended by Jackson (1966).

CAUSES OF DEATH FROM PERITONITIS

Throughout this chapter on peritonitis and its complications, there have been so many references to mortality rates that one may easily overlook the fact that patients rarely die of acute peritonitis; they die of pathologic or physiologic abnormalities that have been initiated by peritonitis. This is not to deny that there will be an occasional patient whose infection is resistant to antibiotic and surgical treatment and who will die in a few days of overwhelming septicemia that must be attributable directly to his peritonitis. Much more commonly, however, death will result from the combination of the sequelae and later complications of peritonitis. This discrepancy implies that any further lowering of the mortality rate ascribed to peritonitis must depend upon improvements in the detection and treatment of complications rather than of the primary disease.

We have seen that the peritoneum itself is remarkably resistant to infection and reacts violently against the slightest contamination. It will not, however, be able to overcome the effects of persistent soilage, so that surgical control of intestinal leakage is absolutely essential for survival.

With control of sepsis, either by natural means or with the aid of antibiotics, and with the elimination of intestinal leakage by surgery or spontaneous sealing, the patient with peritonitis has overcome two major obstacles to survival but many more remain. There is the spendthrift depletion of water, electrolytes, and other blood constituents that are lost into the peritoneal cavity and other extracellular spaces without regard for the total body economy. Patients with perfect control of sepsis and leakage may quickly expire from the effects of fluid loss. Fluid replacement essential for survival must be accurately administered, for imprecise management in this regard may lead to the iatrogenic complications that are just as lethal.

If not recognized, the "high-output respiratory failure" syndrome may lead to death within a few hours after operation, whereas adequate treatment may reverse the process quickly and completely. The later respiratory complications described by Moore and others represent a current frontier of our understanding and, indeed, their development may actually be a valuable sign of persistent uncontrolled peritonitis rather than a detached and autonomous sequela.

One of the most important causes of late death following peritonitis is intestinal obstruction. It is interesting to dissect the causes of death in intestinal obstruction in the same manner as for peritonitis. Here again we conclude that mortality results from fluid and electrolyte loss, toxemia (in strangulating obstruction), and finally starvation in the last analysis, but not from obstruction itself. Nevertheless, the relief of obstruction is essential for survival following peritonitis.

Finally, the resolution of suppurative peritonitis by abscess formation demonstrates in a convincing way the ability of the peritoneal cavity to effectively manage and control infection and contamination. Once the septic products have been enclosed in a pyogenic membrane, the healing of peritonitis may proceed, even though the patient may die of effects of the undrained abscess.

The position of renal failure and cardiac failure as causes of death in peritonitis is not clear at this time. Lower-nephron nephrosis and tubular-cell necrosis are known to occur, but the low blood pressure due to fluid shifts and hypovolemia may have more to do with their development than any toxemia or septicemia. Likewise, there is no satisfactory proof of direct toxic effects upon the heart, though heart failure may occur as the result of inadequate management of fluid or pulmonary complications of peritonitis.

The purpose of this brief summary is simply to emphasize the point that just as the mortality rate in peritonitis is attributable to complications rather than to the basic disease, in a similar way successful treatment of peritonitis demands a flexible approach and alertness to the subsequent appearance of secondary lesions in diverse organs and systems. Successful management of complications is relatively simple if they are detected early; detection is basically a question of being aware of the possibilities and of searching for them diligently in the patient who is not recovering normally. The causes of suppurative peritonitis are well understood and the methods of dealing with those causes are largely standardized. Overall success in management of peritonitis has come now to depend upon the surgeon's ability to recognize that the critical surgical illness does not end as the patient leaves the operating room, but only after the last complication has been treated.

REFERENCES

Altemeier, W. A.: The bacterial flora of acute perforated appendicitis with peritonitis. Ann. Surg., 155:517, 1938.

Altemeier, W. A., and Culbertson, W. R.: Complications of Appendectomy. In Artz, C. P., and Hardy, J. D. (eds.): Complications in Surgery and Their Management. 2nd ed., Philadelphia, W. B. Saunders Company, 1967, p. 564.

Artz, C. P., et al.: Further studies concerning the pathogenesis and treatment of peritonitis. Ann. Surg., 155:756, 1962.

Baker, W. J., and Ritter, K. J.: Complete surgical decompression for late obstruction of the small intestine with reference to a method. Ann. Surg., 157:759, 1963.

Barnard, H. L.: Address on surgical aspects of subphrenic abscess: delivered before the surgical section of the Royal Society of Medicine, January 14, 1907. Brit. Med. J., 1:371, 429, 1908 (cited by Boyd, 1958)

Barnett, W. O.: Experimental strangulated intestinal obstruction: a review. Gastroenterology, 39:34, 1960.

Barnett, W. O., and Hardy, J. D.: Observations concerning the peritoneal fluid in experimental strangulated intestinal obstruction: The effects of removal from the peritoneal cavity. Surgery, 43:440, 1958.

Befeler, D.: Proctoscopic perforation of the large bowel. Dis. Colon Rectum, 10:376, 1967.

Berliner, S. D., et al.: Use and abuse of intraperitoneal drains in colon surgery. Arch. Surg., 89:686, 1964.

Berry, R. E. L., and Sanislow, C. A.: Clinical manifestations and treatment of congestive atelectasis. Arch. Surg., 87:153, 1963.

Boley, S. J., et al.: Pathophysiologic effects of bowel distention on intestinal blood flow. Amer. J. Surg., 117:228, 1969.

Boyd, D. P.: The anatomy and pathology of the subphrenic spaces. Surg. Clin. N. Amer., 38:619, 1958.

Boyd, D. P.: The subphrenic spaces and the emperor's robes. New. Eng. J. Med., 275:912, 1966.

Brown, D. W.: Lung-liver radioisotope scan in the diagnosis of subdiaphragmatic abscess. JAMA, 197:728, 1966.

Burke, J. F.: Discussion of paper by Noon, G. P., et al.: Clinical evaluation of peritoneal irrigation with antibiotic solution. Surgery, 62:73, 1967.

Burke, J. F., et al.: High output respiratory failure: an important cause of death ascribed to peritonitis or ileus. Ann. Surg., 158:581, 1963.

Burnett, W. E., et al.: The treatment of peritonitis using peritoneal lavage. Ann. Surg., 145:675, 1957.

Byrne, R. V.: Localized perforated diverticulitis. Arch. Surg., 88:552, 1964.

Carter, R., and Brewer, L. A.: Subphrenic abscess: a thoracic-abdominal clinical complex. The changing picture with antibiotics. Amer. J. Surg., 180:165, 1964.

Clairmont, P., and Ranzi, E.: Kasuistischer Beitrag zur Operativen Behandlung des subphrenischen Abszensis. Wien. Klin. Wschr., 18:653, 1905.

Cohn, I.: The "toxin" in closed-loop strangulation obstruction. Bulletin of the New York Academy of Medicine, 40:863, 1964.

Cornell, W. P., et al.: A new nonoperative technique for the diagnosis of penetrating injuries to the abdomen. J. Trauma, 7:307, 1967.

Curtis, A. H.: A cause of adhesions in the right-upper quadrant. JAMA, 94:1221, 1930.

Davis, C. E., et al.: Subphrenic space infection—reassessment. Ann. Surg., 168:1004, 1968.

Drye, J. C.: Intraperitoneal pressure in the human. Surg. Gynec. Obstet., 87:472, 1948.

Dudrick, S. J., et al.: Long-term total parenteral nutrition with growth, development, and positive nitrogen balance. Surgery, 64:134, 1968.

Epstein, M., et al.: Pneumonococcal peritonitis in patients with postnecrotic cirrhosis. New Eng. J. Med., 278:69, 1968.

Fonkalsrud, E. W., et al.: Neonatal peritonitis. J. Ped. Surg., 1:227, 1966.

Goldstein, H. S., et al.: Drains at the suture line. Surgery, 60:908, 1966.

Grigsby, W. P.: Surgical treatment of amebiasis. Surg. Gynec. Obstet., 128:609, 1969.

Hermreck, A. S., and Thol, A. P.: The adrenergic drugs and their use in shock therapy. Current Problems in Surgery. Chicago, Year Book Medical Publishers, Inc., July, 1968.

Hunt, T. K. and Hawley, P. R.: Surgical judgment and colonic anastomoses. Dis. Colon Rectum, 12:167, 1969.

Jackson, J. B., and Elem, B.: Resolution of pelvic ab-

scess using indwelling catheter. Surg. Gynec. Obstet., 122:119, 1966.

Kiser, J. L., et al.: Colon perforations occurring during sigmoidoscopic examinations and barium enemas. Missouri Med., 65:969, 1968.

Krizek, T. J., and Davis, J. H.: Acute chylous peritonitis. Arch. Surg., 91:253, 1965.

Levy, E.: Pathognomonic triad of retrorectal abscess: the surgical approach. Dis. Colon Rectum, 8:61, 1965.

Lillehei, R. C., et al.: Treatment of septic shock. Mod. Treat., 4:321, 1967.

MacLean, L. D., et al.: Treatment of shock in man based on hemodynamic diagnosis. Surg. Gynec. Obstet., 120:1, 1965.

Magillian, D. J., Jr.: Suprahepatic abscess. Arch. Surg., 96:14, 1968.

McCarthy, J. D., and Picazo, J. G.: Bile peritonitis: diagnosis and course. Amer. J. Surg., 116:664, 1968.

Mogil, R. A., et al.: The infraclavicular venipuncture: value in various clinical situations including central venous pressure monitoring. Arch. Surg., 95:320, 1967.

Moore, F. D., et al.: Post-Traumatic Pulmonary Insufficiency (Pathophysiology of respiratory failure and principles of respiratory care after surgical operations, trauma hemorrhage, burns and shock). Philadelphia, W. B. Saunders Company, 1969.

Moore, H. D.: Subphrenic abscess. Ann. Surg., 158:240, 1963.

Morris, P. J.: Diagnostic paracentesis of the acute abdomen. Brit. J. Surg., 53:707, 1966.

Nathan, C., and Achsner, E. W. A.: Retroperitoneal operation for subphrenic abscess. Surg. Gynec. Obstet., 37:665, 1923.

Netterville, R. E., and Hardy, J. D.: Penetrating wounds of the abdomen: analysis of 155 cases with problems in management. Ann. Surg., 166:232, 1967.

Noon, G. P., et al.: Clinical evaluation of peritoneal irrigation with antibiotic solution. Surgery, 62:73, 1967.

Ochsner, A., and DeBakey, M. E.: Subphrenic abscess: collective review and analysis of 3608 collected and personal cases. Int. Abstr. Surg., 66:426, 1938.

Ochsner, A., and Graves, A. M.: Subphrenic abscess: analysis of 3372 collected and personal cases. Ann. Surg., 98:961, 1933.

Pollard, J. J., and Nebesar, R. A.: Angiographic diagnosis of benign diseases of the liver. Radiology, 86:276, 1966.

Pontoppidan, H., et al.: Acute respiratory failure in the surgical patient. Advances in Surgery. 4:163–254, 1969.

Rodkey, G. V., and Welch, C. E.: Surgical management of colonic diverticulitis with free perforation or abscess formation. Amer. J. Surg., 117:265, 1969.

Saksena, D. S., et al.: Bacteroidaceae: anaerobic organisms encountered in surgical infections. Surgery, 63:261, 1968.

Sandusky, W. R.: Use of antibiotics and chemotherapeutics in surgery. Current Problems in Surgery. Chicago, Year Book Medical Publishers, Inc., October, 1964.

Shear, L., et al.: Peritoneal transport of antibiotics in man. New Eng. J. Med., 272:666, 1965.

Shepard, J. A.: Surgery of the Acute Abdomen. Baltimore, Williams & Wilkins Company, 1968.

Sherman, N. J., et al.: Subphrenic abscess: a continuing hazard. Amer. J. Surg., 117:117, 1969.

Skillman, J. J., et al.: Peritonitis and respiratory failure after abdominal operations. Ann. Surg., 170:122, 1969.

Smith, G. A.: Intestinal obstruction: tube decompression. Bull. N. Y. Acad. Med., 40:871, 1964.

Spiro, R. H., and Hertz, R. E.: Colostomy perforation. Surgery, 60:590, 1966.

Stahl, W. M.: Resuscitation in trauma: the value of the central nervous pressure monitoring. J. Trauma, 5:200, 1965.

Stajano, C.: Cited by Stanley, 1919.

Stanley, M. M.: Gonococcic peritonitis of the upper part of the abdomen in young women. Archit. Med., 78:1, 1946.

Stevenson, E. O. S., and Ozeran, R. S.: Retroperitoneal space abscesses. Surg. Gynec. Obstet., 128:1202, 1969.

Thomas, C. S., and Brockman, S. K.: The role of adrenal corticosteroid therapy in escherichia coli endotoxin shock. Surg. Gynec. Obstet., 126:61, 1968.

Thoroughman, J. C., et al.: Spreading organisms by peritoneal lavage. Amer. J. Surg., 115:339, 1968.

Vasko, J. S., and Tapper, R. I.: Surgical significance of chylous ascites. Arch. Surg., 95:355, 1967.

Veith, F. J., et al.: Diagnostic peritoneal lavage in acute abdominal disease: normal findings and evaluation in 100 patients. Ann. Surg., 166:290, 1967.

Watkins, G. L., and Oliver, G. A.: Management of perforative sigmoid diverticulitis with diffusing peritonitis. Arch. Surg., 92:928, 1966.

Welch, C. E.: Intestinal obstruction. Chicago, Year Book Medical Publishers, Inc., July, 1958.

Welch, C. E., and Hedberg, S. E.: Complications in surgery of the colon and rectum. In Artz, C. P., and Hardy, J. D. (eds.): Complications in Surgery and Their Management. Philadelphia, W. B. Saunders Company, 1967, p. 577.

Westfall, R. H., et al.: Barium peritonitis. Amer. J. Surg., 112:760, 1966.

Wilmore, D. W., and Dudrick, S. J.: Cannula sepsis (letter). New Eng. J. Med., 277:433, 1967.

Wright, L. T., et al.: An evaluation of Aureomycin in peritonitis. Surg. Gynec. Obstet., 92:661, 1951.

Yeager, G. H., et al.: Terramycin in peritonitis: experimental and clinical. Ann. N. Y. Acad. Sci., 53:319, 1950.

Zintel, H. A., et al.: Influence of antibiotics and sulfonamides on the mortality and bacteria of experimental peritonitis. Surg. Gynec. Obstet., 91:742, 1950.

CHAPTER 19

STRANGULATION OBSTRUCTION

by WILLIAM O. BARNETT, M.D.

William O. Barnett is a Mississippian who studied at the University of Mississippi and the University of Tennessee College of Medicine. After his residency training at Baltimore City Hospital and subsequent military service, he entered surgical practice in Jackson, joining the surgical staff and faculty of the University of Mississippi Medical Center, when it opened in 1955. Applying the practical common sense approach derived from boyhood on a farm, he became an outstanding teacher and clinician and is currently Professor of Surgery. His original contributions toward a better understanding of strangulation intestinal obstruction and peritonitis have been widely acknowledged.

SMALL-BOWEL STRANGULATION

DIAGNOSIS

There are no absolute diagnostic criteria, short of laparotomy, by which the presence of strangulated bowel can be established with finality. Nevertheless, the appearance of certain findings should arouse a strong suspicion that compromise of intestinal circulation may have occurred and that appropriate therapeutic measures should, therefore, be instituted.

In most cases of simple bowel obstruction the pain is intermittent and crampy. The appearance of severe and steady abdominal pain may herald the transition from simple to strangulation obstruction. In those patients who exhibit abdominal pain of a degree sufficient to necessitate the administration of narcotics, the possible presence of strangulation must be suspected. This is also true in those patients with obstruction who appear to be seriously ill. Abdominal tenderness and rebound tenderness constitute findings which should arouse concern over the status of intestinal circulation. The same is true for localized abdominal pain or a localized abdominal mass in the patient with obstruction. Strong evidence favoring strangulation is established by the aspiration of dark or bloody peritoneal fluid. Passage of bloody material per rectum or the occurrence of manifestations characteristic of shock suggests a transition toward strangulation. Demonstration of an external hernia that resists reduction constitutes a suspicious situation. The same is true for elevation of the temperature above 100.5° F. or pulse rate above 110 per minute in the patient with obstruction.

PREOPERATIVE PREPARATION

CENTRAL VENOUS PRESSURE

In the critically ill patient with strangulation obstruction, severe deficiencies of various components of the circulating blood volume occupy a prominent position among the various pathophysiologic changes characteristic of the condition. In many instances it is necessary to give large volumes of blood and electrolyte solutions over relatively short periods of time. This may be necessary in poor-risk, elderly patients with borderline cardiovascular reserve, and it is especially under these circumstances that constant monitoring of the central venous pressure can serve as a valuable adjunct during preoperative preparation. A low CVP indicates that the heart is not pumping at maximal capacity, whereas a

477

normal or elevated value suggests that the myocardium is working to a maximal degree and that additional intravenous infusion would be likely to precipitate heart failure and pulmonary edema.

Central venous pressure may be adequately evaluated by cannulation of either the upper or the lower caval system. We prefer to utilize one of the branches of the superior vena cava because of a lesser inclination toward thrombophlebitis and clot formation. Blind puncture of the subclavian vein with the insertion of a continuous, indwelling polyethylene tube works nicely under certain circumstances, but this procedure may be fraught with complications, such as pneumothorax or intrapleural hemorrhage from injury to the subclavian artery. Another approach consists of dissecting out the cephalic vein along its course between the deltoid and pectoralis major muscles. This requires considerable effort toward location of a comparatively deep structure and may be attended by considerable technical difficulty. The attractiveness of this approach is further limited by frequent occurrence of anatomic variation and, rarely, total absence of the cephalic vein.

We feel that the external jugular vein provides the most efficient route of access to the upper caval system. It is a large vein that can usually be delineated visually without necessitating a cut-down. Prolonged intravenous therapy can be administered with a less than average threat of catheter dislodgement. Plastic tubing sets with disposable needles, available commercially, facilitate the placement of indwelling venous catheters. The tip of the catheter should be advanced until it rests within the innominate vein or the superior vena cava. Blood samples for laboratory analysis should be withdrawn at this point. A bottle of lactated Ringer's solution is connected to a three-way stopcock with the aid of plastic tubing, in order to prevent clotting in the indwelling tube. The third component of the stopcock is connected to a glass manometer of the variety usually found on a spinal-tap tray. The base of the manometer should rest on a level with the atrium of the heart to assure the accuracy of the zero point. We consider a venous pressure value of 8 to 12 cm. of saline the optimal level and strive to accomplish this before surgery. Actually the *trend* toward an upward or downward movement of CVP is probably more dependable in the appraisal of preoperative status than is any single reading (Fig. 19–1).

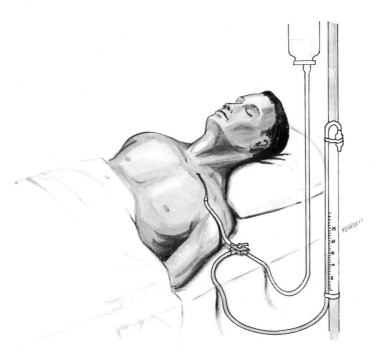

Figure 19-1. Simple bedside apparatus for monitoring central venous pressure.

INTRAVENOUS FLUID AND ELECTROLYTE ADMINISTRATION

Hartwell and Hoguet were among the first to call attention to the vital role of fluid and electrolyte replacement in the management of bowel obstruction. Their paper from the experimental laboratory was published in 1912, but clinical application was not widespread until the 1930's. Observed over the past 30 years, the significant reduction in the mortality rate of patients with simple obstruction is probably related more to this one factor than to any other aspect of management. Depletion of body fluids occurs at a rapid rate in the patient with obstruction because of the inability of the distended bowel to absorb. This situation predisposes to continuing fluid loss through vomiting and through the nasogastric tube. There is, of course, a continuation of normal water loss through the skin, kidneys, and lungs. Additionally, the patient with strangulation obstruction loses significant volumes of fluid into the peritoneal cavity as a result of irritation by bacteria and their products.

There are no specific methods by which precise fluid requirements for the individual case can be ascertained. It is necessary, therefore, to depend upon various clinical parameters for monitoring periodic evaluations concerning the progress of fluid replacement. These include the venous pressure, hematocrit, pulse rate, and urinary output. It has been estimated that when early x-ray signs indicative of obstruction appear, the fluid deficit will be approximately 1500 ml. When the obstruction is well established and there is a history of vomiting, this value will approach 3000 ml. In advanced obstruction, especially when strangulation has supervened, 4000 to 6000 ml. of fluid may be necessary to satisfy the losses (Berry, 1959).

In the usual case of bowel obstruction, pure water loss does not occur. Vomited fluid and nasogastric aspirate contain large concentrations of salts, incurring additional losses to the body economy. In the majority of instances, acid and alkaline ions are lost with equal frequency, so that severe deviations from the normal blood pH are not common. A balanced electrolyte preparation, such as Hartmann's solution, is satisfactory replacement therapy in the absence of significant acid-base derangements. Several balanced electrolyte solutions are commercially available and are entirely satisfactory in the management of the patient with obstruction. When there is deviation of the blood pH toward acidosis, a one-sixth molar sodium lactate solution is useful for repair. When alkalosis exists, good results are usually obtained after the administration of normal saline solutions. Potassium chloride should be given in significant quantities only after adequate urinary output has been established.

BLOOD TRANSFUSION

Blood loss into the infarcted segment of bowel may or may not assume major proportions in gangrenous bowel obstruction. In mesenteric arterial occlusion, for instance, the resulting bowel gangrene may be of a dry type because of a complete arrest of incoming arterial flow. Blood loss is slight under these circumstances, and dark peritoneal fluid is present only to a minimal degree. On the other hand, abnormalities of circulation involving mesenteric veins usually result in massive infarction of intestinal segments with extensive sequestration of blood in the altered bowel and in the peritoneal cavity or hernia sac. As the pressure of the neck of a hernia sac or an adhesion increases across a loop of bowel, the vein is usually occluded before the artery, permitting continued inflow of blood long after outflow has ceased. A series of experimental studies in animals concerning shock in strangulation obstruction revealed that blood administration was necessary in all instances in order to restore normotensive levels and to keep the animals alive (Barnett et al., 1963). The total quantity of blood to be given and the rates of administration are best coordinated with hemoglobin levels, hematocrit, venous pressure, urinary output, and pulse rate.

INDWELLING TUBES

A Miller-Abbott or some similar long tube is passed into the stomach and immediately connected to suction. We believe that the long tube will accomplish just as much as the shorter, Levin tube if one is fortunate enough to accomplish passage of the tip through the pylorus. It is important that gastric decompression be as nearly complete as possible before attempting the induction of anesthesia.

An indwelling catheter should be placed in the urinary bladder early in the course of management of the patient harboring strangulated bowel. Peritoneal irritation may produce bladder irritation to a degree sufficient to precipitate urinary retention with extreme bladder distention. Hourly recording of the urinary output serves as a valuable guide concerning the status of fluid replacement, which can usually be considered to have reached an acceptable level when urinary output reaches 30 ml./hour.

PERITONEAL TAP AND INSERTION OF CATHETER

The more severe pathophysiologic changes and higher mortality rate seen in strangulation obstruction, when compared to the simple variety, are primarily related to two factors. The first is blood loss, but this can be readily corrected by transfusion. The second and more serious difference concerns the gangrenous segment of bowel that generates and releases toxic material into the peritoneal cavity, resulting in general body tissue exposure to gram-negative bacteria and their endotoxins. In the absence of thorough preoperative fluid and electrolyte resuscitation it becomes necessary for the surgeon to evaluate the relative advantages of an immediate operation in strangulation obstruction as opposed to a delayed operation with continuing exposure to toxic materials from the dead bowel segment. There are disadvantages to both approaches that probably account for the mortality rate in excess of that seen in simple obstruction.

The effectiveness of preoperative elimination of the lethal properties of gangrenous bowel segments up to 30 cm. in length has been clearly established by recent studies in the laboratory (Barnett et al., 1968). This was accomplished by the intraperitoneal administration of cephalothin. By this therapeutic approach, then, it is possible to neutralize the toxic effects, the second major difference between simple and strangulated intestinal obstruction. This should allow ample time for preoperative preparation of the patient without the accompanying risk of irreversible changes resulting from prolonged bacterial exposure.

Encouraging results have thus far been obtained when intraperitoneal cephalothin has been given to patients both with intestinal obstruction and with peritonitis resulting from other causes (McMullan and Barnett, 1969).

Technique

The procedure of intraperitoneal insertion of a polyethylene tube should be initiated only after the stomach and urinary bladder have been emptied. Under local anesthesia a small transverse incision is made just above the umbilicus (Fig. 19–2). After the creation of a small fascia defect in the linea alba, a blunt, 14-gauge, 3 3/8-inch needle is inserted through the peritoneum (Fig. 19–3). The needle is altered only by filing the tip away to eliminate the point. We consider this to be an important protective measure against inadvertent puncture of the distended bowel. The needle is aimed in a lateral direction to the side opposite any existing scars. It should describe an angle of about 45 degrees with the surface of the abdomen. Once the peritoneum has been punctured, and after the obturator has been removed from the needle, it is frequently, but not always, possible to aspirate fluid. The characteristics of this material may be of assistance in assessing the status of intra-abdominal disease. Polyethylene tubing with an internal diameter of 0.034 inch and an outer diameter of 0.050 inch is then passed through the needle into the peritoneal cavity, and the needle is withdrawn. Tubing this size fits snugly onto the end of a 20-gauge needle.

Antibiotics

A solution comprised of one liter of isotonic saline and 5 gm. of cephalothin is connected to the intraperitoneal catheter. The rapidity with which the solution is infused into the peritoneal cavity is adjusted to the comfort of the patient. We have found that a cephalothin solution of this concentration can be given rather rapidly without evidence of peritoneal irritation. It should be completed within a five- to six-hour period of preoperative preparation. One gram of kanamycin is administered in the first liter of intravenous fluid.

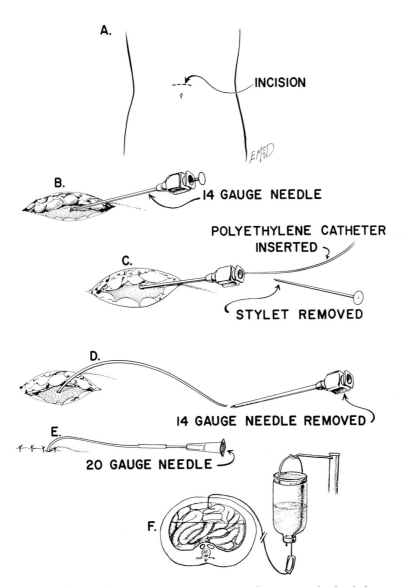

A.

INCISION

B.

14 GAUGE NEEDLE

POLYETHYLENE CATHETER
INSERTED

C.

STYLET REMOVED

D.

14 GAUGE NEEDLE REMOVED

E.

20 GAUGE NEEDLE

F.

Figure 19-2. Technique for preoperative, intraperitoneal insertion of polyethylene catheter.

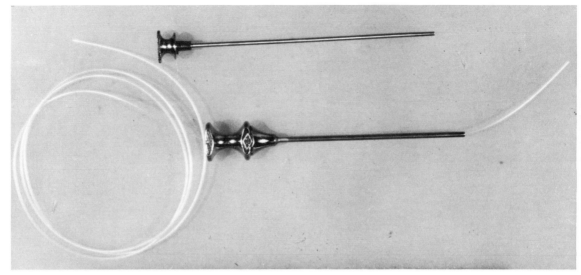

Figure 19-3.   Blunt 14-gauge needle used for intraperitoneal insertion of plastic tubing.

ANTI-ENDOTOXIN AGENTS

Gram-negative endotoxins constitute a threat to the patient with contamination of the peritoneal cavity that may indeed precipitate an irreversible shock picture with fatal consequences (Barnett et al., 1963). Several agents have been shown to exert a protective effect under these circumstances (Lillehei et al., 1958). For clinical use we currently prefer methyl-prednisolone sodium succinate (Solu-Medrol). It is probable that the earlier the agent is given during the course of the illness, the more favorable the outcome. An intravenous infusion of 250 mg. is given immediately, and an additional dose of 125 mg. is administered four hours later by means of the same route.

HEART FAILURE

Many cases of strangulation obstruction are observed in older individuals with borderline cardiac function who are likely candidates for some degree of heart failure during the stresses and strains of this severe illness. A base-line electrocardiogram should be obtained early in the course of management. Digitalization should be resorted to when there is evidence of edema, rales in the chest, venous distention, or an elevation of the central venous pressure.

OPTIMAL TIME FOR SURGERY

It is highly probable that five to six hours of intensive preoperative therapy can be used to advantage before initiating surgery for strangulation obstruction. We believe that this approach is reliable only when a high level of antibiotic is being maintained in the abdomen by continuous intraperitoneal infusion. Before operation the central venous pressure should be in the range of 8 to 12 cm. of saline, and the laboratory values should be as near normal as possible. It is encouraging when the urinary output has reached a level of at least 30 ml./hour. The hemoglobin should be 12 gm. per 100 ml. or above. The intraperitoneal level of cephalothin should be high, and preoperative intravenous kanamycin should be given. Complete preoperative preparation also includes an anti-endotoxin agent, and digitalization should be accomplished when indicated.

OPERATIVE PERIOD

THE INCISION

Entry into the peritoneal cavity can be gained with greater ease and less chance of inadvertent bowel laceration if the site of the incision is placed well away from old abdominal scars. When gangrenous bowel is suspected, the incision must be of sufficient length to afford thorough inspection of the entire intestinal tract. We have achieved excellent exposure with the use of a paramedian incision with lateral retraction of the intact rectus muscle. This incision provides for a strong closure of the abdominal wall, an important consideration in view of the extended periods of abdominal distention often observed in the postoperative period.

WITHDRAWAL OF GANGRENOUS BOWEL SEGMENTS

After the peritoneal cavity has been opened, the first effort should be directed toward thorough and complete aspiration of all free fluid. In the presence of strangulation this material varies from a pink color to dark red in many instances. In advanced cases it may actually be black attended by a foul odor.

The next objective concerns location and withdrawal of the gangrenous bowel segment from the peritoneal cavity onto the abdominal wall. This, of course, terminates continuing exposure of the peritoneal surface to toxic substances emanating from the altered bowel.

IRRIGATION OF THE PERITONEAL CAVITY

Thorough irrigation of the peritoneal surfaces yields additional benefits in removing residual layers of toxic fluid substances that may remain after initial aspiration (Fig. 19–4). The abdominal cavity should be repeatedly flooded with warm saline solution until the aspirate evidences no stain or discoloration. There is strong experimental evidence and considerable clinical support for the efficacy of irrigation of the contaminated peritoneal cavity (Barnett and Hardy, 1958).

BOWEL VIABILITY

Thorough examination of altered bowel must be carried out after the release of intestinal obstruction so that segments evidencing irreversible changes may be revealed. Particular care must be employed during the operative release of an incarcerated inguinal hernia, since early division of the external ring will allow the bowel to escape into the peritoneal cavity before adequate examination has been carried out. When this mishap occurs, it is frequently possible to grasp the questionable segment and withdraw it again through the inguinal opening for observation. This maneuver failing, the surgeon

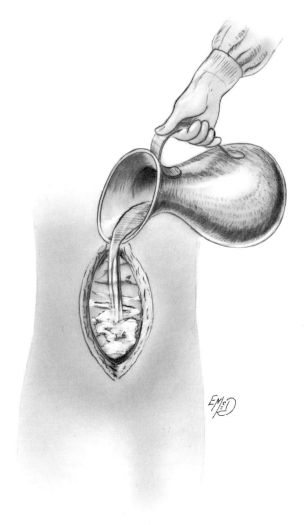

Figure 19-4. Irrigation of peritoneal cavity with warm, isotonic saline is useful in removing discolored fluid and particulate matter.

must make an abdominal incision, so that the exact status of the bowel can be established. The ability of ischemic, traumatized bowel to resume its normal appearance and characteristics is indeed remarkable.

Following the release of the obstructing agent, warm moist packs should be applied to the bowel for at least 10 minutes, after which a decision concerning its viability should be made. Survival of the segment in question is virtually assured if the intestine resumes a pink color, exhibits pulsating vessels in the mesentery, presents a bright, glistening surface, shows no evidence of damage to the serosal surface, and demonstrates a capacity to transmit peristaltic waves. On the other hand, the capacity for survival can be seriously challenged when a dark blue or black color persists, the serosal surface is dull and without luster, mesenteric vessels no longer transmit pulsation, and there is no evidence of peristalsis. Unfortunately, the criteria upon which bowel viability is based are not always positive and clear-cut. Improvement in the status of bowel circulation may be observed following operative decompression if the segment of bowel is found to be distended. Reduction in intraluminal pressure eliminates considerable resistance to blood flow with subsequent beneficial results. Inordinately long periods of examination and pondering should be avoided in arriving at a decision concerning the advisability of intestinal resection. If the capacity for survival is still in doubt after 10 to 15 minutes of examination and observation, intestinal resection should be carried out without further delay. The disastrous consequences which can be expected to follow prolonged peritoneal exposure to gangrenous bowel far outweigh the disadvantages of an intestinal resection performed in the absence of ironclad indications.

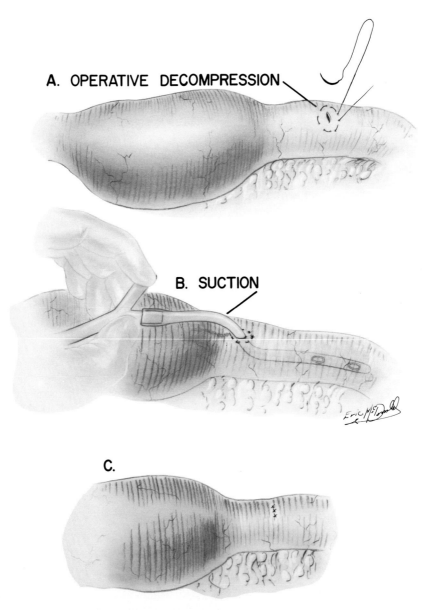

Figure 19-5. Method used for operative decompression of bowel. *A,* Purse-string suture around enterostomy site. *B,* Aspiration using rubber catheter. *C,* Closure of enterostomy site.

OPERATIVE DECOMPRESSION OF THE BOWEL

Small-bowel decompression carried out during laparotomy provides several advantages, among which are increased ease of abdominal closure, improved circulation to the bowel wall, and decreased effort during respiration in the postoperative period. A site is selected in normal bowel, just proximal to the area of gangrene. The site of the enterostomy can be resected along with the dead bowel, and the normal bowel holds sutures much more efficiently than nonviable intestine (Fig. 19–5).

BOWEL RESECTION AND ANASTOMOSIS

Resection of nonviable bowel is initiated by systematically clamping and dividing the mesentery that supplies the involved segment. When the mesentery is not large or excessively thick, free ties usually suffice. In the presence of a thick, fat mesentery, a transfixing suture provides a more secure ligature. Care must be taken in order to avoid undercutting the mesentery supplying normal bowel and thus unnecessarily sacrificing excessive amounts of intestine. Clamps are then applied to each extremity of the gangrenous segment, but well onto normal bowel. The site on the bowel wall used for enterotomy and operative decompression should be included with the resected specimen. Application of the clamps should be made with great care, so that the mesenteric surface is divided at a distance not far removed from adequate circulation. There is minimal collateral circulation within the wall of the human intestine. To "clean off" the mesentery to a point excessively far from the line of the anastomosis predisposes to ischemia and anastomotic leakage. The clamps should be applied at an angle of about 45 degrees from the mesenteric to the antimesenteric surface. Again, this is recommended in order to assure adequate circulation to the antimesenteric surface.

The bowel is now divided on top of the angled clamps after occluding clamps have been placed at each extremity of the specimen to be resected in order to prevent the spillage of luminal content at the time of division. Rubber-shod, noncrushing clamps should be placed at least 12 inches from the divided bowel ends. In our experience, the open anastomosis is preferable for the small bowel. The crushing clamps are now removed from the proximal and distal divided bowel, and diligent effort should be exerted in clamping and tying bleeders which are usually evident. This decreases the chances for an anastomotic hematoma, another factor that tends to weaken the freshly constructed anastomosis.

The first suture line is started at the mesenteric side of the bowel where 000 suture of iodized intestinal chromic catgut is passed through the mucosa, through one side of visceral peritoneum as it folds down to become the mesentery, through the corresponding fold of visceral peritoneum on the opposite divided bowel, and then through the adjacent mucosa. Recently acquired experimental evidence strongly suggests that iodized catgut affords greater protection against leakage when the anastomosis is carried out in the presence of a contaminated peritoneal cavity (Varner and Barnett, 1969). A similar suture is passed through both ends of the divided bowel on the opposite side of the mesentery, and the free ends are tied together. The two mesenteric surfaces are now snugly approximated by tying the needle-bearing ends of the suture, which places another knot on the opposite mucosal surface. Each suture is then carried in a lateral direction as a continuous lock stitch. The suture is now carried to the serosal surface and completed as a Connell stitch, after which the anastomosis is completed by the placement of a row of interrupted Lembert sutures of 000 cotton. Closure of the mesenteric defect with a continuous chromic catgut suture completes the anastomosis (Fig. 19–6).

POSTOPERATIVE PERIOD

It is our practice to continue the monitoring of central venous pressure into the postoperative period as a guide for the intravenous administration of fluids. The urinary bladder catheter is maintained in place so that hourly urinary output can be measured and recorded. Blood plasma electrolyte levels should be followed with frequent laboratory determinations, so that impending deficiencies may be suspected early and corrected. In the average 70 kg. individual

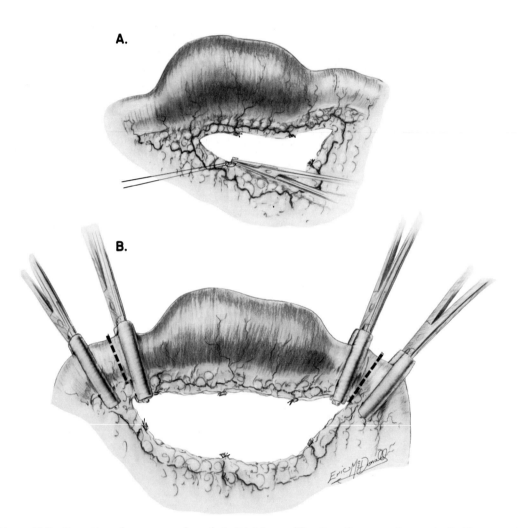

Figure 19-6. Resection of gangrenous bowel. *A*, Division and ligation of mesenteric vessels. *B*, Clamps applied for bowel removal. *C*, Angle sutures placed and tied to close mesenteric defect.

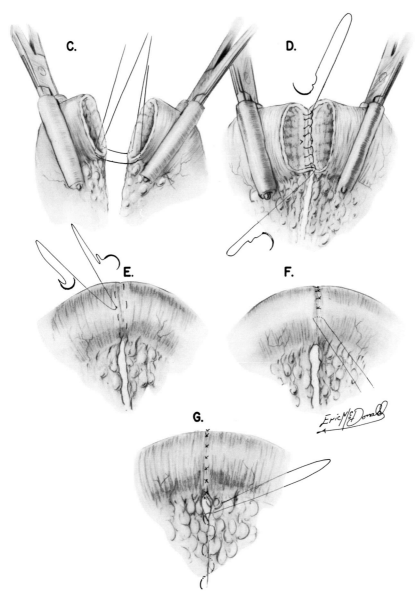

Figure 19-6. *Continued.* *D*, Each suture is carried laterally as a continuous lock stitch. *E*, Anteriorly the mucosal sutures are completed as Connell sutures and tied together. *F*, Serosal layer of 000 cotton completes the bowel anastomosis. *G*, Closure of mesenteric defect.

we would expect to give about three liters of intravenous fluid per 24 hours, but this must be regulated according to CVP and urinary output levels. Intraperitoneal infusion of cephalothin is continued into the postoperative period. Four grams of the antibiotic are dissolved in 500 ml. of isotonic saline and dripped into the peritoneal cavity through the indwelling polyethylene catheter every eight hours. Fluid administered intraperitoneally should be considered in relation to the volume given intravenously, since the latter amount may necessitate a compensatory reduction. Intraperitoneal antibiotics are continued for 72 hours during the postoperative period. In the severely ill patient with widespread peritoneal contamination, it is also our practice to inject 0.5 gm. of kanamycin intramuscularly for four days. Methylprednisolone sodium succinate (Solu-Medrol) is continued intravenously in the amount of 125 mg. per 24 hours for three days after operation.

COLON STRANGULATION

DIAGNOSIS

In the patient with intestinal obstruction, preoperative differentiation between large- and small-bowel blockage can be made with considerable accuracy. Distinction between the two is specifically related to x-ray findings concerning the flat and upright abdominal film. With small-bowel obstruction it is common to find dilated proximal loops, air-fluid levels, and minimal to no air within the colon. The patient with colon obstruction may or may not evidence the findings consistent with small-bowel obstruction. This factor is related to the presence or absence of a competent ileocecal valve.

In a review of 105 cases of colon obstruction, an incompetent ileocecal valve allowing reflux into the small bowel was present in 51 per cent (Barnett and Little, 1965). The dilated colon resulting from obstruction can usually be observed all the way down to the site of luminal occlusion. Characteristic findings suggestive of volvulus in the various divisions of the colon provide valuable diagnostic clues (Fig. 19-7). Instances in which some doubt remains concerning the presence and level of large-bowel obstruction can be readily clarified by the use of a barium enema.

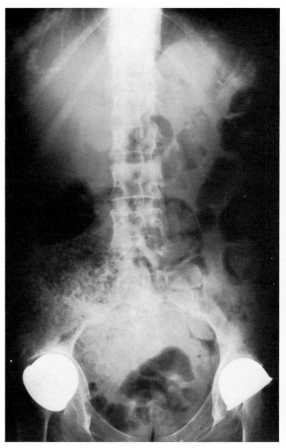

Figure 19-7. X-ray appearance of volvulus of the cecum.

The patient with colon obstruction usually appears seriously ill. Abdominal pain is almost uniformly present. Nausea and vomiting, constipation proceeding to obstipation, and failure to pass gas per rectum are characteristics of the condition. Advanced degrees of abdominal distention are to be expected with colon obstruction; however, closed-loop involvement of relatively short segments, as a result of a competent ileocecal valve, may result in significant distention without generalized abdominal distention. When the obstructing process has extended to strangulation, the patient usually appears acutely ill. Direct and rebound tenderness are usually present, and a localized mass is commonly found. Manifestations suggestive of shock are common in the patient with gangrenous colon obstruction. Elevated temperature and rapid pulse rate are to be expected. It may be concluded that the patient with strangulated colon obstruction usually provides abdominal findings consistent with the establishment of an acute abdomen, and the necessity for operative intervention is readily apparent.

MANAGEMENT

Intensive resuscitative measures are mandatory during the preoperative period if the critically ill patient with strangulation obstruction of the colon is to be afforded maximal opportunity for survival. It is our practice to follow the course of preoperative management outlined above in detail for the preoperative preparation of the patient with strangulation of the small bowel.

Upon opening the peritoneal cavity the initial concern is to locate the involved segment of colon and relieve the obstructing mechanism. In our experience, the most common cause of strangulation of the colon is volvulus (Barnett and Little, 1965) (Fig. 19-7). Thorough irrigation of the peritoneal cavity should be carried out when con-

tamination with dark fluid exists. If bowel viability can be established after reduction of the obstruction, then the course of management is that of simple obstruction. On the other hand, gangrenous colon must be totally removed from the peritoneal cavity. There is a circumstance, especially after reduction of volvulus, in which small, patchy areas of discoloration on the colon wall suggest possible irreversible, ischemic changes. When these areas are small and limited in number, it is safe to invert the questionable site with interrupted, nonabsorbable sutures and thus avoid resection (Fig. 19-8).

Gangrenous changes involving the cecum and right colon are best dealt with by means of right colon resection followed by ileotransverse colostomy. We favor the use of iodized chromic catgut for the inner layer of anastomosis involving unprepared bowel and in the presence of peritoneal contamination. When a gangrenous process involves the transverse colon or sigmoid colon, bowel resection is followed by the establishment of a colostomy, with the plan to return at a later time under elective conditions for reestablishment of colon continuity.

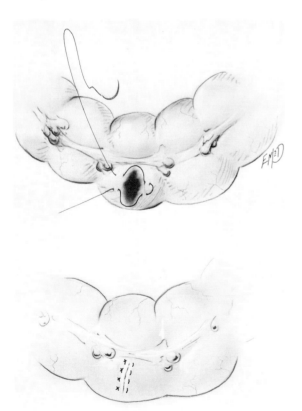

Figure 19-8. Use of interrupted mattress sutures to invaginate small necrotic area of bowel.

REFERENCES

Barnett, W. O., and Hardy, J. D.: Observations concerning the peritoneal fluid in experimental strangulated intestinal obstruction: The effects of removal from the peritoneal cavity. Surgery, 43:440, 1958.

Barnett, W. O., and Little, B. R.: Obstruction of the large bowel. Southern Med. J., 58:1493, 1965.

Barnett, W. O., Oliver, R. I., and Elliott, R. L.: Elimination of the lethal properties of gangrenous bowel segments. Ann. Surg., 167:912, 1968.

Barnett, W. O., Truett, G., Williams, R., and Crowell, J.: Shock in strangulation obstruction: Mechanisms and management. Ann. Surg., 157:747, 1963.

Berry, R. E. L.: Obstruction of the small and large intestine. Surg. Clin. N. Amer., 39:1267, 1959.

Hartwell, J. A., and Hoguet, J. P.: Experimental intestinal obstruction in dogs with special reference to cause of death and treatment by large amounts of normal saline solution. JAMA, 59:82, 1912.

Lillehei, R. C., and MacLean, L. D.: The intestinal factor in irreversible shock. Ann. Surg., 148:513, 1958.

McMullan, M. H., and Barnett, W. O.: The clinical use of intraperitoneal cephalothin. Surgery, 67:432, 1970.

Varner, J. E., and Barnett, W. O.: The use of iodized catgut for contaminated intestinal anastomosis. Surg. Forum, 20:402, 1969.

CHAPTER 20

HIGH-OUTPUT GASTROINTESTINAL FISTULA

by JAMES D. HARDY, M.D.

The individual with a severe gastrointestinal fistula surely qualifies as a critically ill surgical patient. Few other surgical conditions require more diligent and imaginative management to restore the patient to health. Vigorous supportive measures must be combined with wisely conceived surgical intervention where essential. The mortality rate remains substantial.

ETIOLOGY

The majority of gastric or intestinal fistulas are secondary to operation. Other causes include trauma, inflammatory processes, intestinal obstruction, neoplasms, and foreign bodies. Even when the fistula is secondary to operation, infection or chronic disease of the involved bowel or neoplasia is often an important contributing factor.

Fistulas of the gastrointestinal tract may be internal or external. Internal fistulas may involve two adherent loops of bowel, the bowel and the urinary tract or the biliary tract, or the bowel and the aorta. However, it is the external or enterocutaneous small bowel fistula which will be considered here. External fistulas in our hospital have followed a variety of operations, including lysis of adhesions, resection of strangulated small bowel, choledochojejunostomy, feeding jejunostomy, ileoproctostomy, pelvic exenteration, hysterectomy, transvaginal uterine operations, entero-enterostomy for regional enteritis, and still other procedures.

Gastric fistulas usually follow an anastomosis, and here a relative ischemia of the gastric remnant may at times be a factor. Gastric injury may follow splenectomy, vagotomy, or penetrating trauma, and an occasional fistula is due to a perforating ulcer or neoplasm.

A duodenal fistula is most commonly produced by a leak at the stump following a Billroth II distal subtotal gastrectomy. In fact, this is the most frequent cause of death associated with this operation. The cause of stump dehiscence may be insecure closure, obstruction at the gastrojejunostomy, or adhesions involving the proximal loop or volvulus of this loop. The stump fistula is an end fistula, and its management has been considered easier and the prognosis more favorable than in the side fistula. The duodenal side fistula usually follows a Billroth I anastomosis, closure of the duodenum following exploration of the ampulla of Vater, a choledochoduodenostomy, trauma during other operations such as nephrectomy, leakage following closure and drainage of a duodenal ulcer, or penetrating or blunt trauma. The principal difference between the management of the duodenal end fistula and the duodenal side fistula is that after a good drainage tract has been established and the peritonitis has subsided, the patient with the end or stump fistula and a gastrojejunostomy can usually be fed by mouth.

Fistulas of the jejunum or ileum usually follow surgical operations either upon the gut itself or upon adjacent organs. Some fistulas are produced by trauma. Since the mesenteric small bowel has much greater mobility than the stomach or duodenum, small bowel fistulas may drain through a previously prepared drainage site, through the wound itself, into the vagina following hysterectomy or uterine instrumentation, into the bladder, or even spontaneously through the abdominal wall, as is seen occasionally in regional enteritis or in other types of inflammatory processes.

Fistulas of the colon are not commonly associated with massive fluid losses, but occasionally serious losses occur with fistula of the right colon. Colonic fistulas usually follow operation, trauma, inflammatory process, and neoplasia. If the fistula develops distal to the cecum, a proximal colostomy with effective drainage of the leaking area and antibiotic therapy will commonly permit survival, unless overwhelming peritoneal contamination has already occurred. Colon perforation with spontaneous fistula formation through the abdominal wall has followed granulomatous colitis, diverticulitis, and carcinoma, in the writer's personal experience.

Gastrointestinal fistulas usually close spontaneously if the patient is well-managed otherwise and if there is no distal obstruction.

PATHOPHYSIOLOGY

In general, the higher the fistula is in the alimentary tract, the more serious is the outlook. This is because (1) proximal fistulas are likely to be associated with greater fluid and electrolyte losses, (2) a long segment of proximal intestine is not available for food absorption, (3) the fistulous drainage has a greater digestive capacity, and (4) excision or bypassing of the fistula to reduce nutritional losses and to control the infection is less feasible with a gastric or duodenal fistula than with lower small bowel fistulas. Nevertheless, the severe bacterial contamination from colon spillage renders colonic fistulas extremely serious in some instances.

FLUID LOSSES

The high-output external gastric or intestinal fistula is usually described as one from which the drainage exceeds 500 ml. per 24 hours. However, in actual practice a volume of less than one liter is of little consequence from the standpoint of fluid and nutritional loss. Some high small bowel or duodenal fistulas may put out 6 or more liters per 24 hours, rendering continuous fluid therapy a stark necessity. Thus, the first and most threatening complication of a high-output small bowel fistula is water and

salt depletion. Clearly, a patient who loses six liters from the fistula, plus perhaps a liter of urine, would lose seven kilograms or 15.4 pounds that day, assuming that fluid was not simultaneously given by vein. However, as the patient becomes more dehydrated he often loses less fluid from the fistula and secretes less urine, prior to the development of the shock that will surely ensue unless fluid replacement is adequate. In general, the fluid loss from duodenal and small bowel fistulas is a balanced loss, and neither acidosis nor alkalosis presents a major problem initially.

The fluid loss at the fistula site may represent only a portion of the alimentary tract loss. Peritonitis with associated paralytic ileus may result in the pooling of large volumes of fluid in the stomach and small bowel and thus introduce the hazard of pulmonary aspiration.

NUTRITIONAL DEFICITS

Even if the water and electrolyte requirements are met effectively, the patient's general condition will inexorably decline because of caloric and protein deprivation unless adequate nutritional intake can be achieved. The minimal requirements of the average afebrile adult patient at bed rest are approximately one gram of protein and 30 calories per kilogram of body weight. Fever usually increases catabolism and caloric requirements, and most patients with serious alimentary tract fistulas exhibit sepsis at some point in the course of their illness. The effects of progressive starvation are comprehensive and adversely affect the function of virtually all organs of the body. They reduce the capacity of the patient to resist bacterial invasion, and pneumonitis is a major contributing cause of death in many patients with intestinal fistulas and peritonitis.

Fortunately, there are several possible ways of feeding the patient with a gastric or intestinal fistula, and these will be considered later.

SKIN EROSION

In the case of a duodenal or high small bowel fistula, the pain caused by skin erosion can be the most distressing symptom that the patient experiences. Gastric fistulas (e.g., a gastrostomy) do not usually produce severe skin erosion, even when the body surface surrounding the gastrostomy tube is wet continually. This is because acid-pepsin is not as erosive to the skin as is duodenal or upper jejunal drainage; the bile-activated pancreatic trypsin in the upper small bowel will often produce marked excoriation and ulceration around the fistulous site unless special care is taken to protect the skin. Fistulas of the lower ileum or colon cause much less skin irritation than do duodenal or upper jejunal defects.

INFECTION

A simple external jejunal fistula, from a loop of bowel adherent to the wound and sealed off from the rest of the peritoneal cavity, presents no great problem if distal obstruction does not exist. The fistulous drainage escapes promptly to the outside and a minimal area of peritoneum is contaminated. There is little infection, and continuing serious sepsis does not precipitate a potentially disastrous situation. Actually, a patient in this condition is usually afebrile; his white blood count is essentially normal, and a rapid pulse is more likely to reflect inadequate fluid replacement than infection.

In sharp contrast, the duodenal stump blowout that is diagnosed late has often already resulted in widespread contamination of the upper abdomen. Furthermore, for several days the drainage route will not be sealed off from the rest of the peritoneal cavity, and contamination of the upper and perhaps the lower abdomen will continue. Even when the chemical and bacterial peritonitis has receded, after the drainage tract has become walled off and continuous contamination of the free peritoneal cavity has ceased, localized collections of infected material or frank abscesses may persist beneath the diaphragm or liver, among loops of bowel, in the gutters or in the pelvis, or pylephlebitis may have produced multiple intrahepatic abscesses. Moreover, continued intraperitoneal sepsis prolongs intestinal ileus, and under these circumstances nutrition must be achieved solely by the intravenous route. Thus, major infection gravely complicates the management problems of an enteric fistula.

Minor infection along the drainage tract, or in the form of pyogenic granulomas at the skin surface, is present in most significant fistulas. Furthermore, the presence of infection along the drainage tract of a duodenal fistula substantially increases the possibility of spontaneous or secondary hemorrhage, always a hazard when tissues are exposed to activated pancreatic enzymes. In contrast, a simple pancreatic fistula, from the tail of the pancreas and not containing bile, can be remarkably benign. Stress ulcer bleeding from the stomach or duodenum is a frequent complication of the sepsis which often attends a fistula.

DIAGNOSIS

The diagnosis of a gastric or intestinal fistula is usually made promptly, but it also can be delayed, with serious or even disastrous consequences. If the possible development of a fistula has been anticipated and the operative area drained, the appearance of bile-stained material or small bowel contents will promptly suggest the existence of a fistula. However, if the abdomen was not drained at operation, peritoneal contamination and peritonitis may be far advanced before the presence of a fistula is apparent. In general, the onset of abdominal pain, tenderness in excess of that which accompanies the usual operation, fever, tachycardia, and leukocytosis should suggest alimentary tract leakage. If a Billroth II distal subtotal gastrectomy was performed and the patient develops right upper quadrant pain, duodenal stump dehiscence or anastomotic leakage should be suspected, and, if the other evidence is corroborative, the abdomen should be explored and drains inserted.

Even when a drainage tract was prepared at operation, the diagnosis of fistula formation may not be immediately apparent. The first material to emerge from the wound itself, or from a prepared drain site, may appear bloody or purulent and later perhaps serous; this is followed a day or so later by drainage of what is obviously small bowel contents. If the fistula is in the stomach, it may be noted that oral intake of liquids promptly increases the volume of loss from the fistula; this would also be true of a duodenal or high jejunal fistula. In some instances the patient will state that gas escaped from the fistula, a very important sign. If doubt remains, the patient may be given charcoal or indigo carmine by mouth, and discoloration is then noted in the drainage. However, this test does not identify the actual location of the fistula, and it would not necessarily identify a duodenal stump fistula. Thus, barium or other radiopaque media can be given by mouth or injected into the drainage tract to aid in identifying the level of the fistula.

MANAGEMENT

The management of most gastric, duodenal, or more distal small bowel fistulas consists of adequate external drainage plus vigorous supportive measures. Many fistulas close without operative intervention other than for adequate drainage, but operative attack upon the fistula itself constitutes an important phase of total therapy when indicated.

NONOPERATIVE MEASURES

PRELIMINARY ASSESSMENT

The surgeon may first see the patient at any one of the various stages of the development and course of a gastrointestinal fistula, and his preliminary evaluation of the total clinical situation is very important. The prognosis will depend upon how long the fistula has existed, its level, the volume of fluid loss, the degree and extent of peritoneal contamination, and the age and general state of health of the patient. The young person who was in good nutrition originally can usually withstand the effects of a high-output fistula longer than the elderly patient whose nutrition may have been poor initially. However, major sepsis is poorly tolerated by any patient. The following questions are important in the prognosis: Is the patient dehydrated, and is sepsis apparent? Do findings suggest intra-abdominal suppuration and abscesses? Are there associated problems such as other injuries, if the fistula resulted from trauma, or are organs other than the alimentary tract free of disease? In particular, is renal function satisfactory?

The nature of the fistula itself is most important. The volume of fluid loss should be noted, and also whether or not the fistula appears to be well drained as evidenced by absence of pain and sepsis. The duration of a high-output fistula will suggest the probable degree of nutritional depletion, in addition to the evidence obtained on physical examination. The plasma electrolyte measurements will disclose the state of salt adequacy or depletion, relative to the volume of remaining extracellular fluid.

The level of the fistula should be identified with roentgen studies, and the presence or absence of distal obstruction should be determined if possible.

Finally, the condition of the abdominal wall surrounding the fistula should be noted.

FLUID AND ELECTROLYTE THERAPY

The most immediate therapeutic necessity in the patient with a high-output gastrointestinal fistula is to maintain fluid and electrolyte balance and prevent shock due to dehydration. This is achieved by weighing the patient at least daily, and every 12 hours if the volume of fistulous drainage is very large or if its collection and measurement is incomplete. Rapid changes in body weight are due to water retention or loss. However, fluid sequestered in the bowel or in the surrounding peritoneal cavity, and thus physiologically unavailable to replenish the plasma and interstitial fluid volumes, would not be detected as "lost" by weight measurements alone: additional data are required to detect dehydration under these circumstances. Moreover, whereas almost complete collection of the fistulous drainage can be achieved when the tract emerges on the abdominal wall, the writer once managed a high-output small bowel fistula that drained into the vagina, secondary to hysterectomy. In this instance it was impossible to collect all the copious fluid which escaped through the fistula. Nevertheless, the most accurate possible measurement of losses should be attempted to aid in fluid therapy, to protect the skin, and to promote the general comfort of the patient.

Nasogastric suction, initiated to prevent gastric distention in the presence of peritonitis, may aspirate several liters a day in addition to losses through the fistula.

The adequacy of the volume of fluid and electrolyte replacement is determined by the hourly urine output, blood pressure, pulse rate, physical evidence of hydration (condition of tongue, skin turgor, eyeballs), body weight, and measurements of the plasma electrolytes, hematocrit, and BUN (blood urea nitrogen). Since huge fluid shifts and losses may occur in the presence of a high-output fistula, the patient should be examined every two or three hours to determine whether the intravenous fluids ordered are adequate and are actually being administered and whether the device used to collect the drainage is functioning properly or requires corrective action. The volume of fluid to be replaced should equal the fistulous and other drainage, plus 1000 ml. to provide for urine and perhaps another 1000 ml. for insensible loss if the patient is febrile. Drainage from any source, as well as urine volume, should be replaced with electrolyte solution. The adequacy of *volume* replacement is determined by urine flow, vital signs, and the physical examination. The *composition* of the fluid to be administered is determined by serial measurements of the plasma sodium, chloride, potassium, magnesium, calcium, and bicarbonate concentrations. Serum electrolyte concentrations should be measured daily if indicated.

The fluid loss from a gastric fistula contains large amounts of hydrochloric acid, as well as some sodium and potassium. The acid-base derangement produced will tend toward metabolic alkalosis, and there will be a gradual tendency toward hypokalemia and hyponatremia. Accordingly, an isotonic sodium chloride solution, which contains a physiologic excess of chloride relative to the chloride content of plasma, is very useful in fluid replacement. Once urine flow has been restored, potassium supplementation in the amount of 3 to 6 gm. of potassium chloride (13.6 mEq.K per gram of KCl) in a liter of fluid should be employed as necessary, as indicated by the plasma potassium level.

Duodenal and small bowel fistulas usually exhibit balanced losses, and neither marked alkalosis nor acidosis develops. Late in the course of the fistula, however, a tendency toward metabolic acidosis may be noted. A balanced electrolyte solution should be used in whatever volume required.

When the fistula has existed for many days or even several weeks, the possibility of calcium or magnesium deficits should be considered. Actually, tetany is typical of a deficiency of either ion, and when tetany occurs in the absence of alkalosis or hypocalcemia, a magnesium deficiency should be suspected. Serum magnesium determinations are now readily available, but clinically significant magnesium deficits are uncommon except in patients with severe and prolonged alimentary tract fluid losses.

Should marked hyponatremia and hypochloremia exist and symptoms of water intoxication develop, the infusion of 500 ml. of 3 per cent sodium chloride solution, repeated as required, is recommended. However, hyponatremia and hypochloremia may be due to a water excess as well as to a salt deficit, and the proper diagnosis should be established on clinical grounds such as body weight measurements or the presence of overt edema. Incidentally, the patient may gain liters of excess fluid before this fluid retention is apparent on physical examination. Actually, if good renal function exists, these organs will usually excrete water or salt, as required, to maintain normal electrolyte balance so long as the intake of water and salt is adequate.

NUTRITIONAL MAINTENANCE

Body tissue catabolism should be minimized by introducing calories and nitrogen by all available routes. In fact, the efficacy of nutritional therapy can prove to be the crucial factor in the survival of a patient who must exist for weeks with a high-output small bowel fistula. Even if the fistula is in the midjejunum, theoretically permitting use of the proximal jejunum for some feeding, intestinal ileus due to peritonitis and sepsis may preclude oral intake.

The most available route is usually the intravenous one. Each liter of fluid administered should contain some calories in the form of 5 or 10 per cent dextrose (1 liter of 5 per cent dextrose = 50 g. carbohydrate, or 200 calories), and it is also useful to administer protein hydrolysates (protein = 4 calories per gram) and perhaps 5 or 7 per cent alcohol (approximately 7 calories per gram). These nutrients should be given in a drip throughout the 24 hours to reduce spillage in the urine and to minimize solute diuresis, which has a tendency to produce dehydration. Even 1500 calories per day will significantly retard body protein mobilization.

Recently, interest in intravenous hyperalimentation has been renewed through the outstanding investigations of Dudrick and Rhoads (see Chapter 30). After introducing a catheter into the superior vena cava, a hypertonic solution is slowly infused over the entire 24 hour period. In this way both calories and nitrogen are introduced, and it has been demonstrated that complete nutritional support of the patient can be thus achieved for prolonged periods of time.

USE OF THE ALIMENTARY TRACT

If fluid losses from a small bowel fistula do not appear to be substantially increased by oral intake, a low residue diet relatively high in calories and protein should be tried. The bowel proximal to the fistula will absorb some foodstuffs, and some food may pass the fistula and be absorbed in the distal bowel. We have not been convinced that oral intake of a low residue diet significantly retards the rate of closing of the fistula, and a significant amount of nitrogen and calories can often be introduced in this way (see Cases 1, 2, and 4).

If the fistula is from the stomach, it may be possible to pass a tube into the upper small bowel and feed through it (see Case 3). Otherwise, a feeding jejunostomy may be performed after the peritonitis and associated ileus have subsided.

Each patient should be carefully evaluated to determine the routes available for nutrition.

PROTECTION OF THE SKIN

If the patient is seen as soon as the fistula begins draining externally, a temporary ileostomy bag can be applied at once. This will permit complete collection of the fistulous drainage and protect the skin from maceration and erosion. If the skin has already developed a fiery red appearance and areas of desquamation or more severe erosion are in evidence when the patient is first seen, it may be necessary to insert a catheter into the tract for continuous suction temporarily, while the skin is kept dry with a heat lamp and karaya powder is applied to initiate healing of the surrounding skin (Fig. 20-1). This may be facilitated by placing the patient face down on a split mattress and allowing the fistula to drain directly into a receptacle beneath. As soon as the condition of the skin permits, the temporary "disposable" ileostomy bag can be applied with ileostomy glue, dermatome glue, or an adhesive spray. Each of these measures may be variously effective under different circumstances.

In some patients the external opening of the fistula may be so situated that an ileostomy bag cannot be made secure. Here the most effective catheter suction possible

Figure 20-1. Management of skin in small bowel fistula. The skin should be protected from the erosive action of the fistulous drainage by the various measures described in the text. Wherever possible, a disposable ileostomy bag is used to collect the drainage for measurement and to further protect the skin.

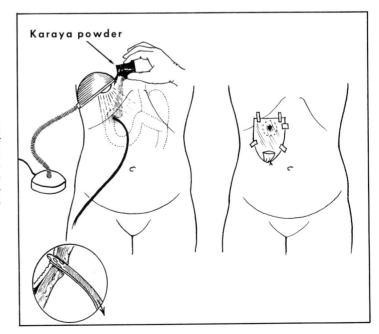

should be continuously maintained, and the surrounding skin should be protected with adhesive spray, karaya powder, and other available measures. Aluminum paste or zinc oxide ointment will protect the skin fairly well, but both soil clothes and bed linen. The most important requirement is that the effectiveness of the measures used for skin protection must be reassessed frequently throughout the 24 hours. With proper diligence the skin excoriation can be prevented or abolished in most instances. As mentioned earlier, less skin digestion occurs when fistulas are located below the jejunal level.

MANAGEMENT OF INFECTION

The most important step in the management of infection is to provide optimal external drainage, by surgical intervention if necessary. If ready egress for the fistulous drainage is provided, the drainage tract will hopefully become walled off, and the free peritoneal cavity will no longer be continuously contaminated. When additional contamination has ceased, the peritoneum may be able to cleanse itself completely. Prior to this, the existing peritonitis should be treated with nasogastric suction, broad spectrum antibiotics, and intravenous fluids. In some instances abscesses will form and will require surgical drainage. These collections may be subdiaphragmatic, beneath the liver, among loops of bowel, in the pelvis, or elsewhere. The possibility of liver abscess formation should be considered when a septic type of fever associated with jaundice is present or when no purulent collection is found at the more readily accessible sites. A liver abscess of significant size may be demonstrated by scintiscan or selective arteriograms. Subdiaphragmatic collections may be identified by chest x-ray, chest fluoroscopy, or by simultaneous lung and liver scintiscans. In our experience the subdiaphragmatic abscess has most often been on the right and has been drained through the bed of the eleventh rib. A left subdiaphragmatic abscess can be drained in a similar fashion, but we have usually preferred to drain it through a left subcostal incision, leaving a large Foley catheter in the abscess cavity extending out between the eleventh and twelfth ribs. If continued drainage is not provided until the infection

has cleared and the space has closed, whichever side is involved, the abscess may form again and operative drainage may have to be repeated. Of course, once an organism has been cultured, bacterial sensitivities should be determined and specific antibiotic therapy instituted. If an abscess is detected by rectal examination, it should be drained through the rectum.

Infection within the abdomen and along the drainage tract may cause blood vessel erosion and bleeding that can be very difficult to control. Pyogenic granulomas at the surface may require excision.

In some patients the peritoneal soilage is so extensive and the subsequent infection so massive, the body defenses are overwhelmed.

OPERATIVE INTERVENTION

It has been emphasized previously that prompt and effective external drainage is essential in the management of gastrointestinal fistulas wherever they occur. Of course, leakage from the stomach, small bowel, or colon does occur from time to time, and the patient survives even in the absence of external drainage. However, this incurs a much greater risk of major morbidity or death than does operation to establish good drainage, if this has not already been provided at a previous operation.

Operative attack upon the fistula represents an important aspect of the total approach to the comprehensive management of gastrointestinal fistulas. The majority of fistulas will close if external drainage is adequate, if there is no distal obstruction, and if the patient is supported vigorously with the measures previously outlined. However, in some patients it will become apparent that success is probably not to be achieved without additional operative measures. Experienced surgical judgment is required under these circumstances, and in each instance the tactics must be decided upon by the merits of the case under consideration. The patient is usually gravely ill, and operative intervention entails a high risk of further morbidity or even death.

The following possible operative procedures may be employed under selected circumstances, with the full realization that the operation may not be successful and is used only because lesser measures have proved inadequate. Definitive operative intervention is usually rendered mandatory when fluid losses by fistula and nasogastric suction, if required, remain severe, when peritoneal contamination continues despite previous drainage, when massive hemorrhage develops, when no significant segment of the alimentary tract is available for enteric alimentation, and when intravenous alimentation has not proved sufficiently effective. Except perhaps in the immediate postoperative period, when alimentary tract disruption may rarely be corrected before peritonitis has developed, definitive operation is not usually attempted until several weeks of high-output fistula drainage have passed, often with substantial depletion of the patient's total physical resources. If a downhill course appears inexorable on nonoperative management, operation may offer a promising alternative. In the absence of intra-abdominal infection, operative intervention may be performed much earlier in the course of the illness and may greatly shorten the period of hospitalization. In contrast, anastomoses performed in the presence of gross intraperitoneal infection are attended by a high incidence of disruption.

THE STOMACH

It has been mentioned that fistulous drainage from the stomach may be due to ischemia, trauma (as during splenectomy), anastomotic imperfection, or other causes. If well drained, the small gastric fistula may be expected to close. This is particularly true of injury incurred during splenectomy, of perforation by a penetrating missile, or by a perforated ulcer. Anastomotic leakage may also cease, but the surrounding inflammation may produce jejunal obstruction by adhesions that may eventually require operation for lysis.

In contrast, complete anastomotic separation or extensive gastric necrosis may require radical measures, and even these may not suffice. If at exploration the anastomosis is found to be almost completely separated and if serious infection did not exist at the previous operation, one should suspect relative ischemia of the gastric remnant. The prognosis under such circumstances will be grave indeed, but restoration of alimentary tract continuity has been successful in an occasional case. If the previous operation was a Billroth I distal subtotal gastrectomy and the anastomosis is widely disrupted, the gastroduodenal closure should be completely divided, a Foley catheter should be inserted into the lateral wall of the duodenum several centimeters from the duodenal stump, and the stump closed with sutures. The catheter should be led out through a stab wound in the right upper quadrant of the abdomen to ensure prolonged duodenal decompression. External drainage of the previous anastomotic area should also be performed. The distal portion of the gastric remnant should now be excised back to a point at which brisk bleeding occurs; the remaining gastric segment should then be joined to the jejunum as a Billroth II anastomosis. A feeding jejunostomy should be performed at the same operation. A successful outcome may not be achieved, but these heroic operative maneuvers are justified because of the gravity of the situation.

If extensive ischemic necrosis of almost the entire gastric remnant is found (this may occur when most of the arterial supply was ligated at the first operation), the only recourse may be to excise the necrotic gastric pouch and anastomose a loop of jejunum to the esophagus. This anastomosis should be drained, antibiotics should be instilled, and a feeding jejunostomy should be performed.

If a Billroth II distal subtotal gastrectomy had been performed previously and wide separation of the anastomotic suture line has occurred, additional stomach should be resected and a new gastrojejunostomy performed at a more distal point.

We had one patient who developed a gastric fistula following splenectomy, and the surgeon believed that he had ligated a portion of the stomach wall with the vasa brevia. Accordingly, when the drainage continued after three months and the drainage tract had become fibrotic and sealed off from the free peritoneal cavity, the fistulous tract was excised, the stomach was closed through healthy gastric wall, and prompt healing occurred.

It is to be reemphasized that conservative management should be given an adequate trial, since in the presence of infection any new anastomoses may fail to heal. Operation is usually employed only when other measures have failed.

THE DUODENUM

A very common cause of duodenal fistula is a blowout of the duodenal stump following a distal Billroth II subtotal gastrectomy. If well drained, these fistulas almost always close in due course, especially if there is no significant obstruction of the afferent or proximal loop. Fortunately, the patient can be fed readily through the gastrojejunostomy as soon as effective external drainage has permitted the peritonitis to subside. A useful preventive measure, if the duodenal closure is in any way unsatisfactory at the original operation, is to insert a #16 Foley catheter into the lateral wall of the duodenum to permit external decompression for a week to ten days postoperatively. Occasionally the duodenal defect is actually visualized when operation is performed to initiate external drainage of a suspected stump fistula. There is no particular contraindication to placing several sutures through the defect, since such sutures have sometimes halted further fistulous drainage. However, in the presence of established peritonitis one is not justified in placing much confidence in this kind of closure.

The duodenal side fistula, if fairly large, presents a different problem from that posed by the stump fistula. Here there is no previously constructed gastrojejunostomy available for feeding, and maintenance of the patient during closure of the fistula will be more difficult. It may be possible to pass a nasogastric tube beyond the fistula, or a feeding jejunostomy may be performed. After the usual nonoperative course of management (except for establishing external drainage if not already present) has been given full trial, a Billroth II distal subtotal gastrectomy may be considered. If this is done, a tube should be left in the distal loop for feeding, or a feeding jejunostomy should be performed for feeding in the event of a leak at the anastomosis.

The activated pancreatic digestive enzymes in the duodenal drainage always pose the threat of arterial erosion and hemorrhage.

The anastomotic fistula, secondary to gastroduodenostomy or gastrojejunostomy, was considered previously.

JEJUNAL FISTULA

A substantial period of conservative management, combined with good external drainage and supportive therapy, should wisely precede operative intervention for a jejunal fistula. The surgical procedure usually takes the form of an entero-enteros-

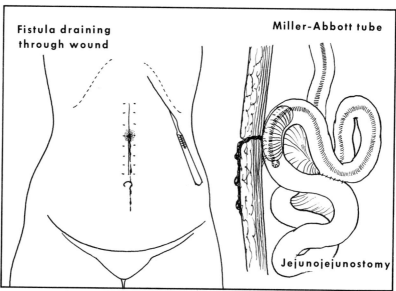

Figure 20-2. Bypass of small bowel fistula. If the site of the fistula is involved in a matted mass of inflamed bowel, one may elect to bypass the fistula to gain time and to improve nutrition. Eventually, however, the fistula should usually be totally excised, with restoration of normal gut continuity. An alternative maneuver is to divide the bowel proximal to the fistula, to invert the distal stump, and to anastomose the proximal bowel end-to-side to the bowel distal to the fistula (Fig. 20-4).

tomy around the fistula (Fig. 20-2), with excision of the bypassed fistula when the general condition of the patient has improved; an excision of the fistula, with end-to-end anastomosis; or a division of the jejunum through healthy bowel proximal to the fistula, inversion of the distal stump, and anastomosis of the proximal end of the jejunum end-to-side to the colon. This may deprive the patient of a considerable segment of useful small bowel, and at some point in the future, when health has been regained and infection abolished, it may be desirable to restore total continuity of the residual intestine (see Case 4).

When operating for a jejunal fistula, it is useful to pass a long Miller-Abbott type tube into the gut proximal to the fistula, so that the proximal gut can be distinguished from the bowel distal to the fistula. Otherwise, extensive adhesions and chronic inflammation may render orientation difficult.

If it is elected to excise the fistula, and to perform primary end-to-end anastomosis, a long tube pulled into the small bowel distal to the anastomosis may serve to maintain patency to beyond this point. In some patients there is very little residual peritoneal reaction at the time of reexploration, but in others there remains a surprising degree of residual inflammation accompanied by chronic edema, thickening, and foreshortening of the small bowel. Under these circumstances there is a considerable risk of anastomotic leakage, and external drainage of the anastomosis should be provided. At other times, when a chronic fibrotic tract has formed providing immediate egress of bowel contents to the outside, the peritoneal cavity may be found remarkably free of inflammation, and complete excision of the fistula with primary anastomosis will usually be successful.

ILEAL FISTULA

The management of an ileal fistula is not greatly different from that of a low jejunal fistula. In each instance it may be possible to use the proximal bowel to achieve a degree of food intake, after the establishment of good external drainage has alleviated peritonitis, and fluid losses are often substantially less than with a high jejunal fistula. Moreover, the lower the fistula is situated in the gut, the more successful direct operative management is likely to be, whether by bypass, complete excision, or by exclusion of the fistulous portion with anastomosis of the end of the divided healthy ileum to the side of the colon. After the inflammatory reaction has subsided and the bowel not involved in the fistula itself has become normal, excision of the fistula may be feasible, as has been successfully accomplished in several of our patients.

COLONIC FISTULA

A colonic fistula is usually not a high-output fistula, as noted previously, but a few words regarding operative management of this lesion are in order. A fistula of the colon is usually managed by proximal colostomy and effective drainage of the leaking bowel, or by exteriorization of the fistulous segment itself. While substantial fluid losses may at times occur from external drainage of right colon contents, fluid balance problems are uncommon in the chronic colonic fistula, and infection becomes the major consideration. Once the peritonitis and associated paralytic ileus have subsided, the patient with a well managed colonic fistula can eat normally. As with other types of fistulas, the colonic fistula can prove fatal or it can be relatively innocuous.

ILLUSTRATIVE CASES

CASE 1. HIGH-OUTPUT JEJUNAL ENTEROCUTANEOUS FISTULA TREATED WITHOUT OPERATION

A 70-year-old retired clergyman was seized with cramping abdominal pain on 4/4/69, and a laparotomy was performed on 4/5/69 in his community hospital with the provisional diagnosis of small bowel obstruction. He had undergone a 70 per cent distal subtotal Billroth II gastric resection in 1954 for peptic ulcer disease and cholecystectomy for gallstones in 1964. At operation the intestinal obstruction was found to be due to adhesions accompanied by gut strangulation, and at least five feet of small bowel was resected. One week later the wound separated and required reclosure, but following this second operation drainage through the wound between the sutures continued. It was soon apparent that a high-output small bowel fistula existed, which was draining from one to three liters every 24 hours. At this point, on the 16th postoperative day, the patient was transferred to the University Hospital.

Evaluation revealed that skin excoriation around the

wound was modest, but that the wound itself was grossly infected. The patient was moderately febrile but not markedly "toxic." He had passed some flatus per rectum, which indicated absence of complete obstruction distal to the fistula. A barium study disclosed that only four to five feet of small bowel remained, and that the fistula appeared to be in about the midportion of the residual small bowel.

It was elected to support the patient vigorously with intravenously administered alimentation, and to correct the minor abnormalities found in the serum electrolytes. On the whole, his hydration had been well maintained by his referring physician. Various additional roentgen studies did not reveal evidence of a subdiaphragmatic or other intraperitoneal abscesses. He clearly still had some peritonitis, as reflected by moderate generalized abdominal tenderness and diminished peristaltic activity. The possibility of operation to bypass or to resect the fistula had to be weighed against the fact that (1) many small bowel fistulas close spontaneously in the absence of distal obstruction and that (2) the sacrifice of any portion of the short length of remaining small bowel could lead to small bowel insufficiency. Fortunately, it was apparent during the first 72 hours of observation that the patient's general situation would permit several weeks of nonoperative management: he was not seriously depleted, his fever was declining owing to antibiotic therapy, he was passing more flatus per rectum, it was not difficult to maintain fluid balance, catheter suction at the fistulous opening was protecting the skin and measuring the volume of loss, some intravenous nutrition was being achieved, and it appeared likely that soon oral food intake could be initiated.

By the seventh day after admission the evidence of peritonitis had abated, and the patient's fever had subsided. He was taking liquid nourishment orally, having bowel movements, and the fistulous drainage had decreased. The appearance of his abdominal wound, through which the fistula had been draining, had improved and stabilized, and frank evisceration had become much less of a threat. Clearly, the total progress was in the direction of recovery, and this favorable outcome continued.

He was allowed to return to his community hospital on 5/9/69, 34 days after the initial operation which had been followed by the anastomotic fistula. He was eating satisfactorily, and drainage from the fistula had decreased markedly. It ceased entirely several days later.

Comment

Case 1 illustrates a fistula which followed bowel anastomosis, and one which was unrecognized for a number of days. Peritonitis developed prior to the establishment of free external drainage through the wound, but the peritoneum gradually overcame the infection with the aid of antibiotics and cessation of intraperitoneal leakage. Intraperitoneal abscess was suspected on the basis of the fever, but major collections were not identified by physical examination or roentgen studies, and the infection present gradually subsided without operative intervention.

Once the ileus secondary to peritonitis had receded concomitantly with the clearing of the peritoneal infection, peristalsis returned, flatus was passed per rectum, and oral intake was initiated despite continued but steadily declining drainage from the fistula. This supplemented the nutrition achieved by the intravenous route. The patient had a severe infection of the laparotomy wound, through which the fistula was draining, but frank evisceration did not occur in our hospital.

Operative management was considered unwise from the outset because previous operations had left the patient with perhaps only four feet of small bowel, in the middle of which was the fistula. Regardless of what the surgeon may hope to find at laparotomy for the management of a small bowel fistula, the adhesions and inflammation may be found to be so dense and severe that injured bowel may have to be resected to salvage the patient's life. Therefore, our plan was to avoid operation in this patient if at all possible, and fortunately nonoperative management proved successful.

CASE 2. ENTEROVAGINAL FISTULA TREATED BY PRIMARY RESECTION

A 58-year-old housewife was admitted to the University Hospital on 12/15/58 with a mass in the pelvis that was tentatively diagnosed as a fibroid tumor. She was febrile and anemic. At laparotomy on 12/24/58 a degenerating and necrotic uterine fibroid with many adhesions was found, and a difficult total abdominal hysterectomy with salpingo-oophorectomy was performed. *Escherichia coli* organisms were cultured from the mass removed, and the patient continued to run a considerable fever postoperatively. There was a serious wound infection.

On the 13th postoperative day a large amount of purulent material was drained through the vagina at the vaginal cuff; this material had a fecaloid odor. Within 24 hours the drainage had definitely changed in appearance to resemble small bowel contents, and a barium study subsequently disclosed a fistula in the low jejunum or upper ileum. The fever gradually subsided after drainage of the pelvic abscess through the vagina was instituted, despite the fact that the small bowel injury had probably been present since the operation on 12/24/58. The enterovaginal fistula continued to drain copiously, producing excoriation of the skin of the perineum. It was not possible to achieve quantitative collection of the drainage through the vagina, but it was estimated at 1000 to 2000 ml per day. No particular difficulty was experienced with the maintenance of fluid and electrolyte balance, and the patient was able to take a liquid diet by mouth.

The Surgical Service was consulted regarding definitive management. It was apparent that the partially separated and previously infected lower abdominal midline wound was becoming clean, and that the maturing enterovaginal fistula was no longer associated with significant peritonitis. The patient was almost afebrile, although she still exhibited tachycardia. There was copious small bowel drainage through the vagina, marked excoriation of the surrounding skin, and no apparent trend toward a reduction in the size of the intestinal defect or in the volume of fluid loss. It was decided that laparotomy should be performed with the objective of either bypassing or excision of the fistula. A long Miller-Abbott tube was passed far into the small bowel to facilitate identification of loops proximal and distal to the fistula at operation.

Laparotomy was performed on 1/12/59 through the previous lower midline incision. The granulating wound was not grossly infected and the peritoneum was incised. The peritoneal cavity was essentially clean, but there was an inflammatory mass in the pelvis that involved several loops of small bowel and that had doubtless caused the symptoms of incomplete small bowel obstruction which had existed several days earlier. In due course the loop of small bowel adherent to the vaginal cuff was identified, and the remainder of the gut was retracted and packed away. Since there was no drainage into the peritoneal cavity itself, and no resulting bacterial contamination and infection, it was considered safe to dissect the involved loop of ileum free of the vagina and to resect the involved gut segment with primary anastomosis (Fig. 20-3). The defect in the intestine, approximately 2.5 × 1.5 cm. in size, was on the antimesenteric border, and it was resected with a 4-cm. margin of uninvolved bowel on each side. This loop of bowel was then placed in a position far removed from the pelvis. A catheter drain was passed from the abdomen into the vagina and was removed several days following operation.

The Miller-Abbott tube was removed on the fourth postoperative day, oral intake was initiated, and recovery was uneventful.

Comment

This patient presented a relatively simple situation. The small bowel fistula followed an operation, which is frequently the case. Associated infection and peritonitis developed but subsided after the fistula began to drain freely through the vagina without further intraperitoneal spillage, illustrating the remarkable capacity of the peritoneum to cleanse itself once further bacterial contamination has been halted. The associated wound infection and partial separation may have been secondary to the development of the fistula or they may have been due to the infection found at the original gynecologic operation. The fistula was classified as a "high-output" fistula, since a loss of one to two liters occurred daily; however, this volume was not sufficient to cause a serious problem in the maintenance of fluid and acid-base balance, and, in fact, the patient was able to take a liquid diet after the initial peritonitis and paralytic ileus had subsided. Operation was performed, after it appeared that the peritoneal reaction had cleared, to reduce the volume of fluid loss and especially to halt further excoriation of the skin

Figure 20-3. Excision of chronic ileovaginal fistula. When the fistula drains directly and immediately to the outside, through the skin or through the vagina as seen here, the peritonitis usually subsides and the fistula can be excised with primary anastomosis. This may substantially reduce fluid and nutritional losses, as well as shorten the hospitalization required.

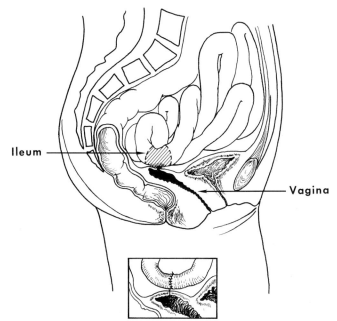

Ileum

Vagina

of the perineum. It was feasible to resect the fistula, with primary gut anastomosis. There was no postoperative complication and the patient was discharged from the hospital on the eleventh postoperative day.

CASE 3. GASTRO-JEJUNAL ANASTOMOTIC FISTULA FOLLOWING BILLROTH II GASTRIC RESECTION

A 49-year-old housewife underwent a Billroth II sub-total gastrectomy on 3/3/58 for massive hemorrhage from a giant gastric ulcer. Her postoperative course was never really smooth, and she exhibited fever and tachycardia on the first postoperative day. However, no other special changes were noted initially, except that her postoperative abdominal pain seemed somewhat excessive; also, it was noted on the second postoperative day that she was jaundiced (serum bilirubin 6 mg. per 100 ml.). The explanation for the jaundice was not clear, but by the fifth postoperative day she exhibited marked abdominal distention, this despite the fact that she was passing flatus and having bowel movements. In fact, she had developed diarrhea. On the seventh postoperative day, 3/10/58, she began to complain further of severe right-sided abdominal pain, associated with an increase in the pulse rate to 130 per minute. The white cell count was 25,000 cells/cu. mm. Intraperitoneal abscess was suspected by her surgeon, and she was explored through the healing midline scar on 3/11/58. A large quantity of old blood was aspirated from the peritoneal cavity, accounting for the multiple transfusions which had been required postoperatively, and it was found that the gastrojejunal anastomosis had leaked anteriorly. Additional sutures were placed through this friable tissue, and the abdominal wound was then closed and drainage provided.

After this second operation she continued to be extremely ill, as evidenced by a spiking fever, rapid pulse, sweating, and an anxious appearance. The urine output remained satisfactory but the jaundice increased (serum bilirubin 21 mg. per 100 ml.). Moreover, on March 16, it was apparent that small bowel contents were extruding between the wound sutures. It was concluded that the anastomosis had again broken down and had produced a fistula. Drainage from this source was profuse, being several liters per day. Catheter sump suction was maintained at the fistulous opening, and the skin was fairly well protected from erosion. It was considered possible, presently, to pass a long tube through the nose and thence into the upper jejunum, and the fistulous drainage and nutritive solutions were introduced into the small bowel in this manner.

The patient exhibited numerous episodes of mild hypotension, and vigorous efforts were required to prevent and to correct dehydration, hyponatremia, and hypokalemia. Furthermore, it was suspected that intraperitoneal abscesses existed, but operative intervention was never required. With continuous nurse and physician care, antibiotics, fluid and nutritional support, and protection of the skin, she eventually recovered. She was discharged from the hospital on 4/7/58, her 35th postoperative day.

Comment

This case illustrates the very serious clinical situation produced by anastomotic leakage following gastrectomy. The old blood found in the peritoneal cavity at the second operation was doubtless due to incomplete technical hemostasis at the first operation. Furthermore, this blood provided an excellent culture medium which probably supported intraperitoneal infection and may have contributed to the breakdown of the gastrojejunostomy. The jaundice could have been due to liver dysfunction, to common duct compression, or to proximal or afferent loop obstruction. However, it was most likely due to hemolysis and absorption of blood from the peritoneal cavity or to the absorption of bile that had escaped through the fistula. In any event, the development of jaundice following gastric resection, and associated with pain, fever, and leukocytosis, should always suggest intraperitoneal leakage of bile from the duodenal stump or the anastomosis.

The sutures placed in the leaking gastrojejunal anastomosis at the second operation, in the presence of almost certain infection, would not have been expected to hold, although the maneuver was worth trying. But in view of the fact that the anastomosis had leaked once, the abdominal drainage provided should have been much more extensive. As it was, the recurrence of the fistula was again not perceived promptly, in this case not until bile-stained fluid had forced itself between the skin sutures and the patient was in a very critical condition.

As is usually necessary, the supportive therapy provided for this patient was excellent and unceasing. The success in passing a long tube through the leaking gastrojejunostomy into the upper jejunum, which permitted feeding and return of the fluid aspirated at the fistulous opening, probably made the difference in saving this patient's life. Nevertheless, she very nearly died. In retrospect, one might speculate that the surgeon had been wise at the second operation not to resect the entire anastomosis in the presence of certain bacterial contamination. Although feeding was achieved through the long tube in this case, usually less oral nutritional intake can be attained by a patient with an anastomotic fistula than with a duodenal stump fistula.

CASE 4. MULTIPLE JEJUNAL FISTULAS SECONDARY TO GUNSHOT WOUNDS; SURVIVAL WITH MULTIPLE OPERATIONS OVER THIRTEEN MONTHS

A 23-year-old man was admitted to the University Hospital on 9/7/67, 16 days after having received a 30-30 rifle bullet wound that had traversed the abdomen. Immediately following injury he had been operated upon in his community hospital, and multiple gut perforations were closed. However, soon thereafter small bowel contents began to emerge from both the entrance and exit wounds on the abdomen, the skin became severely excoriated, and the wound closure became infected. Always slender, the patient had rapidly become almost emaciated in the absence of oral intake or effective intravenous alimentation. However, his fever was minimal. He was severely dehydrated, and the fluid losses from the multiple fistulous sites were substantial.

After several days of evaluation, intravenous hyperalimentation, and blood transfusions, it appeared unlikely that the patient would be saved unless the multiple jejunal fistulas could be corrected or ameliorated by operative intervention. He was very thin, weak, listless, and depressed. Food intake was limited, fluid and electrolyte maintenance was difficult, and the abdomen was severely excoriated and extremely tender and painful. On 9/18/67, a left subcostal incision was made in the hope that the fistulous areas could be bypassed in an area of the abdomen that was relatively clear of peritonitis. A Miller-Abbott tube had previously been passed to facilitate identification of the proximal small bowel. The left upper quadrant was indeed relatively free of reaction, but the lower abdomen was found to be the site of dense inflammatory adhesions containing scattered pockets of pus. It was clear that bypass would not be feasible, unless one were to anastomose a five-foot segment of jejunum to the colon. The segment of lower jejunum containing the fistulas was eventually identified and resected, and the Miller-Abbott tube was pulled through the anastomosis and advanced to the ascending colon.

The immediate postoperative course was reasonably satisfactory, but on 9/22/67, the fourth postoperative day, brownish fluid was seen emerging from a drain site in the right lower abdomen, and within 24 hours this fluid had taken on the unmistakable appearance of small bowel contents: the fistula had recurred. During this period the daily fluid requirements approached six liters, and overall maintenance and nursing care represented a huge expenditure of professional time.

By 11/5/67, almost seven weeks after the previous laparotomy in September, it was generally agreed that the patient was steadily losing ground and would eventually die if successful operative intervention could not be achieved. Again a bypass was planned, this time through a right subcostal incision made on 11/8/69. The entire small bowel was found to be markedly thickened, shortened, and friable. Indeed, it was only a few feet in length. Dissection was most difficult, but again the fistulous site was resected with primary anastomosis. The Miller-Abbott tube introduced preoperatively was advanced to the cecum. With the exception of postoperative bleeding, which necessitated reopening of the wound to ligate a bleeder, the early postoperative course was reasonably smooth, considering the patient's severely depleted condition. Unfortunately, a moderate amount of small bowel drainage appeared on 11/12/67, signalling leakage at the anastomosis. However, this was less than formerly, and occasional bowel movements occurred.

At this point it was believed that further operation was out of the question, and the application of all possible supportive measures was redoubled. His weight had declined from a normal level of 120 lbs. to 74 lbs. In the ensuing weeks, oral and intravenous nutrition were given great emphasis, at a time when fluid and electrolyte balance was maintained only with great effort. He experienced an acute brain syndrome due to water intoxication, a period of frank psychosis, phlebitis with abscess formation from cutdowns, bronchopneumonia, decubitus ulcers, morphine addiction (with recovery), and marked jaundice. Fortunately, renal failure did not develop. He became so weak that it was considered inadvisable to get him out of bed, and on many occasions it appeared that he would surely die. Nevertheless, his weight curve finally began an upward trend, and by the end of January, 1968, he weighed 90 lbs. At this time he was allowed to go home, and was kept under the closest supervision by his family physician and the County Health Nurse.

He maintained himself fairly well at home but was usually immobilized on a bed through which the fistulous drainage from the several sites fell into a basin underneath. Rehabilitation had certainly not been achieved. He was therefore readmitted to the University Hospital on 9/7/68 for still another operative attack upon the fistula. It was believed that the inflammatory reaction in the peritoneal cavity would have disappeared except at the fistula site. A Miller-Abbott tube was again passed and allowed to advance to the fistulous opening beneath the abdominal wall. At laparotomy the peritoneal cavity was found completely free of reaction and the remaining small bowel appeared normal except at the site of the fistula. Accordingly, the normal gut was divided just proximal to the fistula: the proximal end was anastomosed to the side of the right colon, and the distal end was simply closed by inversion using two rows of sutures (Fig. 20-4). The small bowel extending from the ligament of Treitz to the colon was approximately four feet in length. The patient's postoperative course was very smooth, and he began having bowel movements promptly. The drainage from the fistulous openings in the lower abdomen declined to a minimal volume, and the skin excoriation healed in a very short time. He did have multiple stools, with proctitis and excoriation of the perianal skin, but this was gradually brought under control. His general health improved rapidly and he was eventually allowed to return to work with his weight almost normal.

The patient, of course, continues to survive on only several feet of small bowel. He has an almost equal amount of serviceable small bowel excluded from the functioning alimentary tract, and should long-term nutritional defects develop, this defunctionalized distal small bowel could be reinserted into the functioning alimentary tract.

Comment

This case exemplifies the extraordinary supportive effort which may be required to salvage the patient with a high-output small

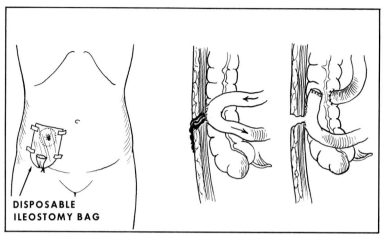

Figure 20-4. Exclusion of high-output small bowel fistula by enterocolostomy. The ileum was divided just proximally to the fistula, the distal stump was inverted, and the proximal ileum was anastomosed to the right colon. Prompt rehabilitation was achieved.

bowel fistula. The most critical phase of this patient's illness lasted five months, but he really was still in jeopardy until after the third major operation in the University Hospital, approximately one year following his original admission. The frequent failure of intestinal anastomoses performed on inflamed bowel, in the presence of peritonitis, was exemplified by the anastomotic dehiscence which occurred with the first two resections of fistulas. In contrast, when the third operation was performed almost a year later, through a clean peritoneal cavity and joining nondiseased bowel, healing occurred at once and the patient was promptly rehabilitated.

CASE 5. HIGH-OUTPUT POSTOPERATIVE JEJUNAL FISTULA WITH FATAL COMPLICATIONS

A 24-year-old previously healthy man was admitted to his community hospital on 12/18/69 with signs and symptoms of small bowel obstruction, probably secondary to adhesions from an appendiceal abscess which had occurred several years before. At laparotomy adhesions were lysed and the bowel was decompressed by enterotomy. Postoperatively he did not respond well and assisted ventilation was required for four to six hours. The blood pressure fell to 50/40 and the next day his temperature rose to 106° temporarily and he became incoherent. Blood cultures grew out *E. coli,* and the patient remained septic and mentally obtunded.

He was transferred to the University Hospital on 12/25/69 in a semicomatose condition with rectal temperature of 106° F. The blood pressure was 110 systolic but the pulse rate was 140. The abdomen was

markedly distended. A small amount of drainage was emerging from a defect in the center of his laparotomy wound, through which a small drain had previously been inserted. A gloved finger gently introduced through this tract released a large volume of gas and extremely foul smelling drainage. It was clear that the patient had either a low small bowel or colonic fistula, and his condition was judged to be extremely critical.

Immediate therapy consisted of improved drainage through the abdominal wall, reduction of fever with a cooling blanket, further blood cultures to determine bacterial sensitivities, nasogastric suction, meticulous measurement of fluid losses including urine output, massive broad spectrum antibiotics, daily weights, and protection of skin around the fistula by application of a disposable ileostomy bag. Intravenous hyperalimentation was planned after the immediate emergency had passed. Operative intervention was considered out of the question for the time being.

These several measures did produce a reduction in the body temperature, and his condition stabilized somewhat over the next several days. The fistula actually drained less than a liter per day.

Unfortunately, on the fifth day the patient began to bleed massively from the fistulous tract and required multiple transfusions. This hemorrhage, from "stress ulcer" or erosion of arteries along the drainage tract, was considered to be more than could be tolerated by this extremely ill patient. It was decided to reopen the old incision, attempt to halt the bleeding, to exteriorize the bleeding bowel, and to drain the abdomen. If bleeding was from a stress ulcer, vagotomy and pyloroplasty with oversewing of the bleeding site would be performed.

At laparotomy on 12/31/69 the abdomen was found to contain huge amounts of pus. Lumps of feces impregnated with barium had eroded through the cecum and right colon and were freely exposed to the peritoneal cavity. A short loop of jejunum had been incarcerated beneath an adhesion, or beneath a loose retention suture, and necrosis had occurred. This jejunal segment was resected (the inner row of continuous sutures were iodized catgut). The entire right colon was removed, leaving an ileostomy and the exteriorized proximal end of the right colon. No operation was performed on the stomach, since the upper small bowel contained no blood. The entire abdomen was cleansed gently and multiple drains were inserted. Postoperatively the endotracheal tube was left in place to assist ventilation during the following 24 hours.

The most remarkable feature of the next few days was the huge fluid losses through the nasogastric tube and ileostomy — at times almost seven liters per 24 hours, including urine volume. Moreover, since the patient was sweating profusely and continuously, the insensible fluid loss probably amounted to 1 to 2 liters per day. Oliguria developed from time to time, doubtless due to dehydration, but because of frequent measurements of plasma electrolytes and body weights, serious renal dysfunction was avoided. The fact that he continued to have bloody bowel movements per rectum, the cause of which was uncertain, posed a special problem. Since there was no bleeding from the ileostomy or nasogastric suction tube, a specific bleeding diathesis seemed unlikely. Hypovolemia was usually first reflected in the development of dyspnea and oliguria, and additional blood, plasma, or an electrolyte-containing solution was given as required. Large amounts of brownish, foul smelling fluid continued to escape from the three abdominal drainage routes that had been provided at operation. A program of intravenous hyperalimentation was activated.

Unfortunately, a major crisis developed on 1/3/70, the third postoperative day. Rather massive blood loss began through both the nasogastric tube and the ileostomy, in addition to the previous loss per rectum from the defunctionalized colon. This upper gastrointestinal hemorrhage seemed most likely to be due to stress ulceration in the stomach, in the duodenum, or both. The patient was severely obtunded, but not actually comatose. The lungs exhibited some evidence of pneumonitis, but the arterial blood gas values were reasonably satisfactory.

Further operative intervention was not feasible, but it was clear that measures would be essential to stop the blood loss believed to be coming from the stomach or duodenum. A program of anticholinergic drugs plus the instillation of milk and antacids every two hours through the nasogastric tube was initiated. The stomach was aspirated completely prior to each new instillation. The volume of nasogastric suction loss had diminished during the previous 24 hours, but the possibility of sudden vomiting and pulmonary aspiration in a desperately ill and obtunded patient prompted discussion of prophylactic tracheostomy for insertion of a cuffed tracheostomy tube. However, it was decided not to perform tracheostomy because (1) he did not need it for respiratory support, (2) he was cared for by experienced nurses who would empty the stomach periodically and avoid the pooling of significant volumes which might be suddenly vomited, and (3) the tracheostomy site would almost surely become infected in the presence of so much other infection, and this would lead to further pulmonary sepsis.

This antiulcer program did appear to be helpful over the next 12 hours. The bleeding from the stomach and from the ileostomy, which was assumed to have traversed the small bowel and thus reflected good small bowel mobility and decompression, declined and the clinical situation was believed to have stabilized. However, at 1:30 A.M. of the fourth postoperative day the patient abruptly vomited a large volume of foul smelling material, completely different in character from any material obtained by nasogastric tube or ileostomy over the previous two days. Pulmonary aspiration and hypoxic cardiac arrest occurred. He was resuscitated and the lungs were cleared through the quickly inserted cuffed endotracheal tube. Even so, this further complication, in addition to all the previous ones, proved to be the final one, and the patient died nine hours later.

At autopsy, it was found that the bleeding into the stomach had had no free communication with the ileostomy. The hemorrhage from the stomach, lower ileum, and defunctionalized colon had all represented separate lesions. The small bowel was moderately distended, friable, edematous, and matted in tight loops despite the fact that the Miller-Abbott tube left through it at operation was still lying as far distal as the mid-ileum. This tube had never drained a significant volume, in contrast to the auxillary nasogastric tube that had been inserted, and the reason was now clear: the small bowel was packed with a semisolid material which may at one time have been blood, but which was no longer grossly recognizable as such because of digestion. This was the type of material that had suddenly been regurgitated from the upper reaches of the jejunum into the stomach and then vomited, which resulted in pulmonary aspiration. The small bowel anastomosis had remained intact, although whether it would have held until firm healing had occurred, in the presence of a diseased bowel wall and surrounding infection, was doubtful. Finally, despite the fact that the peritoneal cavity had been thoroughly aspirated of purulent fluid at operation, it was again filled with large volumes of foul smelling pus. While much similar material had drained from the drain sites over the previous three days, it was obvious that the overwhelming bacterial contamination had produced additional sepsis with great rapidity.

Comment

In reconstructing the train of events that led to the death of this patient with a high-output jejunal fistula, it would appear that, as usually happens, a fistula secondary to operation was the initial complication. In all probability, the loop of jejunum was caught in a retention suture at the time of wound closure in his community hospital. This gave rise to intra-abdominal sepsis, severe fever, and paralytic ileus. The large masses of inspirated barium feces lay in the right colon and gradually eroded through its anterior wall, which could have been rendered relatively ischemic by surrounding infection and a continuously precarious circulatory stability. Whatever the reason that the barium deposits eroded through the colon wall, and the writer has observed such a complication on several occasions, this was probably the complication that placed the patient beyond salvage, because of the overwhelming intra-abdominal contamination produced.

This patient exhibited the great fluid outpouring which may occur into the alimentary tract in the presence of peritonitis with ileus, since the bowel wall itself becomes involved in the inflammatory process. Although the "infection-oliguria-stress ulcer" syndrome did not develop in its entirety, since oliguria was always corrected promptly by appropriate colloid or electrolyte solution therapy, the infection and alimentary tract bleeding were the major problems which led to the patient's death. Although pulmonary aspiration was a final episode, as it frequently is in the extremely debilitated patient, this young man would not have aspirated had he not already been virtually comatose from massive sepsis.

Thus, the patients who succumb to gastrointestinal fistulas die from infection, massive and inadequately replaced fluid losses, hemorrhage, renal failure, liver failure and malnutrition—in most instances. The overall therapeutic approach must be directed toward the prevention of these major complications.

THE OUTLOOK IN GASTROINTESTINAL FISTULA

The prognosis in a given patient depends upon the wide variety of factors outlined earlier. The fact remains that the mortality rate for alimentary tract fistulas remains substantial. Of 68 patients who developed fistulas of the stomach or intestine in the Hospital of the University of Mississippi, 17 died, or an overall mortality rate of 25 per cent. However, the death rate has definitely shown a downward trend in recent years. In few other circumstances is greater and more persevering supportive therapy required, but such treatment, combined with the judicious use of surgical intervention, can save many lives that would otherwise be lost.

REFERENCES

Bowlin, J. W., Hardy, J. D., and Conn, J. H.: External alimentary tract fistulas: Analysis of seventy-nine cases with notes on management. Amer. J. Surg., 103:6, 1962.

Chapman, R., Foran, R., and Dunphy, J. E.: Management of intestinal fistulas. Amer. J. Surg., 108:157, 1964.

Edmunds, L. H., Jr., Williams, G. M., and Welch, C. E.: External fistulas arising from the gastro-intestinal tract. Ann. Surg., 152:445, 1960.

Hardy, J. D.: Small bowel fistulas and ileostomy, In Manual of Preoperative and Postoperative Care. Philadelphia, W. B. Saunders Co., 1967.

Miller, H. I., and White, R. L.: Postoperative small bowel fistulas. Review of 28 cases. Amer. Surg., 32:60, 1966.

Miller, H. I., and Dorn, B. C.: Postoperative gastro-intestinal fistulas. Amer. J. Surg., 116:382, 1968.

West, J. P., Ring, E. M., Miller, R. E., and Burks, W. P.: A study of causes and treatment of postoperative intestinal fistulas. Surg. Gynec. Obstet., 113:490, 1961.

CHAPTER 21

FULMINANT ULCERATIVE COLITIS: TOXIC MEGACOLON, PERFORATION, AND HEMORRHAGE

by WILEY F. BARKER, M.D.

Wiley F. Barker was born in New Mexico and graduated from Harvard University and Harvard Medical School, having been elected to both Phi Beta Kappa and Alpha Omega Alpha. Following surgical residency training at Peter Bent Brigham Hospital and U.C.L.A., his distinguished career in teaching, practice, and research resulted in his being promoted to full Professor of Surgery at U.C.L.A. in 1964. He has served American surgery in numerous capacities. The surgical management of ulcerative colitis has constituted a field of special scientific endeavor.

Among the cataclysmic occurrences in medicine few are more dramatic than fulminant colitis, which may be characterized by hemorrhage, perforation, rapid deterioration, and prostration, or by a pattern of extreme colonic dilatation now commonly known as toxic megacolon. This fulminant process may develop from the first symptom and become life-threatening within weeks. On the other hand, it may arise during the course of a long-standing chronic illness but may follow just as florid a course.

It is a variable disease. It would be misleading to imply that special complications occur only with certain pathologic diagnoses. The clinical manifestations of the disease, rather than the pathologic pedigree, at times will dictate the course of management.

PATHOLOGIC CLASSIFICATIONS

Patients with the generic classification of ulcerative colitis have always been thought to follow a highly unpredictable course. This stems from a classic Hunterian error.[*] There are sufficient clinical similarities between idiopathic mucosal ulcerative colitis and transmural or granulomatous colitis (pain, debility, diarrhea—often bloody—and distention) and sufficient pathologic similarities (ulceration and acute and chronic inflammation) so that until the mid-sixties there had not been a general attempt to separate the two disease entities.[†]

Lockhart-Mummery and Morson (1960, 1964) were among the first to distinguish these lesions clearly. Wolf and Marshak (1962) have contributed excellent radiologic criteria for the diagnostic distinction between them. Turnbull, Schofield, and Hawk (1968) have also provided a simplified pattern of characteristics (Table 21-1).

---

[*]John Hunter, who developed both syphilis and gonorrhea after inoculating himself with material from a chancre, caused the medical world to believe for a considerable period of time that the two diseases were one.

[†]This entity is also known by a score or more of aliases, such as Crohn's disease of the colon, enterocolitis, segmental colitis, ileocolitis, and granulomatous colitis, to name just a few.

Table 21-1. Criteria for Distinguishing Granulomatous (Transmural) Colitis from Idiopathic Colitis*

Mucosal Colitis	Transmural (Granulomatous, Crohn's) Colitis
Mucosal	
Diffuse	Often segmental, asymmetrical
No normal mucosa in diseased bowel	Normal mucosa common between ulcers
Ragged pseudopolyps common	Edematous, "pillow" mucosa, but no pseudopolyps
Serositis rare except in peritonitis	Fiery red serositis common
Inflammatory masses rare	Inflammatory masses common
Strictures rare: commonly neoplastic	Inflammatory masses common
Fistulas to abdominal wall and genitourinary tract rare	Abdominal wall, genitourinary, enteroenteric, and perineal fistulas common
Shortening of colon common	Shortening of colon rare
Small bowel involvement rare, never extensive	Small bowel involvement common
Enlarged mesenteric lymph nodes rare	Enlarged mesenteric lymph nodes common
Mucosa alone involved in inflammation (except in perforated colon with peritonitis)	All coats of colon involved (i.e., "transmural")
Granulomas never seen	Granulomas common, but not always found (bowel wall more common than lymph nodes)
Fissures never	Deep, transmural fissures frequent and characteristic
Fibrosis in submucosa only	Fibrosis transmural, irregular, and disproportionate
Lymphedema never	Lymphedema usual
Crypt abscesses frequent	Crypt abscesses sometimes seen but not usual

*Modified from Turnbull, Schofield, and Hawk (1968).

The criteria in Table 21-1 are not fully acceptable to all pathologists, but they offer the clinician a chance to explain the clinical behavior of the two diseases on pathologic grounds. One of the problems presented by this classification is the difficulty in finding typical granulomata and giant cells in some specimens that might otherwise clearly be classified as transmural colitis. As many as 25 to 50 per cent of patients may not have specific granulomata (Lockhart-Mummery and Morson, 1964). Also, Marshak (1969) has observed that not all segmental colitis is granulomatous colitis, although one of the gross characteristics of granulomatous colitis is its segmental pattern. Ischemic colitis may mimic the appearance of segmental colitis but it rarely occurs in a fulminant form. The term granulomatous colitis, therefore, may not always refer to exactly the same group of patients as transmural colitis.

Extension of inflammation through all layers of the bowel may be found in acute and fulminant cases. This automatically establishes the process as "transmural," but the disease does not necessarily have any of the other characteristics of the usual transmural granulomatous lesion and may otherwise be much more nearly the pure mucosal disease.

Other pathologic processes and pharmacologic influences may alter the course of early colitis and produce a "toxic megacolon" in such a way that the criteria for classification are not present.

Case report

The patient was a 25-year-old woman with a three-month history of mild lower abdominal distress and diarrhea, occasionally bloody. Three weeks before admission to the hospital she developed epigastric pain, which was thought by means of x-ray diagnosis to be due to an ulcer of the duodenum. Large doses of antacids and antispasmodics were prescribed. She eventually developed distention and then, just before admission to the hospital, severe distention, diminution of stools, and a serious toxic status. She entered the hospital with the classic appearance of a patient with toxic megacolon. Results of sigmoidoscopy were normal with the exception of a mildly hyperemic mucosa. She was operated upon after a short period of supportive therapy.

At operation the terminal ileum and ascending and transverse colon were greatly dilated. The serosa of the proximal colon was covered with fine arborizing vessels. The splenic flexure appeared normal. The terminal ileum was dilated and thinned out. There were submucosal hemorrhages on the antimesenteric edge and there was none of the gross thickening consistent with the usual granulomatous lesion. The surgical specimen showed ulcers that extended deep to the submucosa and a chronic inflammatory process with fibrosis penetrating all coats of the bowel, even though the bowel was greatly thinned out. Granulomata were present, but no giant cells were identified. There was only moderate lymphatic enlargement and there were no granulomata in the lymph nodes. Some lesions of periarterial cuffing were believed to represent periarteritis.

The clinical course in this patient was certainly consistent with that of a toxic megacolon secondary to mucosal disease, but the gross appearance was that of a transmural lesion. The microscopic lesions were probably more consistent with the granulomatous transmural disease. In retrospect it would seem that this patient had early segmental granulomatous and transmural disease of the right colon, although Sparberg (1967) has reported a similar case apparently due to mucosal colitis. His patient's acute symptoms were misinterpreted as being those of a duodenal ulcer. The use of antacids and anticholinergics may have precipitated the syndrome of toxic megacolon.

Determining the pathologic nature of the disease does not influence the decision to operate, but it may modify the extent of the operative procedure. That is, it would not be appropriate to resect minimally involved or apparently normal bowel in granulomatous colitis, whereas in mucosal colitis, removal of the entire colon may be necessary. Similarly, it may be better to preserve the ileum in mucosal colitis and to resect it, even if it is only slightly diseased, in granulomatous colitis.

CLINICAL TYPES

Approximately one-sixth of the colectomies performed at the U.C.L.A. Hospital have been for true emergency situations arising from fulminating colitis. Toxic megacolon is a special syndrome of fulminant colitis, which occurs in approximately two to four per cent of patients (Judd, 1969; Thomford et al., 1969). According to Turnbull (1968), one-fourth of the colectomies for mucosal colitis and one-sixth for transmural colitis are performed for toxic megacolon.

There are 26 patients in the emergency series at the U.C.L.A. Hospital. They represent the most seriously ill patients in our series, but not included are many chronically ill patients who came to operation on an urgent but not emergency basis. These 26 patients are presented in Table 21-2 in which the most compelling indication for operation is matched with the pathologic diagnosis.

This table indicates only the most important aspect of the disease that created the emergency. Several patients with toxic dilatation also had severe bleeding, and some with major hemorrhage might also have been designated as intractable and toxic.

There were only four patients in this series with free intraperitoneal perforations, although this complication was suspected in half the patients with toxic megacolon, many of whom proved to have walled-off perforations. Some of the many patients with toxic megacolon showed characteristics of both diseases, but lacked sufficient specific criteria for accurate classification.

All of the patients in this series were critically ill. In assessing the gravity of the illness, no single presenting complaint is a determining factor. Fifteen patients were female and 11 were male. The age span was between 11 and 70 years with an average age of 27. Table 21-3 shows the age distribution more accurately. The pulse rates upon admission ranged from 72 to 170 per minute, with an average rate of 120. There were only three patients whose pulse rates were under 100 at the time they were admitted for emergency operation; all three of these patients survived. The temperature range at the time of crisis was from 37 to 41° C.

White counts also varied. There were only three patients with less than 10,000 white cells per cubic millimeter. The highest count numbered 39,000; the average count was 15,600. The hemoglobin on admission varied, depending a great deal on how many transfusions had been administered recently. The figures ranged from 8.0 to 13.3 gm., with an average of 11.5 gm.

TABLE 21-2. Fulminant Colitis: Operative Indications and Pathologic Diagnoses

			Pathologic Diagnosis	
	Mucosal	*Transmural*	*Unclassified*	*Total*
Toxic megacolon	10	0	2	12
Toxicity and intractability	2	0	0	2
Free perforation	4	0	3	7
Hemorrhage	0	4	1	5
Total	16	4	6	26

TABLE 21-3. Distribution by Age of Patients with Severe Ulcerative Colitis

Age Groups	Number of Patients
10–15	4
16–20	4
21–25	6
26–30	5
31–35	4
36–40	0
41–45	0
46–50	0
51–55	2
56–60	0
61–65	0
66–70	1

These patients were in serious nutritional disability, often with peripheral edema. The average total protein was 5.3 gm. Several patients had only 4.1 gm. of total protein. The albumin-globulin ratio was rarely normal and usually reversed. There were only three patients who came to emergency operation with over 6 gm. of total protein and none over 7 gm.

These gross clinical observations show nothing specific other than evidence of seriously ill patients who have nutritional disturbances.

Although some of the six unclassified patients might fall into the category of transmural colitis when evaluated by other pathologists, there were only four clear-cut diagnoses of granulomatous disease. During a separate period, a substantial number of patients with granulomatous disease of the colon, many of whom were quite ill, came to operation because of the urgency of chronic sepsis, fistula formation, and debility, but since they were not emergency patients they are not included in this series. Also excluded are a comparable number of patients with inexorable debility due to mucosal colitis.

SPECIFIC LESIONS

TOXIC MEGACOLON

Dilatation of the colon due to either dynamic ileus or distal obstruction is common to many acute, intra-abdominal conditions. Marshak first used the term "megacolon" in ulcerative colitis in 1950. Madison and Bargen described a segmental dilatation of the colon in 1951, and, subsequently, many others have written extensively on this topic.

The term toxic megacolon does not have clearly defined limits. The clinician may ascribe toxic megacolon to any patient who is quite ill, has a silent abdomen, and has some dilatation of the colon. Almost all patients with acute colitis, however, have a certain degree of dilatation. The radiologist is more inclined to restrict the term to extreme dilatation of the colon, particularly the transverse colon, although sometimes the ascending colon and sigmoid are also involved; some radiologists are loath to make this diagnosis unless intramural air can be seen in the colon (Figs. 21-1 and 21-2).

The pathogenesis of toxic megacolon is not clear. The most obvious possibility is a toxic paralysis of the muscle, sometimes abetted or precipitated by atropine or opiates. Deterioration of the myenteric plexuses has been suggested as a cause (Bockus et al., 1958). Mechanical or physiologic overstretching of the muscle fibers may contribute to the condition, as, for instance, when the syndrome is precipitated by a barium enema. In at least one of our patients, necrosis of the muscle of the intestinal wall was present, as described by

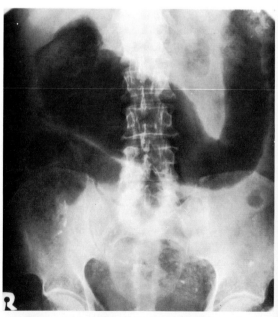

Figure 21-1. Flat film of the abdomen showing dilatation of the ascending and transverse colon. The patient was a 70-year-old man diagnosed as having mucosal colitis, and treated successfully by means of a total colectomy.

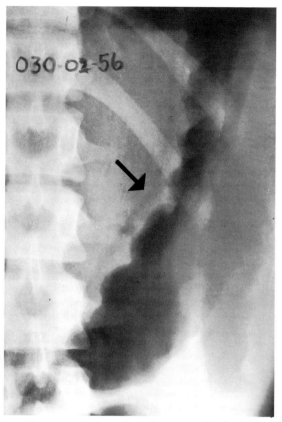

Figure 21-2. An enlarged portion of a flat film of the abdomen showing dilatation of the left transverse and descending colon (arrow). The wall is greatly thickened with some subserosal air. The thickening of the wall and "fingerprinting" suggest Crohn's form of transmural colitis, but the pathologic pattern was typical of mucosal colitis. This 17-year-old girl was treated by means of a two-stage total colectomy. The first stage, subtotal colectomy and ileostomy, was followed by extensive sepsis.

Hickey in 1963. Whether this necrosis allows the distention to occur or whether it is a result of the overdistention is debatable. Total recovery of normal architecture and of intestinal motility in some patients argues against necrosis as the primary cause.

Toxic megacolon has been commonly believed to be restricted to mucosal forms of colitis. Turnbull (1968), however, has cited its common occurrence in transmural

disease, although the question remains as to whether this transmural disease is secondary to the changes of overdistention or really represents the primary pathologic process of granulomatous colitis. In this series there was no clear diagnosis of Crohn's disease among the 12 patients with toxic megacolon (Table 21-4).

Toxic megacolon has also been encountered in acute amebic colitis.

Management

It is generally recognized that surgical management of toxic megacolon has many hazards, serious morbidity, and considerable mortality. For this reason, the internist prefers conservative measures initially, and, indeed, in a variable but significant number of patients with toxic megacolon, recovery does occur with conservative measures. Some of these patients later require colectomy.

MEDICAL TREATMENT. The conservative measures that should be applied initially include rest, antibiotics, and nasogastric suction with a long tube if one can be passed. Restoration of blood volume, of hemoglobin and serum protein levels, and of electrolyte balance is critical. The use of steroids is controversial. If the patient is not already receiving steroids, it is common practice for the gastroenterologist to use either an adrenal steroid or ACTH in an attempt to produce a remission. Some physicians believe that even when a patient is inevitably going to surgery, steroids should be added to prepare him for operation, but there is no evidence that this is effective. No atropine or anticholinergic drugs of any kind, no opiates, and no barium enemas should be administered, since all of these have been implicated in precipitating toxic megacolon (Smith et al., 1962).

Once a patient is started on this regimen, which must be carried out with vigor, failure to improve or even slight deterioration should be considered an urgent reason for

TABLE 21-4. Results of Operation for Toxic Megacolon

	Total Colectomy	Subtotal Colectomy	Hemicolectomy
Survived	3	4°	2
Died	1	2	0

°One patient was not operated on for fulminant colitis and is not properly a part of this series.

operation (Goligher et al., 1967). The surgeon should be brought into consultation early for such a patient.

The immediate results of medical therapy are less favorable when viewed in the light of the late results reported by Crile and Thomas (1968). Only 13 per cent of patients treated medically were fully rehabilitated, and 73 per cent died in two to nine years, whereas substantially all the survivors of surgical treatment were fully rehabilitated.

SURGICAL TREATMENT. It is commonly accepted that total proctocolectomy in one or two stages is a curative operation in the *elective* treatment of colitis. Total colectomy and ileostomy in toxic megacolon, however, is attended by a serious mortality rate. The addition of a resection of the perineal colon is often too much for the sick patient. The pelvic colon is left as a mucous fistula. When a toxic megacolon has perforated freely, it is clear that resection of the colon in the area of perforation is necessary, and failure to do so is usually lethal. Walled-off perforations without generalized peritonitis present a different problem and are best left undisturbed (Turnbull, 1968). They represent deep ulcerations whose base is actually an adjacent serosal surface (Garnjobst and Hardwick, 1968).

Most surgeons have reported a mortality rate of from 10 to 35 per cent for total colectomy in the presence of toxic megacolon. Most of these deaths are related to contamination, either established or iatrogenic (Turnbull, 1968). Some form of surgical therapy other than the usual radical colectomy must be considered in some cases.

Operation cannot be deferred in the patient with a free perforation, and the "risk" of sepsis here must be accepted since it already exists. On the other hand, to create peritoneal sepsis by breaking into walled-off perforations in an as yet uncontaminated peritoneal cavity is a serious error. The following alternatives, therefore, seem possible:

ILEOSTOMY ALONE. An ileostomy is made in the right lower quadrant without resection of the colon. The distal ileum is exteriorized as a mucous fistula and a large catheter is introduced through it into the cecum. The colon can be decompressed through this catheter.

The drawback of this procedure is that it is difficult to construct a good permanent ileostomy unless the ascending colon has been mobilized. Furthermore, it may not be possible to drain and deflate the transverse colon and sigmoid through a catheter in the terminal ileum and ascending colon.

CECOSTOMY. Cecostomy is perhaps the simplest of all the procedures, but, again, it may not succeed in decompressing the transverse colon and the sigmoid colon. Lyons (1960) and Klein et al. (1960), who have advocated this procedure, note that on occasion full remission of the disease occurs and no further operative procedure is required. If further operation is required, however, the presence of the cecostomy may complicate the formation of a proper ileostomy because of sepsis in the flank, although sometimes the site of the cecostomy may be used successfully as the site of the proposed ileostomy.

LOOP ILEOSTOMY AND COLOSTOMY. Turnbull (1968) has advocated the following course. The abdomen is explored through a lower midline incision and if there are no free perforations, ileostomy and colectomy are performed. The colon is first deflated, however, through a large tube placed in the rectum before operation and guided by intra-abdominal manipulation into the appropriate part of the colon to allow the decompression. The contents of the dilated proximal colon can often be gently emptied into the distal colon and so deflated by way of the tube. The bowel wall therefore becomes thicker and less fragile before attempts are made to mobilize it.

If on the other hand, there are walled-off perforations or if the small bowel is intimately adherent to the colon, only a loop ileostomy in continuity is made along with a "blow-hole" colostomy in the transverse colon to decompress the colon. This "blow-hole" colostomy is performed by making a short epigastric incision over the most likely presenting point of the transverse colon, and as the colon rises into the wound the edges are sutured to the structures of the belly wall. The wound is closed and the ileostomy is matured. Only then is the colon deflated by means of an incision. When it is deflated, the colon becomes redundant and the edges rise into the wound where they can be carefully sutured to the skin.

When free perforation is present, mobilization and exteriorization of the bowel should be performed.

ILEOSTOMY AND HEMICOLECTOMY. As a general principle in ileostomy and colectomy, the ileostomy is made as soon as the right colon has been mobilized, so that the procedure may be terminated at any time by closure of the abdomen, with exteriorization of the amount of colon that has been mobilized. Failure to do this may result in the need to attempt a good ileostomy in haste under conditions of serious stress, lightened anesthesia, and hypotension. In our series two patients were treated by ileostomy, and, after mobilization of the right colon, this portion of bowel was exteriorized. Deflation and amputation left only the mucous fistula as a transverse colostomy. A better permanent ileostomy is created with the ascending colon out of the way. There is minimal contamination associated with the division of the ileum alone.

The ascending colon, which has been the most common site of free perforations in our experience, is removed by this procedure. This partial colectomy may be all that need be done at this time. The bowel that is mobilized is the portion that is easiest to handle. The most difficult area to mobilize and the one most subject to iatrogenic injury, the splenic colon, is left for later removal. Table 21-4 gives a summary of our results in the management of toxic megacolon and free perforation. One patient bled postoperatively from the mucous fistula and in one patient the mucous fistula perforated, leading to extensive complications of intraperitoneal abscess.

Role of Steroids

Marx and Barker (1967) stated that there was no qualitative difference in the degree of complications among comparable groups of patients with unclassified ulcerative colitis, treated with or without steroids. Our belief now is that steroids in mucosal disease may have a more deleterious effect than they do in granulomatous disease.

Two patients who had mucosal colitis (one in this series and one in our previous experience) and who were on steroid therapy suffered exsanguinating hemorrhage from gastritis or a gastric ulcer. At least two other patients with mucosal colitis suffered spontaneous perforations of the small bowel while on steroid therapy. These major complications may have been related in part to severe sepsis, but this pattern, fortunately infrequent, seems to be restricted to the combination of mucosal disease and steroid therapy.

Three of the eight patients in this group with toxic megacolon died after operation, and of the four who were not on steroids only one died. If the patient is not already on steroids or ACTH, these drugs should not be added to the regimen in order to "build him up." If they are added to the regimen in order to try to avoid an operation, operation should quickly follow unless prompt remission is obtained. The brief use of steroids under these circumstances does not seriously increase morbidity; it does, however, intangibly but undoubtedly blunt the sharpness of many of the clinical criteria important in recognizing surgical catastrophes.

FREE PERFORATION

Although the discovery of perforation was feared to some degree in almost every case of toxic megacolon, it was much more common to find only walled-off perforations. Some patients not classified as having toxic megacolon may have been decompressed by free perforations, which implies that toxic megacolon may have been present before the free perforation.

Free perforations were encountered in eight patients, of whom only four survived. Free perforation demands resection or at least exteriorization of the involved portion of colon. The treatment of intraperitoneal sepsis and its complications is discussed in detail in another chapter of this book. Our methods of treatment include the use of generous intraperitoneal lavage and débridement, antibiotics both systemically and by catheter infusion into the peritoneal cavity, and all other general supporting measures. Drains into areas of potential abscess should be left in place for long periods of time; Turnbull (1968) recommends 21 days. The surgical drainage of abscesses that develop after such a gross contamination must be performed carefully in order to avoid creating a defect in fragile bowel wall that may lead to the development of intestinal fistula.

HEMORRHAGE

Hemorrhage of sufficient quantity or anemia severe enough to require transfusions is standard in this group of patients. Exsanguinating hemorrhage, however, was the principal cause for operation in only four patients, all of whom incidentally had granulomatous transmural colitis. In addition, six other patients had serious hemorrhage added to their other primary indications. The volumes of blood given were often in the range of 10 to 20 units per day for several days. Operation should be considered for a chronically or acutely ill patient who requires more than five units to replace acute blood loss.

When hemorrhage is a major indication for operation, anything short of total colectomy is hazardous because bleeding may continue from the rectosigmoid segment. When such an operation seems to be of a greater magnitude than the patient can tolerate, control of the bleeding may be accomplished by means of division of the inferior mesenteric artery. Bleeding continuing or arising from the rectal segment after less than total colectomy may be treated by iced saline irrigations or by irrigation with thrombin solution, if a mucous fistula exists. Uncontrolled bleeding from such a segment may force an abdominoperineal resection earlier than otherwise planned.

When acute and life-threatening situations, such as toxic dilatation, free perforation, or acute exsanguinating hemorrhage, occur, one must remember that the patient who has not had a protracted period of suffering with the distresses of chronic colitis may not accept the compromise of a permanent ileostomy as freely as does the patient who has a long history of disease.

GENERALIZED TOXICITY

In two patients systemic toxicity and hemorrhage served as indications for operation, but dilatation of the colon had not reached a degree sufficient to warrant the diagnosis of toxic megacolon. Both of these patients survived. Their course was relatively benign in contrast to the hectic complications experienced by those patients in whom the disease had been allowed to progress to the stage of specific indications, such as perforation, exsanguination, or toxic megacolon.

PRESERVATION OF THE RECTUM

Total proctocolectomy is advised when the diagnosis of mucosal colitis is certain and when the patient can tolerate the operation in one stage; it is mandatory regardless of the diagnosis, if hemorrhage from the rectosigmoid segment is a major risk.

On the other hand, preservation of the rectum may be advised when active rectal disease is not found and segmental granulomatous colitis is suspected, as well as when the patient with either toxic megacolon or free perforation does not seem able to tolerate the addition of the pelvic dissection to the abdominal colectomy, even when the dissection can be done completely from within the abdomen.

The creation of an ileoproctostomy under these emergency conditions is an unwarranted risk.

COMPLICATIONS

The most obvious complications to be expected have already been mentioned but may properly be discussed separately.

Many of the complications are those generally expected in critically ill patients, but some are either specifically identified with ileostomy or with the two forms of disease for which the operation is performed. Intraperitoneal sepsis has been mentioned and is discussed elsewhere in detail. *Subcutaneous* wound infections are also common, and it is desirable to leave the wound open for delayed or delayed primary closure when serious contamination has been encountered.

Failure of a wound to heal well can be attributed to serious nutritional deficits and, perhaps, to steroid therapy. The failure to use retention sutures in these critically ill patients was associated with dehiscence in two of nine patients. Ehrlich and Hunt (1968) have recently advocated the use of large quantities of vitamin A (50,000 units three times a day for five days) as a specific means of restoring the delayed wound healing of steroid therapy to normal.

Venous thrombosis has been a common problem in ulcerative colitis (Graef et al., 1966). One patient in the series died of pulmonary embolism in part, but at least three others suffered infarcts.

Two patients who experienced major postoperative intestinal *hemorrhage* developed the hemorrhagic diathesis after a massive transfusion of blood, but their deaths were due, at least in part, to the initially uncontrollable gastric hemorrhage that required the transfusions.

Spontaneous perforation of the small bowel was observed in one patient in this series (see earlier discussion) and has been observed in other patients.

Acute renal failure and suppurative cholangitis were also encountered. Severe electrolyte disturbances were common, and one patient died of cardiac complications when severe hyperkalemia followed a protracted period of hypokalemia without recognized renal failure.

Several patients experienced intestinal obstruction due to adhesive bands. More specific dysfunction (serositis) or cicatrization is no more common than in any other operation for mucosal or transmural colitis.

OTHER TYPES OF ACUTE COLITIS

Necrotizing enterocolitis of the newborn is an unrelated lesion. It often develops in children in whom some episode of shock or poor perfusion has occurred. It is characterized by vomiting, distention, toxicity, and the accumulation of intraluminal gas. Intramural gas is a characteristic but not routine finding. Prompt surgical therapy is necessary for survival (Stevenson et al., 1969).

Part of the clinical picture that occurs with untreated megacolon of *Hirschsprung's disease* is enterocolitis, which may be mistaken for a toxic dilatation due to ulcerative colitis. Resection of the dilated colon under these circumstances would not be preferable, for if it were decompressed it might be possible to use it later after resecting the aganglionic distal segment.

The finding of "toxic dilatation" in a young child who has suffered constipation and distention since birth would therefore best be treated by less radical procedures than total colectomy until normal ganglion cells can be proved to be present throughout the distal bowel.

Amebic colitis does at times come to medical attention initially as toxic megacolon (Wruble et al., 1966; Faegenburg et al., 1967). Two patients have been seen at U.C.L.A., one an adult and one a child, both of whom died. The characteristics of this disease include extensive muscle necrosis and serious pericolitis, a combination that makes surgical intervention most hazardous (Fig. 21-3). Since a specific etiologic agent is responsible and relatively specific therapy is available, operation should be restricted to preventing further distention and to correcting existing overdistention. Early loop ileostomy and decompression by rectal tube or by "blow-hole" colostomy would seem ideal. The risk of chronic amebic wound sepsis at the site of a colostomy might be feared as a possible complication of colostomy.

In some parts of the world where fulminant amebic colitis is common, it is common practice to use antiamebic therapy before submitting any patient to surgery, except when an immediate threat to life exists (Doxiades, 1968). It is not clear whether the remissions seen when the amebic etiology cannot be proved are caused by a specific effect on a cryptic amebiasis or whether the nonspecific inflammatory reaction is responsible.

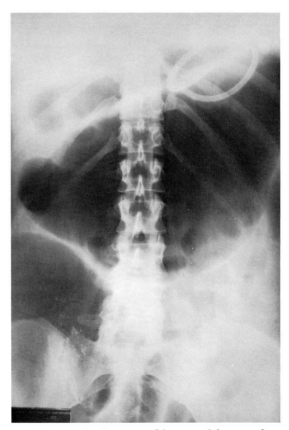

Figure 21-3. Extensive dilatation of the ascending and especially the transverse colon in a 41-year-old woman with toxic dilatation due to amebiasis. The patient had Pseudomonas septicemia. She died following ileostomy and colectomy. Extensive peritonitis and intestinal necrosis were encountered at operation.

REFERENCES

Bockus, H. L., et al.: Ulcerative colitis I. Classification of types—clinical behaviour—life history—prognosis. In Avery Jones, F., (ed.): Modern Trends in Gastroenterology, New York, Paul B. Hoeber, Inc., 1958, pp. 296–314.

Crile, G., Jr., and Thomas, C. Y., Jr.: The treatment of acute toxic ulcerative colitis by ileostomy and simultaneous colectomy. Gastroenterology, 54(Supple.):811, 1968.

Doxiades, T.: Personal communication, 1968.

Ehrlich, H. P., and Hunt, T. K.: Effects of cortisone and vitamin A on wound healing. Ann. Surg., 167:324, 1968.

Faegenburg, D., Chief, H., Mandel, P. R., and Ross, S. T.: Toxic megacolon in amebic colitis. Report of a case. Amer. J. Roentgen., 99:74, 1967.

Ferguson, L. K., and Stevens, L. W.: The surgery of complications of ulcerative colitis. Gastroenterology, 11:640, 1948.

Garnjobst, W., and Hardwick, C.: Toxic dilatation in ulcerative colitis. Hazard of intraoperative contamination. Amer. Surg., 34:519, 1968.

Goligher, J. C., deDombal, F. T., Graham, N. G., and Watkinson, G.: Early surgery in the management of severe ulcerative colitis. Brit. Med. J., 3:193, 1967.

Graef, V., Baggenstoss, A. H., Sauer, W. G., and Spittell, J. A., Jr.: Venous thrombosis occurring in nonspecific ulcerative colitis. A necropsy study. Arch. Intern. Med., 117:377, 1966.

Hickey, R. C., Tidrick, R. T., and Layton, J. M.: Fulminating colitis with colonic wall necrosis. Arch. Surg., 86:764, 1963.

Judd, E. S.: Current surgical aspects of toxic megacolon. Surgery, 65:401, 1969.

Klein, S. H., Edelman, S., Kirschner, P. A., Lyons, A. S., and Baronofsky, I. D.: Emergency cecostomy in ulcerative colitis with acute toxic dilatation. Surgery, 47:399, 1960.

Lockhart-Mummery, H. E., and Morson, B. C.: Crohn's disease (regional enteritis) of the large intestine and its distinction from ulcerative colitis. Gut, 1:87, 1960.

Lockhart-Mummery, H. E., and Morson, B. C.: Crohn's disease of the large intestine. Gut, 5:493, 1964.

Lyons, A. S., Edelman, S., and Baronofsky, I. D.: The place of fecal diverting procedure in the surgical treatment of ulcerative colitis. Ann. Surg., 151:169, 1960.

Madison, M. S., and Bargen, J. A.: Fulminating ulcerative colitis with segmental dilatation of the colon; report of one patient. Proc. Mayo Clin., 26:21, 1951.

Marshak, R. H.: Ulcerative and granulomatous colitis, at U.C.L.A. Seminar in Surgery, Feb. 26, 1969. Unpublished.

Marshak, R. H., Lester, L. J., and Friedman, A. J.: Megacolon; complication of ulcerative colitis. Gastroenterology, 16:768, 1950.

Marx, F. W., Jr., and Barker, W. F.: Surgical results in patients with ulcerative colitis treated with and without corticosteroids. Amer. J. Surg., 113:157, 1967.

Smith, F. W., Law, D. H., Nickel, W. F., Jr., and Sleisenger, M. H.: Fulminant ulcerative colitis with toxic dilatation of the colon: Medical and surgical management of eleven cases with observations regarding etiology. Gastroenterology, 42:233, 1962.

Sparberg, M., and Knudsen, K. B.: Fulminant ulcerative colitis with a normal rectum. Amer. J. Dig. Dis., 12:923, 1967.

Stevenson, J. K., Graham, C. B., Oliver, T. K., Jr., and Goldenberg, V. E.: Neonatal necrotizing enterocolitis. A report of twenty-one cases with fourteen survivors. Amer. J. Surg., 118:260, 1969.

Thomford, N. R., Rybak, J. J., and Pace, W. G.: Toxic megacolon. Surg. Gynec. Obstet., 128:21, 1969.

Turnbull, R. B., Jr., Schofield, P. F., and Hawk, W. A.: Nonspecific ulcerative colitis. In Welch, Claude E., (ed.): Advances in Surgery. vol. 3, Chicago, Year Book Medical Publishers, Inc., 1968, pp. 161–225.

Wolf, B. S., and Marshak, R. H.: Granulomatous colitis (Crohn's disease of the colon); roentgen features. Amer. J. Roentgen., 88:662, 1962.

Wruble, L. D., Duckworth, J. K., Duke, D. D., and Rothschild, J. A.: Toxic dilatation of the colon in a case of amebiasis. New Eng. J. Med., 275:926, 1966.

CHAPTER 22

ENDOCRINE EMERGENCIES

by JAMES D. HARDY, M.D., F.A.C.S. and CARLOS M. CHAVEZ, M.D., F.A.C.S.

Carlos M. Chavez was born in Lima, Peru, and there completed his medical school training with special experience in both anatomy and pathology. He later served fellowships at Massachusetts General Hospital, Methodist Hospital in Houston, and the University of Mississippi Medical Center. He is deeply versed in all phases of angiology, and his special interest in the endocrine organs came initially through angiographic studies directed toward delineation of their anatomic, pathologic, and functional characteristics.

Endocrine crises are met on all general surgical services. The purpose here is to examine briefly a variety of endocrine crises and to present appropriate management (Fig. 22-1). Certain of the conditions to be considered are apt to be far more severe and life-threatening than others, but under special circumstances any one of these states of endocrine dysfunction can prove hazardous if not fatal.

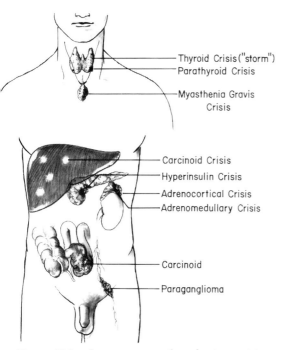

Figure 22-1. Some causes of endocrine crisis.

Thyroid Crisis("storm")
Parathyroid Crisis
Myasthenia Gravis Crisis
Carcinoid Crisis
Hyperinsulin Crisis
Adrenocortical Crisis
Adrenomedullary Crisis
Carcinoid
Paraganglioma

THYROID CRISIS (STORM)

Thyrotoxic crisis represents a major medical emergency. The clinical phenomena are related in some way to increased amounts of circulating thyroid hormones. It has been suggested that the symptomatology represents the net result of an increased sensitization of the tissues to endogenous catecholamines, but this disputed hypothesis does not explain the entire picture. A relative adrenocortical insufficiency has also been postulated. Thyroid crises may occur spontaneously in patients with pre-existing thyrotoxicosis, and it also occurs following thyroidectomy or other operation in patients with hyperthyroidism.

Nelson and Becker (1969) reviewed 21 patients with thyroid crises who had been treated over a period of 19 years at Charity Hospital in New Orleans. In only two instances had the crisis followed an operation, and they attributed this low incidence to the effectiveness of antithyroid drugs in rendering most patients euthyroid prior to surgery. Sixteen patients had died and 13 had been autopsied. Pulmonary infection had been a common complicating factor and, if not present originally, respiratory distress was a prominent feature of the multiple organ decompensation complex that was likely to develop. All patients exhibited objective evidence of thyroid hyperactivity. Their youngest patient was 20 and the oldest 73 years, but we have observed thyrotoxic crisis in childhood.

SIGNS AND SYMPTOMS

The patient typically exhibits tachycardia, tremor, agitation, sweating, fever, dyspnea, disorientation, and, later, delirium. Heart failure may develop. When the patient with a goiter presents such clinical findings either before or after operation, the presumptive diagnosis of impending thyroid crisis should be made and acted upon, unless some other adequate explanation for the symptoms exists.

TREATMENT

The principles of therapy have been examined by Ingbar (1966), Schottstaedt and Smoller (1966), Thompson and Fry (1964), and Waldstein (1960). In thyroid crisis it may be possible to discern different aspects of the disorder that require specific treatment. The overproduction of thyroid hormones should be suppressed to the extent possible. Decompensation of organ systems such as those of respiration and circulation represents an additional aspect of the syndrome. Still another consideration is the disease or diseases that may have precipitated the crisis, if it did not follow operation.

General therapeutic measures include bedrest, sedation, oxygen administration, and control of excessive fever with a cooling blanket. Antithyroid drugs that may be helpful are methimazole (Tapazole) and propylthiouracil (PTU). Either of these agents may be given orally, methimazole in doses of 20 to 30 mg. every six hours and PTU 200 to 300 mg. every six hours. A stomach tube may be necessary in the uncooperative or unconscious patient. Iodides should also be given to block the release of preformed thyroid hormone and, to a lesser degree, to interfere with hormone synthesis. Sodium iodide may be given by intravenous drip at a rate of 1 gm. every six hours.

The important role of endogenous catecholamines in producing the clinical manifestations of thyroid crisis has often been emphasized. Thus, both reserpine and guanethidine have been used to suppress adrenergic effects. Reserpine may cause release of stored catecholamines, but it also blocks their effects. It should be given in doses of approximately 2 mg. intramuscularly every four to six hours as needed to control agitation and tachycardia. Guanethidine is also effective in blocking the release and thus the effects of catecholamines, and may be given orally in a dose of 100 to 200 mg. every 24 hours. This drug does not have the sedative effect of reserpine. We have used reserpine in the management of severe thyrotoxicosis bordering on thyroid storm, but we have not been convinced that this drug is as valuable for this purpose as it has been reported to be. Furthermore, large doses have effects that may render interpretation of the patient's true condition difficult. If morphine is used for sedation it should be used in multiple small or moderate doses.

The need to support various organ systems that may be failing has been mentioned. The failure of the heat-regulating system may permit severe hyperthermia, and this is prevented by artificial cooling of the patient. Cardiac failure, often high-output in type, is treated by digitalization. Cardiac arrhythmias should be controlled by appropriate drug therapy (see Chapter 27), including propanolol (Das and Krieger, 1969). Since hepatic failure as manifested by jaundice has often occurred, a slow but continuous intravenous drip of glucose and water-soluble vitamins is advisable to maintain caloric intake and glycogen reserves, with whatever protection of the liver this can afford. Respiratory insufficiency in the extremely weak or comatose patient should be treated with positive pressure-assisted ventilation with an oxygen-rich mixture, using an indwelling nasotracheal tube or, less optimally, tracheostomy with a cuffed tube. Bronchodilators may be helpful.

The value of glucocorticoid therapy remains in doubt, but this hormone has been recommended for the treatment of thyroid storm. Indeed, at one time it was suggested that thyroid crisis represented, in net metabolic effect, acute adrenocortical insufficiency. In practice, however, whereas large doses of hydrocortisone on the order of 500 mg. every 24 hours may have been helpful in some cases, this treatment alone will not abolish all the physiologic derangements seen in thyroid crisis. Therefore, we view corticoid therapy as simply another modality that may be beneficial in the overall management of severe hyperthyroid crisis.

If infection is found or suspected in the patient with thyroid crisis, appropriate antibiotic coverage should be combined with other measures that may be indicated for dealing with the infection problem effectively.

Unfortunately, the mortality rate among patients with full-blown thyroid storm remains high regardless of what therapeutic measures are employed. Thus, every effort should be made to avoid this complication by early and effective treatment of recognized thyrotoxicosis.

CASE STUDY (1). FATAL THYROID CRISIS FOLLOWING LAPAROTOMY FOR INTESTINAL OBSTRUCTION IN A THYROTOXIC PATIENT

L. B., a 52-year-old Negro housewife, was admitted to University Hospital on August 24, 1959, with a three-month history of nervousness, a 10 to 12 lb. (4.5 to 5.4 kg.) weight loss, and swelling of the neck. Examination disclosed a diffuse goiter and chest x-ray revealed a left superior mediastinal mass. The BMR was +65, but the 131-iodine uptake was only high normal. Administration of 100 mg. of propylthiouracil every eight hours and reserpine 1.25 mg. daily was begun. Evidence of thyrotoxicosis fluctuated from time to time, and, in general, control was considered to be unsatisfactory for several reasons. Thus, on April 8 she was given 25 mc. of I^{131} orally and was discharged on April 15, 1960.

She was readmitted to the Emergency Room on April 30 with a two-day history of cramping epigastric pain of sudden onset and no bowel movement for two days, with nausea and vomiting. Physical examination revealed abdominal tenderness with obstructive peristalsis. Roentgenograms demonstrated distended small bowel. Atrial fibrillation was present, with a pulse rate of 208 per min., and the oral temperature was 100° F. (37.8° C.). She was digitalized and received sodium iodide intravenously every eight hours. When the signs of small bowel obstruction grew worse, operation was judged mandatory.

At laparotomy on April 30, markedly distended and pregangrenous small bowel was liberated by dividing multiple adhesions. In the immediate postoperative period she was critically ill with a pulse rate of 140 per min. and a rectal temperature of 104° F. (40.0° C.), which was reduced with a cooling blanket. A reserpine drip was started, but after 1 mg. had been given the blood pressure declined and the drug was stopped. Sodium iodide and Solu-Cortef were given intravenously but to no avail. An endotracheal tube was inserted for better ventilation in the now semicomatose patient. Later, large amounts of norepinephrine had to be instilled to maintain a detectable blood pressure. By the morning of May 3, however, it was possible to halt the vasopressor support, with maintenance of a good blood pressure and adequate urine output. Nevertheless, she was still severely obtunded. Unfortunately, late that afternoon the blood pressure and urine output declined rapidly over a 30-minute period and cardiopulmonary arrest occurred. All measures at resuscitation were unavailing.

COMMENT

This patient was never adequately controlled from the time her hyperthyroidism was first discovered. It was distressing that emergency laparotomy, for release of pregangrenous small bowel, had to be performed before the radioactive iodine could have rendered her euthyroid. She died from a complex state of metabolic exhaustion at a time when the attending physicians had begun to believe she would survive. The cause of death in thyroid storm is still unknown, the mortality rate is high, and the best management consists of prevention.

PARATHYROID CRISES

HYPERPARATHYROID CRISIS

Our knowledge of serum calcium regulation and the complex role of calcium in the body economy continues to develop. Newer information includes the discovery of thyrocalcitonin, the intimate relationship of serum calcium levels to gastric acid secretion, and "parathormone" secretion by lung, kidney, and skin malignancies. All these considerations are of much interest and importance in surgical practice. Nevertheless, it is the specific problems of severe hypercalcemia or crisis precipitated by a functioning parathyroid adenoma and the severe hypocalcemia that often follows removal of a large functioning adenoma that will be considered here.

THE SYNDROME OF HYPERCALCEMIA

An increased serum calcium level may produce a variety of clinical manifestations resulting from its effects on different systems. The retarded neuromuscular transmission is only the accentuation of the usual physiologic effect of this ion. Action upon the gastrointestinal tract will result in constipation owing to the decrease in gastrointestinal motility. Vomiting may be troublesome, as may be pruritus. Associated pancreatitis may complicate the picture (Cope et al., 1957; Fink and Finfrock, 1961). Fatigue, lethargy, and disturbances of behavior, including frank psychosis, may be the predominant features of this syndrome because of profound neurologic effects. Diagnosis is often greatly delayed owing to the nonspecific nature of these symptoms.

Hypercalcemia may be found in a variety of conditions that affect the absorption, transport, mobilization, and utilization of this ion. In addition to parathyroid gland hyperactivity, other conditions associated with various degrees of hypercalcemia include the milk-alkali syndrome, vitamin D intoxication, multiple myeloma, and sarcoidosis. Furthermore, lymphomas and malignant epithelial cell tumors of various organs may produce parathormone-like substances that cause hypercalcemia. For example, carcinoma of the lung, kidney, bladder, pancreas, breast, and intestine may rarely produce hypercalcemia, even though no distant or bone metastases are demonstrable. Hypercalcemia has also been observed in hyperthyroidism and occasionally in Cushing's disease. Thus the finding of an elevated serum calcium level requires a careful differential diagnosis.

Elevation of the serum calcium to a level high enough to produce hypercalcemia crisis is most commonly found in three conditions: (a) parathyroid adenoma or hyperplasia, (b) disseminated carcinoma with bone metastases, and (c) nonparathyroid parathormone-secreting malignant tumors. Renal impairment with elevation of the BUN and creatinine levels is most commonly found in patients with hypercalcemic crisis due to primary hyperparathyroidism, and is usually absent in the other two conditions. Prerenal azotemia accompanying dehydration is frequently seen with hypercalcemia of any origin. An important point is that hypercalcemia is rarely found associated with hypophosphatemia except in hyperparathyroidism (and with parathormone-secreting tumors), though the serum-phosphorus level is being accorded less and less significance in the diagnostic requirements of hyperparathyroidism as well.

The patient whose serum-calcium level is found elevated on routine screening should be carefully studied to identify the precise cause. It was once considered almost essential for the diagnosis of hyperparathyroidism that the adult patient excrete more than 300 mgm. of calcium in the urine per 24 hours on a dairy-free diet, but we have had patients with renal stones and a functioning parathyroid adenoma whose calcium excretion was normal. Actually, the operative procedure itself is attended by such minimal morbidity and mortality rates that the risk of operation is no greater and perhaps less than that of leaving a functioning parathyroid adenoma.

In some patients with normocalcemia, operated upon because of calcium-containing renal stones and perhaps an increased calcium excretion, a parathyroid tumor has been found.

In addition to measurements of serum-calcium and serum-phosphorus values, alkaline phosphatase, and urine calcium excretion, other methods for identifying the presence of a functioning parathyroid adenoma include actual immunoassay measurement of the serum-parathormone levels, selenium isotope scans, selective arteriography, barium swallow to demonstrate compression of the esophagus, and actual palpation of the tumor. However, the tumor is usually too small or too soft to palpate and the other methods are fairly gross. Therefore, for practical purposes the diagnosis is usually made on the basis of the serum-calcium and serum-phosphorus values.

Management of Hypercalcemia

Most patients with functioning parathyroid adenomas that produce severe hypercalcemia will have had the tumor for quite some time. In our experience, the magnitude of the elevation in serum calcium is more or less directly proportional to the size of the tumor but, of course, disparities do occur. Parathyroid crisis, with serum-calcium levels of above 18 mg. per 100 ml. or 9 mEq./l., is usually associated with a tumor that is one or more centimeters in size and may weigh many grams. When the serum calcium level exceeds 18 mg. per 100 ml., dangerous symptoms of parathyroid crisis should be anticipated if they are not already present.

TEMPORARY MEASURES TO CONTROL HYPERCALCEMIA. Several methods for lowering the serum-calcium level have been described, most of them successfully used in particular situations and individually advocated by those who found them effective in their experience. A low-calcium diet is invariably used to decrease intake of the ion. The use of the disodium salt of ethylenediaminetetra-acetic acid (EDTA) as a chelating agent has found little application. Its effect is transitory and is not free of toxic effects (Anglem, 1966). Actinomycin D has been found to inhibit hypercalcemia induced experimentally by the administration of large doses of parathormone or vitamin D (Eisenstein and Passavoy, 1964; Rasmussen and

Hawker, 1964), but there is as yet little evidence that it is valuable clinically. Thyrocalcitonin may eventually prove to be of value in the treatment of the acute crisis of hypercalcemia (Buckle et al., 1969).

The effectiveness of inorganic phosphate and sulfate solutions in the treatment of acute hypercalcemic conditions has been stressed by Latimer (1968). The phosphate solution acts by exceeding the solubility of calcium phosphate, a displacing phenomenon. It acts rapidly with a prolonged effect, but it causes the inconvenience of extraosseous calcium deposits and, if not well controlled, severe hypocalcemia may result. The sulfate solution, however, acts upon the kidneys to increase the excretion of calcium. It is less rapid in action (3 hours) and may produce hypomagnesemia by promoting renal excretion of magnesium.

Hydration alone may control the situation and, if not, should certainly be employed with any of the agents mentioned. If renal function is adequate, forced fluids are helpful. Glucocorticoids control hypercalcemia if it is not of excess parathormone origin.

Hemodialysis or peritoneal dialysis is also a valuable adjunct in the emergency treatment of hypercalcemic crisis. A calcium-free dialysate will rapidly produce a transfer of serum calcium to the dialysing solution and its elimination, thus lowering the plasma concentration of this ion.

OPERATIVE TREATMENT. The definitive treatment for hyperparathyroidism is surgical. With the introduction of several of the nonoperative measures to treat acute hypercalcemia, emergency parathyroidectomy is not frequently performed at the present time, and operation can be performed after appropriate preparations have been made. Exploration of the neck should be carefully done, identifying all four parathyroid glands, since approximately 10 per cent of parathyroid adenomas are multiple. The search is best achieved in a bloodless field, using sutures to retract the thyroid gland and making positive identification of each parathyroid gland by taking a tiny piece for biopsy. The gland should not be denuded of its blood supply, which enters a small hilum on the medial aspect. Traction on a fine suture passed through the lateral margin of the parathyroid gland facilitates the snipping off of a tiny sliver for microscopic identification. If no tumor is found at the time of exploration

and the parathyroid glands are not enlarged, an anterior mediastinal exploration should be done through the neck incision, though at times it may be necessary to divide the sternum.

If the tumor cannot be located, an operative arteriogram may disclose its position. The adenoma will most often involve one of the lower parathyroid glands, and it may be imbedded in the superior aspect of the thymus. It may rarely be situated within the tissue of the right or left thyroid lobe, and subtotal thyroidectomy has been advocated when the adenoma is not found elsewhere. Actually, in some patients, elements of the thymus gland extend upward to lie against the lower poles of the thyroid gland. It is not at all rare to find a parathyroid gland in a cervical extension of the thymus gland. We had one patient who had four normal parathyroid glands in the neck, and a huge (31,000 mg.) adenoma in the mediastinum at the level of the eighth rib posteriorly (Hardy et al., 1964). The venous blood draining from the tumor had a strong "parathormone" effect on bioassay (Hardy and Eraslan, 1963). Rarely, the patient may have only three parathyroids. A normal gland weighs from 30 to 40 mg.

Removal of a large functioning adenoma is occasionally followed by a precipitous fall in the serum-calcium level within 24 hours, producing "hypoparathyroid crisis."

HYPOPARATHYROID CRISIS

ETIOLOGY

On surgical services, severe hypocalcemia most often follows injury to the parathyroid glands during thyroid surgery or the excision of a functioning parathyroid adenoma.

Hypoparathyroidism Following Thyroid Surgery

It has been estimated that about 2 per cent of patients undergoing thyroid surgery will develop symptoms of tetany postoperatively. Hypoparathyroidism is more frequent following total thyroidectomy, but it is occasionally seen also after subtotal thyroidectomy when it is usually temporary. To prevent the occurrence of permanent hypoparathyroidism, a careful dissection and close inspection of the thyroid to be excised is necessary.

Biopsy and frozen section examination of any likely structure should be performed if necessary to avoid removal of normal parathyroid tissue. However, with experience one learns to recognize the normal parathyroid glands in the operative field with accuracy.

Hypoparathyroidism Following Parathyroid Surgery

Excision of a functioning parathyroid adenoma is often followed by varying degrees of temporary parathyroid hypofunction and hypocalcemia. In these cases the sudden fall in the serum-calcium level may be caused by a longstanding suppressive action of the functioning adenoma upon the remaining parathyroid glands. Time is required for the remaining "normal" parathyroid glands to resume adequate physiologic activity. However, the hypocalcemia seen in these cases may also be the result of preoperative bone demineralization: the sudden shift of calcium from the serum into bone that follows the removal of the functioning adenoma produces hypocalcemia. This, however, is temporary and the calcium levels return to normal when a balance between bone and serum is re-established. A return of alkaline phosphatase to normal values is a good index of adequate bone mineralization.

The removal of a parathyroid adenoma, and perhaps excessive tissue excised with biopsies taken of the remaining glands, may combine to produce hypocalcemia, when excision of the adenoma alone might not have done so. Subtotal resection of the normal-appearing glands is practiced by some groups (Paloyan et al., 1969), but we currently preserve all but the smallest sliver of the normal glands. However, diffuse hyperplasia of all four parathyroid glands may require subtotal resection of each.

SYMPTOMS AND SIGNS OF HYPOPARATHYROIDISM

The clinical manifestations of hypoparathyroidism are related to the effects of hypocalcemia. Low serum-calcium levels increase neuromuscular excitability, which in its early stages gives rise to the premonitory symptoms of tingling of the face, fingers, and toes. At this stage or even earlier a positive Chvostek's sign is usually present. If the hypocal-cemia is not relieved, carpopedal spasm usually develops and becomes increasingly prominent. When severe manifestations of hypocalcemia develop, respiration may become difficult, with laryngeal stridor that may be followed by laryngeal spasm, and, rarely, asphyxia if prompt treatment is not instituted. Besides these respiratory problems, the development of tonic muscular contractions or frank convulsions may complicate the clinical picture still further. Rarely, a patient may go into stupor and coma without the development of seizures, tonic contractions, or convulsions (Kreisler et al., 1969).

DIAGNOSIS

A presumptive diagnosis can be made by the history of operation and clinical examination of the patient. Positive Chvostek's and Trousseau's signs should prompt the measurement of the serum-calcium level. Of course, metabolic or respiratory alkalosis can aggravate or precipitate tetany, as may hypomagnesemia: these possibilities should be excluded.

TREATMENT

The initial and usually the most important therapy in this crisis is the intravenous administration of calcium. The most immediate response is obtained with the intravenous injection of ionized calcium chloride in a 10 per cent solution. The administration of 3 to 5 ml. of this solution is usually followed by dramatic improvement in the patient's condition. This preparation, however, is highly irritating and precautions should be taken to avoid extravasation during the injection. A less toxic and more commonly used preparation, but less rapid in action (10 to 20 minutes), is calcium gluconate, also supplied in a 10 per cent solution. The parenteral therapy should be continued until the patient is able to take calcium orally. Calcium lactate given orally in a dose of 3 gm. every four hours will relieve the symptoms in most patients, with adequate amounts of vitamin D. Vitamin D has a delayed action and is not useful in the acute state but only in those cases requiring prolonged treatment. A brief course of parathormone extract may be useful for severe cases. Occasionally the hypocalcemic state is remarkably protracted, requiring prolonged therapy. Of course, if all parathyroid tissue has been destroyed, the condition will be permanent; but even the most severe hypoparathyroid states tend to improve with time, as the body adjusts to a chronically low serum calcium level. However, severe hypocalcemia should be treated appropriately.

In a permanent hypoparathyroid state following total thyroidectomy, adequate thyroid replacement will raise the plasma calcium level and it also improves bone sensitivity to vitamin D.

CASE STUDY (2). HYPOPARATHYROIDISM SECONDARY TO SUBTOTAL THYROIDECTOMY FOR DIFFUSE TOXIC GOITER

F. Mc., a 25-year-old Negro construction worker, had been well until July, 1968, when he developed the usual signs and symptoms of thyrotoxicosis and had a diffuse toxic goiter without exophthalmos. Hyperthyroidism was confirmed with BMR + 39, 131-iodine thyroid uptake 48 per cent, and serum PBI 14.3 mcg./ml. After prolonged treatment with propylthiouracil he underwent subtotal thyroidectomy on March 10, 1969. The operation was routine and was judged to have been uneventful. Both recurrent nerves were exposed and the parathyroid gland beneath the right superior pole was identified and preserved. Otherwise, care was taken to protect other parathyroid glands by the usual inspection of the gland to be removed and by leaving the posterior capsule on both sides.

The patient did well until the day following operation when a positive Chvostek's sign was noted and subsequently the patient complained of numbness and tingling in his face and hands and "tightness" in most of his musculature. The serum calcium level was found to be 6.5 mg. per 100 ml. and the serum phosphorus level was 5.1 mg. per 100 ml. Large amounts of intravenous calcium gluconate were required, with oral calcium lactate in divided doses, to suppress the symptoms of calcium deficiency. Vitamin D was given in a dose of 100,000 units I.M. for five days and then 50,000 units per day by mouth. Even so, the symptoms were managed only with unusual difficulty and the serum calcium level remained low.

Careful study of the tissue removed at operation disclosed only one parathyroid gland, found beneath a remnant of fatty ectopic thymic tissue situated well up on the gland.

The patient required vigorous calcium therapy for almost five months. At this time the serum calcium level was still in the range of 7 to 8 mg. per 100 ml. and he still had a positive Chvostek's sign. However, he had himself discontinued his calcium therapy and was asymptomatic.

COMMENT

The cause of the severe hypoparathyroidism that followed subtotal thyroidectomy in this patient was never fully explained. The operation was performed by an experienced surgeon. One parathyroid gland was definitely identified and preserved; one was excised, buried in innocent-appearing fatty ectopic thymic tissue well up on the gland. The posterior portion of the capsule was left behind on both sides.

It is possible that the patient had less than the usual number of parathyroid glands or that for some reason the function of the residual glands was subnormal. Radioiodine therapy for hyperthyroidism may increase the risk of post-thyroidectomy hypoparathyroidism, and we and others have encountered such circumstances (Hartemann et al., 1969). As regards blood supply, we found that in dogs it was virtually impossible to produce hypoparathyroidism by ligating blood supply to these glands, so long as they were not separated from small vessels at the hilum of the gland.

The clinical course of this patient was fairly typical of severe postoperative hypoparathyroidism. A great deal of intravenous calcium gluconate, oral calcium lactate, perhaps even parathormone initially, and vitamin D may be required to control severe symptomatology during the first days or weeks. As time passes, however, the remaining parathyroid tissue functions more actively, the body adjusts to a chronically low serum calcium level, and symptoms recede even though a positive Chvostek's sign may remain. Even if this sign does not persist overtly, it may be brought out by unusual needs for calcium such as in pregnancy or by stressing the patient with an intravenous infusion of EDTA.

ADRENOCORTICAL CRISIS

ACUTE ADRENOCORTICAL INSUFFICIENCY

Acute adrenocortical insufficiency is now rare. The availability of complete replacement therapy and its effective use have abolished shock due to hypoadrenocorticism following most operations upon the adrenal glands themselves. Nevertheless, adrenocortical crisis still occurs on surgical services, and its very low incidence renders it especially hazardous because this possible cause of metabolic collapse may not even be considered until too late. When the typical picture follows adrenal resection, adrenocortical insufficiency will be suspected and treated appropriately in most instances. However, pre-existing hypoadrenocorticism may not have been suspected if the patient was not known to have adrenal hypofunction. This may have been produced by adrenal metastases from a malignant tumor, chronic cortisone therapy for a condition such as arthritis, idiopathic Addison's disease, tuberculosis of the adrenal glands, or acute hemorrhage into these organs.

A previously undiagnosed pituitary tumor or insufficiency such as Sheehan's syndrome may be responsible for diminished or absent ACTH response to external stress. Unfortunately, in many patients the true cause of the fatal cardiovascular collapse is disclosed only at autopsy.

Acute adrenocortical crisis results from an abrupt disparity between the metabolic need for glucocorticoids and the amount of these hormones available. Thus, severe metabolic stress, as imposed by operation or sepsis, may produce acute adrenocortical insufficiency even when the hormone supply available was adequate during health. Bilateral total adrenalectomy will of course produce shock in the absence of adequate replacement therapy. The adrenal gland opposite the one containing a resected functioning cortical tumor may have undergone atrophy, because its normal ACTH stimulus from the anterior pituitary had been chronically suppressed by corticoids from the tumor; in this circumstance, adequate transoperative and postoperative replacement therapy is essential.

If acute adrenocortical insufficiency is to develop following an operation, it will usually be manifest during the first 72 hours.

CLINICAL FINDINGS

The patient most often exhibits apathy or restlessness, weakness, anorexia, and at times nausea and vomiting. Abdominal pain and diarrhea may appear but tachycardia, fever, and hypotension are the prominent warning signs. The plasma electrolyte levels as well as the blood glucose and urea nitrogen levels are usually normal, since the time has been insufficient to permit significant change. To be sure, chemical measurement of the plasma and urinary steroid values would be helpful, but these determinations are time-consuming and are not to be depended upon in the acute situation. However, the total eosinophile count in the peripheral blood may be indicative: after most major operations the total count falls almost to zero in the presence of normal adrenocortical activity. If significant numbers of eosinophiles are still present in the peripheral blood, adrenocortical insufficiency should be suspected.

TREATMENT

The most important requirement is to suspect that acute adrenocortical insufficiency may exist, for this will lead to appropriate therapy. Even if the diagnosis should be wrong, the short-term administration of cortisone or hydrocortisone has no serious side effects and to fail to give such therapy when needed can result in circulatory collapse, coma, and death. Therefore prompt treatment is indicated as soon as adrenocortical insufficiency is suspected.

Prophylactic therapy in connection with adrenal or other surgery consists of giving 300 mg. of hydrocortisone in divided doses the day of operation, 200 mg. the next day, 100 mg. on each of the next two days, and then slowly tapering off. The steroid therapy should be given by intravenous drip, as well as intramuscularly (see Case 3).

If acute failure is suspected as the cause of the shock that the patient exhibits, a vasopressor drug should be used initially in a saline drip to raise the blood pressure. Simultaneously, 100 mg. of hydrocortisone should be placed in 500 ml. of saline solution and administered at a brisk rate. Thereafter, 100 mg. are administered intravenously over each six-hour period. For additional security, 50 mg. of cortisone acetate may be given intramuscularly every six hours. In general, hypotension caused by adrenocortical insufficiency is promptly reversed by appropriate steroid replacement therapy.

Subacute adrenocortical insufficiency is met occasionally, as for example in patients whose replacement therapy was tapered off too abruptly following operation. This syndrome is characterized by mental torpor and weakness associated with a rise in the BUN and a decline in the plasma sodium level. Here again, appropriate electrolyte and steroid replacement therapy effectively corrects the metabolic derangements.

The patient who has once exhibited adrenocortical insufficiency should be warned that infection or other stress may or can precipitate the condition again in the future. At all times he or she should carry a card that indicates the need for corticosteroid therapy in case of acute illness.

CASE STUDY (3). ADRENOCORTICAL CRISIS FOLLOWING BILATERAL ADRENALECTOMY

P.D., a 48-year-old white schoolteacher, was admitted to University Hospital on September 5, 1960, with the clinical diagnosis of Cushing's syndrome. However, this diagnosis had not been suspected until almost 10 years after she had begun changing from doctor to doctor in an effort to find the cause of her easy bruisability and extremely poor and prolonged healing of even minor scratches and lacerations. Brownish pigmentation frequently persisted long after abrasions had healed. In recent months she had developed headaches, mild hypertension, mild hirsutism, and increasing weakness and fatigue. The legs were very spindly and the trunk relatively obese. The diagnosis of hyperadrenocorticism was confirmed by an extremely marked increase in the urinary excretion of both 17-kerosteroids and 17-hydroxysteroids following ACTH stimulation.

Initial therapy consisted of pituitary irradiation (4000 R.), but there was little improvement and bilateral adrenalectomy was performed on October 26, 1962.

Postoperatively the steroid replacement therapy consisted of 100 mg. of hydrocortisone by intravenous drip over each six-hour period. The patient's course was uneventful until 11:55 A.M. the day following operation, when she was found to have a blood pressure of 60/?, though she was alert and quite comfortable otherwise. Shortly thereafter the blood pressure became unobtainable. It developed that the intravenous drip had infiltrated earlier that morning, and she had received virtually no steroid therapy for approximately five hours. This was promptly corrected, and a firm policy was then established that 50 mg. of cortisone acetate would be given intramuscularly, every six hours, along with the intravenous drip. In this way the patient would receive replacement therapy that should be adequate even if the intravenous route failed.

COMMENT

The cause of shock in adrenocortical insufficiency is far from clear. In acute crisis, following only hours after operation, little change in blood volume or electrolyte concentrations and distribution will have occurred. Webb and coworkers (1968) demonstrated diminished myocardial contractility in hypoadrenocorticism, and an effect upon peripheral vasculature and its resistance has long been postulated.

HYPERADRENOCORTICISM CRISIS

It is not often that a true acute crisis is seen in states of excessive production of adreno-cortical hydroxycorticosteroids. Of course, severe metabolic derangements, debility, and eventual death may occur as a late result of Cushing's disease or primary aldosteronism. However, the following case does present one of the urgent crises that may develop in connection with hyperadrenocorticism.

CASE STUDY (4). SEVERE ADRENOCORTICISM WITH CUSHING'S SYNDROME AND PSEUDO-TUMOR CEREBRI

M. H., a 16-year-old white schoolgirl, was admitted to University Hospital on March 24, 1963, with a chief complaint of increased appetite, increased weight gain, and leg cramps. Physical examination revealed a well-developed obese white female with moonlike facies, purplish abdominal striae, severe facial acne, pubic hair to the umbilicus, and increased hair all over the body. No abdominal masses were palpable. The tentative diagnosis of Cushing's disease was further substantiated by a positive 24-hour dexamethasone suppression test. Initially the 17-ketosteroid excretion was 37.5 mg. and the 17-hydroxysteroid excretion was 27.6 mg. Twenty-four hours later the 17-KS excretion was 25 mg. and the 17-hydroxysteroid excretion was 20.5 mg. The fact that both levels were reduced by dexamethasone suggested bilateral adrenocortical hyperplasia.

An intravenous ACTH stimulation test was performed on April 12, the day prior to scheduled adrenalectomy. However, the test was followed by headache and drowsiness, and later that afternoon she had a grand mal seizure. At that time the serum calcium level was reported at 4.2 mEq./l. and blood pressure was 160/100. The stimulus for the seizure was considered to be water retention caused by the ACTH, with cerebral water and salt imbalance and cerebral edema.

She became comatose and tracheostomy was performed to permit artificial pulmonary ventilation during periods of apnea. Cautious lumbar puncture a few days later revealed very high cerebrospinal fluid pressure and minimal fluid was removed. A diagnosis of "pseudo-tumor syndrome" was made, and multiple supportive measures were employed. By April 30 she had improved considerably with careful electrolyte balance and anticonvulsant therapy.

On June 24 the patient underwent total bilateral adrenalectomy with transplantation of adrenal tissue to the sartorius muscle in the upper thigh bilaterally. Postoperatively she did well. Steroid replacement therapy was given initially, with ACTH, but eventually the transplants supported her needs (Hardy and Langford, 1964).

She was readmitted on October 14, 1963, with a pancreatic pseudocyst that was drained internally into the stomach. Postoperatively she had a possible pulmonary infarct from deep vein thrombosis in the lower extremities, but anticoagulants were employed and she was discharged in good condition one month later.

COMMENT

This case illustrates the complex fluid and electrolyte derangement termed "pseudo-tumor cerebri," which may develop at times of increasing or decreasing corticosteroid levels. It produced deep coma in this patient, with apnea for a period of time when life was sustained with an automatic ventilator and cuffed tracheostomy tube. Bilateral upper thigh transplants of her hyperplastic adrenal tissue survived, as proved by later biopsy, and these eventually supported her entire adrenocortical requirements following total intra-abdominal adrenalectomy. A pancreatic pseudocyst developed from mobilization and elevation of the tail of the pancreas to permit excision of the left adrenal, and it was drained into the stomach without recurrence.

PHEOCHROMOCYTOMA

HYPERTENSIVE AND HYPOTENSIVE CRISES

The term pheochromocytoma is often applied indiscriminately to any tumor secreting catecholamines, whether in the adrenal gland or elsewhere. However, we prefer to designate as pheochromocytomas those chromaffin neoplasms that arise in the adrenal medulla and usually produce both epinephrine and norepinephrine. In contrast, we designate as paragangliomas those extra-adrenal lesions that arise from the sympathetic chain anywhere from the neck to the urinary bladder and produce largely norepinephrine. This differentiation has practical diagnostic value because if the urine contains increased amounts of both epinephrine and norepinephrine, the tumor is probably situated in one or the other adrenal or both; if the increased catecholamine content of the urine consists almost entirely of norepinephrine, the tumor may lie anywhere along the sympathetic chain but probably not in the adrenal. Most of the catecholamine-producing tumors are benign but an occasional one is malignant and metastasizes, usually to the liver but at times to retroperitoneal structures and veins.

The pathophysiology associated with these chromaffin tumors is a result of their elaboration of excessive amounts of catecholamines. The hypertension produced is either episodic or sustained. Early in the course the excessive elevations of blood pressure are classically intermittent or paroxysmal, but later on the hypertension may become sustained with renal damage. If the hypertension has become fixed, the pheochromocytoma may not be clinically detected unless all patients with otherwise unexplained hypertension undergo a measurement of the 24-hour excretion of catecholamines in the urine. We have found no patient with a significantly functioning chromaffin tumor who did not exhibit an increased content of catecholamine in the 24-hour urine specimen, though the rare exception may exist. In other words, the tumor actually produces a sustained basal elevation in the output of catecholamines every 24 hours, even though this increase may not be sufficient at any given time to raise the blood pressure markedly. Paroxysmal hypertension due to an abrupt increase in the output of catecholamines by the tumor may occur spontaneously or be precipitated by a variety of stimuli such as straining at stool, obstetric labor, palpation of the abdomen, manipulation of the tumor at operation, and, in past years, a "provocative" histamine injection test. At present the histamine provocative test and other measures designated to precipitate an attack for diagnostic purposes are no longer used because they pose the hazards associated with severe hypertension, such as acute left heart failure or stroke. The accurate measurement of catecholamines in the urine now affords a far safer and more accurate means of diagnosis.

SIGNS AND SYMPTOMS

Severe headache, palpitations, and profuse sweating have long been recognized as the acute manifestations of pheochromocytomas. Other associated symptoms are abdominal pain, nausea, and vomiting, and these are manifestations of the gastrointestinal symptomatology associated with this picture. Flushing and pallor of the face, neck, and extremities occur intermittently and are due to the vasomotor changes produced by the release of catecholamines. During the acute attacks the patient is usually apprehensive and irritable. Retrosternal pain which may simulate attacks of angina are referred to by some of these patients, but some of them may also present true angina as a result of the hypertensive crises, especially in those with underlying coronary disease. Hypovolemia and reduced red cell mass may develop.

DIAGNOSIS

Certain diagnostic considerations were presented previously, and measurement of the urinary excretion of catecholamines is the most important requirement.

The clinical findings are mainly those of the pressor amine syndrome, with elevated blood pressure and the collateral symptomatology derived from the release of catecholamines. Incidentally, the individual who has prominent and dilated veins on the dorsum of the hands will rarely be found to have a pheochromocytoma. Occasionally the patient presents with the symptoms or roentgenologic signs of a space-occupying lesion, and in a small number of cases the tumor is met as an incidental finding at the time of abdominal exploration or autopsy.

Functioning chromaffin tumors may produce an elevated basal metabolic rate, glucosuria and hyperglycemia, findings which have at times been attributed erroneously to hyperthyroidism. Presumptive diagnostic evidence is achieved by relief of an attack of paroxysmal hypertension by intravenous phentolamine (Regitine). The administration of 5 mg. intravenously by rapid drip will cause a fall in blood pressure, owing to blockage of the catecholamines. When the test is positive for pheochromocytoma the blood pressure should decrease within three or four minutes. This decrease in blood pressure lasts for several minutes before returning to pre-test values. The patient should be observed carefully during this test to prevent a sudden and precipitous fall in the blood pressure, with undesirable hypotension, and some clinicians no longer use the test. In the patient with underlying coronary disease, this fall in blood pressure could precipitate a myocardial infarction. Again, the most reliable and safe diagnostic test for pheochromocytoma is the measurement of catecholamines in a 24-hour urine specimen, the normal value being less than 400 mcg. A variation of this study is determination of the urinary excretion of vanillylmandelic acid (VMA), a by-product of catecholamine metabolism. The normal urinary VMA content is from 0.7 to 6.8 mg. per day, but this value may be influenced by a number of factors not related to catecholamine production by a tumor. It is not as reliable as the direct measurement of epinephrine and norepinephrine in blood and urine. The blood and urine values are especially likely to be elevated during and just after an attack.

Intravenous pyelogram will demonstrate displacement of kidney or ureter by the tumor in some cases, but more specific data are likely to be obtained with a catheter aortogram or selective arteriogram to show the presence of the tumor. The previous reluctance to perform angiography to identify the presence of a pheochromocytoma, for fear of precipitating a severe attack, has been largely dispelled by reports such as that of Rossi et al. (1968). He reviewed 99 patients reported in the literature and found the procedure safe, except when the translumbar approach was used. No fatalities had followed the use of the catheter technique with modern contrast media.

TREATMENT

The definitive treatment for pheochromocytoma is removal of the tumor or tumors whenever possible. For maximum safety during operation, it is advisable to employ drug therapy to control the hypertension. The use of phentolamine, an alpha-blockading agent, to control marked elevations of blood pressure before and during operation has been most valuable in the management of chromaffin tumors (Hardy et al., 1962). However, the long-term use of phentolamine for the nonoperative management of patients with nonresectable malignant lesions has not been conspicuously successful. The use of an oral preparation of phenoxybenzamine (Dibenzyline) has proved to be fairly effective in the chronic management of inoperable chromaffin malignancy, as well as in the control of attacks prior to surgery. Recently, propranolol, a beta-blockading agent, has been found useful in preventing cardiac arrhythmias during surgery (Glenn and Mannix, 1968), but this drug can produce alarming circulatory side effects in some patients. Lidocaine hydrochloride and a beta-blockading drug such as propranolol, as well as phentolamine (Regitine) should be available at all times during the operation to prevent serious arrhythmias or hypertensive crises during manipulation of the tumor. We keep a Regitine drip prepared and ready for immediate infusion.

Dibenzyline is now being used to prepare patients for operation, the dose being 10 to 30 mg. a day by mouth (Shields, 1969). This agent causes vasodilatation and its use must be accompanied by adequate blood replacement to fill the previously constricted vascular bed. With the use of this agent, emergency operation for chromaffin tumor crisis should rarely be necessary. Death may occur in acute crisis as a result of acute left heart failure with pulmonary edema, stroke, convulsions with respiratory failure, or profound shock after the hypertension.

HEMORRHAGE INTO THE TUMOR

Hemorrhage into the pheochromocytoma has occasionally been described and can be very serious. The hemorrhage may occur during treatment or as a consequence of aortography (Delaney and Paritsky, 1969; Rossi et al., 1968). Of the 5 cases reported by Delaney and Paritzky, only one survived. These patients usually present as cardiac or abdominal catastrophies (Huston and Stewart, 1965). Again, phentolamine or phenoxybenzamine may be used to control severe hypertension, and blood transfusion and if necessary a norepinephrine drip may be required to treat abrupt and prolonged hypotension.

Shock Following Tumor Removal

In some patients, removal of the functioning chromaffin tumor is followed abruptly by marked hypotension, especially if no preparatory drug therapy such as Dibenzyline, with blood replacement, was employed for several days preoperatively. The principal cause of the hypotension is actually a blood volume deficit in a patient whose vascular bed is no longer chronically constricted. Accordingly, blood should be transfused until the arterial blood pressure is satisfactory or until the central venous pressure has begun to rise. Transfusion will prove effective in most patients, but in the occasional case a slow drip of norepinephrine may be required temporarily to permit time for physiologic adjustments. Digitalization may rarely be indicated, and the intravenous infusion of hydrocortisone to combat a relative adrenocortical insufficiency has apparently been useful at times.

In actual practice, using a combination of blood transfusion and at times temporary pressor amine drip, we have had no serious difficulty in managing postresectional hypotension effectively. Furthermore, with increased awareness of the need for blood transfusion we now rarely encounter hypo-

tension following resection of a pheochromocytoma.

CASE STUDY (5). FUNCTIONING PARAGANGLIOMA WITH HYPERTENSIVE CRISES COMPLICATING PREGNANCY WITH POSTRESECTIONAL HYPOTENSION

O. H., a 21-year-old Negro housewife, was referred to University Hospital on December 3, 1960, for control of eclampsia and severe hypertension. She was six months pregnant and gave a history of convulsions with delivery of her first child, 17 months previously.

The blood pressure varied markedly, from time to time, being in the range of 280/150 on numerous occasions. There were frequent episodes of tachycardia and cold sweat. When significant renal disease had been excluded, the possibility of pheochromocytoma began to be seriously considered. Meanwhile, the patient had a severe attack while in the x-ray department, with prostration, systolic blood pressure 300 mm. Hg, marked tachycardia, severe headache, and profuse cold sweat—with a decline in symptoms in a few minutes. Another attack was precipitated by palpation of the abdomen.

At this point the catecholamine levels were reported to be markedly elevated in both blood and urine, and operation was scheduled for December 19. Although the risk of loss of the fetus was fully appreciated and discussed, the consensus was that the mother would otherwise likely die from the disease either before or during delivery. There was no displacement of the kidneys on intravenous pyelogram, abbreviated because of the pregnancy, and chest x-ray disclosed no evidence of an intrathoracic neoplasm. Thus, the location of the chromaffin tumor remained in doubt.

Laparotomy was performed through a midline abdominal incision. Both adrenal glands were noted to be normal in size and appearance. However, at the junction of the aorta and left common iliac artery was found a solid oval mass, 8 × 5 cm., which had not been palpable preoperatively because of the enlarged uterus. Large veins drained into both the mesenteric and caval systems, and the left ureter was intimately fused with the tumor over a distance of several centimeters.

Regitine (phentolamine) had been available for use in case severe hypertension developed during operation, but the blood pressure remained stable. However, on removal of the tumor the blood pressure fell to "zero." Since blood loss had been more than replaced, a norepinephrine drip was started. Several attempts to stop the drug during the evening and the next day were followed by absence of detectable blood pressure and complaints from the patient that she was dying. We believed that we had transfused far more blood than could possibly have been lost at operation, and central venous pressure monitoring had not become common as a guide to the adequacy of transfusion at that time. Therefore, we continued the norepinephrine drip until it was finally possible to discontinue it 48 hours following operation. Meanwhile, she had been aborted of a dead fetus on the first postoperative day. Her subsequent course was uneventful, with the blood pressure 120/80.

COMMENT

This patient had classic signs and symptoms of chromaffin tumor crises. The diagnosis was established preoperatively with catecholamine measurements in blood and urine, and operation was performed, in spite of the pregnancy, to save the mother. Since the neoplasm did not rest in the adrenal gland but arose from the sympathetic chain at the brim of the pelvis, it was designated a paraganglioma rather than a pheochromocytoma.

At the time this patient was operated upon we did not fully appreciate the fact that a markedly reduced blood volume may develop in the patient with a functioning chromaffin tumor. Therefore, when what appeared to be an adequate volume of blood had been transfused, a norepinephrine drip was used to maintain a blood pressure sufficient to sustain life. In a subsequent patient, however, we measured the blood volume preoperatively, found it low, and transfused a large volume of blood postoperatively, using central venous pressure measurements for guidance. Full veins appeared in this patient with transfusion, whereas none had been visible preoperatively, and norepinephrine was not required. Again, prominent distended veins are rarely observed on the forearms and hands of the patient with a functioning chromaffin tumor, prior to its resection. In a still later instance, we employed preoperative Dibenzyline therapy to prepare a patient with recurrent malignant paraganglioma with adequate blood replacement (Sjoerdsma, et al., 1965). However, in this case it proved impossible to resect the invasive tumor.

Thus, postresectional hypotension is now perceived to be largely the result of a disparity between the now dilated vasculature and the available blood volume. Adequate transfusion, with central venous pressure monitoring, will usually preclude the need for a vasopressor drug postoperatively.

HYPERINSULIN CRISES

The hallmark of hyperinsulinism is hypoglycemia. The fall in the blood glucose level is usually episodic, and when it approaches 50 mg. per cent the patient may lose consciousness. In fact, some patients exhibit symptoms at blood glucose levels higher than this, but others become remarkably tolerant of quite low blood glucose levels.

Hyperinsulinism is perhaps the most common overall cause of hypoglycemia. It is most often a result of insulin or sulfonylurea overdosage in diabetic patients, for functioning islet cell tumors secreting insulin are relatively rare. Hypoglycemia is also met in liver failure, hepatoma, pituitary insufficiency, and adrenocortical insufficiency. It is also produced by large retroperitoneal fibromas that may elaborate an insulin-like substance. Idiopathic hypoglycemia occurs with some frequency in children but less often in adults.

In the following discussion we shall deal solely with hyperinsulinism caused by hyperplasia or functioning beta-cell adenomas of the islets of Langerhans. Incidentally, such tumors also occur in other mammals such as dogs and cattle.

SYMPTOMS AND SIGNS

The classic Whipple's triad is still the most important clue in the diagnosis of an insulinoma. It consists of the clinical manifestations of hypoglycemia, coming on long after eating or fasting, a blood sugar level below 50 mg. per 100 ml., and relief of symptoms by the administration of glucose. Nervous tissues are extremely dependent on glucose for their function, and consequently the most striking manifestations of prolonged hypoglycemia are usually neurologic. Irreversible brain damage may occur after repeated episodes of hypoglycemia (Laroche et al., 1968; Williams et al., 1969).

After a long period of starvation (overnight fasting) or unusual exercise, a dramatic hypoglycemia may occur in these patients. Nervous system symptoms include nervousness, irritability, erratic behavior, and sometimes aggressive tendencies. Other symptoms are related to the sudden release of epinephrine from the adrenal medulla, a compensatory attempt to restore the normal glucose balance through glycogenolysis. These symptoms consist of palpitations, headache, profuse sweating, tachycardia, and generalized weakness. Such patients are usually apprehensive and manifest hunger. Convulsions may occur and in severe cases coma will ensue. Hypoglycemia may simulate many neurologic syndromes, and patients with hyperinsulinism have not infrequently been diagnosed initially as having a functional psychosis.

DIAGNOSIS

An adequate history is of great importance. Rarely, it is possible to palpate a tumor in the abdomen. The workup for insulinoma, when suspected, should include multiple fasting blood sugar determinations, a glucose tolerance test, and an L-leucine sensitivity test. The tolbutamide test, combined with measurement of the plasma insulin level, has proved to be of particular value in the diagnosis of insulinoma. The glucagon test is also valuable. Tolbutamide causes release of insulin into the plasma and aggravates the hypoglycemia. Plasma insulin levels can now be measured with considerable accuracy. Angiography may suggest the presence of a tumor in the pancreas. In children, the differential diagnosis between insulinoma and idiopathic hypoglycemia may be extremely difficult, since the responses to the tests mentioned are similar in both conditions. However, it helps to know that insulinomas are more frequent beyond the age of four, whereas idiopathic hypoglycemia is more common under that age.

Islet cell tumors are usually benign. In a series of 154 cases reported by Laroche et al. (1968) the tumor was benign in 118 (89 per cent) and malignant in 14. In the 118 patients with benign tumors, the lesion was solitary in 111 (94 per cent) and multiple in the rest. In this same series, 63 per cent of the tumors were located in the body or tail of the pancreas.

TREATMENT

The medical management of this condition is far from adequate. The acute crisis is best treated by oral or intravenous glucose administration. Frequent meals are mandatory. Usually the patient is aware of the condition and carries candy or sugar-containing food with him, which he ingests when prodromic symptoms develop. The definitive treatment consists of the surgical removal of the tumor or tumors. Since approximately 10 per cent of these tumors are multiple, a careful exploration of the pancreas should be carried out in every instance, with extensive mobilization of this organ for proper palpation. Islet tumors are frequently soft and difficult to palpate. Continuous monitoring of the blood sugar levels during the operation is recommended in these patients to assure removal

of all tumor(s). Blind distal pancreatectomy has been advocated by various authors, from 75 per cent to 90 per cent of the pancreas being resected, and we have used it ourselves. In one series of 33 patients in which the tumor was not identifiable by the surgeon, 15 were found to contain an adenoma in the specimen resected (75 per cent distal pancreatectomy) (Laroche et al., 1968). A Whipple procedure has only rarely been performed. Distal pancreatectomy may provide adequate treatment for cases in which islet cell hyperplasia is responsible for the syndrome.

Medical management consists of a low leucine diet, in addition to oral and intravenous glucose. ACTH and cortisone may prove useful as insulin antagonists. Diazoxide, a hyperglycemia agent of the thiazide group, may reduce the hypoglycemia attacks.

Diazoxide inhibits beta-cell secretion of insulin and stimulates glycogen degradation in the liver and reduces glycogen synthesis. All these actions increase circulating glucose. The drug is administered in a dose of 12 mg./kg. per 24 hours in 4 divided doses. Since it causes fluid retention, a diuretic agent should also be employed.

The emergency treatment of severe hypoglycemia, whatever its origin, may be accomplished by one or a combination of the following: (1) Intravenous administration of 25 per cent dextrose as a continuous drip with a catheter in a central vein to avoid phlebitis. (2) Subcutaneous administration of ephedrine or epinephrine, the latter given in 1.0-mg. doses. A principal effect of these drugs is to mobilize glucose from the liver. (3) Glucagon, given in a 5-mg. dose intravenously slowly, will increase the hepatic output of free glucose. (4) Diazoxide, 5 mg./kg. of body weight by mouth. (5) Steroids (prednisone) have been used with limited beneficial effect.

These measures provide only temporary relief but are invaluable in the treatment of acute crisis.

The Operation

PREOPERATIVE PREPARATION. The night prior to operation the patient is given a continuous infusion of 10 per cent dextrose in water containing 100 mg. of hydrocortisone, and immediately prior to operation an additional 75 mg. of hydrocortisone is given intramuscularly. The steroid is helpful in maintaining adequate blood sugar levels through gluconeogenesis.

POSTOPERATIVE CARE. Frequent postoperative blood glucose determinations should be performed. After 2 to 3 hours the glucose infusion may be stopped and the glucose levels measured. Removal of the tumor will result in a marked rise in blood glucose about 1 to 3 hours following the operation, and the hyperglycemia should persist for days if all functioning tumor has been excised.

When the tumor is malignant and metastases cannot be removed, the long-term management of the hypoglycemia poses a serious problem. Cortisone therapy has been helpful, and the intravenous infusion of glucagon in hospitalized patients has also elevated the blood sugar level. We are presently treating with diazoxide the patient whose case study follows.

CASE STUDY (6). HYPERINSULINISM DUE TO MALIGNANT ISLET CELL TUMOR

J. H., a 53-year-old white carpenter, was first admitted to University Hospital on September 8, 1966. He had been well until 1958 when he developed duodenal ulceration. In 1961 he began having episodes of hunger, lethargy, and confusion, which came on at no particular time of the day. He found that these symptoms were relieved promptly by food intake. On Thanksgiving Day, 1962, an unusually severe attack occurred, and in his community hospital his blood sugar level was found to be 17 mg. per 100 ml. A 340-gm. pancreatic islet cell tumor was removed shortly thereafter, with considerable difficulty because of marked vascularity and substantial blood loss, and the lesion was later diagnosed by the Armed Forces Institute of Pathology as a low-grade malignant insulinoma. Hypoglycemic symptoms were relieved following removal of the tumor.

In February, 1966, the patient developed an episode of weakness and fainting associated with hematemesis and melena. A bleeding duodenal ulcer was managed by vagotomy and pyloroplasty, plus gastroenterostomy.

Upon first admission to University Hospital in September, 1966, with weight loss and multiple abdominal complaints, he exhibited marginal ulceration and recurrence of hypoglycemia. A selective celiac axis arteriogram disclosed evidence of a well-vascularized tumor in the pancreas, apparently a recurrence of the malignant insulinoma that had been excised in 1962. In view of the evidence of recurrent peptic ulceration, plus a high rate of gastric acid secretion, samples of serum, gastric juice, and urine were assayed for excessive gastrin activity, but were negative.

The patient was admitted to the University Hospital once again on July 17, 1967, with a low hemoglobin level and symptoms of peptic ulcer. Two days later, at 5:30 A.M., he developed excruciatingly severe abdominal pain and went into shock, believed to be due to perforated ulcer. At emergency laparotomy it was found that the marginal ulcer demonstrated on previous roentgenogram had perforated into the anterior abdominal wall. A large tumor was present in the head of the pancreas. All things considered, it seemed wise to halt further peptic ulcer complications by performing a total gastrectomy and this was done. Although a definite increase in serum gastrin content had not been demonstrated, the patient had had ulcer problems for nine years, he was secreting large amounts of gastric juice and hydrochloric acid, he had a malignant islet cell tumor, which had recurred, and some islet cell tumors produce multiple hormones. Finally, follow-up of Whipple's patients whose insulinoma had been excised revealed a significant incidence of late peptic ulceration (Markowitz et al., 1961). In addition, the highly vascular tumor in the head of the pancreas, approximately 6 cm. in diameter, was excised to the extent possible. The histologic diagnosis was again malignant islet cell carcinoma, with perineural and lymphatic invasion and direct extension to the gastric wall. The patient had an uneventful postoperative course.

Except for an attack of serum hepatitis he did fairly well at home, being able to serve as town constable until the spring of 1970 when symptoms of hypoglycemia and tumor recurrence again appeared. For example, either he or his wife had to stay awake and see that he ate every three hours, or he would pass into hypoglycemic coma. Celiac axis arteriograms again demonstrated recurrence of the insulinoma and now the liver scan reveals possible evidence of metastases. He wishes to avoid another operation, if at all possible, and he is being treated with Diazoxide and a diuretic, plus multiple feedings, to control his symptomatology.

CARCINOID CRISES

Carcinoid tumors arise from Kulchitsky cells and secrete serotonin (5-hydroxytryptamine). The most frequent location, by far, is in the digestive tract. The appendix is the site most commonly involved, but the tumor may arise at any level of the gastrointestinal tract and even outside it, such as in the bronchus, ovary, and thyroid. However, 95 per cent of the argentaffin mass is located in the gastrointestinal tract. Appendiceal and rectal carcinoids are usually solitary and rarely metastasize (Peskin, 1969). The areas most commonly involved in the spread of the tumor are the lymph nodes and liver.

MALIGNANT CARCINOID SYNDROME

Episodic attacks of flushing, dyspnea, bronchospasm, and hemodynamic alterations that may result in vasomotor collapse are the most common findings associated with this syndrome. Hyperperistalsis and diarrhea, cyanosis, presence of telangiectasia, edema of the extremities, and right heart valvular disease are other frequent manifestations.

The occurrence of the carcinoid syndrome in connection with alimentary tract carcinoids is associated with the presence of liver metastasis, except for primary rectal carcinoids (Peskin and Kaplan, 1969; Tumalder et al., 1968). Under ordinary circumstances (and in the absence of hepatic metastases) the 5-hydroxytryptamine is inactivated in a deamination process by mono-amino oxidase. This is carried out predominantly in the liver but to a minor degree in the lungs.

The characteristic symptom complex has long been attributed solely to the large amount of circulating serotonin produced by the tumor, but recent evidence indicates that there are additional biochemical aspects of the carcinoid syndrome that make the problem more complex than was initially thought. It appears, for example, that carcinoid tumors may produce other biologically active peptides such as kininogen and histamine.

The diagnosis is most securely established by measurement of 5-hydroxyindole acetic acid (5-HIAA) in the urine, which in normal persons is excreted in amounts of 2 to 10 mg. daily.

TREATMENT

For isolated lesions, ample local excision is all that is necessary. The cure rate is high, 60 to 75 per cent, even with local nodal metastasis. Palliative procedures such as hepatic lobectomy are justifiable, since substantial amelioration of symptoms may occur in many cases, lasting for considerable lengths of time (Wilson and Butterick, 1959).

Drug therapy is unsatisfactory except for temporary control of the symptoms. Methysergide maleate, alpha-methyldopa, hydrazine, and cyproheptadine (antiserotonin agents) have been used satisfactorily for symptomatic relief. Chemotherapeutic drugs and radiotherapy have yielded poor results.

General anesthesia is preferred, with careful monitoring of blood pressure, and spinal and epidural block should be avoided. Vascular collapse and death have been reported during the induction of anesthesia. Methoxamine has proved to be a safer pressor agent than other drugs.

nia, and for this reason this disease has usually been excluded from the endocrine gland disturbances. Nevertheless, there remains the belief that the thymus must elaborate some substance that causes, or is related to, the development of myasthenia gravis. Myasthenia gravis, acquired agammaglobulinemia, and aregenerative anemia are all possible autoimmune diseases that have been linked with thymic disorders. However, a direct relationship of cause and effect is not consistently present, and, consequently, removal of the thymus is not always followed by disappearance or even alleviation of the manifestations of these conditions.

Myasthenia gravis usually produces a generalized weakness, but at times the muscular involvement can be quite localized. Symptoms may appear spontaneously but often follow activity of the muscles involved. A common and early manifestation is ptosis of the lids as a result of weakness of the oculopalpebral muscles. Impairment of speech, or of swallowing, or of walking may on occasion be the presenting symptom.

The muscular manifestations in myasthenia are considered to be caused by alterations in the neuromuscular conduction mechanisms, a result of a defect in the acetylcholine system. The course of the disease is marked by remissions and exacerbations, but there is a gradual progression of the muscular involvement. Nearly 25 per cent of the patients with myasthenia will have spontaneous remission of the symptoms, which may last from months to many years. Of 220 patients with generalized myasthenia reported by Harvey (1963), 32 per cent died of the disease from three months to 25 years after the onset of the disease. In some other series, however, the mortality rate is considerably greater than this.

The exact relationship between myasthenia and thymoma has not been clearly established. Myasthenia patients have associated thymomas in approximately 30 per cent of the cases. Furthermore, patients with thymomas and myasthenia will usually die from the effects of myasthenia rather than from the effects of tumor growth (Shields, 1969).

MYASTHENIA GRAVIS CRISES

MYASTHENIA CRISIS

No definite endocrine dysfunction has been established in the etiology of myasthe-

This acute problem is a result of accentuation of muscular weakness to a degree that threatens life. This results from loss of tone of the pharyngeal muscles, leading to pulmonary aspiration, and when the intercostal and other respiratory muscles are involved the result will be respiratory failure. These patients may present symptoms related to inadequate breathing or difficulty in swallowing. An early symptom preceding serious respiratory problems is that of a weak cough owing to the inability of the thoracic muscles to contract adequately. This respiratory muscle fatigue becomes progressive until it reaches critical levels.

This crisis may also develop in patients undergoing surgery for thymomas. In one of our patients, an acute respiratory insufficiency developed in the immediate postoperative period following partial removal of a malignant (invasive) thymoma. Immediate endotracheal intubation with assisted ventilation and administration of acetylcholinesterase drugs were effective in controlling the patient's condition. It was interesting to note that preoperatively this patient had had no symptoms to suggest myasthenia gravis (see Case 7).

TREATMENT

In myasthenia crisis the establishment of an adequate airway is of paramount importance. As an immediate measure, mouth-to-mouth or face-mask ventilation may be essential until nasotracheal or endotracheal intubation or tracheostomy can be performed, if required. Intermittent positive pressure ventilation is thus instituted and specific therapy started. Since the swallow-mechanism is also affected by compromise of the pharyngeal muscles, nasogastric intubation may be necessary for feeding purposes and administration of medications as well. Edrophonium (Tensilon), neostigmine methyl sulfate (Prostigmin), or pyridostigmine bromide (Mestinon) may be used parenterally in the acute situation, the latter in doses of 60 mg. every four hours, with close observation of the patient's reaction. This dose may be increased, if necessary, until a positive response is obtained. Atropine should be given simultaneously (up to 1.0 mg. I.M.). Administration of potassium has been observed to help these patients by mechanisms that have not been clearly established, and it should be considered in the plan of therapy.

CASE STUDY (7). RESPIRATORY FAILURE FOLLOWING EXCISION OF ANTERIOR MEDIASTINAL TUMOR (THYMOMA)

M. B., a 49-year-old white man, had a chest x-ray performed following an accident in July, 1959, and an anterior mediastinal mass was found. He was admitted to the University Hospital on May 7, 1960, for diagnosis and management of the asymptomatic chest lesion. It was suspected of being either a teratoma or thymoma, and thoracotomy was performed on May 13. The operation itself was uneventful, but spontaneous respiration did not return postoperatively. A frozen section examination of the excised mediastinal mass (7.5 × 6 × 5 cm.) revealed that it was an encapsulated thymoma, and the possibility of myasthenia gravis was suspected despite the absence of suggestive symptoms preoperatively. An injection of Tensilon produced spontaneous respiratory activity, and this was still further supported by Prostigmin, 1.0 mg., and atropine, 0.4 mg.

COMMENT

Although the patient remained asymptomatic for some months on appropriate medication for his myasthenia gravis, he died on July 11, 1961, of complications of the disease.

REFERENCES

Anglem, T. J.: Acute hyperparathyroidism: A surgical emergency. Surg. Clin. N. Amer., 46:727, 1966.

Brantigan, C. O., and Katase, R. Y.: Clinical and pathological features of paragangliomas of the organ of Zuckerkandl. Surgery, 65:898, 1969.

Buckberg, G. D., and Mulder, D. G.: Thymectomy for myasthenia gravis: Principles of surgical management. Amer. Surg., 33:797, 1967.

Buckle, R. M., Mason, A. M. S., and Middleton, J. E.: Thyrotoxic hypercalcemia treated with porcine calcitonin. Lancet, 1:1128, 1969.

Cope, O., Culver, P. J., Mixter, C. G., Jr., and Nardi, G. L.: Pancreatitis, a diagnostic clue to hyperparathyroidism. Ann. Surg., 145:857, 1957.

Das, G., and Krieger, M.: Treatment of thyrotoxic storm with intravenous administration of propanolol. Ann. Intern. Med., 70:985, 1969.

Delaney, J. P., and Paritzky, A. Z.: Necrosis of a pheochromocytoma with shock. New Eng. J. Med., 280:1394, 1969.

Eisenstein, R., and Passavoy, M.: Actinomycin-D inhibits parathyroid hormone and vitamin D activity. Proc. Soc. Exp. Biol. Med., 117:77, 1964.

Fink, W. J., and Finfrock, J. D.: Fatal hyperparathyroid crisis associated with pancreatitis. Amer. Surg., 27:424, 1961.

Glenn, F., and Mannix, H., Jr.: The surgical management of chromaffin tumors. Ann. Surg., 167:619, 1968.

Hanes, F. M.: Hyperparathyroidism due to parathyroid adenoma, with death from parathormone intoxication. Amer. J. Med. Sci., 197:85, 1939.

Hardy, J. D., and Eraslan, S.: Parathyroid hormone activity in venous drainage of functioning intrathoracic parathyroid adenoma. Surgery, 54:752, 1963.

Hardy, J. D., and Langford, H. G.: Surgical management of Cushing's syndrome: Including studies of adrenal autotransplants, body composition, and pseudotumor cerebri. Ann. Surg., *159*:711, 1964.

Hardy, J. D., McPhail, J. L., and Gallagher, W. B., Jr.: Pheochromocytoma: Shock following resection; notes on mechanism with catecholamine measurements in case during pregnancy. JAMA, *179*:107, 1962.

Hardy, J. D., Snavely, J. R., and Langford, H. G.: Low intrathoracic parathyroid adenoma: Large functioning tumor representing the fifth parathyroid, opposite eighth dorsal vertebra with independent arterial supply and opacified at operation with arteriogram. Ann. Surg., *159*:310, 1964.

Harrison, T. S.: The treatment of thyroid storm. Surg. Gynec. Obstet., *121*:837, 1965.

Hartemann, P., Leclere, J., Duc, M., Schweitzer, M., and Purchelle, J. C.: Tetanie après traitement de l'hyperthyroidie par l'iode radio-actif. Ann. Endocr. (Paris), *30*:77, 1969.

Hartsuck, J. M., and Brooks, J. R.: Functioning beta islet cell tumors. Preoperative tests and surgical approach. Amer. J. Surg., *117*:541, 1969.

Harvey, A. M.: Myasthenia Gravis. *In* Beeson, P. B., and McDermott, W.: Textbook of Medicine, 11th ed. Philadelphia, W. B. Saunders Co., 1963, pp. 1455–1460.

Huston, J. R., and Stewart, W. R. C.: Hemorrhagic pheochromocytoma with shock and abdominal pain. Amer. J. Med., *39*:502, 1965.

Ingbar, S. H.: Management of emergencies. IX. Thyrotoxic storm. New Eng. J. Med., *274*:1252, 1966.

Kelly, T. R., and Falor, W. H.: Hyperparathyroid crisis associated with pancreatitis. Ann. Surg., *168*:917, 1968.

Kleppel, N. H., Morton, H. G., and LeVeen, H. H.: Hypercalcemia crisis and pancreatitis in primary hyperparathyroidism. JAMA, *192*:916, 1965.

Kreisler, B., Dinbar, A., and Tulcinsky, D. B.: Postoperative atetanic hypocalcemic coma. Report of a case. Surgery, *65*:915, 1969.

Laroche, G. P., Ferris, D. O., Priestley, J. T., Scholz, D. A., and Dockerty, M. B.: Hyperinsulinism. Surgical results and management of functioning islet cell tumors. Review of 154 cases. Arch. Surg., *96*:763, 1968.

Latimer, R. G., Rees, V. L., and Peterson, C. N.: Hypercalcemic crisis treated with inorganic phosphate solution. Amer. J. Surg., *116*:669, 1968.

Lehman, J., and Donatelli, A. A.: Calcium intoxication due to primary hyperparathyroidism. Ann. Intern. Med., *60*:447, 1964.

MacLeod, W. A. J., and Holloway, C. K.: Hyperparathyroid crisis. A collective review. Ann. Surg., *166*: 1012, 1967.

Markowitz, A. M., Slanetz, C. A., Jr., and Frantz, V. K.: Functioning islet cell tumors of the pancreas: 25-year follow up. Ann. Surgery, *154*:877, 1961.

Nelson, N. C., and Becker, W. F.: Thyroid crisis: diagnosis and treatment. Ann. Surg., *170*:263, 1969.

Paloyan, E., Lawrence, A. M., Baker, W. H., and Straus, F. A., II: Near-total parathyroidectomy. Surg. Clin. N. Amer., *49*:43, 1969.

Payne, R. L., and Fitchett, C. W.: Hyperparathyroid crisis: Survey of the literature and a report of two additional cases. Ann. Surg., *161*:737, 1965.

Peskin, G. W., and Kaplan, E. L.: The surgery of carcinoid tumors. Surg. Clin. N. Amer., *49*:137, 1969.

Rasmussen, H., and Hawker, C.: Actinomycin-D and the response to parathyroid hormones. Science, *144*:1019, 1964.

Rossi, P., Young, I. S., and Panke, W. F.: Techniques, usefulness and hazards of arteriography of pheochromocytoma. JAMA, *205*:547, 1968.

Schottstaedt, E. S., and Smoller, M.: "Thyroid storm" produced by acute thyroid hormone poisoning. Ann. Intern. Med., *64*:847, 1966.

Shields, T. W.: The thymus gland. Surg. Clin. N. Amer., *49*:61, 1969.

Sjoerdsma, A., Engleman, K., Waldmann, T. A., Cooperman, L. H., and Hammond, W. G.: Pheochromocytoma: Current concepts of diagnosis and treatment. Ann. Intern. Med., *65*:1302, 1965.

Smith, L. C., Bradshaw, H. H., and Holleman, I. L., Jr.: Hyperparathyroid crisis: A surgical emergency. Amer. Surg., *29*:761, 1963.

Thompson, N. W., and Fry, W. J.: Thyroid crisis. Arch. Surg., *89*:512, 1964.

Tumalder, O. C., Horn, R. C., Jr., Eisenstein, B., Arminski, T. C., Wilson, G. S., and Lucas, R. J.: Carcinoid tumors of the rectum. A review of 40 cases. Arch. Surg., *97*:261, 1968.

Waldstein, S. S.: A clinical study of thyroid storm. Ann. Intern. Med., *52*:626, 1960.

Webb, W. R., and Degerli, I. W.: Myocardial metabolism. Effects of adrenalectomy and acute cortisol replacement. J. Surg. Res., *8*:73, 1968.

Williams, C., Jr., Bryson, G. H., and Hume, D. M.: Islet cell tumors and hypoglycemia. Ann. Surg., *169*:757, 1969.

Wilson, H., and Butterick, O. D.: Massive liver resection for control of severe vasomotor reactions secondary to malignant carcinoid. Ann. Surg., *149*:641, 1959.

CHAPTER 23

ACUTE AORTO-ILIAC OCCLUSION

by JAMES D. HARDY, M.D.

Acute occlusion of the terminal aorta represents a major surgical emergency. If the obstruction is complete and is not relieved in a few hours, the patient may die. If the occlusion involves only one iliac artery, the involved leg will usually be lost unless blood flow can be restored. These dire effects of acute aorto-iliac occlusion are in marked contrast to the relatively benign course that may accompany gradual aorto-iliac occlusion, in which time permits the development of increased collateral circulation. Such collateral pathways often protect at least the buttocks and thighs, and even the lower legs and feet may exhibit remarkably little ischemic change.

Total aorto-iliac occlusion must be relieved promptly because, first, the severe ischemia will produce tissue necrosis with profound metabolic changes, often leading to hypotension and renal shutdown (Provan et al., 1966). Second, the sluggish and virtually absent arterial flow will permit extensive sludging and thrombosis in the smaller vessels of the leg, precluding restoration of good tissue perfusion even if the main arterial trunks are later freed of thrombus.

Thus the plan of management and the prognosis in the given patient will be determined by a wide spectrum of factors that include the cause and duration of the occlusion when the patient is first seen; the extent of the occlusion; age; the overall metabolic state; associated diseases such as cardiac, pulmonary, and renal insufficiency; and the total experience of the physicians in charge. Although it may be difficult to decide to operate on such a critically ill patient, the stark alternatives of probable death, or at least the loss of one or both legs at a high level, should render the decision for surgical intervention clearly appropriate in most instances.

ETIOLOGY

The existence of acute aorto-iliac occlusion is usually apparent, but the cause of the acute occlusion may not be so readily apparent. The most common causes of acute obstruction of the aorto-iliac outflow tracts are as follows:

1. Embolism from the left side of the heart.
2. Acute thrombosis of a vessel previously narrowed by atherosclerosis.
3. Acute thrombosis of an abdominal aortic aneurysm.
4. Dissecting aortic aneurysm.
5. Blunt trauma to the abdomen with injury to a previously diseased (atherosclerotic) aorta.
6. Acute occlusion of an aorto-iliac outflow tract secondary to operative intervention to relieve high-grade incomplete obstruction, or to remove an infected aortic prosthesis.

The most dramatic of these is the saddle embolus at the aortic bifurcation, secondary to either atrial fibrillation or a mural thrombus in the left ventricle following myocardial infarction. The most common cause is abrupt occlusion of a previously narrowed atherosclerotic arterial channel, at times in association with an abdominal aortic aneurysm as noted (Fig. 23-1).

DIAGNOSIS

An accurate diagnosis of acute aorto-iliac occlusion can usually be made on clinical grounds alone. A previously asymptomatic patient, or one who had limited evidence of intermittent claudication, will exhibit severe ischemia of one or both legs, depending upon whether the terminal aorta itself

535

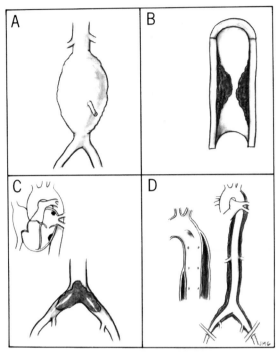

Figure 23-1. Acute aorto-iliac occlusion is most often due to *A*, terminal thrombosis of an aneurysm, *B*, thrombosis of a vessel chronically narrowed by atherosclerosis, *C*, embolism from the left atrium or left ventricle or, *D*, dissecting aneurysm of the aorta.

or one or the other of the iliac outflow tracts has been blocked. If the occlusion is due to embolization from the left side of the heart, the patient will usually give a history of rheumatic heart disease or previous myocardial infarction. The presence of atrial fibrillation, or electrocardiographic evidence of a previous significant myocardial infarction on the electrocardiogram, will offer strong confirmatory evidence.

Usually the patient suddenly experiences either severe pain or numbness and, later, paralysis of the legs. However, some patients have very little pain but experience numbness from the beginning, which persists. As a rule, however, the patient will have severe pain in the extremities, which are blanched and exhibit very poor if any capillary refill. The femoral pulse is absent and the veins are collapsed. When muscle power is lost, the extremity is in serious jeopardy and is approaching a state of tissue necrosis. Pulsations in the abdominal aorta can usually be palpated above the umbilicus, confirming the obstruction between there and the leg. If the opposite femoral pulse is present, the obstruction clearly is in the common or ipsi-

lateral iliac artery, and does not involve the aorta. However, when both femoral pulses are absent, the occlusion may extend all the way to the renal arteries, occasionally even above this level. For, once the outflow of the lower aorta is completely occluded by the embolus, propagating thrombosis may extend in both directions.

If the patient is relatively young and the possibility of atherosclerotic occlusion or thrombosed aneurysm is slight, especially if there exists the history of rheumatic heart disease with atrial fibrillation, aortography is rarely needed for an accurate diagnosis. On the other hand, if the patient is elderly and if there is not strong evidence of previous myocardial infarction or rheumatic heart disease, aortography may be indicated to identify the probable cause of the obstruction. For example, if one side remains open and the iliac outflow tract on this open side is shown to be grossly diseased with marked tortuosity of the vessels, one may conclude that there is little likelihood of successfully removing the obstruction on the other side through a simple femoral incision under local anesthesia, and that laparotomy is required. However, these considerations will vary with each case and must be decided according to the merits of the specific situation.

If aortography is elected, it is often preferable to approach the aorta from a translumbar route, rather than to introduce the catheter into a femoral artery to perform a retrograde aortogram.

A number of additional considerations should be kept in mind as the clinical evaluation proceeds. For example, the signs and symptoms are closely related to the level and extent of arterial obstruction. The presence of varying pulses, now absent but later present, should suggest the possibility of a dissecting aneurysm. The occlusion of major arteries is often confused with paralysis due to a possible neurologic lesion, especially by those who rarely encounter acute arterial occlusion. Moreover, the ischemia of the legs not infrequently results in marked neural deficits and, at times, in a prolonged ischemic neuritis even after the blood flow has been restored. Acute arterial occlusion may also be confused with acute venous occlusion, since venous occlusion may be associated with severe arteriospasm, which abolishes the femoral pulse. However, by and large, acute venous occlusion is associated with cyanosis and swelling of the leg. In contrast, immediately after acute arterial occlusion the leg is not swollen but is cold and even cadaveric in appearance if the patient is white. Here the veins contain little blood and capillary refill is extremely sluggish or absent. Finally, severe spasm of the leg arteries may be secondary to vasospastic agents such as ergotamine derivatives. We treated a nurse who had what initially appeared to represent acute aortic occlusion, but when the femoral arteries were exposed under local anesthesia, to remove the obstructing material in retrograde fashion, we found the femoral arteries in such spasm that they were only 2 to 3 mm. in diameter, approximately the size of a wooden match. Furthermore, the femoral arteriograms identified what appeared to be complete obliteration of arterial branches below this level. Several days later, however, when we had diagnosed the cause of the patient's difficulty as ergotamine poisoning due to a headache prescription, during which time we had used parasympathetic block and eventual sympathectomy in an effort to save the legs from extensive necrosis, the femoral and foot pulses were readily palpable. Following cessation of ergotamine medication she had no further arteriospasm, but the ischemia had been so severe that she had erythema and hyperesthesia of the feet with causalgia for many months thereafter.

Therefore, although the diagnosis of acute aortic occlusion is readily achieved in most patients, in other circumstances the formulation of an accurate diagnosis of the cause and the extent of the involvement can be very difficult indeed.

MANAGEMENT

The diagnosis of acute aorto-iliac occlusion demands prompt action. The conclusion that acute obstruction exists, as well as the differential diagnosis of the extent and probable cause of the occlusion, has been considered previously. A review of several important general considerations will be followed by a survey of the management of each of the most important causes of acute aorta-iliac occlusion.

GENERAL CONSIDERATIONS

The first consideration in any approach to operation is that of the general state of the patient's health. The individual who has experienced acute aorto-iliac occlusion may have serious disease elsewhere, often of the heart. If the patient is young, the cardiac lesion may represent mitral stenosis with atrial fibrillation, in which instance appropriate digitalization and other supportive cardiac therapy may be indicated. In addition, heparinization of the patient will not prevent operation as soon as appropriate, for either the heparin can be neutralized with protamine at the time the incision is made, or, if only femoral incisions are to be employed, heparinization may be allowed to continue during operation. The rationale for heparinization is to reduce the probability of additional thrombus formation in the heart and to maintain patency of the smaller vessels in the legs during the period that their blood flow is minimal prior to operation. Some clinicians prefer to give low molecular weight dextran intravenously, in addition to or in lieu of heparinization. Paravertebral sympathetic block has also been employed to give the maximum diameter of vessels to the legs, and especially to the skin of the legs to prevent skin sloughs that would permit bacterial invasion. Further general supportive measures include the administration of diuretics and the correction of hypoxia, acidosis, and electrolyte derangements. Positive pressure ventilation and other approaches may be employed to correct pulmonary edema. Longstanding atrial fibrillation probably will not respond to drug therapy, but it may be possible later on to convert to a regular rhythm by use of electroshock. Nevertheless, we would not generally attempt electroconversion prior to operation for a saddle embolus.

CLINICAL JUDGMENT

While the above general measures are being initiated to prepare the patient for the minimal operative intervention compatible with the requirements of the given situation, a number of considerations are important in reaching a sound clinical judgment. First, the young person whose aorto-iliac occlusion is due to an embolus from the left atrium will probably do well with either the retrograde femoral or the abdominal approach, assuming that severe cardiopulmonary insufficiency does not already exist and hopefully assuming that no further embolization will occur to vital structures, such as the brain or the mesenteric arterial vasculature or elsewhere, immediately preceding or following the operative procedure. The lower aorta and iliac vessels are not involved with atherosclerosis or aneurysm, and retrograde removal of the embolus through bilateral femoral arterial approaches is usually achieved. An almost equally good result may be anticipated in the patient whose embolus arose from the left ventricle. If marked atherosclerotic changes are not present in the lower aorta and iliac arteries, prompt retrograde embolectomy should be successful. In marked contrast, the patient who has severe atherosclerotic occlusive disease of the legs, with very poor arterial runoff, which may in fact have precipitated the iliac occlusion, may well have a poor prognosis. Furthermore, occlusion secondary to atherosclerosis and thrombosis often occurs in the very elderly patient with other problems and the illness may prove fatal. The patient who is admitted with a previous stroke, who is in advanced heart failure, or who has an elevated BUN secondary to advanced renal failure also has a poor prognosis.

The clinical circumstances in the given case will determine whether the surgeon can approach and remove the aorto-iliac obstruction from the bilateral femoral arterial approach under local anesthesia (see Case 2), or whether he must undertake the more serious transabdominal approach. If there is high-grade obstruction of the iliac arteries with marked atherosclerosis and tortuosity, it will frequently be impossible to introduce the balloon-tipped catheters from below, and the only appropriate approach is through the abdomen. Even here, however, the success of the abdominal approach in relieving the aorto-iliac occlusion will depend upon the quality of the arterial runoff in the branches of the femoral artery below. There will be scant success from removing thrombotic or embolic material from the lower aorta if the runoff into the legs is inadequate to permit the aorta and iliac arteries to remain open postoperatively.

Finally, it must be acknowledged that there is the occasional debilitated elderly patient whose total condition has so deteriorated that the inevitably fatal outcome must be accepted and operative intervention withheld.

Clearly, the surgeon will be faced on different occasions by a wide range of possible factors that will be integrated into his carefully formulated diagnosis, preoperative preparation, and operative approach. Although removal of the clot by the transabdominal operation is effective and widely used, it does subject the patient to greater risk than does the retrograde femoral approach through the groin under local anesthesia. The current availability of high-quality balloon-tipped catheters has enhanced the effectiveness of this approach, and it has the merit of a high success rate and a low risk of death or serious complication. Again, this technique permits the continued use of heparin throughout the operative period and postoperatively. However, when the patient is heparinized, we prefer to leave a drain in the groin incisions for 24 to 48 hours to reduce the incidence of hematomas, which will at times occur despite the most careful attention to hemostasis at operation.

Regardless of whether the approach selected in the given case is retrograde through the femoral arteries or by laparotomy, certain equipment is highly useful and should be on hand. First, the usual array of noncrushing vascular clamps should be available. At a minimum, several bulldog clamps, two Crafoord clamps and two Satinsky clamps may be needed. The balloon-tipped catheters of Fogarty will almost invariably be useful, and several sizes as well as replacements for those which become defective should be ready (Fogarty, 1967). The common femoral arteries should be opened transversely so that transverse closure with interrupted fine sutures will produce no reduction in intraluminal diameter. If the femoral vessels are diseased, as they usually will be in older patients, special care must be exercised to include all layers of the arterial wall in the sutures. No more than three sutures are ordinarily required, following introduction of the balloon-tipped catheters, and we prefer to place all three sutures before tying them down individually. Any distal thrombus in the femoropopliteal channel is removed first and heparin injected by catheter into the distal segment. Following this, the embolic and thrombotic material is removed from the proximal vessels. This sequence is recommended because, if the proximal channel is cleared first, it may thrombose again while attention is turned to the distal segment, though this is unlikely if systemic heparinization has been employed. Since the femoral approach should be through the common femoral arteries and not through the superficial femoral artery, the profunda femoris and the superficial femoral will often need to be clamped. If it is not necessary to occlude both the superficial femoral and profunda femoris arteries below the level of the bifurcation, a certain amount of collateral flow to the leg may be maintained throughout the procedure by placing the clamp above the femoral bifurcation. With appropriate maneuvers, using gentle clamps or the thumb and forefinger (Figure 23-2), the amount of blood lost with each passing of the balloon-tipped catheter can be substantially reduced. Even so, a considerable amount of blood may be lost during the cleansing of the arteries of the thrombotic material or embolus, and at least a liter of crossmatched blood should be available for transfusion if required.

Bleeding from the lumbar arteries can

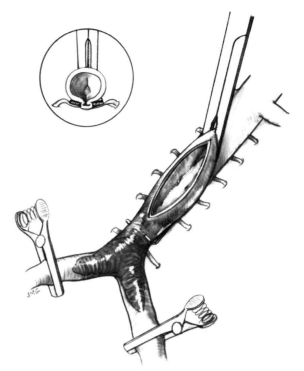

Figure 23-3. Control of lumbar artery bleeding during aortotomy. By placing a suitable clamp as shown, the aorta and lumbar arteries can be gently but adequately compressed to permit aortotomy and thromboembolectomy with minimal blood loss.

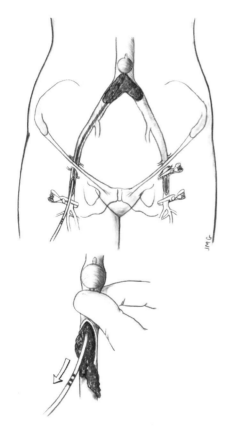

Figure 23-2. Retrograde removal of saddle embolus. By appropriate compression with thumb and forefinger the blood loss can be substantially reduced as the balloon-tipped catheter is passed proximally, the balloon then inflated, and the clot then extracted by drawing the inflated balloon downward.

prove troublesome with the aortotomy in the abdomen, and various maneuvers have been employed to reduce this blood loss during embolectomy or thrombectomy. It is usually possible to minimize or abolish this flow by placing clamps in such a manner that they cross the aorta and occlude the lumbar arteries along the posterior wall of the aorta, while leaving the aortic lumen free for the intra-aortic maneuvers that may be required (Figure 23-3). In this way, exposure of the lumbar arteries for individual control becomes unnecessary, though temporary occlusion of the inferior mesenteric artery may be required. Of course, the bleeding may be so limited in older patients that the best policy is simply to dissect rapidly and to accept a certain amount of bleeding for the few minutes that are required to clear the aorta and the iliac arteries.

Regardless of what maneuvers are employed, damage to the arterial intima should be minimized. For example, the balloons on the balloon-tipped catheters can be inflated so firmly that the intima of the vessels in the lower leg can be damaged and may even be partially avulsed, predisposing to subsequent thrombosis. This clearly should be avoided. Furthermore, when the arterial walls are being compressed against the catheter to reduce blood loss while the catheter is being inserted and withdrawn, the pressure should be gentle enough to reduce bleeding but at the same time not so severe as to injure the intima as the catheter is passed along the vessel. With respect to the number of "passes" which should be made with the catheter, if intimal damage is to be avoided, we try to limit the number to three but of course the effort must be continued until all clot has been removed and arterial flow restored.

SPECIFIC TYPES OF OCCLUSION

EMBOLISM FROM LEFT ATRIUM OR VENTRICLE

Embolism from the left atrium or the left ventricle often produces the most dramatic example of acute aorto-iliac occlusion (Edwards et al., 1966). Even here, however, although the term "saddle embolus" gives a graphic characterization of the pathology involved, the occlusion of one or the other iliac may be incomplete. Or, it may be complete initially and incomplete thereafter, or it may be incomplete and later become complete. This is the type of acute aorto-iliac occlusive disease that is most amenable to removal by prompt surgical intervention.

The general measures to be employed for the correction of heart failure, pulmonary edema, hypoxia, acidosis, and other metabolic problems were outlined previously. Following rapid preparation of the patient, we prefer to attempt first the bilateral femoral retrograde approach under local anesthesia using the balloon-tipped catheters (Ravdin and Wood, 1941). Again, if the patient has been heparinized previously there is no risk in leaving the patient heparinized for the operation, since any bleeding that occurs will be under direct vision in a superficial position in the upper thigh. Both femoral arteries are exposed, so that the introduction of the catheter on one side will not dislodge material into the opposite leg, in which it might embolize to small arteries and be more difficult to remove. The catheter is then passed up one or the other femoral artery to a length that places it well within the aorta. The balloon is inflated with the appropriate amount of saline solution and the catheter is then drawn downward, slight compression of the transverse femoral arteriotomy being maintained between the thumb and forefinger to reduce blood loss. As the clot extrudes it is likely to be followed by a gush of blood that must be controlled promptly. Again, the blood loss at femoral arterial embolectomy or venous thrombectomy is likely to be greater than anticipated, and at least a liter or more of crossmatched blood should be available.

After the embolus has been removed from one side, the catheter should be passed up the other femoral artery and the iliofemoral outflow tract on that side likewise cleared of embolus and propagating thrombus. After both the proximal and distal arterial channels have been cleared of obstruction, the transverse femoral arteriotomies are closed with interrupted 4-0 or 5-0 sutures of silk or synthetic material passed through all layers.

At this stage good distal pulses should have been restored, and a member of the operating team should expose the feet and check the dorsalis pedis and posterior tibial pulses. The absence of these pulses may reflect long-standing occlusion of the popliteal artery or its branches, or it may reflect arteriospasm. On the other hand, absence of the pulses may signify the presence of residual embolus or thrombus farther down the leg. One should not hesitate to perform an arteriogram on the operating table or, if imperfection is detected postoperatively, in the recovery room. Prompt attention to this additional obstruction, if it exists, will be rewarded in many instances with an excellent blood flow to the distal extremity and foot (see Case 1). Above all, success in restoring good arterial blood flow is the result of relentless pursuit of this objective. Every surgeon of experience has been successful in restoring blood flow only after several attempts, in the occasional patient. If the general condition of the patient permits, every effort should be made to remove all obstructing material. Otherwise, at best the patient may have intermittent claudication later and he may lose his leg or even his life.

Following operation, systemic heparinization is continued or low molecular weight dextran is infused. We prefer the latter. If the dextran is used, we usually give 500 ml. during the operation and over the the first several hours thereafter, another 500 ml. over the next 12 hours, and then 500 ml. dripped in slowly over a 12-hour period for each of the next three days. We do not have experimental studies to support this particular use of low molecular weight dextran, but we and others believe it does reduce the incidence of postoperative thrombosis in various types of peripheral arterial operations (Foster et al., 1966). It is not without hazard, however, since it may promote bleeding through fabric prosthesis if given in excess, and a marked augmentation of blood volume can embarrass cardiopulmonary function.

Assuming that the saddle embolus from the left heart has been removed, a next consideration is whether mitral stenosis, if present, should be corrected by closed-finger fracture at the same operation. By and large, we prefer to postpone an attack upon the mitral valve for several reasons. First, the diagnosis may be incomplete, and there may be disease of the aortic valve also. In addition, we prefer that the patient be as well-prepared as possible, so that with the use of cardiopulmonary bypass we can correct at one operation all the intracardiac defects that may need attention.

A major hazard in the patient with atrial fibrillation and embolization is that additional emboli may occur while the patient is still in the hospital. Therefore, we often employ cardioversion to produce a regular rhythm, if this can be accomplished. However, it is after cardioversion that some patients will throw emboli, and the patient must be carefully observed for some time thereafter. In addition, long-term anticoagulation therapy is indicated in most patients, in our judgment.

If the bilateral femoral approach is not successful, we have no hesitation in placing the patient under general anesthesia for the transabdominal approach. For if gangrene of the legs threatens, the metabolic trauma of laparotomy will be far less than subsequent bilateral high thigh amputation. These patients are usually critically ill and an experienced anesthesiologist should be in attendance even when the operation is performed under local anesthesia using the bilateral femoral approach.

If the transabdominal approach is required, the small bowel should be placed in a bag over the right side of the midline incision. The aorta is exposed upward to the point at which a good pulsation is noted, and downward to permit control of the common iliac arteries. It is not usually necessary to dissect the iliac arteries off the iliac veins, for a clamp can simply be placed down across each iliac artery from above. Even though a small amount of vein wall might be included in the clamp, gentle compression will cause no injury to the vein and time is saved. All possible arteries should be cleared of embolic material and associated thrombus.

ATHEROSCLEROTIC AORTO-ILIAC DISEASE WITH ACUTE THROMBOSIS

The most common cause of acute aorto-iliac occlusion is atherosclerosis. The patient may have experienced virtually no symptoms in the past, only to be seized with sudden severe pain in one or both legs, associated with coldness and pallor that are secondary to abrupt cessation of adequate arterial flow. Occasionally this is because of the abrupt occlusion of an abdominal aortic aneurysm, or an iliac aneurysm (see Case 3), but more often it is due simply to final intraluminal thrombosis in the presence of long-standing atherosclerotic occlusive disease of the terminal aorta or one of the iliac arteries. This situation contrasts sharply with that which we considered in connection with the abrupt embolism which follows heart disease. Although many of the patients with atherosclerotic occlusive disease and thrombosis will have coronary artery disease and may have electrocardiographic evidence of previous myocardial infarction, in general their overall state of health may be more stable than that of the patient who has experienced embolization from heart disease. On the other hand, whereas one can be reasonably certain of restoring good blood flow to the legs if prompt operation is performed in the younger patient with mitral stenosis and embolization, the restoration of good blood flow to the legs is not nearly so certain of achievement in the patient with advanced atherosclerotic occlusive disease. This is due to the fact that the patient with occlusive disease and thrombosis frequently has advanced disease of the arteries farther down in the legs. Therefore, even if one is successful in removing the occluding material in the lower aorta or the iliac arteries, the flow to the legs may not be adequate to permit a bypass graft, perhaps from the aorta to the femoral artery, to remain open. Furthermore, extraction of the clot through the retrograde femoral approach will not often be successful. First, much of the material in the lower aorta and common iliac arteries is securely anchored to the vessel wall and does not represent a recent deposit of loose embolus. Second, the common and external iliac arteries may be quite tortuous and so nearly occluded in spots that the catheter cannot be passed from the femoral arteries upward into the aorta. Thus most of these patients will require the transabdominal approach.

Nevertheless, these patients are in no less jeopardy from acute occlusion of the arterial flow to the legs than are younger patients who may have mitral stenosis and embolization. The surgeon has the responsibility of attempting to restore adequate blood flow to the legs by every means possible, and a first consideration is the quality of the runoff in the legs. Therefore, if angiographic visualization of the femoral arteries was not achieved preoperatively, we now expose these vessels and perform arteriograms, first removing distal thrombus if necessary. In general, a bypass is more expeditiously accomplished than is extensive aorto-iliac thrombectomy. However, the lower aorta and common iliac arteries should be cleared if possible, to improve blood supply to the lower colon and pelvic structures through the hypogastrics. An open profunda femoris artery is usually adequate to insure continued patency of a bypass graft.

If the surgeon finds that final occlusion of an aneurysm by thrombus is the cause of the acute occlusive disease (see Case 3), the aneurysm should be resected. One of the more difficult problems to be anticipated is the need to resect a thrombosed aneurysm when the blood flow to the lower extremity is already extremely precarious. The 30 or 40 minutes required for resection of the aneurysm and replacement with a graft may permit clotting of vital residual vasculature in the leg despite the most assiduous attempts at heparinization. In such instances one cannot utilize general heparinization, since the interstices of the graft might fail to clot. However, by preclotting the graft and then heparinizing the patient, with additional heparin instilled distally, it will usually be possible to insert the graft and maintain distal runoff to keep the graft open postoperatively. Again, operative arteriography to identify occlusion of vessels that can be corrected to improve the runoff in the legs should be employed when indicated. If possible, good foot pulses should be established by the end of the operation. This gives a firm baseline against which to check the condition of blood flow in the legs postoperatively. It is always unsafe to assume that "arteriospasm" is the cause of failure to palpate foot pulses. Although it is often true that the spasm of the vessels is present and will relax postoperatively, only with an arteriogram can one exclude the presence of thrombotic or embolic material that should be removed with the balloon-tipped catheters during the operation. Following the operation, maintenance of blood volume will do much toward maintaining good pulses. If an extremity is precariously vascularized, as compared with its opposite member, the undervascularized extremity will be the first member to exhibit cyanosis and coldness and later pallor if cardiac output is diminished. Even if the graft does not become occluded, the blood volume may be inadequate to permit good cardiac output with adequate perfusion of the extremity.

If bilateral aortofemoral bypass is required, flow to one leg should be restored as soon as feasible, since considerable cross circulation occurs from one leg to the other through pelvic collaterals. If thrombotic material is to embolize from the proximal aorta through the bypass, this will usually occur in the leg to which the bypass has been opened first. However, by proper flushing and cleansing of potentially embolic material, distal embolization can be prevented in most instances.

OPERATIVE ALTERNATIVES WHEN LAPAROTOMY IS CONTRAINDICATED

In the occasional patient, the total clinical situation will be so precarious that laparotomy is not indicated. When this occurs, several alternatives are available for revascularizing an extremity in the presence of iliac artery occlusion. These include a cross-over graft from the opposite femoral artery (McCaughan and Kahn, 1960), when flow to only one leg is blocked and the opposite femoral artery has a good pulse (see Case 4). This bypass can be done under local anesthesia. In one of the cases to be described the cross-over graft remained patent beneath the skin of the abdominal walls for months and, when it finally became occluded, sufficient collateral had developed that the patient maintained adequate perfusion of the leg and it remained asymptomatic.

A second alternative is an axillo-femoral bypass (See Chapter 24, Figure 1) (Blaisdell and Hall, 1963; Lewis, 1961). Here again, the entire operation can be performed under local anesthesia in a precariously ill patient. The Dacron prosthesis extends from the axillary artery to the common femoral artery on the involved side, and the operation can be done bilaterally.

DISSECTING ANEURYSM

Occlusion of the terminal aorta or the iliac outflow tracts by a dissecting aneurysm is not particularly common, but it does occur. The most important consideration is to appreciate the nature of the aortic disease, since dissecting aneurysms usually arise in the thorax. To be sure, very occasionally there is a dissecting component of an abdominal aortic aneurysm, but this is rare.

The diagnosis of dissecting aneurysm is usually apparent from the nature of the pain, which begins in the chest or posteriorly between the shoulder blades and progresses downward. The pain is frequently accompanied by a loss of cervical or arm pulsations, and a special feature is that pulses may be present at one time and then disappear and then perhaps reappear. The blood pressure in the two arms may be unequal, since the dissection often begins in the aortic arch, though it may begin anywhere in the aorta and especially just above the aortic valve. Having suspected the diagnosis on the basis of clinical symptoms, an aortogram can be performed, preferably through the right axillary artery, and the dissecting aneurysm can thus be identified. It is not uncommon that the dissecting aneurysm producing intra-abdominal symptomatology is diagnosed at laparotomy. Occasionally the diagnosis is made through a femoral arteriotomy performed for the retrograde removal of a supposed saddle embolus. Although to make the diagnosis in this way poses no special problem, finding a dissecting aneurysm at laparotomy places the surgeon in a position from which he can achieve little and the critically ill patient has thus been subjected to a major operation. The proper approach is to identify the most proximal site of dissection by aortography and then to perform thoracotomy to reconstitute the vessel wall at this point, usually with a Dacron graft (Austen et al., 1967; DeBakey et al., 1967). This corrective procedure is usually performed using left heart bypass to preserve flow to the abdominal viscera. However, this is associated with some risk, since retrograde perfusion through a femoral artery may well result in further dissection or inadequate perfusion of important viscera. Actually, nonoperative management, using antihypertensive drugs, has proved successful in many cases in which surgical intervention was not mandatory to re-establish arterial flow to important viscera (Harris et al., 1967; Wheat and Palmer, 1968).

ACUTE AORTO-ILIAC OCCLUSION SECONDARY TO BLUNT OR OPERATIVE TRAUMA

BLUNT TRAUMA

In the rare circumstance, blunt trauma to the lower abdomen may result in sufficient damage to arteries previously diseased by atherosclerosis that severe occlusion may develop. It is not always appreciated that the lower extremities will tolerate a much shorter period of ischemia when acute occlusion occurs, in contrast to the situation that exists when occlusion has occurred gradually and extensive collateral circulation has developed. Therefore, even if the major arterial trunks are cleared of obstructing material, advanced metabolic changes and even tissue necrosis, with loss of capillary vasculature, may develop if the arrest of arterial flow is prolonged. Judicious heparinization may be indicated, but if anticoagulants are used care must be exercised to avoid hemorrhage from pelvic fractures and related injuries.

POSTOPERATIVE AORTO-ILIAC THROMBOSIS

Postoperative occlusion of the aorto-iliac outflow tract, or a bypass graft from the aorta to the femoral artery, is rare in clinics with a large experience, but many such operations are now performed by surgeons without special experience in vascular procedures. However, even the most experienced vascular surgeon will occasionally realize that the runoff in the leg is so precarious that occlusion of the aorto-femoral bypass may occur. In such situations the alternative means the loss of one leg, possibly both legs, and thus the risk of postoperative thrombosis is accepted.

The usual cause of occlusion of blood flow to the legs following operation involving the distal aorta and the iliac outflow tract is a technical imperfection involving the graft, or inadequate runoff in the legs. No imperfection in the graft itself, in either the proximal anastomosis or the distal anastomosis, should be accepted. If the suture line is not completely satisfactory in every way, it should be taken down and repeated, assuming that other factors permit. It is often unwise to perform endarterectomy on the femoral artery to give a larger lumen. This increases the hazard of thrombosis at the femoral end of the graft, and at times it leaves an insecure suture line for union of the graft with elements of the femoral artery. Rather, if plaques are present in the common femoral artery it will usually be preferable to place the graft to a point more distal in the artery. Another cause of failure of the aortofemoral bypass, aside from technical imperfections, is thrombosis or embolization into the distal extremity. For example, if the operation is slow and time-consuming with prolonged occlusion of blood flow to the involved leg or legs, every effort should be made to maintain excellent anticoagulation in the distal extremity. Otherwise, extensive thrombosis in the capillary bed or even the larger channels may occur, and subsequent efforts to remove this thombus will not be successful in restoring the runoff present preoperatively. Unfortunately, if the bypass does not remain open and clotting occurs, the thrombus may extend into the femoral artery and the patient will have even less perfusion of the leg than he had preoperatively. Under these circumstances prompt reoperation may be mandatory but, unfortunately, extensive small vessel occlusion will at times preclude restoration of good leg perfusion. Experienced judgment and operative technique are vital to success in such circumstances.

CASE STUDY (1). ACUTE LEFT ILIAC ARTERY OCCLUSION WITH AORTO-ILIAC BYPASS AND DISTAL EMBOLISM

H. K., a 61-year-old businessman, was suddenly seized with severe pain in the left leg while at work on January 7, 1970. Although he had had mild claudication in the leg on brisk walking in the past, the new symptoms were so severe that he recognized a major emergency and had himself driven immediately some 150 miles to University Hospital. On arrival it was found that the entire left leg was cold and cadaveric and without sensation. Surprisingly, however, he could still bear some weight on the extremity.

The electrocardiogram was normal, excluding the probability of embolism secondary to atrial fibrillation or mural thrombus from an old myocardial infarction, and it appeared most likely that absence of all leg pulses on the left was due to final thrombosis of a previously narrowed iliac outflow tract. Pulses in the right leg were excellent. Translumbar aortogram disclosed complete occlusion of the left common iliac artery with no visible re-entry below. Operation was initiated by exposure of the left common femoral artery and femoral arteriography, which demonstrated patency of this vessel. Next a laparotomy was performed, and a Dacron bypass was placed from the left common iliac artery above the level of occlusion to the left common femoral artery. Because of the gravity of the threat to the left leg, a left lumbar sympathectomy was also performed to reduce possible arteriospasm and afford maximum leg perfusion from the bypass in the early postoperative period. A good pulse was produced in the femoral artery distal to the bypass and the wounds were closed.

Unfortunately, in the recovery ward it was discovered that, while the left popliteal pulse was adequate, the pulses in this foot were weak. In view of the fact that there were virtually no atrophic changes in the left foot, it appeared likely that these channels had been open prior to the iliac occlusion. Therefore, a percutaneous femoral arteriogram was performed and partial occlusion of the popliteal artery at its trifurcation was demonstrated, possibly due to embolic material. The patient was told that, while the leg was safe, he might later have intermittent claudication in the calf and foot unless the occluding material could be removed. He agreed to reoperation and under local anesthesia old thrombotic material, obviously having embolized from above, was removed with a balloon-tipped (Fogarty) catheter to produce excellent pulses in the foot.

COMMENT

This case emphasizes the pursuit and diligence that may be necessary to achieve the best possible revascularization. Under certain precarious circumstances the limited but adequate perfusion of the left lower leg and foot might have been accepted. However, since the patient was in good general health, the second operation was performed to achieve complete rehabilitation.

CASE STUDY (2). ACUTE THROMBOSIS OF RIGHT ILIAC ARTERY CLEARED RETROGRADE WITH BALLOON-TIPPED CATHETER IN CRITICALLY ILL PATIENT

C. C., a 63-year-old white man, was referred to University Hospital on April 24, 1970, with marked dyspnea due to advanced obstructive pulmonary emphysema and increasing pain in the right leg that had first developed 48 hours earlier. The pulseless right leg was pale, cold, and numb, but some motor power persisted. He had an abdominal aortic aneurysm and an aneurysm involving the left external iliac and common femoral arteries. His general condition was very poor owing to dehydration, chronic malnutrition and emphysema. The ECG exhibited neither atrial fibrillation nor significant previous myocardial infarction. It appeared possible that (a) thrombus had embolized from the abdominal aortic aneurysm to the right iliac artery, (b) thrombosis in this aneurysm had simply extended into the right common iliac artery, or (c) a previously narrowed segment somewhere in the right iliac outflow tract had become thrombosed. Despite the odds against restoring good blood flow by the retrograde femoral approach under local anesthesia, his general physical condition was too poor for laparotomy and the retrograde attempt was elected.

At operation a short transverse incision was made in the right common femoral artery, and it was found to be filled with recent thrombus. A Fogarty catheter was used to clear large amounts of clot from the distal artery and then heparin was instilled. Next the catheter was passed proximally to a length that placed it in the aorta. It was then drawn downward, and several passes were rewarded by removal of both old and recent thrombus and restoration of good arterial flow and pulsations. The arteriotomy was closed with three interrupted silk sutures, and a good posterior tibial pulse was present postoperatively, with complete recovery from the advanced ischemia changes in the leg.

COMMENT

This case represents one instance in which the critical condition of a patient with an abdominal aortic aneurysm prompted the attempt to restore blood flow to the right leg using local anesthesia and the retrograde femoral approach. It was successful. Many times, however, the iliac arteries of such patients will not permit retrograde passage of the catheter into the aorta, not to mention the hazard of dislodging thrombus from within the aortic aneurysm.

CASE STUDY (3). ABRUPT RIGHT ILIAC ARTERY OCCLUSION DUE TO THROMBOSIS OF ANEURYSM WITH RESECTION UNDER LOCAL ANESTHESIA BECAUSE OF HYPOXIA AND HYPOTENSION

D. B., a 60-year-old male hotel clerk with marked kyphoscoliosis and chronic obstructive pulmonary emphysema, was admitted to University Hospital at 4 P.M. on December 12, 1961, in extreme dyspnea with cyanosis, rectal temperature 104° F. (40° C.) and blood pressure 60/? mm. Hg. The chest x-ray disclosed right lower lobe pneumonia. Antibiotics, digitalis, and a Neo-synephrine drip were begun. Soon after admission the patient developed pain in his right leg that rapidly became worse, and the right leg was noted to become pale and cold and was pulseless. The left leg was normal. The surgical service was consulted and it was clear that no major operative procedure was possible in this severely cyanotic and desperately ill man. Nevertheless, to avoid gangrene and loss of the leg, exploration of the right femoral artery under local anesthesia was the elected procedure for retrograde removal of iliac thrombus or embolus with catheters. This could not be achieved but, since the patient was quite thin, the local anesthesia and the incision were extended upward to permit direct inspection of the right iliac artery. A moderate-sized aneurysm of the common iliac artery was found and was replaced with a Dacron graft, the right hypogastric artery being sacrificed.

The leg was revascularized, and the patient recovered from pneumonia and was discharged on December 22.

COMMENT

This man exhibited one of the hazards of hypotension in an older person. Previously narrowed arteries—cerebral, coronary, extremity, or elsewhere—may thrombose completely when blood pressure and blood flow are reduced. In the present instance the occluded iliac aneurysm was approached under local anesthesia with relative ease, since the patient was very thin. There was some concern that the graft might become infected from the organisms producing the pneumonia, but the subsequently isolated pneumococcus proved quite sensitive to intravenous penicillin therapy.

CASE STUDY (4). ACUTE THROMBOSIS OF RIGHT ILIAC ARTERY TREATED BY FEMOROFEMORAL CROSS-OVER BYPASS

L. G., an 85-year-old white woman, was referred to University Hospital on September 19, 1965, with a cold right leg. She had been active and ambulating until one week previously when she had been hospitalized for pneumonia in her community hospital. The symptoms in her leg had developed only a few hours prior to the present admission, but pain had been followed by numbness and now sensation was absent below the knee. The right femoral pulse was absent but the left femoral pulse was fairly good. The ECG confirmed atrial fibrillation. Although embolization might have caused right iliac artery occlusion, it seemed more likely that thrombosis had produced the severe leg ischemia.

In view of her weakness from recent pneumonia and her advanced age, laparotomy was considered to be contraindicated, despite the fact that she would clearly lose the leg if arterial blood flow could not be improved. However, in view of the rather good left femoral pulse, we elected to operate under local anesthesia and, if even the profunda femoris was found to be patent on the right, to perform a 10-mm. Dacron end-to-side cross-over femoral to femoral graft. The right profunda femoris was indeed patent, though the superficial femoral artery was chronically occluded.

Following operation there was no pulse in the right foot because of occlusion of the superficial femoral artery, but the color and warmth of the right leg were improved and venous filling had clearly increased. Power and sensation returned, and in a few days she was able to walk on the leg. The graft, readily palpable beneath the atrophic skin of the abdominal wall, remained pulsatile for almost a year, at which time it became occluded. However, by that time the collateral circulation had improved to the point that no leg symptoms had developed to announce cessation of flow through the prosthesis. It was simply found occluded at one of her regular visits to her local physician.

COMMENT

This woman experienced abrupt occlusion of the right iliac artery following hospitalization for pneumonia, as did another patient (see Case 3). The obstruction may have been caused by embolization, since she did have atrial fibrillation, but on the basis of findings at operation the most likely etiology was final thrombosis of a previously narrowed right iliac outflow tract. When we elected to tunnel a femoral to femoral bypass beneath the skin, to revascularize the right leg while avoiding laparotomy in a weakened and otherwise debilitated 85-year-old woman, we were unaware of previous reports of the successful use of this procedure (McCaughan and Kahn, 1960). It served admirably in this case, and the more extensive axillofemoral bypass was not required.

CASE STUDY (5). OCCLUSION OF LEFT ILIAC ARTERY BY BLUNT TRAUMA

W. M., a 19-year-old Negro male, was admitted to University Hospital at 5:50 A.M. on September 26, 1970, with a cool and pulseless left leg and a pelvic fracture. Two hours earlier his pulpwood truck had turned over on a slippery wet road, pinning him to the ground by pressure on his pelvis anteriorly. He did not go into shock or lose consciousness before or after the truck was removed to release him.

After bladder and urethral injury by the pelvic fracture had been excluded, an aortogram was performed that revealed complete occlusion of the left external iliac artery (Fig. 23-4). Since there was no evidence of significant blood loss, it was assumed that arterial damage with intimal prolapse and thrombosis had produced the obstruction. It was suggested by some that a Fogarty catheter should be introduced through the left femoral artery under local anesthesia and the offending thrombus thus removed. However, the surgeon in charge elected to expose the iliac artery by laparotomy.

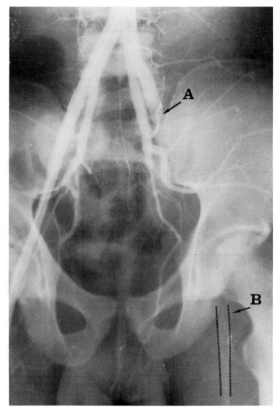

Figure 23-4. The left external iliac artery was not opacified over much of its length. At operation the vessel was found to have been completely severed by external blunt trauma, with retraction and thrombosis and minimal bleeding.

At operation it was found that the severe blunt trauma had caused complete division and retraction of the intima and media, the adventitia remaining intact. The ends of the artery were freshened and closed with 4-0 silk, after the proximal and distal thrombus had been removed.

REFERENCES

Austen, W. G., Buckley, M. J., and McFarland, J., De Sanctis, R. W., and Sanders, C. A.: Therapy of dissecting aneurysms. Arch. Surg., 95:835, 1967.

Blaisdell, F. W., and Hall, A. D.: Axillary-femoral artery bypass for lower extremity ischemia. Surgery, 54:563, 1963.

DeBakey, M. E., Henley, W. S., Cooley, D. A., Morris, G. C., Jr., Crawford, E. S., and Beall, A. C., Jr.: Surgical management of dissecting aneurysms of aorta. J. Thorac. Cardiov. Surg., 49:130, 1965.

Edwards, E. A., Tilney, N., and Lindquist, R. R.: Causes of peripheral embolism and their significance. JAMA, 196:133, 1966.

Fogarty, T. J.: Catheter technique for arterial embolectomy. J. Cardiov. Surg., 8:22, 1967.

Foster, J. H., Killen, D. A., Jolly, P. C., and Kirtley, J. H.: Low molecular weight dextran in vascular surgery:

prevention of early thrombosis following arterial reconstruction in 85 cases. Ann. Surg., *163*:764, 1966.

Hardy, J. D.: Surgery of the Aorta and Its Branches. Philadelphia, J. B. Lippincott, 1960.

Harris, P. D., Malm, J. R., Bigger, J. T., and Bowman, F. O.: Follow-up studies of acute dissecting aortic aneurysms managed by antihypertensive agents. Circulation, 35:(Suppl. 1) 183, 1967.

Lewis, C. D.: A subclavian artery as a means of blood supply to the lower half of the body. Brit. J. Surg., *48*:574, 1961.

McCaughan, J. J., Jr., and Kahn, S. F.: Cross-over graft for unilateral occlusive disease of the iliofemoral arteries. Ann. Surg., *151*:26, 1960.

Provan, J. L., Fraenkel, G. J., and Austen, W. G.: Metabolic and hemodynamic changes after temporary aortic occlusion. Surg. Gynec. Obstet., *123*:544, 1966.

Ravdin, I. S., and Wood, F. C.: The successful removal of a saddle embolus of the aorta, eleven days after acute coronary occlusion. Ann. Surg., *114*:834, 1941.

Wheat, M. W., Jr., and Palmer, R. F.: Drug therapy for dissecting aneurysms. Dis. Chest, *54*:372, 1968.

Willman, V. L., and Hanlon, C. R.: Safer operation in aortic saddle embolism: Four consecutive successful embolectomies via the femoral arteries under local anesthesia. Ann. Surg., *150*:568, 1959.

CHAPTER 24

INFECTED ARTERIAL GRAFTS

by JAMES D. HARDY, M.D., and J. HAROLD CONN, M.D.

J. Harold Conn was born in Oklahoma and graduated from the University of Oklahoma Medical School in 1943. He served his surgical residency at the McKinney Veterans Administration Hospital and, in 1955, became Chief of the Surgical Service at the Jackson Veterans Administration Center. Dr. Conn has long had a special interest in arterial surgery and has published widely in this field. A versatile technical surgeon, he has made a rich contribution through instruction and stimulation of medical students and house officers. His extensive experience with vascular surgery makes him well qualified to discuss the etiology and management of infected arterial grafts.

The development of arterial substitutes has greatly improved the treatment of many arterial diseases. However, all arterial grafts and especially the fabric prostheses are subject to certain complications, which on occasion can be catastrophic. These complications include thrombosis, infection, and disruption of the graft with hemorrhage. At times these problems are actually interrelated, and the patient's limb or life may be placed in the most serious jeopardy. The specific complication primarily to be considered is infection, but sepsis often leads to hemorrhage, graft removal and possible amputation. Fortunately, sepsis is not common following arterial surgery, but when it occurs it represents a most formidable menace.

INCIDENCE OF GRAFT INFECTION

The incidence of graft infection is variously reported from 0 to 6 per cent. Certainly, in any large series of patients some infections will have occurred, though the greater the care exercised in preventing infections, the lower will be the infection rate. A set routine of unchanging nursing personnel who realize the gravity of wound contamination—plus meticulous preoperative, operative, and postoperative care and technique by an experienced surgical team—will result in a low incidence of infection. Staphylococci and coliform bacteria are the organisms most often involved.

GENESIS OF GRAFT INFECTION

It is probable that infection has its genesis in wound contamination at operation in most instances. It is impossible to sterilize the skin completely, and the wound is inevitably open to room air and other sources of contamination for a certain period of time. If the bacterial seeding is minimal, the bacterial defenses of the tissues can usually prevent the development of significant infection.

Other sources of bacterial invasion include lymphatic drainage from infection in the foot, bacteria from the bloodstream, and organisms that enter from the outside when a seroma or hematoma causes skin dehiscence. Subsequent exposure of the graft, perhaps due to excessive length with buckling and necrosis of the overlying skin in the leg, will result in bacterial contamination, as may alimentary tract leakage or urine extravasation within the abdomen.

At times it is difficult to decide whether a false aneurysm developed at the suture line because of infection, or whether the infection developed in the hematoma of the false aneurysm. It is generally believed that autogenous vein grafts are associated with a lower infection rate than are fabric prostheses. This is not really surprising, since the autogenous vein graft is soon incorporated into the patient's own tissues, whereas the fabric prosthesis always remains a foreign body. Infection which develops in association with foreign bodies is notoriously difficult to cure without removal of the offending material. Therefore, most experienced vascular surgeons are less concerned when the patient runs mild fever following the insertion of an autogenous vein graft than if a fabric prosthesis was used. Wylie (1963) has recommended the use of arterial autografts to bridge a contaminated area from which a fabric prosthesis must be removed and flow re-established but, as will be seen, most surgeons prefer to bypass through clean tissue planes when possible, with removal of all graft material from the infected area.

PREVENTION OF INFECTION

Prophylaxis begins well in advance of operation, with elective operation postponed if the patient is febrile. Cutdowns for arteriography should be avoided at sites where an incision is to be made at operation. If a substantial hematoma has developed in the inguinal region following arteriography, planned aortofemoral or femoropopliteal anastomosis adjacent to the hematoma should at times be delayed. Unless arterial surgery is mandatory to save the leg, infection in the foot should be cleared up before operative intervention. Otherwise, bacterial contamination of the graft may occur through the lymphatic route postoperatively. Furthermore, every effort should be made to avoid injury to the skin of the feet and legs, through which infection might gain entry.

The patient should be carefully bathed the night before or the morning of the operation, and at operation itself the most careful preparation of the entire operative field and beyond is carried out. After this we prefer to apply a transparent plastic material over the entire prepared area.

Dissection in the inguinal area is particularly· important. Transsection of multiple lymphatic channels draining the lower leg will permit seromas and often prolonged drainage, which offers a culture medium for at least the minimal numbers of bacteria that are always present in the air of the operating suite. It is preferable to make the skin incision and then spread the tissues vertically to expose the femoral artery. Alternatively, divided lymphatics should be meticulously ligated, to prevent postoperative drainage. Gentleness in retraction will protect fat and muscle from excessive pressure necrosis, thus minimizing the amount of devitalized tissue, and hemostasis should be perfect. Incidentally, subsequent patient annoyance is avoided if the anterior cutaneous and saphenous sensory branches of the femoral nerve are preserved.

In the abdomen, the fabric prosthesis should be carefully protected from the gut by interposition of omentum, retroperitoneal tissues, or elements of the sac when the graft is used to replace an aneurysm. When other pathologic conditions such as gallstones or colon neoplasm are met unexpectedly at operation for aorto-iliac disease, it is the safer course to leave the nonarterial pathology for a subsequent operation. However, we have necessarily removed the gallbladder or performed vagotomy-pyloroplasty on numerous occasions, in association with aneurysm resection, without resulting infection.

As for the operative technique *per se*, careful suture lines with synthetic suture material should prevent postoperative hematomas or false aneurysms, with the risk of further hemorrhage and infection. Good hemostasis permits the avoidance of drains, which always offer a theoretical route for bacterial invasion. If drains are inserted, they should not extend all the way to the graft, and they should be removed at 24 and no later than 48 hours. Drains should generally be avoided but at times they are indicated both to allow blood to escape and to indicate whether or not a generalized ooze is continuing.

The graft itself should be of the proper length, not too long and not too short. If the graft is too long, it will tend to buckle. In the abdomen this may cause thrombosis of the graft, and in the leg it may cause necrosis of the overlying skin and subsequent infection. If the graft is too short, excessive tension is placed on the suture lines and anastomotic defects with early or late hemorrhage may occur. When feasible, an autogenous vein graft is preferred to a fabric prosthesis, especially when potential bacterial contamination exists at the time of operation.

Finally, we believe the operation should be performed as expeditiously as possible, to minimize the time that the open wound is exposed to contamination from all sources — room air, instruments, and defective gloves.

Prophylactic Antibiotics

We use prophylactic antibiotics, usually penicillin and streptomycin, routinely in all major vascular cases. It is acknowledged that there are those who feel that antibiotics are unnecessary, but we feel that the penalty for infection is so severe that the patient deserves the benefit of all feasible prophylaxis available. Specifically, we do not give prophylactic antibiotics preoperatively, but we do instill penicillin and streptomycin in and around the graft and in the rest of the wound at operation, before closing. We also give antibiotics immediately postoperatively by injection, and as soon as possible by mouth, for the first 4 or 5 days following the operation.

With the precautions outlined, infections have been rare on the private service of the senior author.

DIAGNOSIS OF GRAFT INFECTION

The probability that infection exists will usually be apparent. The systemic signs include fever, leukocytosis, tachycardia, and perhaps night sweats. Localized pain is often a prominent feature. If the infection is situated in, or extends to, a site accessible to physical examination, then tenderness, erythema, heat, and swelling may precede a purulent drainage. An abdominal mass may be palpated in the abdomen. The time interval between operation and overt infection ranges from a few days, to weeks, months, or years. As will be seen later, the time of onset is of some importance in planning management. If the infection occurs early, the entire graft is probably involved, since fibrosis has not occurred around the graft to limit spread. In contrast, late infection may have been confined to one end or the other, more often the inguinal site in aortofemoral grafts. If the prosthesis is occluded, infection may have propagated through the thrombus. If there is wound drainage, a positive culture may be obtained. The blood culture may also be positive, especially if fever is accompanied by chills.

When the infection is within the abdomen, diagnosis may be much more difficult. An aortogram may disclose a false aneurysm at the aortic suture line. Urinary symptoms may increase the possibility that an intravenous pyelogram or retrograde pyelography will disclose displacement of urinary tract structures by false aneurysm or hematoma. Shaw and Baue have emphasized that apparent ureteral strictures caused by false

aneurysm or purulent collections usually regress after the compression has been relieved.

Unfortunately, infection may be very difficult to diagnose in the patient with infection around the proximal end of an aortic prosthesis. Here a high index of suspicion must be exercised to prompt adequate management before massive hemorrhage occurs, with loss of limb or life.

Late hemorrhage from an anastomosis may indicate infection but not necessarily. However, if the hemorrhage is associated with infection, bleeding will almost invariably recur, and prompt definitive management is essential to prevent possible disaster.

MANAGEMENT OF THE INFECTED GRAFT

The basic principles for management of the infected graft are (1) maintenance of adequate blood flow to the extremity involved; (2) interruption of blood flow through the infected graft, with instillation of antibiotics through draining sinuses or along limbs of the graft, and (3) operative removal of the infected graft.

MAINTENANCE OF ADEQUATE BLOOD FLOW TO EXTREMITY

The major hazard of an arterial graft infection is that it threatens limb and even life. Except for infected grafts in the midthigh, which occasionally have been salvaged by drainage and intensive local and systemic antibiotic therapy, most infected grafts must be removed. If the graft is already occluded, it can be removed without reducing distal blood flow, and insertion of a second graft can be wisely delayed until all risk of infection has passed. Similarly, collateral flow may be such that the graft can be removed without intolerable distal ischemia. However, when the blood flow through the graft is essential to survival of the part perfused, its removal will produce gangrene unless an alternate pathway has first been established. Remarkable ingenuity has been marshalled to provide such alternative pathways, as shown in Figures 24-1 to 24-6, redrawn from Fry and Lindenauer (1967) in most instances. The new bypass must be placed through unhave to be removed, and an alternative by-pass should be planned.

If bleeding from one or the other of the anastomoses has occurred, especially if there is an associated break in the overlying skin with a sinus tract, the graft must be considered infected and it will almost invariably bleed again. The patient, the nursing staff and members of the patient's family should be carefully instructed regarding steps to take if fresh bleeding occurs. We have a patient whose wife saved his life by applying hard pressure, as instructed, to the supra-clavicular sinus leading from a carotid-subclavian fabric bypass infected by staphy-lococci (see Case 1).

Since renewed hemorrhage could prove disastrous, the patient cannot safely leave the hospital once blood has emerged from a sinus tract leading to the graft. Although the bleeding usually occurs at one of the anastomoses of a fabric graft, we had a pa-tient (see Case 2) in whom the hemorrhage was through the interstices of the middle of the graft, into an adherent loop of small bowel.

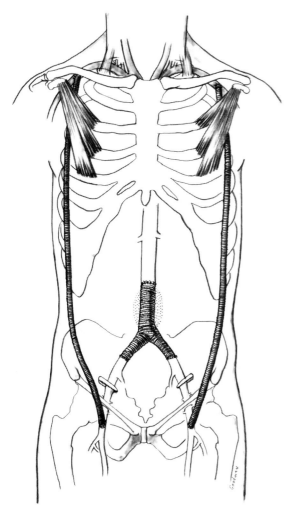

Figure 24-1. Bilateral axillofemoral bypass grafts. Infection of aortic fabric prosthesis.

infected tissue planes. In general, infection involves either the proximal or the distal anastomosis, but any part or all of the graft may be involved.

WHEN MUST THE GRAFT BE REMOVED?

There is great temptation to procrastinate, or to attempt to get by with less than defini-tive measures, when the graft remains patent and provides important blood flow to distal tissues. For example, when the graft has buckled and eventually eroded through the skin, with visible exposure of the fabric, it must be considered infected, and it is rarely possible thereafter to cover the prosthesis satisfactorily and safely with a split-thickness skin graft or a full-thickness flap. It will

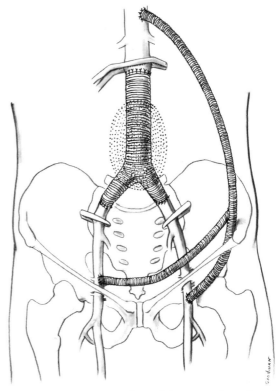

Figure 24-2. Aortofemoral bypasses for infected aortic fabric graft.

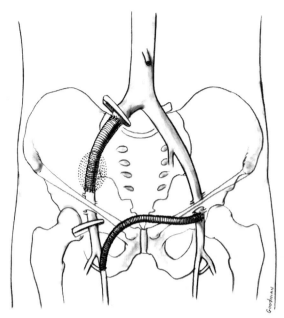

Figure 24-3. Femofemoral bypass for infected right iliac fabric graft.

If operation is for control of anastomotic hemorrhage, at which time the graft must be removed, a new bypass should first be provided through clean tissue planes and these wounds closed; the infected graft is then removed with suture closure of the sites of the proximal and distal anastomoses. Of course, if it be feasible to ligate the proximal and distal arteries through uncontaminated tissues at sites above and below the anastomoses, this should be done.

LIGATION OF GRAFT AND INSTILLATION OF ANTIBIOTICS THROUGH SINUS TRACT

When a sinus tract extends down to the accessible graft, a catheter should be inserted and appropriate antibiotics instilled every several hours for 5 days. If the antibiotic sensitivities change, the therapy should be altered accordingly.

As noted previously, infected grafts in the midthigh have occasionally been salvaged by adequate drainage and prolonged instillation of antibiotics to which the bacteria were sensitive (see Case 5). This presupposes that a false aneurysm with hemorrhage has not occurred. Furthermore, massive hemorrhage into the thigh is far more readily controlled than is hemorrhage associated with

an aortic or an aortofemoral prosthesis. Therefore, infected grafts within the abdomen should always be removed, and the authors virtually always plan from the outset to remove any infected fabric prosthesis, wherever it is located.

Thus, although the initial step (after providing a bypass) is to halt flow through a nonoccluded graft and thereafter to instill antibiotics beside the fabric graft for from 5 to 7 days, the ultimate aim is to remove the graft and to ligate or oversew the artery at each end, preferably through clean tissue planes.

REMOVAL OF GRAFT

Once a bypass has been placed through clean tissue planes and the infection controlled to the extent possible with antibiotic irrigations and systemic therapy, the graft should be removed. Whereas actual extirpation of the prosthesis is usually easily accomplished, secure closure of the artery proximally and distally, especially the aorta, poses a definite hazard. In fact, late dehiscence of the aortic closure is the most common cause of death following removal of an infected aortic prosthesis.

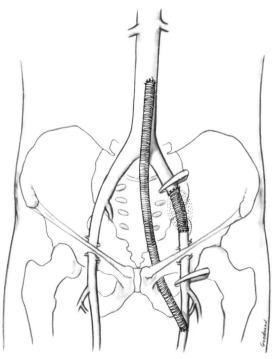

Figure 24-4. Aortofemoral bypass for infected left iliac fabric graft.

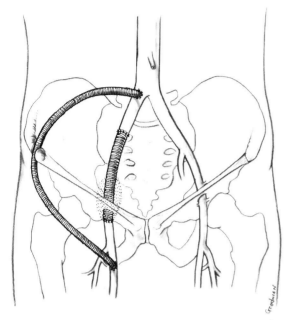

Figure 24-5. Iliofemoral bypass through notch cut in ilium.

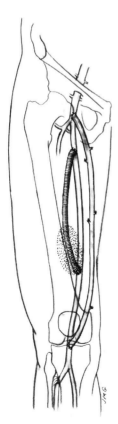

Figure 24-6. Reversed saphenous vein femoropopliteal bypass prior to removal of patent and essential femoropopliteal fabric prosthesis.

MANAGEMENT OF INFECTED GRAFTS AT SPECIFIC LOCATIONS

The plan of attack must be governed by the location of the graft, whether it is essential to the survival of distal tissues, and whether or not emergency operation is required to control hemorrhage.

AORTIC OR AORTOFEMORAL GRAFT

Infection of an aortic graft manifests itself by the general signs of sepsis—fever, tachycardia, night sweats, leukocytosis—and by local signs such as abdominal or back pain or dysfunction of surrounding organs. If the graft extends from the aorta to the femoral arteries, there may exist pain, heat, swelling, and erythema at the groin on the involved side. If the infection has produced hemorrhage within the abdomen the patient may be anemic. The blood culture, repeated several times, may be positive. Displacement or embarrassment of urinary tract structures, or a palpable mass in the flank, should prompt urography and an aortogram, which may disclose a false aneurysm. In contrast to infection in the leg with a femoropopliteal graft, in which hemorrhage can be controlled by pressure or the leg even sacrificed if required to save life, the infected aortic graft must be removed.

Thus, once the diagnosis of infection around the aortic or aortofemoral graft has been made, the steps previously outlined must be taken: (a) a suitable bypass must be provided through clean tissue planes by whichever of the several available techniques is most applicable in the given case (Figures 24-1 and 24-2); (b) antibiotic coverage should be provided for several days, perhaps instilled through a sinus tract or the incision employed to ligate the previously patent prosthesis; and (c) the infected graft should then be removed and the proximal aorta and distal vessel closed securely and covered with available adjacent tissues. Of course, if acute and continuing hemorrhage forces emergency operation, the several steps will have to be completed at the same procedure. If the graft has not been patent, it may be possible to remove it and delay insertion of another graft until all signs of infection have been absent for weeks or months.

The bypass may come from the aorta above the level of the previous graft, from the axillary artery, from the opposite femoral artery beneath the skin of the abdominal wall if the opposite femoral artery is strong and patent, or by other maneuvers presented in the several illustrations.

After a bypass circulation has been provided through clean and uninfected tissues, and after the sinus has been irrigated with appropriate antibiotics for a number of days, the abdominal incision is made and the graft is removed if it has previously become occluded. On the other hand, if the graft has been patent, the next step should be the bilateral exposure of the graft at the femoral areas, the bypass having been established distal to this anastomosis on each side, and the graft then ligated and catheters inserted for instillation of antibiotics through the sinus tract. The ligation of the graft on each side will cause it to clot, and then it can be dealt with more readily later. After irrigation of the sinus tracts with appropriate antibiotics for several days, the formal abdominal laparotomy incision is made and the graft completely removed and the aorta closed. If the graft lies entirely within the abdomen, preliminary operation to occlude the graft is probably not judicious.

When the abdomen is entered for the removal of the infected graft, there may be a temptation to leave a portion of a graft which does not appear to be infected. However, having established a satisfactory bypass to the femoral artery below the level of the insertion of the limb or limbs of the aortofemoral bypass, the entire previous graft should be removed. If the infection is due to a graft that was inserted for removal of an aneurysm, with removal of most of the infrarenal aorta to the iliacs or to the femoral artery, then, of course, the end of the aorta must be closed above. The most serious and often fatal complication of removing the infected aortic prosthesis has been a blowout of the proximal aortic suture line. Various maneuvers have been employed to buttress this aortic closure, including use of surrounding tissue and especially the fascia overlying the spine.

Following removal of the graft and suturing of the aorta, the previously mentioned antibiotic coverage should be continued and the patient should be kept in the hospital for several weeks. Unfortunately, even months later, this aortic infection may recur

and the aortic closure may dehisce with fatal hemorrhage. The most common serious organisms are either staphylococcus, coliform organisms, or pseudomonas.

THE INFECTED FEMOROPOPLITEAL FABRIC GRAFT

The infected femoropopliteal bypass graft has a much less serious connotation than does the aortofemoral bypass, or aortic replacement graft. Life-maintaining viscera are not involved and the leg may be sacrificed if necessary. However, the optimal objective is to salvage the extremity. If the graft has become occluded and the leg is viable, it will of course be possible to remove the graft, close the vessel at each end with appropriate local antibiotic irrigations and systemic therapy, and then allow infection to clear up and place another graft at a later date. Similarly, if the initial graft was inserted for serious intermittent claudication but not for pregangrenous changes, it may be possible to remove the graft without loss of the leg and without a bypass graft. However, if the ischemia for which the graft was initially inserted was so severe as to threaten gangrene, it will usually be necessary to provide an alternate bypass graft if the present original graft is still patent and still supplying the major blood flow to the foot.

A period of nonoperative management is occasionally justified, if massive hemorrhage does not threaten. If the patient and nursing personnel are properly instructed, the danger of exsanguination is not great in the hospital. The infection should be drained, hot wet dressings applied and appropriate antibiotics instilled after sensitivities are obtained. If the graft is occluded, it should be removed and a new graft placed at a later date. Actually, we prefer to use a saphenous vein graft in the leg, when feasible. After the vein has been removed and checked for leakage at its several ligated collaterals, it should be distended with saline to the point of paralysis, achieving maximum diameter.

GRAFTS AT OTHER LOCATIONS

We have not successfully managed infection of a graft in the thoracic aorta. The one patient with such a distressing circumstance was first admitted to University Hospital with intermittent hemoptysis from an aorto-bronchial fistula at the site of an aneurysm. The aneurysm was resected, and replaced with a Teflon graft, though a slight amount of purulent material was present. Massive antibiotic coverage was employed, and the postoperative course was uneventful. Some weeks later, however, the patient rather abruptly exsanguinated, doubtless owing to infection at the suture line.

In the future, we shall provide a bypass through clean tissue planes, and then close the aorta proximally and distally, with removal of the graft. This approach applies to any infected graft, wherever it is situated. A monofilament Dacron suture material is considered preferable to silk, since it provides less of a nidus for persistent infection.

CASE STUDY (1). INFECTION OF LEFT CAROTID LEFT SUBCLAVIAN ARTERY BYPASS

T. S., a 51-year-old airplane mechanic, was well until 1965 when he noted fatigue in the left arm and some dizziness when using a screwdriver with his hands above his head. His physician found the left radial pulse much weaker than the right, with the blood pressure 144/60 in the right arm and unobtainable in the left arm. Arch aortography disclosed occlusion of the proximal left subclavian artery, with left subclavian steal. The left common carotid artery and the innominate and its branches were essentially clear.

At operation in University Hospital on September 22, 1965, a 10-mm. Dacron bypass was placed from the left common carotid artery to the left subclavian artery. The bypass was initially satisfactory, but thrombosed in about one month, with associated staphylococcal infection. It was readily reopened, by removing the thrombus through a small incision in the graft, but the patient was readmitted on November 4, 1965, for massive hemorrhage through a persistent sinus tract. Actually, exsanguination was prevented by his wife, who applied firm pressure over the left supraclavicular space, having been warned of this possibility and carefully instructed as to what to do in case bleeding did occur. At exploration it was found that the hemorrhage had occurred from the center of the graft, where it had been reopened to remove clot previously: the infection appeared to have cleared. Therefore, the graft was again repaired and still not removed—as we would surely do at the present time. He did well thereafter until September 14, 1966, when he returned for evaluation because of a small pustule in the scar, which contained staphylococci. It was clear that, 10 months after the last exploration, the graft was still infected. Furthermore, no pulse could be palpated over the prosthesis. Accordingly, operation was performed, the thrombosed graft removed, and the carotid and subclavian arteries closed by lateral suture. His course thereafter was uneventful, though of course he still had the subclavian steal syndrome and could not work.

COMMENT

A considerable risk was taken by leaving this graft in place when the infection was first discovered. It was not removed, first, because it was functioning; second, any hemorrhage that occurred would presumably be confined and not represent a large volume; third, the site was readily accessible to point pressure control by the alerted family; and, fourth, our policy regarding infection of a fabric prosthesis had not matured to its present stage. At the present time we would usually employ a saphenous vein graft. Furthermore, the diagnosis of staphylococcal infection around a fabric prosthesis, even without hemorrhage, would prompt its removal. We have not yet had a significant infection around a vein graft, and therefore we have not yet forged a policy based on experience: at present each case would be individualized.

CASE STUDY (2). HEMORRHAGE THROUGH WALL OF DACRON GRAFT SECONDARY TO EROSION OF SMALL BOWEL

R. B., a 45-year-old white male, had a left aorto-external iliac Dacron bypass graft in 1961 for complete occlusion of the left common iliac artery. He was readmitted to Veterans Hospital in 1964 because of blockage of the left superficial femoral artery, and another Dacron bypass graft was placed from the left common femoral to the popliteal artery. Symptoms were relieved and he did well until 1965, when he was readmitted with massive bright red bleeding from the rectum. He almost exsanguinated, and was pulseless and without blood pressure. The abdomen was opened quickly without anesthesia and a fistula between the middle of the aorto-iliac graft and the jejunum was found. The bowel had wrapped itself around the fabric prosthesis, and the graft had actually eroded into the lumen of the small bowel. Intestinal fluids had completely dissolved both the organized thrombus in the interstices and the pseudo-intima of this area, allowing blood to pass through the interstices into the lumen of the bowel. The bowel was resected and end-to-end anastomosis accomplished. The graft was allowed to remain in place, covered by available interposed tissues. Unfortunately, the patient had another massive gastrointestinal hemorrhage approximately three weeks later, and on exploration a fistula between the aortic graft suture line and the small intestine was found to be present. The bowel was resutured, and the aortograft suture line was reinforced with silk sutures. The patient developed a jejunocutaneous fistula, continued to do poorly, and eventually expired on April 20, 1965.

COMMENT

This patient might have been saved if the aorto-iliac graft had been removed at the first, and certainly at the second, exploratory operation. Although no further massive hemorrhage occurred, despite the fact that the patent graft remained in place, this dire possibility substantially affected decisions regarding the optimal management of the jejunocutaneous fistula, from which he eventually died.

Optimal management would have consisted of (a) formation of a suitable arterial bypass to preserve blood flow to the left leg; (b) removal of the infected graft, with ligation of the left iliac artery and careful monafilament suture closure of the aorta, with tissue interposition to preserve separation of the bowel and the aortic suture line; and (c) massive antibiotic therapy with agents to which the bacteria were shown to be sensitive.

CASE STUDY (3). SERRATIA MARCESCENS INFECTION OF AORTIC GRAFT, WITH AXILLOFEMORAL BYPASS

J. H., a 62-year-old white man, was first admitted to Jackson Veterans Hospital on May 25, 1968, with a cold, blue, and painful left lower extremity of 24 hours' duration. Past history revealed that a ruptured right internal iliac aneurysm had been ligated and oversewn in a private hospital in Tuscaloosa, Alabama, in June, 1966, and that one month thereafter a ruptured aortoiliac aneurysm had been resected and replaced with a Teflon bifurcation graft at the Veterans Hospital in Birmingham, Alabama. The postoperative course had been uneventful.

A left femoral arteriogram revealed complete block of the left superficial femoral artery, with no run-off but fairly good collateral circulation. A right femoral arteriogram demonstrated large right femoral and popliteal aneurysms. A left lumbar sympathectomy was done, which gave symptomatic relief. He was discharged and returned on July 9, 1968, for resection of the right femoral and popliteal aneurysms with Dacron graft replacement. The postoperative course was uneventful. Urinalysis on this admission showed 70 to 80 white blood cells and cultured *Staphylococcus albus* and diphtheroids.

He was next seen six months later, on January 5, 1969, with a red, tender area over the right femoral incision that had been present for 24 hours. This area spontaneously drained a thick, purulent material that cultured only an abundant growth of *Serratia marcescens*. A repeat culture was predominantly *Serratia marcescens* but also grew *Staphylococcus albus*. The Serratia was sensitive only to kanamycin and gentamicin, so the patient was given kanamycin plus ampicillin and Prostaphlin. The infection cleared rapidly and he was discharged on January 20, 1969. Urinalysis on this admission contained 20 to 30 WBC and cultured Enterococcus, *Pseudomonas aeruginosa,* and *Proteus mirabilis.* He returned to the hospital four days later with recurrence of the right inguinal abscess. Following incision and drainage, his temperature rose to 103° F. (39.4° C.), with chills and fever. A blood culture taken at that time grew a pure growth of *Serratia marcescens*. The right

leg suddenly became ischemic, with severe pain and absence of all pulses, and a lumbar aortogram revealed blockage of the right iliac limb of the aortic bifurcation graft. The patient continued to run a septic course, despite surgical drainage and kanamycin; therefore, the right femoral graft was removed on February 5, 1969. He still remained toxic and nine days later, on February 14, 1969, the entire bifurcation graft was removed and the aorta oversewn immediately below the renal arteries. The graft was surrounded with purulent material that cultured *Serratia marcescens*. A left axillofemoral graft was performed to revascularize the lower extremities. His condition improved markedly, but the right leg remained ischemic and painful. Consequently, a right above-the-knee amputation was done on February 26, 1969. Because of infection, the stump was left open and closed secondarily three weeks later. The patient learned to ambulate with the aid of a walker and was discharged. He did well until May 29, 1969, three and one-half months after the axillofemoral graft, when he was awakened with severe left leg pain. He had been sleeping on his left side at the time. Examination revealed a cold mottled left leg with no pulse in the axillofemoral graft. Left axillary arteriogram demonstrated a complete block of the axillofemoral bypass graft. The left inguinal area was explored, and the graft and femoral artery were found to be thrombosed. The graft was opened anteriorly and all thrombus material and pseudointima removed with a Fogarty catheter. The only patent run-off was the profunda femoris; therefore, the distal end of the graft was re-anastomosed end-to-end to this artery. There was immediate good blood flow, and the left leg and the right thigh stump returned to normal color. After this episode the patient was placed on anticoagulants and has remained on maintenance Coumadin. He returned on November 5, 1969, with right thigh stump pain and temperature of 102° F. (38.9° C.). A small abscess of this area was incised and drained, and again the organism was *Serratia marcescens*. This completely subsided with kanamycin. The axillofemoral graft continued to maintain good blood supply to both lower extremities.

COMMENT

Serratia marcescens, once looked upon as a very innocuous organism, has in recent years been widely reported as a serious pathogen, especially in connection with cardiovascular operations. Clearly, its virulence, manifested by its capacity to invade the tissues and bloodstream and to multiply in the human host, has increased significantly. An axillofemoral graft preserved blood flow to the leg in this patient.

CASE STUDY (4). BILATERAL, AORTOFEMOROPOPLITEAL BYPASS DACRON GRAFT WITH FEBRILE POSTOPERATIVE COURSE, SKIN NECROSIS OVER GRAFT ON LEFT, AND EVENTUAL COVERAGE

T. C., a 65-year-old Negro man who trained bird dogs, was admitted to University Hospital on January 5, 1970, with impending gangrene of the right foot due to ischemia. Aortograms disclosed severe atherosclerotic occlusive disease of the lower aorta and iliac arteries, with poor visualization of the femoral arteries. At operation on January 9, 1970, the femoral artery on each side was found to be inadequate to accept a graft. Therefore, the limbs of the Dacron Y-graft were lengthened by suturing on extensions of 10-mm. Dacron tubing, and bilateral aortofemoropopliteal bypasses were performed. This produced good distal popliteal pulses and substantial improvement of blood supply in the feet. The operation was a long one and the wounds were open to possible contamination for some hours.

The postoperative course was a febrile one, and this disturbing fever persisted for almost 14 days. At first it was believed that pulmonary or urinary tract infection was producing the fever, but, as time passed, the possibility of infection somewhere along the extensive fabric prosthesis received increasing attention. Heavy antibiotic coverage was continued. Cultures of urine and sputum were not remarkable. Gradually, however, the fever declined, and on January 31, 1970, he was discharged from the hospital. At this time he had a very slight superficial infection on the left inguinal incision, but this appeared to be healing steadily.

Unfortunately, when he returned to follow-up clinic, the skin overlying the graft in the left groin now exhibited a 2-cm. area of enlarging necrosis. As this area was observed over the next week or so, more skin necrosis occurred and eventually enlarged to include an area several centimeters in diameter. The graft was not actually visible, but it was pulsating just beneath a layer of granulation tissue. One could not be certain whether or not a sinus tract extended down to the prosthesis. Twice the skin of the upper thigh was undermined under local anesthesia and pulled together with mattress sutures to close the defect. However, each time the closure broke down, leaving a still larger skin defect. Therefore, the patient was readmitted to University Hospital and a skin flap was rotated to fill the defect. This flap eventually became partially necrotic, despite a wide base and virtually no tension, and, finally, a split-thickness skin graft was applied to the prepared site. Despite loss of about 50 per cent of this graft, a sufficient take was achieved to provide eventual coverage after further weeks in the hospital. He now has unlimited exercise tolerance, no skin defect exists, and there is no systemic or local evidence of infection.

COMMENT

This patient had prolonged fever following a tedious operation during which bacterial contamination around a long fabric prosthesis could easily have occurred. Had the graft been situated solely in one leg, we might have been tempted to remove it and accept loss of the leg, especially if hemorrhage had occurred at any time. However, the penalty to one or both legs of removing the bilateral aortopopliteal graft was so large that intensive nonoperative treatment with antibiotic therapy was continued in the absence of definite clinical evidence of actual graft infection. Concern was accentuated when the left limb

of the graft became questionably exposed in the groin. However, skin coverage was finally achieved. Because of the gravity of graft infection, if present, the patient stayed in the hospital for many weeks.

CASE STUDY (5). AORTIC BIFURCATION GRAFT INFECTION SUCCESSFULLY TREATED WITH SURGICAL DRAINAGE AND ANTIBIOTIC IRRIGATIONS

G. B., a 39-year-old white male, was admitted to the Veterans Hospital in February, 1964, for ulcers over the right tibia of five months' duration. These ulcers had increased in size despite intensive treatment by the local physician. Eighteen months prior to admission he had had an ulcer of the left leg, which required one year to heal. There was minimal intermittent claudication of thighs and legs but no impotence. The patient had been involved in a motor vehicle accident 12 years previously, with resultant hemiparesis of right arm and leg.

Physical examination revealed a well-developed, well-nourished white male who appeared older than his chronological age of 39. No femoral or more distal pulses were palpable. The skin was shiny and atrophic bilaterally.

Treatment consisted of saline soaks and antibiotics. The ulcers become clean but showed very little evidence of healing after four weeks. An abdominal aortogram revealed almost complete block at the bifurcation with partial filling of the left common iliac. Attempted (blind) femoral arteriograms were unsuccessful.

At operation on February 14, 1964, bilateral femoral arteriograms showed good run-off in the left extremity but blockage of the right superficial femoral artery, with poor collaterals in the right leg. A bilateral aortofemoral bypass graft using Dacron was performed following endarterectomy of the right profunda femoris artery.

Postoperatively, both lower extremities were warm with both pedal pulses present on the left and a posterior tibial pulse on the right. The ulcers promptly began to heal and finally healed completely with the aid of a split-thickness skin graft. Three weeks postoperatively, the patient spiked a temperature to 103° F. (39.4° C.), with redness and induration over the right femoral incision. Exploration revealed purulent material that cultured gamma Streptococcus. An incision and drainage of this abscess produced about 10 ml. of thin yellow purulent material that was immediately superficial to the Dacron graft. The cavity was thoroughly irrigated with saline solution, was drained, and a PE #90 polyethylene catheter was left in for irrigation. This was irrigated every two hours during the day with kanamycin solution. The wound healed rapidly, the graft continued to function, and there was no recurrence of infection.

COMMENT

This patient, as with others reported in the literature (Whelan), was successfully treated with drainage and antibiotic therapy. The success achieved in our case may have been a result of (a) the superficial nature of the infection, which permitted effective drainage; (b) the relatively nonvirulent organism involved; (c) the fact that almost continuous instillation of appropriate antibiotics was possible; (d) the fact that infection developed soon after operation and was promptly detected because the wound was readily accessible for examination; and (e) the graft itself may not have been involved by the superficial infection.

CONCLUSION

Infection around an arterial graft represents a severe threat to limb or life, and all possible prophylaxis is justified. However, the occasional infection will inevitably occur on any busy vascular service, and an orderly plan of management is imperative. Representative problems have been reviewed and illustrated with case analyses. The treatments used in these patients were not always successful, as happens in clinical practice. Nevertheless, if a carefully conceived plan of management is promptly and vigorously executed, many patients with an infected arterial graft can be treated satisfactorily.

REFERENCES

Blaisdell, F. W., DeMattel, G. A., and Gauder, P. J.: Extraperitoneal thoracic aorta to femoral bypass as replacement for an infected aortic bifurcation prosthesis. Amer. J. Surg., *102*:583, 1961.

Blaisdell, F. W., and Hall, A. D.: Axillary-femoral artery bypass for lower extremity ischemia. Surgery, *54*: 563, 1963.

Carter, S. C., Cohen, A., and Whelan, T. J.: Clinical experience with management of the infected Dacron graft. Ann. Surg., *158*:249, 1963.

Conn, J. H., Hardy, J. D., Chavez, C. M., and Fain, W. R.: Infected arterial grafts: Experience in 22 cases with emphasis on unusual bacteria and techniques. Ann. Surg., *171*:704, 1970.

Diethrich, E. B., Noon, G. P., Liddicoat, J. E., and DeBakey, M. E.: Management of the infected aorto-femoral arterial prosthesis. Surgery. (To be published.)

Foster, J. H., Bergins, T., and Scott, H. W., Jr.: An experimental study of arterial replacement in the presence of bacterial infection. Surg. Gynec. Obstet., *108*:141, 1959.

Fry, W. J., and Lindenauer, S. M.: Infection complicating the use of plastic arterial implants. Arch. Surg., *94*:600, 1967.

Hardy, J. D.: Surgery of the Aorta and Its Branches. Philadelphia, J. B. Lippincott, 1960.

Healy, S. G., et al.: Reconstructive operations for aorto-iliac obliterative disease. New Eng. J. Med., *271*: 1386, 1964.

Hoffert, P. W., Gensler, S., and Haimovici, H.: Infection complicating arterial grafts. Arch. Surg., *90*:427, 1965.

Javid, H., et al.: Complications of abdominal aortic grafts. Arch. Surg., *65*:650, 1962.

Lindenauer, S. M., Fry, W. J., Schaub, G., and Wild, D.: Use of antibiotics in prevention of vascular graft infections. Surgery, *62*:407, 1967.

Mannick, J. A.: Complications of peripheral arterial surgery and their management. Amer. J. Surg., *116*:387, 1968.

Mannick, J. A., Jackson, B. T., Coffman, J. D., and Hume, D. M.: Success of bypass vein grafts in patients with isolated popliteal artery segments. Surgery, *61*:17, 1967.

Mannick, J. A., and Nabseth, D. C.: Axilla-femoral bypass graft: A safe alternative to aortoiliac reconstruction. New Eng. J. Med., *278*:461, 1968.

McCaughan, J. J., Jr., and Kahn, S. F.: Cross-over graft for unilateral occlusive disease of the iliofemoral disease. Ann. Surg., *151*:26, 1960.

Sawyers, J. L., Jacobs, J. K., and Sutton, J. P.: Peripheral anastomotic aneurysms: Development following arterial reconstruction with prosthetic grafts. Arch. Surg., *95*:802, 1967.

Schramel, R. J., and Creech, O., Jr.: Effects of infection and exposure on synthetic arterial prostheses. Arch. Surg., *78*:271, 1959.

Shaw, R. S., and Baue, A. E.: Management of sepsis complicating arterial reconstructive surgery. Surgery, *53*:75, 1963.

Urdaneta, L. F., Visudh-Arom, K., Delaney, J., and Castaneda, A. R.: Use of bilateral axillo-femoral bypass prosthesis for the management of bifurcation grafts: Report of a case with extended follow-up. Surgery, *65*:753, 1969.

Van DeWater, J. M., and Gool, P. G.: Management of patients with infected vascular prostheses. Amer. Surg., *31*:651, 1965.

Veith, F. J., Hartsuck, J. M., and Crane, C.: Management of aorto-iliac reconstruction complicated by sepsis and hemorrhage. New Eng. J. Med., *270*:1389, 1964.

Vollmar, J., Trede, M., Laubach, K., and Forrest, H.: Principles of reconstructive procedures for chronic femoro-popliteal occlusions: Report on 546 operations. Ann. Surg., *168*:215, 1968.

Wylie, E. J.: In discussion of Management of Sepsis Complicating Arterial Reconstructive Surgery, Shaw and Baue, Surgery, *53*:75, 1963.

CHAPTER 25

SEPSIS FOLLOWING KIDNEY TRANSPLANTATION

by

RICHARD L. SIMMONS, M.D.[*],
CARL M. KJELLSTRAND, M.D., and
JOHN S. NAJARIAN, M.D.[*][†]

Richard L. Simmons was elected to Phi Beta Kappa at Harvard University and to Alpha Omega Alpha at Boston University School of Medicine. After extensive residency and postresidency fellowship training at Columbia and Presbyterian Hospital and the Massachusetts General Hospital, he joined the surgical faculty of the University of Minnesota in 1968 as Assistant Professor of Surgery. Tissue transplantation represents his principal research interest.

Carl-Magnus Kjellstrand was born in Sweden and graduated from the University of Lund Medical School in 1962. He took his internship at the Bethesda Lutheran Hospital, St. Paul, Minnesota, and later served as Director of the Artificial Kidney Unit in that institution. At present he is Assistant Professor of Medicine and of Surgery and Director of the Dialysis Unit, University of Minnesota Hospitals, Minneapolis, Minnesota.

John S. Najarian is a Californian who graduated with distinction from the University of California and the University of California School of Medicine. Following his surgical residency at the University of California, he spent three years in tissue transplantation immunology and related research and was named a Markle Scholar in 1964. He became full professor of surgery at California in 1966, and Professor and Chairman of the Department of Surgery at the University of Minnesota in 1967. An accomplished teacher and clinician, he is included among first rank transplantation biologists.

Normally, surgically constructed allografts are rejected with a vigor directly proportional to the degree of genetic disparity between donor and host. In spite of recent progress in clinical histocompatibility typing and matching, circumvention of the immunologic rejection of the clinical allograft is still dependent on the efficacy of the immunosuppressive regimen. Ideally, immunosuppressants temporarily control the immunologic response of the host against the graft until immunologic adaptation takes place and immunosuppression can be withdrawn or reduced to easily tolerated levels. Unfortunately, such an adaptation is seldom complete, and it is only in rare cases that immunosuppression can be completely stopped at any time following successful transplantation. This high degree of chemical immunosuppression during the early post-transplant period combined with the continuation of at least maintenance doses inhibits the ability of the allograft recipient to counteract a number of infectious agents. The incidence of infection following renal transplantation is extremely high and most deaths are due to infections and their complications (Hill et al., 1967). On the other hand, transplant patients do not succumb to every passing organism, so an understanding of those host factors that predispose to infection and death is of prime importance. In this chapter the incidence and natural history of fatal infections in patients treated

[*]Markle Scholars in Academic Medicine.
[†]Supported by Grant #I POI-AM-13083, National Institutes of Health.

559

TABLE 25-1.   Changing Pattern of Survival Following Renal Transplantation

Donors	1963−July, 1967		August, 1967−July, 1969	
	Transplants	Deaths	Transplants	Deaths
Identical Twin	2	0	1	0
Related	33	14	44	2
Unrelated living	1	1	3	1
Cadaver	44°	27°	22†	7†
Total	80	42	70	10

°Three patients received pancreatic transplants with kidney transplants, and three of these patients died.
†Three patients received pancreatic transplants with kidney transplants, and two of these patients died.

with immunosuppressants, the prophylactic measures, diagnostic problems, and treatment are described.

MORTALITY IN TRANSPLANTATION PATIENTS

From the start of the renal transplantation program at the University of Minnesota in 1963 until July, 1969, 150 renal transplants were performed in 140 patients. Ten patients received more than one transplant. Six patients also received a pancreatic transplant in conjunction with the renal transplant as treatment for diabetic renal failure. The program was separated into two phases: (a) those years when renal transplantation was an experimental treatment (1963−July, 1967); and (b) those years since July, 1967, during which renal transplantation has become a truly therapeutic modality. In Table 25-1, the donor of the renal transplant and the number of deaths that occurred are listed for each period. It is apparent from this table that the mortality of transplantation has declined radically recently. In fact, in the last 43 renal transplantations, there were no postoperative deaths.

Of the 52 deaths in this series, 46 were related to septic complication. Table 25-2

shows that these deaths usually occurred in the first three months following transplantation. Of the four deaths not related to sepsis, one was caused by recurrent pulmonary emboli, one by pre-existing disseminated vasculitis, and two patients died many months following removal of the renal transplant while on chronic hemodialysis.

Table 25-3 lists the predominant organism found in the 46 septic deaths. When two or three organisms appeared to be involved in the death, all are mentioned. It is apparent from this table, however, that *Staphylococcus aureus* and *Klebsiella pneumonii* were the most common causes of death in the early postoperative period. Staphylococcal infections are no longer prevalent. Klebsiella, however, remains a persistent problem. The other organisms are, for the most part, opportunistic rather than common pathogens. The gram-positive organisms seem to be easily recognized and eradicated, while the gram-negative organisms, fungi, and protozoans are much more resistant to antimicrobial agents.

Of particular interest is the high incidence of saprophytic organisms that do not commonly cause systemic or fatal infection. Other investigators have reported similar findings. For example, by 1967, the Denver group had identified *Pneumocystis carinii* in the lungs of ten patients who died fol-

TABLE 25-2.   Interval Between Transplant Operation and Septic Death in 46 Patients Following Renal Transplantation

	Number of patients	Time of Death			
		0−3 months	3−6 months	6−12 months	>1 year
1963 to 1967	41	29	5	1	6
1967 to the Present	5	4	−	−	1

TABLE 25-3. Predominant Organisms in 46 Septic Deaths Following Renal Allotransplantation

	Time of Death (Months)			
	0-3	3-6	6-12	>12
Gram positive bacteria				
Staph. aureus	5	1	–	–
Gram negative bacteria				
E. coli	5	–	1	–
Klebsiella	17	2	2	1
Proteus	6	1	–	1
Pseudomonas	9	–	1	–
Bacteroides	1	–	–	–
Other				
Tuberculosis	–	–	–	1
Cryptococcus	–	–	–	1
Nocardia	–	–	–	1
Pneumocystis	–	1	–	1
Aspergillus	2	1	–	–
Candida	3	3	–	1
Cytomegalovirus	3	1	–	–

lowing kidney transplantation (Rifkind et al., 1966). Cytomegalovirus was found in almost half the patients who died following renal allotransplantation (Hill et al., 1967). However, pulmonary insufficiency caused by *Pneumocystis carinii* was considered to be present in only two of the ten patients with the infection, and cytomegalovirus was thought not to be the cause of death in the 30 patients who showed evidence of this virus (Hill et al., 1967). Cytomegalovirus appears to represent a common subclinical infection in patients treated with immunosuppressants (Craighead et al., 1967; Rifkind et al., 1967a). Its significance in relation to other more virulent infections is unknown. *Pneumocystis carinii*, of course, can itself cause severe pulmonary insufficiency and was responsible for two of the deaths in our series. Cytomegalovirus and pneumocystic infections are usually accompanied by other bacterial or fungal invaders (Hill et al., 1967).

Fungal infections were very common in our series, as well as in that of Rifkind (Rifkind et al., 1967b). The pathogens most frequently found in our patient were *Candida albicans* and *Aspergillus fumigatus*. All the patients with aspergillosis were also infected with Candida and one patient with nocardiosis was also infected with *Pneumocystis carinii*, Candida, and cytomegalovirus. Thus, mixed infections with fungal agents and superimposed bacterial infections were frequently the cause of death in these patients treated with immunosuppressants.

Renal failure seldom caused death. The ready availability of hemodialysis can completely prevent death from renal failure. Many of the patients had perfectly adequate renal function at the time of death; however, most of the patients had had multiple rejection episodes requiring increased immunosuppressive medication. The type of infection observed, the elements predisposing to the development of fatal infections, and the problems these infections present to the transplant surgeon are illustrated in the following case study:

CASE 1 (FIG. 25-1)

W. A. was a 20-year-old man with preterminal renal failure due to bilateral hydroureter and hydronephrosis secondary to vesicouteral reflux. Despite suprapubic drainage of the bladder, improvement in renal function was not obtained. The patient was accepted for transplantation when his blood urea nitrogen was 230 mg. per 100 ml. and blood pressure was 200/140. Five hemodialyses were performed prior to renal transplantation from a cadaver donor who had died during open-heart surgery in December, 1965. The patient was placed on prophylactic penicillin and chloramphenicol. At the same time the renal transplantation was carried out, an ileal conduit was fashioned, the ureter of the transplant was anastomosed to the ileal conduit, and bilateral nephrectomy was performed.

Renal function was initially poor, although hemodialysis was not necessary. Initial immunosuppressive drug therapy was 5 mg./kg. of azathioprine, which was maintained for 24 days after transplantation. Renal function deteriorated and BUN rose on the 15th postoperative day. At that time, 6 mg./kg. of prednisone was started and was maintained from the 16th to the 45th day. Thereafter, the prednisone dosage was slowly decreased.

The peripheral leukocyte count fell to less than 3000/mm.[3] between the 22nd and 32nd day. Azathioprine therapy was temporarily discontinued on the 25th day, but was reinstituted and raised to previous levels as soon as the white blood count returned to normal. Renal function improved for a short period of time. However, a second period of leukopenia appeared on the 50th postoperative day necessitating cessation of azathioprine therapy once more. Renal function then slowly deteriorated. As soon as the azathioprine was begun again, leukopenia promptly reappeared. During the second leukopenic episode, a low-grade fever appeared with bilateral basilar lung infiltration. Pseudomonas was found in the urine at that time and penicillin and chloramphenicol were administered. Nevertheless, the patient had difficulty with increasing shortness of breath and a dry, persistent, hacking cough. Crackling rales were heard in both lung fields and yeasts were noted in the urine. Blood cultures on the 62nd postoperative day showed *Candida albicans*. At the same time, it was noted that the patient had hyperglycemia and glycosuria, which were considered to be consistent with the development of steroid diabetes. Steroid dosage was decreased and repeated sputum cultures revealed Pseudomonas and coagulase-positive Staphylococcus, but no Candida. The lung infiltrates

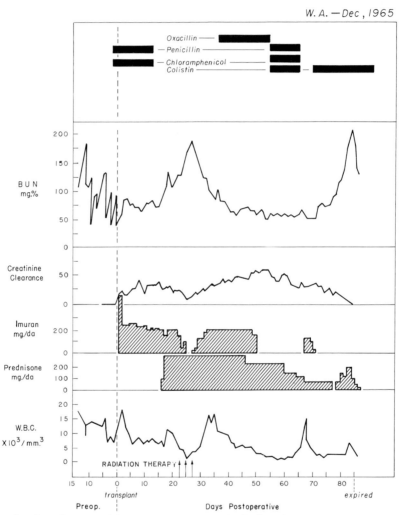

Figure 25-1.   The clinical course of the patient in Case 1, who died on the 85th post-transplant day with candidiasis and aspergillosis. Note the concurrence of rejection and the development of leukopenia, requiring cessation of Imuran on 25th post-transplant day. Note the prolonged leukopenic episode after the 50th day, requiring cessation of Azathioprine therapy, and a severe terminal rejection associated with terminal infections and leukopenia. Both leukopenic episodes were associated with chloramphenicol administration.

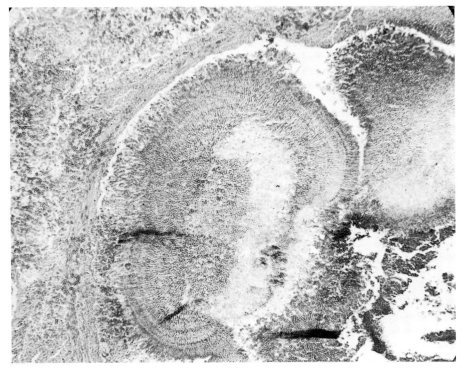

Figure 25-2.   A bronchus filled with the pseudohyphae of *Candida albicans* in the lungs of the patient in Case 1.

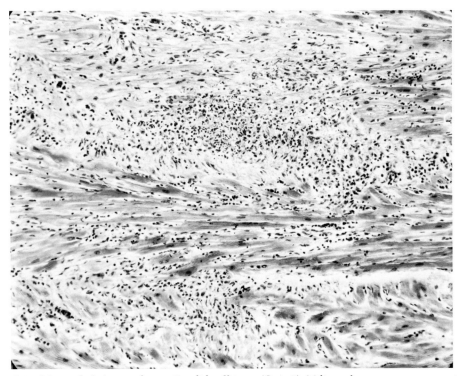

Figure 25-3.   Myocardial abscess due to *Candida albicans* (Case 1). Miliary abscesses were present throughout the body.

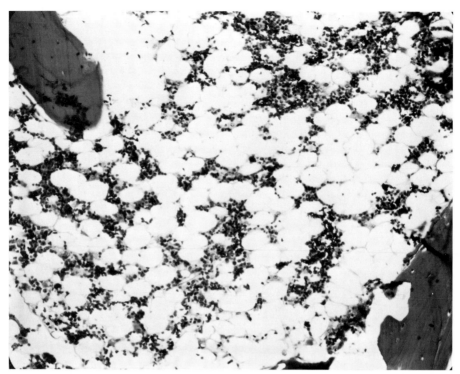

Figure 25-4.   Severe hypoplasia of the bone marrow (Case 1). The patient had multiple episodes of prolonged leukopenia associated with Azathioprine and chloramphenicol treatment.

continued to enlarge and urine cultures on the 70th postoperative day revealed enterococci and *Candida tropicalis.* Four days prior to death, thoracic-duct cannulation was carried out in order to reverse the severe rejection. Three days prior to death, the patient developed upper gastrointestinal bleeding that could not be controlled. He expired on the 86th postoperative day.

Postmortem examination revealed a severe rejection in the transplanted kidney, gastric hemorrhage from diffuse erosions, and multiple Candida abscesses in the lung, peritoneal cavity, thyroid, esophagus, stomach, and heart (Figs. 25-2 and 25-3). The bone marrow was severely hypoplastic (Fig. 25-4). Cytomegalic inclusions and Aspergillus were found in the lung in addition to the Candida pneumonia. Blood cultures at postmortem examination revealed *Proteus mirabilis,* Klebsiella, Pseudomonas, alpha-Streptococcus, and *Candida albicans.*

Comment

This patient illustrates many of the predisposing conditions conducive to the development of systemic sepsis in the transplant recipient treated with immunosuppressants. For example, preoperatively, there was severe vesicoureteral reflux, bilateral hydronephrosis, and a severe urinary-tract infection. Only five hemodialyses were carried out in this severely uremic and hypertensive patient. A single operation was carried out, involving bilateral nephrectomy of the infected kidneys, construction of an ileal

conduit, and renal transplantation. The donor of the renal transplant was an unrelated cadaver who had died during open-heart surgery and consequently had severely damaged kidneys prior to transplantation. Renal function was poor initially, making management of the immunosuppressants difficult, since rejection episodes are hard to detect without a baseline of good renal function. In addition, the azathioprine dosage was maintained at 4 to 5 mg./kg. in a patient whose renal function may not have been able to clear the drug.

A severe rejection episode occurred two to three weeks following transplantation, at which time very high doses of prednisone were begun and maintained for more than 30 days. The high doses of azathioprine accompanied by poor renal function resulted in severe leukopenia and thrombocytopenia. Suspension of azathioprine treatment allowed the bone marrow to recover, but azathioprine was begun again at the previous toxic levels. The second period of azathioprine toxicity and bone marrow suppression appeared. This time bilateral pneumonia also occurred along with a urinary-tract infection. Chloramphenicol may have aggravated the leukopenia and colistin may have further compromised renal function. Meanwhile, the steroid levels had been maintained at dosages sufficient to induce diabetes.

Multiple organisms were cultured at different times from different sites. Candida, however, which was primarily responsible for the pneumonia, was never cultured from the sputum. Neither was Aspergillus, which was responsible for several pulmonary abscesses. This combination of rejection, leukopenia, and severe infection due to organisms not found by routine diagnostic techniques is the most common pattern in patients treated with immunosuppressants dying of overwhelming infection due to opportunistic infectious agents.

CASE 2 (FIG. 25-5)

T. B. was a 36-year-old woman who received a renal allotransplant from her brother in March, 1964. The patient had been known to have albuminuria for six years prior to transplantation. One month before transplantation, the patient developed acute pulmonary edema, which cleared with appropriate therapy. At the time of transplantation, serum creatinine was 14 mg. per 100 ml. and blood pressure was 140/70. No preoperative dialysis was carried out. Bilateral nephrectomy, splenectomy, and cutaneous ureterostomy were performed at the time of transplantation. Azathioprine was started on the day prior to the transplantation and continued postoperatively. Prednisone, actinomycin, and prophylactic radiation therapy to the kidney were begun in the early postoperative period. A wound infection was discovered on the fifth postoperative day.

Although the initial urinary output was good, the creatinine clearance was poor for the first post-transplant week. Soon after the return of good renal function, severe leukopenia and thrombocytopenia appeared, necessitating the cessation of azathioprine therapy. A rejection episode occurred about the same time. Increased steroid doses led to improvement in renal function and a return to normal of the peripheral leukocyte count.

Forty days following transplantation, the patient was noted to have polyuria, glycosuria, and a blood sugar of 320 mg. per 100 ml. Insulin administration was started. Simultaneously with a second rejection episode, fever, dyspnea, and cyanosis appeared. Bilateral pneumonia was diagnosed. Leukopenia (<1000/cu. mm.) was severe. The pneumonia progressed rapidly and death occurred on the 56th post-transplant day secondary to respiratory insufficiency. No pathogens were cultured from the sputum ante mortem.

At postmortem examination, massive bilateral bron-

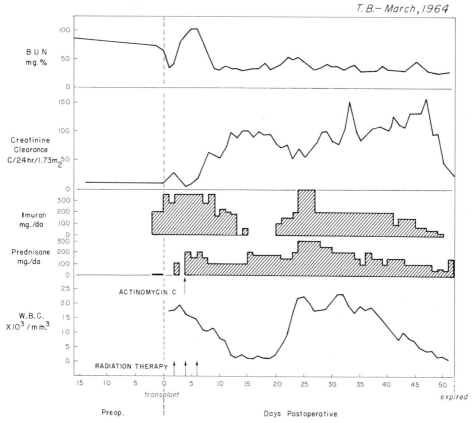

Figure 25-5. The clinical course of the patient in Case 2. Note that early renal function was poor although Azathioprine dosage remained high. Severe leukopenia appeared on the 12th post-transplant day heralding a rejection episode, which did not affect renal function till the 18th day. A second leukopenic episode appeared, associated with terminal rejection and infection. Note that the prednisone dosage was maintained at 100 and 200 mg. per day for the entire two-month period. Aspergillosis was the terminal infection.

chopneumonia was found, with Aspergillus abscesses throughout both lungs. The kidney had been rejected; the marrow was hypoplastic and fat emboli were present. Aspergillosis of the trachea and esophagus was also found. Alpha- and beta-streptococci were grown from the urine.

Comment

This patient represents another case of lethal infection due to a number of organisms. Aspergillus is normally a saprophyte. One factor contributing to the development of this infection was a high initial azathioprine dosage (5 mg./kg.), which was maintained over the first 15 days and then reset at a dose of 4 mg./kg. between the 20th and 40th postoperative days. The steroid dosage was enough to render the patient diabetic. Since azathioprine is partly cleared by the kidneys, this drug may be toxic when initial renal function is poor. Severe leukopenia occurred twice. Additional unfavorable factors included the wound infection, lack of operative dialysis, and a preoperative tendency to pulmonary edema. Once more, routine methods of culture failed to reveal the infecting organism.

PREVENTION OF INFECTIONS IN PATIENTS TREATED WITH IMMUNOSUPPRESSANTS

Review of the deaths due to sepsis following renal allotransplantation reveals that a number of factors seem to predispose to these conditions. Many of these factors are preventable.

PREOPERATIVE FACTORS PREDISPOSING TO LETHAL INFECTIONS

Renal transplantation is a moderate surgical trauma in the presence of severe immunosuppression. A patient should have the best possible fluid and electrolyte balance prior to transplantation. The preoperative status of many patients given transplants early in the experimental phases of renal allotransplantation was less than optimal. Frequently, such patients received neither hemodialysis nor peritoneal dialysis prior to transplantation. Hemodialysis can be carried out for prolonged periods of time with safety and there should be no haste in

performing renal transplantation. Dialysis was inadequate for 20 per cent of the patients in this series who died of infections in the first three months following transplantation. Some patients did not receive dialysis at all. We now give dialysis for all patients twice weekly for at least several weeks prior to transplantation. No postoperative deaths have occurred since this policy has been in force.

More than 50 per cent of the patients who died of infectious diseases in the first few months following transplantation had an active focus of infection at the time of renal transplantation. Most frequently these infections were confined to the urinary tract. Other patients had recurrent septicemia from unknown sources. A few patients had infections at the site of the hemodialysis cannula. Several patients received kidney allografts from cadavers who died with infectious diseases. Renal transplantation need never be performed in the presence of infection. Infected kidneys can be removed electively and the patient allowed to recover fully prior to transplantation. The urinary bladder can be sterilized after nephrectomy with repeated antibiotic irrigations. A voiding cystogram should be performed in the preoperative period in order to detect ureterovesical reflux. If reflux is present, both ureters should be removed down to the level of the bladder in order to obviate reflux in the post-transplant period. If this is impossible, the ureter can be closed from inside the bladder at the time of transplantation. Other sources of infection should be sought by routine preoperative cultures of nasopharynx and throat sputum, urine, stool, and hemodialysis cannula sites. If any source is found, it should be eliminated by the appropriate use of surgical drainage or antibiotic therapy.

One of the most striking findings of our series is that pulmonary complications of uremia preceded the development of fatal postoperative pulmonary infections in 40 per cent of such patients. Uremic pulmonary edema and pneumonia seldom directly preceded the transplantation, but frequently occurred prior to the institution of hemodialysis. It is known that pulmonary congestion and edema can predispose to pulmonary infections and some attention should be paid to improving pulmonary function in the preoperative period if this has been a problem.

OPERATIVE FACTORS PREDISPOSING TO INFECTIONS

Eighty per cent of the patients who died of infectious complications following early renal transplantation had a single-stage operation, consisting of bilateral nephrectomy (with or without splenectomy) combined with the renal transplantation procedure. On occasion, an ileal conduit was constructed at the same time. It is better to minimize the operative procedure in the patient treated with immunosuppressants. If the urinary tract is infected, it is always best to perform the nephrectomy prior to transplantation. Similarly, if urinary diversion is indicated, the conduit should be constructed long before transplantation. We now perform nephrectomy and splenectomy seven to ten days prior to transplantation in all adult recipients of consanguineous kidneys. In recipients of cadaver kidneys, nephrectomy is deferred until the transplant is functioning well. Prior nephrectomy can be performed in any patient with an infected urinary tract or in patients with hypertension unresponsive to medication and dialysis. No postoperative deaths have occurred in the last 43 patients in whom this policy has been followed.

Approximately 30 per cent of the transplantation patients who died of sepsis in this series developed leakage from the urinary tract. The development of a urinary fistula is an almost completely preventable complication. We always perform ureterocystostomy with a submucosal tunneling technique. The bladder is then closed in three layers and Foley-catheter drainage is continued for six days. There have been no urinary fistulas in the 70 transplants performed since August, 1967.

Urinary fistulas inevitably lead to infection. Even with fistulas, wound infections have been found in 70 per cent of patients who died with sepsis. Most such abscesses have been inadequately drained for fear of injuring the kidney. However, the transplanted kidney itself may become infected and removal of the kidney may be necessary for survival. Inadequately drained infections become the source of repeated septicemia. Initially susceptible organisms are replaced by opportunistic organisms as repeated courses of antibiotic therapy are given. Wound infections can be almost completely avoided by eliminating the infections in the patient prior to transplantation, shortening the operative procedure by staging the operation, carefully attending to hemostasis, irrigating the wound with saline to remove devitalized tissue, and carefully closing the wound. We avoid using drains at all times and utilize neomycin and bacitracin wound irrigation. With these techniques, we have encountered only two superficial wound infections in the last 43 renal transplants.

ROLE OF THE RELATIONSHIP BETWEEN DONOR AND RECIPIENT IN THE DEVELOPMENT OF INFECTIONS

It is apparent from Table 25-1 that recipients of cadaver renal transplants do less well than do recipients with living, related donors. This continues to be true despite the use of histocompatibility typing in the selection of cadaver donors. Organs from unrelated donors elicit more frequent and more vigorous rejection reactions. They require more immunosuppressive drugs, more courses of irradiation, and a greater variety of immunosuppressive agents. A vicious cycle is set up in which vigorous immunologic rejection of the graft requires such large doses of immunosuppressive drugs that the patient's resistance even to saprophytic organisms is eliminated. Consequently, if repeated rejection can be avoided, there is little danger that life will be lost due to infection. Rejection can be best avoided by using organs donated by living relatives when possible and carefully matching histocompatibility antigens when organs of unrelated donors are utilized.

ROLE OF IMMUNOSUPPRESSIVE AGENTS IN THE DEVELOPMENT OF INFECTIONS

The immunosuppressive drugs that have been found useful in renal transplantation seriously impair the normal defense mechanisms against a number of infectious agents. The exact mechanisms involved are unclear, but there is no question that this effect is related to the dosage used. Azathioprine doses greater than 4 mg./kg. were maintained for more than 20 days in 50 per cent of the patients who died with infectious complications. Prednisone was maintained at greater than 2 mg./kg. for more than 20 consecutive days in 70 per cent of the patients who died. Several of the patients developed steroid diabetes. Because of the high complication rate associated with large doses of steroids and azathioprine, both in our series and in those reported by others (Hume et al., 1963; Starzl, 1964), we have developed certain guidelines of safe immunosuppression. The single most important principle in the prevention of lethal infection is to sacrifice the kidney whenever it seems that excessive doses of immunosuppressants are required.

The standard immunosuppression regimen consists of pretreatment for two days with azathioprine (5 mg./kg.). This drug is maintained at this level for the first three postoperative days and is then reduced to 4 mg./kg. for three days. By the seventh postoperative day, the dose is cut to 3 mg./kg., and the dose never exceeds that level thereafter. Particular care is paid to the renal function in the early post-transplant period, since azathioprine is partially cleared by the kidney (Starzl et al., 1967). If acute tubular necrosis occurs, the daily dosage cannot exceed 1.5 mg./kg. After the first week, azathioprine dosage is guided by the peripheral leukocyte counts. Any significant fall in the leukocyte count, even if luekopenic levels are not approached, is a signal to reduce the azathioprine dosage. Generally, the drug is not discontinued abruptly, but is reduced to very low levels. Following recovery from leukopenia, azathioprine dosage is gradually increased.

Since azathioprine is partially cleared by the kidney, rejection crises are frequently associated with the development of leukopenia. In fact, leukopenia may herald rejection crises that may not interfere with creatinine clearance for several more days (Figs. 25-1 and 25-5). Consequently, azathioprine dosage must frequently be reduced during the rejection crisis itself. A few patients who died of infectious complications were treated with increased azathioprine dosage during rejection crises. This is scrupulously avoided at present.

Steroid therapy is known to be associated with increased severity and frequency of infectious complications. At present, we administer 1 gm. of methylprednisolone intravenously to adult renal allograft recipients daily for the first three post-transplant days and upon diagnosis of each rejection episode. Prednisone dosage of 1 mg./kg. for recipients of kidneys from related donors is initiated 36 hours before the operation and is reduced gradually over the first three weeks to approximately 0.5 mg./kg. In rejection episodes, prednisone dosage is increased to approximately 2 mg./kg. and reduced at a similar rate. For rejection episodes characterized by progressive deterioration of renal function one or two additional courses of prednisone are given in this way. Thereafter, steroid levels are maintained at approximately 1 mg./kg. until renal function has stabilized and the dose is reduced as soon as possible thereafter. When rejection does not respond to this treatment, steroid therapy is reduced to maintenance levels and the kidney is allowed to be rejected. Progressively increased doses of steroid are not utilized for fear of the development of severe opportunistic infections.

Actinomycin is reserved for rejection episodes that are refractory to other treatments. In these cases, one or two courses (200 micrograms per day, intravenously, for three days) are administered, but no more than this is utilized at any other time.

Local irradiation of the kidney allograft is utilized prophylactically only in recipients of unrelated-donor kidneys in a dosage of 150 R to the kidney every other day for three days. No prophylactic irradiation is given to the recipients of donor-related kidneys. During rejection episodes, 150 R is administered to the kidneys of all patients every other day for three days. The total irradiation dose is restricted to 1500 R in order to prevent the development of severe irradiation nephritis.

Antilymphocyte globulin (ALG) has been utilized recently. This has allowed us to reduce steroid levels somewhat. None of the patients receiving ALG have developed life-threatening infectious complications and no deaths have occurred. Although ALG may reduce local inflammation around certain kinds of experimental infections (Morris et al., 1966), it is not known whether the use of ALG provides a more specific and therefore safer kind of immunosuppression than azathioprine and prednisone. However, mounting experimental data indicate that ALG, like other immunosuppressive agents, renders experimental animals more susceptible to infection. Reduction of the infection rate in our patients is probably due to factors other than the use of ALG. However, the immunosuppressive action of ALG may reduce the incidence of rejection episodes that necessitate increasing doses of steroids, which, in turn, facilitate infection.

The effect of renal function on infection

The maintenance of good renal function is one of the more important factors in minimizing the doses of immunosuppressive agents needed and also allows for the normal elimination of azathioprine (Starzl, 1964). Almost all the deaths due to infectious complications were associated with either acute renal failure or persistent and repeated rejection episodes. In particular, the development of acute tubular necrosis in the early post-transplant period complicates the use of immunosuppressive drugs. About 40 per cent of the patients dying of infectious diseases had severely compromised renal function in the immediate post-transplant period, leading to possible azathioprine overdosage. Acute tubular necrosis at this stage may be circumvented by particular attention to the renal function of the donor during nephrectomy (Najarian et al., 1966), and by avoiding hypovolemia in the recipient. If oliguria does develop, fluid, mannitol, and furosemide are highly effective in increasing the urinary output and creatinine clearance.

It is important to rule out technical errors at this stage. Hyperacute rejection can be recognized by the use of renograms and arteriograms. If the kidney has undergone acute rejection, immunosuppression can be stopped and the kidney removed. The prompt use of these diagnostic procedures also eliminates the need for re-exploration and recontamination of the wound in the search for technical factors contributing to the oliguria. If poor renal function continues as a result of acute tubular necrosis, azathioprine must be severely restricted until renal functional recovery has occurred.

Leukopenia in the development of lethal infections

Ninety per cent of the patients dying with infectious complication during the first three months following transplantation had developed leukopenia (<3000/cu. mm.) at some time during their course. Frequently, the leukopenia was recurrent and associated with heavy doses of azathioprine, acute tubular necrosis, or repeated courses of rejection. Careful observation of the peripheral leukocyte and platelet counts is necessary and azathioprine dosage must be carefully adjusted. The use of other bone marrow depressants (e.g., chloramphenicol) should also be avoided. In the most recent 43 cases, no episode of leukopenia has been associated with severe systemic infection, although leukopenia has heralded a rejection episode on four occasions.

Prophylactic antibiotics and culture routine

Antibiotics not only alter the flora of the host, predisposing to the overgrowth of opportunistic organisms, but they also interfere with the immune elimination of such organisms (Seelig, 1966). The precise role of prophylactic antibiotics in our series is difficult to determine. Certainly, the use of chloramphenicol was associated with leukopenia, which required reduction of azathioprine dosage in a number of patients who died with lethal infections (see Cases 1 and 3). The reduced immunosuppressive levels have permitted subsequent rejection episodes leading to the vicious cycle of rejection and infection. Colistin, likewise, was associated with frequent deterioration of renal function, which was occasionally interpreted as rejection and resulted in higher prednisone dosage. These episodes did not respond to antirejection therapy until the colistin was terminated. At present, we avoid both such antibiotics whenever possible.

Our present practice somewhat limits the use of prophylactic antibiotics. Staphylococcal sepsis was frequently the cause of death in wound infections in the early days of the experimental period. Staphylococcal infections can be almost completely prevented in the postoperative period by the use of prophylactic methicillin for approximately three weeks. We have had no primary staphylococcal infections of any sort in the last 43 patients. Candidiasis, whose portal of entry is primarily the gastrointestinal tract, can be minimized by the use of oral nystatin. Bacitracin and neomycin combinations are utilized for wound irrigations prior to closure. Bladder irrigations with neomycin are used prior to transplantation.

Urine cultures are performed biweekly in the post-transplant period. Whenever colony counts greater than 100,000/cu. mm. are found, specific antibiotic treatment is instituted for urinary-tract infections. Female children are frequently placed on sulfisoxazole as prophylaxis for urinary-tract infections, since they occur very commonly in this group of patients without prophylaxis. No other systemic antibiotic prophylaxis is normally necessary because infectious sources are scrupulously eliminated prior to transplantation.

All fevers, however, indicate that cultures of the nose, throat, sputum, blood, and urine should be performed. Only three episodes of septicemia have appeared in the last 43 patients. The origin of two of these was in urethritis with *E. coli* around the urethral catheter during the first six postoperative days. Both the septicemia and the urethritis responded to appropriate antibiotic therapy and early removal of the urethral catheter. A *Bacteroides melaninogenicus* infection of the teeth and gums was not recognized in one patient prior to transplantation. Postoperatively, multiple episodes of Bacteroides septicemia developed, which responded to appropriate antibacterial therapy. This patient subsequently developed a Bacteroides wound infection in the subcutaneous tissue. All three of these patients are living with perfect renal function at present.

ISOLATION PRECAUTIONS TO PREVENT INFECTION

Isolation precautions have been suggested for the prevention of infections in these patients. Reverse gown, mask, and glove precautions were formally instituted for the first three to six postoperative days. Such measures may have helped prevent the transmission of infection between patients within the transplant area. However, they restrict access to the patient, have psychologic disadvantages, and are probably ineffective against viral, fungal, or endogenous infections. The measures discussed in previous sections have resulted in the absence of fatal infections in the last 43 consecutive renal transplantations. We now institute isolation precautions only when severe leukopenia (<1000/cu. mm.) is present.

LATE OPPORTUNISTIC INFECTIONS IN LONG-TERM SURVIVORS OF RENAL ALLOGRAFTS

It seems possible, therefore, to prevent most of the infectious complications in the first few months following renal allotransplantation by careful attention to the preoperative status, immunosuppression, renal function, and leukopenia. A more difficult group of patients, however, are those who have survived for long periods on immunosuppression and are apparently maintaining satisfactory renal function. These patients may suddenly appear with overwhelming sepsis leading to death. We have encountered eight such cases, one to four years following renal transplantation. Such patients seem to follow a pattern, and it is possible to predict which patients are likely to develop these serious complications.

CASE 3

S. S. was a 14-year-old boy who received a kidney transplant from his mother in October, 1965. The patient had had a previous transplant from an unrelated donor in July, 1965, which was removed because of technical complications. A wound infection that developed at the first transplant site had been drained and had healed well. The first transplant had also been complicated by leukopenia which appeared 18 days following the transplantation, 10 days after the immunosuppression had been stopped.

A thoracic-duct cannula was placed two days prior to the second transplantation. The initial azathioprine dosage of 7 mg./kg. was rapidly reduced to 3 mg./kg. Prednisone was not utilized initially. A rejection episode was diagnosed on the 16th post-transplant day and was associated with leukopenia. At the same time, a Klebsiella urinary-tract infection was discovered. Prednisone and colistin were begun and the response to antirejection therapy was prompt.

A second rejection episode appeared on the 78th postoperative day and prednisone was further increased from maintenance of 0.7 mg./kg. to 3 mg./kg., a dosage which was continued for the following two weeks. At this time it was found that the wound infection in the previous nephrectomy site was still present. Renal function never returned to prerejection levels following this episode, but a creatinine of 1.5 to 2.0 mg. per 100 ml. was maintained.

The patient was readmitted on the 196th post-transplant day with severe leukopenia associated with rejection. The prednisone dosage was increased to 5 mg./kg. and maintained there for the next 35 days. Azathioprine had to be discontinued during this period and the persistent leukopenia militated against its being restarted until the 240th postoperative day. The first transplant nephrectomy site still drained coagulase-positive Staphylococcus.

The patient remained out of the hospital until the 395th day following transplantation, at which time he

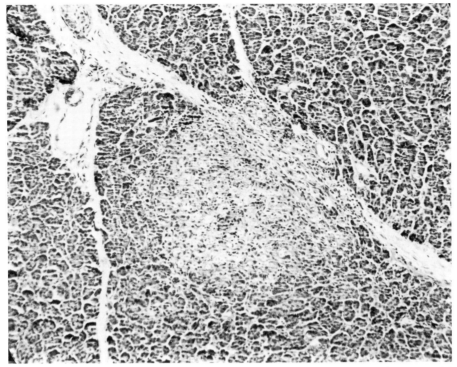

Figure 25-6. Miliary cryptococcal abscess in the pancreas of the patient in Case 3, who survived for more than two years after kidney transplantation. Note the complete absence of inflammatory change.

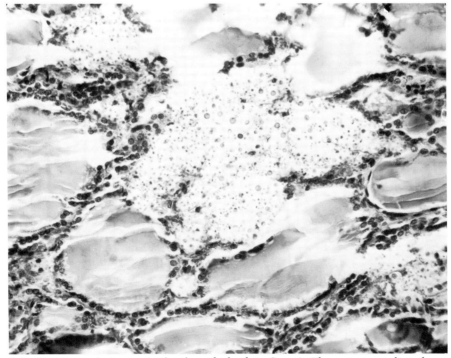

Figure 25-7. Cryptococcal abscess in the thyroid gland in Case 3. The organisms elicited no inflammatory response. Similar lesions were found in all organs.

was readmitted for evaluation of a serum creatinine of 2.3 mg. per 100 ml. The prednisone dosage was increased to 3 mg./kg. per day and was maintained at this level for three weeks. Leukopenia again appeared and for the next three months azathioprine could not be given. The patient was on prophylactic penicillin, ampicillin, and chloramphenicol during this period of time. Around the 500th postoperative day, the patient began having spiking fevers and developed middle-lobe pneumonia. Sputum culture revealed Pseudomonas and coagulase-negative Staphylococcus. In an attempt to treat this infection, penicillin, colistin, and streptomycin were started. The pneumonia was very slow to resolve, but the patient was finally discharged from the hospital on the 594th postoperative day.

On the 710th post-transplant day, the patient was admitted once more for rejection and treated once more with elevated prednisone dosage. The leukocyte count remained normal throughout this episode, but the serum creatinine never dropped below 3.5 mg. per 100 ml. On the 750th postoperative day, the patient was readmitted with severe left chest pain and dyspnea. Sputum culture revealed coagulase-positive Staphylococcus and an unidentified fungus. Chest x-ray revealed multiple small nodules throughout both lungs, and the patient died within four days of admission despite intensive antibiotic therapy.

At postmortem examination, miliary cryptococcosis was found involving the lung, thyroid, liver, kidney, heart, pancreas, spleen, lymph nodes, and bone marrow. There was severe hypoplasia of the bone marrow. No inflammatory reaction to the miliary cryptococcosis was found in the organs involved (Figs. 25-6 and 25-7). The kidneys showed changes consistent with chronic rejection.

Comment

The patient received two kidney transplants. Even following the first transplant, leukopenia developed. His course was characterized by multiple rejection episodes, progressively but slowly deteriorating renal function, multiple episodes of leukopenia, and multiple infections. This course is typical of those patients who survive for more than one year and who ultimately die of infectious complications. Their courses are never smooth, although they have sufficient renal function to maintain life. Such patients should be recognized prior to the development of their terminal infection. The kidney should be allowed to reject and a subsequent transplant performed.

DIAGNOSTIC PROBLEMS ASSOCIATED WITH INFECTIONS IN PATIENTS TREATED WITH IMMUNOSUPPRESSANTS

Essential to the diagnosis of potentially fatal infections in patients treated with immunosuppressants is a high index of suspicion. Any illness, particularly febrile illnesses, should be suspect and the patient admitted for diagnostic study on the basis of minimal symptoms. No symptoms lasting more than a day or so should be attributed to upper respiratory infections of no importance. There are few hard facts on which to base the diagnoses of these infections. Most significant infections, however, are characterized by fever and systemic toxicity. The peripheral white blood count is obviously of little assistance. Routine cultures of the nose, throat, sputum, blood, and urine should be performed whenever fever is present. In the presence of fevers of unknown etiology, particular attention should be paid to the urinary tract and to wounds. Wounds in these patients may reveal hidden infections months and even years after the incision may have seemed to heal.

We have noted the concurrence of infections of the urinary tract, in wounds, and in the respiratory tract with apparent rejection episodes. These rejection episodes themselves may be quite mild and respond to rather short courses of antirejection therapy. Conversely, sudden deterioration of renal function should suggest an occult infection. We cannot explain this concurrence of infection with rejection, but it is undeniably present in a number of patients. It is possible that slight deterioration of renal function leads to relative azathioprine toxicity and a superinfection. More likely the infectious process acts as an adjuvant to the antigens in the transplant that are upsetting the immunologic balance that has been established between donor organ and host. It is also possible that the deterioration of renal function is not a reflection of rejection but of some less specific renal toxic effect of the infection. Nevertheless, complete evaluation of renal function should be carried out when the patient is admitted for local or systemic infections.

Although it is quite clear that the factors previously listed tend to predispose to the development of lethal infection in the patient treated with immunosuppressants, there seems to be no factor that predisposes specifically to one type of infection or another. Urinary-tract infections are usually minor and brought under control without great difficulty. Septicemia seldom appears after the first few weeks of operation and is usually associated with wound infection. The most lethal infections involve the lung.

Most such infections will appear as regional infiltrates on chest x-rays and will be accompanied by symptoms no different from those of other patients with pneumonia.

The prompt choice of proper therapeutic modality in these desperately ill patients depends on precise determination of the etiologic agent responsible for the infection; this may be extremely difficult. Mixed infections are the rule and bacterial infection is present in almost every case of fungal disease. *The diagnostic pitfall here is to treat that organism which is most easily cultured from the sputum.* This may or may not be the organism that is causing the infection, particularly in the patient who is already on antimicrobial therapy. The infecting fungi and protozoa, in particular, are seldom present in the sputum or in the tracheal aspirates. In addition, Rifkind has pointed out that Sabouraud's medium is utilized for isolation of fungi not because of its particular suitability for these organisms, but rather because of its inhibitory effect upon the bacterial flora (Rifkind et al., 1967b). More suitable media are available for each of the common infecting fungi. Thus, it is possible that fungi may not be found by routine techniques. In Rifkind's series, the infecting fungal agent was isolated from the sputum in only six of the 14 patients who died with fungal pneumonias (Rifkind et al., 1967b). In our series, none of the patients who died with fungal diseases was diagnosed by routine techniques.

The pattern of skin tests is of little use in the diagnosis of opportunistic infections. Their development takes too long and delays the institution of therapy. In addition, all delayed hypersensitivity responses may be obliterated in these patients. Patients with known tuberculosis have had negative tuberculin reactions. Even in patients not treated with immunosuppressants, the skin tests for blastomycosis, coccidioidomycosis, and histoplasmosis are frequently negative during the acute disease. One should not be deceived by the use of four skin tests that do not even include the most common fungal agents, which may infect these patients (Candida, Aspergillus, Cryptococcus, and so on) into believing that fungal infections have been ruled out.

When pulmonary infiltrates are present, cultures of sputum and tracheal aspirates should be performed and appropriate antibiotic therapy instituted. If there is no response to therapy, needle biopsy or open pulmonary biopsy should be performed without further delay. Needle biopsy carries the risk of pneumothorax, bronchopleural fistula formation, and contamination of the needle tract. In addition, its yield of positive information is small in these patients because the biopsy is limited to small areas of the lung, whereas multiple organisms may be infecting multiple areas. Therefore, it is frequently necessary to perform open pulmonary biopsy. The antemortem diagnosis was made in only two patients with opportunistic infections; in both cases, open pulmonary biopsy was necessary. When open pulmonary biopsy is performed, a significant piece of involved pulmonary tissue should be taken. If multiple areas are involved, multiple wedges should be taken. Fresh imprints on slides should be made of the lung tissue, and these should be stained with Gram stain, acid-fast stain, silver methenamine, and Giemsa stain (for fungi and *Pneumocystis carinii*). Frozen sections

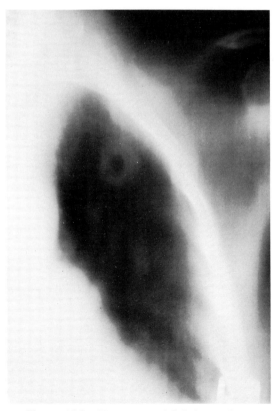

Figure 25-8. Tomogram of left lung of a renal transplant recipient with cavitary lesions of the left upper lobe and several soft nodular infiltrates, which were not apparent on routine x-ray. This upper lobe lesion is characteristic of aspergillosis.

should also be made, since some fungi can be identified on pathologic sections and the typical proteinaceous alveolar infiltrates associated with *Pneumocystis carinii* can be identified. Sections of lung should be cultured both aerobically and anaerobically for bacteria. Multiple media should be utilized for fungal cultures, which should be incubated aerobically and anaerobically for prolonged periods of time.

A few fungal infections have rather typical radiologic patterns, which should raise suspicions. Aspergillus frequently appears in a classic form. The upper lobes are almost uniformly involved and the lesion usually appears as a rounded or oval shadow that is not particularly dense, a portion of which is circumscribed by a thin crescentic line (Orie et al., 1960; Carbone et al., 1964). Cavitation is frequently present. Even in the patient treated with immunosuppressants, the progress of this aspergillosis may be slow. Its early appearance in the upper lobes is classic even though it may later spread to other areas of the lung, with multiple abscesses and cavitation (Fig. 25-8).

The other fungi may present as relatively

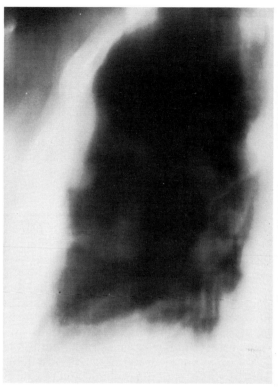

Figure 25-10. Tomogram of the right lung in a renal allograft recipient one year following transplantation. Multiple soft indistinct nodules can be seen, which were not readily apparent on routine chest x-rays. Multiple cultures of pleural effusion and needle lung biopsy failed to reveal the etiologic agent. Open-lung biopsy revealed nocardiosis. At autopsy the patient also had cytomegalic inclusion disease, *Pneumocystis carinii,* and candidiasis in the lung.

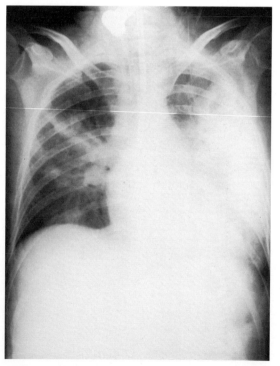

Figure 25-9. Confluent upper lobe abscesses of the left lung and multiple nodular infiltrates of the right in a renal transplant recipient. Patient died with aspergillosis and candidiasis of the lung.

soft, bulky, nodular infiltrates that are not diagnostic one from the other, although the patterns do suggest a nonbacterial origin (Figs. 25-9 and 25-10). The early nodules may be indistinct and require tomography for definition (Fig. 25-10). Two of our patients died of miliary disease, one with tuberculosis, and the other with cryptococcosis. In the patient with tuberculosis, the lungs were not clinically involved, but in the patient with cryptococcosis, multiple miliary nodules were seen on the chest x-ray.

One classic pattern, which is readily recognized and can usually be diagnosed on the basis of the patient's history, physical examination, and chest x-ray, is *Pneumocystis carinii* pneumonia (Rifkind et al., 1966b). This disease may accompany other infections in patients treated with immunosuppressants, but may itself cause respiratory insufficiency and death. These patients

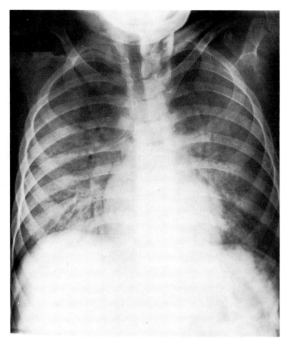

Figure 25-11. Eight-year-old boy with *Pneumocystis carinii.* The air bronchogram and the alveolar infiltrate extending to the periphery of both lungs are characteristic. Open-lung biopsy confirmed the diagnosis. Despite immediate institution of pentamidine therapy, the patient died three weeks later.

usually present with severe shortness of breath, low-grade fever, and a dry, nonproductive cough. The degree of dyspnea far exceeds the other signs of toxicity and there may be cyanosis in the absence of any sputum or fever. On examination, there may be bronchial breathing, but no rales or areas of consolidation. The chest x-ray is almost uniformly diagnostic. There is a uniform bilateral alveolar infiltrate extending from the hilum to the very periphery of the lung (Feinberg et al., 1961). As the infiltrate progresses, an air bronchogram appears caused by the opacity of the remainder of the lung (Fig. 25-11). This pneumonia consists of a thick proteinaceous intra-alveolar exudate composed primarily of the organisms themselves. There is minimal inflammatory change. Severe physiologic arteriovenous shunting results in profound hypoxemia and cyanosis. If recognized early, it can be treated and cured, since it may run an indolent course. The diagnosis is confirmed by either open or closed lung biopsy. The rather time-consuming silver methenamine stain has been replaced by the Giemsa stain on imprints of the fresh lung (Fig. 25-12).

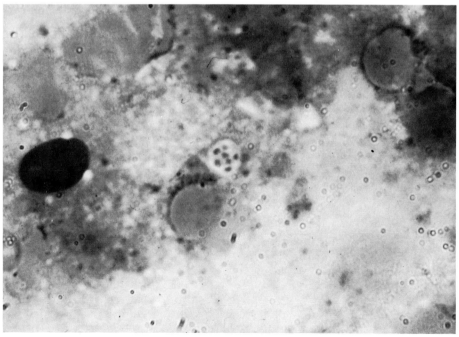

Figure 25-12. *Pneumocystis carinii* organisms within cysts on a lung biopsy imprint (Giemsa stain). Such imprints can be performed immediately at the time of lung biopsy and are diagnostic. (Slide courtesy of B. Berke, M.D.)

NEUROLOGIC COMPLICATIONS OF SEPSIS

Not only are multiple organisms frequently involved in life-threatening infections in patients treated with immunosuppressants, but multiple sites may be involved as well. For example, Rifkind has pointed out that the neurologic manifestations of systemic fungal infections may be due not only to the generalized toxicity involved in any systemic infection, but are also frequently due to fungal abscesses within the central nervous system. Because the CNS manifestations were primarily behavioral and seizure disturbances, specific diagnostic measures were not brought into play to localize the infections prior to death. It is important to bear in mind that pneumonias coincident with neurologic problems are frequently due to fungal diseases, particularly Aspergillus (Rifkind et al., 1967b). The use of arteriogram, brain scan, echogram, and electroencephalogram may be essential in localizing a CNS abscess requiring drainage.

PROBLEMS IN DIFFERENTIAL DIAGNOSIS

Although pulmonary infiltrates usually represent infection, pulmonary emboli, secondary to thrombosis of the common iliac vein, have resulted in one death in our series. Despite the multiple pulmonary infiltrates, no pathogenic organisms could be cultured. If pulmonary biopsy had been performed in this circumstance, the diagnosis would have been made and perhaps the patient could have been saved.

"Transplant lung" refers to a syndrome of arterial hypoxemia of obscure etiology. Minimal physical signs are present and chest x-rays show a variety of patterns ranging from a normal appearance to patchy bilateral pulmonic infiltrate. The classic picture is accompanied by an episode of transplant rejection and a response to the administration of prednisone (Hume, 1968). A number of etiologies have been suggested, such as a diffuse vasculitis or an auto-immune reaction against pulmonary tissue. We have never seen the syndrome. However, the correlation of pulmonary changes with rejection, both of which respond to prednisone, suggests that the rejection episode is accompanied by interstitial pulmonary edema, pulmonary arteriovenous shunting and hypoxemia. Fluid retention, weight gain, and oliguria are frequent consequences of rejection and may result in pulmonary as well as the more obvious peripheral edema. It is important to rule out infection in these patients, since similar syndromes can be produced by *Pneumocystis carinii* (Rifkind et al., 1964).

Obscure fevers, so commonly seen following transplantation, have unfortunately been labeled "transplant fever." Classic rejection episodes are accompanied by fever. With a more efficacious use of immunosuppressive agents and histocompatibility testing, fever is now less often present at these times. Similarly, there is a much lower incidence of nonspecific fevers during the hospital course. Such fevers can usually be related to low-grade urinary-tract infection, allergic reactions to antilymphocytic globulin, or drug sensitivities. They may well be symptomatic of cytomegalovirus infections (Rifkind, 1967a; Balakrishman et al., 1969). Withdrawal of large doses of steroids seems not to be a common cause any more (Hume, 1968), since steroid levels never exceed 2 mg./kg. and are tapered off very slowly. Despite these exceptions, fever still strongly suggests sepsis, and a vigorous campaign of diagnostic procedures to determine the site and etiology of sepsis is uniformly carried out in all such patients.

OTHER INFECTIONS

A number of other infections are common in the recipients in renal transplants. These other infections include herpes zoster, which is usually localized and painful but does not progress to systemic involvement (Rifkind, 1966a). However, recurrent herpes simplex infection has preceded lethal infection in two of the patients in this series.

Hepatitis has been a problem at some centers (Moore and Hume, 1969) presumably as a consequence of multiple blood transfusions received during dialysis, but perhaps as a direct result of transplantation from a cadaver kidney. Fatalities occasionally occur. It is difficult to screen cadaver kidney donors for hepatitis, but we have not encountered hepatitis in the past 70 transplantations.

Jaundice does not necessarily indicate hepatitis. Azathioprine toxicity may present as icterus. In one such patient, reduction of azathioprine dosage led to recovery and increasing azathioprine doses led to a recurrence. No rejection has followed the permanent reduction of azathioprine dosage to very low levels in this patient.

TREATMENT OF INFECTIONS IN PATIENTS TREATED WITH IMMUNOSUPPRESSANTS

The principal aim of the treatment of sepsis in the patient treated with immunosuppressants is to save life. This may necessitate the sacrifice of the kidney by discontinuation of immunosuppression. The latter decision involves a difficult judgment, since one is hesitant to surrender the kidney unnecessarily. It is made doubly difficult since discontinuation of the immunosuppression may well fail to effect a cure in these patients. Such patients may have accumulated an irreversible degree of immunosuppression unresponsive to sacrifice of the kidney, reinstitution of hemodialysis, and appropriate antibiotic therapy. The degree of immunosuppression may be so great that rejection of the kidney may not occur even when immunosuppression is stopped.

However, we must emphasize that not all infections are lethal in these patients. Most localized infections, wound infections, urinary-tract infections, and even bacteremia can be diagnosed readily and antimicrobial therapy instituted. If acute rejection episodes occur simultaneously, antirejection therapy can be instituted at the same time. Both infection and rejection usually improve together. However, in any severe, potentially life-threatening infection (e.g., pneumonia, repeated septicemia), azathioprine should be stopped completely. This is a subtle judgment in the early transplant period when repeated septicemia may occur from an unknown source. We have not had to discontinue immunosuppressive therapy in the three patients with perfect renal function and septicemia, mentioned earlier. The decision is less difficult in those patients who develop infections while chronically rejecting their transplants. It is in these patients that the continual use of repeated courses of antirejection therapy in the face of recurrent infection will lead to the patient's death. This is also true in the patient with renal function that is slowly deteriorating over a period of months and years.

Although it is clear that azathioprine must be discontinued when rejection is present in the face of significant infection, it is less clear how rapidly one should diminish steroid dosage in such patients. Generally, we feel that steroids should be decreased stepwise over a period of three to four days to maintenance levels of approximately 0.2 to 0.3 mg./kg. until the infection is under control.

When immunosuppressants are stopped, an insidious type of rejection may take place. Patients experiencing this should then be placed on a Giovanetti diet in order to stabilize the blood urea nitrogen at low levels. This permits avoidance of dialysis for longer periods. Similarly, the low-potassium diet is necessary to maintain serum potassium levels without dialysis. Hyperkalemia may be a major problem in patients with failing renal function and massive infections. In fact, hyperkalemia is a frequent terminal phenomenon leading to cardiac arrest, and consequently, frequent determinations of serum potassium are necessary. Ion-exchange resins or intravenous glucose, insulin, calcium, and alkalinizing agents may also be needed. Despite such regimens, it is usually necessary to reinstitute hemodialysis when the decision is made to allow rejection to take place. This should be done without hesitation when the usual indications of uremia and hyperkalemia are present. Uremic symptoms should not be allowed to develop.

Most pulmonary infections cause death not by systemic toxicity but by pulmonary insufficiency, hypoxemia, and cardiac death. Great care must be taken to maintain adequate oxygenation of the blood during the period of time before the infection can be brought under control. It is necessary, therefore, to determine arterial blood gases frequently and to maintain the oxygen level within the normal range. Supplementary oxygen may be required, but as the lungs become increasingly stiff and the work of breathing increases, it may be necessary to institute ventilatory support. The principles of respiratory care during relative pulmonary insufficiency have been discussed elsewhere in this volume.

It is not necessary to remove the rejected kidney during this period, since this merely provides another stress to the desperately ill patient. Such wounds frequently become infected after nephrectomy and may themselves be the cause of death. However, the nonfunctioning kidney may become thrombosed and infected and require removal. When this is necessary, the wound should be packed open and treated as an abscess cavity.

ANTIMICROBIAL THERAPY

Antimicrobial therapy is generally based on the results of in vitro sensitivity tests. Such sensitivity tests are usually not available for 24 hours following culturing. Thus, initial therapy in life-threatening infections must be guided by a presumptive diagnosis. A compilation of the sensitivities of various organisms recovered in the local hospital is useful in order to choose the appropriate antibacterial therapy during the period of time before sensitivities have been completed. In this regard, gram smears play an important role in antimicrobial selection. When gram-positive organisms are clearly involved, we frequently select nafcillin (100 mg./kg. per day) because of its high degree of effectiveness toward Pneumococcus, Streptococcus, and methycillin-resistant Staphylococcus. When unspecified gram-negative organisms are involved, chloramphenicol, kanamycin, cephalothin, and ampicillin are frequently utilized. The latter two also have a gram-positive spectrum (Parker, 1969). All of these drugs have severe limitations; for example, Pseudomonas is almost always resistant to all these drugs. It is frequently difficult to rule out Pseudomonas, which is frequently the etiologic agent in these lethal infections. Pseudomonas is, however, more susceptible to polymyxin or gentamicin (Parker, 1969). In cases of overwhelming sepsis due to unknown organisms, we frequently will utilize cephalothin and polymyxin in combination. In all cases, antimicrobial therapy is "tailored," once following identification of the organisms and again when sensitivities are available. Repeated cultures are necessary to treat the rapidly changing flora even after seemingly appropriate therapy is underway.

We avoid kanamycin when life is not threatened, because of the high incidence of deafness in patients who have been uremic and on hemodialysis. Such patients have frequently lost considerable hearing in the

past and hearing can be permanently impaired by kanamycin. We are also reluctant to utilize colistin because of its high incidence of renal toxicity. As mentioned previously, colistin has impaired renal clearance of azathioprine, leading to bone marrow toxicity. When azathioprine is stopped, rejection ensues (Case 1). We also avoid chloramphenicol because of its tendency to aggravate the bone marrow-suppressive qualities of azathioprine (see Cases 1 and 3). Nevertheless, there is no reluctance to use any of these drugs in life-threatening circumstances, when the organisms are sensitive.

Many of the patients with potentially lethal infections have significant impairment of renal function due to rejection, or will develop renal failure secondary to cessation of immunosuppressive therapy. Table 25-4 indicates those drugs which require reduction in dosage during renal functional impairment. In addition, it lists those drugs which are readily removed by hemodialysis. The serum concentration of these drugs must be replenished following hemodialysis. One should not assume that the same drugs that are hemodialysable are also dialyzed peritoneally. Real differences exist in the ability of the two methods to clear these drugs. The entire problem has been extensively reviewed by Kunin (1967). Under some circumstances, serum levels of antibiotics must be obtained in order to check on the therapeutic level and avoid toxicity.

Actual resistance to antibiotic therapy is not the major problem in these patients. Most bacteria are sensitive to available antimicrobials. Inability to diagnose the precise etiologic agent in complicated multiple infections and failure to deliver the antibiotic into sequestered pulmonary microabscesses are greater problems. Lung abscesses due either to fungal or bacterial infection are common, and surgical drainage may be necessary even in these acutely ill patients. This has not been widely practiced in the past, but has been of value in selected immunoincompetent patients (Kilman et al., 1969).

Fungi are responsive in the most part to amphotericin B. Amphotericin is not dialysable by hemodialysis, but is cleared by the kidney. Consequently, loading doses followed by small incremental doses are utilized in patients with renal failure. A

TABLE 25-4. Recommended Dosage for Antibiotics in Renal Failure*

Group	Antibiotic	Recommended dose	
		Serum creatinine 4–10 mg. per 100 ml.	Serum creatinine 10 mg. per 100 ml.
1. Marked reduction in dosage	Tetracycline Oxytetracycline† Kanamycin† Streptomycin† Colistin Polymyxin Gentamycin†	Loading dose followed by standard doses at intervals of 1 to 2 days.	Loading dose followed by standard dose at intervals of 3 to 4 days.
2. Modest reduction in dosage	Penicillin G† Lincomycin Cephalothin†	Loading dose followed by: Standard doses at 4- to 5-hr. intervals Standard doses at 6-hr. intervals Standard doses at 12-hr. intervals	Loading dose followed by: Standard doses at 8- to 10-hr. intervals Standard doses at 12-hr. intervals Standard doses at 24-hr. intervals
3. No reduction in dosage	Chloramphenicol† Erythromycin Methicillin Oxacillin Novobiocin Ampicillin†	Same as in the normal.	Same as in the normal.

*Modified from Kunin, 1967; Schwartz, 1968; and Maher, 1969.
†Drug is readily dialyzed by hemodialysis.

newer fungal agent, 5-fluorocytosine, has been developed. This drug is effective against Candida and Cryptococcus and may well be effective against other fungi as well. The drug is restricted at present to treating recurrent fungal diseases that have not responded to amphotericin (Tassel, 1968). Nocardia is actually a bacteria rather than a fungus, although it is commonly classified among the fungal diseases. It responds readily to sulfadiazine.

Pneumocystis carinii is highly susceptible to pentamadine isethionate. Despite its ability to eradicate the organism, pentamadine is seldom curative in the patient treated with immunosuppressants because of the inability of such patients to eradicate the proteinaceous alveolar infiltrate following the death of the organism. Even when effective, the clinical response is slow. The drug is hepatotoxic and nephrotoxic and may cause hypoglycemia and hypocalcemia.

SUMMARY

Infections are the most common cause of death in recipients, treated with immunosuppressants, of kidney transplants. Such infections can frequently be prevented by careful attention to preoperative, operative, and postoperative details of patient care, and no deaths have occurred in the last 43 consecutive renal transplants in our institution. In particular, attention must be paid to the preoperative preparation of the patient by hemodialysis, eradication of pre-existing infections, prevention of wound infections and urinary fistulas, and postoperative avoidance of excessive immunosuppressive drugs, leukopenia, and renal insufficiency. It is essential to recognize that the patient with chronic and repeated renal rejections requiring prolonged high doses of immunosuppressive drugs with repeated episodes of bone marrow depression is a likely victim of a lethal infection. The early removal of the kidney in patients with this clinical course is necessary to prevent death.

The major diagnostic problem associated with renal infection is identification of the etiologic agent or agents. The infecting organisms are frequently multiple and are not always recognized by routine techniques. Lung biopsy may be necessary to obtain an accurate diagnosis in pneumonia.

Therapy in potentially lethal infections consists of the sacrifice of the kidney by stopping immunosuppression, the institution of hemodialysis when necessary, and the use of the appropriate antimicrobial therapy. Most of the infecting agents are sensitive to available agents, but delay in making the decision to sacrifice the kidney and delay in making the specific diagnosis may lead unnecessarily to a fatal outcome.

REFERENCES

Balakrishman, S. L., Armstrong, D., Rubin, A. L., and Stenzel, K. H.: Cytomegalovirus infection after renal transplantation. JAMA, 207:1712, 1969.

Carbone, P. P., Sabesin, S. M., Sidransky, H., and Frei, E., III: Secondary aspergillosis. Amer. Intern. Med., 60:556, 1964.

Craighead, J. E., Hanshaw, J. B., and Carpenter, C. B.: Cytomegalovirus infection after renal allotransplantation. JAMA, 201:99, 1967.

Feinberg, S. B., Lester, R. G., and Burke, B. A.: The roentgen findings in Pneumocystis carinii pneumonia. J. Radiol., 76:594, 1961.

Hill, R. B., Dahrling, B. E., Starzl, T. E., and Rifkind, D.: Death after transplantation: An analysis of sixty cases. Amer. J. Med., 42:327, 1967.

Hume, D. M.: Kidney transplantation. In Rapaport, F. T., and Dausset, J.: Human Transplantation. New York, Grune and Stratton, 1968.

Hume, D. M., Magee, J. H., Kauffman, H. J., Jr., Rittenbury, M. S., and Prout, G. R., Jr.: Renal homotransplantation in man in modified recipients. Ann. Surg., 158:608, 1963.

Kilman, J. W., Ahn, C., Andrews, N. C., and Klassen, K.: Surgery for pulmonary aspergillosis. J. Thorac. Cardiov. Surg., 57:642, 1969.

Kunin, C. M.: A guide to the use of antibiotics in patients with renal disease. Ann. Intern. Med., 67:151, 1967.

Maher, J. F., and Schreiner, G. E.: Current status of dialysis of poisons and drugs. Trans. Amer. Soc. Artif. Int. Organs, 15:461, 1967.

Moore, T. C., and Hume, D. M.: The period and nature of hazard in clinical renal transplantation. Ann. Surg., 170:1, 1969.

Morris, P. J., Bondoc, C., and Burke, J. F.: Effect of heterologous anti-lymphocyte serum on acute bacterial inflammation. Surg. Forum, 17:74, 1966.

Najarian, J. S., Gulyassy, P. F., Duffy, G., Stoney, R. J., and Braunstein, P.: Protection of the donor kidney during homotransplantation. Ann. Surg., 164:398, 1966.

Orie, N. G. M., DeVries, G. A., and Kikstra, A.: Growth of Aspergillus in the human lung, aspergilloma and aspergillosis. Amer. Rev. Resp. Dis., 82:649, 1960.

Parker, R. H., and Paterson, P. Y.: Antimicrobial agents, selection and use. J. Chron. Dis., 21:719, 1969.

Rifkind, D.: The activation of Varicella-zoster virus infections by immunosuppressive therapy. J. Lab. Clin. Med., 68:463, 1966a.

Rifkind, D., Faris, T. D., and Hill, R. B., Jr.: Pneumocystis carinii pneumonia. Studies on the diagnosis and treatment. Ann. Intern. Med., 65:943, 1966b.

Rifkind, D., Goodman, N., and Hill, R. B., Jr.: The clinical significance of cytomegalovirus infection in renal transplant recipients. Ann. Intern. Med., 66:1116, 1967a.

Rifkind, D., Marchioro, T. L., Schneck, S. A., and Hill, R. B., Jr.: Systemic fungal infections complicating renal transplantation and immunosuppressive therapy. Amer. J. Med., 43:28, 1967b.

Rifkind, D., Starzl, T. E., Marchioro, T. L., Waddell, W. R., Rowlands, D. T., and Hill, R. B., Jr.: Transplantation pneumonia. JAMA., 189:808, 1964.

Schwartz, W. B., and Kassirer, J. P.: Medical management of chronic renal failure. Amer. J. Med., 44:786, 1968.

Seelig, M. S.: Mechanisms by which antibiotics increase the incidence and severity of Candidiasis and alter the immunological defenses. Bact. Rev., 30:442, 1966.

Starzl, T. E.: Experience in Renal Transplantation. Philadelphia, W. B. Saunders Company, 1964.

Starzl, T. E., Marchioro, T. L., Zühlke, V., and Brettschneider, L.: Transplantation of the kidney. Med. Times, 95:196, 1967.

Tassel, D., and Madoff, M. A.: Treatment of Candida sepsis and Cryptococcus meningitis with 5-fluorocytosine. JAMA, 206:830, 1968.

CHAPTER 26

PULMONARY SEPSIS AND DEBILITY

by THOMAS F. NEALON, JR., M.D.

Thomas F. Nealon, Jr., is a Pennsylvanian who graduated from Jefferson Medical College. He received his residency training in general and thoracic surgery at Jefferson and thereafter joined the staff and faculty, being later promoted to full professor. In 1968 he was appointed Director of Surgery, St. Vincent's Hospital and Medical Center of New York, and Professor of Clinical Surgery, New York University School of Medicine. His extensive research and practice in the surgery of thoracic diseases are reflected in the following discussion.

The patient with pulmonary sepsis and debility has at least three major problems—impairment of pulmonary function, infection with its accompanying toxicity, and malnutrition. Each of these is a major problem in its own right and to some degree contributes to the disability created by the other problems. Ideally, all three should be corrected at once. In practice this is not always possible. Furthermore, in different patients the priority of treatment will vary, depending upon the general condition of the patient and the nature and degree of each problem. In instances in which all three problems are severe, the order or priority of treatment is pulmonary disability, sepsis, and debility. This order is the reverse of the order in which the patient can tolerate these problems when they are of considerable magnitude. The patient will be in extremis earliest if poor pulmonary function is not corrected. While debility must be remedied for good healing, sepsis should be cleared prior to this.

Advances in surgical techniques have made it possible to operate on sicker people now than previously. However, some of these efforts will result in patients with this triad of problems. While the present state of the art contributes to the creation of some of these problems, fortunately the techniques developed make it possible to salvage many patients.

In treating patients with these problems one of the most important ingredients is a mature, experienced, well-informed surgeon with an optimistic attitude. He must continually strive to get the patient well, but must be able to differentiate between "doing something" for the patient and carrying out a *definitive* procedure at the *appropriate* time with proper preparation. He must avoid being overwhelmed by the multiplicity of problems.

ETIOLOGY

In the majority of cases the sequence is unresolving pulmonary sepsis, which, because of its chronicity, then causes debility. If the sepsis is not properly treated, it persists with an increase in infection, toxicity, and progressive debility. The problem may begin with (a) a pulmonary abscess, either as an acute infectious process or distal to an unsuspected carcinoma, (b) a middle-lobe syndrome due to enlarged lymph nodes, (c) chronic bronchiectasis, (d) aspiration pneumonitis, (e) pulmonary embolus; (f) empyema, (g) injury, (h) surgery, or (i) acute tracheobronchitis.

PROPHYLAXIS

Prophylaxis is accomplished preoperatively by (1) a careful work-up to properly evaluate the patient's problems, (2) adequate preparation of the patient, (3) treatment of any established infection with definitive antibiotics, (4) correction of any anemia or hypoproteinemia, (5) treatment of any respiratory disability preoperatively, and (6) prompt and proper treatment (surgical or medical) of the pulmonary problem. Definitive treatment of the pulmonary disease is discussed further in this chapter. Many critical illnesses are created by improper or, more commonly, inadequate treatment of one of the etiologic factors listed previously. Proper treatment with adequate preparation is the best prophylaxis.

DIAGNOSIS AND MANAGEMENT

The patient is usually one who has become progressively sicker because of an infection that has advanced out of control until he is quite ill, septic, debilitated, and showing evidence of pulmonary disability. The diagnostic work-up must include an evaluation of the patient as a whole, as well as a careful assessment of the contribution to his condition of impaired pulmonary function, sepsis, and debility.

This is begun with a careful physical examination. The level of his orientation is an indication of his general condition. His color, respiratory rate, depth of respiration, and the effort required to breathe are indications of the patient's pulmonary function. A patient in respiratory difficulty may not be cyanotic, particularly if the gas he is breathing is being supplemented with oxygen. A patient who is cold and sweaty or who is obviously laboring to breathe is probably in respiratory acidosis. If the acidosis is severe the patient most likely has bronchospasm, which contributes further to the impaired ventilation. The examiner may not hear any wheezing in a patient with severe bronchospasm because very little air is moving in or out of the tracheobronchial tree. There must be movement of air through the constricted bronchi to cause audible wheezing. The exact nature of the problem is best assessed by measuring arterial blood gases. If the PO_2 (oxygen tension) is low, the patient is not getting adequate oxygen. This may be due to inadequate gas exchange but is more commonly a result of the shunting of blood through atelectatic lung or of impaired diffusion of the gas across the alveolar membrane due to heart failure or infection. In the majority of cases the PO_2 of the arterial blood can be returned to normal merely by increasing the concentration of oxygen in the ventilating gases. If the PCO_2 (tension of carbon dioxide) is elevated, there is respiratory acidosis due to inadequate pulmonary ventilation. This can be corrected by increasing the volume of ventilation. If the patient is in metabolic acidosis, the possibility of poor tissue perfusion must be considered. The second possibility is that his illness is causing abnormal losses or retention of electrolytes.

Any abnormalities of blood gas values require a careful chest evaluation, including a good physical examination of the chest and x-ray studies as indicated. If there is any evidence of fluid accumulation within the hemithorax, it should be tapped dry and the fluid smeared and cultured for antibiotic sensitivity. At the conclusion of the thoracentesis it is useful to instill antibiotics into the pleural space. The antibiotic is chosen on the basis of the most likely identity of the offending organism. It is good practice to save a specimen of the aspirated fluid in a sealed test tube and leave it available in the patient's room where it can be seen by all physicians involved in his care and can be compared with any fluid aspirated at a later date. A label on the tube should indicate the date of the tap and the amount of fluid aspirated. Changes in the character and quantity of the pleural aspirate are helpful in assessing the patient's course. With the patient's improvement, the aspirate decreases in both consistency and quantity.

The sputum should also be studied for bacteria and their antibiotic sensitivity. Any striking febrile episodes should be an indication to do a blood culture.

The need for support of ventilation is dependent upon the extent to which the ventilation is impaired. If the patient requires only oxygen, then either an oxygen tent or oxygen supplied by a catheter can be used. One should also include humidity, which will thin the bronchial secretions and make them easier to raise (Wells et al., 1963). I have rarely found mucolytic agents necessary to liquefy bronchial secretions. In most instances adequate hydration of the patient is all that is necessary. When this is not sufficient, the addition of specific antibiotic therapy is far more effective than the mucolytic agents.

Intermittent positive pressure breathing will cause the patient to breathe more deeply and help to raise his secretions. The apparatus should be charged with physiologic salt solution to provide a diluent for the bronchial secretions. A bronchodilator should be added if the patient has bronchospasm. Some physicians like to include an antibiotic in the aerosol.

If the patient is having difficulty raising his secretions, nasotracheal aspiration is helpful. If this does not solve the problem, bronchoscopy is indicated. If bronchoscopy must be repeated more than twice, a tracheostomy should be performed.

In extreme cases the patient may require continuous ventilatory support until some of the pulmonary involvement has cleared (Bjork et al., 1957). Indications for support are the inability of the patient to maintain normal gas values in his blood and the patient's labored efforts to breathe. Early in the course of continuous support many physicians attach the ventilator to an endotracheal tube, inserted through either the mouth or the nasopharynx. Such an arrangement is satisfactory only when one is concerned solely with moving the ventilating gas in and out of the patient's lungs. This is not a satisfactory means of removing particulate matter that is invariably present in pulmonary sepsis. It is not possible to aspirate intrapulmonary pus well through an endotracheal tube, regardless of the diameter. This is accomplished much more effectively via a tracheostomy.

After the ventilator is attached, arterial blood should be analyzed for PO_2 and PCO_2, and the volume of ventilation and the oxygen content of the ventilating gases should be adjusted so as to maintain normal blood gas values (Nealon et al., 1966). However, it is unwise to mechanically ventilate with gases containing more than 65 per cent oxygen for long periods of time. Spencer and associates (1966) showed that dogs breathing oxygen-air mixtures under chamber conditions for five to fourteen days showed no ill effects at oxygen tensions below 300 mm. Hg. Oxygen tensions above 250 to 400 mm. Hg regularly produced fatal pulmonary injury in two to six days.

While the improvement in gas exchange made possible by this technique is very valuable, the reduction in the energy requirements expected of the patient may be even more beneficial. Consequently, I prefer to have the patient's ventilation controlled, rather than merely assisted, by the ventilator.

As soon as the tracheostomy is performed a sample of sputum should be taken for identification of organisms and antibiotic sensitivity. Antibiotics should be started immediately. The smear is of some value in choosing an antibiotic. Once the sensitivities are available the choice of antibiotics should be adjusted if necessary. While the patient is quite ill the cultures and sensitivity studies should be checked twice weekly. This will reveal any new bacterial contamination and any change in antibiotic sensitivity. The antibiotics must be changed as indicated by the sensitivity reports.

Good nutrition is a very important part of therapy for this patient. The oral route is preferred whenever available; if he is able to eat he should be encouraged with a full, nutritious diet—a high-caloric, high-protein diet. If there is question as to whether he is eating, the nurses should be asked to check his tray after each meal and record on his chart what he eats. Supplemental feedings are helpful but should not be given at times that will interfere with his next normal meal. Small doses of insulin before meals stimulate eating. The addition of a protein-sparing agent, such as Nilevar, is also helpful. Some physical activity and the correction of any anemia will also stimulate his appetite.

Another effective way to nourish a patient is by means of a feeding tube. A tube can be passed at mealtime and the patient may be fed by means of a gastrostomy feeding. The use of such diets frequently causes diarrhea, often a result of too much carbohydrate in the feeding. Reducing the amount of carbohydrate should stop the diarrhea. Another method is to blenderize a normal meal and dilute it with milk to a satisfactory fluidity for tube feeding.

If the patient is unable to tolerate food by mouth, the intravenous route must be used. It may also be used to supplement the oral route. Intravenous plasma and blood are the most rapid means of preparing a debilitated patient for operation. If prolonged parenteral feeding is necessary, additional calories can be supplied with fat emulsions, concentrated glucose, or intravenous alcohol (Moore, 1967). Recently we have been impressed with the results of infusing a high-caloric mixture over a 24-hour period, as advocated by Dudrick and associates (1969). A plastic catheter is inserted percutaneously via the subclavian vein into the vena cava, using strict aseptic technique. The catheter is sutured in place and should receive regular aseptic treatment to avoid infection. The basic solution consists of 750 ml. of 5 per cent dextrose in 5 per cent protein hydrolysate to which 350 ml. of 50 per cent dextrose has been added. The resultant 1100 ml. of solution contains approximately 5.25 gm. nitrogen, 212 gm. dextrose and 1000 calories. Electrolytes and vitamins are added according to the patient's needs. The solution is administered continuously 24 hours per day at a rate that allows only minimal glycosuria.

If the patient's proteins are low he can be given plasma or albumin intravenously. If his blood volume is below normal or if his proteins are low, any anemia should be treated with blood transfusions. If the blood volume and proteins are normal, anemia should be treated with packed red blood cells.

Frequently a patient who should be convalescing seems to stand still. This is often due to a diminished blood volume or mild anemia that is not recognized. Sometimes a blood transfusion to such patients may substantially increase the rate of convalescence.

Management of the Underlying Pulmonary Sepsis

Ultimately the underlying pulmonary infection must be treated directly. Timing of the operation is very important. The adjunctive measures already discussed will improve the patient but only to a certain point. The surgeon must determine when the maximum improvement possible by these nonmedical measures has been accomplished and then decide whether the patient can tolerate a definitive surgical procedure.

Sometimes if the patient has not improved to the point at which a definitive procedure can be carried out, some adjunctive surgical procedure may be undertaken. The drainage of an infected collection, either by tube or open drainage, may provide sufficient additional response to make the major procedure safer. Purulent collections that are secondary to foci of infection, such as bronchopleural fistulae of severe bronchiectasis, will improve with drainage but will not clear totally until the nidus of infection has been cleared. Ideally, operation should be undertaken when the course of the patient's improvement reaches a plateau.

PULMONARY ABSCESS. This problem may be managed with antibiotics and tracheal toilet. Such treatment should be given an adequate trial. If there is a reasonable response in clearing of the toxicity and diminution of the size of the abscess cavity, one is justified in persisting with this method of treatment for approximately six weeks; if it has not cleared by this time, pulmonary resection is indicated. This operation will occasionally unearth an unsuspected proximal carcinoma that was the cause of the poor response to treatment.

The abscess that does not respond and continues to render the patient toxic is best removed surgically with a pulmonary resection. The response of the toxicity in such a case may be spectacular and very gratifying. Abscesses that must be treated surgically are best treated with pulmonary resection that includes the abscess. If the position or size of the abscess requires the sacrifice of an inordinate amount of pulmonary tissue, the abscess can be treated by open drainage. In such a case the visceral pleura overlying the abscess must be fused to the parietal pleura in a preliminary procedure. Rarely should open drainage be necessary.

MIDDLE-LOBE SYNDROME. An infection in a middle lobe whose bronchus is partially obstructed by enlarged lymph nodes is usually refractory to antibiotics. This is best handled by middle-lobe lobectomy. Care must be taken during operation to avoid spillage into the opposite lung of secretions blocked in the middle lobe. This can be prevented by (a) using a double-lumen endotracheal tube, (b) tying off the middle-lobe bronchus as soon as possible, or (c) frequent aspiration of the bronchus by the anesthesiologist during the operation.

CHRONIC BRONCHIECTASIS. This condition, with large, poorly-drained bronchial spaces, favors the persistence of infection. Preliminary antibiotics, pressure therapy, and postural drainage will improve, but rarely cure, an infection. The problem is best solved by pulmonary resection. All the bronchiectatic tissue need not be removed, since the more severely involved tissue acts as a nidus of infection, feeding the less seriously involved bronchiectatic areas. Removal of the nidus is usually followed by improvement in the remaining areas of bronchiectasis. A word of caution is in order—more often one errs in not removing sufficient pulmonary tissue.

In addition to the steps listed earlier, bronchiectasis requires careful tracheal toilet with pressure therapy, postural drainage, and local and parenteral antibiotics. Improvement is gauged by the quantity and quality of the patient's sputum. Initially, the sputum will become thin but will increase in quantity. The thinning of the secretions will persist and the quantity will gradually diminish. Operation is best withheld until the secretions are maximally reduced.

Anesthesia in such patients is best induced with intravenous agents because the inhalation anesthetics tend to stimulate bronchial secretions, interfering with transfer of the agent across the alveolar membrane.

ASPIRATION PNEUMONITIS. This problem requires aggressive treatment with endobronchial aspiration, antibiotics, and, at times, steroids. If it does not respond, it goes on to abscess formation, the treatment of which is detailed earlier.

PULMONARY EMBOLUS. This is frequently controlled with prophylaxis against further emboli, but in some instances, such as septic emboli, abscesses may develop, which require antibiotics or resection or both.

EMPYEMA. Empyema may occur secondary to pneumonia or following injury or trauma. Fairly rapid response can be obtained by open drainage but the patient is then committed to the presence of a draining fistula in the chest wall for a prolonged period of time. If the patient's condition can be improved to the point at which a resection or decortication can be done, the empyema space can be eliminated with the patient maintaining an intact chest wall. This substantially shortens and simplifies the convalescence.

The toxicity may be controlled preoperatively with intermittent needle aspiration of the pus with repeated thoracenteses at which specific antibiotics can be instilled. Occasionally such a routine can cure empyema. If this proves inadequate, a tube can be inserted for continuous drainage until the patient is ready for the definitive procedure. The decortication allows expansion of the lung to obliterate the space; resection may be necessary to remove the cause of the empyema and avoid a recurrence. The empyema may be due to a bronchopleural fistula. This requires drainage of the empyema and thoracoplasty. All intrapleural dead space must be obliterated if that space is infected.

The offending area can be removed only if the patient's ultimate postoperative condition will leave him with adequate pulmonary tissue to sustain ventilation. After the infection has been controlled within the limits possible with antibiotics and drainage, after debility has been controlled with aggressive nutrition, and after pulmonary function has been improved to a safe level, a definitive operation must be undertaken.

For operation, a high blood level of antibiotic is effected. A high oxygen mixture endotracheal anesthesia is given. The patient's operative course is monitored with arterial blood gas analyses every thirty minutes during operation and in the immediate postoperative period. Particular care must be taken to avoid aspiration of purulent secretions during the operation.

If the patient is unable to maintain normal blood gas values postoperatively, his ventilation must be assisted. If he has not had a tracheostomy, one need not be done at this stage. A nasotracheal or orotracheal tube may be inserted and attached to the mechanical ventilator. The ventilator is adjusted to maintain essentially normal blood gas values. If ventilation must be continued beyond 36 hours a tracheostomy is performed.

The same strenuous measures that were effective in preparing the patient for operation must be continued in the postoperative period.

The utilization of the principles set forth is described in the following case report:

H. G., a 41-year-old woman, was admitted to the hospital in January, 1966. She complained of shortness of breath of three weeks' duration, malaise, and a cough finally productive of foul-smelling sputum. She was known to have had severe bilateral bronchiectasis since she was a child. Ten years prior to this admission she had two pulmonary resections—first of the left lower lobe and then the lingula.

On admission she appeared chronically ill and emaciated. There was flatness over the lower half of her left chest and rales were heard in the base of her right lung. A chest x-ray revealed an air-fluid level posteriorly in her left midlung. A thoracentesis demonstrated foul-smelling purulent material. After preparation with specific antibiotic therapy, an open drainage revealed a large empyema space. This procedure improved her condition considerably and she was discharged in 10 days to continue her convalescence at home.

Her convalescence did not progress at home. She

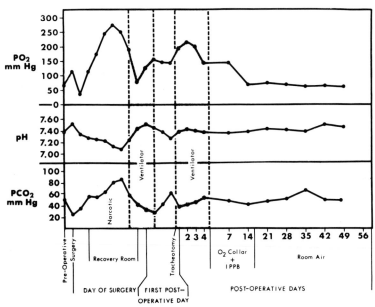

Figure 26-1.   Graph of preoperative and postoperative blood-gas values for the same patient.

developed a bronchopleural fistula and continued to harbor bacteria that could not be treated adequately with antibiotics. Antibiotics were changed several times on the basis of cultures but without lasting results. She was readmitted in May, 1966. A bronchogram demonstrated severe saccular bronchiectasis of the entire remaining left upper lobe and tubular bronchiectasis of the right lower lobe. She was prepared for operation with postural drainage, pressure breathing, antibiotics, and blood transfusions. Her sputum thinned and decreased.

She was operated on on May 16, 1966, and a left upper lobectomy was performed, completing the pneumonectomy. She tolerated the operation without difficulty. She left the operating room in good condition, but in the recovery room she had persistent hypoventilation, made worse by an average dose of an analgesic. She was treated by nasal oxygen, and initial blood gas studies showed a PO_2 of 175, a PCO_2 of 55 and a pH of 7.27. She became more stuporous and four hours after operation it became necessary to ventilate her lungs through a cuffed nasotracheal tube and pressure-regulated ventilation (Fig. 26-1). With this apparatus the patient's condition stabilized (PO_2, 126; PCO_2, 33; and pH 7.51).

The next morning the ventilation was discontinued. The nastotracheal tube was removed after repeated arterial blood gas studies, done over a period of four hours, were within normal limits. That evening the patient began again to accumulate carbon dioxide. Arterial blood studies demonstrated a PO_2 of 147, a PCO_2 of 61, and a pH of 7.27. It was evident that prolonged ventilatory support was necessary. Tracheostomy was performed and she was again attached to the ventilator with good results. Ventilatory support was continued for four days.

For the next week she used an oxygen collar and periodic IPPB. After this she used only IPPB with diminishing frequency. She became careless in the use of this and, without overt clinical evidence, her PCO_2 slowly crept up to 80 and her blood chlorides fell to 60.

Her urinary excretion of chloride increased to compensate for the chronic respiratory acidosis. An increase in the ventilation corrected the acidosis and stopped the urinary excretion of chlorides. The blood chloride level did not return to normal until she was given chloride. With careful management she gradually improved and was discharged on the 95th postoperative day. She procured an IPPB machine and is living comfortably at home, caring for a teen-age son.

REFERENCES

Bjork, V. O., and Engstrom, C. G.: Treatment of ventilatory insufficiency by tracheostomy and artificial ventilation. J. Thorac. Surg., *34:*228, 1957.

Dudrick, S. J., Wilmore, D. W., Vors, H. M., and Rhoads, J. E.: Can intravenous feeding as the sole means of nutrition support growth in the child and restore weight loss in an adult?: An affirmative answer. Ann. Surg., *169:*974, 1969.

Moore, F. D.: Surgical nutrition: Parenteral and oral. *In* Randall, H. T., Hardy, J. D., and Moore, F. D. (eds.): Manual of Preoperative and Postoperative Care. Philadelphia, W. B. Saunders Company, 1967.

Nealon, T. F., Jr., Prorok, J. J., Gosin, S., and Fraimow, W.: Impaired oxygenation with prolonged continuous ventilatory support: Analysis of arterial gases following tracheostomy. Ann. Surg., *164:*558, 1966.

Spencer, F. C., Bosomworth, P., and Ritcher, W.: Fatal pulmonary injury from prolonged inhalation of oxygen in high concentrations. *In* Brown, W. J., and Cox, B. G. (eds.): Proceedings of the Third International Conference on Hyperbaric Medicine. National Research Council publication No. 1404, Washington, D.C., National Academy of Sciences, National Research Council, 1966, p. 189.

Wells, R. E., Perera, R. D., and Kinney, J. M.: Humidification of oxygen during inhalation therapy. New Eng. J. Med., *268:*644, 1963.

CHAPTER 27

LOW CARDIAC OUTPUT AND CARDIAC ARRHYTHMIAS AFTER OPEN-HEART SURGERY

by **GORDON K. DANIELSON, M.D., F.A.C.S.** and
F. HENRY ELLIS, JR., M.D., Ph.D., F.A.C.S.

Gordon K. Danielson, Jr., was born in Iowa and graduated from the University of Pennsylvania, having been elected to Phi Beta Kappa, and from the University of Pennsylvania School of Medicine, having been elected to Alpha Omega Alpha. After internship at the University of Michigan, he returned to Penn for his residency in general and thoracic surgery. He received numerous honors and special fellowships and became Associate Professor of Surgery and Chief of Cardiac Surgery at the University of Kentucky in 1966. He jointed the staff of the Mayo Clinic in 1967 and is currently Assistant Professor of Surgery, Mayo Graduate School of Medicine, University of Minnesota. His scientific writings have been lucid and significant, and he is highly competent in the field of cardiac surgery.

F. Henry Ellis, Jr., was born in Washington, D.C., was elected to Phi Beta Kappa at Yale and to Alpha Omega Alpha at Columbia Medical School. He received his Ph.D. in Surgery at the University of Minnesota. After residency training in general and thoracic surgery at the Mayo Foundation, he joined the staff and became one of the most able members of that illustrious group, being advanced to full professor. In 1970 he became Chief of Cardiovascular Surgery at the Lahey Clinic and Lecturer in Surgery at the Harvard Medical School. His works in thoracic and cardiovascular surgery are recognized throughout the world.

All surgery has benefited from the lessons learned in the management of patients after open-heart surgery. The complex physiologic alterations that follow operations on the sick human organism while the cardiorespiratory system is artificially supported for variable periods with a nonpulsatile, sometimes suboptimal blood flow have demanded of surgeons a thorough grounding in cardiorespiratory physiology, heretofore considered more the domain of the basic scientist. Cardiopulmonary bypass has been likened to a form of controlled clinical shock (Lillehei et al., 1967). The reaction of the body to this stressful situation has been carefully analyzed, and methods have been devised to modify its potentially deleterious effects.

The response of the body under these circumstances is similar to, but often more exaggerated than, its usual response to stress.

There is increased sympathetic nerve activity with an increase in circulating catecholamines and other vasoactive substances. Peripheral arterial resistance increases, particularly in the viscera and skin, resulting in decreased blood flow to these areas. The increased peripheral resistance does not always return to normal at the end of perfusion but may continue for a variable period postoperatively, resulting in increased cardiac work that imposes an added load on the already damaged heart. Cardiac efficiency may be further decreased by the presence of metabolic acidosis. Low cardiac output and cardiac arrhythmias are therefore not unexpected accompaniments of open-heart surgery, although fortunately they are encountered more rarely today than in the early days of the development of this surgical field.

However, the incidence of postoperative

587

low cardiac output and cardiac arrhythmias remains significant under certain circumstances — circumstances in which the management of the patient must be conducted with extraordinary care and precision. These include operations for the repair of acquired valvular heart disease (particularly mitral valve disease), repair of tetralogy of Fallot, and repair of congenital defects in which intracardiac shunting has led to a high pulmonary vascular resistance. In this chapter, discussion will center on the mechanisms involved in the development of these potentially lethal postoperative problems and how they can be recognized and treated.

LOW CARDIAC OUTPUT

DEFINITION

The term "low-output syndrome" has been widely used in the cardiac surgical literature, but it is a poor term because it implies that the cause of the hemodynamic abnormality is unknown and that treatment is nonspecific

and apt to be unsuccessful. In fact, the incidence of the "low-output syndrome" varies inversely with the diligence of those managing postperfusion patients. Furthermore, there is often a mechanical basis for the syndrome. In a recent analysis of early postoperative deaths after open-heart surgery, an identifiable anatomic cause of death was demonstrated in nearly all patients who died manifesting the "low-output syndrome" (Roberts and Morrow, 1967). This places squarely on the surgeon the onus of identifying the cause and correcting it.

This is not to imply that one should expect a normal cardiac output postoperatively after all open-heart operations if no anatomic defect exists. Such is clearly not the case. Barratt-Boyes and Wood (1958) found the average cardiac output of normal resting adults to be 3.5 ($\pm$ 0.7) liters/min./sq. m. Cardiac output measured after various open-heart procedures is less than normal in many patients, particularly after those operations previously alluded to (Table 27-1) (Kirklin and Rastelli, 1967). Cardiac output tends to be lowest on the afternoon of operation and 24 hours later, but it begins to rise toward normal in 48 to 72 hours.

TABLE 27-1. Average Cardiac Output* After Open Intracardiac Operations

Type of Operation†	Cases	Chest Open (½ hr. after bypass)	2 to 4 hrs.	24 hrs.	48 hrs.
		Cardiac Output, Mean (and Range) After Operation			
Repair					
ASD with normal pulmonary vascular resistance	5	3.0 (2.1–3.9)	3.4 (2.4–4.4)	3.0 (2.3–4.0)	3.3 (2.9–3.7)
VSD with normal pulmonary vascular resistance	7	3.8 (3.2–5.3)	3.5 (2.9–4.2)	3.2 (2.7–4.4)	3.4 (2.7–4.4)
VSD with moderately elevated pulmonary vascular resistance	3	3.7 (3.4–4.0)	3.7 (2.9–4.4)	3.0 (1.9–3.6)	2.9 (2.3–3.5)
Tetralogy of Fallot	15	2.5 (2.0–3.5)	2.9 (2.0–5.5)	2.2 (1.6–3.7)	2.5 (1.7–5.2)
Replacement					
Aortic valve with S-E prosthesis	7	2.5 (1.6–3.1)	2.4 (1.4–3.8)	2.8 (2.0–4.5)	3.2 (2.3–4.1)
Mitral valve with S-E prosthesis	12	2.5 (1.1–4.1)	1.7 (1.0–2.6)	1.9 (0.9–3.0)	2.2 (1.2–3.5)

*Normal values = 3.5 ($\pm$0.7) liters/min./sq. m. of body surface.
†ASD = atrial septal defect; VSD = ventricular septal defect; S-E = Starr-Edwards. (From Kirklin, J. W., and Rastelli, G. C.: Low cardiac output after open intracardiac operations. Progr. Cardiov. Dis., *10:*117, 1967. By permission of Grune & Stratton, Inc.)

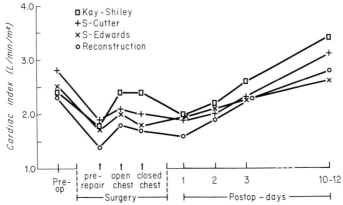

Figure 27-1. Cardiac index before and after open operations on the mitral valve. Note similarity of results regardless of procedure, the lowest indices being measured on the afternoon of operation with a gradual increase to more nearly normal levels at time of dismissal. (From Rouleau, C. A., Frye, R. L., and Ellis, F. H., Jr.: Hemodynamic state after open mitral valve replacement and reconstruction. J. Thorac. Cardiov. Surg., 58:870, 1969. By permission of C. V. Mosby Company)

The lowest values recorded in this study were in patients undergoing replacement of the mitral valve with a Starr-Edwards prosthesis, but a recent detailed analysis of hemodynamics early after open mitral valve operations (Rouleau et al., 1969) showed that cardiac output is depressed regardless of the type of procedure, whether reconstructive or replacement, and is independent of the prosthetic valve design (Fig. 27-1). These findings suggest a common abnormality of mitral valve patients, probably a diseased myocardium. In any case a low cardiac output is the rule rather than the exception after many open-heart procedures, and it is only when cardiac output becomes unduly depressed that specific causes must be sought and appropriate therapeutic measures instituted.

RECOGNITION

While the only precise way to determine cardiac output is to measure it, reliable techniques for the routine performance of such measurements are not yet generally available. The pulse contour method may prove to be a practical technique for easy continuous monitoring of this important variable (Kouchoukos et al., 1969). Careful observation of the patient, however, will usually provide clues to the presence of a low cardiac output. The pale, anxious facies of a restless patient with cold, moist, cyanotic extremities and weakened or absent periph-

eral pulses is familiar to those who have cared for patients after open-heart surgery. It can be known with certainty that cardiac output is reduced when the pulse pressure is diminished and hourly urine output drops. When blood pressure, as measured by Korotkoff sounds, is faint or measurable only by palpation, cardiac output is low even though pressures may be normal as measured by a centrally placed intra-arterial catheter.

Although the clinical picture of profound low cardiac output is usually obvious, minor degrees of this state are best recognized by careful monitoring of certain variables during the first few postoperative days. Such monitoring techniques have become routine in most centers where open-heart surgery is performed, although there is considerable variation in sophistication of the techniques employed. At present, we monitor right atrial pressure, and frequently left atrial and direct arterial pressure, for 24 to 48 hours. The electrocardiogram is monitored constantly on an oscilloscope for three to five days. In patients in whom low cardiac output is likely to develop, urine volume is determined hourly by use of an indwelling urinary catheter. In addition, the usual measures are employed to check the blood pressure by cuff, pulse rate, rectal temperature, and blood loss from drainage tubes. The setup in our intensive care unit is shown in Figure 27-2.

Aided by the techniques just described, careful observation of the patient will usually alert the surgeon to the existence

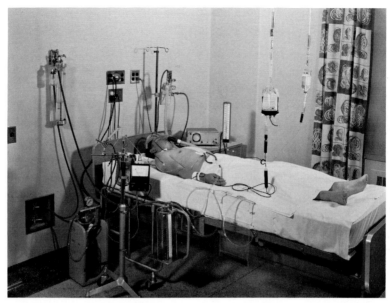

Figure 27-2. Postoperative cardiac intensive care setup. (From Moffitt, E. A., Tarhan, S., and Lundborg, R. O.: Anesthesia for cardiac surgery: Principles and practice. Anesthesiology, 29:1181, 1968. By permission of J. B. Lippincott Company)

of a lowered cardiac output; nevertheless, precise definition of its cause may not be immediately apparent. The remainder of this portion of the chapter will be devoted to this important determination, for proper treatment depends on it. The causes of postoperative low cardiac output can best be discussed under the following broad headings: hypovolemia, cardiac tamponade, residual cardiovascular disease, electrolyte and acid-base disturbances, cardiac rate and rhythm abnormalities, and myocardial dysfunction.

CAUSES

HYPOVOLEMIA

The most frequent cause of low cardiac output in the early days of open-heart surgery was hypovolemia, for it was not known then that blood volume is commonly diminished (Cleland et al., 1966). Blood-volume deficits ranging from 6 to 14 per cent have been measured, and although Litwak and associates (1961) ascribed these deficits to the sequestration of blood in visceral vascular compartments, this concept has not been substantiated by others (Berger et al., 1964; Kloster et al., 1966). Whatever the cause of this phenomenon, there is now ample evidence for the need to augment

blood volume after open-heart surgery, often considerably in excess (500 to 1000 ml.) of measured losses.

Since ventricular filling pressures are primary determinants of cardiac output, knowledge of these pressures, as inferred from atrial pressures, furnishes a guide for safe restoration of blood volume, thus providing for maximal cardiac output. The process of blood-volume restoration is begun in the operating room, the left atrial pressure being raised by transfusion from the pump-oxygenator to a mean of 20 to 25 mm. Hg. This high level of atrial pressure is produced in anticipation of progressive loss of blood and in order to expand the vascular bed maximally with the patient's own blood. Later, further transfusions are administered using right atrial pressure as a guide, or both right and left atrial pressures if the latter is also monitored. Left atrial pressure is usually monitored when it is elevated secondary to mitral valve disease, left ventricular aneurysm, or other diseases of the left side of the heart. It must be remembered that atrial pressure reflects only the status of the downstream ventricle, and reliance on right atrial pressure as a measure of left ventricular function may be misleading and even dangerous (Berglund, 1954).

Although Fishman and associates (1966) have recommended raising left atrial pressures postoperatively even higher (to a mean of 25 to 35 mm. Hg), an arbitrary level cannot be established since different pressure levels are required in different patients to provide for optimal cardiac output. Thus patients undergoing aortic valve replacement often have a good cardiac output at low levels of left atrial pressure (10 to 20 mm. Hg), while patients undergoing open operations on the mitral valve often require elevated pressures (20 to 35 mm. Hg).

Atrial pressures in excess of these levels may result in overstretching of the myocardium (descending limb of Starling's curve) with impairment of cardiac output leading to pulmonary congestion and edema. The degree of elevation of left atrial pressure that may be safely tolerated by the myocardium may be judged in part by the preoperative end-diastolic left ventricular pressure. Thus, if the left ventricle is adapted to elevated diastolic pressures, as in mitral insufficiency, it will tolerate a postoperative elevation of atrial pressure more readily than if it is not, as in tight mitral stenosis. Similarly, the effect of elevated left atrial pressure on the lungs may be judged by the preoperative left atrial pressure. Lungs unaccustomed to elevated venous pressures may develop pulmonary edema at a left atrial pressure of 30 mm. Hg, whereas pressures of 40 to 50 mm. Hg may not produce pulmonary edema in the lungs of a patient with longstanding mitral valve disease.

CARDIAC TAMPONADE

Although it is well known that cardiopulmonary bypass may result in some alterations in the clotting mechanism, which include a reduction in circulating platelets, an increase of circulating fibrinolysins, inadequate neutralization of heparin, and alteration of certain blood-clotting factors (Gans and Krivit, 1962a, 1962b), serious postoperative bleeding problems are fortunately rare. The incidence of reoperation for bleeding at the Mayo Clinic is 3 per cent (Gomes and McGoon, in press). Cardiac tamponade, which clearly depresses cardiac output, usually occurs in association with persistent and excessive postoperative bleeding and is most common after aortic valve surgery and operations for congenital cyanotic heart disease. The diagnosis of cardiac tamponade may be difficult to make, so a high index of suspicion is necessary. The classic signs and symptoms, including a falling blood pressure and a rising venous pressure, may be absent or can equally well reflect the hemodynamic abnormalities of a failing myocardium. According to Fishman and associates (1966), a rising right atrial pressure and a falling left atrial pressure are strongly suggestive of cardiac tamponade.

When bleeding has been excessive and associated with the passage of clots in the drainage tubes, the appearance of low cardiac output must be considered as due to cardiac tamponade until proven otherwise. Sudden diminution of chest tube drainage under these circumstances may be an added clue. These findings demand immediate investigation with syringe irrigation and aspiration of the chest tubes under sterile conditions. If tamponade is not relieved or if bleeding continues, immediate reoperation is mandatory. When it is not possible to identify any specific coagulation deficit, we have found that fresh frozen plasma or fresh whole blood is useful for improving blood coagulation, presumably because of replenishment of labile clotting factors.

Prior to transporting the patient to the operating room, it is prudent to slightly overtransfuse him to avoid the period of hypotension that develops during induction of anesthesia. Rapid reopening of the sternum and careful evacuation of blood and clot from the pericardium usually restore cardiac output dramatically and permanently, even when no specific bleeding site can be identified. Prompt recognition and surgical relief of cardiac tamponade are accompanied by a high survival rate.

RESIDUAL CARDIOVASCULAR DISEASE

A common cause of low cardiac output after open-heart surgery is residual cardiovascular disease. Thus, in patients undergoing attempted closure of a ventricular septal defect, a residual defect of modest size may seriously impair effective cardiac function and jeopardize the patient's recovery. Incomplete relief of obstruction to the right ventricular outflow tract in patients with tetralogy of Fallot can seriously handicap effective cardiac output and lead to right heart failure and death. Incomplete correction of mitral insufficiency by reconstruction techniques or from dysfunction of a prosthetic mitral valve due to paravalvular leak may be poorly tolerated because of the added burden imposed on the postoperative myocardium. If such an anatomic cause of postoperative low cardiac output can be identified, early reoperation should be seriously considered.

Associated untreated or untreatable cardiovascular disease may jeopardize the patient's recovery after open-heart surgery and manifest itself by a low cardiac output. For example, severe elevations of pulmonary arteriolar resistance that do not drop with correction of the underlying congenital cardiac anomaly are poorly tolerated, and concomitant coronary artery disease in patients undergoing aortic valve replacement may impair myocardial function postoperatively (Linhart and Wheat, 1967). Associated valvular disease, particularly untreated tricuspid insufficiency (Kloster et al., 1966), has a deleterious effect on cardiac output after open operations on the mitral valve. In fact, any unrecognized disease of other valves in patients undergoing replacement or repair of a specific acquired valvular lesion may lead to a low cardiac output postoperatively. Accordingly, all patients undergoing open operation for valvular heart disease should have careful preoperative evaluation to exclude associated valvular disease. This does not necessarily mean cardiac catheterization, however, since associated valvular disease can usually be detected and assessed by clinical means. The majority of patients who undergo valve replacements for acquired heart disease at our institution do not have preoperative cardiac catheterizations.

A careful cardiac evaluation at operation is also important. The heart and great vessels are examined and palpated for thrills and other abnormalities. For example, a systolic expansion of the left atrium associated with a systolic thrill on the posterior left atrial wall would indicate significant mitral insufficiency. Pressures are measured in the four cardiac chambers and in the aorta before and after valve repair. Finally, the tricuspid valve is palpated for stenosis and insufficiency prior to cannulation. These measures are useful for excluding associated valvular disease that could result in a low cardiac output postoperatively.

ELECTROLYTE AND ACID-BASE DISTURBANCES

In the early days of open-heart surgery, metabolic acidosis occurred commonly as a result of poor perfusion during operation and low cardiac output after operation (Clowes, 1963; Williams et al., 1965). The deleterious effects of metabolic acidosis on myocardial function, although not accepted by all (Andersen and Mouritzen, 1966), are generally agreed upon by most (Clowes et al., 1960; Darby et al., 1960; Ebert et al., 1962).

Today metabolic acidosis is rarely the primary cause of low cardiac output. When it occurs after open-heart surgery it is more often the result than the cause of low cardiac output, but its successful treatment is vital to restoration of optimal myocardial function. Treatment should coincide with ancillary efforts to improve cardiac output. Artificial ventilation to reduce the additional metabolic demands of the body imposed by the work of breathing is mandatory, since up to 50 per cent of the cardiac output may be required to supply the respiratory muscles in some postoperative patients (Dammann et al., 1963).

Restoration of normal pH can be achieved by the administration of sodium bicarbonate either in a dosage dependent on the measured base deficit or in empiric doses of up to 2 mEq./kg. of body weight. In the first method, base deficit in milliequivalents per liter (Astrup method) multiplied by 0.3 times the body weight in kilograms (representing the extracellular fluid compartment) roughly approximates total extracellular base deficit in milliequivalents. Two-thirds of the calculated dose is given initially, and supplemental doses are given according to the response of the patient and serial determinations of pH, P_{CO_2}, and P_{O_2}. THAM (tris[hydroxymethyl]aminomethane) can also be used for this purpose by infusion of a 0.3 M solution at a rate of 5 ml./kg./hr. Use of this drug has the advantage of avoiding the administration of large amounts of sodium and of providing an osmotic diuretic action; but because of its depressive effect on respiration, patients receiving it should be artificially ventilated.

More commonly today, patients are found to be alkalotic after open-heart surgery. A respiratory alkalosis is imposed during operation by hyperventilation and by the low concentration of carbon dioxide added to the oxygenator. After operation a metabolic alkalosis is at least partially the result of the sodium citrate given in ACD (citric acid, trisodium citrate, dextrose) blood. Alkalosis also has a deleterious effect on myocardial function owing in part to a direct effect on the myocardium (Cook et al., 1965; Wang and Katz, 1965) but more importantly to its effect on potassium balance.

The cations most essential to myocardial function are sodium, potassium, and calcium (Frank, 1964; Holland, 1969; Sarnoff et al., 1966), and the concentrations of all may be altered after open-heart surgery. Hyponatremia is common after cardiac surgery, particularly if hemodilution is used, but moderately altered serum sodium levels are rarely detrimental to cardiac output. If total body sodium is increased, however, retention of water, increase of blood volume, and the danger of pulmonary edema occur. Sodium probably has little primary effect on myocardial contraction except through its interrelationship with potassium and calcium transport across the myocardial cell membrane.

In patients who have had intensive treatment with most diuretics commonly used today, total body potassium is reduced (hypokalemia) even in the presence of normal serum levels (Ebert et al., 1965; Lockey et al., 1966). Potassium diuresis is accentuated by the respiratory alkalosis caused by mechanical ventilatory devices (Flemma and Young, 1964). Urinary loss of potassium continues after operation and often a further shift of potassium into the cells occurs with the improvement in hemodynamics that results (Ebert et al., 1965). This reduction in potassium affects cardiac output primarily because of the cardiac arrhythmias that ensue, which will be subsequently analyzed in detail. In an effort to avoid the complications of a postoperative depression of body stores of potassium, use of digitalis and potassium-losing diuretics is discontinued several days before operation, and potassium supplements are given orally even though serum levels are normal. Sufficient potassium is added to the perfusate to keep the concentration in a physiologic range, and supplemental potassium is given intravenously after operation as indicated. There may be some advantage to administering potassium together with glu-cose and insulin to facilitate its entry into the cell (Moffitt et al., submitted for publication).

The extracellular concentrations of calcium and magnesium have been shown to have a mutually antagonistic effect on myocardial contractility. Guilbault and colleagues (1965) demonstrated that an increased magnesium concentration associated with a low calcium concentration decreases myocardial tonus, whereas the reverse improves contractility. There is also experimental evidence that increased concentrations of calcium improve myocardial function (Vasko and Tapper, 1967). The use of large amounts of citrated blood may cause a decrease in serum calcium and in cardiac output (Carson et al., 1964). Systemic administration of calcium as calcium chloride or calcium gluconate is advisable when multiple transfusions of ACD blood are required postoperatively.

CARDIAC RATE AND RHYTHM ABNORMALITIES

Many arrhythmias adversely affect cardiac output, and a depressed cardiac output predisposes to the development of rhythm disturbances. The entire subject of cardiac arrhythmias and their management will be discussed at length in the section on cardiac arrhythmias.

MYOCARDIAL DYSFUNCTION

Only when every other possible cause of low cardiac output has been excluded or has been effectively treated without benefit should it be assumed that myocardial dysfunction exists. There are many reasons for myocardial dysfunction after open-heart operations. Patients with a history of acquired valvular heart disease of long standing may have a damaged myocardium; this seems to be particularly true of patients with mitral valve and multivalvular heart disease. Associated coronary artery disease has already been mentioned as a possible cause of a damaged myocardium and suboptimal myocardial function.

Even more important, because they are controllable, are the occasions during operation when the myocardium may be injured. Proper protection of the myocardium is important during operation not only to avoid unnecessary cardiac trauma but also to maintain adequate myocardial oxygenation. Although cardiac anoxia is well tolerated for short periods, myocardial function does deteriorate progressively with the duration of anoxia (Sato et al., 1967; Enright et al., 1968; Bolooki et al., 1968). Continuous myocardial perfusion provides the best protection for the heart (Poulias et al., 1965). We have attempted to minimize myocardial ischemia by avoiding it altogether whenever possible and by cooling the perfusate to 30° C. with limitation of the period of aortic cross-clamping to 15 to 20 minutes (Greenberg and Edmunds, 1961). Coronary perfusion is restored and the heart is allowed to recover for 3 to 5 minutes before subjecting it to additional periods of ischemia.

Coronary air embolism is always a potential hazard of operations on the left side of the heart, and its development must be carefully guarded against because it too can seriously impair myocardial contractility (Goldfarb and Bahnson, 1963). Since the right coronary artery is uppermost, it is usually the right ventricle, atrioventricular node, and conduction mechanism that are affected. This is particularly deleterious to the patient with increased pulmonary vascular resistance. A variety of other possible causes of impaired coronary artery blood flow have been suggested, such as antifoam, calcific emboli, fat emboli, and platelet and thrombi aggregates. There is pathologic evidence to support these theories of impaired myocardial circulation during bypass surgery as evidenced by the postmortem demonstration of scattered areas of myocardial necrosis (Morales et al., 1967; Hensen et al., 1969). Although the cause of these changes is uncertain, their scattered distribution and localization to the subendocardial areas clearly suggest some impairment of myocardial perfusion.

Ventricular fibrillation has been employed for a number of years to facilitate operations on the heart, but it too is not without potential hazards. When it is maintained by a constant alternating-current stimulation, it produces immediate and significant deleterious effects on cardiac performance (Reis et al., 1967). Prolonged ventricular fibrillation is known to produce subendocardial infarction in calves (Ghidoni et al., 1969) and is suspected, with or without

an electric current, of producing similar lesions in humans (Najafi et al., 1969). If ventricular fibrillation is induced to facilitate valve replacement or avoidance of air embolism, the fibrillating current should be discontinued after a few minutes, at which time most adult hearts will remain in ventricular fibrillation; the total duration of fibrillation should ideally be kept at a minimum.

Although the various causes that may be responsible for postoperative impairment of myocardial function suggest many prophylactic measures that may be employed during operation, nevertheless an occasional patient exhibits a low cardiac output without obvious cause. Management of these patients is often difficult, and the problem may be insurmountable. Treatment involves support of the myocardium and correction of peripheral vasoconstriction, which impairs perfusion of vital organs.

Digitalis is one of the first pharmacologic agents employed when a lowered cardiac output is thought to be related to myocardial factors. We prefer digoxin (Lanoxin) because of its rapid mode of action and relatively rapid excretion. The parenteral digitalizing dose is estimated on the basis of 0.9 mg. of digoxin per square meter of body surface (1.0 to 1.5 mg. for an adult); half this amount is given initially. One-half of the remaining dose is given orally, intramuscularly, or intravenously in two to three hours and half of the remainder in another few hours according to the response of the heart and under careful electrocardiographic control. Since sudden death has been noted shortly after intravenous administration of additional digoxin when the patient is close to complete digitalization, the oral or intramuscular route is preferred for supplemental doses, particularly in labile postoperative patients. Digoxin given intravenously reaches a maximal effect in three hours, and approximately half the injected dose remains at the end of 24 hours (Kay, 1955). It must be remembered that potassium-depleted patients require less digitalis than normal individuals because they are more sensitive to it.

The maintenance dose of digoxin is roughly one-eighth of the estimated digitalizing dose given twice daily. For patients previously digitalized, adequate blood levels of the drug are reestablished by the cautious administration of 0.125 to 0.25 mg. of digoxin at intervals of two to three hours.

If a digitalis drug alone is ineffective in raising cardiac output, if it is contraindicated, of if a prompt increase in cardiac output is urgent, the beta-adrenergic agent isoproterenol (Isuprel) is preferred because of its combined inotropic effect on the heart and its peripheral vasodilating action. One usually gives it as a continuous intravenous infusion, adjusting the rate of administration to the observed effects and maintaining a systolic pressure of at least 90 to 100 mm. Hg. One milligram in 250 ml. of 5 per cent aqueous solution of glucose gives a concentration of 4.0 μg./ml. With a microdrip administration set, 5 to 15 drops per min. (0.4 to 1.2 μg.) are given according to the response of the heart. An adjustable constant-delivery pump greatly facilitates accurate administration of this potent agent. Toxic effects include tachycardia and premature ventricular contractions.

Some patients who do not improve with isoproterenol therapy will respond favorably to an infusion of epinephrine, 4 mg. in 250 ml. of 5 per cent aqueous solution of glucose. Some patients show less tendency to develop a serious tachycardia after epinephrine than after isoproterenol therapy. In larger doses, the effects of this drug are less cardiotonic and more vasoconstrictive with the result that tissue perfusion is impaired and the myocardium is overburdened (Coffin et al., 1966).

Emphasis has rightly been placed on the need for reversing the peripheral vasoconstriction that occurs as a compensatory response in patients with severe depression of cardiac output. Isoproterenol is an excellent drug for this purpose, as it also has a positive inotropic effect. Trimethaphan (Arfonad) and phenoxybenzamine (Dibenzyline) have also been used. We have had little experience with the last two drugs, but some investigators stress the beneficial effects of the combined use of phenoxybenzamine and massive doses of corticosteroids (Dietzman et al., 1969).

Glucagon has recently been introduced as a drug capable of improving cardiac function in some patients without the danger of arrhythmias that accompany the administration of isoproterenol (Parmley et al., 1969). It is administered intravenously in a dose of 3 to 5 mg. per hour. Other more drastic measures have occasionally been employed, including the use of assisted circulation (Spencer et al., 1965) and hyperbaric oxygen therapy (Yacoub and Zeitlin, 1965). We have relied primarily on digitalis and isoproterenol to support the myocardium, avoidance of vasodilating agents in the presence of hypotension, reduction of the body's oxygen demands and treatment of respiratory acidosis by artificial ventilation, and correction of metabolic acidosis by the administration of sodium bicarbonate.

CARDIAC ARRHYTHMIAS

Arrhythmias constitute one of the most frequently encountered complications in open-heart surgery. All patients can be found, on close monitoring of the electrocardiogram, to have some alterations of cardiac rhythm during and after operation. These may be transient or sustained and range from minor aberrations such as sinus tachycardia and isolated ventricular premature beats to such life-threatening arrhythmias as ventricular tachycardia and fibrillation. The ultimate outcome of the operation in many instances depends on prompt recognition and successful treatment of serious or potentially serious arrhythmias as they develop. Every cardiac surgeon has at some time had the distressing experience of having a patient do well initially, only to lose him subsequently from an uncontrolled disturbance of rhythm. Fortunately, most arrhythmias can now be prevented or controlled by discontinuing the administration of digitalis and other cardiac drugs prior to operation, proper protection of the myocardium during the procedure, and postoperative use of appropriate drugs and electronic pacing devices.

Arrhythmias exert their deleterious effect primarily through a reduction in cardiac output. Slow heart rates decrease total cardiac output even though the heart can partially compensate by an increase in stroke volume. Although normal individuals may do well at heart rates as slow as 60 beats per minute, a rate of 80 beats or more per minute has been found optimal for postoperative cardiac patients. Fast rhythms also decrease cardiac output, primarily by shortening the diastolic filling period and reducing stroke volume. This is particularly important with disk or ball-valve prostheses, as the inertia of the disk or ball becomes a limiting factor at cardiac rates of more than 100 to 110 beats per minute.

Arrhythmia-induced loss of proper synchronization of atrial and ventricular systole as provided in normal sinus rhythm also decreases cardiac output. Studies in normal subjects whose right atrium and right ventricle were paced with a bipolar catheter have shown that levels of cardiac output, aortic pressure, and maximal rate of pressure development in the aorta (dp/dt) are 5 to 15 per cent higher during atrial pacing than during ventricular pacing at identical pacing rates (Benchimol, 1969). However, in patients with heart disease the contribution of atrial systole appears to be of greater significance. In these cases, atrial pacing may give levels of cardiac output that are as much as 20 to 30 per cent higher than those obtained at equivalent rates of ventricular pacing (Benchimol, 1969). These increases can be of critical importance for patients with low cardiac output.

Essential to the prompt treatment of postoperative arrhythmias is their prompt recognition; as mentioned previously, continuous oscilloscopic monitoring of the electrocardiogram is a necessity in the first few postoperative days. Facilities should be available for running electrocardiographic "rhythm strips" when closer study of the cardiac mechanism is desired. Additional refinements that facilitate the management of arrhythmias include the availability of esophageal leads, automatic alarm systems, playback tapes, and remote and telemetry monitoring for ambulatory patients.

Numerous factors are known to be important in the production of postoperative arrhythmias. Clinical experience has shown that hearts with gross myocardial hypertrophy are more prone to develop rhythm disturbances, particularly those related to ventricular irritability. Preoperative arrhythmias such as ventricular premature beats and paroxysmal supraventricular tachycardias are usually present postoperatively as well, often with increased frequency. Advanced myocardial failure predisposes to the development of the low-cardiac-output syndrome, and this increases the likelihood of rhythm disturbances. Coronary artery disease often contributes to arrhythmias, and occasionally the sudden appearance of

a postoperative arrhythmia is the only indication of a "silent" myocardial infarction. Arrhythmias may also be precipitated by such diverse agents as pulmonary emboli, narcotics (Buckley and Jackson, 1961), and the negative phase of artificial ventilation (Pace-Floridia and Galindo, 1968). Knowledge of the preoperative electrocardiogram is important for interpretation of the postoperative tracings, particularly in the presence of atrioventricular conduction disturbances and prior myocardial injury.

Local factors that contribute to postoperative arrhythmias are usually related to cardiac trauma with resultant edema and hemorrhage, particularly when the trauma involves the specialized atrial and atrioventricular conduction systems. Cardiac prostheses, especially mitral and tricuspid caged valves, may stimulate premature ventricular contractions by mechanical impingement on the septum or lateral ventricular wall. Avoidance of oversized prostheses and proper seating of the valves will prevent this complication. Proper protection of the myocardium during the operation and avoidance of prolonged ventricular fibrillation are important for the prevention of arrhythmias as well as for the prevention of the low-output syndrome. These aspects have been discussed in a preceding section.

The profound systemic alterations produced by thoracotomy and cardiopulmonary bypass are also responsible for many postoperative arrhythmias. Hypotension, hypercarbia, hypoxia, fever, hypovolemia, and hypervolemia may all trigger rhythm disturbances. Both acidosis and alkalosis are known to produce alterations in cardiac rhythm and function. Specific predisposing conditions such as atelectasis, respiratory obstruction, hypoventilation, and pneumothorax must be assiduously avoided if possible and vigorously treated when they do occur. For these reasons we have employed assisted ventilation via an endotracheal tube in all patients who are having rhythm problems or low cardiac output postoperatively, particularly those with mitral and multiple valve replacements. The tube may be left in overnight or for several days, depending on the response of the patient. Arterial pH, Po_2, and Pco_2 should be monitored periodically, as arrhythmias caused by abnormalities in these variables often cannot be controlled until normal physiologic values are restored.

One of the most important sources of serious ventricular arrhythmias is hypokalemia, particularly in patients receiving digitalis and diuretics. The prevention of this abnormality has been discussed in detail previously, and the treatment is outlined in the following section.

High levels of catecholamines may be present during and after cardiac operation (Indeglia et al., 1966; Alexander et al., 1969). Their significance in the production of cardiac arrhythmias is unknown, but the effectiveness of propranolol (Inderal), a beta-adrenergic blocking agent, in the treatment of postoperative arrhythmias may be related in part to its ability to antagonize the effects of catecholamines on the heart.

Because many postoperative arrhythmias are related to slow ventricular rates, temporary pacemaker electrodes are being placed prophylactically in an increasing number of patients at the time of operation, particularly those with ectopic foci, slow or unstable rhythms, and mitral or multiple valve replacements. If atrial fibrillation is not present and atrioventricular conduction is intact, one epicardial electrode is placed on the wall of the right atrium and the indifferent electrode is placed in the mediastinal tissues, thus providing for normal atrioventricular synchrony. For other arrhythmias, two wires are placed in the anterior wall of the right ventricle. The distal ends of the electrode wires are led out through the skin lateral to the incision, and an external battery-powered demand pacemaker is activated as needed.

Postoperative pacing is optimally suited for the treatment of bradycardia and advanced degrees of heart block, especially when complicated by ventricular premature beats or bouts of ventricular tachycardia.

Many times the ectopic foci will be suppressed when a satisfactory pacing rate is achieved. If not, antiarrhythmic agents may be used safely without concern that they will extinguish the patient's own pacemaker. Other investigational techniques undergoing clinical trial for suppression of recurrent tachycardias are rapid intracardiac pacing (DeSanctis and Kastor, 1968; Lister et al., 1968), coupled pacing (McNally and Benchimol, 1968b), and paired pacing (McNally and Benchimol, 1968b).

DRUGS USEFUL FOR THE TREATMENT OF POSTOPERATIVE ARRHYTHMIAS

DIGITALIS PREPARATIONS

The cardiovascular effects of digitalis are well known and include a positive inotropic action, depression of atrioventricular conduction, and increased venous tone. For rapid digitalization, slow intravenous administration of digoxin is preferred. Dosage schedules and precautions are described in a preceding section.

ANTIARRHYTHMIC AGENTS

In addition to digitalis, four principal agents are currently used to control postoperative cardiac arrhythmias (Table 27-2): lidocaine (Xylocaine), diphenylhydantoin (Dilantin), quinidine, and procainamide (Pronestyl). All four drugs have a tertiary nitrogen group in the chemical structure, which is thought to be related to their antiarrhythmic properties. All of them depress myocardial conduction, prolong the refractory period, and elevate the threshold of cellular excitability. Further, all have a myocardial depressant effect in

TABLE 27-2. Dosage of Antiarrhythmic Agents for Postoperative Cardiac Patients

Agent	Intravenous Route		Oral Route
	Administration	Usual Adult Dose	
Lidocaine	1.0 mg./kg.	50 to 100 mg.	
Diphenylhydantoin	2 to 4 mg./kg.	100 to 250 mg.	100 mg. q.i.d.
Quinidine			200 mg. q.i.d.
Procainamide			250 to 500 mg. q.i.d.
Propranolol	1-mg. doses	1 to 5 mg.	10 to 20 mg. q.i.d.
Potassium	Slow infusion	40 mEq.	45 to 135 mEq./day

large doses and a peripheral vasodilating effect at all dosage levels. In the postoperative cardiac patient, lidocaine and diphenylhydantoin are preferred when intravenous therapy is necessary because they have a relatively short duration of action and produce less hypotension than equivalent doses of quinidine and procainamide. Quinidine and procainamide are employed primarily in the management of chronic arrhythmias.

In the intact human, lidocaine appears to have a minimal effect on myocardial contraction and arterial pressure at low dosage levels (Harrison et al., 1963). However, studies in which the myocardial circulation is separated from the systemic circulation (Austen and Moran, 1965) show that this agent depresses contractile force and cardiac output at all dosage levels. A suggested explanation for the variations in these findings is that endogenous epinephrine may be potentiated by lidocaine at low dosage levels (Austen and Moran, 1965).

For seriously hypotensive patients, vasopressors should be administered concomitantly with the antiarrhythmic agent in order to avoid potentiation of the hypotension. All of the above antiarrhythmic agents should be avoided in the presence of bradycardia or advanced degrees of heart block, unless the cardiac rate is maintained with temporary electrical pacing or isoproterenol given intravenously. All agents can also cause cardiorespiratory arrest if administered too rapidly or in excessive amounts.

Lidocaine is the drug of choice for rapid control of ventricular arrhythmias ranging from frequent premature beats to ventricular tachycardia. It is only occasionally effective in atrial arrhythmias. The intravenous dose is 1 mg./kg. of body weight, usually given as a single bolus in the amount of 50 to 100 mg. for an average adult. An effect is usually noted within minutes and lasts less than 20 minutes. Because of this short action, a single dose is usually followed by a continuous intravenous drip prepared by placing 1000 mg. of lidocaine in 250 ml. of 5 per cent aqueous solution of glucose (resulting concentration 4 mg./ml.). A microdrip administration set running at approximately 12 drops per minute delivers 1 mg./min. This rate is usually effective but may be safely increased twofold or

threefold if necessary. Administration is facilitated by the use of an adjustable constant-delivery pump, which avoids the difficulties of fluctuations in administration rate caused by changes in position of the patient, the intravenous catheter, or the drip-rate control. Minor side effects include muscular twitching, visual disturbances, and dizziness. Major side effects include hypotension, bradycardia, central-nervous-system depression or excitement, and convulsions.

Diphenylhydantoin has been found effective in various arrhythmias, particularly digitalis-induced ventricular premature beats and supraventricular tachycardias. For intravenous administration, 2 to 4 mg./kg. is given slowly over a period of five minutes. An average dose for postoperative patients is 100 mg., although doses up to 250 mg. may be given cautiously if needed. The effect lasts 10 to 40 minutes (Bigger et al., 1968), and the dose must be repeated intravenously or orally as needed. After oral administration the drug effect peaks in eight hours; the usual dose is 100 mg. given four times daily. Because it may take up to one week to attain an optimal blood level on oral therapy alone, large loading doses (approximately 1000 mg. per day) may be given to establish adequate blood levels more promptly (Bigger et al., 1968). Adverse effects, related to rapid administration and large doses, include decrease in myocardial contractility, increase in atrioventricular block, and cardiorespiratory arrest. Blood dyscrasias, central-nervous-system abnormalities, skin rashes, and gingival hyperplasia may occur with long-term therapy.

Quinidine sulfate is most useful in the management of chronic arrhythmias. The usual dose is 200 mg. given orally every six hours, but some patients may require up to 1600 mg. daily. Gastrointestinal symptoms are common, and some individuals are sensitive to amounts as small as 400 mg. per day. Diarrhea may be controlled by lowering the quinidine dose or by giving 5-mg. doses of diphenoxylate hydrochloride (Lomotil) orally. Toxic effects include hypotension, tinnitus, electrocardiographic changes with widening of the QRS complex, and ventricular fibrillation.

Procainamide is another agent useful in the management of chronic arrhythmias, particularly in patients who cannot take quinidine. The usual dose is 250 to 500 mg. given orally every six hours.

One of the newest drugs for the management of cardiac arrhythmias is propranolol (Krasnow and Barbarosh, 1968; Theilen and Wilson, 1968). This agent's potent beta-adrenergic blocking ability is not possessed by the other antiarrhythmic agents, but it is not certain that this is the mechanism responsible for its action (Cooper and Priola, 1968). Propranolol is particularly useful in digitalis intoxication that presents as paroxysmal atrial tachycardia with block, ventricular premature beats, or ventricular tachycardia. It is also useful for slowing ventricular rates in patients with atrial tachyarrhythmia when digitalis and quinidine are not effective, and it has been used successfully to manage recurring ventricular fibrillation when all other agents have failed (Rothfeld et al., 1968). One milligram may be given intravenously and the dose repeated every 15 minutes for several doses until an effect is noted or until a total of 0.1 mg./kg. has been given. As the duration of action is short (one to three hours), oral administration is started with doses of 10 to 20 mg. given every six hours. Side effects include bradycardia (which can be reversed with atropine), increase in atrioventricular block, and hypotension. Congestive heart failure may be precipitated in patients with borderline myocardial function. The drug is contraindicated in patients with bronchial asthma, in diabetics because it masks insulin reaction, and in patients who are taking reserpine or monoamine oxidase inhibitors.

Intravenously administered potassium is often required to control the common problem of postperfusion hypokalemia and its associated arrhythmias. Even if serum levels of potassium are normal or low-normal, intracellular potassium and total body potassium may be depleted. Administration of supplemental potassium in these circumstances has been found helpful in abolishing frequent premature ventricular contractions and other signs of ventricular irritability, particularly in patients who have been receiving digitalis glycosides. A solution of 40 mEq. of potassium chloride in 100 ml. of 5 per cent aqueous solution of glucose may be given over a two-hour period. This may be repeated one or two times as needed.

It is important to establish that the patient has adequate renal function before supplemental potassium is administered. Potassium excess produces characteristic changes in the electrocardiogram including an increase in amplitude of the T waves, depression of the ST segment, prolongation of the PR interval, decrease in amplitude of the P wave, and widening of the QRS complex. Appearance of these changes dictates cessation of potassium therapy in order to prevent a fatal arrhythmia or asystole. Administration of potassium in the form of elixirs should be begun as soon as oral intake is possible, if continued potassium supplementation is required.

Isoproterenol, exceptionally useful because of its positive chronotropic and inotropic effects and its peripheral vasodilating action, is employed extensively to augment cardiac output and to control arrhythmias associated with bradycardia. This agent may also be used in the emergency treatment of postoperative atrioventricular block until electrical pacing can be instituted. Dosage and administration have been discussed in a preceding section.

Atropine sulfate may be given intravenously or intramuscularly in a dose of 0.5 to 1.0 mg. to suppress excess vagal tone, as either a diagnostic or a therapeutic measure. Glaucoma is a contraindication to its use.

DIRECT-CURRENT COUNTERSHOCK

Cardioversion (direct-current countershock timed with the QRS complex) is useful for the treatment of atrial flutter and other regular supraventricular tachycardias, particularly when these arrhythmias are accompanied by hypotension, thus making it unwise to wait for drug conversion. Atrial fibrillation is usually treated acutely by control of the ventricular rate with digitalis glycosides, but cardioversion is often attempted at a later date when the patient has recovered from operation and all predisposing causes have been corrected. Countershock is used routinely for conversion of ventricular tachycardia and ventricular fibrillation.

Cardioversion is contraindicated for digitalis-induced arrhythmias. Electric discharge is generally ineffective in restoring a normal sinus mechanism, and it may provoke serious or even lethal disorders of the heartbeat (Kleiger and Lown, 1966). The only exception is ventricular fibrillation, when defibrillation is mandatory; success may be achieved if it is employed in conjunction with antiarrhythmic drugs such as lidocaine or diphenylhydantoin.

Cardioversion is relatively atraumatic to the heart, and myocardial enzymes are not released by usual doses of current (Konttinen et al., 1969). Numerous patients are now alive who have received multiple countershocks prior to control of their arrhythmias. It is important to remember that digitalis toxicity may become evident with the conversion of atrial flutter or fibrillation to normal sinus rhythm, and it is therefore desirable to discontinue administration of digitalis glycosides at least 24 hours prior to elective cardioversion (Kleiger and Lown, 1966).

SPECIFIC ARRHYTHMIAS

Therapeutically, postoperative arrhythmias may be arbitrarily divided into three groups: tachycardias, bradycardias, and arrhythmias with normal rates. Each group may be subdivided according to whether the pulse is regular or irregular.

POSTOPERATIVE TACHYCARDIAS

Regular Pulse

Sinus tachycardia, arbitrarily defined as sinus rhythm with a rate of more than 100 per minute, is a usual concomitant of cardiovascular surgery and represents a normal response to fever, trauma, and pain. The rate is generally less than 160 per minute and may vary slightly with respiration. Carotid sinus massage and other measures that increase vagal tone characteristically slow the rate gradually. Other than recognition of this arrhythmia and treatment of any abnormalities that may be contributing to it, no specific therapy is indicated.

Paroxysmal atrial tachycardia and *paroxysmal nodal tachycardia* may be discussed together, since they are clinically indistinguishable and differentiation may not be possible even with an electrocardiogram. The term *"paroxysmal supraventricular tachycardia"* is used to designate either variety. They are characterized by sudden onset and termination, either spontaneously or by measures that augment vagal tone. There often is a history of previous episodes. A special form is associated with accessory atrioventricular conduction (Wolff-Parkinson-White syndrome).

The electrocardiogram demonstrates normal QRS complexes, but the P waves are altered or absent. The base line between P waves is isoelectric, as opposed to the typical sawtooth appearance of atrial flutter. The atrial rate is usually between 160 and 220 per minute, and the ventricles typically contract in a 1:1 ratio with the atria.

Treatment should begin with maneuvers to increase vagal tone, and these alone may be successful. Carotid sinus massage, the Valsalva maneuver, and pharyngeal stimulation with a catheter produce either no effect or a sudden cessation of the arrhythmia. Intramuscular administration of 0.5 to 1.0 mg. of neostigmine (Prostigmin) may be effective, especially if combined with vagal maneuvers 15 minutes after the injection.

Another useful technique employing vagal reflexes is the elevation of systolic blood pressure by intravenous administration of vasopressors. Methoxamine (Vasoxyl), 10 mg., or phenylephrine hydrochloride (Neo-Synephrine), 5 mg., may be diluted in 100 ml. of 5 per cent aqueous solution of glucose and infused rapidly intravenously until the systolic blood pressure reaches 180 mm. Hg.

If reflex maneuvers are not successful in abolishing paroxysmal supraventricular tachycardia, rapid digitalization should be instituted. A careful history should be taken for prior digitalis administration, however, as this arrhythmia may result from digitalis toxicity, discussed in the next paragraph. Reflex maneuvers may then be repeated with an increased probability of success, since vagal tone is augmented by digitalis. Alternate methods of treatment include cardioversion, particularly if the arrhythmia is poorly tolerated and immediate control is necessary, and intravenous administration of propranolol or diphenylhydantoin, if the arrhythmia is due to digitalis toxicity. Quinidine or procainamide given orally is useful as a prophylaxis for recurrent episodes.

Supraventricular tachycardia may be a serious manifestation of digitalis intoxication, especially when accompanied by partial atrioventricular block, and this possibility must be considered whenever this arrhythmia occurs in any patient receiving digitalis. Digitalis toxicity should also be suspected when, in patients with atrial fibrillation, the rhythm becomes regular and progressively rapid as digitalis administration is augmented or as potassium depletion develops. The ventricular rate is often slower than in nondigitalis-induced supraventricular tachycardia, ranging between 70 and 150 per minute. Carotid sinus massage may slow the ventricular rate variably, as opposed to ordinary supraventricular tachycardia. Treatment consists of withholding digitalis, administration of potassium, especially if serum levels are low, and use of propranolol or diphenylhydantoin.

Atrial flutter is one of the more common postoperative arrhythmias, particularly in patients who have undergone mitral valve replacement and in those with pulmonary complications. The sudden appearance of a regular ventricular rate of 150 per minute may be considered atrial flutter until proven otherwise. The electrocardiogram reveals an atrial rate of approximately 300 per minute (range 230 to 360) and, with the usual 2:1 atrioventricular block, a ventricular rate of 150 per minute. There is a typical sawtooth appearance of the base line, which may be nicely demonstrated by increasing the atrioventricular block to 3:1 (ventricular rate 100) or 4:1 (ventricular rate 75) by measures that augment vagal tone. These changes in rate are abrupt and transient and are characteristic for atrial flutter. This arrhythmia is closely related to atrial fibrillation, and patients may shift back and forth between the two rhythms spontaneously or under the influence of drug therapy: flutter to fibrillation with digitalis, and the reverse with quinidine.

Digitalis, often combined with quinidine, is the primary drug used in the treatment of atrial flutter. In addition to its positive inotropic action, digitalis is of value by virtue of its complex effects on atrioventricular conduction, cardiac excitability, and the atrial refractory period. With increasing doses of digitalis, a 2:1 block may be increased to a 3:1 or 4:1 block, but this change is often unstable and difficult to maintain. Occasionally, conversion to normal sinus rhythm occurs directly, but much more often atrial fibrillation supervenes. Conversion of atrial flutter with a

2:1 block to a more favorable rhythm may require large doses of digitalis, bordering on toxic levels. For this reason, cardioversion is now the treatment of choice for atrial flutter in postoperative cardiac patients. The success rate for cardioversion is high and the results are immediate.

Ventricular tachycardia is a serious rhythm disturbance that is nearly always associated with profound hypotension in the postoperative patient. The rate ordinarily is between 140 and 180 per minute, although it may range up to 250 per minute, and it usually progresses rapidly to ventricular fibrillation. It may be preceded by ventricular premature beats, particularly when they are multifocal or occur in runs of two or more. Ventricular tachycardia differs from other types of rapid heart action in having slight beat-to-beat variations (0.01 to 0.03 second) and changes in average rate during an attack or in different attacks in the same individual. The electrocardiogram reveals wide QRS complexes (0.12 second or more) with slight variations in beat-to-beat contour as well as rate. A considerable change in QRS pattern may develop if the attack persists. It is often difficult to differentiate ventricular tachycardia from supraventricular tachycardia with aberrant ventricular conduction. The diagnosis is established if random P waves can be identified or if typical capture beats and fusion beats are seen. More rarely, regular P waves are present when the atria are activated by retrograde impulses. Esophageal leads are particularly useful for detecting P-wave activity in this arrhythmia. A variable first heart sound and irregular cannon waves in the jugular pulse may be identified when atrial activity is dissociated from ventricular depolarization. Carotid sinus massage has no effect.

Digitalis toxicity may be a contributing or precipitating factor, and this arrhythmia can be a toxic manifestation of quinidine or procainamide therapy. Directional reversal of the QRS in alternating complexes (bidirectional alternating tachycardia) carries an especially unfavorable prognosis and particularly suggests digitalis toxicity.

Treatment consists of immediate intravenous administration of lidocaine; if a prompt response is not obtained, cardioversion is performed without delay. When ventricular tachycardia complicates preexisting atrioventricular block, control with lidocaine often results in ventricular arrest. Temporary electrical pacing is then essential for optimal management. When digitalis excess has been a precipitating factor, intravenously administered diphenylhydantoin or potassium, or both, may be effective. Persistently recurring ventricular tachycardia and fibrillation pose an especially difficult problem in management. Propranolol has been used in some cases with success after other antiarrhythmic drugs have failed (Rothfeld et al., 1968). In one of our nonsurgical patients, recurrent bouts of ventricular tachycardia and fibrillation were successfully managed by suppressive electrical pacing combined with propranolol therapy (McCallister et al., unpublished data).

Irregular Pulse

Atrial fibrillation is the most common major arrhythmia occurring after open-heart surgery. Cardiac output is reduced by two mechanisms: (1) loss of atrial contribution to ventricular systole and, of greater importance, (2) inefficient hemodynamics produced by fast ventricular rates.

Atrial fibrillation is characterized by an irregularly irregular rhythm with a pulse deficit when beats recorded at the wrist are compared with audible beats at the cardiac apex. The usual ventricular response in untreated patients is between 90 and 160 beats per minute, but the rate may be much higher in the postoperative patient, particularly when fever and pulmonary complications are present. Vagal stimulation may slow the ventricular rate moderately and transiently.

The basis for diagnosis by electrocardiography is usually straightforward: fibrillation waves varying in amplitude and configuration and having a frequency of 300 to 600 per minute with an irregular ventricular response. At times, when aberrant ventricular conduction (functional bundle-branch block) is present, it may be difficult to distinguish aberrant QRS complexes from ventricular premature beats. Marriott and Sandler (1966) have presented criteria that help distinguish these arrhythmias.

Treatment is with digitalis glycosides, which slow the ventricular rate by direct and vagal influences on the refractory period of the atrioventricular conduction

tissues. The dose and route of administration are governed by the urgency of the situation. Occasionally, when control of the ventricular rate and regression of the precipitating causes are achieved, normal sinus rhythm may spontaneously reappear. Addition of oral quinidine to maintenance digitalis therapy may facilitate this conversion. If atrial fibrillation develops after operation in a patient who was in sinus rhythm preoperatively, drug or electrical cardioversion should be attempted before dismissal from the hospital.

Most patients with mitral and multivalvular disease have been in atrial fibrillation for varying periods prior to operation. If the duration has been relatively short, perhaps less than one year, it has been our practice to attempt to establish a normal sinus mechanism at the conclusion of the operation before closure of the chest. Maintenance doses of digitalis (usually 0.125 mg. twice daily) are begun on the day after operation. The patient will often remain in sinus rhythm for 24 to 48 hours but usually resumes atrial fibrillation as fever and pulmonary problems reach a maximum. This brief interval of sinus rhythm is nevertheless beneficial, as it provides up to 30 per cent increased cardiac output (Benchimol, 1969) when it is needed most in the first hours after operation. Quinidine is often added to the digitalis therapy, and the patient is dismissed from the hospital on this regimen. If he still has atrial fibrillation three months later when all effects of the operation are past, cardioversion is considered advisable to improve hemodynamics and decrease the probability of embolism. The long-term success of cardioversion is related to the preoperative duration of atrial fibrillation and to the functional class of the patient (Morris et al., 1966; Futral and McGuire, 1967). Prophylactic anticoagulant therapy decreases the risk of embolism with cardioversion, particularly in patients with a history of previous embolic episodes (Bjerkelund and Orning, 1969).

Atrial premature beats may produce a rapid irregular rhythm if they are superimposed on sinus tachycardia or other rapid regular arrhythmias. The significance of atrial premature beats lies mainly in their prognostication of possible atrial fibrillation or other atrial tachyarrhythmias. They require no treatment other than perhaps prophylactic digitalization.

Ventricular premature beats constitute the most common disorder of rhythm and are almost invariably seen to some degree in all postoperative cardiac patients. They may be completely benign or they may be a warning sign of myocardial distress. Sporadic, late-coupled premature beats are innocuous and do not require treatment. On the other hand, premature beats increase in clinical significance as they become more frequent, if they have variable coupling, if they occur in runs of two or more, if they are multifocal, or if they fall on the preceding T wave. These findings are ominous and warn of impending ventricular tachycardia or fibrillation. Digitalis toxicity, especially in the presence of hypokalemia, should always be considered a possible cause, particularly when a ventricular premature beat follows each normal beat, producing bigeminy.

Treatment of ventricular premature beats is usually indicated when they are more frequent than 5 to 6 per minute or have the characteristics described above. The first step is to ensure that serum potassium levels are in the normal range. A trial of intravenously administered potassium is often effective, particularly in patients with depleted total body potassium, even if the serum levels are normal. An intravenous drip of lidocaine is then administered at a rate sufficient to control the premature beats. All of the general factors mentioned earlier that influence myocardial irritability should be checked and corrected if abnormal. In particular, blood pH, P_{O_2}, and P_{CO_2} should be measured.

Atrial flutter with a varying degree of atrioventricular block presents as an irregular tachycardia. Therapy is the same as that discussed previously under atrial flutter.

Paroxysmal atrial tachycardia with some degree of atrioventricular block should be regarded as a manifestation of digitalis toxicity until proven otherwise, especially if the P-wave rate is less than 160 per minute. Therapy was considered previously under paroxysmal atrial tachycardia.

Atrioventricular dissociation of the rapid (or usurpation) type presents as a tachycardia that is irregular because of the characteristic capture beats. When it occurs postoperatively, this arrhythmia generally represents digitalis toxicity which is manifested as an enhancement of the automaticity of the atrioventricular node. If the patient has no retrograde atrioventricular conduction, rapid-type atrioventricular dissociation results; if he has retrograde conduction the rhythm becomes nodal tachycardia. Treatment is the same as for digitalis-induced supraventricular tachycardia. Detailed discussions of atrioventricular dissociation appear in the recent literature (Marriott and Menendez, 1966).

POSTOPERATIVE BRADYCARDIAS

Sinus bradycardia, defined as a sinus rhythm at a rate less than 60 per minute, is produced most commonly by a high degree of vagal tone. It may be drug-induced, particularly by digitalis and morphine, or may result from stimulation of vagal reflexes, as by gastric dilation and vomiting. Therapy consists of removing the precipitating factors and, when indicated for hemodynamic reasons, administration of atropine.

Marked slowing of the sinoatrial node or atrial arrest will usually result in an escape *atrioventricular nodal rhythm* at a rate of 40 to 70 per minute. As in sinus bradycardia, this rhythm may be caused by excess vagal tone, especially from digitalis; if so, it is treated accordingly. Nodal rhythm is also commonly encountered when extensive atrial surgery is performed, as in venous transposition (Mustard procedure) for transposition of the great vessels and when the mitral valve is exposed through incisions in the right atrium and atrial septum. The pathophysiology is probably related to trauma to the sinoatrial node and interruption of the internodal tracts (Merideth and Titus, 1968). Treatment is through acceleration of the nodal escape rate with isoproterenol, or by cardiac pacing.

Second-degree atrioventricular block, a more serious problem, may be arbitrarily divided into two types: (1) Wenckebach phenomenon, in which the PR interval is lengthened progressively for several beats until one P wave is not followed by ventricular depolarization (Mobitz type I), and (2) failure of atrioventricular conduction so that only every second (or third or fourth) impulse from the atria is conducted to the ventricles. The dropped beats usually occur in a regular manner resulting in a 2:1 (or 3:1 or 4:1) block (Mobitz type II). Both types of second-degree block may be caused by various drugs and circumstances including digitalis, quinidine, excess vagal tone, and inferior (posterior) myocardial infarction related to occlusion of the right coronary artery. A detailed discussion of the significance of various types of second-degree block is included in the review by McNally and Benchimol (1968a).

Cardiac output is affected when the ventricular rate falls below optimal levels. Normal individuals may tolerate a rate of 40 to 60 per minute well, but this rate is insufficient for postoperative cardiac patients. In addition, second-degree heart block, especially Mobitz type II, may suddenly convert to complete heart block or complete ventricular arrest. For these reasons, when this arrhythmia is present in postoperative cardiac patients, it is desirable to have a demand pacemaker in operation.

Complete (third-degree) atrioventricular block is present when the atrioventricular node and conduction system fail to conduct any impulses to the ventricles. There is no relation between the atrial and ventricular complexes, the first heart sound is variable, and irregular cannon waves are present in the jugular venous pulse. The form of the QRS may be normal if the ventricular focus is in the lower portion of the atrioventricular node or in the upper portion of the septum (bundle of His), but the QRS becomes widened and bizarre when the focus is below the bifurcation of the bundle.

Complete atrioventricular block may result from direct trauma during surgical repair of such lesions as ventricular septal defect and atrioventricular canal in which sutures must be placed near the conduction system. Heart block may also result from hemorrhage into the septum or from other indirect trauma during replacement of the mitral, tricuspid, or aortic valve. Some patients with calcification of the mitral or aortic valve have incomplete (or even complete) bundle-branch block present preoperatively, presumably from damage to the conduction system by calcific deposits. These patients are particularly vulnerable to the development of complete heart block postoperatively, even though no direct manipulations are made in the region of the conduction system.

For example, one patient at the time of operation temporarily developed complete heart block that would persist 5 to 10 minutes every time the apex of the heart was momentarily lifted out of the pericardial sac. At times, complete heart block is evident postoperatively without apparent cause. Fortunately, if direct trauma to the conduction system has not occurred, some type of supraventricular rhythm usually returns after a period of temporary pacing.

Complete heart block in the postoperative period is potentially lethal because of the inadequate rate (30 to 50 beats per minute) and because the idioventricular focus is often labile and vulnerable to drug-induced or spontaneous cessation of activity.

When complete heart block or other bradycardias described above are present at the conclusion of the intracardiac portion of the operation, they are treated by inserting electrode wires into the myocardium and then connecting them to a demand pacemaker as described previously. When complete heart block or serious bradycardia develops postoperatively and epicardial wires have not been previously inserted, an infusion of isoproterenol is started as an emergency measure to increase the idioventricular rate until electrical pacing can be established. We prefer to transfer the patient, whenever feasible, to an image intensifier where a temporary bipolar transvenous electrode is inserted into the apex of the right ventricle. For acute ventricular asystole, external pacing may be established as a temporary measure, or a percutaneous transthoracic pacemaker may be inserted for emergency treatment (McNally and Benchimol, 1968b). Bedside techniques for floating a pacemaker wire into the right ventricle have been employed by some (DeSanctis and Kastor, 1968), and others have used an esophageal electrode for pacing (McNally and Benchimol, 1968b), but we have had only limited experience with either method.

Other forms of bradycardia encountered postoperatively include atrioventricular dissociation of the slow (or default) type and sinoatrial block, both usually due to excess vagal tone, especially from digitalis. Digitalis toxicity in a patient with atrial fibrillation may be manifested as excessive slowing of the ventricular rate, often combined with nodal escape beats and isolated or coupled ventricular premature beats. If digitalis is increased (or serum potassium decreased), the rate may become more regular and rapid, signifying the development of paroxysmal nodal tachycardia, described previously, or ventricular tachycardia. These arrhythmias warn of impending ventricular fibrillation and demand urgent treatment, as previously outlined.

POSTOPERATIVE ARRHYTHMIAS WITH NORMAL RATES

There are many types of arrhythmias with normal rates. Those described in the following paragraphs are of particular significance in postoperative cardiac patients.

Right bundle-branch block is commonly seen after repair of ventricular septal defect, tetralogy of Fallot, atrioventricular canal, and other cardiac anomalies in which a right ventriculotomy is used or in which patches are sutured to the right side of the ventricular septum. This arrhythmia is of no consequence once it is identified and differentiated from possible ventricular arrhythmias. Preexisting bundle-branch block causes no greater operative risk than that of the underlying cardiac pathologic condition, although the incidence of postoperative complete heart block may be somewhat increased, as discussed previously.

First degree atrioventricular block suggests vagal effects but may represent digitalis toxicity; therapy is directed accordingly. The Wolff-Parkinson-White syndrome is often associated with paroxysmal supraventricular tachycardia, discussed previously. If this arrhythmia has been difficult to control preoperatively, consideration should be given to dividing the accessory conduction tissue (Sealy et al., 1969) at the time of cardiac operation.

Other arrhythmias with normal rates include *atrial premature beats*, which are of little consequence in themselves but may warn of an impending major atrial arrhythmia, described previously. *Ventricular premature beats* may be innocuous but can signify serious myocardial distress. Their significance and therapy were discussed previously. *Atrial fibrillation* with a normal ventricular rate may be present postoperatively. Even though the rate is normal, maintenance therapy with digoxin (0.125

mg. twice daily) is begun on the day after operation to prevent the sometimes rapid onset of an uncontrolled ventricular response.

REFERENCES

Alexander, R. W., Kuzela, L., Kerth, W. J., Harrison, J., and Gerbode, F.: Adrenal catecholamine and cortisol secretion during extracorporeal circulation in dogs. J. Thorac. Cardiov. Surg., 58:250, 1969.

Andersen, M. N., and Mouritzen, C.: Effect of acute respiratory and metabolic acidosis on cardiac output and peripheral resistance. Ann. Surg., 163:161, 1966.

Austen, W. G., and Moran, J. M.: Cardiac and peripheral vascular effects of lidocaine and procainamide. Amer. J. Cardiol., 16:701, 1965.

Barratt-Boyes, B. G., and Wood, E. H.: Cardiac output and related measurements and pressure values in the right heart and associated vessels, together with an analysis of the hemodynamic response to the inhalation of high oxygen mixtures in healthy subjects. J. Lab. Clin. Med., 51:72, 1958.

Benchimol, A.: Significance of the contribution of atrial systole to cardiac function in man. Amer. J. Cardiol., 23:568, 1969.

Berger, R. L., Boyd, T. F., and Marcus, P. S.: A pattern of blood-volume responses to open-heart surgery. New Eng. J. Med., 271:59, 1964.

Berglund, E.: Ventricular function. VI. Balance of left and right ventricular output: Relation between left and right atrial pressures. Amer. J. Physiol., 178:381, 1954.

Bigger, J. T., Jr., Schmidt, D. H., and Kutt, H.: Relationship between the plasma level of diphenylhydantoin sodium and its cardiac antiarrhythmic effects. Circulation, 38:363, 1968.

Bjerkelund, C. J., and Orning, O. M.: The efficacy of anticoagulant therapy in preventing embolism related to D.C. electrical conversion of atrial fibrillation. Amer. J. Cardiol., 23:208, 1969.

Bolooki, H., Rooks, J. J., Viera, C. E., Smith, B., Mobinudel, K., Lombardo, C. R., and Jude, J. R.: Comparison of the effect of temporary or permanent myocardial ischemia on cardiac function and pathology. J. Thorac. Cardiov. Surg., 56:590, 1968.

Buckley, J. J., and Jackson, J. A.: Postoperative cardiac arrhythmias. Anesthesiology, 22:723, 1961.

Carson, S. A. A., Morris, L. E., Edmark, K. W., Jones, T. W., Logan, G. A., Sauvage, L. R., and Thomas, G. I.: Acid-base management for open-heart surgery. Circulation, 29:456, 1964.

Cleland, J., Pluth, J. R., Tauxe, W. N., and Kirklin, J. W.: Blood volume and body fluid compartment changes soon after closed and open intracardiac surgery. J. Thorac. Cardiov. Surg., 52:698, 1966.

Clowes, G. H. A., Jr.: Acid-base balance during and after cardiopulmonary bypass procedures. Amer. J. Cardiol., 12:671, 1963.

Clowes, G. H. A., Jr., Alichniewicz, A., Del Guercio, L. R. M., and Gillespie, D.: The relationship of postoperative acidosis to pulmonary and cardiovascular function. J. Thorac. Cardiov. Surg., 39:1, 1960.

Coffin, L. H., Jr., Ankeney, J. L., and Beheler, E. M.: Experimental study and clinical use of epinephrine for treatment of low cardiac output syndrome. Circulation, 33(Supple. 1):78, 1966.

Cook, W. A., Webb, W. R., and Unal, M. O.: Myocardial functional capacity in response to compensated and uncompensated respiratory alkalosis. Surg. Forum, 16:186, 1965.

Cooper, T., and Priola, D. V.: Beta-adrenergic receptor blockade in cardiac therapy. Heart Bull., 17:113, 1968.

Dammann, J. F., Jr., Thung, N., Christlieb, I. I., Little-field, J. B., and Muller, W. H., Jr.: The management of the severely ill patient after open-heart surgery. J. Thorac. Cardiov. Surg., 45:80, 1963.

Darby, T. D., Aldinger, E. E., Gadsen, R. H., and Thrower, W. B.: Effects of metabolic acidosis on ventricular isometric systolic tension and the response to epinephrine and levarterenol. Circ. Res., 8:1242, 1960.

DeSanctis, R. W., and Kastor, J. A.: Rapid intracardiac pacing for treatment of recurrent ventricular tachyarrhythmias in the absence of heart block. Amer. Heart J., 76:168, 1968.

Dietzman, R. H., Ersek, R. A., Lillehei, C. W., Castaneda, A. R., and Lillehei, R. C.: Low output syndrome: Recognition and treatment. J. Thorac. Cardiov. Surg., 57:138, 1969.

Ebert, P. A., Greenfield, L. J., Austen, W. G., and Morrow, A. G.: The relationship of blood pH during profound hypothermia to subsequent myocardial function. Surg. Gynec. Obstet., 114:357, 1962.

Ebert, P. A., Jude, J. R., and Gaertner, R. A.: Persistent hypokalemia following open-heart surgery. Circulation, 31(Supple. 1):137, 1965.

Enright, L. P., Staroscik, R., and Reis, R. L.: Experimental evaluation of methods of protecting the myocardium during prolonged aortic occlusion. (Abstr.) Circulation, 38(Supple. 6):72, 1968.

Fishman, N. H., Hutchinson, J. C., and Roe, B. B.: Controlled atrial hypertension: A method for supporting cardiac output following open-heart surgery. J. Thorac. Cardiov. Surg., 52:777, 1966.

Flemma, R. J., and Young, W. G., Jr.: The metabolic effects of mechanical ventilation and respiratory alkalosis in postoperative patients. Surgery, 56:36, 1964.

Frank, G. B.: Calcium and the initiation of contraction. Circ. Res., 15(Supple. 2):54, 1964.

Futral, A. A., and McGuire, L. B.: Reversion of chronic atrial fibrillation. J.A.M.A., 199:885, 1967.

Gans, H., and Krivit, W.: Problems in hemostasis during and after open-heart surgery. VI. Over-all changes in blood coagulation mechanism. J.A.M.A., 179:145, 1962a.

Gans, H., and Krivit, W.: Problems in hemostasis during open-heart surgery. IV. On the changes in the blood clotting mechanism during cardiopulmonary bypass procedures. Ann. Surg., 155:353, 1962b.

Ghidoni, J. J., Liotta, D., and Thomas, H.: Massive subendocardial damage accompanying prolonged ventricular fibrillation. Amer. J. Path., 56:15, 1969.

Goldfarb, D., and Bahnson, H. T.: Early and late effects on the heart of small amounts of air in the coronary circulation. J. Thorac. Cardiov. Surg., 46:368, 1963.

Gomes, M. M. R., and McGoon, D. C.: Bleeding patterns after open-heart surgery. J. Thorac. Cardiov. Surg. (In press.)

Greenberg, J. J., and Edmunds, L. H., Jr.: Effect of

myocardial ischemia at varying temperatures on left ventricular function and tissue oxygen tension. J. Thorac. Cardiov. Surg., 42:84, 1961.

Guilbault, P., Coraboeuf, E., and Delahayes, J.: Action des ions calcium et magnésium sur l'activité ventriculaire du coeur de mammifère isolé. C. R. Soc. Biol. (Paris), 159:65, 1965.

Harrison, D. C., Sprouse, J. H., and Morrow, A. G.: The antiarrhythmic properties of lidocaine and procaine amide: Clinical and physiologic studies of their cardiovascular effects in man. Circulation, 28:486, 1963.

Henson, D. E., Najafi, H., Callaghan, R., Coogan, P., Julian, O. C., and Eisenstein, R.: Myocardial lesions following open heart surgery. Arch. Path. (Chicago), 88:423, 1969.

Holland, W. C.: Ion distribution and myocardial metabolism as affected by cardiac glycosides. Circ. Res., 15(Supple. 2):85, 1969.

Indeglia, R. A., Levy, M. J., Lillehei, R. C., Todd, D. B., and Lillehei, C. W.: Correlation of plasma catecholamines, renal function, and the effects of dibenzyline on cardiac patients undergoing corrective surgery. J. Thorac. Cardiov. Surg., 51:244, 1966.

Kay, C. F.: The clinical use of digitalis preparations. Circulation, 12:116, 291, 1955.

Kirklin, J. W., and Rastelli, G. C.: Low cardiac output after open intracardiac operations. Progr. Cardiov. Dis., 10:117, 1967.

Kleiger, R., and Lown, B.: Cardioversion and digitalis. II. Clinical studies. Circulation, 33:878, 1966.

Kloster, F. E., Bristow, J. D., Starr, A., McCord, C. W., and Griswold, H. E.: Serial cardiac output and blood volume studies following cardiac valve replacement. Circulation, 33:528, 1966.

Konttinen, A., Hupli, V., Louhija, A., and Härtel, G.: Origin of elevated serum enzyme activities after direct-current countershock. New Eng. J. Med., 281:231, 1969.

Kouchoukos, N. T., Sheppard, L. C., McDonald, D. A., and Kirklin, J. W.: Estimation of stroke volume from the central arterial pressure contour in postoperative patients. Surg. Forum, 20:180, 1969.

Krasnow, N., and Barbarosh, H.: Clinical experiences with beta-adrenergic blocking agents. Anesthesiology, 29:814, 1968.

Lillehei, R. C., Dietzman, R. H., and Bloch, J. H.: Hypotension and low output syndrome following cardiopulmonary bypass. In Norman, J. C.: Cardiac Surgery. New York, Appleton-Century-Crofts, Inc., 1967, pp. 437–456.

Linhart, J. W., and Wheat, M. W., Jr.: Myocardial dysfunction following aortic valve replacement: The significance of coronary artery disease. J. Thorac. Cardiov. Surg., 54:259, 1967.

Lister, J. W., Cohen, L. S., Bernstein, W. H., and Samet, P.: Treatment of supraventricular tachycardias by rapid atrial stimulation. Circulation, 38:1044, 1968.

Litwak, R. S., Gilson, A. J., Slonim, R., McCune, C. C., Kiem, I., and Gadboys, H. L.: Alterations in blood volume during "normovolemic" total body perfusion. J. Thorac. Cardiov. Surg., 42:477, 1961.

Lockey, E., Ross, D. N., Longmore, D. B., and Sturridge, M. F.: Potassium and open-heart surgery. Lancet, 1:671, 1966.

Marriott, H. J., and Menendez, M. M.: A-V dissociation revisited. Progr. Cardiov. Dis., 8:533, 1966.

Marriott, H. J., and Sandler, I. A.: Criteria, old and new, for differentiating between ectopic ventricular beats and aberrant ventricular conduction in the presence of atrial fibrillation. Progr. Cardiov. Dis., 9:18, 1966.

McCallister, B. D., Weidman, W. H., Merideth, J., and Danielson, G. K.: A complex atrial dysrhythmia in a 10-year-old successfully treated with combined demand ventricular pacing and propranolol. (Unpublished data.)

McNally, E. M., and Benchimol, A.: Medical and physiological considerations in the use of artificial cardiac pacing. I. Amer. Heart. J., 75:380, 1968a.

McNally, E. M., and Benchimol, A.: Medical and physiological considerations in the use of artificial cardiac pacing. II. Amer. Heart. J., 75:679, 1968b.

Merideth, J., and Titus, J. L.: The anatomic atrial connections between sinus and A-V node. Circulation, 37:566, 1968.

Moffitt, E. A., Rosevear, J. W., Molnar, G. D., and McGoon, D. C.: Effects of glucose-insulin-potassium solution on metabolism after cardiac surgery. (Submitted for publication.)

Moffitt, E. A., Tarhan, S., and Lundborg, R. O.: Anesthesia for cardiac surgery: Principles and practice. Anesthesiology, 29:1181, 1968.

Morales, A. R., Fine, G., and Taber, R. E.: Cardiac surgery and myocardial necrosis. Arch. Path. (Chicago), 83:71, 1967.

Morris, J. J., Jr., Peter, R. H., and McIntosh, H. D.: Electrical conversion of atrial fibrillation: Immediate and long-term results and selection of patients. Ann. Intern. Med., 65:216, 1966.

Najafi, H., Henson, D., Dye, W. S., Javid, H., Hunter, J. A., Callaghan, R., Eisenstein, R., and Julian, O. C.: Left ventricular hemorrhagic necrosis. Ann. Thorac. Surg., 7:550, 1969.

Pace-Floridia, A., and Galindo, A.: Cardiac arrhythmia induced by negative phase in artificial ventilation. Anesthesiology, 29:382, 1968.

Parmley, W. W., Matloff, J. M., and Sonnenblick, E. H.: Hemodynamic effects of glucagon in patients following prosthetic valve replacement. Circulation, 39(Supple.):163, 1969.

Poulias, G. E., Escobar, G., Beall, A. C., Jr., and De Bakey, M. E.: A comparison of changes in left ventricular contractile force following various methods of myocardial support. Surgery, 57:419, 1965.

Reis, R. L., Cohn, L. H., and Morrow, A. G.: Effects of induced ventricular fibrillation on ventricular performance and cardiac metabolism. Circulation, 35(Supple. 1):234, 1967.

Roberts, W. C., and Morrow, A. G.: Causes of early postoperative death following cardiac valve replacement. J. Thorac. Cardiov. Surg., 54:422, 1967.

Rothfeld, E. L., Lipowitz, M., Zucker, I. R., Parsonnet, V., and Bernstein, A.: Management of persistently recurring ventricular fibrillation with propranolol hydrochloride. J.A.M.A., 204:546, 1968.

Rouleau, C. A., Frye, R. L., and Ellis, F. H., Jr.: Hemodynamic state after open mitral valve replacement and reconstruction. J. Thorac. Cardiov. Surg., 58:870, 1969.

Sarnoff, S. J., Gilmore, J. P., McDonald, R. H., Jr., Daggett, W. M., Weisfeldt, M. L., and Mansfield, P. B.: Relationship between myocardial K^+ balance, O_2 consumption, and contractility. Amer. J. Physiol., 211:361, 1966.

Sato, R., Ogawa, K., Okada, M., Takeda, Y., and Kimura, K.: Studies on the maximal time limit for total occlusion of the coronary circulation by determination of the enzymatic activity level in blood. J. Thorac. Cardiov. Surg., 53:231, 1967.

Sealy, W. C., Hattler, B. G., Jr., Blumenschein, S. D., and Cobb, F. R.: Surgical treatment of Wolff-Parkinson-White syndrome. Ann. Thorac. Surg., 8:1, 1969.

Spencer, F. C., Eiseman, B., Trinkle, J. K., and Rossi, N. P.: Assisted circulation for cardiac failure following intracardiac surgery with cardiopulmonary bypass. J. Thorac. Cardiov. Surg., 49:56, 1965.

Theilen, E. O., and Wilson, W. R.: Beta-adrenergic receptor blocking drugs in the treatment of cardiac arrhythmias. Med. Clin. N. Amer., 52:1017, 1968.

Vasko, J. S., and Tapper, R. I.: Cardiovascular effects of prolonged induced severe hypercalcemia. (Abstr.) Circulation, 36(Supple. 2):257, 1967.

Wang, H. H., and Katz, R. L.: Effects of changes in coronary blood pH in the heart. Circ. Res., 17:114, 1965.

Williams, J. F., Jr., Morrow, A. G., and Braunwald, E.: The incidence and management of "medical" complications following cardiac operations. Circulation, 32:608, 1965.

Yacoub, M. H., and Zeitlin, G. L.: Hyperbaric oxygen in the treatment of the postoperative low-cardiac-output syndrome. Lancet, 1:581, 1965.

CHAPTER 28

RADICAL NECK DISSECTION WITH SLOUGHING, INFECTED FLAPS, EXPOSED VESSELS, AND PHARYNGEAL AND THORACIC DUCT FISTULAE

by JAMES R. CALLISON, M.D., and MILTON T. EDGERTON, M.D., F.A.C.S.*

James R. Callison is a Kentuckian who graduated Alpha Omega Alpha from Vanderbilt Medical School. He served his residency in general surgery at Massachusetts General Hospital and in plastic surgery at the University of Pittsburgh. He became Associate Professor of Surgery and Chairman of the Division of Plastic Surgery, Medical College of Virginia, in 1967. In 1968 he joined the staff at the Johns Hopkins Hospital where he is Associate Professor of Plastic Surgery.

Milton Thomas Edgerton, Jr., was born in Atlanta and graduated from Emory University, having been elected to Phi Beta Kappa. He received his M.D. from Hopkins and, after military service at Valley Forge General Hospital, served his residency years in general and plastic surgery at Johns Hopkins Hospital. Joining the staff, he rose throughout the ranks to become Professor of Surgery (Plastic) in 1962. His scholarly research and writings, together with a rich clinical experience in plastic and head and neck surgery, have made him a world leader in his chosen field.

At the current stage in the treatment of cancer arising in the head and neck region, surgical excision and irradiation remain the principal modalities of therapy. Despite the additive effects of these two modalities in producing a physiologic insult to normal tissues, the quest for improvement in the cure rate has evolved into a more and more frequent wedding of irradiation and radical surgery in the management of oropharyngeal and laryngeal malignancies. This marriage either occurs as a result of a planned "combined" primary therapeutic approach or follows an attempt at salvage after failure of the primary therapy. One consequence of combining surgery with x-ray is an increased incidence of postoperative complications,

with attendant morbidity and mortality. If, indeed, survival rates are improved, the risks of these complications are justified, for recurrent or persistent cancer is eventually 100 per cent lethal. Competent surgeons, forewarned, will always rise to the challenge of these preventable and treatable sequelae of therapy.

Although major surgery within the head and neck area always carries the risk of complications, the most common denominator related to major complications following radical neck or composite oropharyngeal resections is prior irradiation therapy. Suture line breakdown, necrosis of flaps, oropharyngeal fistulae, exposure and rupture of the carotid artery, and serious infections must all be recognized by the surgeon as *resulting from a reduction in tissue circulation to levels that are inadequate to provide sufficient nutrition for cell survival, natural body*

---

*2021 North Central Avenue, Phoenix, Arizona, and the Department of Plastic Surgery, The University of Virginia Medical Center, Charlottesville, Virginia.

defense mechanisms, and the reparative processes of wound healing. This basic concept is the foundation for understanding the deleterious effect of irradiation as well as for formulating prophylactic and management programs for these complications.

Severe infection, necrosis of a flap, or an orocutaneous fistula rarely occurs as a single isolated complication. More commonly, these complications occur in conjunction with, or as a consequence of, another. A sloughing flap invites infection, leading to further tissue breakdown and a fistula. An intraoral suture line dehiscence leads to pooling of salivary secretions, contamination, infection, and subsequent loss of an overlying flap. Each component of the complication makes further demands on tissue physiology which is already taxed to its limit, thereby tipping the balance from healing to necrosis. By the same reasoning, it is unrealistic to expect attention to one component to correct all others; each factor must be treated concomitantly—necrotic tissue must be debrided, dependent pooling of secretions must be drained, and invasive bacteria must be controlled. When wound breakdown seems imminent, first priority therapy should be directed to debridement of nonviable, devascularized tissue. If not debrided, this necrotic conglomerate of proteins and starches provides a favorable environment for bacterial growth and mechanically deters the restoration of wound physiology conducive to repair.

The repetitious theme in the discussion of major complications of radical neck dissections must stress attention to blood supply of tissues, copious irrigations before wound closure, complete debridement of nonviable tissue, drainage of fluid collections, elimination of dead space, splinting of healing wounds, minimizing of foreign bodies in contaminated wounds, and closure of fistulae with healthy vascularized tissues.

IRRADIATION REACTION: IMPLICATIONS IN SURGICAL COMPLICATIONS

Since irradiation is implicated in the vast majority of major complications in head and neck surgery (Habel, 1965), a discussion of the mechanism of its role in these complications is warranted.

Exposing tissues to the high energies of ionizing radiation is simply a method of inducing cellular injury. This is a two-edged sword, for while it induces substantial injury to malignant cells because of their high concentrations of active DNA, ionizing radiation also produces injury to all normal tissues in its path. The response of soft tissue to this injury is similar to the sequence of events set into motion by other forms of injury—inflammation, repair, fibrosis, and cicatrization. These sequelae are related to the degree of injury, and the degree of cellular injury is dose-related. Treatment programs delivering less than 3000 R. to normal tissues are attendant with very little increase in postoperative complications. However, the changes in soft tissues consequent to cancerocidal doses of 5000 R. to 7000 R. produce a marked increase in wound complications (Habel, 1965; Goldman and Friedman, 1969).

The timing of surgical intervention is also an important factor in the incidence of post-irradiation complications. In the early period of irradiation injury (during the two to three weeks following completion of radiation therapy) the tissues are still in their catabolic phase. The inflammatory response manifested externally by erythema and edema of the skin creates a very bloody operative field, with difficult hemostasis and increased risk of hematoma formation in the surgical wound. We have measured the I^{131} capillary skin clearance (method of Kety) during this period of early postirradiation erythema and found it slightly above the normal levels on the opposite side of the face of neck (Edgerton, 1953). In addition, host resistance and cellular immune mechanisms are diminished and appear less able to cope with the inevitable bacterial wound contamination. Thus, infection is more common. Wound healing is delayed by the irradiation effect on fibroblast proliferation. Irradiated oral mucosa is edematous and friable, prone to suture line dehiscence and consequent fistula formation (Grimm, 1968).

By the third week after completion of therapy, the cells surviving irradiation seem to enter a reparative phase. Tissue resistance mechanisms are stronger, wound healing capabilities are improved, and the acute inflammatory response has abated. Again these changes follow the known sequences of wound healing from other forms of injury.

Two to three months following therapy, the

maturation phase of fibrosis develops. Obliterative endarteritis from subendothelial fibrous tissue proliferation produces a reduction in the number of blood vessels and a narrowing in the diameters of those remaining. Hyalinosis is seen in the collagen fibers, and the generalized sclerosis in the subcutaneous connective tissue produces obstruction of lymphatics and consequent edema. The epidermis atrophies with loss of the rete pegs, acanthosis, and parakeratosis; hair follicles and sebaceous glands are destroyed. Oral secretions are diminished as a result of atrophy of mucous glands, producing a dry mouth and possible changes in the bacterial flora. These changes lead again to decreased natural resistance, diminished wound healing capabilities, and an embarrassed circulatory state (Teloh, 1950). Indeed, a state of "chronic ischemia" develops in the entire irradiated field.

Thus, the optimum time for surgical intervention following preoperative radiation therapy is between the third and eighth week after completion of therapy. This has been substantiated clinically by a lower incidence of postoperative complications when excisional procedures have been carried out during this interval, as compared with complication rates following earlier or later surgical procedures (VandenBerg, 1965; Goldman and Friedman, 1969).

FLAP NECROSIS

Integrity of skin coverage of the widely dissected radical neck wound is a prerequisite in the prevention of serious complications. If viable flaps and intact suture lines are maintained, the carotid vessels are protected from rupture, infections are minimized, and most fistulae are prevented. Any fistula that does develop will usually heal spontaneously if no skin loss has occurred. Once the protective barrier of intact skin is broken, the exposed deep tissues are subjected to further injury by desiccation and bacterial invasion. Although major losses of skin flaps are obviously serious complications, minor losses along suture lines or at the corners of flaps should also be recognized for their potential in initiating an ominous chain of events. This minor suture line slough is frequently ascribed to "poor wound healing" when, in fact, this "poor wound healing" is secondary to the necrosis of the tissues expected to accomplish primary healing. Usually such a loss would not have occurred if the flap had not been poorly designed, cut too thin, stretched too far, or sutured too tightly.

ETIOLOGY

Common to all areas of sloughing or necrotic flaps is circulatory insufficiency. The explanation of the role of previous irradiation injury to this vascular insufficiency has already been presented. Many times these added risks must be accepted in order to gain control of the cancer, *but only extraordinary gentleness and attention to detail will produce good healing in heavily irradiated tissues.* The surgeon working in an irradiated field must never forget that the tissue circulation is already embarrassed and cannot afford any technical errors that might further compromise blood supply. Indeed, extra caution is called for, even to the deviation from one's "standard" incisions or techniques, in order to compensate for the vulnerability of this fragile and relatively defenseless irradiated tissue.

Incisions

Considerations in the design of the various incisions advocated for radical neck dissection should include (a) adequate exposure, (b) maintenance of dermal blood supply for primary healing, (c) good coverage of the carotid artery, (d) satisfactory cosmesis, and (e) utilization of needed cervical skin flaps to replace lining or involved skin. Unfortunately, many of the more popular incisions have a trifurcate component in which three flaps join (Fig. 28-1). This design is notorious for poor wound healing at the corners of these flaps (Cramer and Culf, 1969). In addition, this trefoil suture line frequently falls to overlie ligated branches of the carotid vessels, making minor areas of tissue slough a serious threat. When these flaps are designed in cervical skin previously subjected to heavy irradiation exposure, some degree of flap necrosis is predictable. If complications are to be avoided, *the entire plan of reconstruction must be established before any incision is made in the neck to remove the cervical lymphatics.* Failure to coordinate excision with repair has often made necessary the use of a more risky, time-consuming, expensive, and deforming method of repair.

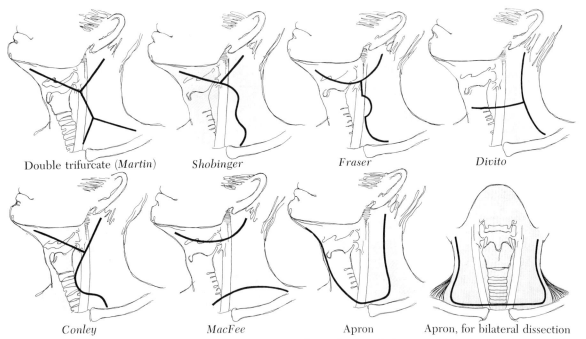

Double trifurcate (*Martin*)   *Shobinger*   *Fraser*   *Divito*

Conley   *MacFee*   Apron   Apron, for bilateral dissection

Figure 28-1. Some of the more popular incisions used in radical neck dissection. The design of many of the incisions is a trifurcate juncture of three flaps. Although the original design of these incisions did not intend that the junction of the three flaps fall to lie over the critical area of the carotid bulb, this tends to occur too frequently, and loss of the corners of these flaps leads to dangerous exposure of the carotid vessel. Modifications of the MacFee incision afford maximum safety in previously irradiated cervical skin. The apron flap is useful in bilateral neck dissection or when cervical skin is needed for intraoral lining.

When special cervical transposition flaps are not needed in the over-all reconstructive plan, the authors advocate the parallel transverse incisions proposed by MacFee (1960) and slightly modified by Grillo and Edmunds (1965) (Fig. 28-2). This bipedicle flap does not compromise exposure, provides secure coverage of the carotid vessels, and gives excellent cosmetic results. Many authors have attested the higher rate of primary wound healing in the irradiated and non-irradiated neck with this incision over others (Stell, 1969; Chandler, 1969). The upper limb incision may be extended into a lip-splitting incision when composite resections demand this exposure. The same incision design can be utilized with safety for subsequent dissection of the opposite side of the neck. When simultaneous bilateral neck dissection is carried out, a large rectangular apron flap, based superiorly along the lower border of the mandible from mastoid to mastoid, has proved most successful. This rectangular flap can also be used in smaller design for unilateral neck dissection or for radical laryngectomy with node dissection (Lipshultz, 1968; Goldman and Friedman,

1969) (Figs. 28-3 and 28-4). These flaps should be designed so that the vertical limbs lie in the lateral neck, posterior to the axis of movement in flexing and extending the neck, thus avoiding late scar hypertrophy.

In neck dissections for cancers of the skin, lip, or buccal mucosa, the platysma should be separated from the skin flap and left on the specimen. However, the additional protection afforded by this muscle to the circulation of the skin flap is of significant benefit in the irradiated patient and may be safely raised with the skin flap in the cases of cancer arising in the other areas of the oral cavity, pharynx, or larynx.

Necrosis at the Margins of Suture Lines

The hemostatic effect of skin sutures is well-known and practiced by all surgeons. However, some surgeons fail to associate this desirable effect with the undesirable corollary of the potential ischemia from skin sutures tied too tightly. Many surgeons still fail to anticipate the predictable edema that occurs during the early postoperative hours

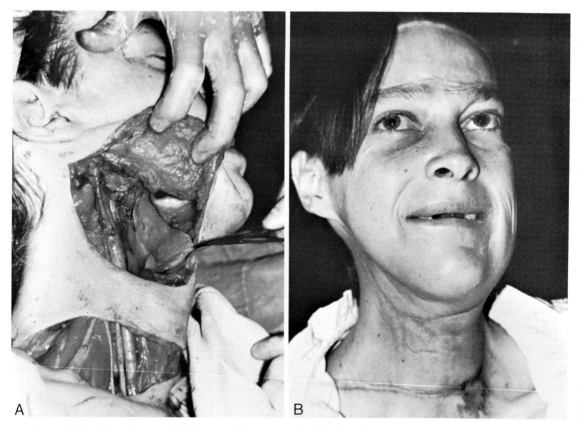

A   B

Figure 28-2.   This 32-year-old diabetic and hyperthyroid white female required emergency resection because of acute hemorrhage from lingual artery in large fungating tongue cancer after receiving 3500 R. to the neck and tongue. Through the parallel neck incisions, total glossectomy, partial mandibulectomy, and right radical neck and left supra-hyoid neck dissection were performed along with total thyroidectomy. Primary reconstruction was achieved with forehead flap and mandibular bar. *A,* Exposure and surgical defect. *B,* Six weeks after surgery. Despite acute radiation effect in cervical skin, primary healing occurred without complications.

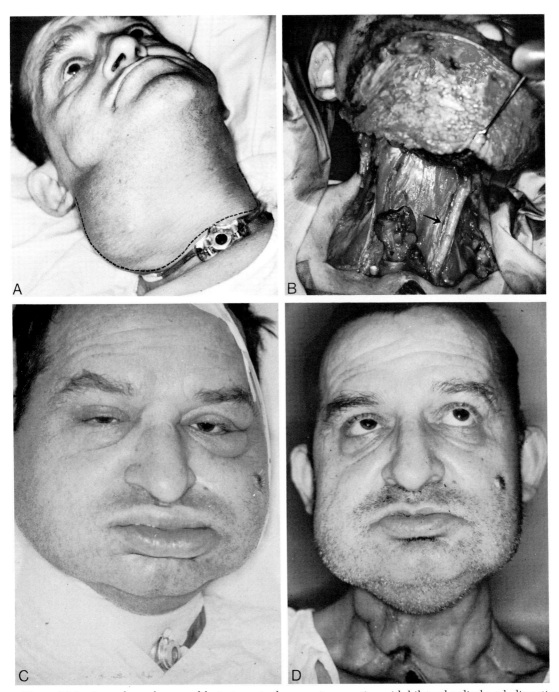

Figure 28-3. Large hypopharyngeal lesion required composite resection with bilateral radical neck dissection. Rectangular apron flap incision gave excellent exposure and primary uncomplicated wound healing, despite massive early postoperative facial edema. *A,* Rectangular flap outlined; preoperative tracheostomy. *B,* Resection field; left jugular vein preserved (arrow). *C,* Massive facial edema on third postoperative day. *D,* Three weeks after operation; note good primary healing and resolution of facial edema.

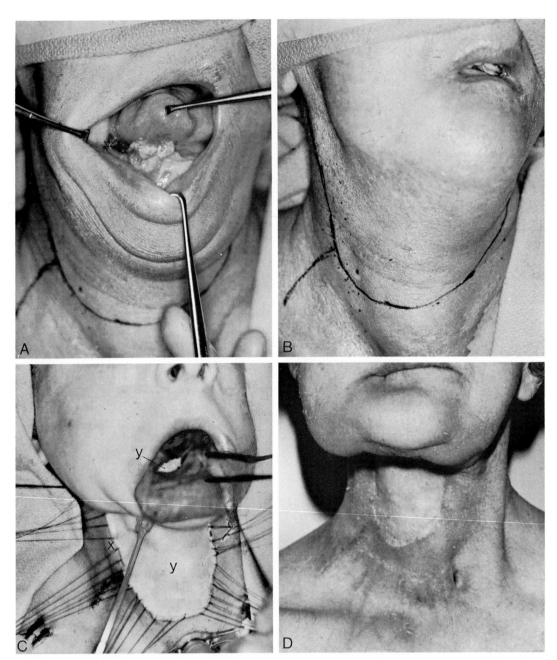

Figure 28-4. This 65-year-old female with squamous cell carcinoma of anterior gingiva and floor of mouth required composite resection of mandible from left canine fossa to right angle, partial glossectomy, and right radical and left suprahyoid neck dissection. Apron flap incision gave good exposure and provided intraoral lining for mandibular reconstruction with iliac bone graft. *A*, Lesion of left anterior gingiva and floor of mouth. *B*, Incision outline. *C*, Flap turned under and sutured to buccal mucosa; split skin graft (*y*) covers donor site and undersurface to tongue; carotid (*x*) covered by cervical skin flaps. *D*, Six weeks after original resection; apron flap has been divided and temporary pharyngostoma closed at three weeks.

and its effect in further compromising the circulation in the tissue encompassed by the skin sutures. These factors are responsible for the majority of problems of marginal suture line slough. Another common villain in marginal necrosis is undue trauma to wound edges during the ablative surgery from too-vigorous retraction, crushing forceps, and electrodesiccation. Smaller technical errors may often be tolerated by normal healthy tissues, but they are critical in a large, thin, irradiated flap. Gentle retraction and handling of the wound margins plus continuous coverage of the reflected flaps with saline-moistened packs will prevent many postoperative problems by abetting early primary wound healing. Flaps should not be acutely folded or kinked backward for long periods during the node dissection; if they are, infarction or ischemia will appear some days later.

Wound Suction Catheters

The use of suction catheters beneath neck flaps has gained wide popularity among many head and neck surgeons. Maintaining apposition of the skin flaps to the remaining deep tissues of the neck prevents formation of "dead space" and collections of fluid beneath the flap. However, caution is advised in placing the catheter beneath the base of a flap and using high negative suction. Such an arrangement has been shown to impede venous and lymphatic drainage, injure the pedicle arterioles, and lead to congestion and infarction of the flap. Suction catheter tips must not lie against major arterial walls or nerve trunks. Sump drains have inherent dangers and are unnecessary in most neck wounds.

Skin Changes in the Elderly

Atrophic and vascular changes similar to those seen in postirradiation skin may occur in certain thin-skinned individuals in senescence. The skin and subcutaneous tissues of such patients demand the same precautionary gentleness of handling as do the tissues of the irradiated patient if postoperative wound breakdown is to be avoided.

Infection in Flaps

Infection incites inflammation. Inflammation leads to local edema, fever, and in-

creased metabolic demands on the tissues. Therefore, the direct toxic effect of invasive bacteria on the survival of tissue is augmented by the consequent inflammation attendant to that infection.

With routine use of postoperative antibiotic therapy in head and neck surgery (as is standard practice with composite resections) streptococcal infections are rare. Pseudomonas and staphylococcal organisms are now the most frequent offenders in serious infections. These necrotizing organisms are usually secondary surface invaders that are commonly cultured from seromas, hematomas, pooled secretions, and dead tissue. Bacterial invasion of the skin is also encouraged by maceration from salivary fistula secretions or excessively wet external dressings. Measures to combat these infections and their sequelae entail removing these "defenseless" culture media. Pooled collections of fluid must be thoroughly drained, seromas and hematomas evacuated, and necrotic tissue rapidly debrided. When this has been accomplished, specific systemic antibiotics have access to the organisms that remain in viable tissues via the bloodstream. In short, "clean the wound so that the leukocytes have a chance."

MANAGEMENT OF FLAP NECROSIS

Salvage Attempts

Because of the serious implications of "impending" flap necrosis, many methods of enhancing flap survival have been explored. The basic requirement for cell survival is an effective circulation of the extracellular fluid environment. This "effective circulation" is dependent upon arterial supply, venous drainage, rate of blood flow, oxygen saturation of the blood, and the metabolic needs of the tissues. Salvage attempts have been based on these pathophysiologic factors.

Hypothermia

Cooling of flaps that exhibit impending circulatory problems may reduce oxygen demands by lowering the metabolic rate (Kiehn and Des Prez, 1960; Sturman, et al., 1969). Cooling also deters edema. Both of these effects have theoretical value but must be balanced against the deleterious effect of vasoconstriction and consequent slowing of the rate of blood flow. Although deeply cyanotic flaps may be brought back to a rosy pink color by use of cracked ice packs, even when kept pink for 10 days the necrosis will usually develop once the hypothermia is discontinued.

Local Vasodilators

Local injections of vasodilators such as histamine have proved effective experimentally in increasing flap survival (Myers and Cherry, 1968). Increase in blood flow has been demonstrated within the stem vessels of pedicle flaps that are based on a specific arterial trunk; peripheral tissue circulation is improved, and hence tissue survival is enhanced in flaps with marginal circulatory reserve (Barisoni and Rangolin, 1967).

Hyperbaric Oxygen

Attempts to temporarily support tissues receiving insufficient oxygenation by the circulatory system through the adjunct of regional hyperbaric oxygen has been demonstrated to be of definite but rather limited benefit in animal experiments (Kernahan, 1965; McFarlane, 1966). However, the application of these experimental findings to humans has not been significantly successful because of the practical problems involved in applying hyperbaric chambers to the head and neck region.

Expanders

Rheomacrodex (low molecular weight dextran) has been demonstrated to exert beneficial effects on capillary circulation by reducing sludging of intravascular cells, stagnation of flow, and thrombosis (Goulian, 1967). Through this effect, its use offers some theoretical benefit in congested flaps having sluggish blood flow, but applications to congested or ischemic human flaps have not produced impressive tissue survivals.

Flap Mechanics

By far the most important and practical effective measures are those which relieve mechanical factors impeding circulation to flap tissues. Kinking, stretching, twisting, and pressure (either negative or positive) — the "KSTP factors" — are the most common surgical errors leading to flap necrosis. These are usually correctable in the early (two to six hours) postoperative period. Judicious release of tension at some point across the flap by removal of a single suture may dramatically relieve edema, congestion, and stagnation of blood flow distal to this line. Transposed or rotated flaps that exhibit persistent impending circulatory insufficiency may necessitate return to their original donor positions. The reopened recipient wound may then be covered with moist sterile gauze, and the sick flap retransposed with success after a few days of recovery and "flap adaptation." It is probable that this "adaptation" is in part due to improved collateral circulation and partly to the flap's conditioning to tolerate more ischemia.

Blistering of a flap is a sign of tissue injury. Blisters form at the interface between tissues whose interstitial circulation is still present and tissues which are nonviable. The tissues beneath a blister are injured, but may survive if adequately protected. Blisters should not be opened or debrided, as the blister fluid provides a protective environment for underlying cells during healing, and systemically administered antibiotic will be found in significant amounts within the blister fluid. However, individual blisters must be observed closely for signs of infection (cloudy fluid or erythema) and must be debrided immediately should infection occur. Debridement and exposure to desiccation may disturb the precarious balance of survival of cells and lead to their death. Protection of such exposed tissues from this desiccation with a Vaseline-impregnated gauze may salvage valuable skin.

Debridement

Nonviable tissue must be debrided. Nothing is gained by watching a clearly demarcated area of necrosis in the hopes that the inevitable problems associated with flap loss may be obviated. Granulations are delayed in the presence of nonviable tissue, while infection is encouraged, thus adding further destructive processes.

Debridement is best accomplished by scalpel and scissors at the bedside and without anesthesia. Then, autobiological debridement, aided by frequent dressing changes of fine mesh gauze, will accurately separate living tissue from dead and stimulate the formation of granulations. It must be remembered that these dressings accomplish their purpose by carrying away debris adherent to the interstices of the gauze at the time of removal. Therefore, the more frequently the dressing is changed, the more rapidly is debridement accomplished. Vaseline-impregnated gauze deters this type of debridement and is used much like wet dressings — only when moisture is desired on the wound surface to prevent crusting and thus promote drainage.

Cleansing of the undermined wound with a small jet spray of one-half strength (1.5%) hydrogen peroxide is often used. Liquefaction of detritus is accelerated, and the copious irrigation with agitation from the hydraulic pressure washes away loose matter.

Special Problems in Debriding Irradiated Areas

Tissue injured by irradiation frequently fails to form granulation tissue and may develop slow progressive waxy necrosis as exposure desiccation leads to further imbalance between nutritional demands and the ability of the circulatory system to respond to these demands. Progressive obliteration of the capillary bed occurs as the irradiation endarteritis of larger arterioles increases. Minute bleeding in the wound is lessened and debridement back to bleeding tissues may be followed by further necrosis unless the wound is immediately covered, preferably by a pedicle flap that will bring its own blood supply and protect these injured cells.

Homografts

The use of refrigerated or freeze-dried split-thickness skin homografts as temporary biological dressings after debridement fulfills two purposes. First, the graft protects the exposed surfaces from drying and from contact with the foreign materials in dressings. Homografts provide a physiologic covering and reconstitute an almost "normal" interstitial milieu for cell nutrition and vascular budding. As such, the surface bacterial population is markedly reduced. Secondly, homografts may be used as a reliable clinical indicator of wound physiology to determine its readiness to accept an autograft or flap. The homografts should be peeled off and replaced at three- to four-day intervals. Evidence of adherence or vascularization of the graft means that debridement is clinically complete, infection is under control, and the tissues are sufficiently healthy to justify fresh autografting.

RESURFACING OF AREAS OF FLAP LOSS

Free Skin Grafts

Many areas of flap loss may be quite adequately resurfaced with free split-thickness skin grafts. Free grafts, placed on a suitable bed, frequently provide a safer, faster, and more simple method of wound closure than does the use of flaps. The grafts do not offer as much protection of exposed major vessels and nerves as flaps, and it is sometimes difficult to obtain a successful take of a free graft adjacent to a salivary fistula. However, a free graft will grow on the wall of a carotid artery, will cover major nerves, and will adhere to the perichondrium of the larynx. Prior irradiation, though deleterious to the graft bed, does not always preclude the use of skin grafts. A free graft, used for a temporary surfacing to "clean up" a wound, will provide some protection against hemorrhage while a distant flap is being delayed. Free grafts may serve as permanent coverings in smaller noncritical areas.

Because of the varying contours and mobility of the neck, some restriction of movement in the postgrafting period is essential if a successful take of the graft is to be obtained. Splints and dressings to achieve this are left to the ingenuity of individual surgeons, *as long as the objective — immobilization — is obtained.* It should be anticipated that some contracture of all free skin grafts occurs. This is related not only to the thickness of the graft but to the rigidity of the underlying bed, the shape of the graft margins (circular versus darted), and the strength of muscles that will tend to stretch the graft postoperatively.

Flaps

Replacement of major surface defects with a flap of skin and subcutaneous tissue having

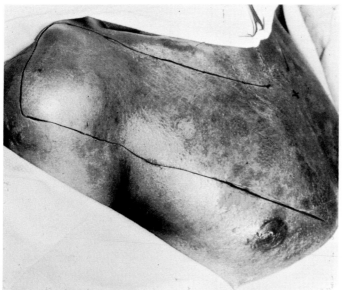

Figure 28-5. The medially based delto-pectoral flap, popularized by Bakamjian, is based on the anterior perforating intercostal vessels at the sternal border. This flap is accessible, usually outside irradiation ports, and can be transferred without delay to surface neck and lower cheek or provide oropharyngeal lining.

its own blood supply is frequently desirable for the following reasons: (a) more secure protection of underlying critical structures, (b) better function, and (c) more acceptable cosmesis. When pedicle flaps are required, it is obvious that local tissue which can be moved immediately without a delay should be selected whenever feasible (Cramer and Culf, 1969). However, previous irradiation therapy portals, prior skin incisions or scars, and previous ligation of stem arterial and venous trunks may limit this selection. Therefore, a surgeon undertaking major head and neck cancer surgery should have a variety of alternative flaps in his armamentarium of reconstruction. *Indeed, only an understanding of all the principles of flap construction will permit him to design the most appropriate flap to fit each individual situation—and to move it into position with minimum delay and maximum safety for his patient.*

With loss of skin after neck dissection, the two sites most readily available for immediate transfer are (1) the skin of the deltopectoral area, and (2) the forehead. The medially based deltopectoral flap popularized by Bakamjian (1965) is based on the first four intercostal spaces, with the perforating branches and tributaries of the internal mammary vessels supplying the pedicle (Fig. 28-5). A large area of skin can be safely transferred by this flap without delay if the pectoral fascia is taken with the flap, and care is taken not to injure the perforating vessels

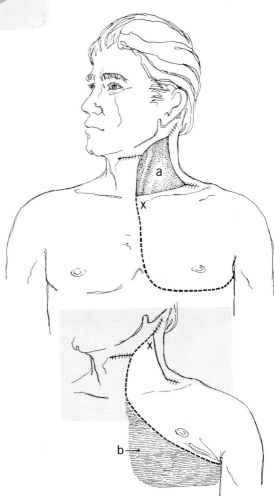

Figure 28-6. Illustration of pectoral chest flap based laterally. *A,* Cervical skin defect. *B,* Donor site defect covered with split skin graft. This flap is also useful to cover parotid cheek defects.

at the sternal border. An attractive feature of this flap is its dependent venous drainage. This flap is usually caudad to irradiation portals used for head and neck cancer.

This same donor area, but based *laterally*, may be used as a large rotation flap for lateral neck defects or the parotid region (Fig. 28-6) (Conley, 1953). Since the stem vascular supply is less definite, a larger base is necessary to this pedicle, incorporating the thoraco-acromial and axillary systems. It provides a large area of skin relatively safely; this flap also has the advantage of producing a pedicle that is away from the opening of the tracheostomy and its secretions.

Smaller defects may be covered with a tubed acromiopectoral flap, based superiorly and laterally (Erdelyi, 1956). When areas of the lower cervical skin are intact, this tubed pedicle has an advantage of spanning this

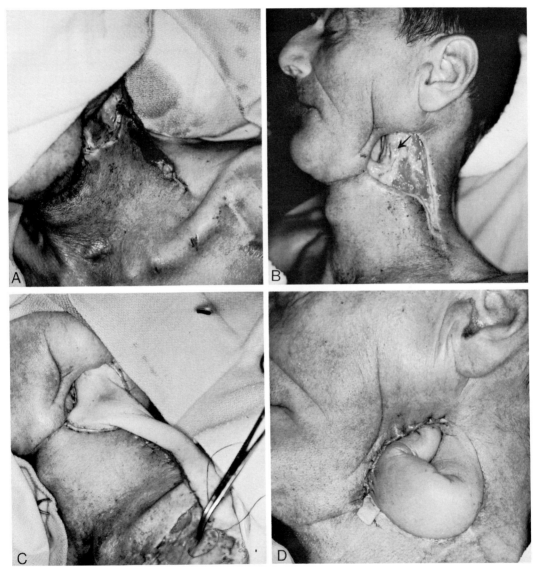

Figure 28-7. This 62-year-old white male developed recurrence of tonsillar carcinoma one year after receiving 6500 R. to the neck and tonsil. Composite resection of tonsil, mandible, and neck was performed through trifurcate incision, with primary closure of oral lining. A, Status when first seen with slough of skin flap and dehiscence of oral lining closure resulted in this large pharyngo-cutaneous fistula. B, Necrotic flaps debrided, carotid artery exposed (arrow). C, Intact skin of lower neck spanned by tubed acromio-pectoral flap to cover carotid bulb and cervical skin defect; pedicle was delayed seven days prior to transfer. D, Three weeks after transfer, base of tube pedicle was turned to supply lining and close fistula.

area to deliver its paddle to a more distant site. The tube also permits ease in turning and rotating the flap (Fig. 28-7).

The vigorous forehead flap of McGregor (1966) will also reach areas of the mid and upper neck. The entire forehead can be utilized without delay if the superficial temporal and posterior auricular vessels are intact. This flap has even been used in the neck after division of the superficial temporal vessels but with a delay of the contralateral superficial temporal and frontal vessels carried out two weeks prior to the transfer (Fig. 28-8). The need for "uphill" venous drainage and the esthetic drawback of the exposed donor site has relegated the forehead a second choice to the deltopectoral area as a donor site for most cervical wounds.

When these two sites are unavailable, an area extending laterally over the posterior superior shoulder can be used, but at least two preliminary delays before transfer of this flap are necessary. Zovickian (1957) described this flap based superiorly on the posterior neck, supplied by the postauricular and greater occipital vessels (Fig. 28-9). The thick fibroadipose tissue in the base of this flap at the nape of the neck posteriorly makes it difficult to rotate acutely unless careful sharp dissection to free the base from the trapezius fascia to the midline is carefully performed. It is a splendid flap to resurface the anterior neck after irradiation necrosis of the larynx has developed.

Jump flaps from the abdomen, carried on the wrist or arm, are time-consuming, fraught with many problems (particularly in the older age group), and are, therefore, to be avoided whenever possible. The lower abdominal flaps described by Shaw can be moved faster than any of the other jump flaps.

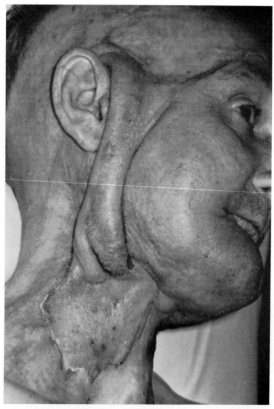

Figure 28-8. Forehead flap used to provide coverage for closure of small pharyngo-cutaneous fistula, following laryngectomy and preoperative irradiation. Superficial temporal artery had been ligated at initial resection. Flap was supplied by postauricular vessel but was delayed two weeks prior to transfer and lined with skin graft to provide pharyngeal lining. Base of pedicle returned to forehead donor site four weeks after transfer.

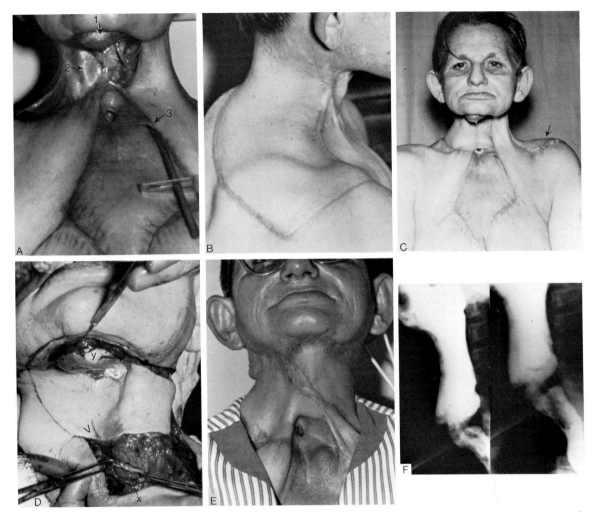

Figure 28-9. Closure of pharyngostoma and esophageal reconstruction using bilateral posterior auricular based shoulder flaps. Large hypopharyngeal carcinoma had been resected with bilateral neck dissection after 5000 R. of irradiation. Cervical skin sloughed and was replaced with bilateral pectoral flaps, which also failed. Coverage was then obtained with split thickness graft, leaving thin unstable surface over right carotid and cervical fascia. *A*, Status when first seen: (1) Base of tongue and pharyngostoma. (2) Carotid and precervical fascia covered with thin epithelial surface. (3) Esophagostomy. *B*, Right shoulder flap delayed two weeks. *C*, Right shoulder flap transferred to replace anterior neck skin, and left shoulder flap delayed (arrow). *D*, Esophageal tube constructed from turn in flaps and tongue (*y*), with left shoulder flap for external coverage. Esophagus (*x*) mobilized for anastomosis with skin tube. *E*, Postoperative photograph after third and final stage of reconstruction. *F*, Barium swallow four months after reconstruction, demonstrating adequate lumen. Stricture prevented at the juncture of the esophagus and skin tube with "V" flap outlined in *D* to break up circular suture line.

OROPHARYNGEAL FISTULAE

The first line of defense against the formation of an orocutaneous fistula is an intact, viable, water-tight closure of the oropharyngeal suture line. Once this defense is broken, it is extremely difficult to prevent the formation of a fistula. Conversely, fistula formation rarely occurs secondary to losses of external skin or suture line dehiscence without a *concomitant or preceding* dehiscence of the intraoral closure.

ETIOLOGY

Since the ablative composite resections for oropharyngeal malignancies necessarily create spatial defects within the oral pharyngeal lining, the closure of these defects primarily usually results in varying degrees of tension on the suture line. The physical structure of the thin mucosa and loose areolar submucosa is particularly vulnerable to these tensile forces produced by postoperative swallowing, jaw movements, or turning of the head. The marked edema that ensues following insult to the mucous membrane further predisposes to breakdown of the suture line by increasing the tension on the sutures, causing them to either cut through or strangulate those tissues which they encompass. The friability of mucous membranes previously subjected to irradiation magnifies the potential risks of all these problems. Tugging on the suture line by motion of the tongue and swallowing in the immediate postoperative period may produce stress forces that are not appreciated under the quiet relaxed state of general anesthesia at the time of closure. Therefore, the mere ability to oppose the margins of the defect following the ablative resection offers little certainty that primary healing will occur. Even when closure results in no postoperative fistulae, healing forces may bind the tongue, palate, jaw, or larynx, so that speech, swallowing, or mastication is disturbed. Factors such as tension on membranes, mobility of parts, edema, and previous irradiation injury must be considered before attempting primary closure. Often it is best to replace the resected lining by additional tissue in the form of flaps or grafts.

Undue tension on closure most commonly is implicated in intraoral or intrapharyngeal wound dehiscence, but other preventable mechanical factors deserve attention. When radical neck dissection is performed and the floor of the mouth is resected with preservation of the mandible, tenting or bridging of the intraoral lining from the superior crest of the remaining mandible to the remaining tongue creates a triangular dead space in the area formerly occupied by the submaxillary gland that is difficult to obliterate. Hematomas, seromas, or saliva accumulating in this space provide rich culture media in which the bacterial contaminants of the mouth will flourish and form a localized abscess leading to fistula formation. The use of postoperative suction catheters to oppose tissue planes and thereby reduce such dead space and resultant collections of fluid is of definite aid in preventing these problems.

Bony prominences of the mandible, intact or partially resected, are likely to produce a pressure type of necrosis on overlying flaps or mucosa unless ample relaxed lining is provided. Any sharp bony prominence should be contoured by a rongeur to accommodate the overlying soft tissues without tension.

Preventive Measures

All oropharyngeal suture lines should be closed in a minimum of two layers, with the second layer further inverting the first to provide more surface contact between the edges. Incisions and closures of cervical skin flaps with a "T" design should be avoided if possible, but when necessary, the tissues beneath the weak juncture of the three converging suture lines should be buttressed first with an adjacent soft tissue or muscle flap.

Preoperative planning of flaps with skin incisions which do not immediately overlie a ligated external carotid artery or an anticipated oropharyngeal closure will reduce danger of postoperative hemorrhage and deter the development of orocutaneous fistulae.

MANAGEMENT OF OROPHARYNGEAL FISTULAE

Drainage

Once an oropharyngeal fistula is established, further undermining of skin flaps must be prevented. Direct dependent drainage with opening of all dead spaces to prevent pooling or further dissection beneath the cervical skin flaps by the oral secretions will avoid secondary complications of infection, skin loss, or erosion of a carotid vessel wall. If the fistulous tract can be kept small by avoiding additional skin loss, spontaneous closure is much more likely to occur, and any subsequent surgical closure will be much easier to accomplish. Attempts at diversion of the oral secretions and the use of sump suction catheters have not proved of value unless needed to protect the entrance of the tracheostomy and prevent atelectasis and pneumonia.

Debridement

Nonviable tissue about a fistula must be debrided either by sharp excision or by dressings *before* healing or contracture can be expected. The more quickly this is accomplished, the more expeditiously will the fistula heal.

Patience

Many small orocutaneous fistulae will close spontaneously if the adjacent skin flaps are healthy. The surgeon should exercise patience when a fistula develops, for early (in the first eight weeks) attempts at resuture of the adjacent tissue will be in vain. The friable inflamed tissues, having already demonstrated their poor wound mechanics and precarious nutritional state, will not hold new sutures under the now added tension necessary to achieve approximation. Only a larger defect will ensue if reclosure is attempted. Much is gained by waiting for secondary healing to attest the healthy state of the tissues and for contracture to reduce the size of the defect. In small defects, obturation of the fistula can sometimes be accomplished by custom-fashioning a soft acrylic or Silastic obturator to fill the defect and reduce drainage while the healing process is maturing. A strip of rubber glove may be fixed to the skin margins with dermatome cement to improve neck hygiene.

Nutritional Losses

The nutritional drain on an individual losing a large volume of salivary juices through a large defect must not be overlooked. Water, electrolytes, and protein losses can be significant in the fluid and nutritional replacement requirements. Measurements from large fistulae have shown that up to 50 gm. of protein may be lost in a period of 24 hours.

Closure of Fistulae

Surgical closure of oropharyngeal fistulae usually demands the introduction of additional lining in the form of flaps. With smaller fistulae in nonirradiated tissues, book flaps of the adjacent skin may be turned inward, based on the subcutaneous tissue and scar. This method requires mature healing of the margins of the fistula, and the amount of flap tissue that can be reflected in this manner is limited. The perifistulous donor site, uncovered by these turn-in flaps, is then covered with a local rotation or distant skin flap. Thus the newly closed oral suture line is backed by healthy tissue with subcutaneous bulk.

Occasionally, adequate oral lining can be obtained from within the oral cavity in the form of tongue flaps, buccal mucosa, or pharyngeal flaps. More commonly, however, the dimensions of the ablative surgery or previous x-ray therapy preclude the safe utilization of only local tissues. For the surgeon who finds himself closing most of his oropharyngeal cancer defects without resort to extraoral pedicle flaps or grafts, there is likely to be an excessive number of local recurrences of cancers or his patients will experience unnecessary binding of functional anatomy and preventable deformity.

Large defects or those in previously irradiated tissues routinely require pedicled flaps for closure. Two surfaces are needed to close all openings—one for internal lining and one for external covering. Although a single flap from the forehead or chest can be lined with a split-thickness skin graft 10 days before transfer (Edgerton, 1964), the skin-graft lining will not permit later bone-graft accommodation through this area, and the skin graft margins may not be lifted to meet tongue or palate as safely as the more versatile pedicle-flap lining. The minimum bulk of a graft lining does make it suitable for buccal, nasal, and palatal defects (Fig. 28-10). Separate simultaneous flaps for internal lining and external covering have proved successful where a secure watertight closure is necessary in the dependent areas of the oropharynx and where mobility of a remaining segment of tongue muscle is crucial to acceptable speech and swallowing.

Flaps for Oral Lining

The three most useful flaps for providing lining for the oropharynx are (1) nasolabial cheek flap, (2) forehead flap, and (3) deltopectoral flap (recently reintroduced and popularized by Bakamjian, 1967). Each of these donor areas has the advantages of being nonhairbearing, usually outside the fields of irradiation, near enough to the tissue defect to be transferred directly and without an intermediate carrier, and of possessing a blood supply of sufficient vigor to permit an immediate transfer without the necessity of a delay.

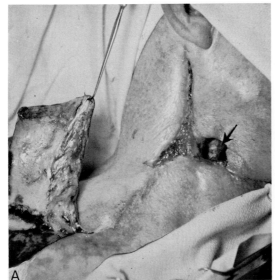
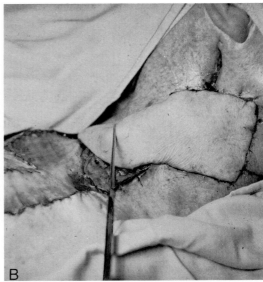
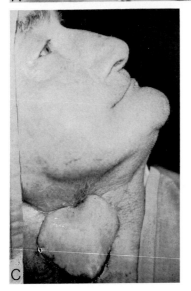

Figure 28-10. Pharyngo-cutaneous fistula occurring at "dangerous" junction of trifurcate incision, following slough of tips of neck flaps and dehiscence of underlying pharyngeal suture line. Patient had composite resection of tonsil and neck dissection after irradiation failure. *A,* Fistula (arrow) and prelined Zovickian delto-postauricular flap. *B,* Flap transposed; skin graft lining tailored for pharyngeal defect. *C,* Base of flap divided and inset with fistula closed.

The nasolabial flap is of particular advantage for defects of the anterior floor of the mouth (Fig. 28-11). Based inferiorly and taken over 1 inch wide, it may be tunneled directly through the cheek. The donor site can be closed primarily, and the temporary fistula in the cheek is usually nonsymptomatic. This flap may be used bilaterally to provide up to 4 square inches of flap lining to the floor of the mouth at the time of initial resection.

A forehead flap can be introduced through the temporal fascia over the zygomatic arch to handily reach the floor of the mouth, base of the tongue, and hypopharynx (McGregor, 1969). It may also be tunneled directly through the cheek in the preauricular area or introduced behind the angle of the mandible to reach lower pharyngeal defects. In either approach, the skin surface falls to lie internally, so that twisting or rotation of the pedicle is unnecessary. When introduced from above, the temporary fistula along the base of this flap is also nonfunctional (Fig. 28-12). A forehead flap can be used as a one-stage island flap by removing the epidermis from the pedicle portion that is to be buried — but this materially increases the risk to its blood supply.

The deltopectoral flap may be based either

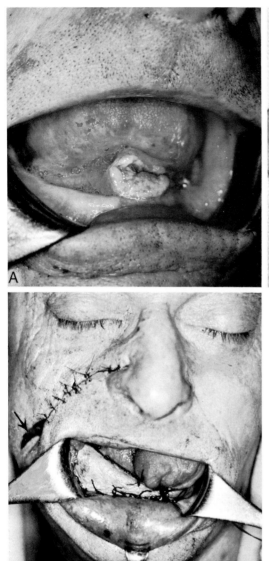

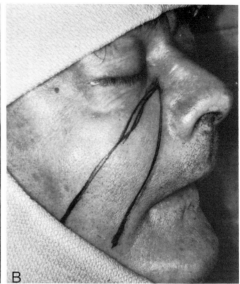

Figure 28-11. Left anterior floor of mouth carcinoma in 61-year-old white male. Defect of resection closed with nasolabial flap. *A*, 2.5 cm. exophytic lesion. *B*, Outline of flap. *C*, Flap tunneled through cheek (arrow) to provide lining of anterior floor of mouth and maintain mobility of tongue; donor site closed primarily. The patient subsequently was fitted with lower dentures.

medially on the sternum or laterally on the deltoid region. It has demonstrated its versatility in usage for defects in either the mucosal lining or the skin from the level of the epipharynx to the lower neck (Fig. 28-13). When introduced for oropharyngeal lining, it does create a temporary dependent fistula (Bakamjian, Culf, and Bales, 1967). Offsetting this minor disadvantage is the deliverance of a large volume of skin and an esthetically acceptable donor site in the male. The deltopectoral flap is also an excellent source for external coverage in the secondary closure of oropharyngeal fistulae.

The tubed deltopectoral flap is also useful to provide oral lining and may be opened on two sides at the time of application in order to provide both internal lining and internal coverage of smaller fistulae (Fig. 28-7).

Other sources of external flap coverage for fistulae have previously been discussed in the section dealing with replacement of flap losses.

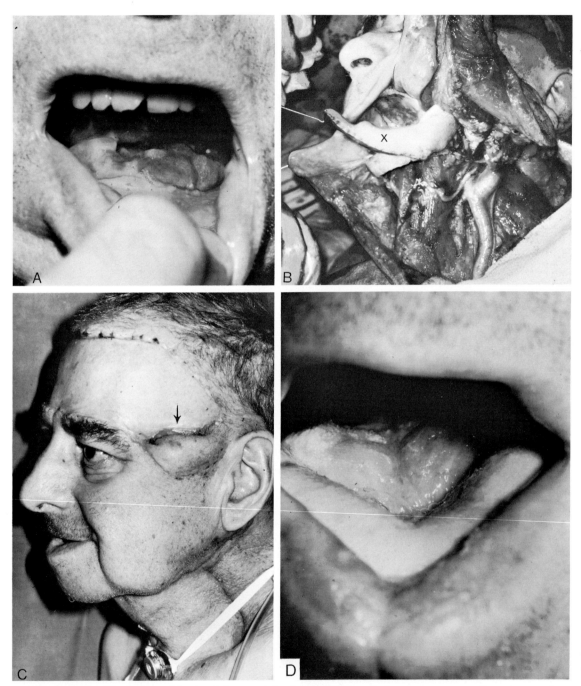

Figure 28-12. Illustration of forehead flap used for intraoral lining. *A*, Large squamous cell carcinoma of anterior floor of mouth and gingiva. *B*, The forehead flap (*x*) has been delivered through the zygomatic foramen to provide lining for immediate bone graft replacement of mandible. Cheek flaps have been reflected by a lip splitting-incision. *C*, Two weeks after resection and reconstruction, the forehead donor surfaced with split skin graft is maturing. The superiorly located temporary fistula along base of flap (arrow) is nonfunctional. *D*, Intraoral photograph of flap over bone graft leaving residual tongue free for better function.

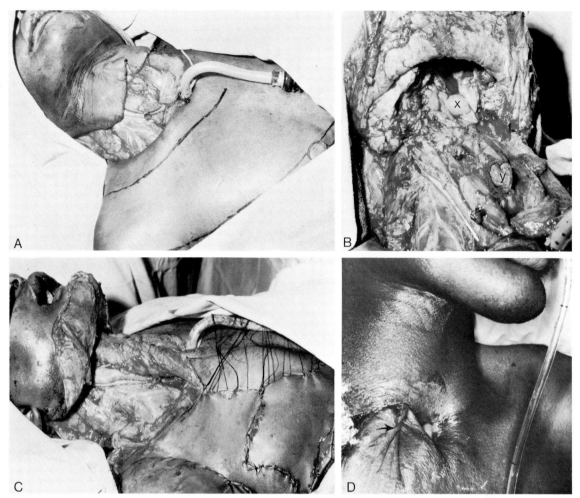

Figure 28-13. Circumferential hypopharyngeal carcinoma requiring laryngopharyngectomy and bilateral neck dissection. Primary reconstruction of pharynx was carried out with medially based deltopectoral flaps. *A*, Large rectangular apron flap incision used for resection. Deltopectoral flap outlined. *B*, Resection bed demonstrating pharynx resected at level of soft palate (*x*) and esophagus (*y*). *C*, Deltopectoral flap has been tubed, skin inside, and sutured to the tongue and nasopharynx. The esophagus is anastomosed end to side into the tube suture line. Donor site of right shoulder is covered with split skin graft. *D*, Three weeks after initial procedure, the apron flap provides external covering of flap and neck. The base of the flap is a temporary controlled fistula (arrow) below the tracheostomy. The feeding tube passes from the nasopharynx through the tubed pedicle flap and into the esophageal anastomosis. Subsequently, it is necessary to divide and close the tube pedicle just below the esophageal anastomosis.

EXPOSED VESSELS — THREATENED RUPTURE

ETIOLOGY

Rupture of the common or internal carotid artery is the most imposing complication to confront the head and neck surgeon. This complication is invariably secondary to other problems, thus compounding the difficulties in management. Exposure of the carotid vessel from loss of cervical skin flaps occurs predominantly in patients with previous irradiation and in those who develop an orocutaneous fistula (Goldman and Friedman, 1969) (Stell, 1969). The radiation effect alters the ability of the exposed tissues to form protective granulations. The concomitant presence of a fistula bathing an exposed vessel with digestive juices further jeopardizes the integrity of the vessel wall. Thus additional tissue necrosis ensues, bacterial invasion adds to the destructive process, and the local wound further deteriorates to end in an exsanguinating hemorrhage.

There are other less common causes of carotid hemorrhage (Conley, 1962). Infections in hematomas may lead to septic breakdown of the vessel wall. Large suction catheters lying directly against the carotid and placed on high negative pressure have resulted in necrosis of a segment of vessel wall. Tumor invasion with secondary necrosis and pseudoaneurysm formation may occur even in the absence of previous surgical intervention, particularly following radiation therapy.

PREVENTIVE MEASURES

The most effective precautionary measure against carotid-artery rupture following surgery is the presence of a viable skin or muscle flap overlying the vessel. For cervical lymph-node dissection, incisions should always be designed with this in mind. Parallel horizontal skin incisions (as urged by MacFee, 1960) or large rectangular-shaped, superiorly based flaps provide the greatest security in this regard (Fig. 28-1).

Various muscle flaps may serve to protect the carotid artery, and their use is especially important when the patient's neck has received prior irradiation. The levator scapulae muscle is most easily used (Fig. 28-14), but the scalenus posterior, sternohyoid, and portions of the trapezius will also reach the artery (Schweitzer, 1962). The levator scapulae is nourished and innervated segmentally in a superior and anteromedial fashion. De-

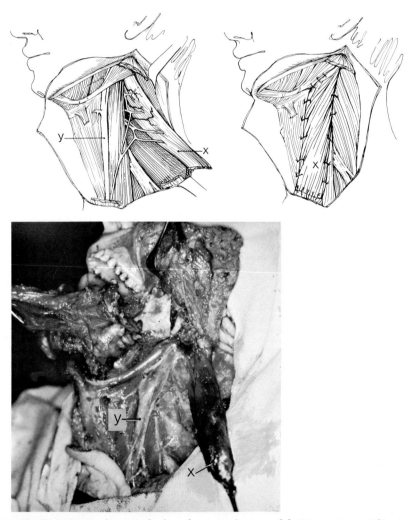

Figure 28-14. The levator scapulae muscle, based superiorly, is useful at times in providing extra coverage for the carotid artery. Blood supply and innervation enter the muscle superomedially in its proximal third. Illustration *A* shows blood supply and innervation; *B*, closure over carotid artery. The photograph *C* demonstrates elevation of the muscle (*x*) to cover the carotid artery (*y*).

tached inferiorly, this muscle can be rotated to cover the carotid at the vessel's most critical area of the bulb and bifurcation where the ligated external carotid stump is left (Staley, 1961). Some authors have advocated free grafts of dermis, denuded of epithelium, be placed over the carotid artery and buried beneath the skin flap to provide additional security in the event of loss of the overlying skin flap (Corso, 1963). Under favorable conditions, these grafts will "take" on the adventitia of the vessels and become vascularized in three to five days. Such a graft is prepared by first removing and discarding 0.010 to 0.012 inch of the epidermis and then utilizing the remaining deep dermis as the graft by suturing it to the strap muscles and levator scapulae to cover the entire length of exposed vessel. However, if mucosal suture line leakage occurs and saliva collects around this dermis, take of the graft is unlikely and necrosis with sepsis may actually add to the danger of hemorrhage. Such a technique is *not* as safe as carotid protection with flaps of skin or muscle that carry their own circulation. Dermal free grafts should be reserved for the reinforcement of wounds that are relatively aseptic—unlike the neck wound in the usual composite resection for oropharyngeal cancer.

MANAGEMENT OF EXPOSED CAROTID VESSELS

Wound disruption associated with significant loss of skin flap and resulting in exposure of the carotid vessel demands immediate and expeditious treatment. The wound must be prepared for coverage as soon as possible. The patient should be immediately moved to a position in the hospital near the nurse's station unless special duty nurses are available. The nursing staff should be instructed how to apply digital pressure to the bleeding point at the moment hemorrhage is detected. Blood should be crossmatched and held in the blood bank until the danger is past. Local measures include debridement of any hematoma or necrotic tissue, even when this further exposes the wall of the vessel. To leave the vessel hidden from view by an overlying necrotic flap will only invite secondary infection and obscure surveillance of a potentially lethal problem. All puddling of saliva or drainage against the artery should

be prevented. In patients with clean wounds and minimal losses of tissue, the flaps may be elevated and advanced for closure without tension, if the neck has not had prior irradiation. However, major wound breakdown requires urgent action and should be covered with a local transposed flap of healthy tissue carrying its own blood supply. In extenuating circumstances, free skin allografts can be used as a biological dressing when immediate flap coverage is not available. "Take" of any skin graft is extremely doubtful in the face of a salivary fistula. Even in the absence of a totally successful "take," the graft may serve as an excellent dressing, protecting the vessel from desiccation, salivary juices, and gross bacterial colonization. The anterior chest and shoulder provide expeditious and secure sources for flap coverage of the carotid area. A vigorous healthy flap can be transferred in the face of a persistently infected bed and will *actually aid in the control of the infection process* if adequate drainage is provided. The designs and sources of flaps for this area have already been described.

CAROTID LIGATION

Morbidity and mortality from ligation of the carotid artery varies in many reports from a 50 per cent stroke rate and 38 per cent mortality to a 23 per cent stroke rate and 12 per cent mortality (Moore, 1969). Actual age plays less of a role in these results than the physiologic age of the patient's vessels and the pattern of the intracranial circle of Willis. There is commonly a warning of impending rupture in the form of a minor bright red bleeding episode, which is easily controlled by pressure. This should prompt the surgeon to perform an elective ligation forthwith. Resuturing the wall of the bleeding carotid will only control bleeding for a few days to be followed by a second bleed. *This should not be attempted without simultaneous use of a muscle flap, since it is rarely if ever successful.*

A 75 per cent stroke rate and 57 per cent mortality in patients whose carotid vessels were ligated while in a clinical state of shock indicate the *importance of restoring blood volume prior to ligation*—or even better, of performing the ligation before exsanguinating hemorrhage occurs (Moore, 1969; Ketchum and Haye, 1965).

Gradual ligation of the carotid vessel over a period of days or weeks results in no less morbidity or mortality than does immediate ligation (Moore, 1969). The vessel must be ligated both superior and inferior to the bleeding point, and the ligated stumps immediately covered with healthy flap tissue.

RECONSTRUCTION

Many attempts at arterial reconstruction by suture, vessel graft, or prostheses in these cases of secondary rupture of the carotid artery have met with little success. The almost invariably infected field condemns prosthetic and autogenous vein grafts. Recently, Stoney and Wylie (1970) have reported successful replacement of the carotid artery (even in the presence of infection) with an autogenous arterial graft obtained from the hypogastric or common iliac vessels in a small series of cases.

Rupture of the Innominate Artery

Erosion of the trachea by an indwelling tracheostomy tube is a well-recognized potential complication. The common metal tracheal tube with a 90-degree curve will frequently cause this pressure and should be replaced by the 45-degree model in all operating rooms. Cases have been reported of rupture of the innominate artery into the trachea anteriorly from these ill-fitting or unusually low-placed metal tracheostomy tubes (Myers and Pilch, 1969). Pressure necrosis of the tracheal or vessel walls from an inflated endotracheal rubber cuff (used for administering positive pressure respiratory assistance) has also been implicated as a causative factor. These complications have been attributed to low placement of the tracheostomy (below the third cartilaginous ring) and failure to deflate the balloon cuff at regular intervals. Even two hours of pressure will cause ulceration of tracheal mucosa, and such postoperative cuffs should be used only in urgent situations. If hemorrhage does result, however, temporary control may be obtained by inflating the balloon and packing the trachea against the posterior wall of the manubrium. Through a median sternotomy, access is then gained to the eroded vessels for repair by resection and direct end-to-end anastomosis (Silen and Spieker, 1965).

THORACIC DUCT FISTULAE

ETIOLOGY

Lymphatic fistulae are encountered in surgery of the head and neck almost exclusively as the result of failure to recognize either the right or left lymphatic chain in the root of the neck during radical neck dissection. The dominant left trunk (thoracic duct), which drains the cisterna chyli, is the most troublesome because of its greater volume of flow. As the lymphatic trunks emerge through the thoracic inlet, they course posterior to the aorta and arch posterior to the internal jugular vein (at times, 5 cm. above the clavicle) to enter the venous system at the junction of the subclavian and internal jugular veins. The anatomy of the thoracic duct varies considerably, frequently consisting of several trunks which may converge to enter either the internal jugular or subclavian vein rather than at the junction of these two. Though thin-walled and clear, the larger significant trunks can be identified with a little care, and the careful ligation of these at the time of division can prevent troublesome postoperative wound problems. The tendency for the skin flaps in this area to bridge from the clavicle to the neck and thereby fail to contour into the excavated cavity leaves a potential dead space behind the clavicular head that contributes to the persistent patency of these channels. The resultant accumulation of pooled chyle beneath the flaps clots poorly and tends to further elevate the flaps. Chyle was noted by Martin (1957) to deter wound healing. He stated, "The chyle infiltrated borders of a wound will always be slow to heal."

The use of suction catheters to oppose the cervical flaps to the deep neck and prevent fluid accumulation reduces the frequency of troublesome lymph fistulae.

MANAGEMENT

Serous drainage from beneath a skin flap which persists for more than seven days can be attributed most often to a lymphatic fistula. This can be confirmed by feeding the patient a fatty meal of Sudan III dye, which will appear in the drainage within approximately two hours (Bressler, 1953).

A light compression dressing to contour the skin flap to the resection bed and obliterate the dead space, in conjunction with

CHARACTERISTICS AND COMPONENTS OF THORACIC DUCT LYMPH

Pressure	@ 7mm. Hg
Flow	@ 100 ml./hr. (1500–3000 ml./day)
Reaction	Alkaline
Fat	2–5.6 gm.% (diet dependent)
Protein	3–6 gm.%
Na^+	130–140 mEq./l.
K^+	3.5–4.5 mEq./l.
Cl^-	90–100 mEq./l.
Lymphocytes	@ 1500 mm.[3]

Figure 28-15. Significant characteristics and components of thoracic duct lymph. Volume losses may reach 1200 cc. to 2500 cc. per day. A persistent major lymphatic fistula will result in severe protein, fluid, and electrolyte losses requiring supplementation.

repeated aspirations or drainage, is usually effective in closing most fistulae. If this is not successful, then the wound must be re-explored, and the leaking duct identified and ligated. When the opening cannot be identified, the open wound is packed, or a muscle flap of one of the adjacent strap muscles is sutured into the area to seal the leak.

Apart from the deleterious effect on flap adherence and wound healing, persistent fistulae result in serious nutritional losses (Fig. 28-15). Depending somewhat on the diet, flow may reach as much as 2000 cc. per day (Lampson, 1948). The milky, watery fluid may contain as much as 5.2 to 5.6 gm. of fat per 100 ml. and 3 to 6 gm of protein per 100 ml. (Klepser and Berry, 1954). This may cause a loss of 100 gm. of fat and 120 gm. of protein, or 1400 calories per day. Weight loss of 5 lb. per week has been observed in some patients with thoracic duct fistulae (Crandall et al., 1943). The potential significance of this nutritional loss was pointed out by Treves in 1898 at Johns Hopkins (before successful suture of a fistula had been carried out) when he commented, "In every case death must follow (in a period of weeks rather than months) from marasmus consequent upon the discharge" (Cushing, 1898). Therefore, detailed attention to replacement therapy is essential in any major lymphatic fistula. A high-protein, low-fat diet, supplemented with vitamins, is indicated along with salt replacement.

OTHER CRITICAL COMPLICATIONS OF RADICAL HEAD AND NECK SURGERY

POSTOPERATIVE AIRWAY OBSTRUCTION

Maintenance of a *secure* airway is a basic responsibility of the head and neck surgeon; yet, each year many patients are lost in the postoperative period following surgery of the oropharynx and neck from complications of airway obstruction.

Not every patient having major surgery of the head and neck will require a tracheostomy, but those involving extensive dissection or resection around the tongue, hypopharynx, or mandibular arch should have a tracheostomy, preferably performed at the initiation of the procedure. Massive lingual edema or a hematoma in the hypopharynx in the postoperative period not only can cause obstruction of the airway, but also can create difficulties in reintubation or in performing a later tracheostomy when a life-threatening crisis demands expediency. Loss of the hyomandibular complex which supports the larynx following resection of the mandibular arch invariably leads to glottic dysfunction and airway problems.

Excessive manipulation of the larynx around an endotracheal tube can lead to postoperative laryngeal edema, particularly whenever the head and neck must be turned, flexed, or extended repeatedly during the operative procedure. When such occurs, a planned tracheostomy is judicious. Injury to the recurrent laryngeal nerve during the ablative surgery is also an indication for tracheostomy.

Accidental dislodgment of the tracheal cannula in the early postoperative period is particularly prone to occur in the fat, short-necked individual. If too short a cannula is used, the tip may slip out of the tracheal stoma to lie in the paratracheal tissues and go undetected by the inexperienced nurse or house officer. Likewise, premature removal or change of the cannula, before a definite tracheocutaneous sinus tract is formed, is extremely hazardous in these thick-necked individuals. Prompt replacement of the tracheostomy tube in a struggling hypoxic patient can be exceedingly difficult. The use of a long cannula secured with sutures to the skin margins for the first three to four days will help obviate these problems as well as lessen the potential constriction of the cervical tissues by the usual cannula tape encircling the neck. Maintaining the latter under proper tension to secure the tracheal cannula yet not jeopardize the cervical flaps can be a problem. Direct suturing of the skin margins to the tracheal stoma, or the use of stay sutures to a tracheal window or flap brought out through the stoma and taped to the skin, facilitates reintubation should the cannula become dislodged in the early postoperative period.

Rarely, an upper mediastinal hemorrhage or abscess may lead to obstruction of the substernal portion of the trachea. The latter can usually be drained from above through the neck, but a median sternotomy affords the most expeditious exposure for a bleeding mediastinal vessel. Temporary control of the bleeding can usually be achieved by packing the wound from the neck as an emergency maneuver while the operating room is being made ready.

Tracheo-esophageal fistula

Just as an ill-fitting or ill-placed tracheal cannula may erode the anterior walls of the trachea and the innominate artery, similar factors can lead to erosion of the posterior wall of the trachea and creation of a tracheo-esophageal fistula. A sudden increase in tracheal secretions or the occurrence of subcutaneous emphysema should elicit a suspicion of a tracheo-esophageal fistula, especially in the patient who has had a tracheal cannula indwelling for a prolonged period of time, or who has required an inflated tracheal cuff balloon. However, it does not necessarily take a prolonged period of time for ischemic pressure to produce necrosis, and, therefore, a fistula may develop early in the postoperative period as well. The use of a 45-degree-angle cannula instead of the customary 90-degree-angle model has significantly reduced the incidence of these serious complications.

Problems of Postoperative Aspiration

All patients requiring ablative surgery of the oropharynx experience some degree of impairment of swallowing. For some, the degree of impairment is such that not only are they unable to handle oral feedings, but even their own salivary secretions pose a constant threat of aspiration. Palatal defects resulting in the inability to seal off the oral from the nasal cavity can alter the normal pressure mechanics necessary to initiate deglutition. Loss of mobility of the tongue from scarring, binding of the tongue from a tight primary closure, or nerve paralysis or resection, interferes with the ability to propel liquids or solids to the posterior pharynx and initiate swallowing. The normal elevation of the larynx during swallowing depends on the support of the hyomandibular muscle and tendinous complex. Injuries to the superior laryngeal nerves may produce hypesthesia of the glottic inlet and predispose to aspiration. Mechanical obstruction from hypopharyngeal strictures may compound the problem. The nasogastric tube has been incriminated as acting as a "wick" to direct secretions into the larynx from its juxtaposition to the glottic inlet as the tube lies in the pharynx.

Not only is aspiration a threat to airway obstruction, but the secondary pneumonia and consequent septicemia are equally as serious in these patients, who frequently have some degree of chronic bronchopulmonary disease. Furthermore, the effectiveness of their cough mechanism is impaired from the surgical procedure and tracheostomy.

Palatal defects should be closed, the tongue freed by skin graft or flaps, the larynx supported, and pharyngeal strictures released whenever these deformities exist. The cervical feeding esophagostomy is gaining popularity as a replacement for the nasogastric tube, not only for its safety advantages, but also for its greater comfort to the patient.

A few patients may be able to overcome these deformities and learn compensatory maneuvers to handle their secretions and oral feedings, but this is not the usual occurrence in the older citizen who incurs significant derangement of his swallowing mechanism. They need all the help they can get to prevent them from becoming oral cripples requiring laryngectomy.

SUMMARY

Complications in head and neck surgery are basically problems in wound healing.

They are more easily prevented than treated. Tissue injury incites inflammation. Nonviable tissue and foreign bodies deter wound healing and invite infection. The metabolic demands of repair require healthy, vascularized tissues. The reparative process culminates in a cicatrix of fibrous tissue, poorly vascularized, nonelastic, and unable to function in the same manner as the tissue which it has replaced. The prevention and management of complications of major surgery of the head and neck entails a thorough understanding of the fundamentals involved in the physiologic response to tissue injury, and reparative process and the application of these fundamentals in methods of reconstruction.

REFERENCES

Bakamjian, V. Y.: A two staged method for pharyngo-esophageal reconstruction with a primary pectoral skin flap. Plast. Reconstr. Surg., 36:173, 1965.

Bakamjian, V. Y., Culf, W. K., and Bales, H. W.: The versatility of the medially based delto-pectoral skin flap and primary reconstruction in head and neck surgery. Trans. of the Fourth International Congress of Plastic Surgery, Oct., 1967.

Barisoni, D., and Ranzolin, G.: The action of kallikrein on tubed pedicle flaps in rats. Brit. J. Plast. Surg., 20:341, 1967.

Bradham, R. R., and Takaro, T.: The nature and significance of the thoracic duct—subclavian vein junction. Surgery, 64:643, 1968.

Bressler, S., et al.: Traumatic chylothorax following esophageal resection. J. Thorac. Surg., 26:321, 1953.

Chandler, J. R., and Ponzoli, V. A.: The use of double transverse incisions in major head and neck surgery. Ann. Otorhinolaryng., 78:757, 1969.

Cheek, H. B., and Rise, E. N.: Carotid artery protection and a new technique. Arch. Otolaryng., 86:179, 1967.

Coleman, C. C.: Local flaps for reconstruction after head and neck tumor surgery. Plast. Reconstr. Surg., 42:225, 1968.

Conley, J. J.: Carotid artery protection. Arch. Otolaryng., 75:530, 1962.

Conley, J. J.: The prevention of carotid artery hemorrhage by the use of rotating tissue flaps. Surgery, 34:186, 1953.

Corso, P. E., and Gerold, F. P.: The use of autogenous dermis for protection of the carotid artery and pharyngeal suture lines in radical head and neck surgery. Surg. Gynec. Obstet., 117:37, 1963.

Cramer, L. M., and Culf, N. K.: Use of pedicle flap tissues in conjunction with a neck dissection. In Gaisford, J. (ed.): Symposium on Cancer of the Head and Neck. St. Louis, C. V. Mosby Company, 1969.

Crandall, L. A., et al.: A study of lymph flow from a patient with a thoracic duct fistula. Gastroenterology, 1:1040, 1943.

Cushing, H. W.: Operative wounds of the thoracic duct. Report of a case with suture of the duct. Ann. Surg., 27:719, 1898.

DeForest, H. P.: Surgery of the thoracic duct. Ann. Surg., 46:705, 1907.

DeVito, R. V.: Horizontal "T" incision for neck dissection. Plast. Reconstr. Surg., 43:538, 1969.

Eade, G. G.: The relationship between granulation tissue, bacteria, and skin grafts in burned patients. Plast. Reconstr. Surg., 22:42, 1958.

Edgerton, M. T.: Reconstructive surgery in treatment of oral, pharyngeal, and mandibular tumors. In Converse, J. M. (ed.): Reconstructive Plastic Surgery. Philadelphia, W. B. Saunders Co., 1964.

Edgerton, M. T., Gee, R., and Hoffmeister, F. S.: Effects of x-ray irradiation on skin capillary clearance. Surg. Forum (American College of Surgeons), 1953.

Erdelyi, R.: Tubular flap procedure for the closure of a large pharyngeal fistula. Brit. J. Plast. Surg., 9:72, 1956.

Fitz-Hugh, G. S., and Sly, D. E.: Elective cervical esophagostomy. Ann. Otol., 76:804, 1967.

Fraser, C. G.: A more plastic incision for radical neck dissection. Plast. Reconstr. Surg., 8:465, 1951.

Frederickson, J. M., and Strahan, R. W.: Esophageal reconstruction for heavily irradiated patients. Arch. Otolaryng., 90:164, 1969.

Goldman, J. L., and Friedman, W. H.: High dose preoperative irradiation in cancer of the larynx. Otolaryng. Clin. N. Amer., 2:473, 1969.

Goulian, D., Jr.: The use of bromphenol blue in the assay of rheomacrodex effect on flap viability. Plast. Reconstr. Surg., 39:227, 1967.

Grabb, W. C., and Oneal, R.: The effect of low molecular weight dextran on the survival of experimental skin flaps. Plast. Reconstr. Surg., 30:649, 1966.

Grillo, H. C., and Edmunds, L. H.: Radical neck dissection after irradiation. Ann. Surg., 161:361, 1965.

Grimm, G.: Plastic operations in tissue damage by irradiation. Acta Chir. Plast. (Praha), 10:303, 1968.

Habel, D. W.: Surgical complications in irradiated patients. Arch. Otolaryng., 82:382, 1965.

Holsti, L. R.: Clinical experience with split course x-ray. Radiology, 92:591, 1969.

Kernahan, D. A., Zingg, W., and Kay, C. W.: The effect of hyperbaric oxygen on the survival of experimental skin flaps. Plast. Reconstr. Surg., 36:19, 1965.

Ketcham, A. S., and Haye, R. C.: Spontaneous carotid artery hemorrhage after head and neck surgery. Amer. J. Surg., 110:649, 1965.

Ketcham, A. S., and Smith, R.: Elective esophagostomy. Amer. J. Surg., 104:682, 1962.

Ketchum, L. D., Ellis, S. S., Robinson, D. W., and Masters, F. W.: Vascular augmentation of pedicled tissue by combined histamine iontophoresis and hypertensive perfusion. Plast. Reconstr. Surg., 39:138, 1967.

Kiehn, C. L., and Des Prez, J. D.: Effects of local hypothermia on pedicle flap tissue. Plast. Reconstr. Surg., 25:349, 1960.

Klepser, R. G., and Berry, J. F.: The diagnosis and surgical management of chylothorax with the aid of lipophilic dyes. Dis. Chest, 25:409, 1954.

Lampson, R. S.: Traumatic chylothorax. J. Thorac. Surg., 17:778, 1948.

Lipshultz, H., and Stetzer, S. S.: Extra radical surgery of the neck. Ann. Surg., 168:901, 1968.

Loeb, M., and McQuarrie, D. C.: Management of simultaneous bilateral radical neck dissection. Surg. Gynec. Obstet., 127:1322, 1968.

Loré, J. M.: Vascular techniques with head and neck cancer. Otolaryng. Clin. N. Amer., 2:515, 1969.

MacFee, W. F.: Transverse incisions for neck dissection. Ann. Surg., 151:279, 1960.

Martin, H.: Surgery of Head and Neck Tumors. pp. 90–91. New York, (Hoeber) Harper, 1957.

Maxwell, E.: Surgical techniques following irradiation of the neck. J. Laryng., 77:872, 1963.

McCall, J. W., Whitaker, C. W., and Hendershot, E. L.: Rupture of the common carotid artery following radical neck surgery in radiated cases. Arch. Otolaryng., 69:431, 1959.

McFarlane, R. M., and Wermuth, R. E.: The use of hyperbaric oxygen to prevent necrosis in experimental pedicle flaps and composite skin grafts. Plast. Reconstr. Surg., 37:422, 1966.

McGregor, I. A.: The temporal flap in intra-oral reconstruction. In Gaisford, J. (ed.): Symposium of Cancer of the Head and Neck. St. Louis, C. V. Mosby Company, 1969.

Moore, O., and Baker, H. W.: Carotid artery ligation in surgery of the head and neck. CA., 8:712, 1955.

Moore, O. S.: Bilateral neck dissection. Surg. Clin. N. Amer., 49:277, 1969.

Moore, O. S., Karlan, M., and Sigler, L.: Factors influencing the safety of carotid ligation. Amer. J. Surg., 118:667, 1969.

Moran, A. G. D., and Leonard, J. R.: Protection of the carotid in radical neck surgery. Brit. J. Surg., 55:648, 1968.

Murphy, W. T.: Complications of radiation therapy. In Artz, C., and Hardy, J. D. (eds.): Complications in Surgery and Their Management. 2nd ed., Philadelphia, W. B. Saunders Company, 1967.

Myers, M. B., and Cherry, G.: Enhancement of survival in devascularized pedicles by the use of phenoxybenzamine. Plast. Reconstr. Surg., 41:254, 1968.

Myers, R. S., and Pilch, Y. H.: Temporary control of tracheal-innominate artery fistula. Ann. Surg., 170:149, 1969.

Nichols, R. T.: Bilateral radical neck dissection. Amer. J. Surg., 117:377, 1969.

Ogura, J. G., et al.: Surgical treatment of carcinoma of the larynx, pharynx, base of tongue and cervical esophagus. Surgery, 52:29, 1969.

Pevow, F. M.: Complications of cervical esophagostomy. Arch. Otolaryng., 90:171, 1969.

Reed, G. F., and Rabuzzi, D. D.: Neck dissection. Otolaryng. Clin. N. Amer., 2:547, 1969.

Royster, H. P.: Complications of surgery for cancer of the head and neck. In Artz, C., and Hardy, J. D. (eds.): Complications in Surgery and Their Management. 2nd ed., Philadelphia, W. B. Saunders Company, 1967.

Schweitzer, R. J.: Use of muscle flaps for protection of carotid artery after radical neck dissection. Ann. Surg., 156:811, 1962.

Shaw, D. T., and Payne, R. L., Jr.: One staged tubed abdominal flaps. Surg. Gynec. Obstet., 83:205, 1946.

Silen, W., and Spieker, D.: Fatal hemorrhage from the innominate artery after tracheostomy. Ann. Surg., 162:1005, 1965.

Silverstone, S. M., Goldman, J. L., and Rosen, H. D.: Combined therapy, radiation, and surgery for advanced cancer of laryngopharynx. Amer. J. Roentgen., 90:1023, 1963.

Staley, C. J.: A muscle cover for the carotid artery after radical neck dissection. Amer. J. Surg., 102:815, 1961.

Stark, R. B.: Immediate complications of head and neck surgery. Surg. Clin. N. Amer., 44:305, 1964.

Stell, P. M.: Catastrophic hemorrhage after major neck surgery. Brit. J. Surg., 56:525, 1969.

Stell, P. M.: Complications encountered in head and neck surgery. J. Laryng., 83:671, 1969.

Stell, P. M.: Transverse incisions for radical neck. Brit. J. Surg., 56:286, 1969.

Stoney, R. J., and Wylie, E. J.: Arterial autografts. Surgery, 67:18, 1970.

Strong, E. W.: Preoperative radiation and radical neck dissection. Surg. Clin. N. Amer., 49:271, 1969.

Sturman, M. J., Terry, J. L., Biggs, J. A., and Bennett, J. E.: The prevention of necrosis in congested tubed pedicles. Plast. Reconstr. Surg., 34:555, 1964.

Teloh, A., et al.: A histopathologic study of radiation injury of the skin. Surg. Gynec. Obstet., 90:335, 1950.

Thompson, N.: The subcutaneous dermis graft. Plast. Reconstr. Surg., 26:1, 1960.

Totter, J. R.: Mechanism of radiation injury. Eneron Health Ser. (Radiol. Health), 33:2, 1968.

VandenBerg, H. J., Jr., et al.: A comparison of wound healing between irradiated and non-irradiated patients after radical neck dissection. Amer. J. Surg., 110:557, 1965.

Wald, A.: High pressure oxygen and flap survival. Surg. Forum, 19:497, 1968.

Warren, S.: Effects of radiation on normal tissue. Arch. Path., 35:323, 1943.

Zovickian, A.: Pharyngeal fistulas: repair and prevention by using a mastoid-occiput based shoulder flap. Plast. Reconstr. Surg., 19:355, 1957.

CHAPTER 29

HEMATOLOGIC CRISES IN SURGERY

by HAROLD LAUFMAN, M.D., Ph.D.*

Harold Laufman was born in Wisconsin and was educated at the University of Chicago and at Rush Medical College, where he was a member of Alpha Omega Alpha. He received his Ph.D. in Surgery at Northwestern and after successive promotions became full professor there in 1962. He served with distinction in the European Theater in World War II, and accumulated a further large clinical experience thereafter. In 1965 he was appointed Director of the Institute for Surgical Studies and Attending Surgeon, Montefiore Hospital, and Professor of Surgery, Albert Einstein College of Medicine. The author of many important publications and the recipient of numerous honors, he has a deep interest in blood problems.

The surgeon's constant encounter with blood as a tissue and as the prime nutrient medium for all body organs requires that his knowledge of its pathologic and physiologic changes be at least as comprehensive as his knowledge of the conditions of other tissues with which he deals. This chapter will consider five of the most critical conditions the surgeon may encounter in relation to either qualitative or quantitative alterations of the blood. These conditions are critical blood transfusion reactions, abnormal bleeding, hemophilia, hematologic reactions to extracorporeal circulation, and hematologic reactions to organ transplantation.

CRITICAL BLOOD TRANSFUSION REACTIONS

EMERGENCY TRANSFUSIONS — CHOICE OF BLOOD

When massive amounts of blood are required for emergency transfusion, it is permissible to use blood from group O, Rh-negative (universal donors). One, two, or even three units of universal-donor blood may be given to sustain life while typing and crossmatching are carried out. If this program is adopted, several basic principles and constraints must be kept in mind:

1. As soon as type-matched blood is available, it should be given in place of the universal-type blood, in order to avoid a possible train of events related to difficulties in crossmatching, which mount as the group O blood exceeds one-half the blood volume. Among these problems are hemolysis, hemoglobinemia, and intravascular agglutination.

2. If more than three units of group-O blood have been administered, reversion to type-matched blood is not advised for at least a week.

3. Universal-type blood should not be used at all if, in the judgment of the surgeon, blood volume can be adequately maintained with a nonblood solution until blood can be obtained by the standard methods of typing and crossmatching. In addition to ABO typing and Rh typing, the Coombs test is used to identify agglutinative antibodies coated on the red cells. The Coombs test becomes more important as multiple transfusions are given.

4. Reactions to "low-titer" universal-donor blood are rare as long as the antibody titer is under 1:200. However, reactions do occur, largely because of a discrepancy in

---

*The author wishes to pay tribute to several collaborators who contributed chapters to the monograph entitled *Hematologic Problems in Surgery,* by Harold Laufman and Robert B. Erichson, from which the material in this chapter was adapted. These collaborators are Parvis Lalezari on Bleeding Problems, Elliott Jacobson on Extracorporeal Circulation, and Kenneth Richards and Frank J. Veith on Organ Transplantation.

635

the agglutinating and immunizing properties of the antibodies.

GENERAL PRINCIPLES

When the surgeon orders blood for transfusion, he makes certain basic assumptions
pertinent to the reliability and responsibility
of the blood bank that supplies the blood.
He can reasonably make the following assumptions: (1) Donors have been properly
screened for hepatitis, malaria, syphilis, and
other diseases transmissible by blood.
(2) Regulations regarding the techniques of
drawing and storing the blood have been
scrupulously followed. (3) The blood is
stored under acceptable conditions and no
longer than a specified length of time.

Blood stored in glass bottles with the usual
acid-citrate-dextrose (ACD) solution undergoes changes that make it unacceptable in
about 14 days. In plastic containers, blood
may not undergo these changes for up to
21 days.

Changes occurring in aged blood include
(1) fall in the pH of the blood; (2) rise in
sodium concentration in the erythrocytes
and fall in sodium content of the plasma;
(3) fall in intra-erythrocyte potassium and
rise in potassium content of the plasma;
(4) increase in cell fragility; and (5) escape
of hemoglobin from cells to plasma.

BANK BLOOD VS. FRESH BLOOD

Besides hemolysis due to aging, even
slight bacterial contamination, as well as the
failure to refrigerate the blood, will result
in hemolysis of the stored blood. Patients
who receive this kind of hemolyzed blood
will experience hypotension and renal
damage similar to or worse than that accompanying mismatched blood transfusion.
Patients in shock or with renal damage react
much more severely to the infusion of slightly
hemolyzed blood than do other patients. In
addition to accentuating the renal damage
in shock patients, overage blood may increase hyperkalemia, hemoglobinemia, and
hemoglobinuria.

Fresh blood is defined as blood that is
infused into a recipient within a few hours
after it is withdrawn from a donor. Whereas
bank blood is ordinarily preserved in citrate
solution, fresh blood may be given by direct

transfusion in silicone-lined tubes without
an anticoagulant. It may be heparinized, it
may be citrated, or it may be collected with a
chelating agent, such as EDTA. In the case
of EDTA treatment, the blood is ion-ex-
changed and lacks platelets.

Reasons for administering fresh blood are
many. Viable leukocytes and platelets may
be obtained by direct transfusion. The proteins in citrated fresh blood, which are
available as normally effective molecules,
including immune bodies, globulin, fibrinogen, and prothrombin, are therefore effective
in treating bleeding problems caused by
deficiencies in these factors. However, unless fresh citrated blood is collected in a
plastic container and used rapidly, most of
the leukocytes and platelets are useless to
the recipient. Heparinized fresh blood is
used if massive transfusion of citrated blood
has given cause for concern over citrate
toxicity.

Untoward effects of blood transfusion
occur in some 5 per cent of recipients. The
complications are categorized as incompatibility, reactions due to bacterial contamination, allergic reactions, reactions
unique to massive transfusion, and leukocyte
immune reactions.

Incompatibility

The most frequent of the critical, acute
transfusion reactions is the one caused by
administration of incompatible blood. It is
estimated to occur in 3 per cent of transfusions. Its manifestations are rapid intravascular hemolysis, oligemic renal failure,
and death.

CAUSES. Red cells are antigenic and,
when introduced into a sensitized individual,
may be rapidly destroyed intravascularly or
more gradually removed extravascularly by
the reticuloendothelial system. Antigens in
the ABO and Rh systems are most often
responsible for severe reactions. Antibodies
to the A and B antigens occur "naturally,"
that is, without known prior exposure to the
antigen. Most other antibodies, including
those in the Rh system, result from prior
exposure to the antigen by means of transfused blood or by fetal-maternal sensitization.

Antibodies present in transfused blood
may also produce a reaction. This is due almost invariably to the administration of
group O blood to a group A, B, or AB indi-

vidual. Reactions are usually, but not invariably, milder than those which occur with the administration of incompatible red cells. The administration of universal-donor group-O blood to patients of blood groups A, B, or AB is generally safe when bloods with high titers of anti-A and anti-B are eliminated.

Incompatible transfusions may result from mistaken identification of recipient or donor bloods, transfusion of the "right bottle to the wrong patient," or inaccurate typing or crossmatching.

MANIFESTATIONS. Symptoms and signs of rapid intravascular hemolysis are characteristically dramatic. Minutes after the start of transfusion the patient develops a flushed face, chest and back pain, fever and chills, tachycardia, and tachypnea.

Plasma and urine samples taken at this time show reddish discoloration and evidence of hemoglobinemia and hemoglobinuria. The patient may have no further untoward effects or he may develop hypotensive shock within hours, followed shortly thereafter by evidence of acute renal failure.

Other laboratory manifestations of hemolysis soon follow. The serum bilirubin rises, reaching its peak three to six hours after transfusion and the serum haptoglobin decreases and remains low for several days. Methemalbumin, the product of albumin binding with hemoglobin, becomes evident in the serum in approximately five hours and persists for one to two days.

Occasionally a patient may have no obvious symptomatology at the time of transfusion only to develop shock and acute renal failure subsequently.

DETECTION OF REACTION IN ANESTHETIZED PATIENTS. Anesthetized patients may show only unexplained diffuse bleeding due to defibrination, a common accompaniment of incompatible transfusion. Other evidence of a transfusion reaction in patients under anesthesia is the appearance of hemoglobinuria or hemolysis.

DIAGNOSTIC MEASURES. When an incompatible transfusion reaction is suspected, the following diagnostic measures should be taken:

1. A sample of recipient venous blood should be carefully withdrawn into a test tube containing anticoagulant, the sample centrifuged, and the plasma examined for the red or yellow discoloration indicative of hemoglobin or bilirubin staining. Hemoglobin is demonstrable in the plasma immediately after an intravascular reaction and persists for approximately eight to twelve hours, depending on the severity of hemolysis. Plasma bilirubin reaches its maximum in three to six hours. Inspection for both pigments may be greatly facilitated by comparison with a pretransfusion sample. Following inspection, quantitative hemoglobin and bilirubin determinations should be performed on the samples.

2. A urine sample should be inspected. Heme pigments may stain the urine red or black. This test must be done promptly, since heme derivatives may be present only very transiently.

3. The blood remaining in the donor bottle and in the donor pilot tube, as well as samples of recipient pre-transfusion and post-transfusion blood should again be typed and crossmatched. When incompatibility exists, retyping of the ABO and Rh groups will usually reveal the offending antigen, but more extensive typing procedures may be required.

TREATMENT. The treatment of transfusion reactions due to incompatibility depends upon what the manifestations are and when they are recognized.

Transfusion should be discontinued at the first sign of an untoward reaction. The patient should be closely observed, with particular attention to blood pressure and urinary output. Hypovolemia should be appropriately treated with compatible blood, plasma, or plasma-volume expander. Hypotensive shock may require the administration of a pressor agent, such as levarterenol.

Acute renal failure due to hemoglobin deposition in nephrons, damaged from shock or other sequelae of the transfusion reaction, is the major factor in morbidity and mortality. Early administration of mannitol, an osmotic diuretic, may prevent this complication. It should be administered when the diagnosis of an incompatible reaction is made; 100 ml. of a 20 per cent aqueous solution should be given intravenously over a five-minute period as often as necessary to maintain a urine flow of 40 ml. or more per hour. No more than 100 gm. should be given within a 24-hour interval. Mannitol should be discontinued as soon as the patient is able to maintain a urine flow of 40 ml. per hour without its use. If the urine flow decreases to less than 30 ml. per hour despite these measures, treatment for acute renal failure must be initiated.

Bacterial Contamination

Blood may become contaminated by bacteria in a variety of ways and may, as a result, cause a reaction in the recipient, ranging from transient fever to shock and death.

Contamination may result from bacteremia in the donor, inadequate sterilization of the blood container or phlebotomy equipment, or the introduction of unsterile cannulas into the donor bottle. Gram-positive organisms that are able to survive and grow during storage at 4° C. are usually saprophytic diphtheroids, which produce fever only. Gram-negative organisms, on the other hand, elaborate a virulent endotoxin, which produces a clinical picture of vomiting, diarrhea, abdominal pain, shock, and renal failure, and the endotoxemia is usually fatal. As little as 50 ml. of blood may produce a reaction. The presence of organisms in the transfusion bottle may be demonstrated by staining a drop of remaining blood. Subsequent confirmation can be obtained by culturing the donor blood at 37° C. and under 30° C., the latter because some of the causative organisms do not grow at body temperature. When the diagnosis is suspected, transfusion should be immediately discontinued. If the donor bottle contains gram-negative organisms, the administration of one or more appropriate antibiotics, such as cephalothin, should be started. Once established, however, the endotoxemia is usually fatal. The only really effective therapy is preventive—observance of meticulous aseptic technique in the handling of blood. Brownish discoloration of blood should be considered a suspicious sign of contamination, and such blood should not be used for transfusion.

Allergic Reactions

Approximately 1 per cent of patients undergoing transfusion have an urticarial or other allergic reaction. Such reactions are usually benign and are treated satisfactorily by discontinuation of the transfusion. Symptoms may be alleviated by the administration of an antihistaminic compound. The reactions are presumably a result of the presence in donor blood of an antigen or antibody whose immunologic counterpart is present in the recipient.

Rarely, allergic reactions assume a more serious, life-endangering form—angioneurotic edema, laryngeal edema, or bronchial asthma—and require therapy with epinephrine or corticosteroids or both, and, occasionally, tracheostomy.

Massive Blood Transfusion

In addition to increasing the incidence of complications that occur with routine blood transfusion, massive transfusion is associated with several additional hazards.

BLEEDING TENDENCY. A bleeding diathesis often accompanies massive transfusion, owing largely to the depletion of platelets and certain clotting factors in stored bank blood. Bank blood is virtually devoid of viable platelets after one day's storage.

The thrombocytopenia may be due in part to factors other than dilution with platelet-poor blood. Individuals undergoing transfusion with normal plasma become thrombocytopenic, and it is possible that a thrombocytopenogenic substance present in normal blood may be partially responsible for the thrombocytopenia of massive transfusion.

The coagulation factors that are labile in stored blood are factors V and VIII. They may therefore be reduced for patients who receive large volumes of bank blood, although this decrease is usually less striking and its contribution to bleeding less important than that of thrombocytopenia.

A reasonable preventive measure, when feasible, is the administration of one unit of fresh blood for every four or five units of stored blood when large amounts of blood must be transfused within a brief period. The fresh blood should be less than six hours old, and preferably less than four, in order to contain a significant number of viable platelets. Treatment of the bleeding diathesis should be aimed at replenishing the missing factors with fresh blood, platelet-rich plasma, or platelet concentrates.

HYPERKALEMIA. The potassium concentration of blood gradually increases during storage from between 3 and 5 mEq. per L to 15 or 20 mEq. per L. This phenomenon is due to the release of potassium from the red cells into the plasma. Massive transfusion may therefore cause hyperkalemia, but this is rarely so except in patients otherwise predisposed to potassium retention, as, for example, those with renal failure. Consequently, an attempt should be made to use relatively fresh blood, preferably blood two to three days old or less, when giving transfusions to patients prone to hyperkalemia.

HYPOTHERMIA. Rapid transfusion of large amounts of cold blood may lower body temperature. Recent studies suggest that this is an important factor in the high incidence of cardiac arrest associated with massive transfusion, occurring in 12 of 25 patients receiving more than 3000 ml. of blood at 50 to 100 ml. per minute. Rapid warming of the blood to body temperature during administration reduced the incidence of cardiac arrest to 6.8 per cent in comparable patients.

ACID-BASE ABNORMALITIES. Massive transfusion may produce metabolic acidosis owing to the gradual acidification of stored blood from a pH of 7, when freshly drawn, to about 6.6 in 21 days. Patients to whom such blood is given often have a pre-existing acidosis associated with diminished tissue perfusion. The condition is then aggravated, rather than helped, by the transfusion. Howland and associates obtained a significant decrease in mortality when patients receiving 20 or more units of blood were given 44.6 mEq. of sodium bicarbonate for every 5 units of blood administered. The acidosis may be transformed after several hours into a metabolic alkalosis, owing to the rapid metabolism of citrate with a resultant excess of sodium ions. The alkalosis reaches its peak on the third post-transfusion day. Correction does not appear to be necessary except when alkalosis of another source, such as that of pyloric obstruction, is thereby increased.

CITRATE INTOXICATION. This is a rare complication of massive transfusion due in part to the calcium-binding property of the citrate in the anticoagulant. It is most apt to occur in patients with liver disease, whose ability to metabolize citrate is impaired. Citrate intoxication is characteristically manifested by muscle tremors and electrocardiographic changes (prolongation of the Q-T interval). Intravenous administration of calcium gluconate effectively prevents or treats citrate poisoning. Accordingly, a good prophylactic measure is the administration of 10 ml. of 10 per cent calcium gluconate for each liter of blood transfused, when blood is given at a rate in excess of 1 unit per five minutes.

Leukocyte Immune Reactions

Reactions due to the leukocyte immune response are listed here, not so much because their manifestations are critical, but because they can be perplexing. Leukocytes are antigenic, and leukocyte antibodies are not uncommon in multiparous females as well as in persons who have had many transfusions. Transfusion of leukocytes into sensitized individuals may cause a reaction characterized by fever and chills. This reaction is usually benign, but it may be severe. The fever occurs within two hours of the start of transfusion and persists for several hours. Leukocyte immune reactions probably account for most recurrent febrile episodes associated with transfusion. Payne was able to demonstrate leukocyte antibodies in 32 of 49 patients with a history of recurrent febrile reactions. The reactions can be prevented in most cases by removal of the buffy coat, which contains the bulk of the leukocytes, prior to transfusion. This procedure should be attempted when blood is to be given to an individual with a history of repeated febrile episodes following blood transfusion.

BLEEDING PROBLEMS

Acute, unexpected bleeding during or shortly after operation in the absence of an accountable surgical source is a vexing problem that may catch the surgeon without a definite plan for management. Under trying and often desperate circumstances, there is neither time nor inclination to run a battery of time-consuming hematologic tests. On the other hand, experience has shown that empiric treatment, such as the administration of fresh blood without the benefit of a hematologic diagnosis, cannot always be depended upon to solve all bleeding problems. In this section a plan of diagnosis and management will be outlined that is designed to cope realistically with bleeding emergencies of uncertain origin during or shortly after surgical operations. The plan is based upon three features: clinical judgment, rapid blood tests, and selective treatment.

CLINICAL JUDGMENT

PREOPERATIVE MEASURES. Pre-existing disorders, congenital or acquired, would presumably be exposed by a thorough history, careful physical examination, and necessary preoperative laboratory tests. Adequate precautions would then be taken to prevent or to meet acute bleeding resulting from the known defects.

In the absence of pre-existing defects, the causes of unexpected bleeding may be narrowed down to some six possibilities: (1) bleeding from a surgical source, (2) fibrinolysis, (3) defibrination, (4) thrombocytopenia from massive bank blood transfusion, (5) anticoagulants and their antagonists, and (6) mixed clotting problems.

CIRCUMSTANCES IMMEDIATELY PRECEDING BLEEDING. Knowledge of these circumstances will help to pinpoint the cause. For example, the administration of more than 5 pints of blood in succession prior to the onset of abnormal bleeding would immediately raise the suspicion of thrombocytopenic bleeding due to massive transfusion of bank blood. Estimation of platelet count may confirm this impression. Treatment, ordinarily successful, can then be carried out with virtually no delay. If, on the other hand, a patient bleeds abnormally after 1 or less than 1 pint of transfused blood, the odds are in favor of hemolysis and intravascular coagulation due to a mismatch. Other circumstances before bleeding include the known administration of anticoagulants and their antagonists. Knowledge of such circumstances is usually sufficient to institute rational specific treatment.

CLINICAL MANIFESTATIONS OF BLEEDING. The combination of careful observation of the character of the bleeding and attention to the patient's response to supportive therapy provides valuable diagnostic information. If the bleeding occurs during operation, the surgeon is usually in a position to recognize its source and to deal with it directly. When hypotension occurs shortly after operation, the possibility of occult bleeding must be given serious consideration.

Bleeding confined to a body space is unlikely to be caused by a hemostatic defect. If the hypotension persists despite good aeration and supportive measures, and if it responds to the transfusion of blood, waxing and waning with the administration and the withholding of blood, the most likely cause is bleeding from the surgical site, and reoperation must be considered. In any case, examination of the patient must not be neglected in favor of examination of the blood.

On pragmatic grounds, it may be assumed that blood loss sufficient to require almost constant transfusion of blood to maintain blood pressure is due to a surgical cause until proved otherwise. Bleeding due to acquired coagulation defects is rarely so rapid as to require constant replacement by transfusion in order to maintain blood pressure. This is not to say that hypotension cannot be caused by bleeding from other causes, such as anticoagulant effects, but generally speaking, blood is not lost as rapidly when the cause is hematologic as it is when the cause is mechanical.

BLEEDING RELATED TO CLINICAL CONDITIONS. Advance knowledge of certain clinical conditions that run a good chance of being complicated by local or general coagulation defects will aid in narrowing down the number of possible causes for bleeding. For example, a likely cause for generalized oozing in a patient with carcinoma of the prostate is fibrinolysis, but in the absence of general fibrinolysis, local bleeding after prostatic surgery may be increased by urokinase present in the urinary tract. After obstetric delivery, severe hemorrhage may be due to such a well known cause as a retained placenta, but it should be known that in the absence of such a pathologic condition, postpartum bleeding may come from obstetric defibrination.

RAPID BLOOD TESTS

Blood testing to identify the cause of bleeding need not be time-consuming nor complicated. Results should be available in 10 to 15 minutes. Test tubes containing 3.8 per cent sodium citrate solution should be kept in readiness at all times in all operating rooms and in the recovery room.

Five simple tests, well known to most laboratory technicians and involving no unusual equipment, will provide virtually all the information required. These are:

1. *Partial Thromboplastin Time (PTT).* This is a sensitive screening test for detection of alterations in coagulation mechanisms, such as previously undiagnosed hemophilia, various coagulation factor defi-

ciencies, circulating anticoagulants, and so on. In our opinion, it should supplant the popular but nonspecific whole-blood clotting-time test when searching for causes of abnormal bleeding.

2. *Rapid estimate of the quantity of platelets.* Hematology technicians can be trained to look at a smear of blood and make a fairly accurate estimate of the platelet count. Platelet counts considerably under 100,000 may well implicate massive transfusion as a cause for bleeding. If the technician does not have the experience to make a rapid estimate, a legitimate platelet count may be done.

3. *Bleeding time.* Bleeding prolonged more than four minutes primarily denotes platelet abnormalities or vascular hemophilia (von Willebrand's disease). Bleeding time is normal in classic hemophilia.

4. *Prothrombin time.* An abnormal test may indicate intravascular coagulation, fibrinolysis, or liver dysfunction.

5. *Thrombin time.* Prolonged thrombin time indicates overheparinization, defibrination, or fibrinolysis.

If the thrombin time is prolonged, *a rapid test to estimate plasma fibrinogen* is valuable. By the simple expedient of serially diluting plasma with saline and adding thrombin to the dilutions, a fibrinogen titer is found. In normal plasma, a good clot forms at dilutions of 1:64 and beyond; in low fibrinogen-titer plasma, a clot will not form at 1:32 or even at higher concentrations.

SELECTIVE TREATMENT

The goal of treatment is to preserve life by stopping blood loss, maintaining vital processes, and eliminating the cause for blood loss. Occasionally these are antithetical, as, for example, when only bank blood is available and it must be used to preserve blood volume in the presence of an already existing platelet deficit caused by an excess of transfused bank blood. Selective treatment depends upon identification of all factors that contribute to the bleeding state.

In general, the *preservation of blood volume* in the presence of bleeding depends upon replacement of the lost blood. However, it is best to postpone one-for-one blood replacement—except in the case of rapid bleeding—until a fairly good idea of the cause of bleeding is determined. If it is possible to delay the administration of blood, certain intravenous fluids, such as normal saline or bicarbonate solution, may be given to preserve urine flow while blood tests are run. Mannitol may be administered to promote renal blood flow and the production of urine. Colloidal solutions that may be used empirically without crossmatching include plasma (which contains clotting factors, but no viable platelets), human albumin, or dextran solution.

Control of bleeding from obvious sources requires more or less standard technical maneuvers known to surgeons of each surgical specialty. Oozing from broad surfaces in an operative field ordinarily can be controlled with pressure packs, usually consisting of laparotomy sponges. It has been demonstrated that the hot pack is less effective hemostatically than one at room temperature or below. The heat not only dilates blood vessels but denatures fibrinogen, thus aggravating the bleeding. Whatever control of oozing this method affords depends solely upon the value of pressure. The appropriate use of such standard methods of surgical hemostasis as ligature, cautery, and clips need not be expounded here. Special hemostatic techniques are used in the various surgical specialties. The employment of absorbable hemostatic substances has a well-defined but limited usefulness.

If a hemostatic defect is demonstrated postoperatively, it is improbable that reoperation for the control of bleeding will be necessary, but the need for reoperation will be predicated upon signs of pericardial tamponade, respiratory difficulties, or other extreme circumstances, such as rapid formation of compressive hematomas and so forth.

Intravascular Coagulation

One cannot expect the administration of blood to have definitive therapeutic value until after specific measures have been taken to counteract the cause of the intravascular coagulation. These measures include such maneuvers as removal of separated but retained placenta and fetus in abruptio placentae, or in septic abortion or missed abortion; neutralization of snake venoms by specific antivenin; control of bacterial invasion in the presence of bacteremia, and, paradoxical though it may seem, heparin for patients in whom bleeding is caused by intravascular coagulation.

Hemolytic Transfusion Reaction

Recognition and management of this condition are discussed on pages 636 and 637.

Fibrinolytic States

As is true in many cases of intravascular coagulation, fibrinolysis is usually a transient condition. Ordinarily, supportive measures to keep the patient alive will often result in control of the fibrinolytic state. If, however, the magnitude of the bleeding is great enough to warrant specific therapy, epsilon-aminocaproic acid (EACA) should be used. EACA is a synthetic amino acid that competitively inhibits the activity of plasminogen and, in high concentrations, inhibits the action of plasmin.

The average adult dose of EACA (commercially available as Amicar) is 5 gm. when given orally, or as a continuous intravenous infusion at the rate of 1 gm. per hour until bleeding is controlled.

Although the availability of EACA has made the treatment of fibrinolytic and other bleeding states gratifyingly successful, its administration is fraught with certain dangers. For example, in the presence of existing intravascular clotting, EACA may cancel out the accompanying fibrinolysis, thus permitting massive propagation of intravascular clotting that could be fatal. Therefore, if intravascular coagulation and fibrinolysis occur together, EACA should be given together with heparin.

Hypofibrinogenemia

Defibrination with or without fibrinolysis may occur during an operation or in the early postoperative period. The relentless ooze is usually, but not necessarily, restricted to the operative field.

Fresh plasma is recommended as the treatment of choice. If commercial fibrinogen is available, it should be given with heparin. Because EACA is often efficacious even when fibrinolysis cannot be demonstrated, it may be given in hypofibrinogenemia. If bleeding is not life-threatening, the passage

of time, usually a few hours, often results in spontaneous control.

Bleeding Following the Use of Anticoagulant Antagonists

Occasionally, the attempted neutralization of heparin effect with protamine sulfate results in a relentless, constant ooze from all incised tissue and puncture holes, which may cause blood loss in amounts capable of producing hypotension within an hour. The first reaction to this situation should be to increase the dose of protamine to twice the original dose. If the dosage of heparin antagonist was adequate (usually 2 mg. of protamine per 1 mg. of heparin administered by slow intravenous injection), recommended treatment for the bleeding is the intravenous administration of heparin from a new vial in the arbitrary dosage of 25,000 units (25 mg.). This injection may be repeated within a half-hour.

In order to avoid this paradoxical condition, it is advisable not to attempt to restore the coagulation mechanism before surgery in patients who have been on either heparin or coumarins. In the dosages that anticoagulant drugs are ordinarily administered, the coagulation time or prothrombin time is not usually carried to infinity. Therefore surgical procedures of most types can be done safely without cancelling a reasonable anticoagulant effect.

Pre-existing Hemostatic Defect

Surgical operation must occasionally be performed for reasons unrelated to an existing hemostatic defect or blood dyscrasia. In the preparation for surgical operation the management of bleeding varies in different coagulopathies, each requiring correction of the identified disorder by a specific plasma factor. In many instances such therapy will suffice without the need for fresh frozen plasma or fresh blood. It is conceivable that the bleeding defect may not be known to the surgeon. Such a situation should be suspected if excessive bleeding appears from the first incision and if all incised tissue and puncture holes bleed excessively. Petechiae may or may not be present. If surgery is not altogether mandatory, the surgical procedure should be discontinued at the first sign of such bleeding. In most instances the specific defect may be treated on the basis of the diagnosis derived from the history and laboratory tests. If no diagnosis has been made, it is best to postpone surgical operation until the specific therapy becomes known.

Mixed Hemostatic Defect or Unexplained Bleeding

When bleeding cannot be ascribed to any of the listed causes — defibrination, fibrinolysis, hemolytic reaction, technical surgical error, excess transfusion with aged bank blood, anticoagulants or anticoagulant antagonists, or pre-existing hemostatic defect — a general plan of treatment that has proved successful consists of combining the treatment for defibrination with that for fibrinolysis. This consists of administering fresh frozen plasma, EACA with heparin, or fibrinogen with heparin or all three. Again, avoidance of volume-for-volume blood replacement is of some importance.

Worthless Measures

It has been argued that the administration of calcium is a worthwhile measure when more than five pints of blood have been given. The true value of calcium in this situation remains unproved. Whatever value calcium might have in the presence of post-transfusion bleeding has been only rarely documented, and appears to be more in support of myocardial function than of hemocoagulation.

It should be self-evident that certain commercially available "anti-hemorrhagic" preparations have no place in the management of unexpected bleeding problems related to surgery. They are mentioned here only because of their unfortunately wide usage. These substances fall into four general categories: vitamins and bioflavinoids ("to prevent excessive capillary permeability"); estrogenic substance and adrenal corticosteroids, which purportedly increase coagulability; lipotropic agents and liver derivatives, which are advertised as aids to clotting; and certain vasoconstrictor substances, such as synthetic "adrenochrome derivatives."

HEMOPHILIA

Improved means of correcting the hematologic defect and maintaining an adequate state of near-normalcy have reduced bleeding dangers in hemophiliacs who must undergo either elective or emergency surgery. Two important requirements for reduction of surgical morbidity in these patients are the preoperative recognition of even mild hemophilia and the control of avoidable factors that might worsen the condition.

DEFINITIONS

Hemophilia A, the classic type of hemophilia is a disease of abnormal bleeding transmitted as a sex-linked recessive trait by heterozygous female carriers to male offspring. The bleeding disorder is caused by a deficiency in the plasma of factor VIII, the antihemophilic factor (AHF).

The extent to which factor VIII is deficient determines the severity of the bleeding disorder. Patients with severe hemophilia have a factor VIII level of under 2 per cent of the normal level. Such patients bleed excessively after minor cuts and bleed spontaneously into the joints, soft tissues, gastrointestinal tract, and urinary tract.

Patients with moderate hemophilia have up to 10 per cent of the normal amount of factor VIII in their plasma. These patients, like those with severe hemophilia, may bleed spontaneously, but especially after minor trauma. Unsuspected hemophilia or occult hemophilia occurs in patients with factor VIII levels between 10 and 25 per cent. The disease may not be recognized in such patients unless a careful history is obtained and laboratory tests are performed.

The occult hemophiliac may reveal no evidence of the disease until severe hemorrhage occurs, occasionally without operation. Among nonsurgical causes of hemorrhage in otherwise unrecognized mild hemophiliacs is the ingestion of aspirin. Kaneshiro and associates demonstrated that ingestion of 1 gm. of aspirin caused a change in bleeding time from $9\frac{1}{2}$ minutes to over 40 minutes in hemophiliacs within two hours after ingestion.

Female carriers who ordinarily exhibit no evidence of abnormal bleeding have factor VIII levels of about 50 per cent of normal.

Hemophilia B, also known as Christmas disease, in honor of a patient's name, and PTC deficiency (plasma thromboplastin component deficiency), is caused by a deficiency of factor IX. Its manifestations are identical to those of hemophilia A, and factor

IX deficiency is inherited in a manner identical to that of factor VIII deficiency. Like hemophilia A, it occurs among brothers, maternal male cousins, and uncles, but not among females or paternal relatives. Hemophilia B is diagnosed by identifying a factor IX deficiency.

Hemophilia B may be congenital or acquired. The acquired form may occur in patients with liver disease and in those receiving coumarin drugs. These anticoagulants deplete the liver of its vitamin-K clotting function.

Von Willebrand's disease is a hereditary coagulation disorder affecting both sexes, which manifests, among other things, a factor VIII deficiency. In addition, platelet dysfunction in the form of impaired aggregation is a component of the disease. Thus, patients with a prolonged bleeding time plus a factor VIII deficiency can be said to have Von Willebrand's disease if the family history is positive. Patients with this disease should be counseled before marriage because the disease is transmitted as a mendelian dominant.

PREOPERATIVE DIAGNOSIS

A personal and family history of easy bruising, and of prolonged bleeding after tooth extractions or other minor trauma, must be sought. Mild hemophilia is usually not suspected unless searched for. It is obviously safer to expose it in the history, confirm it by tests, and treat the patient before operation than to be suddenly confronted with a bleeding emergency of unknown origin toward the end of or after an extensive surgical procedure.

Most hospital laboratories do not perform routine coagulation tests prior to every operation. Perhaps they are not crucial before relatively minor operations if hemophilia is not suspected from the history. On the other hand, every patient scheduled for a major operative procedure, whether or not a suspicious history of bleeding can be elicited, should undergo laboratory studies preoperatively for adequacy of coagulation.

It is generally agreed that the partial thromboplastin time (PTT) is the most sensitive test for factor VIII deficiency. Clotting time may be prolonged, but the test is crude and nonspecific. The bleeding time, prothrombin time, and platelet count are normal in classic hemophilia but should be performed as part of the standard battery of clotting tests because they are useful in detecting other abnormalities of clotting factors.

PREOPERATIVE PREPARATION OF HEMOPHILIAC PATIENTS

Preoperative preparation is directed toward adequate hemostasis during major surgery. Generally speaking, if a minimum factor VIII level of 30 per cent of normal is maintained during operation and for 48 hours thereafter, abnormal bleeding is prevented. The only method of accomplishing this goal in hemophiliacs is by the replacement of deficient factor VIII.

In the postoperative period, maintenance of levels of 15 to 20 per cent is usually sufficient. Ordinarily, therapy is continued until wound healing is fairly complete, that is, for about ten days or two weeks.

For many years, the only available means of providing factor VIII replacement was by the administration of fresh plasma, fresh-frozen plasma, and fresh whole blood. These are still the most readily available preparations, but they have the great drawback of containing relatively low concentrations of factor VIII and therefore are required in large volumes to correct a great deficit. In many instances, the volume required could cause a hypervolemic state and acute pulmonary edema.

Today, hypervolemic problems due to factor VIII replacement have been overcome by the development of factor VIII concentrates. Factor VIII is a plasma globulin that deteriorates rapidly at room temperature.

Two types of factor VIII concentrates are available commercially. One is a cryoprecipitate of human plasma, a by-product of blood-bank fractionation procedures. The main concern with this preparation is the variability in factor VIII yield. As a result, it is recommended that therapeutic dosage be based upon the lowest percentage recovered.

The other factor VIII concentrate is obtained by amino acid precipitation of plasma. Recently Brinkhaus and associates combined cryoprecipitation with polyethylene and glycine precipitation to produce a factor VIII precipitate about 100 times more concentrated than plasma. Whereas older cryoprecipitation methods did not completely separate the fibrinogen fraction from the factor VIII globulin, the newer method removes most of the fibrinogen, yielding a high-potency product relatively free from other blood protein molecules. Another important feature of this preparation is its adaptation to large-scale commercial production. It is available as antihemophilic factor, (AHF, human), method 4. It is assayed for potency and is sterile and pyrogen-free.

Its stability is based on the fact that it is supplied in lyophilized form and must be reconstructed to liquid form before injection.

Regardless of dosage, the half-life of factor VIII after intravenous infusion is 12 to 15 hours.

DOSAGE OF FACTOR VIII CONCENTRATE (AHF HUMAN)

A patient with known hemophilia is prepared for operation by administering a loading dose of factor VIII sufficient to raise the patient's plasma factor VIII level to over 80 per cent of normal. This dose is calculated by the method described by Croom and Hutchin:

If the patient weighs 70 kilograms, has an hematocrit of 45 per cent, and has severe hemophilia, blood volume is calculated by multiplying the weight in kilograms by 8 per cent, and calculating plasma volume:

Blood volume = 70 Kg. × .08 = 5600 ml.

Plasma volume = 100 minus hematocrit × 5600 ml. or .55% × 5600 = 3080 ml.

One unit of factor VIII is defined as the amount in 1 ml. of normal plasma at 100 per cent level. Therefore, to obtain 80 per cent level,

3080 × 80% = approx. 2500 units of factor VIII required.

For the first 48 hours postoperatively, factor VIII levels should be kept at about 40 per cent, and then at 15 to 20 per cent for about two weeks after operation. Injections are given every 12 hours. Ideally, laboratory control of factor VIII levels in the patient's plasma is maintained by obtaining factor VIII assays sufficiently in advance of each infusion to calculate the dose with some accuracy.

As stated previously, the diagnosis of unsuspected hemophilia in patients who bleed excessively after surgical operation or after major trauma should be made before antihemophilic therapy is instituted.

A modified PTT test is used to detect factor VIII inhibitor. This inhibitor occurs in about 5 per cent of severe hemophiliacs. It is important to detect its presence because it neutralizes the therapeutically administered factor VIII, thereby raising the required dosage enormously. Factor VIII inhibitor is detected by the Rodman test, which consists of performing a PTT test on a mixture of the test plasma with an equal amount of normal control plasma. If the PTT of the mixture is more than 30 seconds longer than that of normal plasma, the test plasma contains factor VIII inhibitor.

The surgeon must realize that the calculation of factor VIII dosage may be inaccurate when blood loss is great and after attempts have been made to restore blood volume with fluids or blood. Calculations of blood volume and plasma volume, upon which factor VIII dosage depend, are notoriously inaccurate under these conditions. In this situation, the surgeon may have to depend on his clinical judgment more than on calculations to determine the dosage of factor VIII. Adjustment of the dosage can be made by monitoring factor VIII levels in the patient's plasma and by observing the effectiveness of the treatment.

One important precaution must be realized with administration of factor VIII — the preparation is derived from human plasma and therefore carries the risk of transmitting infectious hepatitis. Croom and Hutchin recommend the routine administration of prophylactic gamma globulin to patients receiving factor VIII concentrate, but admit that this may not be successful in ameliorating the hepatitis.

Until very recently, the factor IX deficiency of hemophilia B could be treated only with stored plasma because factor IX concentrate was not available. Factor IX concentrate is now available under the proprietary name Konyne. It is a complex containing factors II, VII, and X besides factor IX, and is available in a 500-unit size, or the equivalent of 500 ml. of fresh-frozen plasma. A great advantage is that 1000 units can be administered in a volume as low as 40 ml. containing only one gram of protein. It should not be reconstituted and administered in a concentration greater than 50 units per ml.

In factor IX deficiency, administration of 2 units per Kg. of body weight of factor IX concentrate will cause an average in vivo increase in factor IX of 3 per cent in 15 minutes whether the patient is bleeding or not. Factor IX levels should be maintained well above 20 per cent of normal in patients undergoing surgical procedures. With the initial dose, a level of 60 per cent should be sought, making it easier to maintain hemostatic levels later with smaller doses. Post-operative factor IX levels of 20 to 30 per cent appear to be adequate for hemostasis.

Considering the fact that today one can restore the coagulation mechanism of the severest hemophiliac to a condition that will permit the most major surgical operations to be performed with no more risk than to nonhemophiliacs, the risk of infectious hepatitis from the treatment assumes a minor position.

HEMATOLOGIC REACTIONS TO EXTRACORPOREAL CIRCULATION

PRIMING SOLUTIONS

Because of an array of hematologic problems associated with extracorporeal bypass circuits, concentrated efforts continue to be made in several quarters to eliminate, as much as possible, the use of blood for pump-priming. Although fresh blood is still acknowledged to be the ideal priming solution, its procurement and collection present almost insurmountable problems in many institutions, especially those in which several open-heart operations are performed daily.

The main drawback to bank blood as a priming solution is the resultant thrombocytopenia. However, Grindon and Schmidt recently used platelet-poor, 48-hour-old blood for perfusion during cardiopulmonary bypass and compared the postoperative platelet counts with those following the use of whole blood. They reasoned that since the platelets in 48-hour-old blood are wasted, it would be desirable to remove them when they are fresh for use in other patients. It was found that two hours after operation and on the first postoperative day patients who received platelet-poor blood had significantly lower platelet counts than patients who received whole blood, but hemostasis (during or after operations), blood requirements, and mean perfusion time did not differ between the two groups. Moreover, by the second postoperative day there was no longer a significant difference in platelet count.

Although this and other studies indicate that platelet-poor stored blood and whole blood are equally effective as perfusion

fluids for open-heart surgery, all the risks of transfusion complications remain in either case. The most critical risks are hemolysis, intravascular agglutination, and coagulation defects.

As the search continues for suitable substitutes for blood as a priming fluid, each of several currently used fluids has its proponents. Up to the time of this writing, the following solutions have been used with a modicum of success: dextran 40 (Rheomacrodex); 5 per cent dextrose in water; balanced electrolyte solutions or Ringer's solution with or without added sodium bicarbonate; mannitol; albumin; and gelatin solution (Haemacel).

HEMODILUTION TECHNIQUES

Hemodilution techniques have been quite successful, provided the dilution does not exceed a ratio of 1:4, or 20 ml. per Kg. of body weight. Dilutions greater than this may lead to hemolysis. In priming large-volume disc oxygenators, lactated Ringer's solution appears to be superior to 5 per cent glucose in water. With this method the marked decrease in hematocrit is well tolerated and is easily corrected at the end of perfusion by the administration of packed red cells.

HEMATOLOGIC COMPLICATIONS OF BYPASS

HEMOLYSIS. The major cause of hemolysis in pumps is the turbulent mixing of air and blood, especially by the coronary suction system, which returns blood from the cardiotomy site to the pump oxygenator, an action often accompanied by considerable foaming. Since the procedure cannot be stopped at this point, every effort is made to keep foaming at a minimum by using a filter in the system.

PROTEIN DENATURATION. Surface-polarizing forces, acting at the free blood-gas interface in all oxygenators except the membrane type, cause plasma protein denaturation with alteration of the configuration of the protein molecule. In the case of lipoproteins, this may result in the release of lipoid components as "free" lipoid, and eventuate in fat emboli in the microcirculation. Depending upon the gelation potential of denatured globulin molecules that may be adsorbed onto erythrocyte membranes, a variable amount of sludging may lead to occlusion of the microcirculation.

LEUKOPENIA AND LEUKOCYTOSIS. The leukocytes decrease in number with the onset of perfusion, as a result of mechanical trauma to the blood. The postperfusion response is invariably a leukocytosis, which may last over a week in the absence of infection. The proteolytic enzymes released by the leukocyte breakdown during perfusion may play a role in the postperfusion clotting defect.

THROMBOCYTOPENIA. The greatest loss of platelets occurs after the first five minutes of bypass. At the end of the bypass period, platelet counts are approximately 25 per cent of the preoperative levels. Early postoperative platelet-count increases take place for 48 hours, but this is followed by a secondary postoperative thrombocytopenia that may require as long as 10 days to return to normal. A thrombocytosis may then appear for several days. Among the factors contributing to the thrombocytopenia are platelet deposition on foreign surfaces, activation of the coagulation system, direct trauma, improperly cleaned equipment, and transfusion of blood with damaged nonviable platelets. If the thrombocytopenia persists, platelet concentrates, or fresh blood collected in plastic bags, should be administered.

ALTERATIONS IN COAGULATION MECHANISM

The changes in the coagulation system resulting from extracorporeal bypass are multiple. They include reductions in the following components: prothrombin, factors V, VII, VIII, X, and XI, platelets, and fibrinogen. Also, prothrombin time and thrombin time are prolonged. In the fibrinolytic system, a decrease in plasminogen and an increase in activator occur when the blood in the system is heparinized.

Intravascular clotting that occurs during bypass has been ascribed to a combination of processes that are at work simultaneously and include protein denaturation, a depression of plasma coagulation factors, especially factor V, factor VIII, and prothrombin, as well as a decreased rate of thromboplastin generation. Perkins demonstrated that the presence of thromboplastic substances in the plasma at the end of the bypass period may also be a significant cause of intravascular clotting.

A decrease in fibrinogen often occurs during the first five minutes of bypass. This occurrence plus some hemolysis and release of thromboplastin by platelet destruction may also contribute to intravascular coagulation. The resultant bleeding state is considered to be the result of stimulation of plasminogen activator converting plasminogen to plasmin, which, in turn, digests fibrinogen and fibrin. Excessive bleeding of this type can usually be detected as coming from previously dry areas in and around the operative field. Administration of epsilon-aminocaproic acid is advised under these circumstances.

Patients with congenital heart disease commonly have a prothrombin deficiency before surgery that is actually corrected by the operative procedure. Nonetheless, in order to avoid severe decreases in prothrombin levels during bypass, the preoperative administration of vitamin K_1 oxide for several days is usually carried out.

HEPARIN NEUTRALIZATION AFTER BYPASS

Excessive bleeding may accompany attempts at neutralization of heparin after bypass. It may be due to insufficient protamine dosage or to the effects of protamine on fibrinolysis. In general, the longer the period of perfusion, the more likely will be the occurrence of this form of bleeding. Also, a low pH increases the intensity and duration of bypass fibrinolysis, as does low-rate perfusion.

In view of the fibrinolytic complication of protamine neutralization of heparin, the question has been raised about the advisability of the neutralization attempt. It has been suggested that the heparin effect should be allowed to dissipate spontaneously, especially after prolonged bypass, rather than risk protamine fibrinolysis.

In most institutions, however, the problem of post-pump bleeding has been obviated by a series of precautionary and therapeutic measures:

1. Reduce pump time to a minimum.

2. Use protamine in a 2:1 ratio with heparin dosage, rather than 1:1. Do not repeat protamine injection.

3. Use filter for aspirated cardiotomy blood before returning it to the reservoir.

4. Use whole blood, at least for the post-perfusion transfusion, to replenish depleted blood coagulation factors.

HEMATOLOGIC REACTIONS TO ORGAN TRANSPLANTATION

In general, four types of hematologic reactions are related to organ transplantation. These are (1) the nonspecific effects related more to surgical trauma and underlying disease than to the transplant; (2) hematologic effects of graft-host interaction; (3) hematologic reflections of immunosuppression; and (4) organ-specific effects.

NONSPECIFIC EFFECTS

Patients who are recipients of transplanted organs are prone to all of the risks of hematologic changes experienced by other patients who undergo extensive surgical procedures or receive transfusions of blood. These include hemolysis, intravascular agglutination, fibrinolysis, afibrinogenemia, and thrombocytopenia. In addition, patients who may have received steroids preoperatively are prone to sepsis. They exhibit leukopenia, which, as sepsis develops, may become altered to a polymorphonuclear leukocytosis considerably lower than that of normal patients.

GRAFT-HOST INTERACTION

Leukocyte Response

The blood responds to early signs of rejection of an allograft by polymorphonuclear leukocytosis. Later, if the host survives, an abundance of mononuclear forms becomes evident. Sometimes marked eosinophilia occurs during acute rejection. A few days after implantation, neighboring lymph glands contain large pyroninophilic mononuclear cells that later appear in the peripheral blood. When leukopenia occurs in the recipient after transplant, it may be due either to the patient's underlying disease or to immunosuppressive drugs. Cold agglutinins, which may be responsible for leukopenia, have been demonstrated in the serum of recipients undergoing rejection of renal allografts.

Platelet Aggregation

A large percentage of patients demonstrate thrombocytopenia one to three days prior to overt rejection. This is the result of platelet aggregation and thrombi, which remove platelets from effective circulation.

Kahn considers platelet aggregation the most important cause of rejection. Nine months after their operations Kahn's three heart-transplant patients were all alive and well. All received anticoagulants as well as immunosuppressive drugs. Kahn's rationale for administering heparin intravenously every eight hours for the first month and then maintaining the patient on coumarin is based on the fact that platelet aggregation in the small vessels of the heart is one of the earliest signs of rejection. Kahn also performs thymectomy at the time of transplant to lower the lymphocyte level.

IMMUNOSUPPRESSION

Although all the mechanisms underlying rejection are not completely understood, an antigen-antibody reaction is involved in which lymphocytes participate as immunologically competent cells.

Most immunosuppressive drugs are cytotoxic and are capable of producing severe, and sometimes irretrievable, bone marrow suppression. Therefore, patients receiving such therapy must be checked periodically for total and differential leukocyte count, platelet count, and hematocrit. These examinations should be done daily at first, and at least semiweekly when there seems to be no problem concerning rejection. Each of the various immunosuppressive measures carries its own risks of causing hematologic reactions.

Antimetabolites and Alkylating Agents

Purine analogs, such as 6-mercaptopurine and Azathioprine (Imuran) as well as folic-acid antagonists (methotrexate) and alkylating agents (nitrogen mustard) block the appearance of the pyroninophilic immunoblasts until rejection occurs, when the cells increase in number, first in the regional lymph nodes, then in the blood. All the cytotoxic drugs are capable of producing pancytopenia and a bleeding tendency. Toxicity is common, and the occasional idiosyncratic patient may respond with an irretrievable cellular suppression of blood elements.

Corticosteroids

Corticosteroids are known to be lympholytic as well as anti-inflammatory agents. They are frequently used in transplant recipients and the surgeon should be alert for hematologic changes reflecting these actions.

Heterologous Antilymphocyte Serum (ALS)

Injection of ALS produces a rapid fall in peripheral lymphocyte count. An equally serious consequence is the severe thrombocytopenia caused by ALS. Platelet counts of under 50,000/cu. mm. are common without leukopenia. Some batches of ALS have platelet-agglutinating properties that may contribute to the thrombocytopenia. Appropriately cultured and properly absorbed ALS purportedly produces lymphocytopenia and granulocytosis without an associated fall in hematocrit or platelet count.

Surgically Induced Lymphocyte Depletion

Surgical methods aimed at lymphocyte depletion include splenectomy, thymectomy, and thoracic-duct fistula. All these procedures are of questionable value, since the resulting lymphopenia is irregularly produced, and their effects upon host acceptance of allografts remains unconfirmed.

Ionizing Irradiation

In man, whole body irradiation sufficient to achieve efficient immunosuppression uniformly produces fatal bone marrow suppression.

Phytohemagglutinin (PHA)

PHA has recently been advocated as an adjunct to immunosuppressive therapy. It is used along with Azathioprine and steroids. One of its deleterious effects is its tendency to agglutinate erythrocytes. However, adequate absorption, while preventing red-cell agglutination, sometimes causes gastrointestinal bleeding, with resultant anemia, leukoagglutination, and a transient neutrophilic leukocytosis. PHA also stimulates small lymphocytes to undergo metamorphosis to large blast cells and causes a remarkable decrease in the number of nucleated cells in the spleen.

ORGAN-SPECIFIC EFFECTS

The Kidney

The current concept of the role of the kidney in erythropoiesis involves the activity of a kidney-produced hormone, erythropoietin, which controls erythropoiesis by activating a plasma substrate. Extrarenal sources of erythropoietin also exist, as evidenced by the fact that nephrectomized patients still produce red cells, although not in sufficient quantity to prevent hypoproliferative anemia. Decrease in marrow cellularity and reticulocytopenia occur with ablation of kidney function. After successful renal transplantation, a detectable increase in circulating erythropoietin occurs. Early in graft rejection, an accelerated rate of erythropoietic activity may be manifested. As rejection progresses, all the factors that produce anemia in the uremic patient plus the contribution of immunosuppressive drugs lead to the development of anemia in patients with kidney transplants.

In addition, renal disease is sometimes associated with a microangiopathic hemolytic anemia, characterized by arteriolar and capillary thrombi, and occasionally with necrotizing arteritis and fibrinoid arteriolar necrosis. Red cell damage leads to hemolysis. Blood smears contain such bizarre forms as spherocytes, burr cells, and helmet cells. Reticulocyte counts of over 30 per cent, thrombocytopenia, and neutrophilia are common. This same blood and microangiopathic picture is observed in anephric patients during rejection of kidney allografts and is considered to be a characteristic manifestation.

The Liver

Most patients with liver disease of the types which might classify them as candidates for liver transplantation have severe anemia. Associated splenomegaly may be accompanied by depression of all cellular blood elements. Defects in the coagulation mechanism, fibrinolysis, and thrombocytopenia are common among such patients.

Plasma fibrinogen levels fall rapidly during the anhepatic phase and rise rapidly following revascularization of the allograft. Epsilon-aminocaproic acid is ineffective in stemming bleeding during the period of low fibrinogen. All clotting factors assumed to be produced by the liver, such as factors I, II, V, IX, X, and possibly plasminogen, have a half-life of longer than 12 hours. Factor VII has a half-life of four hours. The rapid coagulative defect of the anhepatic stage, therefore, is probably not solely related to the absence of liver function. It is most probably a combination of the release of tissue activators, the failure of the liver to clear the activators, the decline in plasma fibrinolytic inhibitors, and disseminated intravascular agglutination. In other words, the defect is a consumptive coagulopathy associated with pathologic fibrinolysis. For these reasons, among others, operative speed, employment of hypothermia, and gentle handling are essential to successful liver transplantation.

The Spleen

Antihemophilic factor (AHF) has been demonstrated in perfused spleens, and Norman has shown that a transplanted spleen will produce AHF in hemophilic dogs.

The Lung

Lung transplantation may be accompanied by all the general hematologic complications of other organ transplants. The secondary polycythemia of chronic lung disease may one day be treated by removal of the diseased lungs and transplantation.

The Bone Marrow

The bone marrow of genetically related donors has been used by Good as a functioning graft to reverse pancytopenia.

REFERENCES

Critical Blood Transfusion Reactions

Barlas, G. M., and Kolff, W. J.: Transfusion reactions and their treatment, especially with the artificial kidney. JAMA, 169:1969, 1959.

Braude, A. I.: Transfusion reactions from contaminated blood. Their recognition and treatment. New Eng. J. Med., 258:1289, 1958.

Davidsohn, I., and Stern, K.: Blood transfusion reactions; their causes and identification. Med. Clin. N. Amer., 44:281, 1960.

DeGowin, E. L., Greenwalt, T. J., and Merrill, J. P. (Dameshek, W. moderator): Management of an incompatible hemolytic transfusion reaction. Blood, 10:1164, 1955.

Djerassi, I., Farber, S., and Evans, A. E.: Transfusions of fresh platelet concentrates to patients with secondary thrombocytopenia. New Eng. J. Med., 268:221, 1963.

Grove-Rasmussen, M., Lesses, M. F., and Anstall, H. B.: Transfusion therapy. New Eng. J. Med., 264:1034, 1961.

Howland, W. S., Schweizer, O., Boyan, C. P., and Dotto, A. C.: Physiologic alterations with massive blood replacement. Surg. Gynec. Obstet., 101:478, 1955.

Krevans, J. R., and Jackson, D. P.: Hemorrhagic disorder following massive whole blood transfusions. JAMA, 159:171, 1955.

Ludbrook, J., and Wynn, V.: Citrate intoxication. A clinical and experimental study. Brit. Med. J., 2:523, 1958.

Moore, F. D.: Blood transfusions: Rates, routes, and hazards; Effects on blood volume and hematocrit. In Metabolic Care of the Surgical Patient, chapter 14, Philadelphia, W. B. Saunders Company, 1959.

Payne, R., and Rolfs, M. R.: Further observations on leukoagglutinin transfusion reactions with special reference to leukoagglutinin transfusion reactions in women. Amer. J. Med., 29:449, 1960.

Stefanini, M.: Studies on the hemostatic breakdown during massive replacement transfusions. Amer. J. Med. Sci., 244:298, 1962.

Strumia, M. M., Crosby, W. H., Gibson, J. G., II, Greenwalt, T. J., Krevans, J. R., and Gannon, H. T.: General principles of blood transfusion. Transfusion, 3:301, 1963.

Trobaugh, F. E., Jr., and De Cataldo, F.: Management of transfusion reactions. Med. Clin. N. Amer., 43:1537, 1959.

Walter, C. W.: A new technic for collection, storage and administration of unadulterated whole blood. Surg. Forum, 1:483, 1951.

Bleeding Problems

Biggs, R., and MacFarlane, R. G.: Human Blood Coagulation and Its Disorders. Philadelphia, F. A. Davis Company, 3rd ed., 1962.

Cohen, S. I., and Warren, R.: Fibrinolysis. New Eng. J. Med., 264:79-84, 128, 1961.

Conley, C. L.: Blood platelets and platelet transfusions. Arch. Intern. Med. (Chicago), 107:635, 1961.

Glynn, M. F., Movat, H. Z., Murphy, E. A., and Mustard, J. F.: Study of platelet adhesiveness and aggregation, with latex particles. J. Lab. Clin. Med., 65:179, 1965.

Koller, F.: Intravascular clotting and spontaneous fibrinolysis. Acta. Haemat. (Basel), 31:239, 1964.

Laufman, H., and Lalezari, P.: A plan for management of unexpected bleeding problems related to surgery. Mod. Med., Sept. 23, 1968, p. 81.

Linman, J. W.: Principles of Hematology. New York, The Macmillan Company, 1966.

Pechet, L.: Fibrinolysis. New Eng. J. Med., 273:966, 1024, 1965.

Quick, A. J.: Detection and diagnosis of hemorrhagic states. JAMA, *197*:138, 1966.

Quick, A. J.: Hemorrhagic Diseases. Philadelphia, Lea & Febiger, 1957.

Ratnoff, O. E.: Bleeding Syndromes. Springfield, Ill., Charles C Thomas, 1960.

Stafford, J. L.: The fibrinolytic mechanism in haemostasis: A review. J. Clin. Path., *17*:520, 1964.

Stefanini, M., and Dameshek, W.: The Hemorrhagic Disorders. New York, Grune and Stratton, 2nd ed., 1962.

Tocantins, L. M., and Kazal, L. A.: Blood Coagulation, Hemorrhage and Thrombosis. New York, Grune and Stratton, 2nd ed., 1964.

Hemophilia

Aggeler, P. M., Hoag, M. S., Wallerstein, R. O., and Whissell, D.: The mild hemophilias. Occult deficiencies of AHF, PTC and PTA frequently responsible for unexpected surgical bleeding. Amer. J. Med., *30*:84, 1961.

Blombäck, M., Jorpes, J. E., and Nilsson, I. M.: von Willebrand's disease. Amer. J. Med., *34*:236, 1963.

Breckenridge, R. T., and Ratnoff, O. D.: Studies on the nature of the circulating anticoagulant directed against antihemophilic factor; with notes on an assay for antihemophilic factor. Blood, *20*:137, 1962.

Brinkhous, K. M.: Hemophilia-pathophysiologic studies and the evolution of transfusion therapy. Amer. J. Clin. Path., *41*:342, 1964.

Brinkhous, K. M., Shanbrom, E., Roberts, H. R., Webster, W. P., Fekete, L., and Wagner, R. H.: A new high potency glycine-precipitated antihemophilic factor (AHF) concentrate; treatment of classical hemophilia and hemophilia with inhibitors. JAMA, *205*: 613, 1968.

Croom, R. D., III, and Hutchin, P.: Surgical management of the patient with classical hemophilia. Surg. Gynec. Obstet., *128*:793, 1969.

Dallman, P. R., and Pool, J. G.: Treatment of hemophilia with factor VIII concentrates. New Eng. J. Med., *278*:199, 1968.

Horowitz, H. F., and Fujimoto, M. M.: Acquired hemophilia due to a circulating anticoagulant. Report of two cases, with review of the literature. Amer. J. Med., *33*:501, 1962.

Hynes, H. E., Owen, C. A., Bowie, E. J. W., and Thompson, J. H., Jr.: Mayo Clin. Proc., *44*:193, 1969.

Kaneshiro, M. M., Kasper, C. K., Mielke, C. H., and Rapaport, S. I.: Effects of aspirin in hemophiliacs. Paper read at Western Soc. for Clin. Research, cited in JAMA, *207*:1621, 1969.

McMillan, C. W., Diamond, L. K., and Surgenor, D. M.: Treatment of classic hemophilia; the use of fibrinogen rich in factor VIII for hemorrhage and for surgery. New Eng. J. Med., *265*:224, 277, 1961.

Pool, J. G., Hershgold, E. J., and Pappenhagen, A. R.: High-potency antihaemophilic factor concentrate prepared from cryoglobulin precipitate. Nature, *203*:312, 1964.

Rodman, N. F., Jr., Barrow, E. M., and Graham, J. B.: Diagnosis and control of the hemophiloid states with the partial thromboplastin time (PTT) test. Amer. J. Clin. Path., *29*:525, 1958.

Wagner, R. H., McLester, W. D., Smith, M., and Brinkhous, K. M.: Purification of antihemophilic factor (factor VIII) by amino acid precipitation. Thromb. Diath. Haemorrh., *11*:64, 1964.

Webster, W. P., Penick, G. D., Peacock, E. E., and Brinkhous, K. M.: Allotransplantation of the spleen in hemophilia. N. Carolina Med. J., *28*:505, 1967.

Webster, W. P., Roberts, H. R., Thelin, G. M., Wagner, R. H., and Brinkhous, K. M.: Clinical use of a new glycine-precipitated antihemophilic fraction. Amer. J. Med. Sci., *250*:643, 1965.

Whissell, D. Y., Hoag, M. S., Aggeler, P. M., Kropatkin, M., and Garner, E.: Hemophilia in a woman. Amer. J. Med., *38*:119, 1965.

Perfusion

Abbot, J. P., Cooley, D. A., DeBakey, M. A., and Ragland, J. E.: Storage of blood for open heart operations. Surgery, *44*:698, 1958.

Andersen, M. N., and Kuchiba, K.: Blood trauma produced by pump oxygenators. J. Thorac. Cardiov. Surg., *57*:238, 1969.

Atik, M.: Dextrans, their use in surgery and medicine. Anesthesiology, *27*:425, 1966.

Berger, R. L., Iatrides, E., and Ryan, T. J.: The homologous blood reaction of cardiopulmonary bypass. Ann. Thorac. Surg., *4*:542, 1967.

Blombäck, M., Noren, I., and Senning, A.: Coagulation disturbances during extracorporeal circulation and the postoperative period. Acta. Chir. Scand., *127*:433, 1964.

Cooley, D. A., Beall, Jr., A. C., and Grondin, P.: Open heart operations with disposable oxygenators, 5% dextrose prime and normothermia. Surgery, *52*:713, 1962.

DeVries, S. I., Van Geveld, S., Groen, P., Muller, E., and Wettermark, M.: Studies on the coagulation of the blood in patients treated with extracorporeal circulation. Thromb. Diath. Haemorrh., *5*:426, 1961.

DeWall, R. A., Long, D. M., Gemmill, S. J., and Lillehei, C. W.: Certain blood changes in patients undergoing extracorporeal circulation. J. Thorac. Surg., *37*:325, 1959.

Douglas, A. S., McNicol, G. P., Bain, W. H., and Mackey, W. A.: The hemostatic defect following extracorporeal circulation. Brit. J. Surg., *53*:455, 1966.

Dow, J. W., Dickson, J. F., III, Hamer, N. A. J., and Gadboys, H. L.: The shock state in heart-lung bypass. Trans. Amer. Soc. Artif. Intern. Organs, *5*:247, 1959.

Ellison, R. G., McPherson, J. C., Jr., Yeh, T. J., Anabtavic, I. N., and Ellison, L. T.: Metabolic considerations of acid-citrate-dextrose stored blood for extracorporeal circulation. Ann. Thorac. Surg., *2*:540, 1966.

Foote, A. V., Trede, M., and Maloney, J. V.: An experimental and clinical study of the use of acid-citrate-dextrose (ACD) blood for extracorporeal circulation. J. Thorac. Cardiov. Surg., *42*:93, 1961.

Galletti, P. M., and Brecher, G. A.: Heart Lung Bypass, New York, Grune and Stratton, 1962.

Gans, H., and Castaneda, A. P.: Problems in hemostasis during open heart surgery. Ann. Surg., *165*:551, 1967.

Gerbode, F., Osborn, J. J., Melrose, D. G., Perkins, H. A., Norman, A., and Baer, D. M.: Extracorporeal circulation in intracardiac surgery. Lancet, *2*:284, 1958.

Gibbon, J. H., Jr., and Camishion, R. C.: Problems in hemostasis with extracorporeal apparatus. Ann. N.Y. Acad. Sci., *115*:195, 1964.

Grindon, A. J., and Schmidt, P. J.: Platelet-poor blood in open-heart surgery. New Eng. J. Med., *280*:1337, 1969.

Hara, M., Maris, M., Crumpler, J., Corn, B., and Perkins, W. H.: Effect of various priming solutions upon red cell mass, plasma volume, and extra cellular fluid volume of dogs following hemodilution technique of extracorporeal circulation. J. Thorac. Cardiov. Surg., 53:354, 1967.

Jacobson, Elliott: Hematologic changes due to extracorporeal circulation. In Laufman, H., and Erichson, R.: Hematology for Surgeons, Philadelphia, W. B. Saunders Company. In press.

Kaulla, K. N., and Swan, H.: Clotting deviations in man during cardiac bypass: fibrinolysis and circulating anticoagulant. J. Thorac. Surg., 36:519, 1958.

Kendall, A. G., and Lowenstein, L.: Alterations in blood coagulation and hemostasis during extracorporeal circulation. Canad. Med. Assoc. J., 87:786, 1962.

Kirby, C.: Discussion on blood changes. In Allen, J. G.: Extracorporeal Circulation. Springfield, Ill., Charles C Thomas, 1958.

Lee, W. H., Jr., Krumgaar, D., Fonkalsrud, E. W., Schjeide, O. A., and Maloney, J. V.: Denaturation of plasma protein as a cause of morbidity and death after intracardiac operations. Surgery, 50:29, 1961.

Litwak, R. S., Slonim, R., Wisoff, B. G., and Gadboys, H. L.: Homologous blood syndrome during extracorporeal circulation in man. New Eng. J. Med., 268:1377, 1963.

Lobpreis, E. L., Ekkehart, R., Watanabe, Y., and Maloney, J. V., Jr.: A clinical evaluation of fresh and stored heparinized blood for use in extracorporeal circulation. Ann. Surg., 152:947, 1960.

Long, D. M., Sanchez, L., Varco, R. L., and Lillihei, C. W.: The use of low-molecular weight dextran and serum albumin as plasma expanders in extracorporeal circulation. Surgery, 50:12, 1961.

Neptune, W. S., Panico, F. G., and Bougas, J. A.: Clinical use of pump oxygenator without donor blood for priming or support during extracorporeal perfusion. Circulation, 20:745, 1959.

Penick, G. P., Averette, H. E., Jr., Peters, R. M., and Brinkhous, K. M.: The hemorrhagic syndrome complicating extracorporeal shunting of blood: an experimental study of its pathogenesis. Thromb. Diath. Haemorrh., 2:218, 1958.

Perkins, H. A., Osborn, J. J., and Gerbode, F.: The management of abnormal bleeding following extracorporeal circulation. Ann. Intern. Med., 51:658, 1959.

Perkins, H. A., Osborn, J. J., Hurt, R., and Gerbode, F.: Neutralization of heparin in vivo with protamine: a simple method of estimating the required dose. J. Lab. Clin. Med., 48:223, 1956.

Schmidt, P. J., Redin, J. C., Jr., Brecher, A. G., and Baranovsky, A.: Thrombocytopenia and bleeding tendency after extracorporeal circulation. New Eng. J. Med., 265:1181, 1961.

Smith, W. W., Brown, I. W., Jr., Young, W. G., Jr., and Sealey, W. C.: Studies of edglugate-Mg; a new donor blood anticoagulant-preservative mixture for extracorporeal circulation. J. Thorac. Cardiov. Surg., 38:573, 1959.

Woods, J. E., Kirklin, J. W., Owen, C. A., Jr., Thompson, J. H., Jr., and Taswell, H. F.: Effect of bypass surgery on coagulation-sensitive clotting factors. Mayo Clin. Proc., 42:724, 1967.

Zuhdi, N., McCollough, B., Carey, J., and Greer, A.: Double helical reservoir heart-lung machine designed for hypothermic perfusion primed with 5% glucose in water inducing hemodilution. Arch. Surg., 82:320, 1961.

Transplantation

Abaza, H. M., Nolan, B., Watt, J. G., and Woodruff, M. F. A.: Effect of antilymphocytic serum on the survival of renal homotransplants in dogs. Transplantation, 4:618, 1966.

Adamson, J. W., Eschbach, J., and Finch, C. A.: The kidney and erythropoiesis. Amer. J. Med., 44:727, 1968.

Blecher, T. E., Terblanche, J., and Peacock, J. H.: Orthotopic liver homotransplantation. Arch. Surg., 96:331, 1968.

Calne, R. Y., Wheeler, J. R., and Hurn, B. A. L.: Combined immunosuppressive action of phytohaemagglutinin and azathioprine (Imuran) on dogs with renal homotransplants. Brit. Med. J., 2:154, 1965.

Calne, R. Y., Williams, R., Dawson, J. L., Ansell, I. D., Evans, D. B., Flute, P. T., Herbertson, P. M., Joysey, V., Keates, G. H. W., Knill-Jones, R. P., Mason, S. A., Millard, P. R., Pena, J. R., Pentlow, B. D., Salaman, J. R., Sells, R. A., and Cullum, P. A.: Liver transplantation in man—II, a report of two orthotopic liver transplants in adult recipients. Brit. Med. J., 4:541, 1968.

Dacie, J. V.: The Haemolytic Anaemias—Congenital and Acquired, part III. New York, Grune and Stratton, 1967.

Fish, J. C., Sarles, H. E., Remmers, A. R., Tyson, K. R. T., Canales, C. O., Beathard, G. A., Fukushima, M., Ritzmann, S. E., and Levin, W. C.: Circulating lymphocyte depletion in preparation for renal allotransplantation. Surg. Gynec. Obstet., 128:777, 1969.

Good, R. A.: Immunologic reconstitution: the achievement and its meaning. Hosp. Pract., 4:41, 1969.

Groth, C. G., Pechet, L., and Starzl, T. E.: Coagulation during and after orthotopic transplantation of the human liver. Arch. Surg., 98:31, 1969.

Iwasaki, Y., Porter, K. A., Amend, J. R., Marchioro, T. L., Zuhlke, V., and Starzl, T. E.: The preparation and testing of horse antidog and antihuman antilymphoid plasma or serum and its protein fractions. Surg. Gynec. Obstet., 124:1, 1967.

Kahn, D. R.: Quoted in Transplanters' New Hope: Anticoagulants. Med. World News, June 27, 1969, pp. 14-15.

Kashiwagi, N., Brantigan, C. O., Brettschneider, L., Groth, C. G., and Starzl, T. E.: Clinical reactions and serologic changes after the administration of heterologous antilymphocyte globulin to human recipients of renal homografts. Ann. Int. Med., 68:275, 1968.

Kimber, C., Deller, D. J., Ibbotson, R. N., and Lander, H.: The mechanism of anaemia in chronic liver disease. Quart. J. Med., 34:33, 1965.

Lalezari, P. et al.: Development of cold agglutinins following renal transplantation. J. Surg. Res. In press.

Levey, R. H., and Medawar, P. B.: Nature and mode of action of antilymphocytic antiserum. Proc. Nat. Acad. Sci., 56:1130, 1966.

Lichtman, M. A., Hoyer, L. W., and Sears, D. A.: Erythrocyte deformation and hemolytic anemia coincident with the microvascular disease of rejecting renal homotransplants. Amer. J. Med. Sci., *256*:239, 1968.

Lowenhaupt, R., and Nathan, P.: Platelet accumulation observed by electron microscopy in the early phase of renal allotransplant rejection. Nature, *220*:822, 1968.

Marchioro, T. L., Hougie, C., Ragde, H., Epstein, R. B., and Thomas, E. D.: Hemophilia: role of organ homografts. Science, *163*:188, 1969.

Mathé, G.: Bone marrow transplantation. In Rapaport, F. and Dausset, J.: Human Transplantation. New York, Grune and Stratton, 1968.

Medawar, P. B.: Biological effects of heterologous anti-lymphocyte sera. In Rapaport, F. T. and Dausset, J.: Human Transplantation. New York, Grune and Stratton, 1968.

Mowbray, J. F., Cohen, S. L., Doak, P. B., Kenyon, J. R., Owen, K., Percival, A., Porter, K. A., and Peart, W. S.: Human cadaveric renal transplantation report of twenty cases. Brit. Med. J., *2*:1387, 1965.

Norman, J. C., Covelli, V. H., and Sise, II. S.: Transplantation of the spleen: experimental cure of hemophilia. Surgery, *64*:1, 1968.

Norman, J. C., Lambilliotte, J., Kojima, Y., and Sise, H. S.: Antihemophilic factor release by perfused liver and spleen: relationship to hemophilia. Science, *158*:1060, 1967.

Peacock, E. E., Webster, W. P., Penick, G. D., Madden, J. W., and Hutchin, P.: Transplantation of the spleen. Transplantation Proc., *1*:239, 1969.

Pechet, L., Groth, C. G., and Daloze, P. M.: Changes in coagulation and fibrinolysis after orthotopic canine liver homotransplantation. J. Lab. Clin. Med., *73*:91, 1969.

Pierce, J. C., and Hume, D. M.: The effect of splenectomy on the survival of first and second renal homotransplants in man. Surg. Gynec. Obstet., *31*:1300, 1968.

Richards, K., and Veith, F. J.: Hematological effects of organ transplantation. In Laufman, H. and Erichson,

R.: Hematology for Surgeons. Philadelphia, W. B. Saunders Company. In press.

Russell, P. S., and Monaco, A. P.: The Biology of Tissue Transplantation. Boston, Little Brown and Co., 1965.

Rutherford, R. B., and Hardaway, R. M.: Significance of the rate of decrease in fibrinogen level after total hepatectomy in dogs. Ann. Surg., *163*:51, 1966.

Starzl, T. E.: Homograft rejection in patients receiving immunosuppressive therapy. In Experience in Renal Transplantation, Philadelphia, W. B. Saunders Company, 1964.

Starzl, T. E., Groth, C. G., Brettschneider, L., Moon, J. B., Fulginiti, V. A., Cotton, E. K., and Porter, K. A.: Extended survival in three cases of orthotopic homotransplantation of the human liver. Surgery, *63*:549, 1968.

Starzl, T. E., Marchioro, T. L., Porter, K. A., Iwasaki, Y., and Cerilli, G. J.: The use of heterologous anti-lymphoid agents in canine renal and liver homotransplantation and in human renal homotransplantation. Surg. Gynec. Obstet., *29*:301, 1967.

Stremple, J. F., Hussey, C. V., and Ellison, E. H.: Study of clotting factors in liver homotransplantation. Amer. J. Surg., *111*:862, 1966.

Veith, F. J., Luck, R. J., and Murray, J. E.: The effects of splenectomy on immunosuppressive regimens in dog and man. Surg. Gynec. Obstet., *121*:299, 1965.

von Kaulla, K. N., Kaye, H., von Kaulla, E., Marchioro, T. L., and Starzl, T. E.: Changes in blood coagulation. Arch. Surg., *92*:71, 1966.

Webster, W. P., Reddick, R. L., Roberts, H. R., and Penick, G. D.: Release of factor VIII (antihaemophilic factor) from perfused organs and tissues. Nature, *213*:1146, 1967.

Woodruff, M. F. A., and Anderson, N. F.: The effect of lymphocyte depletion by thoracic duct fistula and administration of antilymphocytic serum on the survival of skin homografts in rats. Ann. N.Y. Acad. Sci., *120*:119, 1964.

CHAPTER 30

INTRAVENOUS
HYPERALIMENTATION

by STANLEY J. DUDRICK, M.D. and JONATHAN E. RHOADS, M.D.

Stanley J. Dudrick graduated from Franklin and Marshall College, having been elected to Phi Beta Kappa, and from the University of Pennsylvania School of Medicine with honors. After internship and residency at the Hospital of the University of Pennsylvania, he joined the faculty and is currently Associate Professor of Surgery and Chief of Surgery, University of Pennsylvania Division, Philadelphia Veterans Administration Hospital. His successful development and application of intravenous hyperalimentation has been widely acclaimed.

Jonathan E. Rhoads was born in Philadelphia of a distinguished old Quaker family. He was elected to Phi Beta Kappa at Haverford College and to Alpha Omega Alpha at Johns Hopkins University School of Medicine. When his residency at Penn was completed, he continued on the staff to rise through the ranks to full professor in 1949. His broad leadership qualities led to his being named Provost of the University of Pennsylvania. In 1959 he was appointed John Rhea Barton Professor of Surgery and Chairman of the Department. Dr. Rhoads is one of the deans of American surgery and his varied activities have also included such community responsibilities as President of the Board of Managers of Haverford College and membership on the Philadelphia Board of Public Education. Among his multiple investigative interests has been an enduring search to improve nutritional therapy for surgical patients, and successful intravenous hyperalimentation is the result of almost thirty years of dedication to this goal. For this he and Dr. Dudrick were given the American Medical Association's Joseph Goldberger Award in Clinical Nutrition for 1970.

Although optimal nutrition may be a difficult and, at times, almost impossible goal to achieve in surgical patients with debility or dysfunction of the gastrointestinal tract, the establishment and maintenance of an adequate feeding program may be vital to the successful management of the patient with critical surgical illness. Periods of relative or complete anatomical or functional disruption of the alimentary tract frequently accompany a patient's primary pathological process and may assume primary importance in his clinical course, further compounding existing nutritional problems by precluding adequate enteral feeding. In too many instances, the patient must endure excessive morbidity and may, in fact, succumb not from his primary disease but rather from the complications of secondary starvation.

Maintenance or restoration of nutritional balance is desirable during all phases of diagnosis, therapy, and convalescence in surgical patients. This goal may be accomplished with thoughtful attention to dietary regimens, individualized to the specific needs and conditions of patients, and delivered to the alimentary tract orally or by various feeding tubes whenever feasible; however, when use of the gastrointestinal tract is inadequate, ill-advised, or impossible for prolonged periods of time, nourishment must be provided by parenteral means.

Parenteral alimentation, using routine intravenous feeding regimens, can provide only a fraction of a debilitated patient's nutritional requirements. Peripheral intravenous administration of 5 per cent dextrose solutions within the limits of fluid tolerance (2500 to 3000 ml. per day) provides approximately 500 to 600 calories. In the average resting adult patient, caloric requirements are approximately three times this amount; hence, all of the intravenously administered nutrients are metabolized for energy rather than for tissue synthesis, and the additional energy requirements are met by the catabolism of body glycogen, fat, and protein. If caloric needs are abnormally increased by fever, infection, trauma, or a pathologic process requiring large amounts of high energy substrates for repair, the patient supported by the usual peripheral intravenous ration is receiving only one-fifth to one-third of his nutritional requirements and is clearly subsisting on a starvation diet.

Several approaches to increasing the quality and efficacy of intravenous nutrition have achieved limited clinical success (Beal et al., 1957, and Holden et al., 1957). With the infusion of somewhat hypertonic 10 to 15 per cent sugar solutions within limits of water tolerance, caloric levels of about 2000 kcal. per day have been administered by peripheral vein; however, long-term parenteral nutrition with this technique is accompanied by a prohibitive incidence of thrombophlebitis. The use of intravenous diuretics as an adjuvant to the infusion of isotonic or slightly hypertonic nutritive solutions in quantities of 5 to 7 liters per day has allowed the delivery of up to 2600 kcal per day while promoting the renal excretion of the surplus vehicular water (Rhoads, 1962, and Rhoads et al., 1965). The risks of cardiovascular embarrassment, water overload, and electrolyte imbalance restricted the widespread application of this technique. The use of energy substrates of higher caloric density than carbohydrate, such as alcohol (7 kcal./gm.) and fat (9 kcal./gm.), has also fallen short of expectations (Lehr et al., 1962).* A safe, effective, and stable fat emulsion is currently unavailable for clinical use in this country. The side effects—intoxication, obtundity, and cellular damage—have narrowed the range of the clinical usefulness of alcohol. Thus, the only universally applicable approach to providing adequate nutrition parenterally is to concentrate the nutrients known to be safe and efficacious. The resultant hypertonic solutions must be delivered into the superior vena cava at a constant rate throughout each 24-hour day in order to avoid thrombophlebitis and exceeding the body's capability for metabolizing and excreting water and glucose.

Parenteral hyperalimentation consists of the intravenous administration of suitable carbohydrates, amino acids, and other nutrients in substantial excess of existing requirements for nitrogen equilibrium in order to achieve tissue synthesis and anabolism in patients who have increased nutritional needs. It consists basically of infusing highly concentrated nutrient solutions continuously through an indwelling catheter inserted into an external jugular or subclavian vein and directed centrally into the superior vena cava. The primary aim of the technique is intravenous delivery for long periods of time of essential nutrients in quantities as high as two and a half times the basal requirements. Thereby, positive nitrogen balance and an anabolic state have been achieved during conditions usually associated with a catabolic response (Dudrick et al., 1968). In pediatric patients who require total intravenous feeding during the course of illness, an additionally desired goal is normal growth and development until oral feeding can be resumed (Wilmore and Dudrick, and Wilmore et al., 1968, 1969). In some patients, the achievement of mechanical and secretory bowel rest, while providing all nutrients exclusively by vein, has been a primary or secondary goal of the technique (Dudrick, Long et al., and Dudrick, Wilmore et al., in press).

The beneficial effects of providing adequate nutrition to patients with critical illness or following a major injury or operation have been widely recognized. Even after moderate trauma or an operation, a striking catabolic response occurs in the otherwise healthy and well-nourished patient, manifested by a marked rise in the urinary losses of nitrogen, creatine, sulphur, phosphorus, and potassium and accompanied by significantly increased basal oxygen consumption (Cuthbertson and Tilstone, 1968). As part of the generalized post-traumatic or postsurgical inflammatory response, both protein catabolism and anabolism are accelerated, but catabolism is accelerated to a much greater degree than anabolism (Levenson et al., 1961). Moreover, the body's glycogen stores are quickly mobilized after surgery or injury, and glucose tolerance is somewhat decreased along with a concomitant decrease in plasma amino nitrogen (Green et al., 1949). The administration of intravenous nutrients at increased levels beyond the apparent requirements does not reverse

---

*(See also Symposium on intravenous fat emulsions. Metabolism, 6:591, 1957.)

the excessive urinary losses of nitrogen and other catabolites but results in achievement of a modest positive nitrogen balance in most patients by providing more nitrogen to the body than it is excreting. Thus, theoretically more nitrogen-containing substrates are available for protein synthesis and tissue repair. Although a detailed discussion of the myriad complex catabolic problems associated with serious illness, surgery, and trauma are beyond the scope of this chapter, emphasis must be placed on the fact that it is not uniformly impossible to achieve positive nitrogen balance in patients in the immediate postsurgical or post-traumatic period. On the contrary, many of these patients have been brought into strongly positive balances.

The technique of total intravenous hyperalimentation has proven efficacious in supporting several hundred malnourished infant and adult patients for prolonged periods of time at the University of Pennsylvania Medical Center (Dudrick et al., 1969c). Wound healing, weight gain, fistula closure, remissions of regional enterocolitis and ulcerative colitis, and increased strength, activity, and feeling of well-being have been regularly observed in adults; normal growth and development have been achieved in infants fed exclusively by vein. Some patients with renal failure or impaired hepatic function also have been adequately supported intravenously with essential L-amino acids and hypertonic glucose when feeding by way of the alimentary tract was impossible or was aggravating their clinical courses (Dudrick et al., 1969b). Thus, it is no longer necessary that critically ill patients be nutritionally deprived or subjected to the ravages of starvation because they cannot eat.

PRINCIPLES OF INTRAVENOUS HYPERALIMENTATION

SOLUTION PREPARATION

The basic nutrient mixture is a hypertonic solution (approximately six times isotonic) consisting of 20 to 25 per cent dextrose and 4 to 5 per cent protein hydrolysate and providing 5.25 to 6.0 gm. of nitrogen (32.5 to 37.5 gm. protein equivalent) and 900 to 1000 calories per liter. The solution can be prepared in lots from commercially available products by a manufacturing pharmacist or

in individual units by a physician, pharmacist, or registered nurse using strict aseptic technique (Dudrick et al., forthcoming) (Table 30-1).

In the bulk method of solution preparation in a pharmacy, anhydrous dextrose U.S.P. is added to commercially available 5 per cent protein hydrolysate in 5 per cent dextrose in the ratio of 165 gm. to 860 ml. The resultant solution is sterilized by passage through a 0.22-micron membrane filter and bottled in liter units. Aliquots are taken for bacteriologic and pyrogen testing, and each lot is quarantined pending negative results of these tests in order to ensure the safety of the solution.

In institutions in which such facilities are not readily available, individual units of the base solution can be prepared daily as needed entirely from commercially available parenteral solutions. Using strict aseptic technique and preferably working under a laminar-flow, filtered-air hood, 250 ml. is discarded from a liter bottle of 5 per cent protein hydrolysate in 5 per cent dextrose. To the remaining 750 ml. in the bottle, 350 ml. of 50 per cent dextrose is carefully added from a 500-ml. bottle. Use of 50 per cent glucose from 50-ml. ampules greatly compounds the risk of contamination and is not recommended. The resultant unit of solution so prepared is clinically approximately equivalent to that unit of solution prepared by the bulk method; however, the former unit contains an additional 100 ml. of water while providing slightly less nitrogen, dextrose, and calories.

For the average adult patient without evidence of significant renal, hepatic, or cardiovascular disease, 40 to 50 mEq. of sodium chloride, 30 to 40 mEq. of potassium chloride, and 3 to 4 mEq. of magnesium sulfate are added to each bottle of the base solution. To one bottle of base solution daily, an ampule of water and fat soluble vitamins* is added. Vitamin B_{12}, vitamin K, and folic acid can be added to one bottle of the base solution daily or given intramuscularly intermittently as indicated or desired. Calcium as 10 per cent calcium gluconate and phosphorus as potassium acid phosphate are not given routinely to adults but are added to the regimen as indicated by serum levels of these electrolytes. When calcium and phosphorus are required

---

*MVI, USV, Pharmaceutical Corp., New York, New York, 10017.

TABLE 30-1. Preparation of Hyperalimentation Solutions for Adults

Unit Composition of Base Solution

Bulk Method (Pharmacy)
165 gm. anhydrous glucose U.S.P. +
860 ml. 5% glucose in 5% fibrin hydrolysate

Single Unit Method (Ward or Pharmacy)
350 ml. 50% glucose +
750 ml. 5% glucose in 5% fibrin hydrolysate

Sterilization through a 0.22-micron membrane filter under laminar-flow filtered-air hood

Aseptic mixing technique under laminar-flow filtered-air hood

Volume	1000	ml.	1100	ml.	
Calories	1000	kcal.	1000	kcal.	
Glucose	208	gm.	212	gm.	
Hydrolysates	43	gm.	37	gm.	
Nitrogen	6.0	gm.	5.25	gm.	
Sodium	8	mEq.	7	mEq.	
Potassium	14	mEq.	13	mEq.	

Additions to Each Unit of Base Solution (Average Adult)

Sodium	(chloride)	40–50 mEq.
Potassium	(chloride)	30–40 mEq.
Magnesium (sulfate)		4–5 mEq.

Additions to Only One Unit Daily (Average Adult)

Vitamin A	5000–10,000 U.S.P. units
Vitamin D	500–1000 U.S.P. units
Vitamin E	2.5–5.0 I.U.
Vitamin C	250–500 mg.
Thiamine	25–50 mg.
Riboflavin	5–10 mg.
Pyridoxine	7.5–15 mg.
Niacin	50–100 mg.
Pantothenic Acid	12.5–25 mg.

Optional Additions to One Unit (As indicated by serum studies)

Vitamin K	5–10 mg.	
Vitamin B_{12}	10–30 mcg.	Alternatively may be given intramuscularly in daily or weekly dosages
Folic acid	0.5–1.5 mg.	
Iron (dextriferron)	2.0–3.0 mg.	
Calcium (gluconate)	4.5–9 mEq.	
Phosphate (potassium acid salt)	4–10 mEq.	

Micronutrients such as zinc, copper, manganese, cobalt, and iodine are present as contaminants in hydrolysate solutions but may be given in plasma transfusion once or twice weekly if desired.

parenterally, it is best not to add them to the same bottle, as precipitation may occur. The addition of calcium gluconate and sodium bicarbonate to the same bottle may also result in a precipitate. Iron stores can be replenished most expeditiously by blood transfusion. Iron can also be added daily in minute amounts to the solution or can be given less frequently in depot form intramuscularly. Trace elements are present as contaminants in most intravenous solutions, particularly in protein hydrolysates, and thus are not routinely provided in parenteral form except in infants and in markedly malnourished adults. Micronutrients such as zinc, copper, manganese, cobalt, and iodine can be

given in the solution intermittently as specially prepared additives or can be alternatively provided by the administration of one unit of plasma or albumin twice a week.

Slight alterations of the adult formula are necessary to provide the nutrients required for growth in infants (Dudrick et al., forthcoming) (Tables 30-2 and 30-3). Modification of the average adult formula is also required by patients with liver disease, congestive heart failure, or massive nutritional edema in whom sodium is greatly reduced or restricted. It is also required by patients with hepatic or renal failure in whom special solutions of essential L-amino acids are substituted for the protein hydrolysates in order

TABLE 30-2.   Preparation of Pediatric Hyperalimentation Solutions

Unit Composition of Base Solution

400 ml. 5% Glucose in 5% Fibrin Hydrolysate		160 kcal.	⎰ 20 gm. Hydrolysates
250 ml. 50% Glucose		500 kcal.	⎱ 20 gm. Glucose
650 ml.		660 kcal.	

Additions to Each Unit of Base Solution

Sodium	20 mEq.	Sodium Chloride (2 mEq./ml.)	10	ml.
Potassium	25 mEq.	Potassium Acid Phosphate	13	ml.
Phosphorus	25 mEq.	(2 mEq./ml.)		
Calcium	20 mEq.	Calcium Gluconate 10% (0.45 mEq./ml.)	44	ml.
Magnesium	10 mEq.	Magnesium Sulfate 50% (6 mEq./ml.)	1.2	ml.
Multiple Vitamin Infusion			4	ml.
Vitamin K ⎫ Vitamin B$_{12}$ ⎬ Folic Acid ⎪ Iron ⎭		Added to solution daily or weekly or given intramuscularly	1	ml.
Trace elements		Added to solution daily or given as 10 ml./kg. plasma twice weekly	1	ml.
			75	ml.

BASE SOLUTION	650 ml.
ADDITIVES	75 ml.
FINAL SOLUTION	725 ml. (Given at rate of 145 ml./kg./day = 130 kcal./kg./day

TABLE 30-3.   Comparison of Daily Average Pediatric Nutritional Requirements
with Intravenous Ration

	Oral Recommendations		Intravenous Dose	
Protein	2.5	gm./kg.	4	gm./kg.
Calories	115	kcal./kg.	125	kcal./kg.
Water	150	ml./kg.	125	ml./kg.
Sodium	46	mg./kg.	100	mg./kg. (4–5 mEq.)
Potassium	58	mg./kg.	156–195	mg./kg. (4–5 mEq.)
Chloride	150	mg./kg.	150	mg./kg. (4 mEq.)
Calcium	218	mg./kg.	72	mg./kg. (3–4 mEq.)
Phosphorus	218	mg./kg.	58	mg./kg. (5–6 mEq.)
Magnesium	60	mg./kg.	25	mg./kg. (2 mEq.)
Iron	6	mg./kg.	0.02	mg./kg.
Copper	0.07	mg./kg.	0.022	mg./kg.
Cobalt	–		0.014	mg./kg.
Manganese	0.2	mg./kg.	0.04	mg./kg.
Zinc	0.3	mg./kg.	0.04	mg./kg.
Iodine	0.07	mg./kg.	0.015	mg./kg.
Vitamin A	1500	I.U.	3000–4000	I.U.
Thiamine	0.4	mg.	15–20	mg.
Riboflavin	0.5	mg.	3–4	mg.
Pyridoxine	0.25	mg.	4.5–6	mg.
Vitamin C	30	mg.	150–200	mg.
Vitamin D	400	I.U.	300–400	I.U.
Vitamin E	–	–	1.5–2	I.U.
Niacin	6	mg.	30–40	mg.
Pantothenic Acid	–	–	7.5–10	mg.
Vitamin K	1.5	mg.	1–1.5	mg.
Folic Acid	0.35	mg.	0.5	mg.
Vitamin B$_{12}$	1	mcg.	1	mcg.

to reduce blood urea nitrogen and ammonia and by patients with compromised renal function in whom potassium administration is reduced or omitted. Initially, solution modification may be necessary quite frequently, depending upon the patient's metabolic response to his illness, operation, trauma, or various complications. No single parenteral nutrient mixture can be ideal in all conditions in all patients at all times, and individual requirements must be satisfied appropriately as they arise.

SOLUTION ADMINISTRATION

The final hypertonic solution contains 25 to 30 per cent solute and must be infused continuously at a constant rate throughout each 24-hour day in order to achieve maximum metabolic efficiency and assimilation of the nutrients. In addition, because of the hyperosmolarity (1800 to 2200 milliosmoles per liter), the solution must be delivered into the blood stream through a large-diametered, high-flow vessel such as the superior vena cava. Preferably, infusion is accomplished through an indwelling catheter placed percutaneously into the superior vena cava by way of the subclavian vein (Dudrick and Wilmore, 1968). In neonates and infants weighing less than 10 pounds, percutaneous subclavian catheterization may be difficult and dangerous. Therefore, cannulation of the superior vena cava is best performed by inserting a small polyvinyl or silicone rubber catheter into an external or internal jugular vein by cutdown (Dudrick et al., 1969a). Regular antiseptic care and maintenance of the catheter and its insertion site ensures safe, prolonged infusion (Wilmore and Dudrick, 1969b).

Starting at established levels of water metabolism (2000 to 2500 ml. per day in average adults, 100 ml./kg. per day in infants) and carbohydrate utilization (0.4 to 0.9 gm./kg. per hour), daily infusion is gradually increased to levels of tolerance (3000 to 4000 ml. per day in adults, 130 to 150 ml./kg. per day in infants). The basic guides for safe intravenous hyperalimentation are determinations of weight and fluid balance daily, fractional urine sugar concentration every six hours, serum electrolytes daily until stable and then two or three times weekly, and complete blood counts, blood urea nitrogen, and blood sugar weekly. Occasional determinations of serum osmolality, calcium, phos-

phorus, magnesium, and proteins, and urine specific gravity, osmolality, and electrolytes are helpful in monitoring the status of the patient. Critically ill patients may also have serious cardiovascular, respiratory, or metabolic derangements, necessitating periodic measurements of arterial pressure, central venous pressure, pH, and blood gases.

Occasional adjustment of fluid volume, carbohydrate concentration, nitrogen source, or electrolyte content may be necessary during the clinical course of the critically ill or traumatized patient. Relative glucose intolerance may occur upon starting parenteral hyperalimentation therapy, immediately following trauma, during an operation, in the immediate postoperative period, in premature or newborn infants, in the aged, or in the presence of sepsis. To avoid persistent significant glycosuria, secondary osmotic diuresis, and excessive urine electrolyte loss, glucose is infused at a rate which will not allow quantitative urinary glucose to exceed 2 per cent (greater than 3+ reaction). Ideally, the patient will not excrete any sugar in the urine; however, a trace to 2+ sugar in the urine does not represent a significant percentage of the total sugar administered. Such small amounts of glycosuria will induce a mild diuresis which may be helpful in excreting any excess-administered water, and it will indicate that the patient's tolerance for sugar is not being significantly underestimated.

In the average patient, glucose administration is gradually increased as the normal pancreas increases its output of endogenous insulin in response to the continuous carbohydrate infusion. In all patients with diabetes mellitus, crystalline insulin is given routinely either subcutaneously in evenly divided doses or by equal distribution in the intravenous fluid. Occasionally in nondiabetic patients with relative glucose intolerance, supplemental crystalline insulin may be added to the nutrient solution in amounts of 5 to 25 units per 1000 calories. This addition of insulin is indicated in the presence of elevated blood sugar to encourage more rapid and efficient glucose utilization and positive nitrogen balance in elderly patients with borderline glucose tolerance, in patients with known pancreatic disorders, in the early post-trauma period, and in critically ill, nutritionally depleted patients whose survival seems to depend upon the expeditious achievement of positive caloric and nitrogen balance.

Particularly close attention to potassium administration is essential in order to achieve positive nitrogen and potassium balance and restoration of depleted intracellular stores while maintaining a normal serum potassium level. The usual daily intravenous dose of 40 to 50 mEq. of potassium in the surgical patient is generally not enough to maintain normal serum potassium concentration because of the intracellular movement of this cation associated with anabolism. The obligatory daily excretion of potassium in the urine in the average patient with normally functioning kidneys approximates 40 to 50 mEq. This loss may be increased by additional stress or by the mild diuresis and glycosuria that may accompany glucose infusion. Not only it is necessary to replace the obligatory loss, but it is essential to increase the intake of potassium in order to achieve optimal protein synthesis. Therefore, in order to maintain adequate serum potassium levels and a normal potassium-nitrogen ratio (2.4 to 3.5:1) required for cellular growth and tissue synthesis, potassium must be administered in larger doses than is usually given with routine intravenous therapy. Ordinarily, 40 mEq. of potassium are required for each 1000 calories, and, at times, patients with voluminous losses from the gastrointestinal tract, large open wounds, or extensive burns may require more than 250 mEq. of potassium per day. In the elderly or in patients with compromised kidney function, potassium dosage must be reduced or omitted completely, depending upon the conditions prevailing in the individual patient. In the presence of varying degrees of renal, cardiac, or hepatic failure, particularly close attention must be given to serum chemistry values, urinary output, and the amount of administered potassium in order to prevent serious complications of hypokalemia or hyperkalemia.

Usually, 50 mEq. of sodium are given per 1000 calories, either entirely as the chloride salt or as two-thirds sodium chloride and one-third sodium bicarbonate. Adjustments in the amount and form of sodium administered are sometimes necessary. Compromised function of the heart, liver, or kidneys may dictate significant reduction or even total restriction of sodium in the intravenous ration. For patients with ascites or anasarca, the omission of salt from the regimen may help to promote the movement of large amounts of water and salt accumulated in the extravascular space back into the intravascular compartment for excretion. Each commercial protein hydrolysate preparation contains slightly different amounts of sodium and potassium. These minimal quantities of electrolytes in the different hydrolysate solutions should be known by the physician who uses them.

In patients with marked hypoproteinemia or anemia, albumin or blood are sometimes given early in the course of hyperalimentation in order to restore colloid osmotic pressure and red cell mass to normal levels. In patients with borderline serum protein concentrations, judicious administration of the nutritional solutions alone is often all that is needed to correct the deficiencies. When the circulating blood volume is inadequate to maintain normal cardiovascular dynamics, prompt administration of colloid as blood or albumin is essential to establish homeostasis before instituting parenteral hyperalimentation. Colloid is administered to restore normal osmotic pressure or circulating blood volume and not primarily for nutritional purposes, since the half-life of albumin is too long to be an efficient nutrient. The amino acids, on the other hand, are immediately available for protein synthesis and should not be administered for the purpose of maintaining osmotic pressure. The primary nutritional value of intravenous albumin is to spare the body's labile proteins. Amino acids are preferred for use as substrates in the synthesis of tissue.

SUPERIOR VENA CAVA CATHETERIZATION

Infraclavicular percutaneous subclavian vein puncture has been the best technique for catheterization of the superior vena cava in adults and children weighing more than 10 pounds. Either subclavian vein may be used safely in this technique unless a specific contraindication is present such as ipsilateral thoracotomy, radical neck dissection, clavicular fracture, or radical mastectomy. Despite the theoretical possibility of thoracic duct injury, no evidence of this complication has been observed.

The patient is positioned with his head down 15 degrees (Trendelenburg position) to allow maximal filling and dilatation of the subclavian vein, making it a larger target. The shoulders are thrown back maximally or hyperextended over a rolled sheet placed longitudinally under the thoracic spine. The roll under the spine allows the shoulders to drop posteriorly. With the shoulders then depressed caudally and the head turned maximally to the opposite side, the subclavian vein becomes most accessible.

The skin over the lower neck, shoulder, and upper chest is widely shaved, defatted with ether or acetone, and prepared with 2 per cent tincture of iodine or merthiolate similar to preoperative surgical skin preparation. Using strict aseptic technique with sterile surgical gloves and instruments, the area is draped with sterile towels, and local anesthetic (usually 1 per cent lidocaine) is infiltrated into the skin, subcutaneous tissue, and periosteum at the inferior border of the midpoint of the clavicle. A 2-inch long, 14-gauge needle attached to a 2- or 3-ml. syringe is inserted, bevel down, through the wheal and advanced beneath the inferior margin of the clavicle in a horizontal (frontal) plane with the needle tip aimed for the anterior margin of the trachea at the level of the suprasternal notch (Fig. 30-1, A). With the needle and syringe barrel in a frontal plane and adjacent to the anterior deltoid prominence, the needle will enter the anterior wall of the subclavian vein (Fig. 30-1, B). As the needle is advanced beneath the clavicle, slight nega-

tive pressure applied through the syringe will help to ascertain accurate venipuncture. The needle is advanced a few millimeters further after blood first appears in the syringe to ensure that the entire beveled tip is inside the vein. The patient is asked to perform a Valsalva maneuver; the syringe is removed carefully while the needle is held firmly in place. A 16-gauge, 8-inch long radiopaque catheter is introduced immediately through the needle and threaded its full length into the vein. The catheter should advance easily if the needle tip is entirely within the lumen of the vein and if the original direction of the needle has been maintained. The proximal end of the catheter is attached to a standard intravenous infusion set, and after the catheter is flushed with fluid, the needle is withdrawn and the catheter is secured by a 3-0 silk suture placed lateral to the skin puncture site. At this point, the solution bottle is momentarily lowered below bed level to ensure free flow in both directions, an indication that proper placement of the catheter within the superior vena cava has been accomplished. A broad-spectrum antibiotic ointment is applied to the puncture site, and a sterile gauze dressing is fixed to the skin occlusively with tincture of benzoin and adhesive tape (Fig. 30-1, C). To

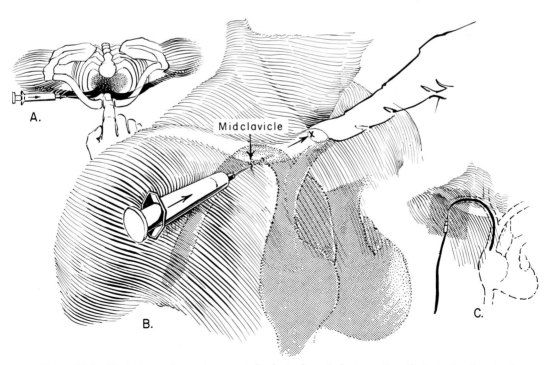

Figure 30-1. Technique of percutaneous infraclavicular subclavian vein catheterization (see text).

prevent accidental disengagement of the intravenous tubing from the catheter and possible air embolism, the tubing-catheter connection is carefully reinforced with adhesive tape. A loop is made in the intravenous tubing and is secured again with tape to guard against accidental traction on the catheter itself. Prior to infusing the hypertonic solution, a chest x-ray should be obtained in order to verify the position of the catheter in the superior vena cava.

The same basic technique may be used with commercially available 8-inch long internal needle and external catheter combinations. The longer needle may be helpful in reaching the vein in large-framed or obese individuals. Catheters may also be threaded into the superior vena cava by way of an external jugular vein. Because of the mobility of the neck and location of adjacent hair-growing areas, the jugular vein puncture site is less comfortable and more difficult to keep sterile and properly functioning than is the subclavian route.

In infants weighing less than 10 pounds, the small subclavian vein and high apex of the lung can make a percutaneous subclavian puncture very difficult and dangerous. Long-term intravenous catheterization in such patients is more wisely achieved by inserting the catheter by way of an external or internal jugular vein cutdown, using a 1-cm. incision at the base of the neck. After proper placement within the superior vena cava, the catheter is secured to the vein, and the proximal end is brought out through a subcutaneous tunnel to a stab wound in the parietal area of the scalp (Dudrick et al., 1969a). The catheter exit site is thereby removed to a point distant from the phlebotomy site, ensuring added safety from infection and mechanical kinking and making catheter maintenance easier here than in the crease of the neck. The neck wound is closed, and the catheter is sutured at the scalp exit site with 4-0 silk. An antibiotic ointment is applied, and the scalp is dressed in a fashion similar to the infraclavicular subclavian catheter site.

If safe, long-term intravenous catheterization is to be achieved, compulsive and meticulous care and maintenance of the catheter is just as important as proper insertion (Wilmore and Dudrick, 1969b). Every two or three days, the intravenous tubing is changed and the dressing over the puncture site is removed. Using aseptic technique and sterile gloves, the area is again defatted with acetone or ether and prepared with tincture of iodine or merthiolate. Antibiotic ointment is reapplied and a sterile occlusive dressing replaced. Withdrawal or administration of blood through the subclavian catheter should be avoided, since these practices significantly increase the possibility of contamination or clotting of the catheter. Antibiotics, heparin, or steroids are not added routinely to the solutions but may be administered through a Y-tubing attached to the intravenous catheter if indicated or desired. Extreme care in adding medications or measuring central venous pressure should be practiced in order to prevent contamination of the solution or tubing.

INFUSION APPARATUS

With ambulatory adult patients, standard intravenous fluid bottles and infusion sets are used to deliver the nutrient solution by continuous gravity drip. Rolling intravenous poles allow ambulation and mobility which are essential for optimal nutrition and rehabilitation. Use of closed, filtered infusion systems provides maximal safety against airborne contaminants which may gain entry into the solution or tubing. Lightweight battery-operated portable pumps will ensure a constant rate of infusion and can be attached to the intravenous pole or directly to the patient, allowing considerable freedom of position and activity.

In infants, the nutrient solution is delivered continuously at a constant rate by means of a peristaltic pump with variable speed controls. Syringe pumps must never be used with nutrient solutions, as the risk of contamination with such pumps is too great. A standard pediatric administration set attached to the reservoir bottle quantitates the infused fluid. Between the pump and the catheter, the infusion tubing is attached to a 0.22-micron membrane filter (Wilmore and Dudrick, 1969a). This in-line final filter protects against transmission of contaminants which may be introduced into the solution or tubing and prevents inadvertent air embolism, since air does not pass through the pores once it has been moistened with the solution. In-line membrane filters may also be used in adult patients, but a larger pore size, 0.45 micron, is necessary in order to permit an adequate rate of infusion. The larger pores theoretically will permit passage of certain very small species of *Pseudomonas* organisms, but in practice these filters have been satisfactory. The filter and administration set are replaced every three days or more often if needed.

COMPLICATIONS

Prevention of infection and sepsis is of utmost importance to the success of long-term intravenous hyperalimentation. The incidence of catheter sepsis is negligible if aseptic and antiseptic principles are conscientiously observed in insertion and maintenance of the intravenous cannula (Wilmore and Dudrick, 1969b). Because the solutions are excellent culture media for many species of bacteria and fungi, meticulous asepsis must also be maintained in solution preparation, additive insertion, and long-term infusion. Should fever occur without an obvious etiology, the solution and tubing are promptly replaced and specimens of the blood and the solution are cultured. If the fever persists following replacement of the solution and tubing, infusion is terminated. The subclavian catheter is removed, and the tip is immediately placed into thioglycolate broth and sent for culture. Depending upon the clinical situation, another catheter may be inserted into the opposite subclavian vein, or administration of isotonic fluid may be started by peripheral vein. Broad-spectrum antibiotic therapy is rarely required. If desired, however, antibiotics may be started at this time and modified when specific sensitivity testing is completed.

The presence of fever or sepsis prior to the institution of intravenous hyperalimentation is not necessarily a contraindication to the use of the technique. In a traumatized or critically ill patient, sepsis actually accentuates the need for adequate nutrition. Antibiotic therapy has already been instituted in many such patients, and, although seeding of the indwelling catheter by circulating microorganisms is a high risk possibility, it has not been a significant problem; resolution of systemic infections has occurred frequently during the period of intravenous hyperalimentation. Whenever the clinician is suspicious that the infectious course of the patient might be caused or aggravated by the superior vena cava catheter, it should be removed and cultured promptly.

Although thrombophlebitis is theoretically a possibility with the use of long-term indwelling catheters and hypertonic solutions, superior vena cava thrombosis has not been observed clinically in over 600 patients. The high blood flow in this vessel assures prompt dilution of the hypertonic fluid if it is administered correctly. Attention to sterility practically eliminates the threat of thrombophlebitis. The rare instances of thrombophlebitis occurred in patients whose catheter tip was misdirected into an internal jugular, external jugular, or axillary vein. If any difficulty is encountered during cannulation of the subclavian vein, the precise catheter position should be confirmed by chest x-ray.

Other complications, such as inadvertent air embolism, catheter embolism, and catheter clotting, can be avoided readily by adherence to principles and techniques previously discussed. A thorough knowledge of the anatomy, coupled with common sense and a strict adherence to the technique of percutaneous subclavian catheterization, should minimize the risk of accidental pneumothorax, hydrothorax, subclavian artery puncture, bleeding, or injury to the thoracic duct or brachial plexus.

Hyperosmolar nonketotic hyperglycemia can be precipitated by infusion of the hypertonic fluid too rapidly, causing marked osmotic diuresis, serum and urine electrolyte aberrations, dehydration, central nervous system irritability, and seizures. The chronic form of this syndrome can occur insidiously when glucose utilization is impaired but not recognized, particularly in the presence of diabetes mellitus, extensive burns, and major trauma, and after intracranial operations. If blood and urine sugar concentrations are not conscientiously monitored in such patients, blood sugar can become markedly elevated with accompanying weakness, listlessness, and, eventually, coma. Treatment of either form of hyperosmolar hyperglycemia consists of judicious infusion of isotonic or half-strength solutions of saline or glucose along with insulin, while obtaining frequent measurements of fluid loss, central venous pressure, electrolytes, and blood sugar. Thorough assessment and understanding of the patient's disease process, his metabolic status, and the established principles of the technique of intravenous hyperalimentation will prevent most of these complications and enhance the benefits of the technique.

In several patients who have shown relative glucose intolerance, plasma insulin levels have been normal or high, perhaps indicating that an inactive form of insulin is also being measured. If exogenous insulin is added to the regimen, glucose utilization significantly improves in most of these patients. Since there is apparently no feedback mechanism in operation to decrease formation and release of endogenous insulin as exogenous insulin is administered, the pancreatic islet cells may eventually increase endogenous production to physiologic limits in response to continuous glucose infusion. Therefore, exogenous insulin administration must be reduced concomitantly in order to prevent hypoglycemia. The dynamic alterations in glucose and insulin metabolism must be frequently monitored by urine sugar and blood sugar determinations in order to permit adjustments in glucose or insulin administration or both. These adjustments are necessary to ensure patient safety. Sudden cessation of hypertonic glucose infusion has occasionally been followed by a prompt hypoglycemic reaction which is thought to result from a delay in the readjustment of endogenous insulin production and output. To avoid this hypoglycemic rebound phenomenon, the patient should be weaned gradually over several hours from intravenous hyperalimentation to oral feeding.

Blood sugar levels have been difficult to control in a few patients, especially those who have latent or overt diabetes mellitus complicated by infections, metastatic carcinoma, or liver damage. In some of these patients, large doses of crystalline insulin fail to elicit the typical response. This apparent insulin resistance can best be managed by decreasing the infused sugar load rather than by increasing the insulin dosage.

Clinical application

Over 600 patients with a variety of diseases precluding adequate nourishment by the gastrointestinal tract have been fed entirely by vein with 2400 to 5000 calories per day from 7 to 275 days. Weight gain and increased strength and activity were regularly observed in all patients despite a wide variety of conditions usually associated with increasing weakness, disability, and deterioration. Strongly positive nitrogen balance has been achieved in patients with intravenous hyperalimentation during preoperative preparation, intraoperative therapy, and postoperative management. Body weight increased as much as 45 pounds in patients fed

entirely by vein, despite clinical courses complicated by prolonged ileus, sepsis, wound disruption, and multiple operative procedures. Prompt healing of previously indolent wounds and sinuses was associated with achievement of the anabolic state. More than 60 previously persistent intestinal fistulas closed spontaneously within 3 to 4 weeks following initiation of total intravenous hyperalimentation. Gastrointestinal secretory and motor activity was minimized while providing adequate nutrition.

Most dramatic has been the normal growth and development of over 50 newborn infants nourished entirely or primarily by intravenous feedings from 7 to 650 days. Despite multiple or complex congenital anomalies of the gastrointestinal tract and repeated operative procedures, a constant and predictable weight gain has been observed in these infants maintained on intravenous hyperalimentation. Wound healing, fistula closure, increased activity, and survival were observed, whereas previously death would have been almost certain.

Parenteral nutrition has been progressively improved in each decade, but rarely until now has a prolonged, sustained, and meaningful state of anabolism been achieved exclusively with intravenous feeding, particularly under conditions ordinarily associated with a catabolic response. The depleted patient with severe disability of the alimentary tract requires increased nutritional support for restoration of body tissues and metabolism. Superimposed on this need are the increased energy and nitrogen requirements resulting from preoperative and intraoperative relative starvation, the postoperative catabolic response, and the accelerated metabolism associated with postoperative complications. By the intravenous administration of adequate basic nutrients, tissue synthesis, weight gain, growth, and development can be achieved to the benefit of patients with complex gastroenteropathy.

Fistula closure is best accomplished by a combination of suction, good nutrition, and bowel rest. Patients with inflammatory diseases of the gastrointestinal tract may gain weight, since total intravenous nutrition minimizes the mechanical and secretory irritation of the bowel which provides optimal conditions for resolution and healing of the diseased viscera. If surgical procedures are eventually undertaken, the patient is in a better nutritional state to resist infection and withstand the stress of anesthesia and operation. Infants with multiple or complex anomalies may grow and develop while reconstructive procedures are staged. Finally, maintenance of the anabolic state in all patients requiring major operative procedures may allow a decreased incidence of operative complications and infections, may reduce duration and cost of patient hospitalization, and may achieve more rapid patient rehabilitation and restoration to productive life.

CONCLUSION

Intravenous hyperalimentation should be considered a primary mode of therapy rather than a modified method of standard intravenous treatment. Every effort should be exerted to ensure strict asepsis and antisepsis in dealing with the nutrient solution, intravenous infusion tubing, the indwelling catheter, and the catheter entrance site. The nutrient solution is an excellent culture medium for bacteria and fungi with direct access to the blood stream. Thorough precautions must be taken to avoid contamination; the possibilities of an infection are greatly minimized by using a closed infusion system to avoid airborne contamination, an in-line membrane filter to ensure solution sterility, laminar-flow filtered-air hoods for mixing and handling solutions and additives, and meticulous technique in the insertion and maintenance of the catheter. The nursing staff must be well-informed and aware of their responsibility to ensure constant continuous infusion of the nutrient solution. The intern and resident staff must be knowledgeable of the expected sugar and electrolyte flux and the possibility of osmotic diuresis with secondary hyperosmolar dehydration. Finally, the surgeon may require the help of a pharmacist, biochemist, psychiatrist, social worker, and physical therapist in order to meet the needs of the critically ill, nutritionally depleted patient. The technique of intravenous hyperalimentation, when properly utilized, offers a new dimension in the care and management of the critically ill patient.

REFERENCES

Beal, J. M., Payne, M. A., Gilder, H., Johnson, G., Jr., and Carver, W. L.: Experience with administration of an intravenous fat emulsion to surgical patients. Metabolism, 6:673, 1957.

Cuthbertson, D. P., and Tilstone, W. J.: Nutrition of the injured. Amer. J. Clin. Nutr., 21:911, 1968.

Dudrick, S. J., Groff, D. B., and Wilmore, D. W.: Long-term venous catheterization in infants. Surg. Gynec. Obstet., 129:805, 1969a.

Dudrick, S. J., Long, J. M., Steiger, E., and Rhoads, J. E.: Intravenous hyperalimentation, Med. Clin. N. Amer. (In press.)

Dudrick, S. J., and Wilmore, D. W.: Long-term parenteral feeding, Hosp. Pract., 3:65, 1968.

Dudrick, S. J., Wilmore, D. W., Steiger, E., Mackie, J. A., and Fitts, W. T., Jr.: Spontaneous closure of traumatic pancreatoduodenal fistulas with total intravenous nutrition. J. Trauma. (In press.)

Dudrick, S. J., Wilmore, D. W., Steiger, E., and Rhoads, J. E.: Reversal of uremia and body wasting with intravenous essential amino acids. Fed. Proc., 28:808, 1969b.

Dudrick, S. J., Wilmore, D. W., Steiger, E., Vars, H. M., and Rhoads, J. E.: The use of carbohydrates and proteolysates for long-term parenteral feeding. In Nahas, G. G. (ed.): Body Fluid Replacement in the Surgical Patient. New York, Grune and Stratton. (Forthcoming.)

Dudrick, S. J., Wilmore, D. W., Vars, H. M., and Rhoads, J. E.: Can intravenous feeding as the sole means of nutrition support growth in the child and restore weight loss in an adult? An affirmative answer. Ann. Surg., 169:974, 1969c.

Dudrick, S. J., Wilmore, D. W., Vars, H. M., and Rhoads, J. E.: Long-term total parenteral nutrition with growth, development, and positive nitrogen balance. Surgery, 64:134, 1968.

Green, H. N., Stoner, H. B., Whiteley, H. J., and Elgin, D.: The effect of trauma on the chemical composition of the blood and tissues of man. Clin. Sci., 8:65, 1949.

Holden, W. D., Krieger, H., Levey, S., and Abbott, W. E.: The effects of nutrition on nitrogen metabolism in the surgical patient. Ann. Surg., 146:563, 1957.

Lehr, H. B., Rhoads, J. E., Rosenthal, O., and Blakemore, W. S.: Use of intravenous fat emulsions in surgical patients. JAMA, 181:745, 1962.

Levenson, S. M., Einhaber, A., and Malm, O. J.: Nutritional and metabolic aspects of shock. Fed. Proc., 20:99, 1961.

Rhoads, J. E.: Diuretics as an adjuvant in disposing of extra water employed as a vehicle in parenteral hyperalimentation. Fed. Proc., 21:389, 1962.

Rhoads, J. E., Rawnsley, H. M., Vars, H. M., Crichlow, R. W., Nelson, H. M., Spagna, P., Dudrick, S. J., and Rhoads, J. E., Jr.: The use of diuretics as an adjuvant in parenteral hyperalimentation for surgical patients with prolonged disability of the gastrointestinal tract. Bull. Internat. Soc. Surg., 24:59, 1965.

Symposium on intravenous fat emulsions, Metabolism, 6:591, 1957.

Wilmore, D. W., and Dudrick, S. J.: An in-line filter for intravenous solutions. Arch. Surg., 99:462, 1969a.

Wilmore, D. W., and Dudrick, S. J.: Growth and development of an infant receiving all nutrients exclusively by vein. JAMA, 203:860, 1968.

Wilmore, D. W., and Dudrick, S. J.: Safe long-term venous catheterization. Arch. Surg., 98:256, 1969b.

Wilmore, D. W., Groff, D. B., Bishop, H. C., and Dudrick, S. J.: Total parenteral nutrition in infants with catastrophic gastrointestinal anomalies. J. Pediat. Surg., 4:181, 1969.

INDEX

Page numbers in *italics* indicate illustrations; (t) indicates tabular information.

667